CONTENTS

CONTRIBUTORS

The following people edited and contributed new chapters to this book:

David Anderson, RGN, RSCN, DipEd, DPSN
Senior Nurse, Smithfield Paediatric Unit,
The Royal Hospitals NHS Trust, London.
Chapter 7

Julie Asquith, RGN, RSCN, DipN(Lond), DMS, ENB 100
Senior Nurse Manager (Paediatrics), Evelina Children's Unit,
Guy's and St Thomas' Hospital NHS Trust, London.
Chapter 28

Jan Barlow, RSCN, RGN
Clinical Nurse Specialist (Child Health)
Scarborough General Hospital, Scarborough.
Chapter 27

Philip Beed, RGN, OND, DPSN
Lecturer/Practitioner in Ophthalmic Nursing
Radcliffe Infirmary NHS Trust, Oxford.
Chapter 23

Chris Betts, RGN, RSCN, DipHSM
Director of Health and Family Services, The Children's Trust,
Tadworth, Surrey.
Chapter 20

Steven Campbell, BNurs, RGN, RSCN, HVCert, DNCert, CertEd, MRSH
Lecturer in Child Health Nursing, The School of Nursing and Midwifery,
University of Southampton, Southampton.
Chapters 1, 3, and 27

Anne Casey, MSc, RSCN, RGN, DipNEd, DipNurs, RNT
Senior Nurse (Research and Development)
Great Ormond Street Hospital for Children NHS Trust, London.
Chapter 9

Frances Clarke, BSc(Hons), RSCN, RN, RNT
Senior Lecturer (Children's Nursing),
University of Northumbria at Newcastle, Newcastle-upon-Tyne.
Chapter 26

Sue Croom, BA, RGN, HVCert, FWTCert, ENB 603
Senior Nurse Lecturer/Practitioner, The Flemming Nuffield Unit,
City Health Trust and the University of Northumbria,
Newcastle-upon-Tyne.
Chapter 19

Philip Darbyshire, PhD, MSc, RSCN, RNMH
Senior Lecturer in Nursing Studies, Department of Nursing and
Community Health, Glasgow Caledonian University, Glasgow.
Chapter 3

Mary El-Rayes, RN, RHV, Dip Health Management
Director
Stillbirth and Neonatal Death Society, London.
Chapter 15

Margaret Evans, BSc(Hons), RGN, RSCN, DipN(Lond)
Macmillan Lecturer in Paediatric Oncology Nursing/Macmillan Paediatric
Consultant, School of Nursing and Midwifery
University of Southampton, Southampton.
Chapter 30

Alison Fielder, RGN, RSCN
Epilepsy Nurse Specialist, The Child Health Directorate,
Southampton University Hospitals Trust, Southampton.
Chapter 31

Hazel Foale, BSc(Hons), RGN, RSCN, DipN(Lond)
Paediatric Ward Sister, Evelina Children's Unit
Guy's and St Thomas' Hospital NHS Trust, London.
Chapter 33

Stuart Gemmell, BSc(Hons), RMN
Community Nurse Therapist
Elizabeth Dibben Centre
Bordon, Hampshire.
Chapter 18

Edward Alan Glasper, PhD, BA, RGN, RSCN, ONC, DN, CertEd, RNT
Professor of Nursing, Director of Child Health Studies
School of Nursing and Midwifery
University of Southampton, Southampton.
Chapter 1

Diane Gow, BA(Hons), RGN, RSCN, RCNT, RNT
Teaching Fellow (Child Health), School of Nursing and Midwifery
University of Southampton, Southampton.
Chapter 16

Tony Harrison, BA(NursEd), RGN, RSCN, RNT
Tutor
Manchester College of Nursing and Midwifery
Tameside, Ashton-under-Lyne.
Chapter 29

Maggie Hicklin, RGN, RSCN
Specialist Clinical Nurse for Paediatric Nephrology
Evelina Children's Unit
Guy's and St Thomas' Hospital NHS Trust, London.
Chapter 25

Louise Hooker, RGN, RSCN, CertHEd, PaedOncCert
Piam Brown Nursing Research Fellow, School of Nursing and Midwifery
University of Southampton, Southampton.
Chapter 29, 30

Maddie Hooton, BSc(Hons), RGN, RSCN, DPSN, CertEd, ENB 405
Lecturer/Practitioner, Faculty of Health, Social Work and Education,
Nursing Department, University of Northumbria at Newcastle,
Newcastle General Hospital, Newcastle.
Chapter 17

Sue Jones, BSc(Hons), RGN, RSCN
Paediatric Emergency Nurse Practitioner
(Chair of the RCN Society of Paediatric Nursing)
Bristol Royal Hospital for Sick Children, Bristol
Chapter 6

Jenny Leggott, RGN, RM, RSCN, ENB 405, ENB 998, MBA
Team Leader for re-engineering the Emergency Entry Process
Leicester Royal Infirmary NHS Trust, Leicester.
Chapter 13

Morag Liddell, RGN, RSCN
Senior Sister, Neonatal Surgical Unit,
The Royal Hospital for Sick Children, York Hill NHS Trust, Glasgow.
Chapter 14

Whaley and Wong's

CHILDREN'S NURSING

Edited by

Steven Campbell

BNurs, RGN, RSCN, HVCert, DNCert, CertEd, MRSH
Lecturer in Child Health Nursing, The School of Nursing and
Midwifery, University of Southampton

Edward Alan Glasper

PhD, BA, RGN, RSCN, ONC, DN, CertEd, RNT
Professor of Nursing, Director of Child Health Studies, School of
Nursing and Midwifery, University of Southampton

Editorial Consultant

Donna L. Wong

PhD, RN, PNP, CPN, FAAN
Nurse Consultant, Saint Francis Hospital Children's Center;
Adjunct Associate Professor, Department of Pediatrics, University of Oklahoma
College of Medicine, Tulsa;
Clinical Associate Professor, University of Oklahoma College of Nursing, Tulsa;
Adjunct Associate Professor/Consultant, Oral Roberts University, Anna Vaughn
School of Nursing, Tulsa

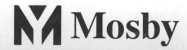 Mosby

Copyright © 1995 Times Mirror International Publishers Limited.

Published in 1995 by Mosby, an imprint of Times Mirror International Publishers Ltd.

Printed by Grafos, S.A. Arte Sobre papel, Barcelona, Spain.

ISBN 0 7234 20718

For full details of all Mosby titles please write to Times Mirror International Publishers Ltd, Lynton House, 7-12 Tavistock Square, London WC1H 9LB, England.

A CIP catalogue record for this book is available from the British Library.

Project Manager:	Tuan Hô
Developmental Editor:	Georgina Massy
Designer:	Lara Last
Production:	Mell Van de Velde
Cover Illustration:	Kevin Palmer
Cover Photograph:	Southampton University Hospitals Trust, Southampton
Publisher:	Griselda Campbell

Noelle Llewellyn, BA, SRN, RSCN, DPSN
Clinical Nurse Specialist, Acute Pain Service
Great Ormond Street Hospital for Children NHS Trust, London.
Chapter 7

Teri Lockyer, RNMH, DPSN, CertEd
Teaching Fellow, School of Nursing and Midwifery
University of Southampton, Southampton.
Chapter 22

Celia Mostyn, RGN, RSCN
Neurology Clinical Nurse Specialist
Great Ormond Street Hospital for Children NHS Trust, London.
Chapter 34

Jean Orr, MSc, BA, RGN, RHV, HVTutCert
Professor of Nursing/Director of School of Nursing, School of Nursing
The Queens University of Belfast, Belfast.
Chapter 11

Christine Patch, BSc, RGN
Nurse Specialist, Wessex Clinical Genetics Service,
The Princess Anne Hospital NHS Trust, Southampton.
Chapter 12

Julie Pearce, BSc(Hons), RGN, ENB 100
Senior Research Fellow (Intensive Care Nursing),
School of Nursing and Midwifery
University of Southampton, Southampton.
Chapter 24

Cath Powell, BNSc(Hons), RGN, RSCN, RHV
Lecturer in Child Health Nursing, School of Nursing and Midwifery
University of Southampton, Southampton.
Chapter 16

Sue Price, MN, RGN, RSCN, DipN, CertEd
Lecturer in Nursing Studies
University of Birmingham, Birmingham.
Chapter 8

Jim Richardson, BA, RGN, RSCN, PGCE
Lecturer in Nursing Studies, School of Nursing Studies
University of Wales College of Medicine, Cardiff.
Chapters 1, 2

Helen Rushforth, BA, RGN, RSCN, DipNSc, RNT
Lecturer in Child Health Nursing
School of Nursing and Midwifery
University of Southampton, Southampton.
Chapter 27

Beth Sepion, BEd(Hons), RGN, RSCN, SCM, OncCert
Lecturer/Practitioner in Paediactric Oncology
Royal Marsden NHS Trust Hospital, Surrey.
Chapter 21

Jeanne Smith, MN, RGN, RSCN, DPSN
Paediatric Emergency Nurse Practitioner
Bristol Royal Hospital for Sick Children, Bristol.
Chapter 6

Eileen Thomas, MA, RGN, RHV
Senior Lecturer, Institute of Public Health Medicine
University of Southampton, Southampton.
Chapter 10

Irene Webber, BA, RGN, RM, RHV, PGCEC(A)
Lecturer in Nursing Studies, School of Nursing Studies
University of Wales College of Medicine, Cardiff.
Chapter 5

Mark Whiting, MSc, BNurs, RGN, RSCN, DNCert, HVCert
Team Leader, Paediatric Home Care and Hospital/Community Liaison
St Mary's Hospital, Parkside Health NHS Trust, London.
Chapter 4

Zoe Wilks, RSCN, RN, Adv Dip Child Devel(Lond)
Senior Sister, The Programmed Investigation Unit
Great Ormond Street Hospital for Children NHS Trust, London.
Chapter 32

Acknowledgements
The editors and publisher gratefully acknowledge the following people for
their assistance with this book.

Margaret Chambers, David Colburn, Judith Ellis, Ann England, Andrea
Ford, Elizabeth Fradd, Penny Guilbert, Caryn Hess, Heather King, Joan
Kirsopp, Margaret Lane, Christine Lappin, Elaine Lawrence, Doreen
MacLean, G McEwing, Joan Ramsey, Amy Salter, Steve Shrimpton, Dr
Stevens, Nicky Torrance, Hannah Tudge, Kathy Wickham, Child Health
Studies Team, School of Nursing and Midwifery, University of Southampton.

FOREWORD

In most professions all too often there is a gulf between theory and its practice and paediatric nursing is no exception. The gulf is perpetuated when theory is taught in a theoretical setting and practice is taught by the practitioner. This inherent gulf has to be bridged by students of nursing and the publication of *Whaley and Wong's Children's Nursing* is a very useful tool to aid such bridge building. It aims to help relate theory and practice in a meaningful way while underlining the importance of the child being cared for by the appropriately qualified children's nurse, with true parental participation as valued members of the team.

This textbook provides a comprehensive overview of children's nursing, covering all aspects of child health care, addressing future needs for education, practice and research development. All the chapters show where care has been improved through research findings, how such findings can act as a catalyst for change and advocate that children's nurses must be at the forefront of these developments. Learning outcomes are clearly identified and a helpful range of further reading is suggested to allow more detailed study following each chapter. It demonstrates immense potential for the future development of children's nursing and innovative practice.

It has a logical organization, encompassing all recent changes in health care and emphasises the move from tertiary to primary health care. It also stresses the important role children's nurses play in health education and discusses common problems which occur in otherwise healthy children.

Children's nurses are required to know and understand the needs of children and their families from neonates to adolescents with a wide variety of conditions both physical and mental. This textbook covers all aspects and core skills required to care for children of all ages. Each chapter has been written by highly skilled competent paediatric nurses including those with an academic background who have brought together a clear vision for the future.

The framework of family-centred care and true parental participation clearly requires a change in attitude, explaining more, valuing their presence, extending parental participation into psychological or emotional involvement in care.

This is one of the most dynamic paediatric nursing books to be published for many years. The contributors have clearly demonstrated the importance of enhancing the care of children. They have also shown how the *UKCC's Scope of Professional Practice* facilitates practitioners in ensuring that practice remains dynamic and is able to adjust, readily and appropriately, to meet changing care needs.

Mary Uprichard OBE, RSCN, RGN, RM, MTD
President, UKCC

Hilary Herron RSCN, RGN
Council Member, UKCC
Former Chair of the RCN Society of Paediatric Nursing

PREFACE

Whaley and Wong's Children's Nursing has been honed to meet the needs of students of paediatric nursing in the UK by 37 specialist contributors. The strengths of this book are its comprehensiveness as well as its combination of the biological and behavioural sciences with an extensive review of sick children's care in all areas of primary, secondary and tertiary health care. Much of the central core of this text is concerned with the creation of child and family-centred cultures within health care settings. To this end we have included much material to reinforce this basic concept of paediatric nursing. Paediatric nurses should not forget that they are advocates for children and their families. Families of young children need advocates and this role development is integral to the paediatric nursing curricula. If information giving is the key to empowerment, this text should help all paediatric nurses in their pursuit of family advocacy.

The mission of children's nursing remains as it always has been "The child first and always". We believe that one area of great importance is the provision of family information. Families of sick or injured children hunger for information and their growing assertiveness in seeking such information is proving challenging to some health care professionals. However, it must be recognized that some families will actively seek out information while others avoid it. We hope the readers of this text will develop strategies which will allow them to become more aggressive in the promotion of health information and opportunistically involve even those families who under normal circumstances would prove passive in the pursuit of information.

It is quite clear that success in research and development will be the driving force for paediatric nurses in the future and the achievements of these nurses in clinical practice, research and education will have to be clearly articulated. Care which is underpinned by these guiding philosophies will be necessary to ensure the highest quality of care. The editors have endeavoured to give this text such a mission; it should perhaps be remembered that the formal education of children's nurses in the UK dates back to 1878 and it was Catherine Jane Wood, an early matron of the Hospital for Sick Children, Great Ormond Street, London, who first said in 1888 "Sick children require special nursing and sick children's nurses require special training". Miss Wood's pronouncement is as true today as it was then and in order to function effectively in a range of therapeutic environments, children's nurses require a special text. This book is that special text and its design has been influenced by the views of UK children's nurses.

The value of children's nursing lies in its commitment to care. This care is predominantly family focused with the emphasis being on partnership. Partnership in care is easier said than done and the role of the paediatric nurse in making this more than a token gesture is invaluable. Such nurses have learned to debate their care in the sometimes harsh economic climate which has prevailed within the UK health sector for some years. These debates are informed and underpinned by a variety of seminal publications which are given due prominence in this new text. Publications such as *The Welfare of Children and Young People in Hospital*, *Parents Staying Overnight in Hospital with their Children*, *The Children's Act*, *Bridging the Gaps*, *Just for the Day*, *Children First* and others are the foundation stones of current caring philosophies for children in need. This text endeavours to be true to their guiding and enlightening approach to child care.

In this text we have conveyed examples of best practice from throughout the United Kingdom and further afield. Clearly, in an increasingly specialist health care arena, it would be impossible to present any text as a panacea, but we hope this new edition will fulfil all its goals as a reader to those students undertaking diplomate and undergraduate programmes in children's nursing.

THE CONTENT OF THE BOOK

This text includes coverage of all the main conditions and care situations that children's nurses will experience during their courses. Its structure is firmly underpinned by research-based information, a strong integrated focus on the family and a logical organization throughout. New chapters written for the UK book include Family-centred Care, Nursing Care in the Community, Emergency Care of the Young Person, and the Child and Surgery. The chapters based on the US authors' work have been adapted to reflect UK populations, cultures, health care, nursing practice, terminology and research base.

STRUCTURE OF THE BOOK

Unit 1: Fundamentals of Children's Nursing provides a comprehensive overview of children's nursing within our multicultural society, reflecting the growing trend towards an increased emphasis on community care.

Unit 2: Health Problems and Health Promotion details each of the stages of childhood development, emphasizing the nurse's role in health promotion. Initial discussion concentrates on the normal health problems expected in otherwise healthy children, providing information on the common occurrence of individual manifestations.

Unit 3: The Child with Special Needs looks specifically at the child and family with special needs, including chronic illness and life-threatening illness.

Unit 4: The Child with Dysfunction contains chapters on the detailed care required by children with serious health problems.

THE FORMAT OF THE CHAPTERS

The chapters are designed to aid effective student learning and to assist readers in quickly finding particular subjects.

Each chapter contains:

Learning outcomes - the main concepts which can be learned from the chapter are outlined in order to reinforce student learning.

Glossary of terms - to highlight and expand on terminology used within the text and to facilitate the reading process.

Boxed highlights - to extract and emphasize important issues and points for the reader, pertinent to the chapter, including boxed information in the form of 'Parent Guidelines' and 'Questions and Controversies'.

Illustrations - there are clear tables, diagrams, and photographs to illustrate the text, and enhance understanding of the text.

Key Points - located at the end of each chapter help the reader to summarize and assimilate key information.

References - to give full citations of the literature and research on which the chapter is based in order to provide the reader with the opportunity to gather further information if required.

Further reading - recommendations for further resources both general and related to specific conditions.

We hope you enjoy using *Whaley and Wong's Children's Nursing*. Should you have any comments about the book, please write to us care of the Publishers - we'll be pleased to hear from you.

S Campbell

E A Glasper

Unit One

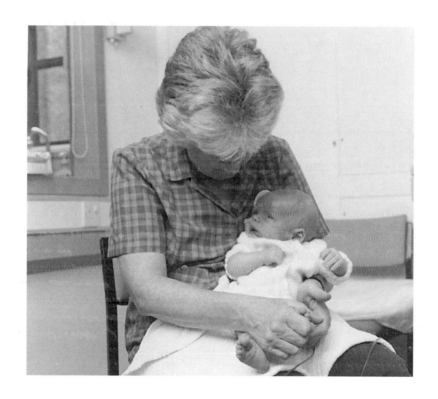

*Fundamentals
of Children's Nursing*

Chapter 1

Perspectives of Children's Nursing

LEARNING OUTCOMES

After studying this chapter you should be able to:

◆ Identify major landmarks in the historical development of children's nursing.
◆ Integrate the social scientific developments in child care into the development of children's nursing.
◆ Understand four important ethical principles: non-maleficence, beneficence, justice and autonomy; and two major schools of ethical thinking: deontology or duty-based ethics and consequentialism.
◆ Articulate arguments for and against the development of generic nurse training.
◆ Identify the advantages and disadvantages of an all-graduate profession.
◆ Identify opportunities for practice development based upon empowerment of families and children.
◆ Articulate innovative research and development in primary, secondary and tertiary care.

GLOSSARY

Loco-Parentis In place of the parent. Usually an adult acting in place of the parent

consequentialism The belief that the morality of a action is to be solely judged from its consequences

generic Characteristics of or belonging to a genus or class; applicable to (any individual of) a large group or class, general, non-specific

advocacy The function of an advocate; pleading in support of

adovate A person who pleads, intercedes, or speaks for another. A person who speaks in favour of

holistic Treating of the whole person including mental and social factors rather than just the symptoms of a disease

hildren's nurses working in all aspects of professional child care are committed to family-centred
care and the need for family advocacy. While advocacy has
been a part of children's nursing since the early days of pro-
fessionalization, the nurse is now *proactive* rather than *reactive*.
The nurse has moved from simply supporting the family or
making a case for them, to a role as guardian of their rights
of independence and freedom of choice.

The medical model has been integral to the historical
development of the profession of nursing. From the time of
Nightingale, nursing has adopted a military hierarchy with
unswerving obedience to the higher ranks, including doctors.
Loyalty, therefore, was considered to be all important and
there was no room for criticism. Today, reflective practice is
a key aspect of modern children's nursing education and has
led to profound change in the manner in which children and
their families are cared for in all arenas of practice.

Increased family involvement in care during the last 30
years has stemmed from an increased understanding of the
welfare of children in hospital and the potential poor consequences of admission to hospital. Consequently, many
children's nurses have questioned the provision of care for
children in hospital. Changes in practice have been driven
by the aspirations of parents to become more involved with
the care of their own children. This is a significant challenge
for the children's nurse.

Western culture regards children as innocent, but vulnerable, individuals. This is reflected in legislation for their protection in most countries. Child care usually is undertaken by
the family. When this falters, society has a legal obligation to
behave *in loco parentis* until the family can resume care or until
the child is out of danger. The Convention on the Rights of
the Child states that 'the family, as the fundamental group of
society and the natural environment for the growth and well
being of all its members and particularly children, should be
afforded the necessary protection and assistance so that it can
fully assume its responsibilities within the community'. The
Convention came into place on 2 September, 1990. On 29
September, 1990, the United Nations' World Summit for
children supported the Convention. This represented the first
worldwide action for its implementation (UNICEF, 1990).
These fundamental innovations set the agenda for the future
welfare of children.

The needs of children should be a high priority in the distribution of resources, even if resources are scarce. Family-
focused nursing care is one aspect of this strategy.

In addressing these issues, it is impossible to cover all of the
areas of importance to children's nursing. The areas which are
covered are addressed superficially, because they represent
major facets of the profession which are the subject of much
debate, research and publication beyond the scope of this
chapter. Therefore, four major aspects are presented here: the
historical background of children's nursing; children's nursing
and ethics; the vision for the future; and education, research,
development and practice.

HISTORICAL ASPECTS OF CHILD CARE

Perceptions of childhood have changed throughout history.
Views about children have varied from inherently evil to inherently good. This has lead to opposing schools of thought in
child rearing practices. De Mause (1974) traced these changing
attitudes from those of Rousseau, who viewed children as inno-
cents, to John Wesley who saw them as sinful and evil.
Rousseau's views had great influence, but were not reflected in
child rearing practices in most of the western world until the
second half of the 19th century. By contrast, the influence of
the puritan, nonconformist, Wesleyan movement was greater.
Wesley believed that children could be saved only through
physical punishment. These attitudes have persisted into the
20th century.

The liberation of children and their families has been gradual
and is far from complete. The development of the care of
children in the United Kingdom can be traced to 1739 and
Thomas Coram, a retired sea captain who spent most of his
working life in the new world. When he returned to London,
he found dying children in the streets and the corpses of babies
on the dung heaps. Coram gained the support of influential individuals and was given a royal charter to open a foundling hospital
in 1739, near the site of the Hospital for Sick Children, Great
Ormond Street. It was a refuge for unwanted children, not a
hospital for sick children as we understand it. Besser (1977)
noted that only 4,400 of the 15,000 children admitted from 1756
to 1760 lived to adulthood. This mortality rate was the result of
childhood infections and ignorance about how infections spread.
Yet, despite these tragedies, the perception of children was
slowly changing. Increasing literacy within industrialized nations
enabled authors, such as Charles Dickens and Charles Kingsley,
to bring attention to such social injustice.

When the Hospital for Sick Children, Great Ormond
Street, opened on 14th February, 1852, it symbolized a
triumph for childhood. The hospital became a model for other
hospitals throughout the world.

Some of the first children's hospitals were created during the
pre-Nightingale era before the Crimean War. Professionalism,
with its inherent military philosophy, epitomized the Nightingale ethic. This 'professionalism' left little room for nonprofessionals, including parents. Thus, the welfare of families
with children in hospital was neglected, and this situation
remained for nearly 100 years. Consequently, strict visiting
hours were established and parents were effectively prevented
from visiting their children. Nurses used the excuse of 'protecting' families from the harsh realities of childhood illness
at a time when childhood mortality was high. These paternalistic attitudes have obstructed children's nurses in their search
for family advocacy.

The education of children's nurses originates from the Victorian children's hospitals, such as those in London, Edinburgh
and Manchester. The motivation behind the development, and
therefore the nature, of this nurse training was to support the

specialist medical interventions. Nurse training (which produced the first registered children's nurses in the 1920s) reflected this medical model.

In the 1950s, social scientists studied the separation of children from their parents and particularly from the parental role (Bowlby, 1951; Robertson, 1958). This interest came from two phenomena: the alteration of the woman's role during the Second World War, and the effect upon children of evacuation to rural areas. These studies had major implications for the children's nurses, but were not acted upon at the time. Indeed, some actions are still to be completed. This may have been attributable to the type of nurse training current at that time, the post-war paternalistic environment of the children's hospitals and the extent to which nurses were able to bring about changes.

The Platt report (Ministry of Health, 1959) (Box 1-1) was influenced by the work of these social scientists (Bowlby, 1951; Robertson, 1958), but the recommendations remained largely ignored through the 1960s. Hawthorne (1976) continued to draw attention to the need for change in children's nursing. Reports about the wide range of child health provision created a further atmosphere of change (Court, 1976). More recently, the Audit Commission Report (1993) has questioned whether these recommendations have been acted upon.

The development of nurse education in the 1970s sought to rebalance medically dominated courses by incorporating greater nursing and social science content. This revised curriculum included aspects of humanism and holism, which are key aspects of conceptual models and frameworks of nursing. Family-centred care suited this approach, but was not developed into a framework of nursing. However, there are important concepts within the notion of family-centred care. Darbyshire and Campbell (see Chapter 3) have outlined some intrinsic difficulties in the notion of family-centred care: these represent major challenges for today's children's nurses. If family-centred care is to develop to its full potential, these issues must be addressed through practical application of this philosophy on the hospital ward.

ETHICS AND CHILDREN'S NURSING

Before children's nurses can address their future needs for education, practice and research, we must consider the purpose of such changes. Change is often accompanied by ethical dilemmas. Children's nurses must be able to deal with these sensitively. Nurses' appreciation of these ethical issues is developing. However, the situations which face children's nurses from day to day are highly complex. For innovation to occur in education, practice and research, therefore, it must carry the hearts and minds of not only the children's nurses, but also the children, their families and the general public. Understanding the ethics of current and future children's nursing practice is central to ensuring their support.

This section identifies some of the important concepts of ethical thinking related to children's nursing. As this is a very

---

◆ BOX I-I

Major reports affecting children's nursing

1994 Department of Health *Doing no harm.*

1994 Department of Health *The Allitt inquiry.*

1993 Audit Commission *Children first—a study of hospital services.*

1993 Thornes R *Bridging the gaps.*

1992 Department of Health *Working together, a guide to arrangements for inter-agency co-operation for the protection of children from abuse.*

1991 Department of Health *Welfare of children and young people in hospital.*

1991 Thornes R *Just for the day–children admitted to hospital for day treatment.*

1989 Department of Health *The Children Act, an introductory guide for the NHS.*

1988 Thornes R *Hidden children–an analysis of ward attenders in children's wards.*

1988 Thornes R *Parents staying overnight with their children.*

1976 Department of Health *Fit for the future: child health services.*

1959 Ministry of Health *Welfare of children in hospital.*

---

concise introduction, only the basic principles are examined. However, a range of further reading is suggested to allow more detailed study.

Modern children's nursing covers many activities that take place in a variety of settings. The increased possibilities in children's care, created by developments in nursing and medical technology, have also brought many ethical dilemmas. For example, what is the extent of the child's right to participate in decisions regarding his or her health care? In the case of life-threatening conditions of childhood, who decides when active interventive care is or is not appropriate? Do children enjoy the same rights as adults in health care concerning confidentiality and self-determination? What is the potential for the child's dependent relationship within his or her family to raise conflicts of interest in the decision making process in difficult ethical situations? These issues, and others, can be clarified and analysed using *ethical frameworks*.

WHAT IS ETHICS?

Most people have a vague idea that ethics is concerned with defining what is 'right' and 'wrong'. However, many other factors affect ethical decisions; good manners, good taste; the United Kingdom Central Council for Nursing, Midwifery and Health Visiting (UKCC) *Code of Professional Conduct* (UKCC,

1992); religious canon; and the law. Therefore, ethics can be seen as the sum of these things; it is concerned with morality, the 'rightness' or 'wrongness' of our actions, and how these affect other people.

These ideas are clearly of central concern to people — throughout human history, moral philosophers have sought to clarify the important issues of ethics (Warburton, 1992). This effort has resulted in the formulation of several important ideas and schools of thought.

Non-maleficence

This is the principle which stipulates that you should cause no harm. This would include both acts of *omission* and acts of *commission*. The *Code of Professional Conduct* (UKCC, 1992) expresses the idea of this principle:

Ensure that no action or omission on your part, or within your sphere of responsibility, is detrimental to the interests, condition or safety of patients and clients. (Clause 2)

This may state the obvious, but with increasingly complex health care technology, the 'obvious' can sometimes be difficult to determine. For example, what *is* harm? Can over-treatment be harmful?

Beneficence

The core of beneficence is in doing that which will produce benefit. This idea is illustrated in the *Code of Professional Conduct* (UKCC, 1992) as:

Act always in such a manner as to promote and safeguard the interests and well-being of patients and clients. (Clause 1)

These ideas of beneficence and non-maleficence are of primary importance to the children's nurse in judging daily situations and in deciding a course of action in difficult situations. These principles are, however, ideals — the 'gold standard'. Therefore, in complex situations involving many factors and conflicting interests, they may not be entirely helpful. This forms the basis of ethical dilemmas.

Justice

Justice is concerned with fairness. We attempt to formally ensure justice or fairness for everyone through our legal system and related structures. *Fairness* can be defined by the degree to which someone's rights are respected and acted upon. *Rights* define what we can fairly expect in our relationships with others and in our daily life. Basic rights for children have been codified in the United Nations Convention on the Rights of the Child (Newell, 1991) This is an area of ethics in which our thinking has evolved greatly in recent years (Archard, 1993). In ethical decision making, the difficulty arises when rights are conflicting. For example, does a child have the right not to be corporally punished or do parents have the right to discipline their children as they see fit? One person's right can often be seen as another person's responsibility.

Autonomy

Autonomy involves our independence as a human being and being allowed to make our own decisions. Respect for the dignity and autonomy of the individual in a health care setting can be seen in the need to obtain consent from the patient before undertaking any treatment or procedure. For the children's nurse, the principle of autonomy is important because, until recently, children were not seen to have the ability to make decisions autonomously. Children vary in their cognitive maturity at different developmental stages; their understanding is often not equivalent to an adult's. Combined with the fact that children are dependent on adults for their well-being, it is obvious how children's autonomy might be compromised in the health care setting. Until recently, as far as the law was concerned children under age 16 could not give consent to medical care. The Children Act of 1989 addressed this situation by enabling children to exercise autonomy in this context if it is clear to their carers that the child has the maturity and insight to appreciate the implications and consequences of any decision he or she might make. Alderson (1990, 1993) has made an invaluable contribution to the current debate on this topic.

Deontology

Deontology is concerned with *duty*: what we should or should not do. Professional codes of conduct, religious rulings, and the legal system tend to be duty based. The *action* is the focus of consideration; the *consequence* of the action is not the concern.

The example Anna in Box 1-2 illustrates the principles of deontology. As far as duty is concerned, the issue is clear. It would be 'wrong' to ignore Anna's express wishes and to approach her parents. The UKCC *Code of Professional Conduct* (1992) requires the nurse to:

protect all confidential information concerning patients and clients obtained in the course of professional practice. (Clause 10)

◆ **BOX 1-2**

Principles of deontology

Fifteen-year-old Anna has come to the Accident and Emergency Unit with a two day history of lower abdominal pain and bloody vaginal discharge. The medical team suspect that she may be having a miscarriage but she has refused to speak to or cooperate with the doctor. While chatting with the children's nurse she admits that she has been sexually active for the last six months and has not been using any form of contraception. The children's nurse explains that Anna will need to undergo further investigations and treatment to preserve her health. This raises the issue of consent for treatment which formally can only be obtained from Anna's parents as she is still legally a minor. Anna reacts very angrily to this – she insists that the nurse may not discuss this issue with her parents.

Although this is a crucially important principle, it gives us little guidance when considering the consequences of fulfilling this duty.

Consequentialism

This ethical school of thought emphasizes the *outcome* or *consequences* of a situation: an action is only 'good' insofar as it produces a 'good' result. This sort of thinking produces the 'white lie'. Although deontological thought condemns any untruth as conflicting with the duty to tell the truth, consequentialist thinking sees such an untruth as being acceptable if it is the means to a 'good' end.

The consequentialist perspective focuses on the end result and feels justified in the means necessary to achieve this aim. Of course, human issues are rarely this black and white. There are always mitigating, as well as complicating, factors which make up the 'shades of grey'! In the case of Matthew (Box 1-3), there are means which the children's nurse can employ to make the means of achieving a 'good' end more acceptable for Matthew.

It can be seen that these two ways of thinking about ethics are focused on two different perspectives. Deontology is concerned with the duty to do good: the nature of the action is the major concern. Consequentialism, on the other hand, is concerned with the *nature* of the outcome produced: by the action, the end is more significant than the means. Clearly, for children's nurses, a combination of these two approaches is useful in thinking about moral aspects of professional issues. One method might be to produce an analysis of the situation by considering the:

- Rights – of everyone involved in the situation and how these interlink.
- Responsibilities – of everyone involved in the situation and how these interlink.
- Consequences – the outcome foreseen for each of the choices of actions considered.

Case study accounts of actual scenarios are a useful way to analyse the ethical implications of a range of child health care dilemmas. Those of Brykczynska, offer interesting topics for consideration (Bryczynska, 1989, 1990, 1991a, 1991b).

◆ BOX 1-3

Consequentialism

Five-year-old Matthew has osteomyelitis in his ulna at his wrist. He will require treatment with intravenous antibiotics for several weeks. He has an indwelling intravenous cannula but this has required changing several times. On one occasion, after several bad experiences, Matthew simply refused to allow a cannula to be resited. In the event he was eventually coerced to allow this procedure to be completed.

This framework of ethical analysis needs to be included in the curriculum of children's nursing courses. Such a framework can be the nurse's firm foundation for analysing all aspects of practice and research in children's nursing.

A VISION FOR THE FUTURE

Health care within the National Health Service and nursing are currently subject to profound change. These changes have important consequences for children's nurses working in all aspects of health care. While these changes are bewildering for some, their impact upon the development of children's nursing is already apparent. Children's nurses have tended to improve the care of their particular patient group in a *reactive* manner, rather than in a *proactive* manner. This past should not be ignored when planning innovations in health care.

Innovation needs to occur in three areas of nursing: *education, practice,* and *research and development.* The emphasis on the 'three Es' (economy, efficiency and effectiveness), mean that planning for the future is not always easy. Darbyshire (1993) was emphatic that 'we must rediscover our passion for and about nursing as a real social force with an ethic of good immovably embedded within it'. It is doubtful that children's nurses have ever lost this passion, but they have been perceived by their colleagues as altruistic, well meaning and caring. Some believe they are passive and somewhat traditional in their attitudes, but this is not a true reflection of reality in the 1990s. Indeed, there is immense potential for the future development children's nursing.

EDUCATION

Unlike most other Western countries, the United Kingdom has maintained separate registers for the different specialty branches of nursing (Glasper, 1995). The normal route to specialization, since the development of Project 2000 diplomate courses, is at pre-registration level. Students tend to be dedicated to one branch of the profession from the start of their course. Under these circumstances, student nurses select their area of specialization (adult, children's, mental health, or learning difficulty nursing, or midwifery) and remain within that specialism for their entire career. As a result, there has been a reduction in the number of available post-registration courses leading to other parts of the register. This rigid approach may cause some students to enter the profession and a particular branch of nursing without true insight into themselves and their specialty. It is more realistic that nurses, like medical students, only choose their final area of specialization after experiencing a variety clinical environments.

GENERIC NURSE

Some senior nurses are increasingly propounding the advantages of generic nursing, as a way to ensure the provision of a cost effective, educated, trained workforce. With the difficulty among nurses holding special registration who wish to work in Europe, the US, Canada and Australia, there might be some support for the generic nurse within the profession.

If the profession does follow the generic route, safeguards must be imposed to protect the existing specialized branches. This may occur through innovative nursing curricula. For children's nursing, this might include suitable clinical experiences in tertiary, secondary and primary health care settings. Generic training might allow newly specialized nurses to practise at a minimum level, and their future promotion could depend upon further education and practice. In part, this already exists in the educational framework and higher award schemes of the professional bodies. Generic registration would then be followed by specialist education and practice in subsequent continuing professional curricula. There is a synergy in these ideas with the UKCC's nurse specialist and advanced practitioner recommendations. Some might argue that children's nursing more easily conforms to specialist and advanced practice, rather than its current pre-registration diploma status.

The integration of nurse education into higher education provides opportunities for the development of innovative curricula which could alter the nature of nursing. The assertion by Biley (1991) that nurse education must adopt progressive strategies is correct. Such progression must be linked to potential improvements in nursing care.

There remains much discussion about the long-term future of the specialist registration. The impact of Project 2000, 're-profiling' and budgetary constraint on the professional development of nursing is the subject of long-term evaluation. It seems likely that there will be a continued decrease in student numbers in the United Kingdom. The Audit Commission Report (1993) has reiterated the call for more registered children's nurses and refutes claims that there is an over capacity of such practitioners.

The debate about the future of children's nursing must be conducted in the public arena. The idea of the specialist register being built upon a generic undergraduate programme at postgraduate diploma or masters level is not without its critics (Glasper, 1993). Some suspect that an all-graduate generic workforce will disadvantage those able, but less academically gifted, individuals who wish to become nurses. However, the general acceptance of the credit accumulation and transfer scheme (CATS), the assessment of prior learning and experiential learning (APL and APEL) should allow students not entering higher education through the normal route to gain access to undergraduate courses. The NVQ, SNVQ and GNVQ schemes will produce a more educated workforce, better equipped to take advantage of opportunities in higher education. Despite the concerns, the number of applicants with appropriate A level passes for the limited undergraduate nursing places in the United Kingdom is such that there is an argument for the abandonment of Project 2000 at diplomate level. The reworking of existing diplomate courses (240 CATS points) into honours degree courses (360 CATS points) would not be difficult and should be encouraged. Currently, a large proportion of Project 2000 diplomate students

intend to continue their studies after registration, and to complete a degree. This belies the thoughts of cynics, who perceived that the uptake of post-registration honours degree courses would be minimal.

Nursing may wish to adopt the Australian approach, where the move from diploma to degree was achieved quickly, with minimal fuss. Many Australian diploma courses were revalidated, with only minor changes, to become degree courses. Under these circumstances, the issue of three-year or four-year degree programmes would need to be resolved. Therefore, it may be possible to develop generic nurse courses and to present these at first degree level.

Nursing is now one of the few non-graduate health care professions in the United Kingdom. Without taking the all-graduate option, it is difficult to encourage raising the profile of nursing as a profession. Children's nursing can follow one of two routes. The first route would convert the existing RSCN courses into a (postgeneric) postgraduate diploma/masters qualification. The second route, an all-graduate children's nursing workforce, is not feasible in the near future. The number of students on the child branch of Project 2000 diplomate courses, as well as the oversubscription applicants for undergraduate child branch nursing degrees, make this feasible in the long term. It is also in line with the development of children's nursing as an academic subject in its own right. Greater cooperation with other professionals, such as health visitors and school nurses, needs to be achieved. The current artificial barriers among these colleagues will slow the development of this important branch of nursing, as well as limit its potential.

MAINTAINING QUALITY

Undergraduate nurse education in the United Kingdom has resulted in many graduate nurses remaining in clinical practice longer than their non-graduate colleagues. It is difficult to explain this fact, but it does allay some of the fear that undergraduates might not wish, nor be able, to practise. Most of these courses, except that in Oxford, have a small number of students — typically about 20 per year. Nurse education based on graduates would require great increases in student numbers. There is a need to ensure that the quality of educational milieus, which have nurtured high-quality graduates, is not undermined by the necessity for large numbers of students. It is normal for degree courses to start at the beginning and finish at the end of the academic year. There is a problem in that all the student nurses will qualify at the same time of year. This does not happen currently with programmed diplomate entry and the relatively small number of undergraduates. Medicine has dealt with this problem by having standard dates for the movement of staff, accompanied by standard promotion through the lower grades. It would be difficult to establish such a national system for children's nurses. If, as a result of the single exit problem, there are periods when no nurses are qualifying, other types of carers will be sought by managers: probably those that are less expensive to employ than a children's nurse.

An all-graduate profession may be in parallel with the advent of health care assistants, possibly at NCVQ level III. Graduate nurses need to be able to supervise, teach, manage, and lead in order to ensure that both health care assistants and families perceive the children's nurse as the expert. The graduate must therefore be equipped with the clinical skills to act as a role model for all professionals involved in child health settings. This approach will avoid the realization of pessimistic predictions that health care assistants will become the true children's nurses, by providing the direct care with the families.

RESEARCH, DEVELOPMENT AND PRACTICE

While undergraduate nursing in the United Kingdom was established at the University of Edinburgh in 1960, the general progress of nurses towards higher education has been long and protracted. Higher education affords nursing students greater levels of professionalism and autonomy. It also establishes a solid research base and structure for continued professional development. However, the recent HEFC (Higher Education Funding Council) research assessment exercise placed nursing research at the bottom of the league of excellence. Marsland (1993) noted the crudity of this exercise when he stated, 'Nothing could be more helpful to our rivals than to have top nursing researchers admitting that the ratings were valid and accurate'. Health care research is highly competitive and funds are won with difficulty. Other professionals, such as social scientists and the professions allied to medicine, are active health care researchers and are suspicious of the entry of nursing into this field. Some professionals have a history of research in child health and if nurses wish to compete they need to have the appropriate research skills. Reflective practice is an appropriate educational strategy through which to achieve this goal. The children's nurse in the 1990s is mainly concerned with improvement and innovation in practice in tertiary, secondary and primary health care.

CHANGING PATTERNS OF RESEARCH

Research methodology in the early years of academic nursing followed those used in the breadth of higher education. With no history of research to draw upon, pioneering nurse researchers were forced to rely on established methods to give them respectability with colleagues from other disciplines. The need for a theory of nursing to support the art and science of nursing, was recognized for many years and was probably responsible for a trend towards esoteric research. Nolan and Grant (1993) viewed this esotericism as 'The manifest failure of the theoretical and research based literature to make substantial inroads into the world of practice' and called it 'the theory–practice gap'. This gap between the researchers (theory) and the innovators (practice) is a source of concern and must be closed as soon as possible. The new nursing courses, such

as Project 2000 and the PREP framework of continuing education, are already helping to reduce this theory–practice gap.

The changes in the funding arrangements for research activity within the National Health Service, under the auspices of Professor Michael Peckham, are designed to ensure that research is linked to practice. This practical approach to health care research runs parallel to the *Health of the Nation* recommendations and its emphasis on the burden of disease, and the promotion of health gain. This approach favours multidisciplinary cooperation. Nursing must look to its practice-based discipline and its various patient groups for research inspiration. Methodologies such as as *evaluation research* and *action research* are useful in involving practitioners and, therefore, have their merits. Action research in particular brings the participating researcher into active involvement in the process of change.

PRIMARY HEALTH CARE

Recent reorganizations in the health service have emphasized the move from tertiary to primary health care. This philosophy is manifest in the government white paper *Working for Patients* and in its subsequent working papers, including the Community Care Act 1992, which have dramatically changed the nature of health care in the United Kingdom. The transition from mechanistic medical care to a greater emphasis on holism is demonstrated in the *Patient's Charter* which establishes the status of patients/parents as consumers of health care. This is an example of an emerging reform which will alter the traditional doctor/nurse/patient power relationships which have bedevilled health care for so long. Patient's charters or other 'bills of rights' are the precursors to advocacy and the empowerment of families. Children's nurses have acted as advocates for families by providing information to promote empowerment. Information is the key to empowerment. There have been some impediments for children's nurses in their quest for family advocacy: chief among these being the vestigial medical paternalism. This approach was said to protect families and children from the true nature of childhood illness, stemming from an era, before antibiotics, when child mortality was high. Reflective practice in nursing is undermining this outmoded approach and leads nurses to become more assertive in practice. Strategies which ensure and promote quality measurement help to create an environment of advocacy and have brought attention back onto parents as *partners* in care. Partnership is now a major theme in children's nursing, especially among community nurses involved with child care. Health visitors, paediatric community nurses and school nurses have led this change of approach, which has thrown out the old role of parents as passive onlookers in the care of their children. This equal partnership in care has developed more slowly within the inpatient sectors of health care. This is changing as a result of the work of Casey (1988) at The Hospital for Sick Children, London. Such partnership now forms a major thread in several diplomate and undergraduate child branch courses in the United Kingdom.

Earlier discharge from hospital, and the growth of surgical day care, have increased the work of the primary health care nurses, in particular. While these changes have been promoted through psychological justification (i.e., the best place for a child is at home), the economic factors have also had a part to play. The cost to both family and to professionals of caring for a sick child at home must continue to be evaluated. The change towards research by nurses in this field will be a prominent feature of the 1990s. Neylon (1993) showed the need for and effect of health promotion for school children, and confirmed the importance of the role of the school nurse, in particular. Studies which promote greater empowerment of a designated patient group will continue to attract funding. Neylon's study showed that health promotion for school-aged children was effective in 75% of cases, and argued for child health interviews as a method of school health education.

SECONDARY HEALTH CARE

Once the 'Cinderella' of child health care, secondary health care has now assumed greater importance. The development of the purchasers – provider 'market', through NHS trusts and health commissions, has been reinforced by the creation of GP fundholders. These GPs are likely to promote the development of secondary care for children to a great extent. Day care units and outpatient departments (OPDs), as well as accident and emergency departments, are re-examining their function in the light of the changes sweeping the health service. Some general practitioners are already insisting on changes in the coordination of referrals to children's outpatients. After years in the wilderness, OPDs are now becoming areas of innovation. An example is the work of Campbell *et al* (1993) in developing the first paediatric nursing development unit at Southampton. These developments complement the findings of the Caring for Children in the Health Services publication *Bridging the Gaps* (Thornes, 1993). This study explored the interfaces between primary and specialist care for children and emphasized the need for sharing of information with families. Such findings support the introduction of family information centres. Children's nurses working in secondary care settings will find the document a useful source of inspiration.

The outpatient department is, for many families, the first contact with the hospital and, in common with the accident and emergency department, is a potential shop window for innovation and change. While publications such as *Bridging the Gap* can promote change, they are generally based on 'best practice' from around the United Kingdom and beyond. However, it is clear that children's nurses do not need to work in well–known prestigious units to be able to promote change. There are good examples of action research in secondary care, often in small units. A team approach to problems can often succeed where single researchers might flounder. Hawthorn's work (1992) in promoting the care of bereaved relatives is a good example. Hawthorn collected data from parents bereaved of their infants, and was able to change the way the hospital's

Chapel of Rest worked and the manner in which parents were counselled at the time of bereavement and subsequently.

The interest in day care has been assisted by The Caring for Children in the Health Services publication *Just for the Day* (Thornes, 1991). This recommends good practice and innovation in the management of children undergoing minor surgical and medical procedures. Increases in available day care for this patient group have important implications for the resourcing of the primary health care team. There is also a need to evaluate the impact of day care upon the family. Such reports provide further impetus for children's nurses in the promotion of innovation among their colleagues.

The reduction in the length of stay for children in hospital has occurred at the same time as the growth in day care, leading to further use of outpatient services. This extra patient volume is a challenge for nurses working in these areas and will need to be monitored. Despite greater use of secondary hospital services, the non-attendance of families is still a major problem but is rarely investigated. GP fundholding will focus attention on this usually ignored, but important problem.

TERTIARY HEALTH CARE

This was formerly, and should still be, the high profile area of children's nursing. The title 'registered sick children's nurse' epitomizes the main direction of the care provided by nursing in the recent past. Some people question whether this title should be used at all. The generic route, which has been discussed, could make the RSCN title redundant and we could see postgraduate diplomas/masters degrees which incorporate the skills of the three groups of children's nurses (children's nurse, school nurse and health visitor).

Despite the move away from inpatient care, many research and development projects are designed to improve the *delivery* of this care. The importance of the clinical nurse specialist is well represented in the UKCC's PREP proposals, and is a key aspect of children's nursing in all aspects of health care. The complexity of tertiary care predisposes it to specialist nurses. The current trend is that children requiring inpatient care are often very sick and require 'high care'. The breadth of the specialties within child health requires a similar supply of skilled nurses. Some would view this as following the medical model and, superficially, this would appear to be the case. However, the unique nursing needs of the families of very sick children make this an organizational necessity. Much innovation has been generated regarding the environment of the hospital and the role of parents. There should be no complacency, however, and research and development bids from nurses working in the tertiary areas needs to be seen at the forefront of their work.

The Audit Commission (1993) identified several problems which are important for children's nursing. These problems include failure to implement the principle of child- and family-centred care in some children's units, a general shortage of RSCNs and children being nursed on adult wards. Innovation designed to deal with the recommendations of these reports will attract research and development monies from a variety of funding agencies. Children's nurses must develop competitive qualities in making applications for funding.

ATTRACTING RESEARCH AND DEVELOPMENT SPONSORSHIP

To attract research and development sponsorship it is necessary to (Glasper, 1993):

• Develop a cogent, clearly defined research question.
• Foster a multidisciplinary research team approach (the project is likely to attract funding if several professional groups are involved).
• Ensure an appropriate research methodology — solicit the support of your local university nursing studies department.
• Be realistic with costings — research always costs in terms of time and money. Research on the cheap will be bad research. If the project is worth doing, it is worth supporting, but first you have to convince the funding body!
• Remember that printing costs money, as does secretarial and computer time.

The replication of research conducted in other units within the United Kingdom or abroad is often underestimated, but may be valuable, especially if a visit to the centre can be arranged beforehand. Such visits to develop research and development are supported by a number of bodies, such as The Florence Nightingale Memorial Fund, the Association of British Paediatric Nurses' Portex Scholarship or the Royal College of Nuring's Cow and Gate Scholarship.

The Department of Health's (1993) *A Vision for the Future* (Department of Health/NHS Management Executive publication,) outlines the renewed strategy for nursing. It is important for children's nurses who wish to promote innovation through research and development. The report highlights the prime focus of clinical practice and urges professionals to work with academic departments towards enhanced care. Recommendations that all units show where care has been improved through research findings will act as a stimulus for change. Children's nurses must be at the forefront of these developments.

KEY POINTS

◆ The historical development of paediatrics influences the current and future nature of children's nursing.
◆ Children's nursing should seek innovative strategies for professional development.
◆ A change to generic nurse education must also include the protection of the specialized branches.
◆ An all-graduate workforce may prevent able, but less academically gifted, people from becoming nurses.

◆ Paediatric nurses should be pre-eminent as reflective practitioners.
◆ Charters for children and families promote advocacy and empowerment.
◆ Partnership is a familiar trend in the philosophy of children's nursing.
◆ Traditionally a 'Cinderella' department, outpatient services are now areas of innovation.

REFERENCES

Alderson P: *Children's consent to surgery,* Buckingham, 1993, Open University Press.

Alderson P: *Choosing for children: parents' consent to surgery,* Oxford, 1990, Oxford University Press.

Archard D: *Children: rights and childhood,* London, 1993, Routledge.

Audit Commission: *Children first—a study of hospital services,* London, 1993, HMSO.

Besser FS: Great Ormond Street anniversary, *Nurs Mirror* 144(6): 31, 1977.

Biley F: The divide between theory and practice, *Nurs* 4: 29, 1991.

Bowlby J: *Maternal care and mental health, Geneva,* 1951, World Health Organization.

Brykczynska GM: A father's right, *Paediatr Nurs* 3(6):25, 1991b.

Brykczynska GM: A question of tolerance, *Paediatr Nurs* 3(4):21, 1991a.

Brykczynska GM: Doing good, *Paediatr* 2(4):8, 1990.

Brykczynska GM: Truthfulness in a paediatric setting, *Paediatr Nurs* 1(7):23, 1989.

Campbell SJ, Lowson S, Glasper EA: Families first, the Southampton Nursing Development Unit, *Paediatr Nurs* 4(8):35, 1993.

Casey A: A partnership with child and family, *Senior Nurse* 8(4):8, 1988.

Court SDM: *Fit for the future: report of the Committee on Child Health Services,* London, 1976, HMSO.

Darbyshire P: Preserving nurse caring in a destitute time (guest editorial), *J Adv Nurs* 18:507, 1993.

de Mause L: *The history of childhood,* London, 1974, Souvenir Press.

Department of Health: *Fit for the future: child health services,* London, 1976, HMSO.

Department of Health: *The Children Act, an introductory guide for the NHS,* London, 1989, DoH

Department of Health: *Welfare of children and young people in hospital,* London, 1991, HMSO.

Department of Health: *A vision for the future,* London, 1993, HMSO.

Department of Health: *Doing no harm,* London, 1994, Medical Devises Directorate.

Department of Health: *The Allitt inquiry,* Report of the Clothier Committee, London, 1994, HMSO.

Department of Health: *Working together, a guide to arrangements for inter-agency co-operation for the protection of children from abuse,* London, 1994, HMSO.

Glasper EA: Funding for the future, *Child Health* 1(4):160, 1993.

Glasper E A: Back to the future. Innovating trends in child health nursing. *Child Health* 1(3):93, 1993.

Glasper E A: The value of children's nursing in the third millenium, *Br J Nurs* 4(1):27, 1995.

Hawthorn A: *Give sorrow words,* London, 1992, RCN Society of Paediatric 8th Birthday Conference.

Hawthorne PJ: *Nurse I want my mummy,* London, 1976, Royal College of Nursing.

Marsland D: Research and destroy, *Nurs Stand* 7(23):45, 1993.

Ministry of Health: *Welfare of children in hospital (Platt report),* London, 1959, Ministry of Health.

Newell P: *The UN Convention and children's rights in the UK,* London, 1991, National Children's Bureau.

Nolan M, Grant G: *Action research and quality of care, J Adv Nurs* 18:305, 1993.

Neylon J: Health promotion for school children, *Nurs Stand* 7(30):37, 1993.

Robertson J: *Young children in hospital, London,* 1958, Tavistock Publications.

Thornes R: *Hidden children—an anlysis of ward attenderss in children's wards,* London, 1988, Caring for Children in the Health Services Consortium.

Thornes R: *Just for the day—children admitted to hospital for treatment,* London, 1991, Caring for Children in the Health Services.

Thornes R: *Bridging the gaps,* London, 1993, Caring for Children in the Health Services Consortium.

Thornes R: *Parents staying overnight with their children,* London, 1988, Caring for children in the Health Services.

United Kingdom Central Council for Nursing, Midwifery and Health Visiting: *Code of Professional Conduct,* London, 1992, UKCC.

UNICEF : *First call for children—world declaration and plan of action from the world summit for children — convention on the rights of the child,* New York, 1990, United Nations Children's Fund.

Warburton N: *Philosophy: the basics,* London, 1992, Routledge.

FURTHER READING

Baylis F, McBurney C: *In the case of children,* Toronto, Canada, 1993, Department of Bioethics, The Hospital for Sick Children.

Bracegirdle KE: A time to die: withdrawal of paediatric intensive care, *Br J Nurs* 3(10):513, 1994.

Brykczynska GM, editor: *Ethics in paediatric nursing,* London, 1989, Chapman & Hall.

Chadwick R, Tadd W: *Ethics and nursing practice: a case study approach,* Basingstoke, 1992, Macmillan.

Charles-Edwards I, Casey A: Parental involvement and voluntary consent, *Paediatr Nurs* 4(1):16, 1992.

Charles-Edwards I: Who decides? *Paediatr Nurs* 3(10):6, 1991.

Ellis P: A child's right to die: who should decide? *Br J Nurs* 1(8):406, 1992.

Glasper E A: Preserving children's nursing in a climate of gerericism, *Br J Nurs* 4(1):21-25, 1995.

Hunt G, editor: *Ethical issues in nursing,* London, 1994, Routledge.

Kuhse H, Singer P: *Should the baby live? — the problem of handicapped infants,* Oxford, 1985, Oxford University Press.

Rumbold G: *Ethics in nursing practice,* London, 1986, Baillière Tindall.

Seedhouse D: *Ethics: the heart of health care,* Chichester, 1988, John Wiley & Sons.

Chapter 2

Cultural, Social and Religious Influences on Child Health Care

LEARNING OUTCOMES

After studying this chapter you should be able to:

◆ Define the key terms introduced in the chapter.
◆ Discuss the influence of culture on the formation of health beliefs and health behaviour.
◆ Demonstrate an appreciation of how culture influences the child's and family's response to ill health and health care interventions.
◆ Discuss the importance of taking cultural and religious factors into account in providing individualized nursing care.
◆ Show an understanding of social influences on the health of children and their families.
◆ Define glossary terms.
◆ Articulate innovative research and development in primary, secondary and tertiary care.

GLOSSARY

acculturation Gradual changes produced in an individual or a culture by the influence of another culture that cause new cultural features to be adopted

culture shock Feelings of helplessness and discomfort in a state of disorientation experienced by an outsider attempting to adapt to a different cultural group

culture The shared beliefs, values and customs developed by a group of people in adaptation to the physical and social circumstances in which they find themselves

ethnicity Shared racial, cultural, social, and linguistic heritage characterized by a shared identity and sense of belonging to a group

ethnocentrism Attitude that one's own ethnic group is superior to other ethnic groups

race Group of people with similar physical characteristics, such as colour, that are transmitted through generations and are sufficient to characterize the group as a distinct human race

role Expected behaviour of individuals in a particular culture

socialization The process by which individuals learn the ways of a given society in order to function within that group

stereotyping Labelling; lack of recognition of differences among individuals within a particular cultural ethnic, or religious group

subculture Smaller group within a culture that possesses many characteristics of the larger culture while contributing its own unique values

transcultural nursing Nursing that focuses on the comparative study and analysis of different cultures to provide culture-specific and sensitive care practices

he future of any society depends on its children. If it is to survive, the society must make provision for their care, nurture and socialization. *Cultural* survival depends on whether the customs and values of the culture are transmitted from one generation to the next through families. The culture into which children are born outlines the roles of their parents, structures their relationships with other people and determines much of the behaviour they acquire. A holistic view of any child requires that nurses develop some understanding of the ways that culture contributes to the development of social and emotional relationships, and influences child-rearing practices and attitudes towards health. An orientation to transcultural nursing includes an awareness of the nurse's own cultural frame of reference and a concerted effort to recognize and appreciate the views and beliefs of the health care recipients to deliver culture-specific and sensitive care.

CULTURE

"*Culture* can be seen as an inherited 'lens' through which individuals perceive and understand the world that they inhabit" (Helman, 1990). Culture differs from both race and ethnicity. *Race* generally refers to a group of people with similar physical characteristics, such as skin colour, that are transmissible by descent and which distinguish it as a particular human type. Classification by race generally includes the following recognized types: caucasoid (white), negroid (black), and mongoloid (yellow). *Ethnicity* refers to a shared racial, cultural, social and linguistic heritage (Martinson, 1989). *Socialization* is the process by which individuals learn the ways (beliefs, values, and behaviours) of a given society in order to function within it (Dobson, 1991).

A culture is composed of individuals who share a set of values, beliefs, practices and information that is learned, integrative, and socially affirmed. Culture is an *ingrained* orientation to life that serves as a frame of reference for individual perception and judgement; people from one culture differ from those in other cultures in the ways they think, solve problems, perceive and structure the world. Culture is, essentially, the way of life of a group of people that incorporates experiences of the past, influences thought and action in the present, and transmits these traditions to future group members. Adaptation is necessary, however, for the culture to survive in an ever-changing world. Consciously and unconsciously, individuals abandon, modify or assume new patterns to meet the needs of the group.

The observable components of a culture, such as material objects (dress, art, utensils and other artefacts) and actions, are sometimes termed the *material, overt* or *manifest culture; nonmaterial covert culture* refers to aspects which cannot be observed directly, such as the ideas, beliefs, customs and feelings of the culture. Related to the larger culture are many *subcultures,* each with an identity of its own.

The culture in which children are reared determines the type of food they will eat, the language they will speak, the behavioural ideals they will follow and the way they will conduct themselves in social roles. To be acceptable members of the culture, children must learn how the culture expects them to behave towards others in the group. In turn, they learn how they can expect others to behave towards them.

Cultures and subcultures contribute to the uniqueness of child members in such a subtle way and at such an early age that children may grow up to feel that their beliefs, attitudes, values, and practices are 'correct' or 'normal', and that those of other cultures are 'deviant' or 'wrong'. A set of values learned in childhood is apt to characterize children's attitudes and behaviour for life.

The manner and sequence of growth and development phenomena are universal and fundamental features of all children. However, the variations in behavioural responses that children display to similar events are believed to be determined by cultural facets. Inborn temperament and modes of behaviour that prompt children to behave in their own preferred and highly individual manner may be in harmony or in conflict with their culture. Forces such as heredity and maturity limit the influence that parents and other social groups may have.

A culture fosters and reinforces behaviours deemed desirable and appropriate, and attempts to suppress or extinguish those at conflict with its norms. For example, some cultures encourage aggressive behaviours; others favour amiability and compliance. Some foster individual resourcefulness and competition; others emphasize cooperation and submission to group interest.

Standards and norms vary from culture to culture and location to location. For example, a practice that is accepted in one area may meet with disapproval in another. The extent to which cultures tolerate divergence from the established norm varies among cultures and subcultural groups. Although conformity provides a degree of security, it is a decided deterrent to change (Mares, Henley and Baxter, 1985).

SUBCULTURAL INFLUENCES

Except in rare situations children grow and develop in a blend of cultures and *subcultures*, (e.g., smaller groups within a culture that possess many characteristics of the larger culture while contributing their own particular values). In a highly populated and complex society such as the United Kingdom, different groups have their own set of standards, values and expectations within the collective ways of the larger culture. Although many cultural differences are defined by geographical boundaries, subcultures are not always restricted by location. Subcultures can even be related to the age stages of development that have traditions, games, loyalties and rules. Age-related subcultures are easily identified in the behaviour of school-age children and adolescents, most often being apparent in children's play activities, as these are less influenced by adults.

Children's membership in a cultural subgroup is, generally, involuntary. They are born into a family with a specific ethnic and/or racial heritage, socioeconomic level, and religious belief.

Although in British society there are numerous subcultures and considerable variations in ways of life, subcultural factors that exert the greatest influence on child-rearing are ethnicity, social class and occupational roles. School and peer-group subcultures are also strong influences in the socialization of children.

Ethnicity

Ethnicity is the classification of divisions of mankind, differentiated by customs, characteristics, language or similar distinguishing factors. Ethnic differences extend to many areas and include such manifestations as family structure, language, dress, dance, food preferences, moral codes, and expressions of emotion. Some behavioural patterns (for example, the traditional role of the father) result from the cultural heritage of the specific ethnic group. Other behavioural patterns reflect the interaction between subcultures, most notably between members of the majority culture and members of minority subcultures (McCall, 1991).

To establish their place in a group, children learn how to adhere to a mode of behaviour that is in accordance with standards distinctive to the group. Children take their cues by observing and imitating those to whom they are exposed. For example, children of a racial minority form a perception of their role as group members by observing the manner in which role models within the subgroup respond to treatment by people outside the subgroup. When they see group members display an attitude of inferiority, they assume this to be the appropriate behaviour. These perceptions are then incorporated into their own self-concept.

It is particularly difficult for persons to attempt to maintain an identity within a subculture while living and conforming to the requirements of the larger culture. Universal customs and language of the dominant culture used in commercial and educational systems are different from those of the minority culture. Often, the values conflict. Consequently, children reared in this environment may be confused about roles and values, and usually adopt those of the more influential or higher-status culture. Youth, in particular, are influenced by the locally dominant group.

Ethnocentrism

Ethnocentrism is the emotional attitude that one's own ethnic group is superior to others, that one's values, beliefs, and perceptions are the correct ones, and that the group's ways of living and behaving are the best way. Ethnic *stereotyping* or labelling stems from ethnocentric views of people. Ethnocentrism implies that all other groups are inferior and that their ways are not in the best interests of the group. This attitude strongly influences the ability of individuals to evaluate the beliefs and behaviours of others objectively, and tends to bias their interpretation and understanding of the behaviour of others. Ethnocentrism is often a largely unconscious process (Richardson, 1993).

Religion

The religious orientation of the family dictates a code of morality and influences the family's attitudes towards education, male and female role identity, and attitudes regarding their ultimate destiny (Fig. 2-1). It may also determine which schools the children attend, the companions with whom they associate, and often their mate selection. In many cultures, the religious beliefs are such an integral part of the culture that it is difficult to distinguish one from the other.

Schools

When children enter school, their range of relationships extends to include a wider variety of peers and a new focus of authority. Although parents continue to exert the major influence on children, in the school environment teachers can have a significant psychological impact on children's development and socialization. The function of teachers is primarily limited to teaching, but, like parents, they are also concerned about the children's emotional welfare. Both parents and teachers must constrain behaviour, and both are in a position to enforce standards of conduct.

Socialization.

Next to the family, schools exert a major influence in providing continuity between generations by conveying a vast amount of culture from older members to younger members. In this

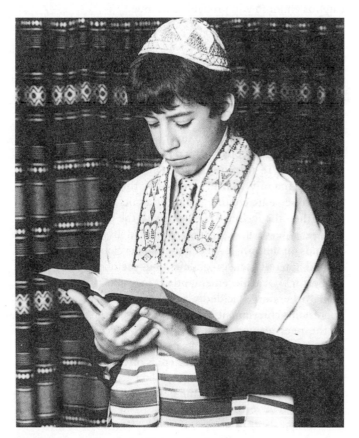

Fig. 2-1 A Jewish boy during his bar mitzvah ceremony.

way, children are prepared to carry out the traditional social roles they are expected to assume as adults. School is the centre of 'cultural diffusion' wherein the cultural standards of the larger group are mediated to the local community. It governs *what* is taught and, to a large extent, *how* it is taught. School rules and regulations regarding attendance, authority relationships, and the system of sanctions and rewards based on achievement transmit to the child the behavioural expectations of the adult world of relationships and employment. School is often the only institution in which children systematically learn about the negative consequences of behaviours that deviate from social expectations. In addition, school provides an opportunity for some children to participate in the larger society in rewarding ways, and often provides avenues for social mobility for both students and teachers. Through education, individuals in lower socioeconomic classes are offered the opportunity for further education and the capacity to move up in the social strata.

Teachers are responsible for transmitting the knowledge and values of the dominant culture; that is, values on which there is broad consensus. They are expected to stimulate and guide the intellectual development of children, their sense of aesthetics, and their capacity for creative problem-solving.

Traditionally the socialization process of school began when the child entered nursery or primary school. With many mothers now working outside the home, this socialization process begins much earlier for many children in a variety of day-care settings. Considering that many mothers work because of economic necessity, this trend towards out-of-home care for children will probably continue.

Peer Cultures

Peer groups also influence the socialization of children. Peer relationships become increasingly important and influential as children proceed through school. Although children are exposed to value systems of their family, ethnic group, and social class, the values imposed by the peer group are especially compelling because children must accept and conform to them in order to be accepted as members of the group. When the peer values are not too different from those of family and teachers, the mild conflict created by these small differences serves to separate children from the adults in their lives and to strengthen the feeling of belonging to the peer group.

The type of socialization provided by the peer group depends on the special subculture that develops from the background, interests, and capabilities of its members. Some groups support school achievement, others focus on athletic prowess, while others are decidedly antithetical to educative goals. Scholastic achievement is strongly related to the value system of the peer groups. Many conflicts between teachers and students, and between parents and students, can be attributed to fear of rejection by peers. There is often a conflict between what is expected from parents regarding academic achievement and what is expected from the peer culture. This is especially pronounced in secondary school.

Although it has neither the traditional authority of the parents nor the legal authority of the schools for teaching information, peer groups convey a substantial amount of information to its members, especially about subjects such as sex and drugs. Children's need for the friendship of their peers brings them into an increasingly complex social system. The world of the peer group is different from the adult world and, through peer relationships, children learn ways to deal with dominance and hostility, and to relate with persons in positions of leadership and authority. Other functions of peer subculture are to relieve boredom and to provide a form of individual recognition that children do not receive from teachers and other authority figures.

The peer-group culture has secrets, mores and codes of ethics with which they promote feelings of group solidarity and detachment from adults. They have traditions and customs that are transferred from 'generation to generation' of school children and that greatly influence the behaviour of the group. These include age-related games and other activities which, as children move from one level to the next, are discarded as older-age activities are adopted.

Biculture

Some children are exposed to the values, role relationships and life-styles of two cultures—a virtual 'straddling' of two cultures. This is sometimes observed in the play group, but usually is not a significant factor until children enter school. Children of two cultures must unlearn some of the established practices of one culture in order to become socialized in the other, especially in role relationships. For example, children from Oriental cultures are taught to look away when scolded; in school, however, the teacher expects direct eye contact—'Look at me when I speak to you'. Children learn new roles and social behaviour more rapidly than their adult counterparts.

An occasional effect of biculture is that children meld the elements of the dominant culture and their minority culture to form a subculture that is uniquely their own.

THE CHILD AND FAMILY

Family life in the United Kingdom is characterized by increasing geographic and economic mobility. There is less reliance on tradition; families are fragmented; and there is limited opportunity to transmit and acquire the traditional and accepted customs of a culture. Consequently, young adults rely to a greater extent on peers and mass media for acquisition of acceptable patterns of behaviour, including child-rearing practices. Each generation, as it adapts to the new, discards the inadequacies of previous generations. This often constitutes a source of confusion and frustration as parents attempt to adjust to rapid changes; tradition and precedent no longer meet the needs and challenges of rapid change that require new approaches and innovation for problem solving. According to Weller (1994), competent parents attempt to determine the comparatively stable, essential components of the culture and to transmit these to their children.

Minority-Group Membership

When minority groups immigrate to another country, a certain degree of cultural/ethnic blending occurs through the process of *acculturation*. This is the process in which gradual changes produced in a culture, by the influence of another culture, cause one or both cultures to become increasingly similar to each other. However, these changes occur with varying degrees in different families and groups. At one time, is was thought that the differences among different cultures would eventually diminish to produce a homogeneous society. However, this does not appear to be the case. Many groups continue to identify with their traditional heritage while adapting to their conceptions of the dominant culture.

Previous studies indicate that children become aware of their racial or ethnic status early in life. They also become aware of discriminatory attitudes of the majority culture towards their group at an early age. The direct effects of discrimination are anger and low self-esteem, which become manifest in a variety of behaviours. Inner conflicts and suppressed hostility that focus children's attention inward may be factors in the failure of many children to achieve in other areas.

CULTURE SHOCK

The term *culture shock* describes the "feelings of helplessness and discomfort and a state of disorientation experienced by an outsider attempting to comprehend or effectively adapt to a different cultural group because of differences in cultural practices, values, and beliefs" (Leininger, 1978). This state occurs with both patients and health care providers who move from one culture to another culture or setting. It can happen to persons who immigrate to a new country (such as refugees) or persons from a subcultural group who must adjust to the ways of an unfamiliar subgroup (such as children entering the school subculture, or patients who enter the hospital subculture). Culture shock is characterized by the inability to respond to, or to function, in a new or strange situation.

Several factors influence the reactions to a new environment. Language barriers, including dialects and jargon (such as medical language) specific to a subcultural group, inhibit effective communication. Habits and customs (such as different role behaviours or etiquette) and differences in attitudes and beliefs are puzzling to the stranger in the new environment. The outsider experiences a sense of isolation and feelings of loneliness. Nurses entering an unfamiliar cultural situation can reduce culture shock by becoming familiar with the cultural groups with which they work and by learning tolerance towards the values, beliefs and customs of these groups.

Immigrants and refugees from cultures in which children are taught to respect and obey their elders, and in which females are considered inferior to males, may have difficulty dealing with the consequences of Western egalitarianism.

CULTURAL/RELIGIOUS INFLUENCES ON HEALTH CARE

Cultural beliefs and practices are an important part of data gathering in the nursing assessment. Nurses continually encounter beliefs and practices that may facilitate or impede nursing interventions, including attitudes towards family planning, food habits and customs that are firmly entrenched in the culture. The language of the patient may be different from that of the larger culture, or there may be regional or ethnic peculiarities in their use of basic English. Subcultural influences, such as religious beliefs and practices, may conflict with standard health practices and therapeutic interventions.

SUSCEPTIBILITY TO HEALTH PROBLEMS

Some groups of people are more susceptible, and others more resistant, to certain illnesses than are people from other groups. An innate susceptibility is acquired through generations of evolutionary changes that take place within constrained or segregated populations. Heredity, general physical status, environmental factors and the proximity to disease are significant factors associated with health problems.

Hereditary Factors

The genetic constitution of individuals influences the degree to which they are susceptible to a specific disorder. It may be the result of an inherent lack of resistance to a disease organism, a trait that is an advantage in one environment a disadvantage in another, or the consequence of intermarriage within a relatively narrow range of geographic, ethnic, or religious restrictions.

Some ethnic or racial groups appear to have a predisposition towards certain diseases. For example, Tay-Sachs disease, characterized by early neurological deterioration and mental retardation, affects primarily Ashkenasi Jewish families, particularly those of Northeastern European origin, while Sephardic Jewish families appear to be no more at risk for the disease than other populations. The incidence of cystic fibrosis is highest in caucasians, almost nonexistent in Orientals, and rare in black families (except where ancestry is mixed). Some selected genetic disorders that are more prevalent in certain populations are listed in Table 2-1.

Common food items and drugs may cause health problems in certain racial groups. For example, persons with glucose-6-phosphate dehydrogenase (G-6-PD) deficiency develop acute haemolytic anaemia after they ingest fava (horse or broad) beans or certain drugs such as aspirin preparations, sulphonamides, or primaquine. This deficiency is found in a large percentage of people around the world, especially those of Mediterranean, African, Near Eastern, and Asian origin.

Sensitivity to food containing lactose is a common hereditary characteristic of several cultural groups, especially southern Europeans, Jews, Arabs, blacks and Asians. Lactose intolerance usually does not become a problem until the child reaches

ETHNIC OR POPULATION GROUP	GENETIC OR MULTIFACTORIAL DISORDER PRESENT IN RELATIVELY HIGH FREQUENCY	ETHNIC OR POPULATION GROUP	GENETIC OR MULTIFACTORIAL DISORDER PRESENT IN RELATIVELY HIGH FREQUENCY
Armenians	Familial Mediterranean fever Familial paroxysmal polyserositis	Jews *Sephardi*	Familial Mediterranean fever Ataxia–telangiectasia (Morocco) Cystinuria (Libya) Glycogen storage disease III (Morocco)
Blacks (African)	Sickle-cell disease Haemoglobin C disease Hereditary persistence of Haemoglobin F G-6-PD deficiency, African type Lactase deficiency, adult β-Thalassaemia	Lebanese	Dyggve–Melchoir–Clausen syndrome
Burmese	Haemoglobin E disease	Mediterranean people (Italians, Greeks)	G-6-PD deficiency Mediterranean type β-Thalassaemia Familial Mediterranean fever
Chinese	α-Thalassaemia G-6-PD deficiency, Chinese type Lactase deficiency, adult	Oriental	Dubin-Johnson syndrome (Iran) Ichthyosis vulgaris (Iraq, India) Werdnig–Hoffman disease (Karaite Jews) G-6-PD deficiency, Mediterranean type Phenylketonuria (Yemen) Metachromatic leucodystrophy (Habbanite Jews, Saudi Arabia)
English	Cystic fibrosis Hereditary amyloidosis, type III		
Finns	Congenital nephrosis Generalized amyloidosis syndrome, V Polycystic liver disease Retinoschisis Aspartylglycosaminuria Diastrophic dwarfism	Polish Portuguese	Phenylketonuria Joseph disease
		Scandinavians (Norwegians, Swedes, Danes)	Cholestasis–lymphoedema (Norwegians) Sjögren–Larsson syndrome (Swedes) Krabbe disease Phenylketonuria
Irish	Phenylketonuria Neural tube defects		
Japanese	Acatalasia Cleft-lip palate Oguchi disease	Scots	Phenylketonuria Cystic fibrosis Hereditary amyloidosis, type III
Jews *Ashkenazi*	Tay–Sachs disease (infantile) Niemann–Pick disease (infantile) Gaucher disease (adult type) Familial dysautonomia (Riley–Day syndrome) Bloom syndrome Torsion dystonia Factor XI (PTA) deficiency	Thai	Lactase deficiency, adult Haemoglobin E disease

Data from Cohen, 1984; Damon, 1969; Der Kaloustian et al., 1980; Ferak, et al., 1982; Goodman, 1979; McKusick, 1988; Tamot, 1974; and Stanbury, 1983.

Table 2-1 Distribution of selected genetic traits and disorders by population or ethnic group.

3 to 5 years of age. However, lactose-intolerant children become uncomfortable with distention, flatus and diarrhoea after ingesting milk or milk products. Well-meaning health workers may unknowingly be responsible for these symptoms in their patients when they offer foods containing lactose.

An example of resistance to disease, or selective advantage, of a population is found in persons who possess the sickle-cell trait. Sickle-cell disease is a classic disorder of black, especially Afro-Caribbean people. Persons with sickle-cell trait are highly resistant to a form of malaria, and in the parts of the world where the organisms are prevalent, there is a high frequency of the trait. However, in an environment where malaria is not a threat, possession of the trait has no advantage and only the negative aspects of the condition remain (e.g., risk of sickle-cell anaemia in offspring).

Physical characteristics

There are observable differences in physical appearance among racial groups. The most obvious are skin and hair colouring and texture. Skin colour is determined by the amount of melanin pigment present in the skin. Persons from countries located near the equator have darkly pigmented skin, which protects it from the year-round exposure to the sun's rays; persons from the northern countries have very light skin, which provides maximum exposure to the sun's rays (necessary for vitamin D metabolism) during the short daylight hours. There can be wide variations in skin colour between these two extremes in terms of geographic origin or from intermixing of dark and light skin colour.

As a consequence of the dark pigmentation, the detection of skin colour changes can be difficult and requires modification of assessment techniques. For example, vasomotor alterations, cyanosis, and jaundice are not easily recognized in very dark or black skin. Variations in the skin colour can alter the appearance of the skin in a given circumstance.

Physical variations (e.g., stature and body build) in newborn infants are often related to racial or ethnic origin. For example, newborn infants of Asian and black parents are smaller than infants of white parentage (David, 1990). Bluish pigmented areas (mongolian spots) on the sacral region are a common observation on Oriental and black infants. Oriental children are usually smaller at all ages, and black children are taller and heavier between ages 5 and 14 than white children of the same age. This difference in stature can lead to misinterpretation of health status and capabilities. In communication and education, a child who is smaller than average may appear precocious and one who is larger might appear to be slow. Expectations determined on this basis can be detrimental to the child.

Socioeconomic Factors

The most overwhelmingly adverse influence on health is socioeconomic status. A higher percentage of lower-class individuals are suffering from some health problem at any one time than are those in any other group. The sum of all aspects of their situation contributes to and compounds health problems;

this includes crowded living conditions and poor sanitation, which facilitate transfer of disease (Townsend *et al.*, 1992).

In the lower classes, relative inaccessibility to health services may inhibit treatment for any but severe illness or injury. Sometimes health care is inadequate because of ignorance. For example, the parents may not have information regarding causes, treatment, outcome of the illness, or preventive measures.

Poverty

A high correlation between poverty and the prevalence of illness has long been observed. Impoverished families suffer from poor nutrition; they have little if any preventive health care and maintenance, and very limited access to health services (Townsend *et al.*, 1992). Health care often ranks low on their list of priorities. Day-to-day needs of food, clothing and lodging take precedence as long as the ailing person feels able to perform activities of daily living.

Families must find care for dependants, such as other infants and small children, or have them accompany them when taking an ill child for care. Preventive care can be delayed indefinitely unless health services are relatively accessible.

Poor nutrition accounts for many health problems in the lower classes. Lack of funds and ignorance result in a diet that may be seriously lacking in essential food substances, especially protein, vitamins and iron. This inadequate diet may lead to nutritional deficiency disorders and growth retardation in children. Unstructured eating patterns and irregularly scheduled mealtimes can also contribute to erratic food intake and a proportionately larger consumption of non-nourishing snacks, which can result in excessive weight gain.

Because of deficient preventive care, dental problems are more prevalent. Poor sanitation and crowded living conditions also contribute to the higher incidence and perpetuation of illness. In general, poor people become ill more frequently and remain ill for longer periods of time than the more advantaged.

Homelessness

Homeless children experience all of the health problems associated with poverty, as well as other types of disorders. Preventive health care, especially dental care, may be lacking. Both delayed growth and overweight problems are common, as are illnesses resulting from exposure to cold and weather conditions. Developmental delays, severe depression, anxiety and learning difficulties have been reported. The erratic, chaotic lifestyle of these children increases their vulnerability to any number of physical and psychosocial problems.

Migration

Migrant families generally suffer more illness, both acute and chronic, than the general population. They are subject to unhealthy environments, poverty and insufficient medical care; their health-seeking behaviour in general is an illness- or injury-orientated recourse to medical care. Affected persons may postpone seeking care for themselves or their children until physical pain or suffering is almost unbearable.

CUSTOMS, BELIEFS AND VALUES

Nurses are becoming increasingly aware of the need to consider cultural differences in patients when providing health care. An understanding of the various beliefs regarding the causation of illness and disease as well as traditional health practices is essential to successful intervention. The more nurses know about the values, beliefs and customs of other ethnic groups, the more able they are to meet the needs of families and to gain their cooperation and compliance.

Compliance with medical therapies is primarily related to accessibility and availability. For example, medications provided by health workers are more likely to be taken than those that must be obtained at a pharmacy or chemist. In addition, medications are often discontinued following self-perceived recovery. Treatment regimens that do not interfere with work or family responsibilities are most likely to be adhered to.

Relationships with Health Care Providers

The manner of relating with health care providers differs considerably among cultural groups. One area of conflict for some nurses is the attitude towards time and waiting that is part of some cultures. The time orientation of some ethnic groups is in the present. These groups are very flexible in their time orientation. For example, a family from this type of group may be late for or miss appointments because other issues take precedence over the appointment, and the family may not communicate this to the health care provider.

In many cultural groups, the mother assumes the responsibility for health care; in others, both parents are involved equally in relationships with health workers. A different approach is apparent in some of the Oriental cultures. For example, the father in South Asian families, as unquestioned head of the family, is traditionally the family member who interacts with persons outside the family unit (including health care providers). Therefore, he is the one who represents the family in health matters.

Usually, a family confers with other members before reaching a decision regarding treatment or hospitalization of a child. In working with families, it is essential for nurses to identify key members—failure to include these significant individuals in teaching can seriously hinder adherence to the plan of care. Nurses should also be aware of any specific attitudes regarding the manner of approach to a child in a given culture.

Some ethnic groups consider a child's admission to the hospital a family affair, with all members gathering to support and console the child and the parents. In others, the family is willing to relinquish the care of the child to the hospital authority without interference. Their visits with the child are short, although intense, but this behaviour may be misinterpreted by the hospital staff as disinterest or abandonment.

Members of all ethnic groups are entitled to be treated with dignity and respect. Family members should be addressed correctly, according to their wishes: many groups consider it an affront to be called by their first name. Stereotyping should not

occur. Persons are individuals who should be evaluated in relation to their cultural standards, needs, and preferences (Fig. 2-2).

Nurses who are members of a majority culture may encounter tension and distrust in a child from a minority culture as a result of the child's learned conception of or relationships with other persons in the majority group. Based on these perceptions, minority children may suspect that nurses have hostile feelings towards them, and thus fear ill treatment. When such children are hospitalized, this feeling compounds the feelings of loneliness, helplessness and retribution that accompany fearful events and separation from families. The reverse situation may be encountered by a nurse from a minority culture attempting to meet the needs of a child who has been conditioned to view the nurse's cultural or ethnic group as inferior.

Communication

Communication is basic to all human relationships, but it may be a source of distress and misunderstanding between persons from different ethnic groups, especially if the languages are different. Ideally, conversations with families who are unable to speak the dominant language are best conducted by a health care worker who speaks the language of the family. If this is not possible, it may be necessary to engage the services of an interpreter. However, use of an interpreter can be a source of misunderstanding if the interpreter is unfamiliar with the medical terminology or if there are no corresponding words in the second language to express the ideas and concepts under discussion.

Some persons with poor or limited language comprehension may simply smile and nod in agreement if they do not understand the questions or directives. It is vital that the family fully understand all the implications of a child's care and management before they sign consent forms for special procedures or assume responsibility for the child's care. It is not uncommon

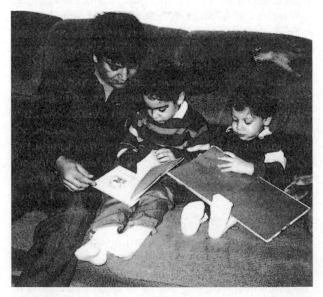

Fig. 2-2 Fathers from many cultures assume an active parenting role.

for an Oriental family to indicate 'yes' when in fact they mean 'no' in order to avoid social disharmony. They tend to use indirectness rather than confrontation, and may become evasive when direct questioning makes them feel uncomfortable.

Eye contact is viewed differently in cultures. It is not uncommon for persons in some ethnic groups to avoid eye contact and become uncomfortable when conversing with health workers. In non-Western cultures, a patient may not look directly into the nurse's eyes, as a sign of respect.

There may be reluctance on the part of families to question or otherwise initiate contact with health professionals. In the Asian cultures, for example, it is considered a sign of disrespect to question those who are viewed as persons of authority (Orque, 1983).

It is necessary to speak slowly and carefully, not loudly, when conversing with families who have poor language comprehension. Many persons are able to read and write English better than they can speak or understand it. Also, the dominant language usually takes over in anxiety-provoking situations, even in persons who are able to communicate satisfactorily under ordinary circumstances.

Terms of address vary among cultures and can create confusion in institutions. For example, in Asian cultures, the family name is given first (in respect for the family) with the given names following. Therefore, all siblings in a family have the same first name (in some families it may be the middle names that are the same).

Although all people share the same basic emotions, there are decided ethnic variations in the way they are expressed. In some cultures (e.g., persons of Latin or Jewish background), emotions are expressed openly and members are accustomed to share their sorrows and joys with family and friends. Conversely, Nordic and Asian groups are more restrained in expressing emotion.

Nurses caring for persons of other cultures will be better able to communicate if they understand the common names used by other cultures to describe symptoms and diseases (Hayward, Woo and Kangesu, 1991), such as 'miseries' (pain) and 'locked bowels' (constipation) in black people.

Food Customs
Food customs and symbolism of various cultural, ethnic, and religious groups have become an integral part of their lives. Special holidays, ceremonies and life experiences such as births, birthdays, weddings and death are often marked by special food items or feasts. In many cultures, specific food practices are followed during pregnancy in the belief that certain foods damage the developing fetus.

The distinctive food customs of ethnic groups are a product of their native environment, determined by availability. Fish is a staple food of persons living near the ocean, such as people from Japan, Polynesia and Scandinavia. Fruit and vegetable preferences are also directly related to the climate in which these grow naturally or can be cultivated. The types of grain that are ethnically associated are also those that grow best in their native lands. For example, rice is the staple grain of the Orient, wheat of the temperate climates of Europe and rye in

Scandinavia. In some cultures, food is highly spiced; in others, foods tend to be bland.

There are several restrictions related to food items. Some have a physiological origin, such as lack of dairy foods in the diets of some persons of African or Asian ancestry who have lactose intolerance. Others have religious restrictions, such as kosher foods and food preparation of the Orthodox Jewish faith and the vegetarian diets of Buddists and Hindus.

Children in a strange environment, such as the hospital, feel much more comfortable when they are served foods to which they are accustomed (Fig. 2-3). The hospital food often tastes strange and bland, especially to children who enjoy the highly seasoned foods of their culture. The family may be concerned that the child is receiving foods appropriate to their culture and beliefs. Where possible, it is advisable to provide children's ethnic foods or to allow families to bring favourite foods that are not available on the hospital menu. Concern for differences in food habits and patterns projects an attitude of respect for the family's ethnic or religious heritage.

HEALTH BELIEFS AND PRACTICES

Nurses encounter people of many different racial and ethnic origins in the process of meeting the health needs of children and families. Some of these families have become so enculturated to the majority culture that their health beliefs and practices are consistent with those of the health care system. There are still many families, however, whose traditional practices and beliefs are an integral part of their daily lives. It is important for health care workers to be aware that 'other people may live by different rules and priorities from those of the health care provider, and these rules and priorities decisively influence health-related behaviour' (Bauwens and Anderson, 1984).

Health Beliefs
Beliefs related to the cause of illness and the maintenance of health are an integral part of the cultural heritage of families.

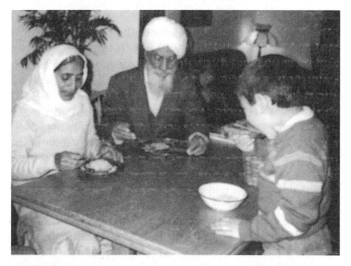

Fig. 2-3 Food customs outside the home can differ significantly from traditional cultural practices.

Often inseparable from religious beliefs, they influence the way families cope with health problems and the way they respond to health care providers. Predominant among most cultures are beliefs related to natural forces, supernatural forces and the imbalance between forces.

Natural forces

The most common natural forces held responsible for ill health, if the body is not adequately protected, include cold air entering the body, impurities in the air, or other natural sources. For example, a parent may overdress an infant in an effort to keep cold wind from entering the child's body.

Some cultures consider behaviour, such as overeating, overwork, anxiety, and inadequate food and sleep, as natural causes of illness. Many cultures consider health to be a state of harmony with nature and the universe, and thus ill health to be a lack of such harmony.

Supernatural forces

High on the list of causes of illness in many cultures, are forces beyond comprehension and logical explanation. Evil influences such as voodoo, witchcraft or evil spirits are viewed in some cultures as causes of adverse health, especially those illnesses that cannot be explained by other means.

Although seldom expressed to health care providers, the belief that a witch can cast a spell or curse over another person at the request of someone who wishes the person ill or dead is found in some cultures.

Imbalance of forces

The concept of balance or equilibrium is widespread throughout the world. One of the most common imbalances supported by the Asian, Oriental and Arab cultures is between 'hot' and 'cold'. A similar belief is reputedly derived from the Hippocratic theory of humoural pathology, which states that illness is caused by an imbalance of the four humours: phlegm, blood, black bile, and yellow bile. 'Hot' and 'cold' describe certain properties and conditions completely unrelated to temperature. Diseases, areas of the body, foods, and illnesses are classified as either 'hot' or 'cold'. In Chinese health belief, the forces are termed *yin* (cold) and *yang* (hot). In order to maintain health and prevent illness, these hot and cold forces must be kept in balance.

Illness is treated by restoring normal balance through the application of appropriate 'hot' or 'cold' remedies. A 'cold' condition such as a respiratory disease is believed to be caused by exposure to cold weather, rain, or cold wind entering the body; it is treated by administration of 'hot' foods, herbs, or drugs.

Health care workers who are aware of this belief are better able to understand why some persons refuse to eat certain foods. It is often useful to discuss the diet with the family to determine their feelings and beliefs regarding food choices. It is possible to help families devise a diet that contains the necessary balance of basic food groups prescribed by the medical subculture, while conforming to the beliefs of the ethnic subculture (Karseras and Hopkins, 1987).

The hot-cold food classification may have adverse effects. For example, newborn infants are often started on evaporated milk formulas. Evaporated milk is considered to be a 'hot' food, while whole milk is viewed as a 'cool' food. Infants tend to develop rashes, which are believed to be caused by 'hot' foods; in such cases, parents may decide to switch to whole milk. However, parents fear that it is dangerous to change too rapidly, so they often feed the child some type of neutralizing substance, which may create additional health problems (Murillo-Rohde, 1980). Such problems might be averted if the family's preference is determined before discharge from the hospital and a formula prescribed that is agreeable to both the family and the practitioner.

Health Practices

There are many similarities among cultures regarding the prevention and treatment of illness. All cultures have some types of home remedies that they apply before seeking help from other persons. Within the ethnic community, folk healers who are endowed with the ability to 'cure' maladies are sought for special situations and when home remedies are unsuccessful. For example, the Asian may consult a herbalist, knowledgeable in medicines, and/or an ethnic practitioner practised in Asian therapies, including acupuncture (insertion of needles), acupressure (application of pressure) and moxibustion (application of heat).

Folk healers are very powerful persons in their community and have the ability to acquire information about an illness without resorting to probing questions. They 'speak the language' of the family who seeks help, and often combine their rituals and potions with prayer and entreaties to a god. They also are able to create an atmosphere conducive to successful management. Furthermore, they exhibit a sincere interest in the family and their problem.

Often it will be found that folk remedies are compatible with the medical regimen and can be used to reinforce the treatment plan. For example, most of the foods contraindicated for a person with peptic ulcer are 'hot' foods and would be avoided because of the person's belief system. Also, aspirin (a 'hot' medication) is an appropriate therapy for 'cold' diseases such as the common cold and arthritis (Murillo-Rohde, 1980). It is not uncommon to discover that a folk prescription has a scientific basis. However, numerous health remedies or preventive practices have no scientific basis, such as use of copper or silver bracelets to protect the wearer. If they do no harm, these practices should be respected.

Health practices of different cultures may also present problems of assessment and interpretation. For example, the Vietnamese practice of 'coining' may produce welt-like lesions on the child's back when a coin, held on edge, is repeatedly rubbed lengthwise on oiled skin to rid the body of the disease (Feldman, 1983). Another such custom is the Old World practice of 'cupping'. A container, such as a tumbler, bottle or jar containing steam is placed against the skin surface to 'draw out the poison' or other evil. When the heated air within the container cools, a vacuum is created that produces a bruise-like blemish on the skin directly beneath the mouth of the container (Asnes and Wisotsky, 1981; Holland and Sweeney, 1985). Both of these remedies can be misdiagnosed as evidence of 'child abuse' by uninformed professionals.

Faith healing and religious rituals are closely allied with many folk-healing practices. Wearing of amulets, medals, and other religious relics believed by the culture to protect the individual and facilitate healing, is a common practice. It is important for health workers to recognize the value of this practice and to keep the items where the family has placed them or nearby. This offers comfort and support and rarely impedes medical and nursing care. If an item must be removed during a procedure, it should be replaced, if possible, when the procedure is completed. The reason for its temporary removal should be explained to the family, and they should be reassured that their wishes will be respected.

Although most subcultures in developed countries have become acculturated to Western medical systems, many still maintain faith in traditional healing practices and practitioners. When the folk practices do not interfere with the welfare of the patient, they need not be discouraged. Often, a compromise can be reached that accomplishes the goal of the nurse while maintaining the dignity and self-esteem of the patient.

RELIGIOUS BELIEFS

Religion influences the lifestyles of most cultures. Among many groups, illness, injury or death is believed to be sent by God as a punishment for sin. Some may believe that health workers will be unable to help a person whom God is punishing and may express a fatalistic attitude toward treatment, stating that it is 'the will of God'. Others view it as a test of strength, as the testing of Job in the Bible, and strive to remain faithful and overcome the conflicts.

Religious affiliation has implications for many health-related functions and procedures. It is comforting to the family of an ill child to have this need recognized and respected. Nurses need to determine if there are any special considerations related to spiritual practices that are important to the family. Dietary restrictions are clarified, especially in denominations in which there may be a number of variations. Where specific religious practices do not interfere with the health of the child or the therapy (such as fasting), the wishes of the family are respected. Family members should be asked whether they want a clergy member present and whether they prefer hospital staff to phone or to do this on their own.

It is also important to determine the wishes of the family regarding baptism, rites or practices related to death, and other religious rituals (such as circumcision, communion or the use of amulets or icons). An important role of the nurse is to be aware of spiritual needs of families and to convey an attitude of concern for this element of the child's care. Religion, which offers families understanding and spiritual support, can be a valuable asset to health care.

IMPORTANCE OF CULTURE AND RELIGION TO NURSES

To begin to understand and deal effectively with families in a multicultural community, it is important that nurses are aware of their own attitudes and values regarding a way of life, including health practices. Nurses, too, are a product of their own cultural background and education; frequently, they and other health care workers are not aware of their own cultural values and how those values influence their thoughts and actions. Those who are aware of their own culturally founded behaviour, are more sensitive to cultural behaviour in others. To recognize that a behaviour may be characteristic of a culture rather than an 'abnormal' behaviour places nurses at an advantage in their relationships with families. When nurses respect the cultural differences of a family, they are better able to determine whether the behaviour is distinctive to the individual or is characteristic of the culture. What appears to be puzzling behaviour may simply be the customary response in the culture (e.g., expression of emotion).

Cultural standards and values, the family structure and function, and past experiences with health care influence a family's feelings and attitudes towards health, their children, and health care delivery systems. It is often difficult for nurses to be non-judgemental and objective in working with families whose behaviours and attitudes differ from or conflict with their own; but if they rely on their own values and experiences for guidance, they will only experience frustration and disappointment. It is one thing to know what is needed to deal with a health problem; it is often quite another to implement a fruitful course of action unless nurses are willing to work within the cultural and socioeconomic framework of the family.

It is beneficial to make an effort to adapt ethnic practices to the health needs of the family rather than to attempt to change long-standing beliefs. To this end, nurses should have a readily available resource file containing pertinent information about the cultural and subcultural characteristics of the community in which they practise (e.g., traditional practices related to infant feeding, the time and manner of weaning, and toilet training). Bridging cultural gaps in health care requires the establishment of a close relationship with the community, and ongoing assessment of one's attitudes and behaviours (and those of other health workers) towards people of other racial or ethnic origins. It is important, therefore, for nurses to assess the patient and family in order to identify how they are similar to, and different from, the patient's cultural and religious background.

KEY POINTS

◆ Nurses have a responsibility to understand the influence of culture, race, and ethnicity on the development of social and emotional relationships, child-rearing practices and attitudes towards health.

◆ A child's self-concept evolves from ideas about his or her social roles.

◆ Primary groups are characterized by intimate contact, mutual support and behaviour constraint among members.

◆ Secondary groups have limited intermittent contact, little mutual support and no pressure for conformity.

◆ Important subcultural influences on children include ethnicity, social class, occupation, poverty, affluence, religion, schools and peers.

◆ Children who live in poverty, who are homeless, or have migrant families suffer from more physical and mental health problems than other children.

◆ Drug response, food sensitivity, disease resistance, physical characteristics, and disease states may demonstrate ethnic or cultural variations.

◆ Cultural beliefs related to the cause of illness and the maintenance of health may focus on natural forces, supernatural forces, or the imbalance of forces.

◆ In planning and implementing patient care, nurses must adapt ethnic practices to the family's health needs, rather than attempt to change long-standing beliefs.

◆ The only way to clearly understand someone's cultural needs, is to ask that person.

REFERENCES

Asnes RS and Wisotsky DH: Cupping lesions simulating child abuse, *J Pediatr* 99:267-268, 1981.

Bauwens E, Anderson S: Social and cultural influences on health care. In Stanhope M, Lancaster J: *Community health nursing*, St Louis, 1984, Mosby–Year Book.

Cohen FL: *Clinical genetics in nursing practice*, Philadelphia, 1984, J.B. Lippincott Co.

Damon A: Race, ethnic group and disease, *Soc Biol* 16:69, 1969.

Der Kaloustian VM, Maffah J, Loiselet J: Genetic diseases in Lebanon. *Am J Med Genet* 7:186, 1980.

David R: Race, birthweight, and mortality rates, *J Pediatr* 116(1):101, 1990.

Dobson S: *Transcultural nursing*, London, 1991, Scutari.

Feldman SS, Aschenbrenner B: Impact of parenthood on various aspects of masculinity and femininity: a short term longitudinal study, *Dev Psychol* 19:278, 1983.

Ferak V, Gencik A, Gencikova A: Population genetical aspects of primary congenital glaucoma, *Hum Genet* 61:193, 1982.

Goodman RM: *Genetic disorders among the Jewish people*, Baltimore, 1979, Johns Hopkins University Press.

Hayward PJ, Woo M, Kangesu E: One solution to the linguistic problems faced by health visitors, *Health Visitor* 64(6):185-197, 1991.

Helman GJ: *Culture, health and illness*, ed 2, London, 1990, Butterworth-Heinemann.

Holland S, Sweeney E: *Vietnamese children and families: the impact of culture*, Washington, DC, 1985, Association for Care of Children's Health.

Karseras P, Hopkins E: *British Asians—health in the community*, London, 1987, Wiley & Sons.

Leininger M: *Transcultural nursing*, New York, 1978, John Wiley & Sons.

Mares P, Henley A, Baxter C: *Health care in multiracial Britain*, Cambridge, 1985, National Extension College/Health Education Council.

Martinson IM: The challenge of culturally diverse pediatric clients. In Feeg V, editor: *Pediatric nursing: forum on the future: looking toward the 21st century*, Pitman, NJ, 1989, Anthony J Jannetti.

McCall J: Ethnic minorities, *Surg Nurs* 4(4):20, 1991.

McKusick V: Mendelian inheritance in man, ed. 8. Baltimore, 1988, Johns Hopkins University Press.

Murillo-Rohde I: Health care for the Hispanic patient, *Crit Care Update* 7(5):29-36, 1980.

Orque MS: Nursing care of South Vietnamese patients. In Orque MS, Bloch B and Monrroy LSA: *Ethnic nursing care*, St Louis, 1983, Mosby-Year Book, Inc.

Richardson J: Transcultural aspects of paediatric nursing. In Glasper EA, Tucker A: *Advances in child health nursing*, London, 1993, Scutari.

Stanbury JB: *The metabolic basis of inherited disease*, New York 1983, McGraw-Hill, Inc.

Tamot B: Genetic polymorphisms and diseases in man, New York, 1974, Academic Press, Inc.

Townsend P, Davidson N, Whitehead M: *Inequalities in health: the Black report and the health divide*, Harmondsworth, 1992, Penguin.

Weller B: Cultural aspects of children's health and illness. In Lindsay B, editor: *The child and family: contempory nursing issues in child health and care*, London, 1994, Baillière Tindall.

FURTHER READING

Ablon J, Ames GM: Culture and family. In Gilliss CL *et al*, editors: *Toward a science of family nursing*, Menlo Park, CA, 1989, Addison-Wesley.

Balarajan R, Raleigh VS: *Ethnicity and health: a guide for the NHS*, London, 1993, Department of Health.

Brink PJ: Value orientations as an assessment tool in cultural diversity, *Nurs Res* 33:198, 1984.

Health Visitors Association Racial Issues Working Party: *Entitled to be healthy: health visiting and school nursing in a multiracial society*, London, 1989, HVA.

Lash ME: Community health nursing in a minority setting, *Nurs Clin North Am* 15(2):339, 1980.

Lipson JG, Meleis AI: Culturally appropriate care: the case of immigrants, *Top Clin Nurs* 7(3):48, 1985.

Lutwak RA, Ney AM, White JE: Maternity nursing and Jewish law, *MCN* 13(1):44, 1988.

Mandelbaum JK: The food square: helping people of different cultures understand balanced diets, *Pediatr Nurs* 9:20, 1985.

O'Brien ME: Transcultural nursing research—alien in an alien land, *Image* 13:37, 1981.

Oberg CN: Pediatrics and poverty, *Pediatr* 79(4):567, 1987.

Ruiz MCJ: Open-mindedness, intolerance of ambiguity and nursing faculty attitudes toward culturally different patients, *Nurs Res* 30:177, 1981.

Stoll RT: Guidelines for spiritual assessment, *AJN* 79:1574, 1979.

Thiederman SB: Ethnocentrism: a barrier to effective health care, *Nurs Pract* 11(8):52, 1986.

Thornton A: Reciprocal influences of family and religion in a changing world, *J Marriage Fam* 47:381, 1985.

Tripp-Reimer T, Lauer G: Ethnicity and families with chronic illness. In Wright L, Leahey M: *Families and chronic illness*, Springhouse, PA, 1987, Springhouse Corp.

Tripp-Reimer T, Brink PJ, Saunders JM: Cultural assessment: content and process, *Nurs Outlook* 32:78, 1984.

Chapter 3

Family-Centred Care

LEARNING OUTCOMES

After studying this chapter you should be able to:

- Relate background theory to the notion of family-centred care.
- Understand the need for empowering and enabling behaviours to promote family-centred care.
- Have respect for the unique quality of each and every family.
- Identify the constituent parts of the framework of family-centred care.
- Understand the potential for family-centred research.
- Define the glossary terms.

GLOSSARY

partnership State of being partners (from partner, one who shares or takes part with another, player on the same side in a game)

empowerment The process of giving power or authority

saturday morning clubs Preadmission programs run for families prior to the admission of a child to hospital

family-centred care Where the needs of all family members are considered during childhood illness

charter A written grant of rights

The notion of family-centred care incorporates the family as the constant in a child's life and the service systems and personnel must support, respect, encourage and enhance the strength and competence of the family (Johnson *et al.*, 1989). Families are supported in giving care and in making decisions by building on the strengths of the individuals and families. The maintenance of the way of life of the family at home and in their community is promoted. The needs of all family members, not the child alone are considered. Family-centred care recognizes diversity among family structures and backgrounds; family goals, aspirations, strategies and actions; and family support, service, and information needs (Ahmann, 1994).

Two processes are required to achieve family-centred care: the enabling and the empowerment of families. Health professionals enable families by creating opportunities and ways for all family members to use their abilities and capabilities and to acquire the new skills and attitudes that are necessary to meet the needs of their sick child and family. Empowerment describes the interaction of professionals with families so that families maintain or acquire a sense of control over their lives and make constructive changes that result from professional assistance that fosters their own strengths, abilities and actions (Dunst *et al.*, 1988). The parent-professional partnership is a powerful mechanism for enabling and empowering families (Casey, 1988; Casey and Mobbs, 1988). Parents serve as respected equals with professionals and have the correct role of deciding what is important for themselves and their family; the professional's role is to support and strengthen the family's ability to nurture and promote its member's development in a way that is both enabling and empowering.

Partnerships imply the belief that partners are capable individuals who become capable by sharing knowledge, skills, and resources in a manner that benefits all participants. Collaboration is viewed as a continuum. Families have the option of being anywhere along that continuum, depending on the strengths and needs of the child, the family and the professionals who are involved (Shelton *et al.*, 1987). The nurse can help every family, including those with a previous history of serious personal and/or family problems, to identify strengths, build on them, and assume a comfortable level of participation.

Children's nurses have been quick to accept the notion of family-centred care, but Wong (1995) argues that nurses in the United States have been slow to implement care which reflects the intrinsic philosophy of "family as patient". This lag has occurred in part because family-centred care requires a shift in orientation regarding provision of services. The philosophy requires stretching beyond clinical practices that have become tradition because of their convenience to the institution and personnel (Ahmann, 1994). Common examples of system-based care are exclusion policies of not allowing family members to stay with their children during a procedure and restricting visiting hours as well as numbers and ages of visitors.

On the other hand, family-centred care requires viewing families as the centre of care, with their input serving as the major determinant of the interventions provided. For example,

exclusion policies are replaced with family-based care, such as parental and child choice regarding separation during procedures, open visiting hours, and no limitations on the ages and numbers of visitors, except at the family's request (Flint and Walsh, 1988). In fact should the word "visitors" ever be used? Family members certainly are not visitors to their child; nurses and other staff are.

Even child-based care is not synonymous with family-based care. For example, the hospital dietary service may provide food selections for children but fail to provide inexpensive meals for parents or consider cultural/religious traditions. Primary nurses may focus on the child's needs, but place little emphasis of the family's concerns.

In your practice, what policies can be considered system-, child-or family-based care? How can those that are not family-based care be changed? What reasons do staff give for preferring system-based care? Compare the community or acute Trust's policies with its mission statement and purpose. In the United States, Hostler (1992) reported that, during visits to 30 leading hospitals in the United States, not one single model of excellence in the implementation of family-centred care was found. Fortunately, models of family-centred care, such as Casey's Partnership model (Fig. 3-1), and the Nursing Mutual Participation Model (Casey, 1988; Casey and Mobbs, 1988; Curley, 1988; Curley and Wallace, 1992), do exist and have documented benefits, such as:

- Families experience greater feelings of confidence and competence and less stress in caring for their children.
- The dependence of families on professional care givers decreases
- Child minding costs decrease
- Professionals experience greater job satisfaction
- Both parents and providers are empowered to develop new skills and expertise

(Curley and Wallace, 1992; Johnson *et al.*, 1992)

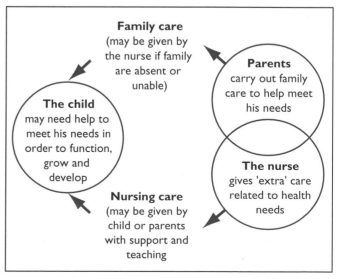

Fig. 3-1 Casey's partnership model for children's nursing. (From Casey, 1988.)

THE CONCEPT OF FAMILY-CENTRED CARE

Within the United Kingdom, the concept of family-centred care, and the desirability of helping parents to be with and to participate in their hospitalized child's care, is widely accepted within children's nursing. The government report, *Welfare of Children and Young People in Hospital* (Department of Health, 1991), is emphatic about this point. A cardinal principle of hospital services for children is "Families with children have easy access to hospital facilities ..." (Department of Health, 1991, p.2). Similarly, "Good child health care is shared with parents/carers and they are closely involved in the care of their children at all time ..." (Department of Health, 1991, p.2). Such participation is not a luxury, it is a necessity.

The first of the cardinal principles mentioned in the Department of Health (1991) guidelines on the Welfare of Children and Young People in Hospital is that "Children are admitted to hospital only if the care they require cannot be as well provided at home, in a day-clinic or on a day basis in hospital" (Department of Health, 1991, p.2). This document supported the use of Paediatric Community Nursing services, which were described as "a very helpful contribution to the support of families caring for sick children at home" (Departmemt of Health, 1991, p.9). Such services have made a substantial contribution to the development of family centred care in the United Kingdom. Where these services exist, many children avoid the need to be admitted, and are also probably discharged earlier. Whiting (1994) noted a substantial increase in the number of such services, in 1981 there were only eight such generalist services, but by April 1993 there were 61. These teams provide continuity of care with their hospital colleagues, enabling and empowering parents and carers to provide appropriate care for their child. Such teams are not part of the every day experience of care within North American Child Health Care. One of the strategies used in North America has been the development of "Care by Parent Units", however, the development of Paediatric Community Nursing Services in this country made such innovations surplus to requirements (Cleary *et al.*, 1986).

The following points provide a useful summary of the three main concepts involved in family-centred care:

- It is an approach to nursing which regards the unit of care as being the family and not just the patient.
- It accepts the family's own definition of what constitutes 'family'.
- The nursing care and environment help to promote the strengths and individuality of the family in order to enable them greater scope for caring for their relative.

These points apply equally to the adult patient and family as to the child. While family-centred care might be more easily applied when working with children, the approach could, and probably should, be adopted in other areas of nursing practice.

COMMUNICATING THE PHILOSOPHY OF CARE

Families need to have a clear idea of the philosophy of the ward into which their child is admitted. If family-centred care is part of this philosophy, but is not clearly defined, then it is not surprising that parents do not fully understand the care or the nature of their involvement (Dearmun, 1992). The Action for Sick Children charter identifies the rights of children in hospital. Wards using such a philosophy have a greater consensus about care. A research-derived definition of family-centred care could form a similar focus.

IMPLEMENTING THE PHILOSOPHY

These perspectives have led children's nurses to a recognition that understanding and adopting family-centred approaches to care are problematic (Robinson, 1987; Rushton, 1990a and b; Campbell and Clarke, 1992; Campbell and Summersgill, 1993). They identified impediments to family-centred care, such as changes in patient populations; staff shortages; professional attitudes; institutional climates' and possible discrepant perspectives to illness, hospitalization and care held by parents and nurses.

Clearly, there is a need for research which sheds more light upon children's nursing's cherished concepts and 'cardinal principles' such as 'family-centred care' and parent participation. Darbyshire (1992) conducted a qualitative research study which examined the questions of how parents understand the experience of staying with their child in hospital and how parents and children's nurses relate in this new era of 'family-centred care'. This study showed that children's nursing may have underestimated the complexity of the concept of family-centred care.

Darbyshire (1992) offered a description of the ways in which nurses both understood and construed the notions of 'parent' and 'family', and revealed that such meanings, previously taken for granted, are in fact problematic. Perhaps before family-centred care can be promoted as a treatment or nursing ideology, more fundamental questions need to be asked such as 'Who are the family in family-centred care?', for, as this particular study showed, this is not as simple a question as it seems, and indeed is a question with profound implications for the 'everyday' practices of all children's nurses.

THE FUTURE OF FAMILY-CENTRED CARE

SOCIALIZATION OF HEALTH CARE PROFESSIONALS

The education and training of health care professionals and their subsequent shared experience at work lead to a common perspective about the world, including the family, especially in relation to care. This makes a shared vision of the needs of families highly likely, probably from the shared socialization, rather than a true knowledge of the families.

Children's nurses believe that they can speak on behalf of the families of sick children. Indeed, this advocacy is a role which has been used to great mutual advantage over recent years, particularly for the disadvantaged. Health professionals need to take care that the advocacy they are involved does not interfere with the enabling and empowerment strategies which they are involved in. Perhaps there are other ways of advocacy, whereby the parents/carers have an opportunity to make their opinions felt as a valued and equal member in the parent-professional relationship. While some of the advocacy has been appropriate there is a need to be sure that the nurse is open to the true needs of the family. For instance, nursing innovations should be proven to be needed by the families, and prioritized according to the families' needs in a scientific manner. There may be more pressing requirements than a change of uniform or of primary nursing in the minds of the families.

Development of the Framework

The framework of shelton *et al.* (1987) is recognized as being pre-eminent in the identification of the elements of family-centred care (American Association of Children's Health Care). Variation of this framework is offered here in order to investigate the potential of the individual factors:

1. Recognition that the family is the constant in the child's life while the service systems and personnel within those systems fluctuate.

There has been a prevailing attitude that within a hospital situation, children's nurses are best placed to give an overall view of a child's state. However, it is common that a family may be cared for by a large number of health professionals over a short period of time. Even when a system of primary nursing is used with an individual child/family, the nurse cares for a group of children while the family remains responsible only for their own child. Currently, the family are seen as visiting the ward for short periods of time. This facet of the framework indicates that it is the ward team who are 'visiting' the family for a short period. In this way, Health Visitors and other community child health nurses may be closer to achieving family-centred care. Illness, for most children, will be only for a short period - perhaps 24 hours of hospitalization. Health care professionals need to regard this as being only of transient importance, compared with the family. As has been stated, perhaps the term "visitor" should not be used for the family and friends visiting the child and family while sick, but is more appropriate for the health professionals who are visiting the child and family mostly for such short periods. Knocking on cubicle doors by health professionals before entering is not just polite, but also a recognition of the privilege of entering the lives of these families.

Parents, carers and families need to be enabled and empowered to remain the constant in the child's life while the child is ill, whether this is at home or in hospital. Open visiting while in the hospital environment is one such strategy as well as the provision of high quality overnight accommodation for family members (Thornes, 1986). If the concept of family is broadened out to what the family says constitutes the family, then facilities for all of the family to visit or potentially stay overnight need to be provided. Currently, children's units in hospitals struggle to offer proper accommodation for a parent of a sick child and this is most probably for the mother (Darbyshire, 1994). Some paediatric oncology units, aware of the problem of maintaining the family and normal life of children on long-term treatment, have introduced week-end visiting in vacant cubicles, for siblings and friends, which has been especially effective for adolescents. Similarly, children are having blood samples taken at home by community nurses for full blood counts before treatment for varying cancers. In this way, the children remain at home longer as well as avoiding unnecessary disruption to their lives if their "count" is too low for treatment.

2. Facilitation of parent/professional collaboration at all levels of health care.

Organizations in this country with the advent of such initiatives as the Patient's Charter are realizing the need for collaboration between client and professional. In the field of Paediatrics, the drive is to provide environments of care which are appropriate for the child and family. Families have a wealth of information about the care of their children whether ill or well. This can become a source of innovation for open-minded health professionals seeking to develop paediatric services.

Health Visitors and other Community Child Health Nurses have responded in recent years to the needs of families by introducing support networks for new mothers, for instance. Materials have been produced for children and their families for the early education of young people in sexual health. These forms of collaboration are in their infancy in the United Kingdom and there is great potential for development.

3. Sharing of unbiased and complete information with parents about their child's care on a continual basis in an appropriate and supportive manner.

The showing of an X-ray to a parent is likely to provide the majority of parents with little or no extra information, but it is the making available of the X-ray which can make all the difference to a family, not for the information, but for the message it gives to the family about access to information. It contributes to a sense of trust. Not all families will want or even need such gestures, but for some it may be all important. Many children's units in hospitals in the United Kingdom, have adopted Casey's partnership model, where some of the interpretations of the model result in care being documented in terms of nurse, shared and parental care. The paper work is in many instances kept at the bottom of the child's bed and is in all cases completed with the active participation of the family. Such access to information contributes to the empowerment of families while their child is ill in hospital.

The establishment of the amount of information the family and the individuals within that family want is an important aspect of this part of the framework. Simply asking whether the family have understood what has been said and whether they wish to know more is a constant within the professional dialogue with families. Some families will want to know very little, leaving all of the decisions to the health professionals, others will want to know everything and be involved in all of the decisions, and there is a continuum between these extremes. This depends greatly upon what information is sufficient to gain the family a sense of control. Constantly checking that the family has sufficient information, as the family become less shocked at the child's admission, for instance, means that the nurse can react to the family's changing need for information.

The language used by health professionals, including the abbreviations, can be a source of exclusion of parents to unbiased information. They need to caution themselves to use language which is assimilable by families with varying education. This is not just the spoken word, but also the written one. Ward rounds need to include families at all times, ensuring that the language even between professionals is comprehended by the families, otherwise this will undermine the inclusion of the family in the ward round.

Children who are suspected of being abused might represent a group in which health professionals believe that communicating 'biased' and incomplete information about investigations may be in the best interest of the child; "We are just going to carry out a few more tests". The prevarication about straight information might make an eventual diagnosis of abuse more shocking to the family. Such openness should then ensure that opportunities for information giving would not be blocked by well-meaning professionals trying to be kind, with the resulting loss of trust by the family. Like all aspects of family-centred care, this facet of the framework requires a multidisciplinary approach.

4. Implementation of appropriate policies and programmes that are comprehensive and provide emotional, spiritual, cultural and financial support to meet the needs of families.

Policies which promote family-centred care need to take into account all of the support which may be necessary for the family. The unique nature of each family leads to the necessity of such policies being flexible as well as comprehensive. The introduction of "Saturday morning clubs" in the United Kingdom has been a useful innovation in the preparation of children and their families for routine and day surgery (Thornes, 1990). This service is comprehensive in that it is available for all families. Flexibility is built in by incorporating health professionals who make the families aware that they are prepared to show respect for the individuality of each family in the preparation of their child for surgery. There is usually a standard presentation of materials related to the surgery of children and subsequently the staff make themselves available for discussion about other aspects of the support needed, whether emotional, spiritual, cultural or financial. In this way, a programme is instigated which allows for all aspects of support to be explored and established prior to the admission of the child for surgery (Glasper and Thompson, 1993). Sim-

ilarly, policies cannot be prescriptive, but also need to take into account the different aspects of support required by the families.

Approaches need to incorporate respect for all aspects of the religious lives of families, such as religious artefacts (Slater, 1993) as well as the cultural context of such religious practices. Normality of reaction to a hospitalized child comes in many forms and is influenced by the cultural, religious as well as emotional reaction to the event. Normal for a family is not the same in every family and there is a need for policies and programmes which are accepting of all reactions to a child's hospitalization, for instance. Such respect for the reactions of a family will allow the more equitable working of a relationship between family and health professional towards resolution of the reaction and constructive reaction to support the sick child. Therefore, children's services need to be cognizant of all aspects of support required by the families of sick children, otherwise they may gather the impression that the system and the individuals which work the system are not interested in their needs. The families need to be empowered to feel that a concern for them is also a concern for the staff. That no concern is too small to be mentioned.

Financial matters are often discarded as a topic for discussion when a child is ill. There seems to be a prevailing attitude to a sick child being so important that money should not be mentioned. However, especially for families of chronically ill children, the burden of having a child ill in hospital can cause division within the family. Some charities, such as the Malcolm Sergent Cancer fund, recognize the extra costs of having a child with cancer and provide grants to support the family. Unfortunately, this is one of only a few charities which help the families of sick children in this way. Similarly, the "Too Dear to Visit" campaign (Action for Sick Children, 1993) has highlighted the costs incurred by families in visiting their sick child in hospital and that financial difficulties of families are far from being eradicated within the health care delivery system.

5. Recognition of family strengths and individuality, and respect of different methods of coping.

A family's response to the crisis of a child being brought into hospital cannot be predicted. Therefore, a service must be able to respond to their reactions in a supportive and non-judegmental manner. This is not just a matter of attitude of the staff, but also of those other families who may witness the coping behaviour of other families in the bays and Nightingale wards of British hospitals and clinics. This is about creating an environment and an attitude in all of the participants, which has respect for each individual's and each family's right to cope in a manner which is right for them. This currently exists for families who are being informed of a serious diagnosis for their child, where they are likely to be taken to a separate room and given time to deal with the knowledge in their own way. It needs to spread to other information, so that a similar respect for the family's need to cope in different ways can be expressed.

The extent of involvement of each family will vary. Each family member comes with their own abilities to care for the sick child, a unique relationship with the child and their own reaction to the hospitalization. The ability of each member of the family to care for the child will depend on all of these issues as well as others, such as the need to earn money for the family. Nurses in particular have highly developed skills in involving family members in the care of their child in an appropriate manner for the child and the individual, which is comfortable for both and which assists in reducing the trauma of hospitalization for the child. Parents, in particular, can feel under great pressure to get over their own reticence to be involved actively in the care of their child. This pressure most usually comes from the child, but nurses need to caution themselves against overenthusiastic involvement of the parents at their expense and potentially at the expense of the relationship of the child and parent.

6. Understanding and incorporating the developmental and emotional needs of infants, children and adolescents, and their families, into health care delivery systems.

Over the past ten years there has been a move away from employing nursery nurses on children's wards to the employment of play workers. Some of these individuals are highly skilled and use a variety of play techniques in order to reduce the trauma of hospitalization. These play therapists, although there are not as yet appropriate courses, carry out play preparation for children of all ages, such as pre-surgery or pre-chemotherapy. They are also involved in dealing with hospital sourced phobias, such as from needles. Play workers are now employed in out-patient departments and are making a major contribution to the environment in these establishments.

Health care delivery systems come in many forms. For instance, some hospitals organize their wards by medical specialty rather than by age group. Children's out-patient departments, similarly, tend to be organized by diagnosis of the child rather than the age of the child. This creates difficulties in creating an environment, both physical and emotional, which supports the developmental needs of the children and young people. Some interest is being expressed in using developmentally specific play modules in order to get around some of these difficulties. The modules, which are effectively trolleys, contain age specific play materials and these can be wheeled to the appropriate children. Decoration of these clinical areas, which used to be predominated by wall papers which were only of interest to the 3 to 8 year old age range, is now age neutral, but calming in nature. In this way the adolescents, in particular are not alienated.

The provision of appropriate environments for adolescents is notoriously difficult within United Kingdom hospitals. These young people tend to be given beds with younger children or placed in side wards away from peer interaction. Some hospitals have created adolescent bays or wards and these are certainly an effective way of providing an appropriate environment for these young people in their transitional years. Working with these young people can be challenging and the skills required to provide sensitive and informed support are no less sophisticated than for the neonate, although the development of courses to inform this practice is at its infancy.

Other environments can be challenging to provide an appropriately supportive environment which takes into account the developmental needs of the child. The provision of play facilities, such as a play pen in a paediatric intensive care unit, is not just about providing a safe and stimulating environment for a young sibling. It makes a statement about the importance attached to such activity when high-technology equipment might indicate otherwise. This is potentially empowering for the family. Other environments where children are a proportion of the client group, such as adult intensive care units, need to make similar provision and are not excused from doing so.

7. Encouragement and facilitation of parent-to-child support.

As has been discussed, the professional-family relationship is about empowering and enabling families to care for their sick child using the skills that they already possess as well as developing new ones in order that they can remain the prime carer. All of this needs to be carried out at an appropriate speed and within comfort limits for the family and the child in question. For some of the children, such as three year olds there will be enormous pressure on the families and the parents in particular for them to carry out the physical care. Nurses need to act in a supportive manner, being alert to the needs of the family in this regard as well as the sick child. Not all families will be able to carry out the care straight away and the nurse will need to work with the child and family to carry out the physical care.

Mouth care is an example of care which families are content to complete for their child with support and explanation from the nursing staff. The carrying out of such care by the parents is supportive for both parties and returns a sense of normality. However, when the procedure becomes painful, then some parents find that they are unable to provide the care preferring to ask the nurses to clean the child's mouth. This is a reasonable request, but the nurse has little chance of success and the importance of mouth care for children with cancer, for instance, is that it can reduce morbidity and even mortality in this group of children.

Care and treatment tends to be led by the needs of the system and there is great potential for further support of the family to the child and vice versa with some imagination on behalf of the care team. For instance, a timetable for a chemotherapy regimen need not be the product of medical and nursing priorities for staffing, but might be family-led. For some families, this might involve chemotherapy being given at times outside those when other family members visit, or might be designed to allow a father, who visits only in the evening, to support the family.

8. Assurance that the design of health care delivery systems is flexible, accessible and responsive to family needs.

In order that health care staff can create an environment which is truly family centred, there is a need for those staff to have some control over the systems in the hospital or in the community. Such control will allow the staff to manipulate the environment to empower and enable the needs of the family to be dealt with in a way which respects their individuality. For instance, traditionally outpatient services are provided as a Monday to Friday, '9 to 5' centralized service. It is highly likely that a family-empowered service would be flexible enough to offer evening and weekend appointments. This would avoid loss of school attendance and earnings, and would enable all the relevant family members to attend. Local clinics might afford better attendance rates, as well as easier access (Campbell *et al.*, 1993). Some hospitals with a large child population have created "drop in" clinics where families who are concerned about their child and feel that they need expert paediatric knowledge can circumvent accident and emergency departments as well as General Practitioners. These facilities are well used by such families and General Practitioners tend to refer children to these facilities.

Generally about the framework

It would be inappropriate to assume that this is an exhaustive framework. However, its use in the United States over recent years would indicate that it is a useful tool on which to base strategies for family-centred care. Further development of the content of the framework needs to be based on active research in an inductive manner, which could be coined 'family-centred research'. This needs to be based on data grounded in the knowledge of the families with sick children receiving the care in hospitals and at home in the United Kingdom.

STRATEGIES

INVOLVEMENT IN MANAGEMENT OF THE WARDS

The role of parent governors is now seen as integral to the state education system. Such involvement is not mirrored in the management of children's units. Day-to-day delivery of a child's care is naturally part of the role of the primary nurse in partnership with the families (Casey, 1988). However, policy decisions about matters such as the organization of a ward traditionally have been made by the nursing and medical professions without formal recourse to the families' views. Such decisions might be related to the design of a cubicle, or to the reallocation of bays by age rather than by diagnosis. Children's nurses certainly have skills which allow them to make informed decisions about such matters, but these decisions are more informative if made with the actual support and critical analysis of participating families.

The selection of such families is a difficult problem. A 'tame' parent, adolescent, or group of parents would not have the impact upon the management of a clinical area that the open-minded and adventurous family-centred care team would wish. An aggressive and opinionated parent could be destructive to the strategy of family involvement. Whereas the choice of these individuals may be influenced by their ability to deal with potential meetings, this assumption should be made cautiously. The family members should be perceived as equal

partners in the management of the clinical area and, although they are unlikely to be formally elected, it is important for them to maintain a representative perspective.

This strategy has already been employed in the children's hospice movement, where parents are seen as essential members of trustee and management committees. The manner in which this involvement affects the service delivered, its responsiveness to the changing needs and expectations of families, requires investigation.

FAMILY INFORMATION

Family information leaflets have been developed at many centres (Glasper and Burge, 1992). Although efforts have been made to ensure such leaflets are family-friendly, these initiatives have been largely professionally led. There is a great deal of potential in the concept of family-led information leaflets.

Family led information might resolve the discrepancy between the professional's view of the family's need for information and their actual needs. The professional may wish to impart information about temperature control, whereas the family may want practical advice on how to cool a child. Without an effective strategy to seek the information needs of families, professionals may continue to make inappropriate assumptions. This will lead to less effective health promotion.

Focus groups may be one means of achieving family-led information. Such groups might consist of experienced and potential users of the service, for the particular issue to be addressed. These ideas can then be taken forward and translated into an information format by experienced practitioners with or without family assistance. It is essential that such material is reviewed by the families to ensure it has fulfilled their needs and that it is in an appropriate form.

These ideas fall within the domain of inductive research. The traditional comments box and patient satisfaction tolls still leave the research agenda with professionals. The voice of the parent is currently forgotten, except when spoken through the mouths of informed nurses - a potentially patronizing approach. In prioritizing the research and innovation needs of a children's unit, there are clearly issues of acceptability, enthusiasm and workload to overcome. There is a balance to be found between the research needs perceived by the establishment and those of the families. Currently, the establishment has a large voice and the monetary power to back it. The use of parental views about need could go some way to redressing this balance.

NURSING EDUCATION

Nursing curricula tend to be based upon theoretical models of care. This is a reasonable way in which to ensure that a full range of nursing perspectives are addressed by the students. However, there are practical choices about the nature and kind of experiences which are again a matter of professional judgement, without recourse to the views of families who are the consumers of the resultant care. This might be redressed by the inclusion of family members in course planning and management teams, although it is difficult to envisage that parents will be motivated to become fully involved in such endeavours in the manner in which they currently operate.

Family-centred care is a dynamic process that can be developed effectively only if families are given full rights of involvement at all levels, through enabling and empowering practices of health professionals and nurses in particular. Currently, there are situations in which some parents are given an opportunity to participate in nursing techniques such as the administration of intravenous therapy, while parents in the same ward are not able to gain adequate pain control for their child. The Framework of Family-Centred Care offers a means by which each nurse, ward and children's unit can assess the extent to which family-centred care is being practised. It also allows the families and nurses to plan developments in partnership.

KEY POINTS

◆ Family-centred care represents a holistic approach to care.

◆ Enabling and empowering families is at the root of family-centred care.

◆ The nature of involvement of families in the care of their child varies from family to family.

◆ Health care staff need to be sure that they have good grounds for believing that they know the needs of families.

◆ The framework of family-centred care is a source of innovation and analysis.

◆ Family-centred research is a way forward for the investigation of care.

◆ Nurses may not have a concrete or appropriate definition of the nature of the family.

REFERENCES

Ahmann E: Family Centered Care: the time has come. *Pediatr Nurs* 20 (1): 52-53, 1994.

Campbell ST, Lawson S, Glasper EA: Familes first, *Paed Nurs* 4(8): 35, 1993.

Campbell SJ, Clarke FM: Ethos and philosophy of Paediatric Intensive Care. In Carter B, editor: *Manual of paediatric intensive care nursing*, London, 1992, Harper Collins.

Campbell SJ, Summersgill P: Keeping it in the family: defining and developing family-centred care, *Child Health* 1:17, 1993.

Campbell SJ, Kelly PJ, Summersgill P: Putting the family first: interpreting a framework for family-centred care, *Child Health* 1:59, 1993.

Casey A: A partnership with child and family, *Senior Nurs* 8(4): 8-9, 1988.

Casey A, Mobbs S: Partnership in practice. Spotlight on Children. *Nurs Times* 84:67-68, 1988.

Cleary J *et al*.: Parental involvement in the lives of children in hospital, *Arch Dis Child* 61(8):779, 1986.

Curley M: Effects of the nursing mutual cooperation participation model of care on parental stress in the pediatric intensive care unit. *Heart Lung* 17 (6): 682-688, 1988.

Curley M, Wallace J: Effects of the nursing mutual cooperation participation model of care on parental stress in the pediatric intensive care unit - a replication. *Pediatr Nurs* 7 (6): 377-385, 1992.

Darbyshire P: *Parenting in public: A study of the experiences of parents who live-in with their hospitalised child, and of their relationships with paediatric nurses*, PhD Thesis, 1992, University of Edinburgh.

Darbyshire P: *Living with a sick child in hospital: the experience of parents and nurses*, Glasgow, 1994, Chapman & Hall.

Dearmun A: Perceptions of parental participation, *Paediatr Nurs* 4(7):6, 1992.

Department of Health: *Welfare of children and young people in hospital*, London, 1991, HMSO.

Dunst C, Trivette C, Deal A: *Enabling and empowering families.* Cambridge, MA, 1988, Brookline Books.

Flint NS, Walsh M: Visiting policies in pediatrics: parents' participation and preferences. *J Pediatr Nurs* 3 (4): 237-246, 1988.

Glasper EA, Burge D: Developing family information leaflets, *Nurs Stand* 6 (25): 24, 1992.

Glasper EA, Thompson M: Preparing children for hospital admission. In Glasper EA, Tucker A, eds: *Advances in child Health Nursing*, London, 1993. Scutari Press.

Hostler S: Personal communication cited in Johnson BH, Jeppson ES, Redburn L: *Caring for children and families: guidelines for hospital*, Bethesda, MD, 1992, Associationfor the Care of Children's Health.

Johnson BH, McGonigel M, Kaufmann R, editors: *Guidelines and recommended practices for individualized family service plan*, Washington, DC, 1989, Association for the Care of Children's Health.

Johnson *et al*, 1992 from p 33.

Robinson CA: Roadblocks to family-centred care when a chronically ill child is hospitalised, *Matern Child Nurs J* 16(3):181, 1987.

Rushton CH: Strategies for Family-Centred Care in the Critical Care Setting, *Pediatr Nurs* 16(2):195, 1990a.

Rushton CH: Family-centred care in the critical care setting: myth or reality? *Children's Health Care* 19(2):68, 1990b.

Shelton T, Jeppson E, Johnson B: *Family-centred care for children with special health care needs*, Washington DC, 1987, Association for the Care of Children's Health.

Slater M: *Health for all our children: achieving appropriate health care for black and minority ethnic children and their futures*, London, 1993, Action for Sick Children.

Thornes R: *Parents staying overnight with their children*, London, 1986, Caring for Children in the Health Services.

Thornes R: *Just for the Day*, London, 1990, Caring for Children in the Health Services.

Whiting M: Meeting needs: RSCNs in the community, *Paediatr Nurs*, 6 (1): 9-11, 1994.

Wong DL: *Whaley & Wong's Nursing Care of Infants and Children*, ed 5, St Louis, MO, 1995, Mosby–Year Book Inc.

FURTHER READING

Algren CL: Role perception of mothers who have hospitalised children, *Children's Health Care* 14(1):6, 1985.

Beuf AH: *Biting off the bracelet: a study of children in hospital*, Philadelphia, PA, 1979, University of Pennsylvania Press.

Cleary J: The distribution of nursing attention in a children's ward, *Nurs Times* (occasional paper) 73(28):93, 1977.

Consumers Association: *Children in hospital: a Which? campaign report*, London, 1980, Consumers Association.

Elfert H, Anderson JM: More than just luck: parents' views on getting good nursing care, *Canadian Nurs* 83(4):14, 1987.

Fagin CM, Nusbaum JG: Parental visiting privileges in paediatric units: a survey, *J Nurs Admin* 8:24, 1978.

Foster RLR, Hunsberger MM, Andersen JJ: *Family-centred nursing care of children*, Philadelphia, 1989, WB Saunders.

Fletcher B: Psychosocial upset in post-hospitalised children: A review of the literature, *Matern Child Nurs J* 10:185, 1978.

Hall DJ: Social and psychological care before and during hospitalisation, *Soc Sci Med* 25(6):721, 1987.

Hardgrove C: Helping parents on the paediatric ward: a report on a survey of hospitals with 'living-in' programs, *Pediatrician* 9:220, 1980.

Gill KM: Nurses' attitudes toward parent participation: personal and professional characteristics, *Children's Health Care* 15(3):149, 1987.

Gubrium JF, Lynott RJ: Family rhetoric as social order, *J Family Issues* 6(1):129, 1985.

Hawthorne PJ: *Nurse I want my Mummy!* London, 1974, Royal College of Nursing.

Johnson BH, Jeppson ES, Redburn L: *Caring for children and families: guidelines for hospital*, Bethesda, MD, 1992, Association for the Care of Children's Health.

Knafl KA, Dixon DM: The participation of fathers in their child's hospitalisation, Issues Comprehensive *Paediatr Nurs* 7(4-5):269, 1984.

McCawley C: Family-centred care: a transatlantic study, *Aust Nurs J* 11:49, 1980.

Merrow DL, Johnson BS: Perceptions of the mother's role with her hospitalised child, *Nurs Res* 17(2):155, 1968.

Monahan GH, Schdake JK: Comparing care by parent and traditional nursing units, *Pediatr Nurs* 11(6):463, 1985.

Morgan ML, Lloyd BJ: Parents invited, *Nurs Outlook* 3(5):256, 1955.

Robinson CA, Thorne S: Strengthening family 'interference', *J Adv Nurs* 9(6):597, 1984.

Robertson J: *Young children in hospital*, ed 2, London, 1970, Tavistock.

Sainsbury CPQ *et al.*: Care by parents of their children in hospital, *Arch Dis Child* 61(6):612, 1986.

Chapter 4

Nursing Children in the Community

LEARNING OUTCOMES

After studying this chapter you should be able to:

◆ Discuss how the nursing role may vary, depending upon the setting in which care is delivered.
◆ Describe the historical development of community nursing services for children in the United Kingdom.
◆ Consider the various contributions nursing staff make to the care of children in the community.
◆ Identify a range of nursing needs which might be experienced by children in non-institutional settings.
◆ Describe the scope of professional nursing practice in relation to the role of the paediatric community nurse.
◆ Define the glossary terms.

GLOSSARY

PCN Paediatric community nurse

BPD Bronchopulmonary dysplasia

CAPD Continuous ambulatory peritoneal dialysis

home care Care delivered to children with health care needs at home for the purpose of promoting and maintaining health

paediatric community nurse A children's nurse specifically educated to provide home care for sick children

paediatric community nurse's forum A special-interest group within the Royal College of Nursing's Society of Paediatric Nursing

Children require nursing care both within and outside of the hospital setting. The sociological context of caring for children and their families in the community differs from that of the hospital. Specifically, the environment of care (i.e., the community) can influence the relationship between the nurse, the child and the family.

Presently, there are an estimated 14 million children under the age of 16 in England and Wales (Audit Commission, 1993). In any one year, approximately 1.2 million children will require admission to hospital; more than 5 million will attend a hospital outpatient department; and approximately 3.5 million will attend a hospital accident and emergency department (Caring for Children in the Health Services, 1987; Audit Commission, 1993). While these figures represent a considerable use of the hospital sector by children and their families, the majority of childhood ill health is actually managed in the community and is provided by the parents with support, when necessary, from the family general practitioner (GP).

The provision of professional nursing support in the community to the families of children with health problems is not common, for several reasons: (1) much childhood illness is episodic and acute, with a sudden onset and an equally rapid resolution of symptoms, and (2) the majority of parents expect nursing needs can and should be met by themselves (Harrison, 1977; Campbell, 1987). This expectation is generally shared both by the parents and by health care professionals from whom they might seek advice. For example, most parents accept that it is their responsibility (or even their duty) to sit with a child who is unwell through a long, restless night; their responsibility to clean up vomit and faeces from a child with gastroenteritis; their responsibility to manage the symptoms of pain or discomfort of pyrexia. In addition, many parents gladly follow instructions from their family GP. This might, for instance, include preparing and administering oral rehydration solutions for a baby with acute gastroenteritis, or applying antibiotic eyedrops for an infant with conjunctivitis (Whiting, 1987).

In the past, if a child required admission to hospital, from the moment the child entered the hospital many of these nursing care responsibilities might have been 'taken away' from parents by nurses who then assumed many aspects of this care - aspects which, prior to admission, the parents undertook at home (Casey, 1988; Brykzynska, 1989). Although it could be argued that some parents believe it is 'right' that the nurse should 'do' these things for the child, many children's nurses have historically been very active participants in the ritual 'de-skilling' of parents. Increasingly, however, parental participation in the care of the hospitalized child has become the accepted norm (Cleary *et al.*, 1986; Casey, 1988). Indeed, the care-by-parent scheme described by Cleary *et al.* offers many excellent examples of the roles which parents can assume when caring for their own child in hospital.

Outside the hospital setting, when the families of sick children receive formal nursing support, the role of the nurse is of teacher/facilitator. In a study of the work of the paediatric community nurse (PCN), 'teaching practical procedures', 'education and support about disease/health processes' and 'support of parents in performing procedures' were the activities most frequently identified (Whiting, 1988).

While nursing care for children in the community is delivered in a variety of settings, including schools, nurseries, clinics and health centres, most care is provided in the family home. The actual setting in which care is delivered is a critical factor in providing care (see Box 4-1).

Box 4-1 illustrates some of the factors which might usefully be considered in relation to the respective roles of the nurse, parent and child when nursing care is delivered in the home. For the nurse who is involved in such care, it is clear that the role is one of *negotiation* and *partnership* with parents. Such care requires careful planning. Indeed, for many PCNs, care planning is undertaken jointly with the parents and child. When children have long-term care needs, they can be formalized in written *collaborative care plans* which are jointly signed by nurse, the parents and child; are shared by all involved in the care; and remain in the child's home.

HISTORICAL CONSIDERATIONS

Prior to the 1950s, the admission of a sick child to hospital was itself considered to be an effective therapeutic stratagem (Oppe, 1971). It has been argued (Graham, 1977) that, because of the adverse social circumstances in the overcrowded cities of Victorian England, hospitalization often saved children's lives. Incremental improvements in sanitation and housing throughout the twentieth century have rendered this approach to paediatric care largely obsolete.

However, until the 1950s, nobody seriously questioned the assumed therapeutic value of hospitalization. Hospitalized children were separated from their families (Robertson, 1958), hospital visiting was often restricted to a few hours each day, and parents were discouraged from 'rooming-in' with their sick child (Ministry of Health, 1959). It was at this time that Bowlby identified a syndrome, called *maternal deprivation*, in young children who had been separated from their mothers (Bowlby, 1951).

Robertson (1958) suggested that children under 4 years of age were particularly vulnerable to the effects of such separation:

If at this crucial stage in his development, when he has such a possessive and passionate need of his mother, and he is blindly trustful of his parents, he is admitted alone to hospital, he experiences a serious failure of that environment of love and security hitherto provided by his family and which we know to be a necessary experience if he is to be a loving, secure and trustful person in later life.

Robertson argued that hospitalization held two main dangers for the child: (1) the traumatic, 'in which the child suffers the shock of losing his mother and multiple other stresses' and (2) the deprivational, 'in which lengthy deprivation of mothering by one person may result in lasting impoverishment of the personality' (Robertson, 1958).

◆ **BOX 4-1**

Nursing the child in his/her own home

Considerations when compared to hospital care
The Child

- The environment is safer for the child. The child knows the layout, where the hazards are and how to avoid accidents!
- The microbiological flora of the home is familiar to the child's defence systems: there is a reduced risk of infection.
- Home represents security, love and warmth. The child knows and feels comfortable with the noises, the smells, the things he or she sees and knows as home. The child has its own toys, and sleeps in its own cot/bed in its own room. Home is usually a happy place.
- When painful procedures such as dressings or injections are required, this might cause the child to associate certain parts of the home (e.g., certain rooms) with pain or trauma. (The nurse needs to be aware of this possibility.)

The Parent

- 'This is my home, my territory, my rules!'
- Parents will generally feel more relaxed, more comfortable, more able to ask questions or even to question what the nurse is doing and why.
- Parents should be able to control/direct many aspects of the interaction between themselves, their child and the nurse.
- While valuing the autonomy which being at home can give, the parent will no longer have immediate access to professional carers, as would have been the case in hospital. This can cause considerable anxiety.
- The nature of the child's nursing needs may be such that he or she must remain in the house throughout the day or night. This means that an adult must be available at all times. Parents may not be able to 'escape' from their own home, even for a few moments.

The Nurse

- The nurse must plan the time of arrival at the child's home to suit the family's needs, rather than, for instance, 'fitting them in' between the complex demands of the busy hospital ward.
- The time that the nurse spends with the child and family is their time, with little likelihood of interruption.
- The nurse is working in somebody else's territory; territory which must be respected. There may be cultural or family rules and values which need to be considered when delivering care.
- The nurse must strike a balance between confidently controlling the delivery of care and accommodating the child and family's need for autonomy within their own home.
- Careful consideration must be given to the environment and facilities available within the home (e.g. for undertaking aseptic procedures).

Bowlby (1951, 1969) contended that illness, in itself, makes children more dependent and increases their need for close contact with the mother. Both Bowlby and Robertson discussed the sequence of 'protest, despair and denial' ('detachment', Bowlby) reactions in children who are separated from their mothers and placed in the care of strangers. This is due to the 'loss of maternal care at a highly dependent, highly vulnerable stage of development' (Bowlby, 1969). It is generally agreed that the most vulnerable children are those aged between six months and four years. Additionally, children of any age who require repeated admissions, or whose condition necessitates a single protracted period of hospitalization are considered to be at risk (Bowlby, 1969; Douglas, 1975; Quinton and Rutter, 1976; Shannon *et al.*, 1984).

Emergent theories of child care, based largely upon the research of Bowlby and Robertson, have been reflected in successive statements of health service policy since the Platt Report (Ministry of Health, 1959) which recommended that:

Children should not be admitted to hospital if it can possibly be avoided. (Paragraph 17, page 5)

Further details concerning how admission might be avoided were included in the recent Department of Health guidance, *The Welfare of Children and Young People in Hospital* (Department of Health, 1991a):

Children are usually treated in their own homes by the primary care services, with help as necessary from elsewhere in the NHS – eg community paediatric nurses – and other agencies such as social services and education departments. (Paragraph 3.13)

SHIFTING THE BALANCE OF CARE

The timing of the work undertaken by Robertson and Bowlby was critical to its impact in guiding the philosophical and political approaches to the care of sick children in the years that followed. Of particular relevance was the fact that the National Health Service was, at that time, in an embryonic form, as hospital and community sectors began to work together to develop more integrated approaches to care provision. While it is important to acknowledge that there have been considerable changes in the care of sick children, and many of the negative aspects of hospitalization have been remedied or improved (Department of Health, 1991a; Audit Commission, 1993), the care of sick children has moved steadily from being almost exclusively the responsibility of the hospital (Oppe, 1971) towards that of the community (Department of Health, 1991a; British Paediatric Association, 1991; Caring for Children in the Health Services, 1993; Audit Commission, 1993). This is perhaps best illustrated by the significant reduction in the average length of hospital stay for children as described by the Audit Commission in 1993 (see Fig. 4-1). Many children are now admitted to hospital for a relatively short period of assessment and acute care, before being discharged to the care of their parents. However, despite widespread acceptance that admission to hospital should be avoided, the total number of children admitted to hospital per annum has shown a steady and sustained increase for as long as statistics have been collected (Hill, 1989; Henderson *et al.*, 1992; Audit Commission, 1993) (see Fig. 4-2).

This trend of increasing child admissions to hospital has been accompanied by increases in outpatient, and accident and emergency attendances by children (Department of Health, 1993a) and a sustained reduction in the number of GP consultations (OPCS, 1994).

These changes in the patterns of uptake of health services by children have occurred for several reasons, including:

- Increasing car ownership and mobility of the population, in general, creating greater accessibility to hospitals.
- Epidemiological changes in the patterns of childhood disease and, in particular, the decline in acute infectious disease (other than respiratory infections [Wyke *et al.*, 1991]) which has reduced the necessity for GP consultations (OPCS, 1994).
- Closer collaboration between primary and secondary care sectors as the National Health Service has developed, resulting in significant increases in GP referral rates to hospital paediatric departments (Department of Health, 1993a).
- Shifting patterns of childbirth from home to hospital confinement, as identified by the Court Report (Department of Health and Social Security, 1976) and discussed in detail by the Department of Health Expert Maternity Group (1993b) has increased the familiarity of new parents with the hospital sector and may legitimize the use of the hospital, even when the presenting problem might be more appropriately dealt with in the primary care sector. Many of the medical conditions accounting for the increase in admission rates, particularly with very young babies, seem to reflect a shift towards hospital in the management of conditions which have historically been managed in the community (Hill, 1989; Henderson *et al.*, 1992 OPCS, 1994).

- Increasing mobility of the population generally has resulted in significant geographical isolation of the parents of young children from their own parents and extended families. Consequently, much of the experiential knowledge of the extended family is not available. This has been compounded by the overall reduction in the size of the average family to the extent that parents are often no longer able to draw upon knowledge gained from nursing an older sibling though a period of acute illness at home.
- In the past 20 years, there has been a steady increase in the use of GP deputizing services, perhaps most significantly in the inner cities. In addition, particularly for larger practices, complex 'cross-cover' arrangements have been established. Consequently, parents who attempt to arrange an out-of-hours consultation for an acutely ill child are likely to be faced with a GP they have never met before. For some parents, this specific factor increases the likelihood that they will bypass the GP system and go directly to the hospital. For example, an analysis of the Kensington and Chelsea and Westminster Family Health Services Authority *Directory of General Medical Practitioners* (July 1992) found that almost 90% of listed practices used a 'commercial deputizing service' for out-of-hours cover. A further 5% of GPs participated in complex on-call cover systems covering two or more practices.
- Many GP surgeries, which previously allowed patients to be seen without any prior arrangement, now operate on formal appointment systems, particularly for non-urgent consultations.
- These factors may contribute to the fact that many parents use the accident and emergency department of the local hospital, both when their child is acutely ill and when symptoms have appeared throughout several hours or days. Many, who might previously have consulted their GP, now either take the child directly to the hospital or

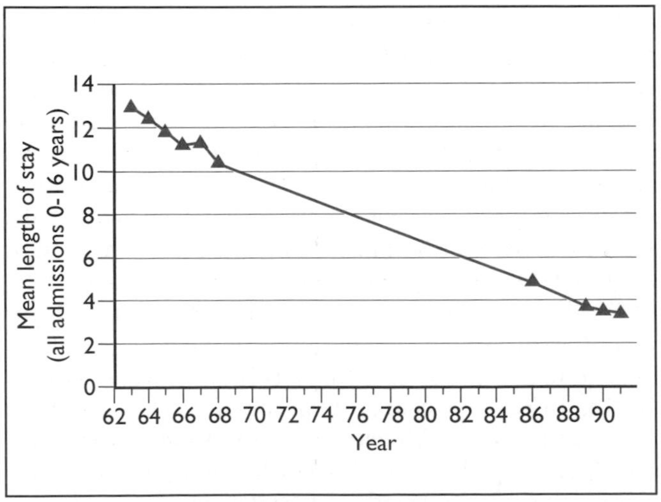

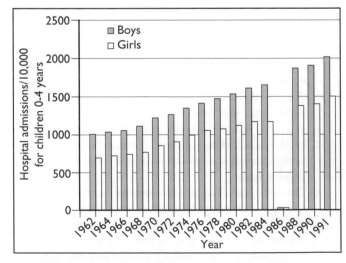

Fig. 4-1 Mean length of hospital stay for children. (Source of data, Audit Commission, 1993.)

Fig. 4-2 Total number of hospital admissions for children per annum. (Source of data, Audit Commission, 1993.)

dial 999. This pattern of usage of accident and emergency departments is illustrated in the serial analysis of admissions to the Queen's Medical Centre in Nottingham (Wynne and Hull, 1977; Hutchison *et al.*, 1987).

• An additional factor concerns what happens to children once they arrive at the hospital. Despite the reduction in the general number of children's hospital beds over the past 30 years, the significant decreases in the average length of hospital stay for children has resulted in an overall increase in bed availability. Fig. 4-2 shows that there has been a twofold increase in the number of child admissions to hospital during this period. This increase in admission rates was already well established by the time of the Court Report (Department of Health and Social Security, 1976), which suggested that part of the increase might 'reflect a greater readiness to admit children to hospital for short periods'. A detailed study of admissions across the Oxford region between 1975 and 1985 (Hill, 1989) identified a doubling of admissions within that period and its author suggested: 'the increase in admissions was due to lower thresholds for admission resulting in part from the increased availability of beds because of diminishing lengths of stay'. This is supported by the large numbers of children who are admitted to hospital for short periods, possibly for intensive observation and treatment, followed by a rapid discharge.

The use of hospital facilities by children is considerable, illustrating the need for close collaboration and integration of primary (community) care and secondary (hospital) care. While the need for such integration has been apparent since the hospital and community sectors were brought together as a result of the National Health Service Act of 1946, it was not until the publication of the Court Report (Department of Health and Social Security, 1976) that significant strategic impetus was given specifically to coordinating the disparate children's services.

The changes in the patterns of hospitalization of children described above have been accompanied by significant developments in the provision of services in the community for sick children. From a medical perspective, this has included, for instance, the introduction of vocational training for GPs (including the requirement for training in hospital paediatrics), and the development of the role of the consultant community paediatrician (Department of Health and Social Security, 1976; BPA, 1991). In 1993, a working party of the British Paediatric Association suggested that a radical rethink of the approach to inpatient and outpatient paediatric medicine was needed (BPA, 1993). The working party argued that much of the current inpatient provision for children should be replaced by a national network of children's day care service centres (CDCSC). If such a strategy were to be adopted, the role of community paediatricians would have to undergo dramatic change.

The most important development in nursing provision for children in the community has been the dramatic expansion in the availability of paediatric community nursing services, particularly since the early 1980s (Whiting, 1988; Whiting/ Royal College of Nursing, 1994).

NURSING IN THE COMMUNITY

Before discussing paediatric community nursing in detail, it is helpful to consider the development of the three principle community nursing services: district nursing and health visiting and, to a lesser extent, school nursing.

District nursing, health visiting and school nursing are major services in the United Kingdom. Within England alone there are, in whole time equivalents (Department of Health, 1993c):

• 9,739 district nurses
• 5,346 registered and enrolled nurses assisting them
• 10,371 health visitors
• 2,387 school nurses

In England, in 1990-1991, district nurses made professional contact with 3.2 million people (but only 76,000 children) and health visitors made professional contact with 3.7 million people, including 2.25 million children under the age of five (Department of Health, 1993c).

DISTRICT NURSING

It is generally accepted that the roots of the present district nursing service lie in the pioneering work of William Rathbone who, in 1859, engaged the services of a hospital trained nurse to help care for his dying wife at home. Following his wife's death, the nurse was employed by Rathbone to care for the sick poor people in the city of Liverpool (Rathbone, 1890). By 1874, a National Association for 'providing trained nurses for the sick poor in London and elsewhere' had been founded and, in 1887, Queen Victoria's Jubilee Institute for Nurses was established as the first formally organized district nursing scheme. During the next 50 years, district nursing services expanded steadily, being organized on a local basis by either voluntary agencies or local authorities (Stocks, 1960). It was not until the National Health Service Act of 1946 that community nursing could be considered to be a universally available service for the provision of nursing care in the community. The Act placed formal responsibility upon local health authorities 'for securing the attendance of nurses on persons who require nursing in their own homes.'

Much of the early work of the district nurse was concerned with the care of sick children in the community (Stocks, 1960; Baly, 1987). More recent studies, however, have indicated that children now form only a very small part of the district nurse's caseload (OPCS, 1982).

HEALTH VISITING

The history of health visiting has been reviewed in considerable detail by While (1985). As with district nursing, the predecessors of modern health visitors can be traced to the middle of the nineteenth century. One of the most significant features of nineteenth century England was the mass movement of the population from the countryside into the growing cities. The consequences of this for the poor – living in overcrowded, squalid and disease ridden circumstances – were devastating. Infant mortality in England in the mid-19th century was in the order of 150 deaths per 1,000 (Graham, 1977). In 1890, for instance the main causes of infant deaths in England and Wales were inanition (malnutrition), 19,490 deaths; convulsions, 18,140 deaths; bronchitis, 16,160 deaths; diarrhoea, 11,390 deaths (Graham, 1977). The same circumstances which had prompted William Rathbone's philanthropic activities in Liverpool, led to the establishment of the Manchester and Salford Sanitary Reform Association in 1852 (While, 1985), though it was not until 1862 that a fulltime visitor was first appointed. From 1862-1890, five more sanitary visitors were appointed. Their role was principally one of teaching and counselling, rather than of practical nursing. At this time, no previous nursing experience was deemed necessary for the visitors, whose title changed to 'health visitors' 1900. Thus, the development of health visiting was the product of two factors: (1) an increased recognition of the need for sanitary reform, and (2) the philanthropic activities of middle class Victorian women.

The Statutory Rules and Orders of the Local Government Act (1929) provided for a qualification and standard training for health visitors. The National Health Service Act of l946 required that all health visitors must be qualified. As with district nursing, the National Health Service Act placed responsibility on the Local Health Authorities to provide a health visiting service. The Act stated:

It shall be the duty of every local health authority to make provision in their area for the visiting of persons in their homes by visitors to be called 'health visitors' for the purpose of giving advice as to the care of young children, persons suffering from illness and expectant or nursing mothers, and as to the measures necessary for the spread of infection. (Part III, section 25)

Clark's (1981) extensive review of health visiting practice noted that the work of health visitors was predominantly concerned with the provision of services to young children and their families. However, health visiting practice is focused on the needs of the healthy child as outlined in the description of health visiting practice by the Council for the Education and Training of Health Visitors (CETHV) in 1977 which stated, 'the professional practice of health visiting consists of planned activities aimed at the promotion of health and the prevention of ill-health.'

The Court Committee (Department of Health and Social Security, 1976) discussed the role of various members of the primary health care team in caring for the sick child in the community, and concluded that although mothers may seek advice on the care of a sick child from the health visitor, only rarely do health visitors undertake any practical nursing care with children. Davis (1985) claimed:

There is an increasing muddle over who does what in the community...but because paediatric community nursing is not apparently regarded as a speciality in its own right, some of the work is being done by district nurses, some by health visitors and some by midwives. This cannot be sensible and perhaps accounts for the fact that often the wrong children are kept at home and the wrong ones admitted to hospital.

The Court Committee (Department of Health and Social Security, 1976) recommended the appointment of specialist child health visitors with joint responsibility for the promotion of health and the management of paediatric nursing problems in the community. However, this approach was not followed and subsequent guidance has emphasized the necessity for nurses who provide care for children in the community to be appropriately trained in the care of sick children (Department of Health, 1991).

SCHOOL NURSING

Strehlow (1987) has reviewed the history of the school nursing service in detail, paying particular attention to developments subsequent to the 1981 Education Act, within which specific responsibility was placed upon the local educational authorities to ensure that children requiring 'special educational provision' be 'educated in ordinary schools'. The Act has significant implications for children who have continuing health needs, who might previously have been denied the option of mainstream education, but who may now be integrated within it. This issue has also been addressed by the Education Reform Act (1993). Although the role of the school nurse is principally health education and health surveillance, the potential contribution of school nurses to the needs of such children must be acknowledged. Indeed, school nurses play a strong role in the care and support of children with chronic physical disease. Despite this, it is clear that the school nurse's involvement in the care of the child who is acutely ill, or whose medical condition necessitates exclusion from school, is likely to be limited.

PAEDIATRIC COMMUNITY NURSING

Development

The existence of specific community nursing services for children was first formally acknowledged in the Report of the Ministry of Health (1954), in which developments in Rotherham, Exeter and part of Birmingham were noted.

As a result of a 'high infant death rate in the Winter of 1948-1949' (Gillet, 1954a), a paediatric community nursing service was introduced in 1949, in Rotherham. The district nurses, who were appointed to this scheme, were primarily involved in the management of acute paediatric problems, specifically in children with infectious respiratory diseases and gastroenteritis. These nurses had undertaken a 'postgraduate course covering children's diseases' (Gillet, 1954b).

The first recorded appointment of Registered Sick Children's Nurses (RSCNs) in the care of children in the community was in the Paddington Home Care Unit, established in 1954 (Lightwood, 1956). The Paddington team has included both RSCNs and paediatric medical staff, since its inception (Oppe, 1971).

A 'domiciliary nursing service for infants and children' was formally established in Birmingham in 1955 (Smellie, 1956). Initially, district nurses, who were already in post, were seconded for a week to the children's hospital prior to appointment. By the mid-1960s, however, the RSCN qualification was considered necessary for the nursing staff (Robottom, 1969).

Most of the initial literature about the development of these paediatric community nursing services placed emphasis upon the acute nature of the nurses' work, and was rather disease-oriented in its approach (Gillet, 1954a; Smellie, 1956; Lightwood, 1956). Furthermore, much of this literature was written by paediatric medical staff and appeared in medical journals.

Early developments in paediatric community nursing were acknowledged in the Platt Report (Ministry of Health, 1959) which suggested that 'the extension of such schemes should be encouraged'. Despite this, no further schemes were established for the next 10 years. During this time, however, in both Birmingham and Paddington, a gradual shift was reported in the nature of the casework away from acute care and towards the care of children with chronic health problems (Boorer, 1970; Howell, 1974, Jenkins, 1975).

In 1969, further paediatric community nursing schemes were introduced in Southampton and in Edinburgh. The Southampton scheme was originally intended to provide a nursing follow-up service to children who had undergone surgery in a newly built daycase unit (Atwell *et al.*, 1973). By 1976, although the principal role in the follow-up of daycases remained, a more long-term caseload of chronic paediatric patients had been identified (Gow, 1976).

The paediatric community nursing team at Edinburgh Sick Children's Hospital was based in the outpatient department of the hospital. The work of this team has always been concentrated in the care of children with chronic medical problems, such as cystic fibrosis, asthma and diabetes mellitus (Campbell, 1987).

A 'paediatric home nursing scheme' was established in Gateshead in 1972 (Hally *et al.*, 1977), by appointing four district nurses, who each gained three weeks of paediatric 'experience/training to enable them to care for children in the home' (Hally *et al.*, 1977). However, it was emphasized that a paediatric qualification for nurses within the team was desirable. No further record of this service is found in the literature beyond 1978. Two further PCN schemes were established in

the 1970s: Oxford in 1975 (Smith *et al.*, 1984), and Brent in 1976 (Smith, 1977).

Each of these schemes developed in response to a locally identified need. From the reports referred to above, it appears there were wide variations in the clinical roles of the nursing staff within the schemes.

By 1981, there were only eight PCN schemes in the United Kingdom. However, throughout the 1980s and early 1990s, there has been a dramatic expansion in the availability of services (Whiting, 1988; Lessing and Tatman, 1991). This expansion in provision has included both the introduction of large numbers of PCN teams whose work could be best described as generalist and the emergence of several specialist roles for PCNs. By April 1994, there were 92 generalist PCN teams and 57 specialist teams (Whiting/Royal College of Nursing, 1994).

As the number of schemes increased during the 1980s, patterns began to emerge in the nature of the caseloads and in the range of clinical practices undertaken by the nurses. A survey of all generalist teams which had been established up to 1988 found much common ground regarding sources of referral, broad categories of nursing need, underlying medical diagnoses and nursing activities undertaken (Whiting, 1988). The survey also noted important variations in the geographical base (hospital or community setting) and line of management (within acute or community units) of the nursing team.

Scope of generalist role

While the work of the specialist practitioner is important (indeed it is only by virtue of the availability of access to specialist support that much of the work of the PCN has evolved), for the purposes of this particular text the separation of roles is not deemed to be appropriate. Specialist practice has therefore been absorbed within the overall account of paediatric community nursing practice.

The work of paediatric community nurses can be considered under seven broad headings, each of which describes a specific area of nursing provision (Box 4-2).

◆ BOX 4-2

The work of the paediatric community nurse

- Neonatal (and post-neonatal) care.
- Caring for children with acute paediatric nursing needs.
- Supporting children undergoing planned surgery.
- Supporting families of children who have long-term nursing needs arising from physical disease processes.
- Follow-up and support of children requiring emergency treatment (surgery, trauma and orthopaedics).
- Supporting the families of children with disability.
- Supporting families who are caring for children during the terminal phase of their lives.

It is not feasible to provide a comprehensive description of every possible area of nursing need addressed by PCNs in the United Kingdom. However, each of the following sections contains examples of both the nursing need and the type of support and care that is being provided by PCNs somewhere in the UK. These examples are intended to provide insight into some of the areas of current practice and to provide some indications of likely areas of service development in the foreseeable future.

Neonatal (and Post-Neonatal) Care

Within this section, the discussion of paediatric community nursing provision for neonates has been restricted to those areas of clinical practice which relate specifically to neonatal care. Clearly, some neonates have nursing needs which might also occur in older children (e.g., acute gastroenteritis, inguinal herniae or cystic fibrosis) and some neonates have nursing needs which have more long-term consequences (e.g., congenital cardiac disease, congenital alimentary tract atresia or neuro-developmental problems). Such needs will be considered elsewhere in this chapter, rather than under the somewhat exclusive heading of 'neonatal care'.

Community nursing support services for premature babies in the UK have existed for many years. The Manchester Community Special Baby Care Service, for example, was established in 1945 (Couriel and Davies, 1988). However, the dramatic development of neonatal paediatrics has resulted in the survival of a large population of medically fragile babies. The demands made by these babies go far beyond those which might have previously been provided in the hospital special care baby nursery or in a community special care baby service.

Increasingly, babies weighing less than 1500 g or even 1000 g at birth are surviving (Marlow *et al.*, 1987). It has been shown that these babies are major users of health care services. Morgan (1985), for instance, found that 53% of a sample of 111 infants weighing less than 1500 g at birth were readmitted to hospital during the first year of life. A second sample of 216 full-term infants born in the same hospital found only 9.7% of these infants were readmitted in the same period. Furthermore, for the very premature infant, complex problems arising particularly from the immaturity of the respiratory and gastrointestinal systems have resulted in many babies spending much of their first year of life in hospital.

Bronchopulmonary dysplasia (BPD) provides a useful example of the problems which can arise for such babies and the level of support which might be required in order to effect transfer from hospital to home.

Advances in the medical care of babies of below 30 weeks gestation, particularly in terms of the management of respiratory function, have resulted in significant improvements in survival (Royal College of Physicians of London, 1988). Many such babies subsequently develop BPD, however, and require long-term respiratory support with continuous low-flow oxygen supplementation. The introduction of programmes for the provision of domiciliary oxygen therapy to such babies is a major step forward. However of equal, if not greater significance, is the need to provide the parents with the necessary professional support networks which will allow the baby to be transferred home (Brooten *et al.*, 1986; Sleath, 1989; Scott, 1990; Silverman, 1992) as an alternative to long-term hospitalization. In addition, the potential impact of such support in terms of reducing the morbidity experience and readmission to hospital is an issue of great interest (Couriel and Davies, 1988; Zahr and Montijo, 1993).

A second area of particular relevance in the care of the neonate is in the management of physiological jaundice which, in terms of diagnostic measurement of serum bilirubin levels and the therapeutic treatment of hyperbilirubinaemia, has historically been almost exclusively the responsibility of the hospital. Earlier in this chapter, the shift from home to hospital confinement was noted. During the 1980s and 1990s the average length of post-natal hospital stay has shown a steady and sustained decline (Department of Health, 1993b). The introduction of rapid discharge protocols in many obstetric units has led to a situation in which neonates with physiological jaundice are presenting in increasing numbers in the community, rather than on the post-natal ward. It seems rather ludicrous that neonates should be returned to hospital for diagnostic investigation and treatment when there is a growing body of evidence that for many babies this can be safely undertaken in the community (Slater and Brewer, 1984; Eggert *et al.*, 1985; Hartsell, 1986).

Caring for Children with Acute Paediatric Nursing Needs

The management in the community of children with acute medical problems is an area of tremendous interest (Whiting, 1988; Dryden, 1989). Earlier in this chapter, it was noted that acute medical admissions account for the majority of the increase in the rate of childhood hospitalization of the past 40 years. Two primary reasons for admission are infections of the respiratory tract and asthma (Henderson *et al.*, 1991). The extent to which paediatric community nurses are providing care to such children is not clear (Whiting, 1988). However, there is considerable demand for the support of parents by professionals with skills such as those of RSCNs. The stated aims of many PCN services suggest that this area of practice should be high on the agenda (Fradd, 1992; Tatman *et al.*, 1993). The potential role of RSCNs in supporting children in the community who have various conditions, such as gastroenteritis, recurrent urinary tract infections, and respiratory tract infections (including pneumonia), otitis media, constipation, and febrile convulsions is considerable, in both preventing admission and in facilitating earlier discharge.

As noted earlier, much of the work of early PCN teams involved the care of acutely ill children. However, the increasingly earlier discharge from hospital of children with more long-term needs and the demand for the provision of nursing support to such children in the community, has resulted in significant diminution of PCNs' contribution to the care of the acutely ill, even to the extent that this now represents perhaps the greatest area for potential development of the PCN in the future. If such development is to succeed, however, it demands both a recognition of the particular skills that are required of the nurse working with the parents of an acutely ill child in the community and the establishment of effective working relationships between the nurse and the primary health care team.

The caseload of the Paddington Home Care Team has changed over the past 40 years. Although the team also includes registrar grade paediatric medical staff, very little of the current caseload could be described as 'acute paediatric'. This is rather surprising, particularly when the Paddington Team (in common with many others which have been established since 1954) have always aimed for 'the avoidance of admission of children to hospital beds' (Lightwood, 1956). Another factor worth noting at this point is that in the first year of operation of the Paddington Team, 60% of referrals were made directly to the team by the local GPs. In 1993-1994, only six referrals were made by GPs.

The extent to which a team of PCNs might be expected to realize the aim of avoiding admission of acutely ill children to hospital might depend upon many factors (Box 4-3).

◆ BOX 4-3

Avoidance of hospital admission

Factors for Consideration

Size and skills/knowledge base of the team and other demands made by the caseload upon those resources: It is essential that members of the PCN team are able to respond to the demands which might be made by the families of children who are acutely unwell. If parents are expected to care for sick children at home, then they need to feel supported in this. Parents need to know what to expect of the nursing team, how to contact a nurse, how quickly a nurse will respond to a telephone call, and what skills the nurse has to offer when she/he arrives. Even if the child has reached the recuperative phase of an episode of illness, the support of parents in the management of symptoms may require a wide range of nursing skills.

Hours the service is available: Some teams provide 24-hour, 7-day cover, though most operate a daytime-only service. Others, particularly where only one nurse is employed, operate on an 'office hours only' basis, from Monday to Friday.

Mechanisms for gaining access to a nurse: While most teams have an answerphone in their base office and collect their messages at set times each day, others can be accessed at all times via a mobile telephone or radio pager service.

Availability of medical backup for the nurse: Before the nursing team take on the care of an acutely ill child at home, clear mechanisms should be in place for accessing medical support. This might be provided by the GP or by hospital- or community-based paediatric medical staff. Depending upon local circumstances and the particular problems faced by the child, medical care might be provided in the child's home or he/she might be brought to the doctor.

Supporting Children Undergoing Planned Surgery

Although planned surgery for many children might require overnight hospitalization or a longer stay, much of the 'cold' surgery of childhood can be safely undertaken as day surgery (Caring for Children in the Health Services, 1991). A major component of the reduction in the average length of hospital stay for children can be accounted for by revolutionary changes in surgical and anaesthetic practices, and in the overall organizational approach adopted in the care of children after surgery (Department of Health, 1991a; Audit Commission, 1993). In many centres, children are no longer admitted to hospital one or even two days prior to surgery, as was the case in the past, and procedures which might historically have resulted in a five or more nights' postoperative stay in hospital now result in discharge on the same day as the operation (Atwell and Gow, 1985).

While paediatric day case surgery in the UK has its roots in the work of Nicoll at the turn of the century (Nicoll, 1909), the day surgical unit based at Southampton General Hospital has been pioneering on two important fronts: (1) in extending the range of procedures which can be safely undertaken as day surgery in children, and (2) in establishing the benchmark for the provision of postoperative support to children and their families in the community (Atwell and Gow, 1985; Gow and Ridgway, 1993).

It is important, however, to note that for many children in the UK, day surgery is undertaken with absolutely minimal postoperative community support built into the schedule of care (Caring for Children in the Health Services, 1991). A further concern for the families of children who undergo day surgery relates to the rapid, almost conveyor-belt systems, whose existence is deemed to be essential for the smooth running of daycase services in some centres. The need to establish support systems for the families of children undergoing planned surgery is absolutely paramount. This must include effective preoperative preparation (Bates and Broome, 1986), adequate preparation and advice giving prior to discharge (Harrison, 1977) and the provision of skilled professional support — including both practical/clinical expertise and insight into the psychological and emotional needs of parents and children after the child arrives home (Gow and Ridgway, 1993).

The overall role of PCNs in supporting children undergoing planned surgery is one of tremendous potential, incorporating (as it does in centres of excellence) elements of preoperative preparation, predischarge advice and reassurance, and postdischarge support.

Supporting the Families of Children with Long-term Nursing Needs Arising from Physical Disease Processes

This area represents the central focus for much of the work of paediatric community nurses. Although the PCNs initial care of such children might involve either performing practical nursing procedures or demonstrating and teaching those procedures to the child or carer(s), the long-term role of the PCN often becomes more supportive and educative in nature (Whiting, 1991) as the family assumes the responsibility for carrying out the procedures. The range of procedures which might be involved are listed in Box 4-4.

The role of the PCN regarding children with chronic disease has been reviewed by many authors; notably, Sinclair and Whyte (1987), Campbell (1987), Whiting (1988), and Gow and Ridgway (1993). Extensive literature now exists in the United Kingdom describing the nursing role in supporting the families of children with a range of specific medical conditions as listed in Box 4-5.

A recurrent theme in paediatric community nursing practice is the tremendous pressure created for many families by the responsibility of caring for children whose medical condition makes great demands of the family (Harrison, 1977; Sinclair and Whyte, 1987; Jennings, 1992; While, 1994). Many PCNs consider it to be central to their role with such families, to provide a level of support which helps to dissipate that pressure.

Follow-up and Support of Children Requiring Emergency Treatment (Surgery, Trauma and Orthopaedics)

An extensive range of PCN activities can be considered under this heading.

◆ BOX 4-4

Possible 'nursing' procedures that may be undertaken by the child and/or the child's family

- Use of drug delivery inhaler/nebulizer devices (e.g., for asthma).
- Applying wet-wrap dressings (e.g., for eczema).
- Finger-prick blood sampling and giving injections (e.g., for diabetes).
- Giving suppositories and/or enemas (e.g., for constipation).
- Preparing and administering intravenous antibiotics (e.g., for cystic fibrosis) and cytotoxic chemotherapy.
- Tracheal suction, changing tracheostomy tubes.
- Taking blood from established central venous lines (e.g., Port-a-caths, Hickman lines, Vascu-ports) and phlebotomy.
- Intravenous cannulation (e.g., for haemophilia).
- Feeding via parenteral lines, nasogastric tubes and gastrostomies.
- Monitoring oxygen saturation.
- Overnight ventilation.
- Continuous ambulatory peritoneal dialysis (CAPD).
- Renal dialysis.
- Administering chelating agents (e.g., for thalassaemia or sickle-cell disease).
- Administering home oxygen therapy.
- Administering blood and blood products.
- Establishing and maintaining infusions of narcotic agents.

Emergency surgery

For children who require admission to hospital followed by emergency surgical intervention, the possibility that community nursing support at home might facilitate early discharge is an important consideration. The term 'hospital at home' is being used with increasing frequency in describing nursing care of this order (Marks, 1991).

Emergency admissions to hospital are generally more disruptive to normal family life than when a child's admission to hospital is planned. Consequently, the possibility of early discharge may be particularly welcome. Careful and comprehensive predischarge planning is important in ensuring that the incidence of predictable and potentially avoidable postoperative problems is minimized (Department of Health, 1994). In addition, it is imperative that the family fully appreciates the implications of facilitated early discharge in terms of the commitment that adult members of the family will need to make in bearing most of the responsibility for meeting the child's needs.

The care of children who have undergone appendicectomy provides a useful illustration of the potential for early discharge. For children whose surgery has been uncomplicated, the availability of nursing support to the family in the community should allow for discharge from hospital around 36 to 48 hours post surgery. In supporting the families of children who are discharged from hospital in this manner, the PCN must recognize the demands that this will place on the family, and must be aware of, and sensitive to, the holistic needs of the child. Close and continuing liaison with the hospital surgical team and the family GP is particularly important in such circumstances.

Traumatic injuries

As noted above, approximately 3.5 million children attend accident and emergency departments each year. Nearly 2 million of these attendances are the result of an accident. Approximately 120,000 accidents to children each year result in hospital admission (Child Accident Prevention Trust,

---

◆ BOX 4-5

Selected UK literature regarding specific aspects of paediatric community nursing practice

Condition	Literature
Asthma	(Whiting, 1991)
Cancer and leukaemia	(Patel, 1990, Beardsmore and Alder, 1994)
Constipation	(Keating, 1990)
Chronic nutritional failure/ intestinal disease	(Stapleford, 1989; Holden, 1991)
Cystic fibrosis	(Sidey, 1990; Stephenson, 1989)
Diabetes	(McEvilly, 1991)
Tracheostomies	(Jennings, 1989)

1989). In the United Kingdom, one child in seven will attend a hospital accident and emergency department each year as a result of an accident. In addition to preventing admission of children who present with paediatric medical problems, the PCN team can also provide a useful adjunct to the accident and emergency service for children who have sustained minor injuries, including burns or scalds, injuries which have required suturing, and injuries where further dressings are required (Glucksman *et al.*, 1986). Providing continuing wound care in the child's home offers the following advantages:

- Less anxiety and stress for the child (and parents) undergoing painful nursing procedures.
- Increased opportunities for health education, using the combined foci of the wound and, in many instances, the home setting (which accounts for approximately 40% of all childhood accidents, and a higher percentage in the pre-school child [Department of Trade and Industry, 1994b). The prevention of childhood accidents is a key target of the government's *Health of the Nation* strategy (Department of Health, 1991b) and provides a useful illustration of the potential role of the PCN as a health educator.

Emergency orthopaedic problems

Many children are admitted to hospital each year as an emergency with problems of orthopaedic origin (Audit Commission, 1993). Fractures of the femur provide a useful example of the type of support which PCNs can provide.

Children who have sustained femoral fractures occupy more bed nights than any other emergency surgical condition (Henderson *et al.*, 1992). The management of children with femoral fractures in the community is not a new phenomenon (Powell, 1972; Holmes *et al.*, 1983), though it is far from commonplace.

In the care of adults with femoral fractures, stabilization of the fracture by internal fixation and the provision of enhanced nursing support in the community has increasingly been utilized in facilitating rapid discharge (Marks, 1991). In the Peterborough Hospital at Home scheme, for instance, the availability of nursing support in the community has facilitated a reduction in mean length of hospital stay from 25.5 to 8.2 days (Pryor and Williams, 1989).

For children, with growing bones, internal fixation of femoral fractures is not appropriate. External fixation using either skin traction or skeletal traction is the usual method of stabilization of the fracture. While external traction of this order clearly requires the child to be bed-bound (for several weeks in many instances), it is not always necessary for the bed to be in hospital!

Careful discharge planning, involving the hospital team, PCNs, the child's family and the local ambulance service, is absolutely essential if early discharge is to be effected (Department of Health, 1994). Several factors are of particular importance, as shown in Box 4-6.

◆ BOX 4-6

Home care of a child with a femoral fracture: factors for consideration

- The parents must feel confident that they are capable of managing the child's pain or discomfort without recourse to continuous professional support.
- If the child has a Thomas splint or Steinman pin *in situ*, parents need to be taught how to participate in the care for these, before the child goes home. Parents may also need to learn how to reapply bandages/skin traction.
- The fracture must be stable, and capable of withstanding the journey between hospital and home.
- The family must understand and be committed to the absolute necessity for the bed-bound child to have immediate access to an adult 24-hours per day.
- The family should have access to a telephone and should be aware of arrangements for emergency contacts throughout the 24-hour day.
- The PCN team should confirm that the home can accommodate a hospital bed, traction frame, or both. This will include details of room sizes, door widths and any stairs/lifts to be negotiated.
- Arrangements for outpatient treatment should be made, including ambulance bookings for return journeys to hospital for X-rays and orthopaedic medical follow-up.

Supporting the Families of Children with Disabilities

The most extensive survey to date of childhood disability in Great Britain estimated that there were 360,000 disabled children — just over 3% of all children under 16 years of age (OPCS, 1989).

Many of these children present with problems in the early days of life. Some problems are apparent on visual assessment of the newborn child; others are brought to the attention of health care professionals as a consequence of parental self-reporting or routine health screening and surveillance.

The provision of support to the families of these children is generally coordinated from local child development or special needs teams. The role of the PCN is usually concerned only with children who have discrete, identifiable nursing needs. The definition of the boundaries of practice for the PCN will depend upon local custom and protocol, though the PCN can expect to work closely with colleagues within the child development team.

Where practical, and where other nursing needs are apparent in the early days of life, the PCN may form an integral part of a complex support team for the family. This might include the community midwife, health visitor, GP, paediatrician and other professionals, depending upon the nature of the child's problems.

Supporting Families who are Caring for a Children during the Terminal Phase of their Lives

Nearly 10,000 children die each year in the United Kingdom. Of these, approximately 40% are newborn babies, 45% die suddenly or unexpectedly (for instance as a result of an acute illness or an accident) and the remaining 15% die more slowly, as a result of a degenerative or life threatening disease. Within this latter category, approximately 400 children die each year from cancers, 300 from other major organ failure and 800 from degenerative conditions and severe physical disability (BPA/King's Fund/NAHA, 1988). There is, in addition, a small but increasing population of children who die as a consequence of HIV disease (Duggan, 1993).

Several research studies have indicated that the families of many dying children express a preference for the terminal phase of the child's life, and the inevitable death, to occur at home rather than in hospital (Martinson *et al.*, 1986, Lauer *et al.*, 1983; Edwardson, 1983). However, each of the studies identified the enormous psychological and emotional pressures which can be generated within a family who have chosen to care for a dying child at home.

The role of the PCN in supporting such families is multifaceted and serves perhaps as the best illustration of the breadth and complexity of that role.

Palliative care and the management of pain, incontinence, constipation, diarrhoea, vomiting, anorexia, immobility, bleeding, anaemia, convulsions, or hyperpyrexia may all form part of the complex demands which are faced jointly by the child, family and health care team (Patel, 1990; Beardsmore and Alder, 1994). The PCN takes on a key role as family advocate and information giver, linking with the family and a complex array of fellow professionals. In this way, two primary objectives can be achieved: (1) the child is able to live as complete and fulfilling and 'normal' a life as possible, for as long as possible, and (2) the inevitable death occurs in a place of the child's and family's choice.

In striving to achieve these dual objectives, the PCN plays a key role in recognizing and responding to the psychological and emotional impact upon every member of the family. However, caring for a dying child at home makes demands which go far beyond the psychological pressures, and which inevitably permeate all aspects of family life. There may be considerable financial consequences, with one or both parents being required to alter their normal work patterns or to give up work altogether. The physical demands of lifting, positioning and caring for a child whose mobility is often reduced, combined with sleepless nights, sheer physical exhaustion, and simply 'having to be brave' for the child and any siblings, may prove to be overwhelmingly tiring.

The PCN needs to be acutely aware of these potential problems, to anticipate the need for providing the principle carers with timely respite from direct care responsibilities (if they will accept such respite), and to utilize a range of possible alternatives including home-based respite care (provided by other family members, the PCN or other professional or voluntary support agencies), short stays in hospital or the use of formal respite facilities.

The period around the child's death is inevitably traumatic. Careful anticipation and planning by the PCN and other members of the health care team can help alleviate some of that trauma, however. While the death of a child is almost always a distressing event, there is a great deal that can be achieved for both child and family by providing skilled, sensitive nursing care in the child's home, where the child is surrounded by family, friends, and familiar toys, games and comforts during the final days of life.

KEY POINTS

- ◆ Hospitalisation can have a negative psychological effect upon young children.
- ◆ The development/expansion of paediatric community nursing services allows for the provision of a viable alternative to hospitalization children with a wide range of nursing needs.
- ◆ Paediatric community nursing services first appeared in the UK in 1954. There has been a marked expansion in service provision during the 1980s and 1990s.
- ◆ Although district nurses, health visitors and school nurses have historically provided services to many children in the community, the needs of the child with health care deficits are, in many instance s, best met by registered children's nurses.
- ◆ Paediatric community nurses are involved in a broad spectrum of activity including care of the neonate, caring for children following surgery, supporting the families of children with disability with disability, caring for children who are experiencing both short-term and more long-standing health deficits, and supporting families who are caring for a child during the terminal phase of their lives.
- ◆ Children should be cared for in their own homes where possible.
- ◆ Children who require frequent admissions to hospital are considered to be at risk.
- ◆ There has been a dramatic expansion in the availability of paediatric community nursing services.
- ◆ The development of paediatric day surgery has been underpinned by the availability of paediatric community nurse.
- ◆ The work of the paediatric community nurse includes children with both acute and chronic illnesses.

REFERENCES

Atwell JD, Burn JMB, Dewar AK, Freeman NV: Paediatric day-case surgery, *Lancet* 2(7834):895, 1973.

Atwell JD, Gow MA: Paediatric trained district nurse in the community: expensive luxury or economic necessity? *BMJ* 291(6489):227, 1985.

Audit Commission: *Children first: a study of hospital services*, London, 1993, HMSO.

Baly ME: *A history of the Queen's Nursing Institute*, Beckenham, 1987, Croom Helm.

Bates TA, Broome M: Preparation of children for hospitalization and surgery: a review of the literature, *J Pediatr Nurs* 1(4):230, 1986.

Beardsmore S, Alder S: Terminal care at home—the practical issues. In Hill L, editor: *Caring for dying children and their families*, London, 1994, Chapman and Hall.

Boorer D: Home nursing in Birmingham, *Nurs Times* 66(24):741, 1970.

Bowlby J: *Maternal care and mental health*, Monograph Series, No 2, Geneva, 1951, World Health Organization.

Bowlby J: *Attachment and loss. Volume 1: Attachment*, London, 1969, Hogarth Press.

British Paediatric Association/British Association of Paediatric Surgeons: *Children's attendance at accident and emergency departments*, London, 1986, BPA/BAPS.

British Paediatric Association/King Edward's Hospital Fund for London/National Association of Health Authorities: *The care of dying children and their families*, Birmingham, NAHA, 1988.

British Paediatric Association: *Towards a combined child health service*, London, 1991, BPA.

British Paediatric Association: *Flexible options for paediatric care*, London, 1993, BPA.

Brooten D *et al.:* A randomized clinical trial of early hospital discharge and home follow-up of very-low-birth-weight infants, *New Eng J Med* 315(15):934, 1986.

Brykczynska GM: *Ethics in paediatric nursing*, London, 1989, Chapman and Hall.

Campbell M: Children with ongoing health needs, *Nurs Third Series* 23:871, 1987.

Caring for Children in the Health Services: *Where are the children?*, London, 1987, National Association for the Welfare of Children in Hospital.

Caring for Children in the Health Services: *Just for the day*, London, 1991, National Association for the Welfare of Children in Hospital.

Caring for Children in the Health Services: *Bridging the gaps*, London, 1993, Action for Sick Children.

Casey A: A partnership with the child and family, *Senior Nurs* 8(4):8, 1988.

Clark J: *What do health visitors do? A review of the research 1960-1980*, London, 1981, Royal College of Nursing.

Child Accident Prevention Trust: *Basic principles of child accident prevention: a guide to action*, London, 1989, CAPT.

Cleary J, Gray OP, Rowlandson PH, Sainsbury CPQ, Davies MM: Parental involvement in the lives of children in hospital, *Arch Dis Child* 61(8):779, 1986.

Couriel JM, Davies P: Costs and benefits of a community special care baby service, *BMJ* 296(6628):1043, 1988.

Council for the Education and Training of Health Visitors: *An investigation in the principles and practice of health visiting*, London, 1977, CETHV.

Davies J: Paediatric trained district nurse in the community (letter), *BMJ* 291(6497):547, 1985.

Department of Health and Social Security: *Fit for the future — the report of the Committee on Child Health Services*, (Chairman—SDM Court), London, 1976, HMSO.

Department of Health: *The welfare of children and young people in hospital*, London, 1991a, HMSO.

Department of Health: *The health of the nation: a consultative document for health in England*, London, 1991b, HMSO.

Department of Health: *Outpatients and ward attenders: financial year 1992/3*, London, 1993a, HMSO.

Department of Health: *Changing childbirth (Part 1: Report (of the Expert Maternity Group)*, London, 1993b, HMSO.

Department of Health: *Health and personal social services statistics for England*, London, 1993c, HMSO.

Department of Health: *Hospital discharge workbook: a manual on hospital discharge practice*, London, 1994, HMSO.

Department of Trade and Industry: *Home and leisure accident research: 16th annual report home accident surveillance system (1992 data)*, London, 1994, HMSO.

Douglas JWB: Early hospital admission and later disturbances of behaviour and learning, *Devel Med Child Neurol* 17:80, 1975.

Dryden S: Paediatric medicine in the community, *Paediatr Nurs* 1(8):17, 1989.

Duggan C: A family affair: multidisciplinary care for children and families with HIV and AIDS, *Child Health* 1(1):33, 1933.

The Education Act, London, 1981, HMSO.

The Education Reform Act, London, 1993, HMSO.

Edwardson SR: The choice between hospital and home care for terminally ill children, *Nurs Res* 32(1):29, 1983.

Eggert LD *et al.:* Home phototherapy treatment of neonatal jaundice, *Pediatr* 76(4):579, 1985.

Fradd E: Working with the specialists, *Community Outlook* 2(6):29, 1992.

Gillet JA: Children's nursing unit, *BMJ* i:684, 1954a.

Gillet JA: Domiciliary treatment of sick children, *Practitioner* 172:281, 1954b.

Glucksman E *et al.:* Home care team in accident and emergency, *Arch Dis Child* 61(3):294, 1986.

Gow MA: Domiciliary paediatric care in Southampton, *Queen's Nurs J* October:192, 1976.

Gow MA, Ridgway G: The development of a paediatric community nursing service. In Glasper EA, Tucker A, editors: *Advances in Child Health Nursing*, London, 1993, Scutari Press.

Graham S: Little victims—sick children in the Victorian era, *Nurs Times Supple*, London, 1977, Macmillan.

Hally MA *et al.:* Paediatric home nursing scheme in Gateshead, *BMJ* 1(6063):762, 1977.

Harrison S: *Families in stress*, London, 1977, Royal College of Nursing.

Hartsell MB: Home phototherapy, *J Pediatr Nurs* 1(4):282, 1986.

Henderson J *et al.:* Conditions accounting for substantial time spent in hospital in children aged 1-14 years, *Arch Dis Child* 67(1):83, 1991.

Hill A: Trends in paediatric medical admissions, *BMJ* 298(6686):1479, 1989.

Holden C: Home parenteral nutrition, *Paediatr Nurs* 3(3):13, 1991.

Holmes SJK, Sedgwick DM, Scobie WG: Domiciliary Gallow's traction for femoral shaft fractures in young children—feasibility, safety and advantages, *J Bone Joint Surg* 65B(3):288, 1983.

Howell M: *Domiciliary care of sick children in Birmingham—its history and development* (Paper presented to a NAWCH conference), October, 1974.

Hutchison TP, Durojaiye L, Madeley RJ: Improved primary care does not prevent the admission of children to hospital, *Arch Dis Child* 62(6):645, 1987.

Jenkins SM: Home care scheme in Paddington, *Nurs Mirror* 140(8):68, 1975.

Jennings P: Tracheostomy care—learning to cope at home, *Paediatr Nurs* 1(7):13, 1989.

Jennings P: Coping strategies for mothers, *Paediatr Nurs* 4(9):24, 1992.

Keating M: Constipation, *Community Outlook* December:4, 1990.

Kensington and Chelsea and Westminster Family Health Services Authority: *Directory of general medical practitioners*, 1992.

Lessing D, Tatman M: Paediatric home care in the 1990s, *Arch Dis Child* 66(8):994, 1991.

Lauer ME *et al*: A comparison study of parental adaptation following a child's death at home or in the hospital, *Pediatr* 71(1):107, 1983.

Lightwood R: The home care of sick children, *Practitioner* July (177):10, 1956.

Marks L: *Home and hospital care: redrawing the boundaries*, London, 1991, King's Fund.

Marlow N, D'Souza SW, Chiswick M: Neurodevelopmental outcome in babies weighing less that 2001 g at birth, *BMJ* 294(6587):1582, 1987.

Martinson IM *et al.*: Home care for children dying with cancer, *Res Nurs Health* 9(1):11, 1986.

McEvilly A: Home management on diagnosis, *Paediatr Nurs* 3(5):16, 1991.

Ministry of Health: *Report of the Ministry of Health*, London, 1954, HMSO.

Ministry of Health: *The welfare of children in hospital—report of the committee (chairman—Sir H Platt)*, London, 1959, HMSO.

Morgan MEI: Late morbidity of very low birthweight infants, *BMJ* 291:171, 1985.

The National Health Service Act, London, 1946, HMSO.

Nicoll JH: The surgery of infancy, *BMJ* ii:753, 1909.

Office of Population Censuses and Surveys: Dunnell K, Dobbs J: *Nurses working in the community*, London, 1982, HMSO.

Office of Population Censuses and Surveys: Bone M, Meltzer H: *The prevalence of disability among children*, OPCS Surveys of Disability in Great Britain—report 3, London, 1989, HMSO.

Office of Population Censuses and Surveys: *Morbidity statistics from general practice 1991/92*, Series MB5, No 3, London, 1994, HMSO.

Oppe TE: Home care for sick children, *Br J Hosp Med* 5(1):39, 1971.

Patel N: The child with cancer in the community. In Thompson J, editor: *The child with cancer: nursing care*, London, 1990, Scutari Press.

Powell HDW: Domiciliary Gallows traction for femoral shaft fractures in young children, *BMJ* ii:108, 1972.

Pryor GA, Williams DRR: Rehabilitation after hip fractures: home and hospital management compared, *J Bone Joint Surg* 71-B(3):471, 1989.

Quinton D, Rutter M: Early hospital admission and later disturbances of behaviour: an attempted replication of Douglas' findings, *Devel Med Child Neurol* 18(4):447, 1976.

Rathbone W: *Sketch of the history and progress of district nursing for its commencement in 1859 to the present date*, London, 1890, Macmillan.

Robertson J: *Young children in hospital*, London, 1958, Tavistock.

Robottom BM: The contribution of the children's nurse to the home care of children, *Br J Med Ed* 3(4):311, 1969.

Royal College of Physicians of London: *Medical care of the newborn in England and Wales*, West Midlands, 1989, Cradley Print Cradley Heath.

Scott D: Home oxygen for preterm infants, *Midwife Health Visitor Community Nurs* 26(6):219, 1990.

Shannon FT, Ferguson DM, Dimond ME: Early hospital admissions and subsequent behaviour problems in 6 year olds, *Arch Dis Child* 59(9):815, 1984.

Sidey A: Co-operation in care, *Paediatr Nurs* 2(3):10, 1990.

Silverman M: Domiciliary oxygen therapy for children, *J Royal College Physicians London* 26(2):125, 1992.

Sinclair H, Whyte D: Perspectives on community care for children. In Barnes J, editor: *Recent advances in nursing (16): children's nursing*, Essex, 1987, Longman Group.

Slater L, Brewer MF: Home versus hospital phototherapy for term infants with hyperbilirubinaemia: a comparative study, *Pediatr* 73(4):515, 1984.

Sleath K: Breath of life, *Nurs Times* 85(44):31, 1989.

Smellie JM: Domiciliary nursing service for infants and children, *BMJ* i:256, 1956.

Smith JP: Brent's integrated paediatric nursing unit, *Nurs Mirror* 145(5):22, 1977.

Smith MA, Strang S, Baum JD: Organisation of a diabetic clinic for children, *Practical Diabetes* 1(1):8, 1984.

Stapleford P: Formula feeding, *Paediatr Nurs* 1(4):14, 1989.

The Statutory Rules and Orders of the Local Government Act, London, 1929, HMSO.

Stephenson K: Giving antibiotics at home, *Nurs Stand* 3(30):24, 1989.

Stocks M: *A hundred years of district nursing*, London, 1960, Allen & Unwin.

Strehlow M: *Nursing in educational settings*, London, 1987, Harper and Row.

Tatman MA *et al.*: Paediatric home care in Tower Hamlets: a working partnership with parents, *Quality Health Care* 1(2):98, 1993.

While AE: *Health visiting and health experience of infants in 3 areas*, unpublished PhD Thesis, University of London, 1985.

While AE: Personal communication, London, 1994.

Whiting M: Options in the care of acute childhood illness, *Nursing* 23(23):865, 1987.

Whiting M: *Community paediatric nursing in England in 1988*, unpublished MSc Thesis, University of London, 1988.

Whiting M: Caring for a child with asthma using Orem's Self-Care Model. In While AE, editor: *Caring for children: towards partnership with families*, Kent, 1991, Edward Arnold.

Whiting M/Royal College of Nursing: *Directory of paediatric community nursing services*, London, 1995, RCN.

Wyke S, Hewison J, Russel I: Children with cough: who consults the doctor? In Wyke S, Hewison J, editors: *Child health matters*, Milton Keynes, 1991, Open University Press.

Wynne J, Hull D: Why are children admitted to hospital? *BMJ* 2(6095):1140, 1977.

Zahr LK, Montijo J: The benefits of home care for sick premature infants, *Neonatal Network* 12(1):33, 1993.

Chapter 5

Reaction of the Child and Family to Illness and Hospitalization

LEARNING OUTCOMES

After studying this chapter you should be able to:

◆ Describe the usual reactions of children, of differing ages, to hospitalization.
◆ Consider appropriate nursing strategies to prevent or minimize the negative effects of hospitalization.
◆ Understand the need to inform and support parents/carers of the hospitalized child.
◆ Become familiar with several pain rating scales and pain management strategies suitable for use with children of varying ages.
◆ Consider the use of play in a hospital setting.
◆ Consider the nursing contribution to making the period of hospitalization a positive experience for children and their families.
◆ Construct an appropriate discharge plan.
◆ Define the glossary terms.

GLOSSARY

analgesia Absence of pain without loss of consciousness

anaclitic depression Maternal deprivation syndrome

ATC Around the clock

autonomy Self direction, independence

cognitive Mental awareness and functioning

Cutaneous stimulation Touching or stimulating the skin

drug tolerance Clinical need to increase the drug dosage in order to attain the same desired effect

egocentric Self centred

ICU Intensive care unit

IM Intramuscular

IV Intravenous

narcotic Legal term for any substance causing psychological dependence

narcotic addiction Behavioural pattern of overwhelming involvement with obtaining and using a narcotic for its psychic effects rather than for medical reasons

negativism A state of expressing denial, refusal

non-pharmacological Refers to therapies excluding drugs

opioid Natural or synthetic analgesic with morphine-like actions

pharmacological Durg related

physical dependence Adaptive physiological state that occurs when a drug is taken in increasing amounts and that is manifest by development of withdrawal symptoms

play therapy A technique used by specially trained therapists to interpret the behaviour of emotionally disturbed children

SC Subcutaneous

therapeutic play A nondirective activity which allows children to express and deal with their concerns and fears

time structuring Formulating a time table or schedule of the day's events

lness and hospitalization constitute a stressful experience for children and their families. It is often the first crisis children must confront. Children, especially during the early years, are particularly vulnerable to the crises of illness and hospitalization because: (1) stress represents a change from the usual state of health and environmental routine, and (2) children have a limited number of coping mechanisms to resolve the stressful events. Children's reactions to these crises are influenced by their developmental age; previous experience with illness, separation, or hospitalization; available support system; their innate and acquired coping skills; and the seriousness of the diagnosis.

This chapter focuses on various aspects of illness and hospitalization in children in order to assist nurses in providing the quality of care that promotes optimum resolution of the crisis, and positive growth from the experience for the entire family unit.

STRESSORS AND REACTIONS RELATED TO DEVELOPMENTAL STAGE

Children's understanding of, reaction to, and method of coping with illness or hospitalization are influenced by the significance of individual *stressors* (events that produce stress) during each developmental phase. These include separation, loss of control, bodily injury, and pain.

SEPARATION ANXIETY

The major stress from middle infancy throughout the preschool years, especially for children ages 15 to 30 months, is separation anxiety, also called *anaclitic depression*. The principal behavioural responses of these children to the three phases of separation anxiety are summarized in Box 5-1 (Robertson, 1979).

During the phase of *protest*, children cry loudly, scream for the parent, refuse the attention of anyone else, and are inconsolable in their grief. They may continue this behaviour for a few hours to several days. Some children may protest continuously, ceasing only from physical exhaustion. If a stranger approaches them, children will initially protest even louder.

During the phase of *despair*, the crying stops. The child is much less active, is disinterested in play or food, and withdraws from others. The child looks sad, lonely, isolated, and apathetic. The major behaviour characteristic is depression, a result of increasing hopelessness, grief, and mourning.

The third phase is *detachment*, sometimes also called *denial*. Superficially, the child appears to have adjusted to the loss. The child becomes more interested in the surroundings, plays with others, and seems to form new relationships. However, this behaviour is the result of resignation and is not a sign of contentment. The child detaches from the parent in an effort to escape the emotional pain of desiring the parent's presence. The child copes by forming shallow relationships with others, becoming increasingly self-centred, and attaching primary importance to material objects. This is the most serious phase,

since reversal of the potential adverse effects is less likely to occur once detachment is established. However, the separations imposed by hospitalization are temporary, children are remarkably resilient, and permanent ill effects are rare.

EARLY CHILDHOOD

Separation anxiety is most evident during the ages of six to 30 months and is the greatest stress imposed by hospitalization. If separation is avoided, young children have a tremendous capacity to withstand any other stress. Children in the

---

◆ BOX 5-1

Manifestations of separation anxiety in young children

Phase of Protest

Observed behaviours during later infancy
  Cries
  Screams
  Searches for parent with eyes
  Clings to parent
  Avoids and rejects contact with strangers
Additional behaviours observed during toddlerhood
  Verbally attacks strangers (e.g., 'Go away')
  Physically attacks strangers (e.g., kicks, bites, hits, pinches)
  Attempts to escape to find parent
  Attempts to physically force parent to stay
Behaviours may last from hours to days
Protest, such as crying, may be continuous, ceasing only with physical exhaustion
Approach of stranger may precipitate increased protest

Phase of Despair

Observed behaviours
  Inactive
  Withdraws from others
  Depressed, sad
  Uninterested in environment
  Uncommunicative
  Regresses to earlier behaviour (e.g., thumb-sucking, bed-wetting, use of dummy, use of bottle)
Behaviours may last for variable lengths of time
Child's physical condition may deteriorate from refusal to eat, drink, or move

Phase of Detachment

Observed behaviours
  Shows increased interest in surroundings
  Interacts with strangers or familiar caregivers
  Forms new, but superficial, relationships
  Appears happy
Detachment usually occurs after prolonged separation from parent; rarely seen in hospitalized children
Behaviours represent a superficial adjustment to loss

toddler stage demonstrate more goal-directed behaviours. For example, they may verbally plea for their parents to stay and physically attempt to secure or find them. They may demonstrate displeasure on the parents' return or departure by having temper tantrums; refusing to comply to the usual routines of mealtime, bedtime, or toileting; or regressing to more primitive levels of development.

In general, the protest behaviours of preschool children are more subtle and passive than those seen in younger children, and include refusing to eat, difficulty sleeping, crying quietly for their parents, continually asking when they will visit, or withdrawing from others. They may express anger indirectly by breaking their toys, hitting other children, or refusing to cooperate during usual self-care activities.

LATER CHILDHOOD

School-aged children may display increased need for parental security and guidance, especially those who are struggling with the crisis of school adjustment. Middle and late school-aged children may react more to the separation from their usual activities and peers, than to absence of their parents. Their high level of physical and mental activity frequently finds no suitable outlets in the hospital environment. Feelings of loneliness, boredom, isolation, and depression are common. It is important to recognize that such reactions may occur more as a result of separation than from concern about the illness, treatment, or hospital setting.

School-aged children may need and desire parental guidance or support from other adult figures, but may be unable or unwilling to ask for it. Cultural expectations to 'act like a man' or to 'be brave and strong' bear heavily on these children, especially males, who tend to react to stress with stoicism, withdrawal, or passive acceptance. Often the need to express hostile, angry, or other negative feelings finds alternative outlets, such as irritability and aggression towards parents, withdrawal from hospital personnel, inability to relate to peers, rejection of siblings, or subsequent problems in school.

For adolescents, separation from home and parents may be a welcomed and appreciated event. However, loss of peer-group contact may be a severe emotional threat because of loss of group status, inability to exert group control or leadership, and loss of group acceptance.

LOSS OF CONTROL

One of the factors influencing the amount of stress imposed by hospitalization is the amount of control that persons perceive themselves as having. Lack of control increases the perception of threat and can affect children's coping skills (LaMontagne, 1984). Hospital experiences may temporarily slow development or even permanently retard it.

TODDLERS

Toddlers are striving for autonomy, and this goal is evident in most of their behaviours — motor skills, play, interpersonal relationships, activities of daily living, and communication. When their egocentric pleasures meet with obstacles, toddlers react with negativism, especially temper tantrums. Any restriction or limitation of movement, such as the simple act of laying toddlers on their back, can cause forceful resistance and noncompliance.

Loss of control also results from altered routines and rituals. Toddlers rely on the consistency and familiarity of daily rituals to provide a measure of stability and control in their complex world of growing and developing. Hospitalization or illness severely limits their sense of expectation and predictability, since most details of the hospital environment differ from those of the home.

Toddlers' main areas for rituals include eating, sleeping, bathing, toileting, and play. When the routines are disrupted, difficulties can occur in any or all of these areas. The principal reaction to such change is regression. Although regression to earlier forms of behaviour may seem to increase toddlers' security and comfort, in reality it is very threatening for them to relinquish their most recently acquired achievements.

Enforced dependency is a chief characteristic of the sick role and accounts for the numerous instances of toddler negativism. The effects of the sick role are most severe in instances of chronic, long-term illnesses or in those families who foster the sick role despite the child's improved state of health.

PRESCHOOLERS

Preschoolers also suffer from loss of control caused by physical restriction, altered routines, and enforced dependency. However, their specific cognitive abilities, which make them feel omnipotent and all-powerful, also make them feel out of control. This loss of control in the context of their sense of self-power is a critical influencing factor in their perception of and reaction to separation, pain, illness, and hospitalization.

Preschoolers' egocentric and magical thinking limits their ability to understand events, because they view all experiences from their own self-referenced perspective. Without adequate preparation for unfamiliar settings or experiences, preschoolers' fantasy explanations for such events are usually more exaggerated, bizarre, and frightening than the facts. One typical fantasy to explain the reason for illness or hospitalization is that it represents punishment for real or imagined misdeeds. The response to such thinking is usually feelings of shame, guilt, and fear.

Preschoolers' cognitive ability is also concrete. Explanations are understood only in terms of real events. Purely verbal instructions are often inadequate for them, because of their inability to abstract and synthesize beyond what their senses tell them. When combined with their egocentric and magical powers, they can interpret any message according to their particular past experiences. Even with the best preparation for a procedure, they may misconstrue the details.

Transductive reasoning implies that preschoolers deduct from the particular to the particular, rather than from the specific to the general, or vice versa. For example, if preschoolers' concept of nurses is that they inflict pain, preschoolers will think that every nurse (or everyone wearing a similar uniform) will also inflict pain.

SCHOOL-AGED CHILDREN

Because of their striving for independence and productivity, school-aged children are particularly vulnerable to events that may lessen their feeling of control and power. In particular, altered family roles; physical disability; fears of death, abandonment, or permanent injury; loss of peer acceptance; lack of productivity; and inability to cope with stress according to perceived cultural expectation may result in loss of control.

Many routine hospital activities usurp individual power and identity. Dependent activities, such as enforced bed rest, use of a bedpan, inability to choose a menu, lack of privacy, help with a bed bath, or transport by a wheelchair or stretcher can be a direct threat to their security. However, when children are allowed to exert a measure of control, regardless of how limited it may be, they generally respond very well to any procedure. For example, some of the most cooperative, satisfied, and contented patients are school-aged children who help make their beds, choose their schedule of activities, assist in procedures, and help the nurses care for the younger children. An increased sense of control usually results from a feeling of usefulness and productivity.

Illness itself may also cause a feeling of loss of control. One of the most significant problems of children in this age group centres on boredom. When physical or enforced limitations curtail their usual abilities to care for themselves or to engage in favourite activities, school-aged children generally respond with depression, hostility, or frustration. Keeping a normally active child on bed rest is no small challenge. However, emphasizing areas of control and capitalizing on quiet activities, particularly hobbies such as building models or collecting specific objects, promote their adjustment to physical restriction. Nursing judgement regarding selection of a room-mate is one of the most important contributing factors to children's overall adjustment to illness and hospitalization.

ADOLESCENTS

Adolescents' struggle for independence, self-assertion, and liberation centres on the quest for personal identity. Anything that interferes with this poses a threat to their sense of identity and results in a loss of control. Illness, which limits their physical abilities, and hospitalization, which separates them from the usual support systems, constitute major situational crises.

The patient role fosters dependency and depersonalization. Adolescents may react to dependency with rejection, uncooperativeness or withdrawal. They may respond to depersonalization with self-assertion, anger or frustration. Regardless of which response they manifest, hospital personnel generally tend to regard them as difficult, unmanageable patients. Parents may not be a source of help because these behaviours serve to further isolate them from understanding the adolescent. Although peers may visit, they may not be able to offer the type of support and guidance needed. Sick adolescents often voluntarily isolate themselves from age-mates until they feel they can compete on an equal basis and meet group expectations. As a result, ill adolescents may be left with virtually no support systems.

Loss of control also occurs for many of the reasons discussed for school-aged children. However, adolescents are more sensitive to potential instances of loss of control and dependency than younger children. For example, both groups seek information about their physical status and rely heavily on anticipatory preparation to decrease fear and anxiety. However, adolescents react not only to what information is supplied, but also to how it is conveyed. They may feel very threatened by others who relate facts in a derogatory manner. Adolescents want to know that others can relate to them on their own level. This necessitates a careful assessment of their intellectual abilities, previous knowledge and present needs. It may also require the nurse's willingness to learn the adolescent's language.

REACTION TO BODILY INJURY AND PAIN

Fears of bodily injury and pain are prevalent among children. Recent research documents that young children, including newborns, react to painful stimuli. In caring for children, nurses must appreciate the concerns related to bodily harm and children's reactions to pain at different developmental periods. Developmental considerations related to children's understanding of illness and pain are summarized in Table 5-1.

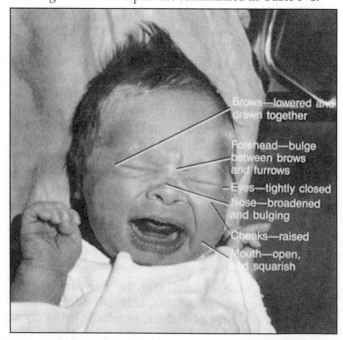

Fig. 5-1 Facial expression of physical distress is the most consistent behavioural indicator of pain in infants.

INFANTS

There is marked variability in measures of distress, especially initial cry and heart rate, which may decrease in some infants. The most consistent indicator of distress is a facial expression of discomfort (Fig. 5-1). Body movements include squirming, writhing, jerking, and flailing. Children who react less intensely than others may still be experiencing significant discomfort.

Infants less than six months of age seem to have no memory of previous painful experiences, and react to a potentially stressful situation with less apprehension and fear than older children. However, after this time, children's response to pain is influenced by their recall of prior painful experiences and the emotional reaction of parents during the procedure. Older infants react intensely with physical resistance and uncooperativeness. Distraction does little to lessen their immediate reaction to pain, and anticipatory preparation, such as showing them the equipment, tends to increase their fear and resistance.

TODDLERS

Toddlers' concept of body image, particularly the definition of body boundaries, is very poorly developed. Intrusive experiences, such as examining the ears or mouth or taking a rectal temperature, are very anxiety producing. Toddlers may react to such painless procedures as intensely as they do to painful ones.

COGNITIVE STAGE (AGE)	CONCEPT OF ILLNESS*	CONCEPT OF PAIN†
Preoperational thought (2 to 7 years)	*Phenomenism:* Perceives an external, unrelated concrete phenomenon as the cause of illness; e.g., "being sick because you don't feel well" *Contagion:* Perceives cause of illness as proximity between two events that occurs by "magic"; e.g., "getting a cold because you are near someone who has a cold"	Conceives of pain primarily as physical, concrete experience. Thinks in terms of magical disappearance of pain. May view pain as punishment for wrongdoing Tends to hold someone accountable for own pain and may strike out at person
Concrete operational thought (7 to 10+ years)	*Contamination:* Perceives cause as a person, object or actional external to the child that is "bad" or "harmful" to the body; e.g., "getting a cold because you didn't wear a hat" *Internationalization:* Perceives illness as having an external cause but as being located inside the body; e.g., "getting a cold by breathing in air and bacteria"	Conceives of pain physically; e.g., headache, stomach-ache Able to perceive psychological pain; e.g., someone dying Fears bodily harm and annihilation (body destruction and death) May view pain as punishment for wrongdoing
Formal operational thought (13 years and older)	*Physiological:* Perceives cause as malfunctioning or nonfunctioning organ or process; can explain illness in sequence of events *Psychophysiological:* Realizes that psychological actions and attitudes affect health and illness	Able to give reason for pain; e.g., fell and hit nerve Perceives several types of psychological pain Has limited life experiences to cope with pain as adult might cope despite mature understanding of pain Fears losing control during painful experience

*Data from Bibace, R., and Walsh, M.E.: 1980. † Data from Hurley, A., and Whelan, E.G.: 1988.

Table 5-1 Children's developmental concepts of illness and pain.

Memory, physical restraint, parent separation, emotional reactions of others, and lack of preparation partially determine the intensity of the behavioural response. In general, toddlers continue to react with intense emotional upset and physical resistance to any actual or perceived painful experience. Behaviours indicating pain include grimacing, clenching their teeth/lips, opening their eyes wide, rocking, rubbing, and aggressiveness, such as biting, kicking, hitting, or running away. Unlike adults, who usually decrease their activity when in pain, young children typically become restless and overly active.

By the end of this age period, toddlers usually are able to communicate about their pain. Although they have not developed the ability to describe the type or intensity of the pain, they usually are able to localize it by pointing to a specific area.

PRESCHOOLERS

Concepts of illness begin during the preschool period and are influenced by the cognitive abilities of the preoperational stage. Preschoolers differentiate poorly between themselves and the external world. Their thinking is focused on externally perceived events, and causality is based on the proximity of two events. Consequently, children define illness according to what they are told or are given external evidence of, such as, 'You are sick because you have a fever'. The cause of illness is seen as a concrete action the child does or fails to do, such as, 'Catching a cold because you go out into cold weather' (Perrin and Gerrity, 1981); consequently, it implies a degree of responsibility and self-blame. Another explanation may be based on contagion, that the proximity of two objects or persons causes the illness; for example, 'A person gets a cold when someone else with a cold gets near him' (Bibace and Walsh, 1980).

The psychosexual conflicts of children in this age-group make them very vulnerable to threats of bodily injury. Intrusive procedures, whether painful or painless, are threatening to preschoolers, whose concept of body integrity is still poorly developed. Preschool children may react to an injection with as much concern for withdrawal of the needle as for the actual pain. They fear that the intrusion or puncture will not reclose and that their 'insides' will leak out.

Concerns of mutilation are paramount during this age period. Loss of any body part is threatening, but preschool boys' fears of castration complicate their understanding of surgical or medical procedures associated with the genital area, such as circumcision, repair of hypospadias or epispadias, cystoscopy, or catheterization. Their limited comprehension of body functioning also increases their difficulty in understanding how or why body parts are 'fixed'. For example, telling preschoolers that their tonsils are to be removed may be interpreted as 'taking out their voice'.

Preschoolers respond more favourably to preparatory interventions, such as explanation and distraction, than younger children. Physical and verbal aggression are more specific and goal directed. Instead of showing total body resistance, preschoolers may push the offending person away, try to secure the equipment, or attempt to lock themselves in a safe place. Much more thought is evident in their plan of attack or escape.

Verbal expression, in particular, demonstrates their advanced development in response to stress. They may verbally abuse the attacker by stating, 'Get out of here' or 'I hate you'. They may also use the more cunning approach of trying to persuade the person to give up the intended activity. A common plea is, 'Please don't give me an injection; I'll be good'. Some statements are not only attempts to avoid the event but also evidence of children's perceptions about the experience.

Attempts to be comforted may also be evident through behaviours such as clinging to a parent, wanting to be held, or refusing to be left alone. It is important to recognize the need for support from others during a time of stress. Admonishing children to act grown-up or encouraging them to do things by stating, 'I know you can do it yourself', deprives them of the support they are requesting and increases their own feelings of guilt and shame.

SCHOOL-AGED CHILDREN

Fears of the physical nature of the illness surface at this time. School-aged children may be less concerned with pain than with disability, uncertain recovery, or possible death. Girls tend to express more and stronger fears than boys, and previous hospitalizations may have no effect on the frequency or intensity of these fears (Aho and Erickson, 1985). Because of their developing cognitive abilities, school-aged children are aware of the significance of different illnesses, the indispensability of certain body parts, potential hazards in treatments, lifelong consequences of permanent injury or loss of function, and the meaning of death. A major concern of hospitalized school-aged children is their fear of not being well again. They generally take a very active interest in their health or illness.

The school-aged child defines illness by a set of multiple concrete symptoms, such as signs of a cold, and views the cause as primarily germs or bacteria. The 'germs' have a powerful, almost magical quality, so that in the child's mind, illness can be prevented by avoiding people with the germs (Perrin and Gerrity, 1981). There is also the idea of contamination, which is similar to that seen in the younger age group; for example, the illness occurs because of physical contact or because the child engaged in a harmful action and became contaminated (Bibace and Walsh, 1980). Consequently, feelings of self-blame and guilt may be associated with the reason for becoming ill.

School-aged children begin to show concern for the potential beneficial and hazardous effects of procedures. Besides wanting to know if a procedure will hurt, they want to know what it is for, how it will make them better, and what injury or harm could result. For example, these children fear the actual procedure of anaesthesia. Unlike preschoolers, who fear the mask and the strange surroundings, school-aged children fear what may happen while they are asleep, whether they will wake up, and if they may die. Preadolescents also worry about the procedure itself, particularly one that will result in visible changes in body appearance.

Intrusive procedures of a nonsexual nature, such as routine physical examination of the ears, nose, mouth, and throat, are generally well tolerated. However, concerns for privacy become evident and increasingly significant. Examination of, or procedures performed on, the genital area, are usually very stressful for them, especially for preadolescents who are beginning pubertal changes.

By the age of nine or ten, most school-aged children show less fright or overt resistance to pain than younger children. They generally have learned passive methods of dealing with discomfort, such as holding rigidly still, clenching their fists or teeth, or trying to act brave by the 'grin-and-bear-it' routine.

School-aged children verbally communicate about their pain in respect to its location, intensity, and description. Children eight years and older use a wide variety of words and phrases, such as hurting, sore, burning, stinging, aching, and 'like a sharp knife' (Tesler *et al.*, 1989).

School-aged children also use words as a means of controlling their reactions to pain. For example, these children may ask the nurse to talk to them during a procedure. Some prefer to participate in a procedure, whereas others choose to distance themselves by not looking at what is happening. Most appreciate an explanation of the procedure and seem less fearful when they know what to expect. Others try to gain control by attempting to postpone the event. A typical request is, 'Give me the needle when I am finished with this'. Although the ability to make decisions does increase their sense of control, unlimited procrastination results in heightened anxiety. When choices are allowed, such as selection of the injection site, it is best to structure the number of possible sites and to limit the number of 'procrastination' techniques.

The visible composure, calmness, and acceptance of school-aged children often masks their inner longing for support. It is especially important to be aware of nonverbal clues, such as a serious facial expression, a half-hearted reply of 'I'm fine', silence, lack of activity, or social isolation, as signs of the need for help.

ADOLESCENTS

Injury, pain, disability, and death are viewed primarily in terms of how each affects adolescents' views of themselves in the present. Any change that differentiates the adolescent from peers is regarded as a major tragedy. For example, diseases such as diabetes mellitus often present a more difficult adjustment period for children in this age group than for younger children because of the necessary changes in the adolescent's life-style. Conversely, serious, even life-threatening illnesses that entail no visible body changes or physical restrictions may have less immediate significance for the adolescent. Therefore, the *nature* of bodily injury may be more important in terms of adolescents' perception of the illness than its actual degree of severity.

Adolescents' rapidly changing body image during pubertal development often makes them feel insecure about their bodies. Illness, medical or surgical intervention, and hospitalization increase their existing concerns for normalcy. They may respond to such events by asking numerous questions, withdrawing, rejecting others, or questioning the adequacy of care. Frequently, their fear for loss of control and body image change is demonstrated as over-confidence, conceit, or a 'know-all' attitude.

Because of sexual changes, adolescents are very concerned about privacy. Lack of respect for this need can cause greater stress than physical pain.

Adolescents react to pain with much self-control. Physical resistance and aggression are unusual at this age, unless the adolescents are totally unprepared for a procedure. They are able to describe their pain experience and to use any of the pain assessment tools developed for adults. However, they may be reluctant to disclose their pain unless the nurse is willing to listen closely and observe physical indications, such as limited movement, excessive quiet, or irritability. They may also believe that the nurse knows how they feel; thus, they may see no need to ask for analgesia (Favaloro and Touzel, 1990).

SUBSEQUENT EFFECTS OF HOSPITALIZATION

Children not only react to the stresses of illness and hospitalization during admission, but may demonstrate temporary behavioural changes following discharge, especially children under four years of age (Box 5-2). These effects result from: (1) separation from significant people, (2) a lack of opportunity to form new attachments, and (3) a strange environment.

◆ BOX 5-2

Post-hospital behaviours in children

Young Children

Some initial aloofness towards parents; may last from a few minutes (most common) to a few days

Frequently followed by dependency behaviours:

  Tendency to cling to parents

  Demand parents' attention

  Vigorously oppose any separation (e.g., staying at preschool or with a babysitter)

Other negative behaviours include:

  New fears (e.g. nightmares)

  Resistance to going to bed, night waking

  Withdrawal and shyness

  Hyperactivity

  Temper tantrums

  Food finickiness

  Attachment to blanket or toy

  Regression in newly learned skills (e.g., self-toileting)

Older Children

Negative behaviours include:

  Emotional coldness, followed by intense, demanding dependence on parents

  Anger towards parents

  Jealousy towards others (e.g., siblings)

STRESSORS AND REACTIONS OF THE FAMILY OF THE HOSPITALIZED CHILD

The child is an integral member of the family unit. Consequently, hospitalization of the child affects other members of the family and the way the family functions.

PARENTAL REACTIONS

Parents' reactions to illness in their child depend on a variety of influencing factors (Box 5-3).

Initially parents may react with *disbelief*, especially if the illness is sudden and serious. Following the realization of illness, parents react with *anger, guilt*, or both. They tend to search for self-blame about why the child became ill or to project anger at others for some wrongdoing. Even in the mildest of illnesses, parents question their adequacy as caregivers and review any actions or omissions that could have prevented or caused the illness. When hospitalization is indicated, parental guilt is intensified.

Fear, anxiety, and *frustration* are common feelings expressed by parents. Fear and anxiety may be related to the seriousness of the illness and the type of medical procedures involved. Feelings of frustration are often related to lack of information about procedures and treatments, unfamiliarity with hospital rules and regulations, a sense of unwelcomeness from the staff, or fear of asking questions. Much frustration can be alleviated in a paediatric unit where parents participate in their child's care and are regarded as the most significant contributors to the child's total health.

Parents eventually may react with some degree of *depression*. The depression usually occurs when the acute crisis is over, such as following hospital discharge or complete recovery.

SIBLING REACTIONS

Siblings' reactions to a sister's or brother's illness or hospitalization include anger, resentment, jealousy, and guilt. Various factors have been identified that influence the effects of the child's hospitalization on siblings:
- Fear of contracting the illness.
- Younger age.
- Close relationship to sick sibling.
- Out-of-home residence during period of hospitalization.
- Minimum explanation of the sick child's illness.
- Perceived changes in parenting, such as increased parental anger.

NURSING CARE OF THE HOSPITALIZED CHILD AND THE FAMILY

Children and their families require competent and sensitive care to minimize the potential negative effects of hospitalization and also to promote positive benefits from the experience.

> ◆ **BOX 5-3**
>
> ### Factors affecting parents' reactions to their child's illness
>
> Seriousness of the threat to the child
> Previous experience with illness or hospitalization
> Medical procedures involved in diagnosis and treatment
> Available support systems
> Personal ego strengths (coping abilities)
> Previous coping abilities
> Additional stresses on the family system
> Cultural and religious beliefs
> Communication patterns among family members

Interventions should focus on: (1) eliminating or minimizing the stressors of separation, loss of control, and bodily injury and pain for children; and (2) providing specific supportive strategies for family members, such as fostering family relationships and providing information.

PREVENTING OR MINIMIZING SEPARATION

The primary nursing goal is to prevent separation, particularly in children under five years of age. However, this is not always possible, and measures to minimize the effects of separation must be implemented. In such cases continuity in nursing care assumes even greater importance.

PARENT PARTICIPATION AND 'ROOMING-IN'

Prevention of separation requires rooming-in facilities in paediatric hospital settings. Although some health facilities provide special accommodations for parents, the concept of 'rooming-in' can be instituted anywhere. When hospital staff genuinely appreciate the importance of continued parent-child attachment, they foster an environment that encourages parents to stay. When parents are included in the care planning and made to feel as if they are a contributing factor to the child's recovery, they are more inclined to remain with their child and have more emotional reserves to support themselves and the child through the crisis.

Some may be under such great emotional stress that they need a temporary reprieve from total participation in caregiving activities. Others may feel insecure in participating in specialized areas of care, such as bathing the child after surgery. Individual assessment of each parent's preferred involvement is necessary to prevent the effects of separation while supporting parents in their needs, as well.

With life-styles and sexual roles changing, some fathers may assume all or some of the usual mothering roles in the household. In this case, it may be the father - child relationship that requires preservation. The father, or other carer (as appropriate), would need to be included in the plan of care and respected for the contribution they make.

One of the potential problems with continuous parent visiting is neglect of the parent's need for sleep, nutrition, and relaxation. After a few days, parents can become exhausted but feel obligated to stay. Encouraging them to leave for brief periods, arranging for sleeping quarters on the unit but outside the child's room, and planning a schedule of alternating visiting with the other parent or with a family member can minimize the stresses for the parent.

Nurses need to work in partnership with parents to determine the appropriate contribution that each will make to the care of the child.

STRATEGIES TO MINIMIZE THE EFFECTS OF SEPARATION

When separation cannot be prevented, numerous strategies can be employed to minimize the effects. Ideally, a named nurse is assigned to meet the child's needs and he or she will require the parents' assistance in compiling a thorough, detailed nursing history that specifically identifies the child's established daily routine. Usual daily activities, such as food preparation and method of feeding, help establish a complementary schedule of caregiving practices. It also helps the parent feel as if he or she is participating in the child's care, but through another person.

The nurse caring for the child must have an appreciation of the child's separation behaviours. As discussed earlier, the phases of protest and despair are normal. If detachment behaviours are evident, the nurse maintains the child's contact with the parents by frequently talking about them, encouraging the child to remember them, and stressing the significance of their visits, telephone calls, or letters.

Separation may be equally as difficult for parents, especially when they do not understand the behaviours of separation anxiety. Helping parents recognize that separation behaviours are normal and expected can decrease their anxiety and may ease their fears about leaving their child. Explaining to parents how the child reacts after they leave may also be helpful. Many parents think the child cries for hours after they leave, whereas in reality the child may cry for a few minutes but settles down when comforted by someone else.

The young child's ability to tolerate parental absence is very limited. Therefore parental visits should be frequent. For example, it is better for parents to visit three times a day for short periods than once a day for an extended time. This may necessitate that each parent visit at different times to lessen the length of separation. When parents cannot visit, the presence of other significant people can be comforting for the child (Fig. 5-2).

If parents leave after the child falls asleep, they still need to communicate their absence. The parents of a five-year-old boy solved this problem by devising a sign; on one side they drew a picture of a telephone and on the other a hamburger. Before they left, they turned the sign to the appropriate side to tell the child when he awoke that they were out using the telephone or eating.

Familiar surroundings also increase the child's adjustment to separation. If parents cannot room-in, they should leave favourite home articles with the child, such as a blanket, toy, bottle, feeding utensil, or article of clothing. Since young children associate such inanimate objects with significant people, they gain comfort and reassurance from such possessions. They make the association that if the parent left this, the parent will surely return. Placing an identification band on the toy lessens the chances of its being misplaced and provides a symbol that the toy is experiencing the same needs as the child. Other momentos of home include photographs and tape recordings of family members reading a story, singing a song, saying prayers before bedtime, relating events at home, or taking a 'talking walk' through the home. Some units allow pets to visit, which can be a special event for a child and can have therapeutic benefits.

Older children also appreciate familiar articles from home, particularly photographs, a radio, a favourite toy or game, and the usual pyjamas. It is reported that about half of school-aged children have a special object to which they formed an attachment in early childhood and that this is a normal and healthy phenomenon (Sherman *et al*, 1981). Therefore such treasured or transitional objects can help even older children feel more comfortable in a strange environment.

Helping children maintain their usual non-home contacts also minimizes the effects of separation imposed by hospitalization. This includes continuing school lessons during the illness and confinement, visiting with friends either directly or through letter writing or telephone calls, and participating in extracurricular projects whenever possible.

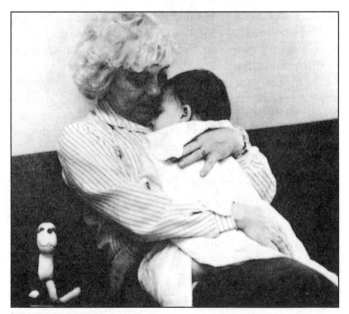

Fig. 5-2 When parents cannot visit, other significant persons, such as a grandparent, can provide comfort to the hospitalized child.

For extended hospitalizations, youngsters enjoy personalizing the hospital room to make it 'home' by decorating the walls with posters and cards, rearranging the furniture (when possible), and displaying a collection or hobby.

MINIMIZING LOSS OF CONTROL

Feelings of loss of control result from separation, physical restriction, changed routines, enforced dependency, magical thinking, and altered roles within the family or peer group. Although some of these cannot be prevented, most of them can be minimized through individualized planning of nursing care.

PHYSICAL RESTRICTION

Younger children react most strenuously to any type of physical restriction or immobilization. Although some restraint, such as immobilizing an extremity for maintenance of an intravenous line, is frequently necessary, most physical restriction can be prevented if the nurse gains the child's cooperation.

For young children, particularly infants and toddlers, preserving parent-child contact is the best way to decrease the need for, or stress of, restraint. For example, almost the entire physical examination can be done in a parent's lap, with the parent hugging the child, for procedures such as otoscopy. For painful procedures, the parents' preferences for assisting, observing, or waiting outside the room are assessed.

Environmental factors also influence the need for physical restraint. Keeping children in cots may not represent immobilization in a concrete sense, but it certainly limits sensory stimulation. Increasing mobility by transporting children in wheelchairs, carts, wagons, or on stretchers or beds provides them with mechanical freedom.

In some cases, restraint or isolation is necessary for recovery. Whenever possible, restraints should be removed to allow the child some period of supervised freedom, such as during the bath or when parents visit. When restraints or isolation cannot be discontinued, such as with severe burns, the environment can be manipulated to increase sensory freedom. For example, moving the bed towards the door or window; opening window blinds; providing musical, visual, or tactile toys; and increasing interpersonal contact can all substitute mental mobility for the limitations of physical movement.

ALTERED ROUTINES

Children's response to loss of routine and ritualism is often demonstrated in problems with activities such as feeding, sleeping, dressing, bathing, toileting, and social interaction. Although some regression is to be expected in all these areas, sensitivity to the special needs of children can minimize the negative effects. For example, loss of appetite and marked food preferences are common in ill or hospitalized children. (Suggestions for feeding sick children are discussed in Chapter 8).

Although regression is expected and normal, nurses also have the responsibility of fostering children's optimum growth and development. Hospitalization can become a significant opportunity for learning and advancing. For example, extended hospitalization for long-term chronic illness or situations of failure to thrive, abuse, or neglect represent instances in which regression must be seen as an adjustment period, to be followed by plans for promoting appropriate developmental skills.

One technique that can minimize the disruption in the child's routine is *time structuring*. It involves scheduling the child's day to include all those activities that are important to the nurse and child, such as treatment procedures, schoolwork, exercise, television, playroom, and hobbies. Together, the nurse, parent, and child then plan a daily schedule with time and activity written down (Fig. 5-3). This is left in the child's room, and a clock or watch is available for the child's use. Whenever possible, a calendar is also constructed with special events marked, such as favourite television programmes, visits by friends or relatives, events in the playroom, and holidays or birthdays. If specific changes in treatment are expected (e.g., 'beginning physiotherapy in two days'), these are added.

ENFORCED DEPENDENCY

The dependent role of the hospitalized patient imposes tremendous feelings of loss on older children. Principal interventions should focus on respect for individuality and the opportunity for decision making. When decision making is geared towards the patient, nurses can feel threatened by a sense of lessened control.

Promoting children's control involves maintaining independence, and the concept of *self-care* can be most beneficial. Self-care refers to the practice of activities that individuals personally initiate and perform on their own behalf in maintaining life, health, and well-being (Orem, 1985). Although self-care is limited by the child's age and physical condition, most children beyond infancy can perform some activities with little or no help. Whenever possible, these activities are encouraged in the hospital.

ERIC'S DAILY SCHEDULE:		
7:00AM	- Breakfast, watch T.V, brush teeth, wash up	3:00PM - Tutor, (M,W,F) Study time (T,Th)
9:00	- Bathroom, dressing change	4:00 - Physiotherapy
		5:00 - Dinner
10:00	- Rest, T.V, snack	6:30 - Dressing change
11:00	- Physiotherapy	7:00 to - T.V, reading, snack, 9:00 friends visit
12:00P.M	- Lunch	
1:00	- Playroom, Quiet, play, rest, friends visit	9:00 - Brush teeth, wash up
		9:15 - Bedtime

Fig. 5-3 Time structuring is an effective strategy for normalizing the hospital environment and increasing the child's sense of control.

LACK OF UNDERSTANDING

Loss of control can occur from feelings of having too little influence on one's destiny, as well as from sensing overwhelming control or power of fate.

Most children feel more in control when they know what to expect, because the element of fear is reduced. Anticipatory preparation and providing information help greatly to lessen stress and prevent lack of understanding (Adams, Gill, McDonald, 1991).

ALTERED FAMILY AND SOCIAL ROLES

In addition to the effects of separation on family roles, loss of parenting, sibling, and offspring roles may affect each family member differently. One of the most common reactions of parents is specialized and intensified attention towards the sick child. The other siblings may regard this as unfair, and may interpret the parents' attitude towards them as rejection. Such responses place unique burdens on ill children. For example, the ill child may feel obligated to play the sick role in order to meet parents' expectations, especially children who have had limited physical ability and regain normal health status, such as following corrective heart surgery. Parents, as well, may be unable to perceive the child's recovery and therefore need to continue the pattern of overprotection and indulgent attention.

Ill children may also feel jealousy and resentment from other siblings. Because of their singular position in the family, they may be denied the companionship of their brothers and sisters. Rivalry between siblings tends to be greatest in the sibling who is nearest the ill child's age. Without an understanding of the interpersonal dynamics between siblings, parents are likely to blame the well children for antisocial behaviour.

Illness may also result in children's loss of status within either their family or social group. For example, illness in the oldest child may temporarily terminate special privileges as 'big' brother or sister. The hospitalized adolescent loses rank within the peer group.

MINIMIZING BODILY INJURY

Beyond early infancy, all children fear bodily injury from any of mutilation, bodily intrusion, body image change, disability, or death. In general, preparation of children for painful procedures decreases their fears (Broome, Endsley, 1987). Manipulating procedural techniques for children in each age group also minimizes fear of bodily injury. For example, since toddlers and young preschoolers are traumatized by insertion of a rectal thermometer, axillary temperatures or electronic temperature probes can effectively be substituted. Whenever procedures are performed on young children, the most supportive intervention is to do them as quickly as possible and maintain parent-child contact.

Because of young children's poorly defined body boundaries, the use of bandages may be particularly helpful. For example, telling them that the bleeding will stop after the needle is removed does little to relieve their fears, whereas applying a small plaster usually provides much reassurance. The size of bandage is also significant to children in this age group. The larger the bandage, the more importance is attached to the wound. Using successively smaller surgical dressings is one way of their measuring healing and improvement. Prematurely removing a dressing may cause them considerable concern for their well-being.

Children may fear bodily injury from a variety of sources. Use of strange equipment for examination, unfamiliar rooms or awkward positions can be perceived as potentially hazardous. In addition, thoughts and actions can be imagined sources of bodily damage. For older children, masturbation or sex play may be perceived as powerful weapons of potential destruction. Therefore, it is important to investigate imagined reasons, particularly of a sexual nature, for illness. Since children may fear revealing such thoughts, using projective techniques such as drawing or doll play may demonstrate previously undisclosed misconceptions.

Older children fear bodily injury of both internal and external origins. For example, school-aged children are aware of the heart's significance and may fear the actual procedure as much as the pain, the stitches, and the possible scar. Adolescents may express concern for the surgery, but may be much more anxious about the resulting scar.

Children can grasp information only if it is presented according to their cognitive development. The example of a seven-year-old who interpreted the doctor's statement of 'there's oedema in your belly' as 'there's a demon in your belly' is proof of the necessity to choose words carefully and re-evaluate the child's understanding of the message (Perrin and Gerrity, 1981).

When children are upset about their illness, their perception can be changed by: (1) providing a somewhat different and less negative account of the disease or (2) offering an explanation that is characteristic of the next stage of cognitive development (Bibace and Walsh, 1980). An example of the first strategy is reassuring a preschool child who fears that, after a tonsillectomy, another sore throat means a second operation. Explaining that once tonsils are 'fixed' they do not need fixing again can help relieve the fear. An example of the second strategy is to explain that germs made the tonsils sick and even though germs can cause another sore throat, they cannot cause the tonsils to ever be sick again. This higher level explanation is based on the school-aged child's concept of germs as a cause of disease.

PAIN ASSESSMENT

Pain assessment is a critical component of the nursing process. Unfortunately, health professionals, including nurses, tend to underestimate the existence of pain in children (Richardson, 1992). Several studies have documented the enormous disparity between medication practices with children and adults. One reason for inadequate management of pain is a lack of understanding of what pain is — a personal phenomenon that *cannot* be experienced by another individual. Therefore, defining pain in terms of another's perceptions is inappropriate and inaccurate. An operational definition that is useful in clinical practice is: *pain is whatever the experiencing person says it is, existing whenever the person says it does* (McCaffery and Beebe, 1989). This definition implies a very important attitude towards patients — *that they are believed*. It includes both verbal and nonverbal expressions of pain.

FALLACIES AND FACTS

Children are undertreated for pain for many complex and interrelated reasons, including professionals' misconceptions about pain; the complexities of pain assessment, particularly in nonverbal children; and the lack of information regarding currently available pain reduction techniques. Several fallacies continue to flourish because of incorrect knowledge about pain in infants and children, despite these fallacies having been disproved by current research on paediatric pain (Table 5-2).

PRINCIPLES OF PAIN ASSESSMENT IN CHILDREN

Since pain is both a sensory and an emotional experience, using several assessment strategies provides qualitative and quantitative information about pain. One approach to pain assessment in children is QUESTT (Baker and Wong, 1987):

- Question the child.
- Use pain rating scales.
- Evaluate behaviour and physiological changes.
- Secure parents' involvement.
- Take cause of pain into account.
- Take action and evaluate results.

Question the child

Children's verbal statements and descriptions of pain are the most important factors in assessing pain. However, young children may not know what the word 'pain' means and may need help in describing it using familiar language. Therefore, using a variety of words to describe pain, such as 'ouch', 'feel

FALLACIES	FACTS
Infants and children do not feel pain or feel pain less than adults do.	Neonates and infants demonstrate physiological, behavioural, and biochemical indicators of pain (Anand, Phil, and Hickey, 1987; Shapiro, 1989). Children's sensitivity to pain actually *decreases* with age. Younger children tend to rate procedure-related pain higher than older children do (Wong and Baker, 1988).
Children cannot tell where they hurt.	Children beyond infancy can accurately point to the body area or mark the site on a drawing. By age 3 years, they can use simple pain scales (e.g., faces) (Wong and Baker, 1988).
Children always tell the truth about their pain.	Children may be frightened by an injection and not admit having pain to avoid one. Because of constant pain, they may not realize how much they are hurting. Because of egocentric thinking, children and adolescents may believe that others know how they are feeling and so not ask for analgesia. (Favaloro and Touzel, 1990).
Children tolerate pain better than adults and become accustomed to pain or painful procedures.	Children may not demonstrate decreased behavioural signs of discomfort with repeated painful procedures.
Behavioural manifestations of pain reflect pain intensity.	Behavioural manifestations do not necessarily correlate with pain intensity. Developmental level, coping skills, and temperament influence children's behavioural responses to pain (Wallace, 1989).
Narcotics are dangerous drugs for children. They cause addiction and respiratory depression.	Narcotics (opioids) are no more dangerous for children than they are for adults. Addiction from narcotics (opioids) used to treat pain is extremely rare in adults, and no reports substantiate this fear in children. Reports of respiratory depression in children are rare.

Table 5-2 Fallacies and facts about children and pain.

funny', or 'hurt', is necessary. Older children also benefit from using simple words to describe pain. Suggested questions for obtaining information about children's experiences with pain are presented in Box 5-4. Asking children to locate the pain is also helpful, and play can provide other means for helping children to reveal discomfort.

When asking children about pain, the nurse must remember that they may deny pain because they fear receiving an injectable analgesic or because they believe they deserve to suffer as punishment for some misdeed. They may also deny pain to a stranger, but readily admit it to a parent.

Use a pain rating scale

Pain rating scales provide a subjective quantitative measure of pain. Although various pain scales exist (Table 5-3), not all of them are appropriate for young children. For the most valid and reliable pain intensity rating, a scale is selected that is suitable to the child's age, abilities, and preference. Scales using facial expressions are readily accepted by children and can be used by very young children better than other scales (Wong and Baker, 1988).

It is best to use the same scale with children to avoid confusing them with different instructions. Ideally, children should be taught to use the scale before pain is expected, such as preoperatively. Familiarizing children with the scale facilitates its use when children are actually in pain.

◆ **BOX 5-4**

Pain experience inventory

Questions for Parents

Describe any pain your child has had before.

How does your child usually react to pain?

Does your child tell you or others when he or she is hurting?

How do you know when your child is in pain?

What do you do to ease discomfort for your child when your child is hurting?

What does your child do to get relief when hurting?

Which of these actions work best to decrease or take away your child's pain?

Is there anything special that you would like me to know about your child and pain? (If yes, have parent[s] describe.)

Questions for the Child

Tell me what pain is.

Tell me about the hurt you have had before.

What do you do when you hurt?

Do you tell others when you hurt?

What do you want others to do for you when you hurt?

What don't you want others to do for you when you hurt?

What helps the most to take away your hurt?

Is there anything special that you want me to know about you when you hurt? (If yes, have child describe.)

From Hester N, Barcus C, 1986.

PAIN SCALE/DESCRIPTION	INSTRUCTIONS	RECOMMENDED AGE
FACES Pain Rating Scale (Nix, Clutter and Wong, 1994; Wong and Baker, 1988): Consists of six cartoon faces ranging from smiling face for "no pain" to tearful face	Explain to child that each face is for a person who feels happy because there is no pain (hurt) or sad because there is some or a lot of pain. Face 0 is very happy because there is no hurt. Face 1 hurts just a little bit. Face 2 hurts a little more. Face 3 hurts even more. Face 4 hurts a whole lot, but Face 5 hurts as much as you can imagine, although you don't have to be crying to feel this bad. Ask child to choose face that best describes own pain. Record number under chosen face on pain assessment record.	Children as young as 3 years.

| 0 | 1 | 2 | 3 | 4 | 5 |

(cont.)

Table 5-3 Pain rating scales for children.

Oucher (Beyer, 1989): Consists of six photographs of child's face representing "no hurt" to "biggest hurt you could ever have"; also includes a vertical scale with numbers from 0 to 100; scales for African-American and Hispanic children have been developed (Villarruel and Denyes, 1991) and validated (Beyer, Denyes, and Villarruel, 1992).

Photographs: Explain to child that face at bottom has "no hurt"; second picture, "just a little bit of hurt"; third picture, a "little bit more"; fourth picture, "even more hurt"; fifth picture, "pretty much hurt"; and last picture "biggest hurt you could ever have". Ask child to choose face that best describes own pain.

Numbers: Explain to child that 0 means you have "no hurt"; 0 to 29, "little hurts", 30 to 69, "middle hurts"; 70-99, "big hurts", and 100, "biggest hurt you could ever have." Ask child to choose any number between 0 and 100, not just numberss pictured on Oucher, that best describes own pain.

Children 3–13 years; use numeric scale if child can count to 100 by 1s and identify larger of any two numbers (as in original instructions), or by 10s (Jordan-Marsh and others 1994); otherwise use photographic scale

Numeric Scale: Use straight line with end points identified as "no pain" and "worst pain"; divisions along line are marked in units from 0 to 10 (high number may vary.)

Explain to child that at one end of the line is a 0, which means that a person feels no pain (hurt). At theend is a 10, which means the other person feels the worst pain imaginable. The numbers 1 to 9 are for a very little pain to a whole lot of pain. Ask child to choose number that best describes own pain.

Children as young as 5 years, provided they can count and have some concept of numbers and their values of more or less

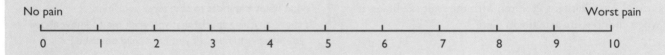

No pain   Worst pain

0   1   2   3   4   5   6   7   8   9   10

Poker chip tool: Uses four red poker chips placed horizontally in front of child.

Tell child, "These are pieces of hurt." Beginning at the chip nearest child's left side and ending at the one nearest child's right side, point to chips and say, "This (the first chip) is a little bit of hurt and this (the fourth chip) is the most hurt you could ever have." For a young child or for any child who does not comprehend the instructions, clarify by saying, "That means this (the first chip) is just a little hurt this (the second chip) is a little more hurt; this (the third chip) is more hurt; and this (the fourth chip) is the most hurt you could ever have." Ask child, "How many pieces of hurt do you have right now?" Children without pain will say they don't have any. Clarify child's answer by words such as "Oh, you have a little hurt? Tell me about the hurt." Elicit descriptors, location, and cause. Ask the child, "What would you like me to do for you?" Record number of chips selected.

Children as young as 4 to 4.5 years, provided they can count and have some concept of numbers

Table 5-3 Pain rating scales for children (continued).

Word Graphic Rating Scale (Tesler and others, 1991): Uses descriptive words (may vary in other scales) to denote varying intensities of pain

Explain to child. "This is a line with words to describe how much pain you may have. This side of the line means no pain and over here the line means worst possible pain. " (Point with your finger where "no pain" is, and run your finger along the line to "worst possible pain," as you say it.) "If you have no pain, you would mark like this." (Show example.) "If you have some pain, you would mark somewhere along the line, depending on how much pain you have." (Show example.) "The more pain you have, the closer to the worst pain you would mark. The worst pain possible is marked like this." (Show example.) "Show me how much pain you have right now by marking with a straight, up-and-down line anywhere along the line to show how much pain you have right now." With a millimetre ruler, measure from the "no pain" end to the mark and record this measurement as the pain score.

Children as young as 5 years, although words may need explanation; words shown below were used with children ages 8 to 17 years

| No pain | Little pain | Medium pain | Large pain | Worst possible pain |

Visual Analogue Scale. Uses 10 cm horizontal line with end points marked "no pain" and "worst pain"

Ask child to place a mark on line that best describes amount of own pain. With a centimetre ruler, measure from the "no pain" end to the mark and record this measurement as the pain score.

Children as young as 4-5 years; vertical or horizontal scale may be used (Walco and Ilowite, 1991)

Colour Tool (Eland, 1993): Uses markers for child to construct own scale that is used with body outline.

Present eight markers to child in a random order. Ask child, "Of these colours, which colour is like... ?" (the event identified by the child as having hurt the most). Place the marker away from the other markers. (Represents severe pain.) Ask child, "Which colour is like a hurt, but not quite as much as ...?" (the event identified by the child as having hurt the most). Place the marker with the marker chosen to represent severe pain. Ask child, "Which colour is like something that hurts just a little?" Place the marker with the other colours. Ask child, "Which colour is like no hurt at all?" Show the four marker choices to child in order from the worst to the no-hurt colour. Ask child to show on the body outlines where they hurt, using the markers they have chosen. After child has coloured the hurts, ask if they are current hurts or hurts from the past. Ask if child knows why the area hurts if it is not clear to you why it does.

Children as young as 4 years provided they know their colours, are not colour blind, and are able to to construct the scale if in pain

Table 5-3 Pain rating scales for children (continued).

Evaluate behaviour and physiological changes

Behavioural changes are common indicators of pain and are especially valuable in assessing pain in nonverbal children. Children's behavioural responses to pain change with age and follow a developmental trend (Box 5-5). However, children vary widely in their responses and may exhibit behaviours at one age that are more typically seen at a different age. In addition, temperament affects coping style, and children with more positive moods may appear to be in less pain than they actually are. Children who use passive coping behaviours (offering no resistance, cooperating) may rate pain as more intense than children who use active coping behaviours (resisting, attacking). Cultural background may also play a role in children's pain responses, although the influence appears slight (Abu-Saad, 1984). Unfortunately, nurses often make judgements about pain based on behaviour, which results in some children receiving inadequate pain medication (Wallace, 1989).

One of the most valuable clues to pain is a change in behaviour and vital signs after administration of an analgesic. Improved behaviour (e.g., less irritability, cessation of crying) and decreased pulse, respirations, and blood pressure provide important evidence of pain. Often, the change in vital signs is attributed to the depressant effect of opioids, when in reality the return to more normal physiological functioning is due to pain relief.

Secure parents' involvement

Parents know their child and are sensitive to changes in behaviour. However, little documentation exists on parents' ability to recognize pain in their children. Some parents may never have seen their child in severe pain and may equate certain responses, such as irritability or withdrawal, with discomfort. However, others are aware that certain behaviours signal pain, because the child has acted similarly during previous painful events. In addition, parents usually know what comforts their child, such as rocking, stroking, or talking.

Take cause of pain into account

When children exhibit behaviours or other clues that suggest pain, reasons for discomfort should be investigated. Pathology may give clues to expected intensity and type of pain. For example, pain associated with vaso-occlusive crises in sickle cell disease is severe. Pain caused by bone marrow puncture is typically greater than the discomfort associated with a venepuncture.

A golden rule to follow in pain assessment is: Whatever is painful to an adult is painful to an infant or child until proved otherwise.

Take action and evaluate results

The reason for assessing pain is to relieve it. Total pain relief should be the goal, with the combined use of pharmacological and nonpharmacological interventions. Regardless of the type of pain intervention, evaluation of the results is essential. No single pain reduction technique is effective for all children.

◆ BOX 5-5

Developmental characteristics of children's responses to pain

Young Infants
Generalized body response of rigidity or thrashing, possibly with local reflex withdrawal of stimulated area
Loud crying
Facial expression of pain (brows lowered and drawn together, eyes tightly closed, mouth open and squarish)
Demonstrates no association between approaching stimulus and subsequent pain

Older Infants
Localized body response with deliberate withdrawal of stimulated area
Loud crying
Facial expression of pain and/or anger (same facial characteristics as pain but eyes may be open)
Physical resistance, especially pushing the stimulus away *after* it is applied

Young Children
Loud crying, screaming
Verbal expressions of 'Ow', 'Ouch', or 'It hurts'
Thrashing of arms and legs
Attempts to push stimulus away *before* it is applied
Uncooperative; needs physical restraint
Requests termination of procedure
Clings to parent, nurse, or other significant person
Requests emotional support, such as hugs or other forms of physical comfort
May become restless and irritable with continuing pain
All these behaviours may be seen in anticipation of actual painful procedure

School-Aged Children
May see all behaviours of young child, especially *during* painful procedure but less in anticipatory period
Stalling behaviour, such as 'Wait a minute' or 'I'm not ready'
Muscular rigidity, such as clenched fists, white knuckles, gritted teeth, contracted limbs, body stiffness, closed eyes, wrinkled forehead

Adolescents
Less vocal protest
Less motor activity
More verbal expressions, such as 'It hurts' or 'You're hurting me'
Increased muscle tension and body control

Data from Craig et al., 1984; and Katz et al.,1980.

Directions:

1. Record time of administering drug and assess analgesic effect 30 minutes later and then hourly.
2. State 'Reason for drug administration' in behavioural terms, e.g., 'child says he hurts' or 'child crying and irritable'.
3. Use column 'Reason for drug administration' to record behaviour during reassessment, e.g., 'child says he feels better' or 'child playing'.
4. Use pain rating scale if child understands its use and only when child is awake. Name of scale: _____
   Rating: No pain = _____ and Worst pain = _____.
5. Suggested guidelines for safe minimum respiratory rates for children receiving opioids are 10 to 16 breaths/minute. Consider child's age (with age, respiratory rate decreases) and physiological status (shallow respiration, decreased oxygen saturation, decreased consciousness) when evaluating respirations.

Date	Time	Drug administered	Reason for administration	Pain rating	Respirations	Signature

Fig. 5-4 Pain assessment record.

Therefore, a pain assessment record is used to monitor the effectiveness of the interventions (Fig. 5-4).

PAIN MANAGEMENT

Relief of pain is a basic need and right of all children, yet doctors and nurses are often reluctant to order and administer analgesics and lack knowledge of well-documented approaches to pharmacological pain control.

Effective pain management requires that health professionals be willing to try several interventions to achieve optimum results. Basically, pain-reducing methods can be grouped into two categories: nonpharmacological and pharmacological. Whenever possible, both should be used; however, nonpharmacological measures should not be considered substitutes for analgesics.

NONPHARMACOLOGICAL MANAGEMENT

Several nonpharmacological techniques exist for lessening the perception of pain and, when used with analgesics, can enhance these drugs' effectiveness. However, nonpharmacological strategies can also produce a cooperative child who continues to suffer 'in silence' (Zeltzer, Jay, and Fisher, 1989). Therefore, nurses must carefully evaluate the effectiveness of the intervention in truly reducing pain and avoid setting an expectation of passive acceptance. Aside from this risk, nonpharmacological methods are extremely safe and most are independent nursing functions.

Nonpharmacological interventions include *general strategies* that are effective with most children, especially those who can benefit from explanations. However, *specific nonpharmacolog-ical strategies* are more effective with certain children than with others (Box 5-6). Experimentation with several strategies that are suitable to the child's age, pain intensity, and abilities is often necessary to determine the most effective approach. Where appropriate, it is best to use a strategy already familiar to the child and family.

Children should learn a new strategy *before* pain occurs or before it becomes severe. To reduce the child's effort, instructions for a strategy, such as distraction or relaxation, can be audiotaped and played during a period of discomfort.

PHARMACOLOGICAL MANAGEMENT

Using pharmacological methods to control pain requires attention to four 'rights': right drug, right dose, right route, and right time. Although nurses may not prescribe the medication, knowledge of these essential principles assists in optimally implementing analgesic prescriptions and discussing with other practitioners possible strategies to improve pain control. In addition, observing for side effects of the drugs and using supportive approaches with children when administering the drug are important nursing interventions.

USE OF PLAY TO MINIMIZE STRESS

Play is one of the most important aspects of a child's life and one of the most effective tools for managing stress. Since illness and hospitalization constitute crises in the child's life and often involve overwhelming stresses, playing out fears and anxieties gives the child a means to cope with these stresses.

Play is the 'work' of children. It is essential to their mental,

◆ BOX 5-6

Guidelines for nonpharmacological pain management

General Strategies

Form a trusting relationship with child and family.

Express concern regarding their reports of pain.

Take an active role in seeking effective pain management strategies.

Use general strategies to prepare child for painful procedure (see Chapter 8).

Prepare child before potentially painful procedures but avoid 'planting' the idea of pain. For example, instead of saying:

'This is going to (or may) hurt', say 'Sometimes this feels like pushing, sticking, or pinching and sometimes it doesn't bother people. You tell me what it feels like to you'.

Use 'nonpain' descriptors when possible (e.g., 'It feels like intense heat' rather than 'It's a burning pain').

This allows for variation in sensory perception, avoids suggesting pain, and gives child control in describing reactions.

Avoid evaluative statements or descriptions (e.g., 'This is a terrible procedure' or 'It really will hurt a lot').

Stay with child during a painful procedure.

Encourage parents to stay with child, if child and parent desire; encourage parent to talk softly to child and to remain near child's head.

Involve parents in learning specific nonpharmacological strategies and assisting child in their use.

Educate child about the pain, especially when explanation may lessen anxiety (e.g., that child's pain is expected after surgery and does not indicate something is wrong; reassure that child is not responsible for the pain).

For long-term pain control give child a doll, which becomes 'the patient' and allow child to do everything to the doll that is done to the child; pain control can be emphasized through the doll by stating, 'Dolly feels better after the medicine.'

Specific Strategies

Distraction

Involve parent and child in identifying strong distractors.

Involve child in play; use radio, tape recorder, record player; have child sing or use rhythmic breathing.

Have child concentrate on yelling or saying 'ouch' by focusing on 'yelling loud or soft as you feel it hurt; that way I know what's happening.'

Use humour, such as watching cartoons, telling jokes or funny stories, or acting silly with child.

Relaxation

With an infant or young child:

Hold in a comfortable, well-supported position, such as vertically against the chest and shoulder.

Rock in a wide, rhythmic arc in a rocking chair or sway back and forth, rather than bouncing child.

Repeat one or two words softly, such as 'Mummy's here'.

With a slightly older child:

Ask child to take a deep breath and 'go floppy like a rag doll' while exhaling slowly, then ask child to yawn (demonstrate if needed).

Help child assume a comfortable position (e.g., pillow under neck and knees).

Begin progressive relaxation: starting with the toes, systematically instruct child to let each body part 'go limp' or 'feel

heavy', if child has difficulty with relaxing, instruct child to tense or tighten each body part and then relax it.

Allow child to keep eyes open, since children may respond better if eyes are open rather than closed during relaxation.

Guided imagery

Have child identify some highly pleasurable real or pretend experience.

Have child describe details of the event, including as many senses as possible (e.g., 'feel the cool breezes', 'see the beautiful colours', 'hear the pleasant music').

Have child write down or record script.

Encourage child to concentrate only on the pleasurable event during the painful time; enhance the image by recalling specific details, such as reading the script or playing the record.

Combine with relaxation.

Positive self-talk

Teach child positive statements to say when in pain (e.g., 'I will be feeling better soon', 'When I go home, I will feel better', 'Relaxing will make me hurt less').

Thought-stopping

Identify positive facts about the painful event (e.g., 'It does not last long').

Identify reassuring information (e.g., 'If I think about something else, it does not hurt as much').

Condense positive and reassuring facts into a set of brief statements, and have child memorize them (e.g., 'Short procedure, good veins, little hurt, nice nurse, go home').

Have child repeat the memorized statements whenever thinking about or experiencing the painful event.

Cutaneous stimulation

Includes simple rhythmic rubbing; use of pressure, electric vibrator; massage with hand cream, powder, or menthol cream; application of heat or cold, such as an ice cube on the site before giving injection or application of ice to the site opposite the painful area (e.g., if right knee hurts, place ice on left knee).

A more sophisticated method is transcutaneous electrical nerve stimulation (TENS) (use of controlled low-voltage electricity to the body via electrodes placed on the skin).

Behavioural contracting

Informal — may be used with children as young as four or five years:

Use stars or tokens as rewards.

Give uncooperative or procrastinating children (during a procedure) a limited time (measured by a visible timer) to complete the procedure.

Proceed as needed if child is unable to comply.

Reinforce cooperation with a reward if the procedure is accomplished within specified time.

Formal — use written contract, which includes the following:

Realistic (seems possible) goal or desired behaviour.

Measurable behaviour (e.g., agrees not to hit anyone during procedures).

Contract written, dated, and signed by all persons involved in any of the agreements.

Identified rewards or consequences are reinforcing

Goal can be evaluated.

emotional and social well-being. As with their developmental needs, the need for play does not stop when children are ill or when they enter the hospital. On the contrary, play in the hospital serves many functions (Box 5-7). Of all hospital facilities, no room probably does more to alleviate the stressors of hospitalization than the playroom. In this room, children temporarily distance themselves from the fears of separation, loss of control, and bodily injury. They can work through their feelings in a nonthreatening, comfortable atmosphere and in the manner most natural for them. They also know that the boundaries of this room are safe from intrusive or painful procedures, strange faces, and probing questions. The playroom becomes a sanctuary of peace and safety in an otherwise frightening environment.

Children in various age groups require different types of play facilities. Infants and toddlers need maximum safety, whereas school-aged children and adolescents benefit most from group recreation.

DIVERSIONAL ACTIVITIES

Almost any form of play can be used for diversion and recreation, but the activity should be selected on the basis of the child's age, interests, and limitations.

When supervising play for ill or convalescent children, it is best to select activities that are simpler than would normally be chosen according to the child's developmental level. Also, special consideration must be given to the child who has limited movement, has a restricted extremity, or is isolated. Toys for isolated children must be capable of being disposed of or disinfected after use.

Toys

Parents of hospitalized children often ask nurses about the types of toys that would be best to bring for their child. Most want to bring new ones to cheer and comfort the child and assuage their own guilt feelings. The nurse should tell the parents that small children need the comfort and reassurance of familiar things, such as the stuffed animal the child hugs for comfort and takes to bed at night. These are a link with home and the world outside the hospital.

EXPRESSIVE ACTIVITIES

Play provides one of the best opportunities for encouraging emotional expression, including the safe release of anger and hostility. Nondirective play that allows children freedom for expression can be very therapeutic. Therapeutic play, however, should not be confused with the psychological technique of play therapy. *Play therapy* is reserved for use by trained and qualified therapists who use the technique as an interpretative method with emotionally disturbed children. *Therapeutic play*, on the other hand, is a very effective nondirective modality for helping children deal with their concerns and fears; at the same time, it often helps the nurse to gain insights into their needs and feelings (Clatworthy, 1981).

◆ **BOX 5-7**

Functions of play in the hospital

Provides diversion and brings about relaxation

Helps the child feel more secure in a strange environment

Helps to lessen stress of separation and the feelings of home sickness

Provides a means for release of tension and expression of feelings

Encourages interaction and development of positive attitudes towards others

Provides an expressive outlet for creative ideas and interests

Provides a means for accomplishing therapeutic goals

Places child in active role and provides opportunity to make choices and be in control

---

Tension release can be facilitated through almost any activity. With younger ambulatory children, large-muscle activity such as use of tricycles and wagons is especially beneficial. Much aggression can be safely directed into games and activities that involve pounding and throwing. Bean bags are often thrown at a target or open receptacle with surprising vigour and hostility.

Creative expression

Drawing and painting are excellent media for expression. The child needs only to be supplied with the raw materials, as children usually require little direction for self-expression; however, older children may be given some direction in what to paint or draw. For example, they may be asked to draw the hospital room or draw what they like or do not like about the hospital.

Dramatic play

Dramatic play is a well-recognized technique for emotional release, allowing children to re-enact frightening or puzzling hospital experiences. Through the use of puppets, replicas of hospital equipment, or some actual hospital equipment, children can play out the situations that are a part of their hospital experience.

In planning any play activities, the nurse must not forget that the reason for the child's hospitalization always takes precedence over other considerations, including the need for play. Play must be scheduled around medical needs and any limitations imposed by the child's condition. For example, small children may eat paste and other creative media; therefore a child who is allergic to wheat should not be given finger paint made from wallpaper paste or play dough made with flour. A child on a restricted salt intake should not play with modelling dough, since salt is one of its major constituents. Treatment schedules, and the institution's rules and policies must also be considered. At home, the play programme should be planned around the therapy regimen.

MAXIMIZING POTENTIAL BENEFITS OF HOSPITALIZATION

While hospitalization generally represents a stressful time for children and families, it also presents an opportunity for facilitating positive change within the child and among family members. Therefore, nursing interventions must also focus on maximizing the potential benefits of the experience.

FOSTERING PARENT - CHILD RELATIONSHIPS

The crisis of illness or hospitalization can mobilize parents into more acute awareness of their children's needs. For example, one school-aged child who was diagnosed with a serious physical condition commented to the nurse that he 'enjoyed' the hospital because it was the first time that he had seen so much of his parents. He expressed concern over discharge because he anticipated the loss of the intensified love and attention.

Hospitalization provides opportunities for parents to learn more about their children's growth and development. When parents are helped to understand children's usual reactions to stress, such as regression or aggression, they are not only better able to support the child through the hospital experience but also may extend their insights into childrearing practices following discharge.

Difficulties in parent - child relationships that may result in feeding problems, negative behaviour, and enuresis may decrease during hospitalization. The temporary cessation of such problems sometimes alerts parents to the role they may be playing in propagating the negative behaviour. With assistance from health professionals, parents can restructure ways of relating to their children to foster more positive behaviour.

Hospitalization may also represent a temporary reprieve or refuge from a disturbed home. Typically abused or neglected children's dramatic physical and social improvement during hospitalization is proof of the growth potential of this experience. Hospitalized children temporarily are able to seek support, reassurance, and security from new relationships, particularly with nurses, hospitalized peers, and others.

PROVIDING EDUCATIONAL OPPORTUNITIES

Illness and hospitalization represent excellent opportunities for children and other family members to learn more about their bodies, each other, and the health professions. For example, during a child's admission for a diabetic crisis, the child may learn about the disease; the parents may learn about the child's needs for independence, normalcy, and appropriate limits; and each of them may find a new support system in the hospital staff.

During extended hospitalization, special tutoring can help children advance their studies and concentrate on difficult subjects. The child's relationship with a tutor can foster a more positive attitude towards school and learning.

PROMOTING SELF-MASTERY

The experience of facing a crisis, such as illness or hospitalization, coping successfully with it, and maturing as a result of it constitutes an opportunity for self-mastery. Younger children have the chance to test out fantasy vs. reality fears. They realize that they were not abandoned, mutilated, castrated, or punished. In fact, they were loved, cared for, and treated with respect for their individual concerns. For older children, hospitalization may represent an opportunity for decision making, independence, and self-reliance. They are proud of having survived the experience and may feel a genuine self-respect for their achievements. Nurses can facilitate such feelings of self-mastery by emphasizing aspects of personal competence in the child and not acknowledging uncooperative or negative behaviour.

PROVIDING SOCIALIZATION

Hospitalization may offer children a special opportunity for social acceptance. Lonely, asocial, sometimes delinquent children find a sympathetic environment in the hospital. Children who are physically deformed or in some other way 'different' from their age-mates may find an accepting social peer group. Although this does not always spontaneously occur, nurses can structure the environment to foster a supportive child group. For example, judicious selection of a roommate can help children gain a new friend and learn more about themselves. Forming relationships with significant members of the health care team, such as the doctor or the nurse, can greatly enhance the child's adjustment in many areas of life.

Parents may also encounter a new social group in other parents who have similar problems. Nurses can encourage parents to discuss their concerns and feelings collectively. They can also refer parents to organized 'self-help' groups or can use the help and support of recovered hospitalized patients.

SUPPORTING FAMILY MEMBERS

Optimal paediatric care requires that the nursing assessment and care plan includes family members who are normally involved in the care and support of the child (Wright and Leahey, 1984). Resources can then be targetted to achieve the best outcome.

Support involves an acceptance of cultural, socioeconomic, and ethnic values. Parents need help in accepting their own feelings towards the ill child. If given the opportunity, parents often disclose their feelings of loss of control, anger, and guilt. They often resist admitting to such feelings, because they expect others to disapprove of behaviour that is less than perfect.

PROVIDING INFORMATION

One of the most important nursing interventions is to provide information on all aspects of care (Kanneh, 1990).

For many families, the child's illness is their first contact with the hospital experience. Often, parents are not prepared for the child's behavioural reactions to hospitalization. Nurses can provide parents with information about normal behavioural responses, hospital routines, and about what to expect and what is expected of them. Nurses can also help family members become more adept at seeking information about their child's condition by asking questions that elicit meaningful information (Box 5-8). In giving information, nurses need to be alert to information overload.

Parents also need to be aware of the effects of illness on the family and strategies that prevent negative changes. Specifically, parents should keep the family well informed and communicating as much as possible. They should treat all the children as equally and as normally as before the illness occurred. Discipline, which initially may be lessened for the ill child, should be continued to provide a measure of security and predictability. When ill children know that their parents expect certain standards of conduct from them, they feel certain that they will recover. When all limits are removed, they fear that something catastrophic will happen.

Helping parents understand and expect post-hospitalization behaviours in the sick child is also necessary. Parents who do not expect such reactions may misinterpret them as evidence of the child's 'being spoiled' and may demand perfect behaviour at a time when the child is still reacting to the stress of illness and hospitalization. If the behaviours, especially the demand for attention, are dealt with in a supportive manner, most children are able to relinquish them and assume pre-crisis levels of functioning.

Nurses should also forewarn parents of the reactions of siblings to the ill child — particularly anger, jealousy, and resentment. Older siblings may deny such reactions because they provoke feelings of guilt. However, everyone needs outlets for emotions, and the repressed feelings may surface as problems in school, with age-mates, as psychosomatic illnesses, or in delinquent behaviour.

Parents need to know that siblings may also require information and support, and may wish to be allowed to participate in caring for their sick sibling, as appropriate. Sibling fears of illness and feelings of guilt and rejection may also need to be addressed.

PREPARATION FOR HOSPITALIZATION

The rationale for preparing children for the hospital experience and related procedures is based on the principle that fear of the unknown (fantasy) exceeds fear of the known. Therefore, decreasing the elements of the unknown results in less fear. When children do not have paralyzing fear to cope with, they can then direct their energies towards dealing with the other unavoidable stresses of hospitalization and benefit optimally from the growth potential of the experience.

For children past infancy and early toddlerhood, in-hospital and/or home preparation for hospitalization reduces children's stress (Stewart, 1984; Price, 1991).

Ideally, preparatory procedures should be:
- Planned by the hospital staff before any child's admission to the hospital.
- Appropriately designed for each child's developmental age.
- Sufficiently individualized to account for different children's previous experience with hospitalization, present reason for admission, and available support system.

TIMING OF PREPARATION

If tours are arranged for individual children, the parents should be included and possibly the well siblings. Pre-hospital admission programmes should be scheduled for the time of day when staff members are most available and most treatment procedures are completed. No firm consensus exists on the timing of the event. Some authorities recommend preparing children four to seven years of age about one week in advance so they can assimilate the information and ask questions. For older children, the time may be longer. However, for young children, who may begin to fantasize about what they observed, one or two days before admission is sufficient time for anticipatory preparation (Petrillo and Sanger, 1980). Other research has found that children of age five to 12 years prefer to know about impending hospitalization from several weeks to a few minutes before the event, suggesting that the optimum approach is one that is individualized for each child (Ross and Ross, 1984). The length of the session should be suited to the children's attention span — the younger the child, the shorter the programme.

SETTING OF THE TOUR

The setting of the tour should avoid any frightening aspects of the hospital environment and should typically include an inpatient room, the playroom, the parents' waiting room, the nurses' station, and any other areas deemed appropriate (e.g., dining room). Children who are undergoing serious surgery requiring special postoperative care may be taken to visit the intensive care unit. Children scheduled for special tests, such as cardiac catheterization or cystoscopy, are sometimes shown these areas. Young children may respond better to shorter tours that concentrate on the areas of most concern, such as the paediatric unit, playroom, and recovery room. In any case, throughout the tour, the nurse (or other guide) must be alert to signs of concern or fear in the children. Strange noises, sights, sounds, and smells that are routine to hospital personnel can be frightening to children.

PREPARATORY MATERIALS

The most suitable type of presentation for children includes a variety of preparatory materials, including films, lecture, demonstration, and play, depending on the developmental level. For example, a puppet show may re-enact the basic steps of hospitalization — admission procedures; preparation for and recovery from surgical treatment. The main focus of each scene is the use of concrete actions and models to familiarize the family members with what will occur. The puppets talk about children's common fears — pain, anaesthesia, and parent separation. The *intent* of what is conveyed greatly surpasses the sophistication of the materials used.

OPPORTUNITY FOR DISCUSSION

Any type of preparatory programme needs to provide ample opportunity for discussion both before and after the tour. During the tour, family members are encouraged to ask questions and to familiarize themselves with the environment by sitting on a bed, riding in a wheelchair, or handling the equipment in the special rooms. Ideally, the tour should also be an opportunity for meeting the appropriate nursing staff. The nursing staff should be introduced to the children by name. Introducing them to one specific nurse, such as the sister or charge nurse, or clinical specialist, helps them feel more comfortable in knowing who is available for questions or concerns during the hospital stay.

PRE-HOSPITAL COUNSELLING BY PARENTS

In many situations the preparation of children for hospitalization is left up to parents. Parents may abdicate this responsibility for a variety of reasons. For example, they sometimes think the child is too young to understand or is better off not knowing beforehand; often, they are unable to prepare the child because of their own lack of knowledge and understanding.

Professionals can help parents prepare their children by adequately informing them of the specific details of hospitalization and related procedures, through both direct discussion and written material. Many hospitals develop their own pamphlets, books and photograph albums for this purpose. Nurses

working with these parents should also assess their level of anxiety regarding the impending hospitalization, to prevent emotional contagion to the child.

HOSPITAL ADMISSION

The preparation that children require on the day of admission depends on their pre-hospital counselling. If they have been prepared in a formalized programme, they will usually know what to expect in terms of initial medical procedures, inpatient facilities, and nursing staff. However, pre-hospital counselling does not preclude the need for support during procedures such as drawing blood, x-ray tests, or physical examination. For example, undressing young children before they feel comfortable in their new surroundings, can be very upsetting. Causing needless anxiety and fear during admission may adversely affect the nurse's establishment of trust with these children. Therefore, nursing assistance during the admission procedure is vital, regardless of how well prepared any child is for the hospitalization. In addition, spending this time with the child gives the nurse an opportunity to evaluate understanding of subsequent procedures, such as surgery (Fig. 5-5). Admission procedures for children are outlined in Box 5-9.

NURSING ADMISSION HISTORY

The nursing admission history refers to a systematic collection of data about the child and family that allows the nurse to plan individualized care. One of the main purposes of the history is to assess the child's usual health habits at home, in order to promote a more normal environment in the hospital. Therefore, questions related to activities of daily living are a major part of the assessment. Adaptations of the Roper, Logan and Tierney model are commonly seen in paediatric units (Aggleton, Chalmers, 1986; Newton, 1991).

Once the data are collected, they must be applied to the nursing process and communicated to other staff. It makes little sense to assess a child's home routine if none of this knowledge is integrated into the plan of care. Most nursing units have provisions for care plans in which specific information about the child's habits and needs are recorded.

PHYSICAL ASSESSMENT

The nurse and paediatrician should cooperate during the physical examination the child undergoes on admission to hospital, in order to avoid duplication of procedures. For example, when the nurse is present to support the child psychologically, the opportunity can also be used to observe the child's body for any bruises, rash, signs of neglect, deformities, or physical limitations.

PLACING THE CHILD

The minimum considerations for room assignment are age, gender, and nature of the illness. Ideally, however, room selection should be based on a variety of developmental and psy-

---

◆ **BOX 5-9**

Guidelines for admission

Preadmission

Guidelines for Emergency Admission

Assign a room based on developmental age, seriousness of diagnosis, communicability of illness, and projected length of stay.

Prepare room-mate(s) for the arrival of a new patient; when children are too young to benefit from this consideration, prepare parents.

Prepare room for child and family, with admission forms and equipment nearby to eliminate need to leave child.

Admission

Introduce named nurse to child and family.

Orient child and family to inpatient facilities, especially to assigned room and unit; emphasize positive areas of paediatric unit.

Room: explain call light, bed controls, television, etc.; direct to bathroom, telephone, etc.

Unit: Direct to playroom, desk, dining area, or other areas

Introduce family to room-mate and his or her parents.

Apply identification band to child's wrist, ankle, or both (if not done).

Explain hospital regulations and schedules (e.g., visiting hours, mealtimes, bedtime, limitations [give written information if available]).

Perform nursing admission history.

Take vital signs, blood pressure, height, and weight.

Obtain specimens as needed and order needed laboratory work.

Support child and perform or assist practitioner with physical examination (for purposes of nursing assessment).

Lengthy preparatory admission procedures are often impossible and inappropriate for emergency situations.

Unless an emergency is life-threatening, children need to participate in their care to maintain a sense of control.

Focus on essential components of admission counselling, including:

Appropriate introduction to the family

Use of child's name, not terms such as 'love' or 'dear'

Determination of child's age and some judgement about developmental age (if the child is of school age, asking about the grade level will offer some evidence for concurrent intellectual ability)

Information about child's general state of health, any problems that may interfere with medical treatment (e.g. sensitivity to medication), and previous experience with hospital facilities

Information about the chief complaint from both the parents and the child

Guidelines for Admission to Intensive Care Unit

Prepare child and parents for elective ICU admission, such as for postoperative care after cardiac surgery.

Prepare child and parents for unanticipated ICU admission by focusing primarily on the sensory aspects of the experience and on usual family concerns (e.g., persons in charge of child's care, schedule for visiting, area where family can wait).

Prepare parents regarding child's appearance and behaviour when they first visit child in ICU.

Accompany family to bedside to provide emotional support and answer questions.

Prepare siblings for their visit; plan length of time for sibling visitation; monitor siblings' reactions during visit to prevent them from becoming overwhelmed.

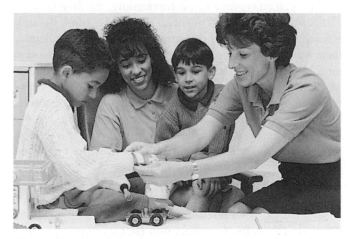

Fig. 5-5 The initial admission procedures allow the nurse to begin knowing the child and assessing his or her understanding of the hospital experience (Courtesy of Southampton University Hospitals Trust).

chobiological needs. Determining compatible room-mates, both for the children and for rooming-in parents, greatly influences the growth potential from the hospital experience.

NURSING CARE DURING SPECIAL HOSPITAL SITUATIONS

In addition to a general paediatric unit, children may be admitted to special facilities, such as a day hospital, an adolescent unit, an isolation room, or an intensive care unit. Some admissions are unexpected and frequently constitute medical emergencies. Such situations require special preparation of the child and family and nursing care interventions based on an awareness of the child's needs and the unique stressors associated with these hospital facilities.

DAY HOSPITAL

The concept of a day hospital is to provide needed medical services for the child while eliminating the necessity of overnight admission. Among the benefits of a day hospital are: (1) minimization of the stressors of hospitalization, especially separation from the family; (2) reduced chance of infection; and (3) economic saving. Admission to the day hospital usually is for surgical or diagnostic procedures, such as insertion of tympanostomy tubes, hernia repair, adenoidectomy, tonsillectomy, cystoscopy, or bronchoscopy.

Because of the limited contact with the child, nursing admission procedures are extremely important. Ideally, each child and family should receive pre-admission counselling, including a tour of the facility and a review of the expected day's procedures. However, when this is not possible, surgery should be scheduled to allow some time for children to become acquainted with their surroundings and for nurses to assess, plan, and complement appropriate teaching.

Discharge instructions must also be explicit (Thornes, 1991).

ADOLESCENT UNIT

In recent years, there has been increased awareness of children's needs based on developmental considerations. To meet the unique needs of adolescents, special units have been developed that provide privacy, increased socialization, and appropriate activities for these young people (Kuykendall and Dunne, 1981). These units provide more flexible routines and activities, such as more group activity, wearing of street clothes, provisions to leave the adolescent unit temporarily, and access to the items so critical to teenagers — telephones; record, compact disc and tape players; video recorders and televisions. Because adolescents' food habits are rarely limited to the three traditional meals a day, a ready supply of snacks should be available. However, the most important benefit of these units is increased socialization with peers. In addition, staff members usually enjoy working with this age group and are well suited to establishing the trust so essential for communication.

ISOLATION

Admission to an isolation room increases the stressors typically associated with hospitalization. There is further separation from familiar persons, additional loss of control, and added environmental changes, such as sensory deprivation and the strange appearance of visitors. These stressors are compounded by children's limited understanding of isolation. Preschool children have difficulty understanding the rationale for isolation because they cannot comprehend the cause-and-effect relationship between germs and illness. They are likely to view isolation as punishment. Older children understand the causality better, but still require information to decrease fantasizing or misinterpretation. When a child is placed in isolation, preparation is essential for the child to feel in control.

All children, but especially younger ones, need preparation in terms of what they will see, hear, or feel in isolation. Therefore, they should be shown the mask, gloves, and gown, and should be encouraged to 'dress up' in them. Playing with the strange apparel lessens the fear of seeing 'ghost-like' people walk into the room. Before entering the room, nurses and other health personnel should introduce themselves and let the child see their face before donning a mask. In this way, the child associates them with significant experiences and gains a sense of familiarity in an otherwise strange and lonely environment.

When the child's condition improves, appropriate play activities should be provided to minimize boredom. Rather than dwelling on the negative aspects of isolation, the child can be encouraged to view this experience as challenging and positive. For example, the nurse can help the child look at isolation as a method of keeping others out and letting only special people in. Children often think of intriguing signs for their doors, such as 'Enter at your own risk' or 'Many have entered but few have left.' These poster-like signs also encourage people 'on the outside' to talk with the child about the ominous greetings.

EMERGENCY ADMISSION

One of the most traumatic hospital experiences for the child and parents is an emergency admission. The sudden onset of an illness or the occurrence of an injury leaves little time for preparation and explanation. Sometimes the emergency admission is compounded by admission to an intensive care unit or the need for immediate surgery. However, even in those instances requiring outpatient treatment, the child is exposed to a strange, frightening environment and to people who often inflict pain. Thus, every medical emergency requires psychological intervention to reduce the fear and anxiety frequently associated with the experience.

Lengthy preparatory admission procedures are often inappropriate for emergency situations. In such instances, nurses must focus their nursing interventions on the essential components of admission counselling (see Box 5-9) and complete the process as soon as the child's condition is stabilized.

Unless an emergency is life-threatening, children need to participate in their care to maintain a sense of control. Because accident and emergency departments are frequently hectic, there is a tendency to rush through procedures in order to save time. However, the extra few minutes needed to allow children to participate may save many more minutes of useless resistance and uncooperativeness during subsequent procedures. Other supportive measures include ensuring privacy, accepting various emotional responses to fear or pain, preserving parent-child contact, explaining all events before or as they occur and personally remaining calm.

INTENSIVE CARE UNIT

Admission to an intensive care unit (ICU) can be a particularly traumatic event for both the child and the parents. The nature and severity of the illness, and the circumstances surrounding the admission, are major factors, especially for parents. Parents experience significantly more stress when the admission is unexpected rather than expected. Stressors for the child and family are described in Box 5-10.

The family's emotional needs are very important when a child is admitted to an ICU. The same interventions that were discussed earlier for the stressors of separation, loss of control, and bodily injury and pain, also apply here.

When an ICU admission is expected, such as for postoperative care after cardiac surgery, the child and parents should be prepared for the event. Some units advocate a tour, whereas others use picture books of the unit to familiarize the family with the environment and usual equipment. As much reassurance as possible should accompany the introduction of stressful information.

When parents first visit the child in the ICU, they need preparation for how the child will look and what the child is experiencing, if awake. Ideally, the nurse should provide them with emotional support and answer any questions. If siblings visit, they need the same preparation as parents. Whether they should visit soon after the child is admitted or after the child's condition has stabilized, is controversial. The length of time for sibling visitation should be planned ahead and monitored during the visit to prevent the well child from becoming overwhelmed.

Children admitted to the ICU need their parents' comfort and security, and parents are encouraged to stay with their child. If visiting hours are limited, the schedule should be flexible to accommodate parental needs. With liberalization of visiting hours, many parents think they must stay; nurses need to be sensitive to their needs, suggesting periodic respites from the tense, stressful ICU environment.

Since altered parental roles are a major stress for parents, nurses need to implement interventions to minimize this concern, such as: (1) educating and preparing parents for the expected role changes; (2) identifying ways in which parents can continue to fulfil parenting functions, such as helping with the bath or feeding, touching and talking to the child; and (3) determining new roles, such as helping with procedures. Information sharing can increase parents' sense of control and responsibility, but facts must be conveyed simply, repeated often, and monitored to prevent overwhelming family members. Since medical jargon abounds in a complex environment such as the ICU, unfamiliar terms need to be clarified and simpler terms substituted.

As in emergency admissions, there is a tendency in the ICU to perform procedures quickly and without attention to the child's preparational needs. Therefore, nurses need to remember the special concerns of children in each age group about bodily injury. Explaining each procedure, altering it, whenever possible, to decrease the child's fears, and supporting the child are essential. Giving children an object that symbolizes their courage, such as a 'hero badge' or an 'ICU diploma', helps them face their fears and anxiety. It is a positive memento of an otherwise stressful experience. Because of the numerous procedures performed on the child and the nature of the illness, pain management needs to receive a high priority.

Of particular importance in decreasing fear is ensuring that discussions that do not directly include the family are held where the child and family cannot overhear them. Casual conversation can often be overheard and taken out of context.

Extensive monitoring makes a usual day - night cycle difficult in an ICU. However, some schedule should be established that maintains a similarity to daily events in the child's life. This includes organizing care during normal waking hours, keeping regular bedtime schedules, including quiet times when televisions and radios are lowered or turned off, closing and opening curtains as appropriate, dimming lights, placing a curtain around the bed for privacy and decreased stimulation, and having clocks or calendars in easy view for older children. In particular, staff members must realize the need for quiet and refrain from loud talking or laughing. Equipment noise should be kept to a minimum by turning alarms as low as safely possible, performing treatments requiring equipment at one time, turning off bedside equipment not in use (e.g., suction, oxygen), and avoiding loud, abrupt noises (e.g., clattering

---

◆ **BOX 5-10**

Neonatal/paediatric ICU stressors for the child and family

Physical Stressors

Pain and discomfort (e.g., injections, intubation, suctioning, dressing changes, other invasive procedures)

Immobility (e.g., use of restraints, bed rest)

Sleep deprivation

Inability to eat or drink

Changes in elimination habits

Environmental Stressors

Unfamiliar surroundings (e.g., crowding)

Unfamiliar sounds

  Equipment noise (e.g., monitors, telephone, suctioning, computer printout)

  Human sounds (e.g., talking, laughing, crying, coughing, moaning, retching, walking)

Unfamiliar people (e.g., health care professionals, patients, visitors)

Unfamiliar and unpleasant smells (e.g., alcohol, adhesive remover, body odours)

Constant lights

Activity related to other patients

Sense of urgency among staff

Psychological Stressors

Lack of privacy

Inability to communicate (if intubated)

Inadequate knowledge and understanding of situation

Severity of illness

Parental behaviour (expression of concern)

Social Stressors

Disrupted relationships (especially with family and friends)

Concern with missing school/work

Play deprivation

Data primarily from Tichy AM *et al.*

bedpans, toilet flushing). Such measures can reduce the sensory overload and the sleep deprivation commonly associated with ICU admissions.

Despite the stresses normally associated with ICU admission, a special security develops from being carefully monitored and receiving individualized care. Therefore, planning for transition to the regular unit is essential and should include: (1) assignment of a named nurse on the regular unit who visits before the transfer, (2) continued visits by the ICU staff to assess the child's and parents' adjustment and to act as a temporary liaison with the nursing staff, (3) explanation of the differences between the two units and the rationale for the change to less intense monitoring of the child's physical condition, and (4) selection of an appropriate room, such as one close to the nursing station, and a compatible room-mate.

DISCHARGE PLANNING AND HOME CARE

Most hospitalizations necessitate some type of discharge planning. Often this involves education of the family for continued care and follow-up in the home. Depending on the diagnosis, this may be relatively simple or considerably complex. With the current concern for cost containment and recognition of children's emotional needs, home care for children with technologically complex care, such as youngsters on ventilators, has become increasingly common. Preparing the family for home care demands a high degree of competence in planning and implementing discharge instruction.

ASSESSMENT

Discharge planning for home care must begin with an assessment of the family's desire and capability in assuming care responsibilities. For a discussion of family and home assessment strategies, Chapter 9. In addition to adequate family resources, an investigation of community services, including respite care, is needed to ensure that appropriate support agencies are available. To coordinate the immense task of assessment and to plan implementation, a case coordinator should be appointed early in the discharge programme.

PLANNING

Ideally, preparation for hospital discharge and home care begins during the admission assessment with the establishment of short- and long-term goals for both child and family. For children who require complex care, discharge planning focuses on those skills that parents or children are expected to continue at home.

All families should receive detailed *written* instructions about home care before they leave the hospital, as well as telephone numbers for assistance.

TRANSITIONAL CARE

Once the family is competent in performing the skill, they should be given responsibility for the care. Whenever possible, the family should have a transition or trial period to assume care with minimum supervision. This may be arranged on the unit or during a home visit. Some programmes incorporate a hospital trial into their discharge criteria, necessitating that the family successfully manage this phase before discharge to home.

EVALUATION AND CONTINUING SUPPORT

Evaluation is a critical part of any discharge plan and assumes even more importance in home care of children with complex needs. Factors to consider in home care programmes include the need for subsequent hospitalization, the child's developmental and physical progress, effects of home care on the family, actual vs. expected use of resources by the family and home care team, financial costs and savings, and improved survival.

In most instances, parents need only simple instructions and understanding of follow-up care. However, the often overwhelming care assumed by some families necessitates continued professional support after discharge.

KEY POINTS

◆ Children are particularly vulnerable to the stresses of illness and hospitalization, because stress represents a change from the usual state of health and routine, and because they possess limited coping mechanisms.

◆ Feelings of loss of control are caused by unfamiliar environmental stimuli, physical restriction, altered routine, and dependency.

◆ The three phases of separation anxiety are protest, despair, and detachment.

◆ Fear of bodily pain may be manifested in the following ways: infants – expressions, body movements; toddlers – intense emotional upset, physical resistance; preschooler – aggression, verbal expression, dependency; school-aged children – precise verbalisation of pain, passive requests for support or help, procrastination technique; adolescents – self-control, irritability, limited movement.

◆ Because of their separation from significant people, hospitalized children may lack the opportunity to form new attachments in the strange environment and may exhibit negative behaviours after discharge.

◆ Family reactions are influenced by the seriousness of illness, experience with illness or hospitalization, diagnostic or therapeutic procedures, available support systems, personal ego strengths, coping abilities, additional stresses, cultural and religious beliefs, and family communication patterns.

◆ The following increase the negative effects of a brother's or sister's illness/hospitalization on siblings: fear of contracting illness, their young age, a close relationship with the ill sibling, substitute child-care, minium explanation of the illness, and perceived changes in patenting.

◆ Nursing care of the hospitalization child and family is aimed at preventing or minimizing separation, decreasing loss of control, minimizing bodily injury and pain, using play to lessen stress, maximizing potential benefits of hospitalization, and supporting family members.

◆ Pain assessment includes questioning the child, using pain rating scales, evaluating behaviour and physiological changes, securing parents' involvement, taking the cause of pain into account, and taking action.

◆ Pain management should incorporate both pharmacological and nonpharmacological methods. Pharmacological methods focus on four rights: right drug, right dose, right route, and right time.

◆ The nurse can maximize potential benefits of hospitalization by fostering parent–child relations, providing educational opportunities, promoting self-mastery, and encouraging socialization.

◆ Supporting family members involves listening to parents' verbal and nonverbal messages; providing clergy support; accepting cultural, socioeconomic, and ethnic values; and giving information to families and siblings.

◆ The major goals of pre-hospital preparation are to make the hospital less strange and frightening to parents and children and to establish a positive atmosphere and trusting relationship with a positive atmosphere and trusting relationship with staff and family members.

◆ In preparing families for hospitalization, the nurse should consider small group size and timing of the events, setting of the tour, inclusion of preparatory materials, time for discussion, and pre-hospital counselling for parents.

◆ Emergency admission or admission to a day hospital, isolation room, or intensive care unit requires additional intervention strategies to meet the child's and family's needs.

REFERENCES

Abu-Saad H: Cultural group indicators of pain in children, *Matern Child Nurs J* 13(3):187, 1984.

Adams J, Gill S, McDonald M: Reducing fear in hospital, *Nurs Times* 86(51):62, 1991.

Aggleton P, Chalmers H: *Nursing models and the nursing process*, London, 1986, Macmillan.

Aho AC, Erickson MT: Effects of grade, gender, and hospitalization on children's medical fears, *Dev Behav Pediatr* 6(3):146, 1985.

Anand KJS, Hickey PR: Pain in the fetus and neonate, *N Eng J Med* 317:1321, 1987.

Baker C, Wong D: QUEST: a process of pain assessment in children, *Orthopaed Nurs* 6(1):11, 1987.

Beyer JE, *The Oucher: a user's manual and technical report*, Denver, CO, 1989, University of Colorado.

Beyer JE, Denyes MJ, Villarruel AM: The creation, validation and continuing development of the Oucher: a measure of pain intensity in children, *J Pediatr Nurs* 7(5):335346, 1992.

Bibace R, Walsh ME: Development of children's concepts of illness, *Pediatr* 66(6):912, 1980.

Broome ME, Endsley RC: Group preparation of young children for painful stimulas, *Western J Nurs Res* 9(4):484, 1987.

Clatworthy S: Therapeutic play: effects on hospitalized children, *Child Health Care* 9(4):108, 1981.

Craig K *et al.*: Developmental changes in infant pain expression during immunization injections, *SSoc SSci Med* 19(12):1331, 1984.

Eland JM: Children with pain. In Jackson OB, Saunders RB: *Child Health Nursing, Philadelphia*, 1993, JB Lippincott.

Favaloro R, Touzel B: A comparison of adolescents' and nurses' post-operative pain ratings and perceptions, *Pediatr Nurs* 16(4):414, 424, 1990.

Hurley A, Whelan EG: Cognitive development and children's perception of pain, *Pediatr Nurs* 14(1):21, 1988.

Jordran-Marsh M *et al*: Alternate Oucher form testing gender ethnicity and age variations, *Res Nurs Health* 17:111-118, 1994.

Kanneh A: The need to communicate, *Nurs Standard* 5(5):19, 1990.

Katz E. Kellerman J, Siegal S: Behavioural distress in children with cancer undergoing medical procedures: developmental considerations, *J Consult Clin Psychol* 48(3): 356, 1980.

Kuykendall JW, Dunne M: An adolescent ward, *Nursing* (second series) 24:1040, 1981.

LaMontagne LL: Children's locus of control beliefs as predictors of preoperative coping behavior, *Nurs. Res.* 33(2):76-79, 1984.

McCaffery M, Beebe A: *Pain: clinical manual for nursing practice,* St Louis, 1989, Mosby–Year Book.

Newton C: *The Roper-Logan-Tierney model in action,* London, 1991, Macmillan.

Nix K, Clutter L, Wong DL.: *The influence of the type of instructions in measuring pain intensity in young children using the FACES Pain Rating Scale,* Unpublished manuscript, 1994.

Norris L: Coaching the question, *Nurs* 16(5): 100,1986.

Orem D: *Nursing: concepts of practice,* ed 3, New York, 1985, McGraw-Hill.

Oucher (can't find it)

Perrin EC, Gerrity PS: There's a demon in your belly: children's understanding of illness, *Pediatr* 67(6):841, 1981.

Petrillo M, Sanger S: *Emotional care of hospitalized children,* ed 2, Philadelphia, 1980, JB Lippincott.

Price S: Preparing children for admission to hospital, *Nurs Times* 87(9):46, 1991.

Richardson J: Acute pain in childhood, *Surg Nurs* **vol(issue)**:22, 1992.

Robertson J: *Young children in Hospitals<* London, 1979, Tavistock Publications.

Ross DM, Ross SA: Childhood pain: the school-age child's viewpoint, *Pain* 20(2):179, 1984.

Sparshott M: Pain and the special care baby unit, *Nurs Times* 85(41):61, 1989.

Shapiro C: Pain in the neoate: assessment and intervention, *Neonatal Network* 8(1):7–21, 1989.

Sherman M *et al.* Treasured objects in school-aged children, *Pediatrics* 68(3):379, 1981.

Stewart A: Prepared for parting, *Nurs Mirror* November 7:15, 1984.

Tesler MD *et al.*: Children's words for pain. In Funk SG *et al.*, editors: *Key aspects of comfort: management of pain, fatigue, and nausea,* New York, 1989, Springer Publishing.

Tesler M *et al*: The word-graphic rating scale as a measure of children's and adolescents' pain intensity, *Res Nurs Health* 14:361-371, 1991.

Thornes R: *Caring for children in the health services: just for the day,* London, 1991, NAWCH.

Tichy AM *et al.*: Stressors in paediatric intensive care units, *Pediatr Nurs* 14(1):40, 1988.

Villarruel AM, Denyes MJ: Pain assessment in children: theorectical and empirical validity, *Adv Nurs* Sci 14(2):32-41, 1991.

Walco GA, Illowite NT: Vertical vs horizontal visual analog scale of pain intensity in children, *J Pain Symptom Manage* 6(3):200, 1991.

Wallace M: Temperament: a variable in children's pain management, *Pediatr Nurs* 15(2):118, 1989.

Wong D, Baker C: Pain in children: comparison of assessment scales, *Pediatr Nurs* 14(1):9, 1988.

Wright LM, Leahey M: *Families and chronic illness,* Philadephia, 1984, FA Davis.

Zeltzer LK, Jay SM, Fisher DM: The management of pain associated with paediatric procedures, *Pediatr Clin North Am* 36(4):941, 1989.

FURTHER READING

Childhood Hospital Admission

Department of Health: *Welfare of children and young people in hospital,* London, 1991, HMSO.

Department of Health and Social Security: *The welfare of children in hospital: Platt report,* London, 1958, HMSO.

Eiser C, Hanson L: Preparing children for hospital: a school-based intervention, *Prof Nurs* 5(3):29719.

Hawthorn P: *Nurse—I want my mummy!* The Study of Nursing Care Project Reports, Series 1, No 3, London, 1974, RCN.

Hedgethorn E: Enforced separation, *Nurs Mirror* November 7:18, 1984.

Hopkins J: Hospitalization: the psychotherapist's view, *Nurs Times* October 19:42, 1983.

Jolley J: Timmy goes to hospital, *Nurs Times* March 27:27, 1985.

Jolley J: The child's adaptation to hospital admission, *Nurs* 34:40, 1989.

Jolley J: *The other side of paediatrics,* London, 1981, Macmillan.

Kiely T: Preparing children for admission to hospital, *Nurs* 33:42, 1989.

MacCallum IJ: A child in hospital: the needs of the parents, *Nurs Series 3,* 20:594, 1983.

Muller DJ *et al.*: *Nursing children: psychology, research and practice,* London, 1992, Chapman & Hall.

National Association for the Welfare of Children in Hospital (now Action for Sick Children): *NAWCH Charter for Children in Hospital,* London, 1984, NAWCH.

Royal College of Nursing: *Paediatric nursing—a philosophy of care,* RCN Issues in Nursing Health 10, London, 1992, RCN.

Robbins M: Sharing the care, *Nurs Times* 87(8):36, 1991.

Rodin J: *Will this hurt? Preparing children for hospital and medical procedures,* London, 1983, RCN.

Rutter M: *Maternal deprivation reassessed,* ed 2, Harmondsworth, 1981, Penguin.

Swanwick M: Play as a coping mechanism, *Nursing* Series 3, (39):1154, 1985.

Webb J, Cleaver K: The child in casualty, *Nurs Times* 87(15):27, 1991.

Pain Assessment and Relief

Beyer JE, Wells N: The assessment of pain in children, *Ped Clin N Am* (6):837, 1989.

Gurono MA, Reisinger CL: Patient controlled analgesia for the young paediatric patient, *Paed Nurs* 17(3):251, 1991.

SELECTED BOOKS FOR CHILDREN

Althea: *Going into hospital,* London, 1986, HarperCollins.

Althea: *I go to hospital,* London, 1977, Brightstar Books, Souvenir Press.

Chapter 6

Emergency Care of the Young Person

LEARNING OUTCOMES

After studying this chapter you should be able to:

◆ Identify major landmarks in the historical development of children's nursing.
◆ Describe the reasons why children attend Accident and Emergency departments.
◆ Discuss the need for a specialized environment for care.
◆ Identify the nature and causes of accidents in childhood.
◆ Discuss the care of the bereaved family.
◆ Describe the priorities of care for the acutely ill child.
◆ Discuss the altered physiological processes that may be involved
◆ Discuss alternative methods of managing the emergency care of the sick child, such as telephone triage.
◆ Identify and discuss the importance of the role of the emergency paediatric nurse practitioner.
◆ Define the glossary terms.

GLOSSARY

A&E Accident and emergency

Anaphylaxis An unusual or exaggerated allergic response of an organism to foreign protein or other substance

Apnoea Temporary cessation of breathing

Birth asphyxia Inability to breathe at birth

Cyanosis Bluish discolouration of the skin and mucous membranes

Birth asphyxia Inability to breathe at birth

Hypoxia Deminished availability of oxygen to the tissues

Ischaemia Deficiency of blood in a part due to functional constriction or actual obstruction of a blood vessel

NAI Non accidental injury

RSCN Registered sick children's nurse

RTA Road traffic accident

SIDS Sudden infant death syndrome

Triage Assessment of the patient's priority needs for care

Trauma Injury or emotional shock

CARE OF THE CHILD AND FAMILY IN THE ACCIDENT AND EMERGENCY DEPARTMENT

Every year, approximately one in four children under the age of 16 will attend an accident and emergency (A&E) department in the United Kingdom. This comprises between 20-30% of all cases admitted to the A&E department. Many of these children will be less than five years of age; a high proportion of them will be under the age of two years.

Injured children account for the majority of child attendees in A&E. Most have relatively minor injuries, but a few sustain major injuries. Accidents are the most common cause of death in children over one year old in the United Kingdom and cause 700 child deaths annually. A further 10,000 children per year sustain injuries leading to a permanent disability. At least 20% of all children's admissions to hospital are as the result of accidents.

Fifteen to twenty per cent of A&E attendees will have medical problems. These will range from children who are seriously ill and in need of urgent treatment, to those whose injury or illness might easily be managed by the primary health care team. In the latter group are also those children whose parents either want a 'second opinion', are worried that their child is acutely unwell, or are not registered with a general practitioner (GP). Most medical problems will be found in children under the age of five, with those under-two predominating.

A lesser proportion of child accident and emergency cases will present with non-traumatic injuries or surgical conditions, such as appendicitis, phimosis, hernia or torsion. A smaller percentage of children, particularly adolescents, attend with symptoms related to alcohol, drug or solvent abuse, or following attempts at deliberate self-poisoning or self-harm. Non-accidental injuries or incidents of abuse may be found throughout the whole spectrum of child A&E attendees (Box 6-1).

◆ **BOX 6-1**

Categories of attenders

TRAUMA – injured children account for 60-70% of all attenders.

MEDICAL – 15-20% will have medical problems ranging from the seriously ill to the less acute.

SURGICAL – a small percentage will attend with non-traumatic injuries or conditions requiring surgical intervention.

BEHAVIOURAL/PSYCHIATRIC – A lesser number of children, particularly adolescents, will attend with symptoms of some form of substance abuse or self-harm attempts.

NON-ACCIDENTAL INJURY OR ABUSE – May be found throughout the whole spectrum of attenders.

The A&E department is not merely the provider of emergency care for the sick or injured child — it is also the dynamic interface between primary and secondary care providers, and may actually serve as a source of primary health care for some vulnerable groups, such as travelling families, homeless families, and those living in temporary accommodation. The ever changing face of contemporary health care provision dictates that the traditional divisions that have existed between these two sources are no longer an appropriate basis for planning current and future health care provision for children and their families (Thornes, 1993).

The function of the A&E as the interface between primary and secondary, or specialist, care is vitally important. The report *Bridging the Gaps* (Thornes, 1993) stresses the need for prompt and effective communication between all providers, but especially between care providers and families.

THE ENVIRONMENT FOR CARE

Most children will be treated in the A&E of a district general hospital, as there are very few dedicated paediatric casualty departments. As approximately one-third of all patients seen in A&E departments are children, there needs to be special provision for their care. Planning the environment for care can make all the difference to the child's successful treatment. There must be separate provision for the reception and treatment of sick and injured children and their families, with suitable decor and furniture, and appropriate equipment and resuscitation facilities. The first impressions of the department are important, and if the child is welcomed in to an area that has been decorated with pictures and toys that are familiar and contemporary, fears may be allayed and successful communication and treatment enhanced.

There must be nappy changing facilities, room for push chairs, and consideration of family-centred care. Distressed parents should have the use of a private room with access to a telephone. Trolleys and furniture should be child-size, both for safety and for reassurance. It is essential that plenty of toys and books are available for entertainment, distraction and preparation for procedures.

APPROACHES TO CARE

In addition to a suitable environment for care, experienced and qualified medical and nursing staff are vital. The minimum requirement is at least one RSCN or RN (child) in every department (DoH, 1991a). Their remit should be to raise awareness of the unique needs of the child, to set standards for care, to educate staff and parents, and to be actively involved in research and health promotion (Box 6-2).

THERAPEUTIC PLAY

The accident and emergency department may be the child's first contact with hospitals and health care workers. The potentially negative effects of hospitalization may be ameliorated by

---

♦ **BOX 6-2**

Minimum requirements for children in A&E

- Separate waiting area with play facilities
- Separate treatment area, suitably decorated and equipped
- Private room for distressed parents
- At least one RSCN trained nurse on staff
- A consultant paediatrician to have responsibility for liaison with the consultant in A & E medicine concerning general arrangements for children
- A liaison health visitor to facilitate communication between the department and the community

Reproduced from Morton and Phillips (1992) and supported by the joint statement on children's A & E attendances produced in 1988 by the BPA, BAPS and CSA.

♦ **BOX 6-3**

The effects of hospitalization

- Regression to an earlier developmental stage
- Depression and restlessness
- Appetite disturbances
- Sleep disturbances
- Urinary and faecal incontinence
- Bed-wetting
- Hypochondria

From Chambers M (1993)

---

the skilful use of therapeutic play (Box 6-3). Therapeutic play can decrease anxiety and distress, and is essential for emotional care (Chambers, 1993). Children naturally use play as part of their normal growth and development, and for self expression and communication. In preparing children for medical procedures, directed play, such as performing a technique on a doll or puppet, will familiarize the child with the procedure and lessen anxiety caused by fear of the unknown. Body outline or calico dolls may be useful for this purpose.

CHILDREN AND THEIR ACCIDENTS

Minor accidents in childhood are a normal part of the maturation process, but many of the more serious accidents have a known cause, and can therefore be prevented. The age, gender, developmental level and socioeconomic circumstances of the individual may determine the likelihood of an accident being encountered. At all ages, and for most types of accidents, boys are more likely to have accidents than girls; a fact proven by virtually all studies (Mead, Sibert, 1991). The only exception to this is during the first year of life. More boys than girls are involved in fatal road traffic accidents (RTAs), have more accident-related hospital admissions, and more boys visit A&E for this reason (Avery and Jackson 1993). Accidents are the most common cause of death among toddlers and older children, and attendance at A&E following accidents increases with age. In the infant and toddler age group, the majority of accidents occur in the home; a smaller proportion occur on the road and during sports and leisure activities. As the child becomes older, the focus of accidents shifts from the home to sports and leisure activities, including organized sports and gymnastics at school (Box 6-4).

Social class is the single most relevant factor in childhood accidents, with variations between social class being greater in childhood accidents than for any other 'disease' or for any other age group (Avery and Jackson, 1993). Children in social class 5 are five times more likely to be killed in accidents than children of social class 1. These differences are further emphasized in certain classes of accidents, where socially deprived children are at increased risk. The only type of accident to be equally distributed throughout the social classes is poisoning.

NON-ACCIDENTAL INJURY AND ABUSE

All staff working with children need to be alert to indicators of child abuse. Staff in A&E have a significant role in identifying the child whose injuries may have been non-accidental or who may have been subject to other forms of abuse. Recognizing the abused child is not always easy and in a busy A&E department it is essential that local child protection policies and procedures are strictly observed (RCN, 1994). Non-accidental injuries (NAIs) should be managed in the community under the guidance of the community paediatrician, and in partnership with the family, but with the child's interests as

---

♦ **BOX 6-4**

Children and their accidents: key facts

Nearly one half of all deaths in children between ages of 10-15 years are due to accidents

Three children die every day as the result of an accident.

120,00 children are admitted to hospital every year after an accident.

Every year, one in five children requires hospital every year or GP treatment for accident-related injury.

More than one half of the fatal accidents to infants and young children under five years happen in the home.

The child pedestrian death rate in the UK is one of the highest in Europe.

At all ages, and for most types of accidents, boys have a higher death rate than girls.

---

the focus of concern (The Children Act, 1989). Where suspected cases are referred to the A&E department, appointments should be made in advance so the child's and family's needs can be met without interfering with seriously ill patients and accident victims.

As the majority of children who have been abused are dealt with by the primary health care team, the average A&E department may now receive fewer suspected cases of abuse. The assessment skills and intuitive judgement of a dual-qualified children's and A&E nurse are paramount in identifying vulnerable children whose illness or injury raises concern.

THE POISONED CHILD

Accidental poisoning is the most common cause for presentation to the A&E and accounts for about 40,000 attendances per year in England and Wales (Morton and Phillips, 1992). Less than half of these cases need to be admitted for observation or treatment. Poisoning, unlike other types of childhood accidents, occurs with similar frequency across all social classes.

The inquisitive and oral nature of the most vulnerable age group (one- to three-year-olds), coupled with their apparent lack of discrimination to unpleasant tastes, may be a causative factor. Accidental poisoning usually occurs when the child is unsupervised. An increased incidence of poisoning is sometimes found in households where there are stressors such as a new baby, concomitant serious illness in a family member, or anxiety or depression in a parent.

Common substances that are accidentally ingested by children include drugs (prescribed and non-prescribed), household products and plants (Box 6-5). With the introduction of child-resistant containers, the number of admissions for poisonings related to analgesics has decreased (Box 6-6). Mead and Sibert (1991) provide a comprehensive picture of the aetiology of poisoning and a discussion of commonly ingested substances (Box 6-7).

Some children attending A&E, particularly adolescents, may have acute or chronic behavioural problems. They may present as having intentionally overdosed or self-harmed in some other way. Nurses must have a full understanding of the drugs and

---

◆ BOX 6-5

Commonly ingested substances

- Paracetamol and other analgesic drugs
- Anxiolytics
- Cough medicines
- Oral contraceptives
- Vitamins
- Bleaches
- Detergents
- Disinfectants
- Petroleum distillates

◆ BOX 6-6

Key points in poisoning

Many ingestions of non-toxic substances do not require gastric evacuation or admission.

Gastric evacuation using ipecacuanha is safe and effective in the conscious child.

Activated charcoal is indicated for certain poisons.

Gastric lavage is contraindicated for ingestion of household products or corrosive substances.

Advice should be sought from a Poisons Centre.

Children who have poisoned themselves intentionally or who have abused drugs or solvents, should be referred to Child and Adolescent Psychiatry.

Consider poisoning as the cause of obscure, serious symptoms such as coma.

Adapted from Morton and Phillips (1992)

◆ BOX 6-7

Substances of low toxicity when ingested

MEDICINES
Antibiotics
Antacids
Calamine
Oral contraceptives
Vitamins (without iron)
Zinc oxide creams

HOUSEHOLD PRODUCTS
Chalks and crayons
Emulsion and water paints
Fabric softeners
Plant foods and fertilizers
Silica gel
Toothpaste
Wallpaper paste

PLANTS
Begonia
Honeysuckle
Mahonia
Cacti
Cotoneaster
Rowan
Spider plant
Cyclamen
Sweet Pea

Reproduced from Mead and Sibert (1991)

substances that are prone to abuse by this age group; for example, alcohol, marijuana, cocaine, crack, ecstasy, heroin, and volatile agents such as lighter fluid and glues. A sympathetic and non-judgemental approach provides support at the time of crisis and may encourage the individual to seek further help.

THE SUDDEN DEATH OF A CHILD IN A&E

The death of a child is always a devastating event, but this is compounded when the death is sudden and unexpected. Care must extend beyond that needed for the child, to the emotional and psychosocial care of the parents and family. Such care should focus on providing empathy, support and practical advice. Bereavement care starts at the time of death and an appreciation of this will help family members begin to grieve. The emergency nurse will not have the opportunity to witness the resolution of the parents' and family's grief, and will have to cope with the raw emotions of shock, disbelief, anger, denial and sorrow that accompany the sudden death of a child. Compassion, sensitivity and sincere concern will do much for these parents and other family members when they begin the therapeutic road to managing their bereavement.

If resuscitation is attempted in the A&E, it is vital that one member of staff is delegated to stay with and support the parents. The parents should be offered the privacy of a room located near the resuscitation area. In some instances, parents may wish to be present during resuscitation attempts. Current research suggests that this may be beneficial in enabling the parents to come to terms with the event, regardless of the outcome. In this case, staff will need to offer support and explanation of what may be perceived as threatening and invasive treatment.

If the child is already dead when brought to the department, or if it becomes obvious that resuscitation efforts may fail, staff will need to give the family an honest and clear indication of what has happened or is likely to happen. There is a fine line between being honest and being blunt. Do not give false hope or use words that are designed to soften the blow, but which may not be understood by a frightened and anxious parent. The word 'dead' is a harsh word, but is more helpful if sensitively expressed, than euphemisms like 'passed away' or 'lost'. Consideration of cultural and religious needs must be met and appropriate resources mobilized to offer the grieving parents spiritual help and support. The emergency nurse should be aware of the differences in the normal grief responses of various cultural groups and should be prepared to facilitate expression of their feelings.

Experienced children's nurses often lack confidence about the skills they have to care for a bereaved parent. Empathy, listening skills, and reaching out in response to pain and distress, achieve more than words. Nurses should avoid the desire for a solution; the problem cannot be solved, but the presence of nursing support will be instrumental in helping the parents to cope. Following the initial reaching out, helping can begin to be more structured (Wright, 1986).

Before the parents see their child, emergency equipment should be cleared away, all invasive devices removed, and all signs of blood or body fluids dealt with. Wherever possible, the body should be taken to a private room away from the public, where the parents should be able to express their grief in privacy, but with skilled nursing support nearby.

Account should be taken of the parents' wishes in the observance of death (Department of Health, 1991a) and, when the parents have been able to come to terms with the death, they should be encouraged to see their child and to hold him or her. Viewing the child is important to grief resolution, but it is equally important that parents should not be forced to do this against their wishes. The parents may wish to be involved in washing the child and choosing clothes for the child to be dressed in. A lock of hair or a photograph may be taken, or in the case of an infant, hand and foot prints. Even if the parents do not wish this at the time, such things should be securely stored with the patient's notes in case the parents request them later

Parents should be allowed to spend as much time as they need with their child, and may sometimes need to be given 'permission' to leave, but should have the opportunity to return and view their child at a later stage. The nursing approach needs to be consistent and, where possible, continuity of personnel should be ensured. Visiting needs and parental requests for specific toys or clothes to be placed with the child should be documented, and the parents should be given the name and telephone number of the nurse who will facilitate their visits. Before the parents leave the department, practical issues such as funeral arrangements, death certificates and post-mortem examination should be discussed. Even if arrangements are not able to be made at the time, the parents may be given the contact numbers of those who can best help them. Prompt liaison with the GP and health visitor should be made, as they will need to visit the family at home and will be an ongoing source of support.

SUDDEN INFANT DEATH

Sudden infant death syndrome (SIDS) is defined as 'the sudden death of an infant or young child, unexpectedly by history, in which a thorough post-mortem examination fails to demonstrate an adequate cause for death' (Beckwith, 1969). Sudden infant death syndrome (also called 'cot death') was the leading cause of death during infancy after the first week of life until the start of the 'Back to Sleep' campaign in 1993. Recent research by Fleming *et al.* (1990) showed that eliminating proven risk factors such as sleeping position, parental smoking, and thermoregulation of the infant and the environment, could reduce infant mortality.

However, cot deaths do still occur and its management in the A&E department needs to be handled sensitively. Senior nurses can do much to help parents, nurses and medical staff face the emotional distress of these situations by implementing local protocols which ensure that liaison between all agencies (hospital, police, social workers, coroners, GPs and health visitors) is effective and sensitive to the parents' needs. An example is the Avon Infant Mortality Study Team, which comprises neonatologists, research midwives and health visitors who are able to offer intervention and support to the bereaved parents of SIDS victims in the hospital, and later, at home in the community, thereby reinforcing the dynamic interface of care. The team also supports staff who have dealt with these events in A&E (see flowchart, Fig. 6-1).

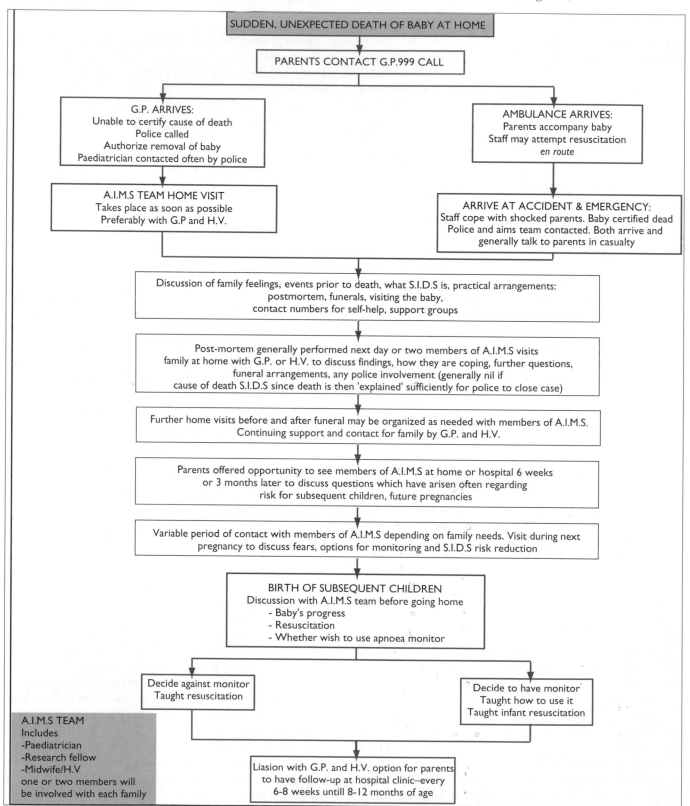

Fig. 6-1 Sudden, unexpected death of baby at home.

STRESS, DISTRESS AND BURNOUT IN THE ACCIDENT AND EMERGENCY DEPARTMENT

Stress is not always a bad thing — it is a message that coping is required (Wright, 1986). Critical incident debriefing is essential after distressing events concerning children in the A&E department, and senior nurses should facilitate this, seeking appropriate professional help where indicated. Nurses need help to ensure they are not burdened with emotion that does not necessarily belong to them, in order to be effective carers and to cope with the next stressful situation. Early recognition of the symptoms of 'burnout' by nurses and their managers can help them recognize the need for help, for time out, or for a change in career (Box 6-8).

PAEDIATRIC TRIAGE

An important aspect of the care of the child in the A&E department is the use of triage to ensure early recognition of life-threatening conditions, as this may be the first step in appropriate treatment (Table 6-1).

◆ **BOX 6-8**

Signs of burnout

- Overconcern and overinvestment
- Fatigue, loss of energy, weariness and exhaustion
- Malaise, aches and pains
- Coughs, colds and headaches
- Nausea, indigestion, diarrhoea and constipation
- Disturbed sleep
- Itching and rashes
- Shortness of breath and wheezing
- Emotionally labile
- Quickly angered
- Avoiding patients and colleagues
- Difficulty in concentrating

FACTOR	NURSING CONSIDERATIONS
Airway	
Large tongue	Airway can easily become obstructed by tongue; proper positioning is often all that is necessary to open the airway.
Smaller diameter of all airways: in 1-year-old child, tracheal diameter is less than child's little finger.	Small amounts of mucus or swelling can easily obstruct the airways: child normally has increased airway resistance.
Cartilage of larynx is softer than in adults	Airway of infant can be compressed if neck is flexed or hyperextended:
Cricoid cartilage is narrowest portion of larynx	provides a natural seal for endotrachea tube: cuffed tubes are not necessary in children less than 8 years of age and may damage airway
Breathing	
Sternum and ribs are cartilaginous: chest wall is soft; intercostal muscles are poorly developed: infants are obligate nose breathers for first 4 weeks of life: increased metabloic rate (about twice that of an adult): increased respiratory demand for oxygen consumption and carbon dioxide elimination.	Infant's chest wall may move inward instead of outward during inspiration (retractions) when lung compliance is decreased: greater intrathoracic pressure is generated during inspiration: anything causing nasal obstructions can produce respiratory distress: respiratory distress increases oxygen demand, as does any condition that increases metabolic rate, such as fever.
Circulation	
Child's circulating blood volume is larger per unit of body weight, but absolute volume is relatively small: 70% – 80% of newborn's body weight is water (compared to 50% – 60% of adult body weight): about one–half of this volume is extracellular	Blood loss considered minor in an adult may lead to shock in child: decreased fluid intake or increased fluid loss can quickly lead to dehydration.
Increased heart rate, decreased stroke volume (cardiac output equals heart rate times stroke volume): cardiac output is higher per unit of body weight	Tachycardia is the child's most efficient method of increasing-cardiac output and is the first sign of shock: CO decreases if heart rate is greater than 180–200 beats per min

From Hazinski MF: *Nursing care of the critically ill child,* St. Louis. 1984. Mosby-Year Book:
Holsclaw DS: Early recognition of acute respiratory failure in children. *Pediatr Ann* .6.57. 1977.

Table 6-1 Paediatric triage: differences in airway, breathing and circulation.

For triage to be effective, it is essential that the nurse has a thorough understanding of the anatomy and physiology of the infant and child, and the developmental differences that may influence management.

The triage nurse must think and act quickly, establishing the critical factors in the incident, and should be able to recognize the seriously ill infant or child in need of urgent treatment or resuscitation. This demands assessment skills and a sound theoretical knowledge base.

Good assessment skills are required, as children have the ability to compensate homeostatically and their vital signs will not immediately reflect the seriousness of their illness. It is important not to focus only on the obvious, because subtle but serious problems could be missed. Above all it is important that no child is refused assessment in A&E, no matter how trivial the complaint may seem.

Children usually demonstrate respiratory signs first and cardiovascular symptoms second, unless the child has undiagnosed congenital abnormalities of the heart. Assessment of peripheral pulses and four-limb blood pressure recordings will be needed if an undiagnosed cardiac problem is suspected.

Respiratory signs and symptoms can be quite subtle at first; therefore, it is important to undress infants and children, and to observe their breathing pattern. Nasal flaring, the use of accessory breathing muscles, and rib recession are early signs that can be hidden by clothing. This may progress to sternal and intercostal recession.

Wheezing and grunting are signs of lower airway problems. Stridor, a barking cough, dysphagia and drooling are signs of upper airway problems. The child whose respiratory effort is severely compromised will demonstrate signs of hypoxia—bradycardia and agitation. Cyanosis is a very late sign – the child will appear pale and waxen before turning blue. The child who is 'head bobbing' or seeking a comfortable position may be struggling to breathe (Table 6-1).

The children's triage nurse should make a quick assessment using observation skills, listening for breath sounds and checking oxygen saturations, and should always be prepared for the apnoeic child who will need an anaesthetist and intubation.

Cardiovascular assessment involves looking at the child's colour and capillary refill. Depression of the nail bed or forehead should result in a return of colour in two seconds; five seconds or more is abnormal. The child with a tachycardia may be demonstrating the first signs of shock, but an increase in pulse rate may also be caused by anxiety or fever. Hypotension is a serious sign and may be an indicator of uncompensated shock.

Level of consciousness should be noted and a quick assessment for hypovolaemia made. Children can become hypovolaemic much more rapidly than adults (Box 6-9). An assessment of the child's skin turgor, and in infants, the fontanelle, is needed. A sunken fontanel is evidence of dehydration and a bulging fontanel is evidence of raised intracranial pressure.

◆ BOX 6-9

Known circulating blood volumes

Neonates = 90ml/g circulating blood volume

Infant = 80ml/g circulating blood volume

Child = 70ml/g circulating blood volume

Adult = 65-70ml/g circulating blood volume

The Glasgow Coma Scale is commonly used to assess neurological function in adults, but an adapted scale should be used to evaluate children's neurological status. The most important part of the assessment of the child's neurological status is the history and evaluation of the level of consciousness. Evaluation of this may be enough to classify the child as an emergency in need of urgent treatment. The AVPU mnemonic (alert, responds to verbal stimuli, responds to painful stimuli, unresponsive) is especially useful in evaluating the preverbal infant or child.

ANAPHYLAXIS

Anaphylaxis is a potentially life-threatening syndrome which is immunologically mediated, and which may lead to shock and cardiovascular collapse if not treated. The most common cause in childhood is allergy to certain foods, such as nuts. The time lapse from onset of symptoms to collapse may be very short (Box 6-10 and Fig. 6-2).

THE CHILD IN NEED OF RESUSCITATION

Cardiac arrest in infants and children is rarely caused by primary cardiac disease. In childhood, most cardiac arrests are secondary to hypoxic events, with underlying causes including birth asphyxia, epiglottitis, inhalation of foreign bodies, bronchiolitis, asthma and pneumothorax. Respiratory arrest may also be secondary to neurological dysfunction such as that caused by poisoning or convulsions.

Whatever the cause of the collapse, by the time of arrest, the child will have experienced a period when hypoxia and respiratory acidosis have occurred, causing cellular damage and necrosis before myocardial damage is severe enough to result in cardiac arrest (Fig. 6-3).

Children who have an out-of-hospital arrest have the worst outcomes, as they often arrive apnoeic and pulseless. While initial resuscitation may be successful, the child may still have a poor chance of long-term, intact neurological survival due to a prolonged period of hypoxia and ischaemia before Cardiopulmonary resuscitation had been commenced. Early recog-

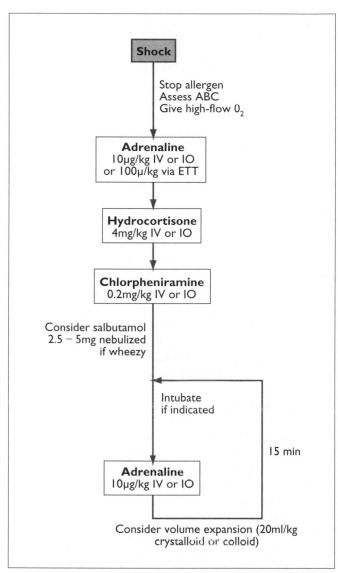

Fig. 6-2 Protocol for the management of anaphylaxis. (ETT, endotrachial tube.)

◆ **BOX 6-10**

Symptoms of anaphylactic shock

- Flushing
- Itching
- Facial swelling
- Urticaria
- Abdominal pain and gastrointestinal upset
- Wheezing and/or stridor

nition of the seriously ill or injured child and extensive public training in basic life support skills could improve outcomes for these children.

The primary role of the triage nurse is early recognition of the seriously ill or injured child whose treatment may need to be prioritized. The use of triage in A&E will also enable staff to ensure that standard 5 of the Patient's Charter is met (DoH, 1991b), namely, that patients in accident and emergency departments are seen immediately and their need for treatment assessed. This is particularly important for children in the A&E whose assessment and care needs to be 'fast-tracked'.

TELEPHONE TRIAGE

Telephone advice has always been given by nurses working in A&E departments; however, it should be governed by policies. Standards and protocols are needed if safe practice is to be established and litigation avoided.

Eighty-nine per cent of households now own a telephone (OPCS, 1992) and many parents will contact a health professional for medical advice for their children via a telephone. Calls to A&E departments concerning children are particularly frequent, and advice given should be based on symptoms,

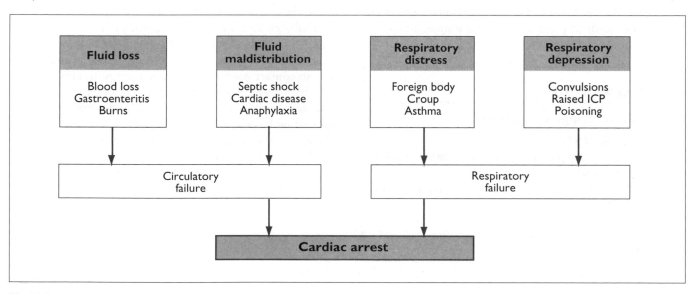

Fig 6.3 Pathways leading to cardiac arrest in childhood (with examples of underlying causes). (ICP, intracranial pressure.)

and not diagnostic, with the provision that the child may be brought to the department at any time if the parent remains concerned.

Using a formal telephone triage system will enhance parental empowerment in the care of their child, and will result in a lesser number of 'inappropriate attendees' to A&E and the GP's surgery. This will ultimately provide a cost effective service which links the primary and secondary health care providers (Box 6-11). In Toronto, where such a scheme is well established, the cost of a paediatric triage call is $10, compared to the $100 cost of a visit to the emergency room. An average of 160 calls per day are received (Glasper, 1993).

However, the implementation of this concept needs to be consistent. There must be a dedicated, experienced children's nurse to run the service at all times. A help line that may not be answered due to other emergencies in the department, is worse than no help line at all. Training programmes for staff will be needed to improve telecommunication skills.

Even if it is not practicable to establish a formal telephone triage system, children's nurses can still play a major role in allaying parental anxieties when telephone requests for help and advice are made. Documentation of name, date of birth and address, and the nature of the problem will enable further communication with, or referral to the primary health care team to be made, if necessary. This will also aid in auditing the efficacy and appropriateness of the advice given.

EMERGENCY NURSE PRACTITIONERS

It has been recognized by nursing and medical staff that a significant proportion of patients attending A&E do not require the services of a doctor (Jones 1989, Howie 1992). Nurses working in minor injuries units have worked informally as nurse practitioners for many years, while major A&E departments have successfully researched the scope for the role and have formally established nurse practitioner services. Consequently, suitably qualified and experienced nurses are directly meeting the needs of patients, reducing waiting times, and assisting in the reduction in junior doctors' hours.

◆ BOX 6-11

Telephone triage outcomes

Glasper A (1993)
- To prompt the patient to seek immediate medical help, including first aid.
- To direct the patient to a health professional, with less urgency.
- To empower self-care unit.

Specialist emergency departments, such as ophthalmic and paediatric, are different. In ophthalmic casualty departments, the nursing role has always been extended and specialist paediatric casualty departments are beginning to establish the role. In Nottingham, for example, 5% of patients attending are assessed and treated to conclusion by an emergency nurse practitioner (ENP) (Kobran and Pearce, 1991).

An ENP has been defined as, 'An A&E nurse who has a sound nursing practice base in all aspects of A&E nursing, with formal post basic education in holistic assessment, in physical diagnosis, in prescription of treatment and in the promotion of health' (RCN, 1993, page 1).

As the role develops, and confidence grows, the ENP role will expand naturally. One study of 5,000 patients in a major A&E found that the ENP treated 10% of patients and this resulted in a 50% reduction in waiting times for patients who actually needed to see the doctor (Burgess, 1992).

Children's nursing has evolved from the institutionalized paediatrics of the early 19th century to the family-centred care environment of today. The immense scope for an ENP role in a specialist children's casualty department is exciting. The main limitation is the lack of dual qualified staff, those who are both RSCN and A&E trained or experienced.

PRIMARY CARE IN A&E

Patients have been traditionally categorized by medical and nursing staff as 'appropriate' or 'inappropriate' attendees. Throughout the literature, blame is apportioned to patients, and they are viewed as deviant for their perceived misuse of A&E departments.

Any member of the general public can refer himself or herself to A&E at any time of the day or night. Since the inception of the NHS, this continued open access policy has diminished medical control (because the public, and not the medical staff, decides who attends) (Sbaih, 1993).

In inner city areas, families prefer to use A&E for primary health care, particularly if the emergency department is part of a specialist children's hospital. One study in London (Bedford *et al.*, 1992) found that 96% of patients had been seen by a community midwife and 89% by a health visitor. Parents knew how to contact community services, yet only 11% of those attending A&E required admission to hospital.

Community liaison health visitors and established communication links between the interfaces of care are essential. The experienced children's nurse in A&E has much to offer families. The integration of hospital care and a community paediatric nursing service will improve the provision of health care to children both currently, and in the future (Thornes, 1993).

KEY POINTS

- The use of triage will improve patient outcomes and ensure early recognition of life-threatening injuries and disorders.
- Nurses working in A&E departments need to appreciate the physiological, cognitive, psychological and emotional differences in children — they are not 'mini adults'.
- The emergency care of children should take place in a safe and secure environment that is equipped for their care and staffed appropriately.

- The A&E department is a vital part of the dynamic interface between primary and secondary care providers.
- Standards of care should be set and monitored by experienced children's nurses.

REFERENCES

Avery J, Jackson RH: *Children and their accidents,* London, 1993, Edward Arnold

Beckwith JB: Epidemiology. In Bergman AB, Beckwith JB and Ray CG: *Sudden infant death syndrome,* Washington, 1969, Washington University Press.

Bedford H *et al.*: Use of an east end children's accident and emergency department for infants: a failure of primary health care?, *Quality Health Care* 1: 29, 1992.

Burgess K: A dynamic role that improves the service: combining triage and the nurse practitioner roles in A&E *Prof Nurs* 7(5):301, 1992.

Chambers M: Play as therapy for the hospitalised child, *J Clin Nurs* 2(6):349, 1993.

Department of Health: *Welfare of children and young people in hospital,* London, 1991a, HMSO.

Department of Health: *The Patients' Charter,* London, 1991b, HMSO.

Departments of Health: *The Children Act,* London, 1989, HMSO.

Fleming P *et al.*: Interaction between bedding and sleeping position in the sudden infant death syndrome: a population based case-control study, *BMJ* 301:85, 1990.

Glasper EA: Telephone triage: extending practice, *Nurs Stand* 7(15):34-36, 1993.

Howie P: Development of the nurse practitioner, *Nurs Stand* 6(27):10, 1992.

Jones G: The waiting game, *Nurs Times* 85(41):28, 1989.

Kobran M, Pearce S: The paediatric nurse practitioner, *Paediatr Nurs* 3(5):11, 1991.

Mead D, Sibert J: *The injured child: an action plan for nurses,* London, 1991, Scutari Press.

Morton R, Phillips B: *Accidents and emergencies in children,* Oxford, 1992, Oxford University Press.

OPCS: *General household survey,* London, 1992, Central Statistics Office HMSO.

RCN: *Emergency nurse practitioners: guidance from the RCN,* London, 1993, Society of A&E Nursing and Emergency Nurse Practitioner Special Interest Group RCN.

RCN: *Protecting children: an RCN guide for nurses,* London, 1994, RCN.

Sbaih L: Accident and emergency work: a review of some of the literature, *J Adv Nurs* 18:957, 1993.

Thornes R: *Bridging the gaps: an explanatory study of the interfaces between primary and specialist care for children within the health services,* London, 1993, CCHS, Action for Sick Children.

Wright B: *Caring in crisis,* London, 1986, Churchill Livingstone.

FURTHER READING

Budassi-Sheehy S: *Emergency nursing — principles and practice,* St Louis, 1992, Mosby-Year Book.

Crain EF, Gershel JC, Gallagher EJ: *Clinical manual of emergency pediatrics,* 1992, NY, McGraw-Hill.

Fallis JC: *Pediatric emergencies — surgical management,* Philadelphia, PA, 1991, BC Decker.

Henry J, Volans G: *ABC of poisoning* — drugs, London, 1985, British Medical Journal Publishing Group.

Mead D, Sibert J, editors: *The injured child: an action plan for nurses,* London, 1991, Scutari Press.

Morton RJ, Phillips BM: *Accidents and emergencies in children,* Oxford, 1992, Oxford University Press.

Chapter 7

The Child and Surgery

LEARNING OUTCOMES

After studying this chapter you should be able to:

- Describe the issues which should be explored during the admission assessment.
- Identify some issues which may facilitate postoperative pain management.
- Discuss the role of the parents in preparing children for surgery.
- Identify the different types of pain assessment tools available and consider their relative merits and disadvantages.
- Explore the contribution which the use of premedications may make to the child's overall operative care.
- Discuss the nurse's role in carrying out postoperative observations.
- State the analgesic needs of children undergoing day care surgery.
- Describe the factors which should be considered before electing to use PCA postoperatively.
- Identify the factors to consider prior to discharging children home.
- Evaluate the role of play in the care of children undergoing surgery.
- Define the glossary terms.

GLOSSARY

ADH Antidiuretic hormone

advocate One who speaks for another

analgesic ladder The gradual progression from mild to potent analgesics developed by the hospice movement and now recommended by the World Health Organization

balanced analgesia The use of different analgesic interventions to block or modify the pain pathway simultaneously at several different points in the body

day care surgery Admission to hospital, surgery and discharge home all occuring on the same day

core temperature Central temperature, usually taken per axilla

discharge planning A strategy for follow on care in the community

elective admission Planned admission to hospital

EMLA Eutectic mixture of local anaesthetic

epi-/extradural On or over the dura mater

informed consent The process of providing those concerned, the requisite competence to consent to a procedure in a manner they can readily understand

NCA Nurse controlled analgesia

non pharmaceutical pain management strategies Pain relief management without the use of drugs

NSAID Nonsteroidal anti-inflammatory drug

PCA Patient controlled analgesia

peripheral temperature Skin temperature at periphery (e.g., toe)

pharmacological pain management strategies The use of drugs for pain relief

per os (PO) By mouth, orally (Latin)

postoperative pain Pain which occurs after surgery

pre-emptive analgesia The use of analgesic drugs before a painful event

premedication Drug(s) administered to a patient before a surgical procedure

pro re nata (PRN) According to circumstances (Latin)

rigour Shivering and a sensation of coldness accompanied by a rapid rise in body temperature

systemic Affecting the whole body

For many members of the public, and indeed for many health care professionals, the notions of *surgical procedure* and *pain* are inextricably linked. Indeed, a report published in 1990 stated that despite a high incidence of postoperative pain, patients often have high levels of satisfaction, confirming the notion of pain as an inevitable part of a surgical admission (The Royal College of Surgeons, 1990). Despite increasing literature about paediatric postoperative pain, it has had a distinct lack of influence on clinical practice (McIlvaine, 1989) and there can be little doubt that paediatric postoperative pain remains in many cases a problem for the child, their family and the health care workers. This chapter explores the general principles to consider when caring for children undergoing a surgical procedure, and highlights the issue of pain and ways in which pain assessment and management can be integrated into the holistic care of the child and family.

A positive surgical experience (and effective pain management) for the child and family can be described as a series of strategies that begin when the child is admitted to the ward and end when the child is discharged. In today's health service, these strategies can be extended to include pre-admission preparation at home (in the case of elective surgery), and the vital role community nurses play after the child has been discharged (particularly after day care or short stay surgery).

Admission to hospital can be a stressful experience for both the child and family (see Chapter 5). Even 'routine' or elective admissions, which are planned with the family and thereby minimize disruption and also enable pre-admission preparation (Taylor, 1991), may cause considerable anxiety. If the child is admitted to hospital as a 'surgical emergency', there is little time for the child and family to be physically, psychologically and emotionally prepared for the experience (Muller *et al.*, 1986).

Much of the routine paediatric surgery is carried out at local hospitals by surgical and anaesthetic staff who may have variable experience in the care of children. It is recognized that most of their clinical workload is with adult patients (Audit Commission, 1993). Cooperation between the surgical, anaesthetic and paediatric teams will facilitate the care of the children in this situation. It is equally important that the nurses caring for the child are 'experts' and act as the child's advocate in any discussions with the medical staff (Department of Health, 1991).

ADMISSION TO THE HOSPITAL UNIT

The admission assessment should be structured to reflect the needs of the particular child and family. The aim of the assessment is to systematically identify relevant information in order to negotiate an individualized care plan for the child and family during their stay in hospital.

At the initial admission interview, a detailed nursing assessment should be carried out. This should include information regarding the child's general health prior to admission (Adamson and Hull, 1984), previous admissions to hospital (if any), the reason for the admission and, of course, whether the child is currently receiving any medication or undergoing any treatment for a pre-existing condition. The nurse must ensure that all relevant information is relayed to the medical and anaesthetic staff. Establishing the child's and family's understanding of the reason for the admission is also important, as they may have erroneous ideas which the nurse must explore and address. The notion of the child as a unique member of a family group, and the need to acknowledge and value the role of the child's primary carers, are the main tenets of nursing models which reflect a 'partnership in care' approach (Casey, 1993). However, this approach relies on each of the health care team, the child, and the family to identify their respective roles during hospitalization (Campbell and Summersgill, 1993). Cooperation between child, family and nursing staff is essential for a successful outcome to be achieved (Birch, 1993). It should also be recognized that the child's primary caregivers may initially feel deskilled in their role as carers, due to the stresses of their child's condition and the ward environment. This may be a particular problem when the child has been admitted as a surgical emergency.

During the admission assessment, the nurse should record baseline observations of temperature, pulse and respiratory rate, to establish that the child is well enough to undergo elective surgery, or so that appropriate interventions can be carried out if the child has been admitted as a surgical emergency. Since the prescribing of paediatric drugs is generally based on the weight of the child (Adamson and Hull, 1984), an accurate admission weight should be recorded with the child wearing the minimum of clothing. This figure should be prominently displayed on all the relevant documentation, including the prescription chart, anaesthetic chart, preoperative checklist and fluid balance charts. The nurse should also establish whether the child has any known allergies or sensitivities to drugs, adhesive tapes or wound dressings. This information should also be recorded on the relevant documentation and relayed to the relevant medical and anaesthetic staff.

As part of the admission procedure, some units routinely screen children for the presence of infection. This may include routine urinalysis and obtaining swabs from the nose and throat. The nurse admitting the child must be aware of any outbreaks of infection within the hospital; for example, methacillin-resistant *Staphylococcus aureus* (MRSA), which may require more comprehensive screening programmes. Other investigations may include chest x-ray, full blood count and particular investigations for the proposed procedure. Children from particular ethnic groups may require further haematological investigation; for example, children of Asian, North African, Mediterranean and Afro-Caribbean origins will require assessment of their sickle cell or thalassaemic status (Adamson and Hull, 1984).

The integration of the subject of pain into the admission assessment can, if handled sensitively, be advantageous for everyone. The nurse may obtain information which will facilitate the assessment and management of the child's pain, while the child and family are given the opportunity to discuss their concerns, and are made aware that postoperative pain is not considered to be an inevitable part of the child's surgery.

A comprehensive list of the pain issues to be discussed during the admission assessment is neither helpful nor desirable. The process of gathering information should be *dynamic* and *responsive* to the needs of each child and family; however, a framework may provide a valuable starting point for the discussion. As with many aspects of nursing, effective communication is vital. Eland (1988) suggests that adults may use 141 words to communicate their pain to others, but children may be preverbal or may have limited language skills. It is therefore important to establish the specific word or words that a child and his or her family use to communicate about pain. Common 'pain words' include, 'baddie', 'nasty', 'hurt' or 'owie', but some families may have their own 'pain language' and establishing and using this will facilitate communication. Establishing the 'pain language' may also enable the nurse to discover what painful things have happened to the child in the past. This information may be helpful when explaining proposed procedures to the child, and will also give the nursing staff some knowledge of the child's awareness of the body and its functions. The parents may also be able to provide valuable information about the behavioural cues their child gives when in pain. It is important to establish whether these fall into either of these two categories: (1) pain of acute onset and relatively short duration, and (2) pain of a longer duration. It may also be helpful to establish the pain management strategies which the family use at home. This should include both pharmacological and nonpharmacological interventions. For example, many paediatric nurses have found that perfectly acceptable sweetened paracetamol elixir becomes totally unacceptable if the sugar-free type is used in hospital. Some children may have a set routine for the administration of the medicine, a certain cup to drink from, or a specific spoon. When possible, these routines should be followed; this may improve compliance with analgesic administration. The nonpharmacological pain management strategies which the family use are of equal importance to pharmacological interventions. For example, the child may (or may not) like to be held and cuddled when in pain, or the use of a transitional object may be of crucial importance (Darbyshire, 1985). Certain songs, videos or games may also help maintain continuity in the child's life when admission to hospital has disrupted the normal routine.

When this core of information has been established, the nurse will be in a better position to select the most appropriate pain assessment tool for the child. The nurse can then confirm the appropriateness of the tool, and can educate the child and family about it. The range of analgesic techniques available for the child postoperatively can also be discussed and, where appropriate, education about a particular intervention can also be given (analgesic techniques and patient education will be discussed later in this chapter).

PREOPERATIVE CARE

Fear of the unknown can be a considerable source of anxiety for the child and family. Whenever possible, they should be given a proposed itinerary of events for their admission. This should identify any necessary preoperative investigations, proposed visits by other health care professionals, and a brief outline of their role in the child's care and other specific considerations relevant to the child's procedure. This information may have to be repeated on several occasions, as the child's and family's ability to retain and internalize information may be affected by the stress of the situation. Parental anxiety can 'infect' a child; therefore, the nurse must try to alleviate parental anxiety, to enable them to support and comfort their child (Glasper and Thompson, 1993). It is also vital to ensure the child and family understand the language used when this information is being given; for example, the expression 'nil by mouth' should be explained.

SELECTING A SUITABLE PAIN ASSESSMENT TOOL

Pain assessment tools can be divided into three broad categories: (1) those addressing a child's verbal response or self-report of pain, (2) their behavioural response and (3) their physiological response (Adams, 1989). (See also Chapter 5).

Self-report tools facilitate the child's description of pain. While they cannot be considered absolute measures of pain (due to the subjective nature of the experience), they may be used to estimate the child's needs and respond to them more effectively. Many tools are available, including simple descriptive and numerical rating scales; for example, the Eland Color Tool (Eland, 1988), the Children's Global Rating Scale (Carpenter, 1990), the Wong/Baker FACES pain rating scale (Bieri, 1990; Broome *et al*, 1990; McGrath 1985; Wong and Baker, 1988), the Oucher (Beyer *et al.*, 1992) and the Hester Poker Chip Scale (Hester *et al.*, 1992). All of these tools rely to some extent on the child having a knowledge of size or number concepts and therefore are generally considered more suitable for children over the age of four. The tools also acknowledge that a child's level of cognitive functioning may be altered or impaired due to hospitalization. The crucial factor in the use of self-report tools is to select a tool which is suitable for the child and not to use one tool for all children. It is also important that the nursing staff have a thorough working knowledge of the tool. Many units caring for children of varying ages and abilities elect to use a limited number of tools which broadly address the needs and abilities of the children. This enables the nurses to develop their skills and knowledge in a more structured way, rather than using tools on an *ad hoc* and possibly infrequent basis.

Although behavioural cues may be helpful in the overall assessment of pain, reliance solely on them may lead to erroneous decisions about the child's pain. Many 'pain behaviours' are not unique to the pain experience. For example, a child may cry from pain, but may also cry because the parent has left the ward. Equally, pain may cause a child to adopt a rigid, tense posture, but fear and anxiety may also result in this behavioural response. To minimize the effects of rogue behavioural observations, it is preferable to use tools which assess a variety of behaviours, such as the Children's Hospital of Eastern Ontario Pain Scale (CHEOPS) (McGrath *et al.*, 1985), the Procedure Behavior Rating scale, the Observation of Behavioral Distress scale or the Child Behavior Observation Rating scale (Broome, 1991). For the preverbal child, behavioural assessment tools may be the most appropriate to use, providing their limitations are understood and acknowledged (Beyer *et al.*, 1990).

The child in pain manifests a 'global, non-specific, physiological response', which generally consists of an elevated heart rate, blood pressure and respiratory rate, accompanied generally by a reduction in oxygen saturation and increase in palmar sweating (Gedaly-Duff, 1989). However, other stimuli, such as fear and anxiety may also result in a similar physiological responses. Although it may be appropriate to suggest that the child in pain generally has some degree of fear and anxiety, is the converse also true?

Increasingly, the value of assessing the multidimensional experience of pain, using a combined self-report (where possible), behavioural and physiological approach is being acknowledged. Robertson (1993) describes the testing of the Princess Margaret Hospital Pain Assessment Tool (PMHPAT) a multidimensional tool that assesses the child in pain from a self-report and behavioural perspective.

Baker and Wong describe pain assessment as 'a constant process or (1987). The components of QUESTT are, Questioning the child, Using pain rating tools, Evaluating behaviour, Sensitizing the parents to their valuable role as co-workers and indeed primary workers in some situations in pain assessment, Taking the cause of pain into account, and Taking action to manage pain when it has been identified.

PREOPERATIVE FASTING

The preoperative fasting period can be a stressful time for the child and family. In Western society, it is generally considered that a large part of the parental role is to nurture children. The notion of nurturing and providing food are intrinsically linked, and when the parents' ability to respond to their child's needs is withdrawn, albeit with valid reason, the parent-child relationship can become strained. The importance of being 'nil by mouth' prior to surgery should be explained to the child (where appropriate) and family to encourage their cooperation (Adamson and Hull, 1984). The duration of the preoperative fast remains a relatively contentious issue. Schreiner (1994) states that "Even individuals with the slowest emptying rates will retain only 10% or less of the original liquid within their stomachs after two hours". In practice a three hour preoperative fasting period is appropriate for breast fed infants. Older children and formula fed infants are traditionally given normal diet up to six hours preoperatively and then offered a clear feed three to four hours after this. It is suggested that this practice does not increase the risk of pulmonary aspiration and indeed,

children who have been given a clear glucose feed two to three hours prior to anaesthesia are generally less irritable and thirsty than those who have undergone a prolonged period of fasting (6–8 hours) (Welborn *et al*; 1993). If delays to surgery cause this period to be extended, the child's blood glucose levels should be monitored and appropriate interventions taken to prevent the child becoming hypoglycaemic. For babies and infants, it may be necessary to commence an intravenous infusion preoperatively to maintain adequate hydration and normal blood glucose levels (Whaley and Wong, 1995). The mobile child who is 'nil by mouth' must be clearly identified to prevent the child inadvertently being given food or drinks, which could delay or postpone the operative procedure. A badge which the child chooses may be helpful in this situation.

INFORMED CONSENT

The concept of informed consent has recently become a major issue in paediatric nursing. Dingwell (1989) defines informed consent as providing those concerned with the requisite competence to consent to a procedure in a manner which they can readily understand, while also exploring the implications of all the other options. As the child's and family's advocate, the nurse must ensure that they understand the implications of the proposed procedure and should help empower them to make an informed decision.

The notion of parental and informed consent has become more complex since the publication of *The Children Act* (1989) and the Gillick Case (Gillick v Wisbeech Area Health Authority) (Barnes, 1985). Since the publication of the 1989 *Act*, the emphasis has changed from sole parental consent to a situation of combined parent/child consent. The importance of the child's feelings and wishes must now be more carefully considered. The nurse should encourage the family to discuss the proposed procedure with their child in a full and frank manner, using language and aids (where appropriate) to ensure that the wishes and needs of the child have been explored and addressed.

Informed consent still presents some legal and ethical problems. The principle of consent by a representative parent still continues in paediatrics, due to previous legislation. In many instances, it is still adults, seeking to achieve the optimum care for their child, who sign the consent form (Hendrick, 1991). For the child/parent relationship to emerge undamaged from a period of hospitalization, the parents must therefore be advised of the best options available (Brykczynska, 1987).

PREMEDICATIONS

The use of premedications is a contentious issue. McIlvaine (1989) states that the goals of premedication are to provide perioperative sedation and analgesia (pre-emptive analgesia), to minimize secretions, to maximize haemodynamic stability during induction, and finally (perhaps most importantly) to make the induction experience more tolerable for all concerned. When premedications are used, the most common routes of administration are oral or intramuscular. Usually, one or a combination of the following types of drugs are used: opioids, to provide pre-emptive analgesia and some sedation; anxiolytics or neuroleptics (e.g., trimeprazine or benzodiazepine), to provide sedation; or antimuscarinic drugs (e.g., atropine or hyoscine), to dry bronchial and salivary secretions and to prevent excessive bradycardia and hypotension as a result of the use of inhalational anaesthetic agents. The anaesthetist in charge of the child's perioperative management decides whether or not to use a premedication and what type to use. However, as consumers of health care, children and their parents are becoming increasingly assertive in expressing their needs and wishes to medical staff. The nurse must act as the child and family's advocate, while ensuring they have sufficient knowledge to make an informed decision.

If the child is to have intravenous induction of anaesthesia, the use of local anaesthetic creams, such as eutectic mixture of local anaesthetic (EMLA), may significantly reduce the pain of cannulation.

CHECKING PROCEDURES

Before transferring the child to the operating theatre, a rigorous procedure should be completed to ensure the maintenance of the child's safety. Case notes, x-rays (where appropriate), a signed and valid consent form, an identity bracelet, nursing documentation and, in some cases, a preoperative checklist should be thoroughly checked for any omissions.

The nurse must ensure the child removes all jewellery and hair clips. The use of diathermy to cauterize blood vessels during surgery may cause contact burns on the child if metal objects are not removed. Equally important, all nail polish and makeup must be removed. This ensures that the child can be readily monitored for signs of hypoxia during surgery, which is manifested as blue tinges of the peripheral areas, particularly the nailbeds and lips. The nurse must also check for loose teeth, as these may be very dangerous if they are inadvertently 'extracted' by a laryngoscope or endotracheal tube during intubation.

If the child has a favourite toy or comforter, this should accompany him or her to theatre. Care must be taken that it is returned to the ward to await the child's return from surgery.

TRANSFER TO THE OPERATING THEATRE

Transferring a child from the ward to the operating theatre may be influenced by the type of premedication (if any) the child has been given and the distance to the operating theatre department. Older, non-premedicated children may prefer to walk to the operating theatre. Younger children and those who have received narcotic or sedative premedications will require some assistance. For infants and toddlers, it is probably easier and more reassuring for them to be carried to theatre, preferably by their parent. Where theatre trolleys are used these may be transformed into a 'train', a 'rocket', or a 'ship' rather than an alien trolley. Making

the journey an 'adventure' may help decrease anxiety. Conversely, for adolescents, maintaining their dignity is of great importance. It is unlikely that an adolescent would feel comfortable travelling to theatre in a 'space rocket' (Harris, 1991).

In some institutions, parents accompanying their child to the anaesthetic room remains a contentious issue. However, children's nurses should advocate that any and all children have a fundamental right to have their parent with them during stressful times (Day, 1987). To ensure a positive experience for everyone involved in caring for the child in the anaesthetic room, it is vital that the parents are given adequate preparation by the ward and theatre staff to enable them to help and support their child before he or she is anaesthetized (Coulson, 1988). Preoperative preparation will also enable the parents to know when they should leave the anaesthetic room (Pethen, 1990), and will therefore remove one of the main 'reasons' for excluding parents from anaesthetic procedures.

CARE OF THE PARENTS DURING SURGERY

The parental role enters a state of suspended animation while the child is in theatre. Once the child is anaesthetized, the parents' physical role stops until the child is returned to the ward or recovery area (Muller, Harris and Wattley, 1986). Sitting patiently by an empty bed can be an emotionally draining experience. If parents decide to wait on the ward for their child's return, regular progress reports may help them feel 'in touch' with their child. This time can also be used to encourage parents to use catering and washing facilities in order to prepare themselves for their child's return to the ward (Mitiguy, 1986).

POSTOPERATIVE CARE

The safety of the child during the postoperative period is of paramount importance. Once in theatre, the child's bed area should be prepared for his or her return. Oxygen and suction equipment should be available and working correctly. An appropriately sized airway should be easily accessible. Specific equipment required for the child's care postoperatively should also be collected, including IV stands, drainage bags and holders, nasogastric tubes, or pulse oximeter monitor.

Following transfer from the theatre or recovery area, the child should be returned to bed as quickly as possible.

NURSING OBSERVATIONS

Baseline observations of temperature, pulse, respirations and blood pressure give an indication of the stability of the child's immediate postoperative condition. The use of fundamental nursing skills, observing and listening, in conjunction with frequent recording of the child's vital signs, will enable the nurse to monitor the child's postoperative recovery. The frequency of the recording of the child's observations should reflect the child's general condition (Whaley and Wong, 1995) and should be increased or decreased accordingly. Nursing observations can help to identify postoperative complications such as shock and haemorrhage. Children may also become hypoglycaemic following surgery and in some cases blood glucose monitoring may be indicated. The child may also have become chilled during surgery and may require both peripheral and core temperature monitoring. If there is a significant discrepancy between the core and peripheral temperature, the child may require gradual warming, using 'space blankets', gamgee, extra blankets and for the small child, hats and mittens to reduce this 'gap'.

Depending on the type of surgery performed, routine antibiotics may be prescribed. Initially, these may be administered intravenously and, as the child's condition improves, may then be administered orally. The duration and type of antibiotic therapy will be influenced by the nature of the surgery.

It may also be necessary to give the child a blood transfusion to replace blood lost during the operative procedure. The nurse must be alert to the possibility of adverse reactions to the transfusion, such as elevation in temperature, flushing, and in severe cases, rigors.

PAIN MANAGEMENT

Pain management is traditionally viewed as the administration of analgesia after pain has been identified. Increasingly, the view of this as the optimum regime for postoperative pain management is being challenged by the use of pre-emptive analgesia. As the name suggests, pre-emptive analgesia is the use of analgesic drugs *before* the painful event (or noxious stimuli) which thereby reduces the effect of subsequent noxious stimuli on the individual (Morton, 1993). The hormonal response to injury is reduced and fewer prostaglandins are produced from the damaged tissues. More obviously, the use of central or regional nerve blocks as pre-emptive analgesia may result in greater stability of the child's vital signs during the operative procedure, perhaps an indication that the procedure is having a lessened effect on the anaesthetized child. The value of pre-emptive analgesia remains very controversial and more research is required to confirm its short- and long-term benefits (McQuay, 1992).

In chronic pain management, the use of the World Health Organization's *analgesic ladder* is well documented (Alder, 1990; Watt-Watson and Donovan, 1992). The child is given analgesia at an effective dose and frequency of administration which is appropriate to the level of pain. The child then moves up the 'ladder' and receives stronger analgesia if the pain increases, or moves down the 'ladder' if the pain decreases. In contrast to chronic pain management, innovative postoperative pain management attempts to create *balanced analgesia*, to block or modify the pain pathway simultaneously, at several different points in the body, by using different types of analgesic interventions (Morton, 1993). Although many of these analgesic interventions are outside the nurse's role, it is vital that he or she understands the implications of the various techniques in order to care for the child effectively and to intervene appropriately should analgesia be inadequate.

Wound infiltration with a local anaesthetic solution is a relatively simple procedure performed at the end of surgery prior to closing the wound. This may substantially reduce the child's need for further postoperative analgesia after relatively minor procedures such as herniotomy or pyloromyotomy. However, inadvertent infiltration of muscles may result in higher blood levels of the drug and an increased potential for toxic effects, such as hypotension, bradycardia, agitation, euphoria and respiratory depression.

Peripheral nerve blocks using a local anaesthetic solution can provide postoperative analgesia for up to eight hours. Peripheral nerve blocks are particularly suitable for operations on lower limbs; for example, a sciatic or femoral nerve block, or a peripheral nerve block of the dorsal nerve of the penis for circumcision. A brachial plexus block may be used for surgery on the upper limbs. Temporary paraesthesia rarely occurs as a result of the use of peripheral nerve blocks.

Central nerve blocks distribute analgesia to larger areas of the body. The caudal extradural block is one of the most commonly used central blocks in paediatric practice (Lloyd-Thomas, 1990) and is particularly suitable for surgery involving both lower limbs, the anoperineal region, the urinary tract, or the abdomen below the umbilicus. Again, the use of a local anaesthetic solution can provide postoperative analgesia for up to eight hours, and indeed the duration of analgesia can be extended by combining an opioid (e.g., diamorphine) with the local anaesthetic. Children who have received a diamorphine caudal block should be closely observed for the potential complication of respiratory depression. For this reason, this technique is not suitable for children undergoing day-care surgery. Children may also manifest other side effects of opioid administration, such as nausea, vomiting and urine retention.

Increasingly, following major abdominal, genitourinary or cardiothoracic surgery, a continuous central nerve block may be considered a more effective method of providing pain relief. Extradural (or epidural) infusions enable the perioperative benefits of central nerve blockade to be carried into the postoperative period for as long as considered necessary by the health care team, the child and family. Continuous infusions of local anaesthetic and opioids provide targeted analgesia to the dermatomes affected by the surgical procedure and should enable the child to cooperate more readily with postoperative care, such as physiotherapy and movement. Potential complications of continuous extradural infusions include inadequate analgesia due to postoperative movement of the catheter in the extradural space (resulting in inadequate blockade to the relevant spinal nerves), excessive sedation and respiratory depression due to the effects of the opioid, nausea, vomiting and pruritus, also due to the effects of the opioid. Urine retention can also occur as a result of the opioid or of the local anaesthetic. Technical complications, such as leakage from the insertion site, catheter occlusion, premature removal of the catheter, and catheter disconnection may occur quite readily, possibly as a result of the small gauge catheters which are used for children (Wilson and Lloyd-Thomas, 1993). A continuous infusion in children does not appear to result in the profound hypotensive episodes or altered lower limb sensation and function, which are so typical of obstetric extradural pain management. The nursing care of a child receiving a continuous extradural infusion should focus on the identifation and appropriate intervention of the potential complications, and also in encouraging the family to maintain their role as primary caregivers. Many parents feel extremely apprehensive about holding their child or taking the child out of its cot or bed for a cuddle when an extradural catheter is present. If the extradural infusion is seen to prevent this contact with the family, then the child is not receiving optimum pain management.

The use of systemic opioids for pain management in adults is well documented (Kuhn *et al.*, 1990). This group of drugs is being used increasingly within the postoperative paediatric population (Berde and Burrows, 1993). They should not be perceived as the 'cure all' for postoperative pain in children. The cost - benefit balance must be carefully weighed and meticulous care should be taken at all times to ensure the child does not suffer unwanted side effects of opioid administration (Gourlay and Boas, 1992). Opioids can be administered via the oral, rectal, intramuscular, subcutaneous and intravenous routes. They are usually used for pain management following major surgery and the preferred routes of administration are usually intravenous, subcutaneous and intramuscular.

Administration of intramuscular opioids for postoperative pain management tends, for a variety of reasons, to provide unsatisfactory analgesia in the majority of cases. Children dislike the thought of an injection (Broome, 1985) and may therefore decide to endure their existing pain rather than experience the additional pain of analgesia administration. Indeed, many young children are unable to discriminate between different types of 'hurt' and nurses caring for them are unable to rationalize the need for the intramuscular injection - the children cannot understand that the second 'hurt' will reduce their existing 'hurt' and therefore will not agree to the procedure. Many nurses feel reluctant to give injections to children, and frequently may wait until the child has demonstrated an overt need for analgesia, before contemplating giving the child an injection (Gillies, 1993). This 'wait and see' approach may be successful in a very few instances, but in the majority of cases, the child experiences unsatisfactory pain management because constant blood levels of the prescribed analgesic have not been maintained. Although the intramuscular route is not considered particularly suitable for paediatric pain management, it is important to stress that the technical and information-giving skills of the nursing staff involved may make the process much more tolerable for everyone. When no alternative route for opioid analgesia is available, the nurse must discuss with the child and family whether analgesia (albeit via a less desirable route), is better than no analgesia.

Continuous infusions of opioids provide more constant analgesic drug levels than intermittent intramuscular injections and have been used successfully for postoperative pain management in children (Dilworth and MacKellar, 1987).

However, this technique does not reflect the fact that postoperative pain is not constant and that pain levels may be altered as a result of several factors. Analgesic administration should therefore be equally responsive to provide optimum pain relief. The lack of control which many children experience postoperatively may heighten anxiety, which in turn may lead to increased pain perception and therefore increased analgesic requirements. The administration of intravenous opioids via a patient-controlled analgesia (PCA) pump may be a means to empower certain groups of children in this potentially powerless situation (Fig. 7-1). Selecting suitable children for PCA is the first important step in ensuring the success of the technique. Although chronological age is a major deciding factor it is not the only aspect to consider. The child should also have the cognitive ability to understand how PCA works. This may be simply 'pressing the button, makes the machine give me some medicine which makes my leg/tummy/bottom feel better'. With older children, a more complex explanation may be required. The child must be able to make the cause-and-effect link between pressing the button and opioid administration. Some PCA pumps reinforce this link by 'beeping' whenever the button (or handset) is pressed. It should be emphasized that the child should press the handset *only* when pain relief is required, and that it should be used *every* time he or she needs analgesia, regardless of the lockout interval (the amount of time that must elapse between using the handset and receiving analgesia, and the next dose of analgesia being available). The child must also be physically able to use the handset, as many designs are intended for adult-sized hands and as such, may be virtually impossible for the smaller child to use. Finally, the child and family must be willing to cooperate with the use of PCA. The success of PCA relies not only on the selection and education of suitable children, but also on the programming of the pump, and the responsiveness of the health care team in altering the programming if the technique is not providing adequate analgesia. An imbalance between the demands (the number of times the handset has been used) and the good demands (the number of times analgesia has been administered)

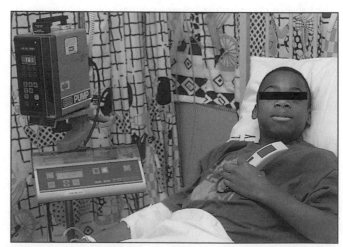

Fig. 7-1 Child using PCA equipment (Courtesy of the Acute Pain Service, The Great Ormond Street Hospital for Children NHS Trust).

may indicate that the pump programming needs to be reviewed; however before changing the programming, the health care team must recheck the child's understanding of PCA and ensure no other factors are contributing to the child's apparent increased analgesic requirement. Some children may be too young, unwilling or unable to cooperate with a PCA regime. These children may benefit from a technique known as nurse controlled analgesia (NCA). NCA takes the equipment and principle of PCA (a flexible method of administering opioids according to the needs of the child) but places the responsibility of administering bolus doses with the nurse, in negotiation with the child's family. Programming of the pump is altered to reflect this and the child is usually given a continuous infusion to create adequate analgesia. Bolus administration is therefore required only before potentially painful procedures or if the child appears to be experiencing increased pain. The lockout interval is substantially increased to ensure the child's safety. A natural development from the idea of nurse-controlled analgesia, is parent-controlled analgesia, but care must be taken to ensure that the optimum programming parameters have been established before the responsibility for bolus administration is invested solely in the parents.

Recently, the use of nonsteroidal anti-inflammatory drugs has become more popular for the paediatric patient. Administration via oral, intravenous, intramuscular routes, but particularly the rectal route, has further increased their suitability for postoperative pain management. This groups of drugs may provide a valuable 'halfway house' between potent opioids and paracetamol.

Paracetamol is often maligned as an analgesic and in many hospitals, its role as an antipyretic appears to have superseded its role as an analgesic. Paracetamol via the rectal or oral route has a valuable role to play in achieving optimum analgesia. Difficulties arise when it is administered on a prn (*pro re nata*) basis, because the blood levels may then fall below therapeutic levels.

The aim of balanced analgesia is to use a combination of analgesic interventions to create the maximum desired effect for the child, with minimum unwanted effects. Therefore, the general rule is to balance opioid with non-opioid interventions, thereby enhancing pain relief. The nursing care of children receiving postoperative analgesia should focus on achieving optimum analgesia, while maintaining safety, and intervening swiftly and appropriately if unwanted side effects occur. Although guidance may be taken from published papers, the guidelines for caring for children should be established locally and should reflect the particular needs of the children, staff and environment. It is imperative that a multidisciplinary approach is taken and that all members of the health care team are consulted before definitive guidelines are created.

Although effective pharmacological pain management is vital for the postoperative paediatric patient, the value of non-pharmacological methods of pain relief should also be considered. More complex techniques such as aromatherapy, reflexology, acupressure and acupuncture may not be appropriate in the immediate postoperative period, and should certainly be undertaken only by qualified personnel. However, postoperative nursing actions also contribute greatly to the child's comfort and quality of life, and thereby reduce anxiety and pain perception. A story, a cuddle or simply someone nearby may be very important to the child following surgery.

FLUID BALANCE

Accurate measuring and recording of the child's fluid balance is very important during the immediate postoperative period. The child may have experienced fluid loss during surgery and as a result of preoperative fasting. However in some cases, the child may retain fluid as a result of the stress response to surgery. Increased antidiuretic hormone (ADH) is secreted from the anterior lobe of the pituitary which then acts on the renal tubules of the kidney, thereby increasing permeability and reducing or preventing the excretion of water. It may be necessary to restrict the fluid intake of children who are experiencing this inappropriate ADH response until the endocrine response has equilibrated (Willatts, 1982).

Charting fluid output postoperatively is also very important if and when replacement fluids are required. Nasogastric aspirate, wound drainage and urinary output may require millilitre-for-millilitre replacement by intravenous fluids. It is very important to ensure the replenishment of vital fluid electrolytes which maybe lost through wound drainage and nasogastric routes.

Urinary output should also be monitored regularly. It is generally considered that a child should have a urine output of between 0.5-1.0 ml/kg of body weight per hour. This is obviously easier to monitor if the child has an indwelling urinary catheter. Urinary retention can present a major postoperative complication, but close observation of the patient can lead to early detection of urinary retention and instigation of corrective therapy.

WOUND CARE

Wound observation and care are also important factors of postoperative care. Changes in the wound such as inflammation, bruising, oozing or bleeding should be reported to the medical staff immediately. Psychologically, both the child and family should be supported by the nurse when the wound is viewed for the first time. This can be a very significant occasion, especially if reconstructive surgery or a stoma is involved. However, the expertise of specialist nurse practitioners can assist both the child and parents in alleviating stress and coping with a new body image.

MOBILIZATION/PHYSIOTHERAPY

The postoperative child is potentially susceptible to many complications associated with restricted mobility. For major surgery, the use of antiembolic stockings may be indicated to reduce the risk of pulmonary embolism due to venous stasis. Skin integrity must be maintained and the child should be monitored at least every two hours to ensure the skin is not becoming reddened. Skin integrity can generally be maintained by assisting the child to change position in the bed every two hours, and by keeping the skin clean and dry. Mobilization should occur gradually and should facilitate the child's return to a state of optimum health. Mobilization and physiotherapy are essential to prevent postoperative complications, such as chest infections. With guidance, most parents will be happy to be involved in theses interventions, and may become extremely proficient in making physiotherapy and mobilization an enjoyable experience for their child, rather than a chore which must be endured.

DISCHARGE PLANNING

Discharge from hospital can often be a daunting prospect for many children and families. Where major or even minor surgery has been performed, the thought of returning home may be associated with a feeling of abandonment. Planned discharges are an ideal way to help alleviate worries and anxieties (Lewer and Robertson, 1987). Indeed, discharge planning must begin at the child's admission. Through consultative planning, many questions, problems and potential problems can be highlighted and addressed at the earliest opportunity. Advice leaflets can also be very effective in smoothing the transition from hospital to home. Detailed instructions regarding outpatient appointments and community support services should also be given (Audit Commission, 1993). If drug therapies are to be continued at home, the nurse must explain the importance of adhering to these therapies. Written instructions should be given to the family about the frequency of administration of the medications and the possible side effects. This information should be readily available as an integral part of the nursing care (Thornes, 1991). The child's general practitioner and referring hospital (if appropriate) should be contacted prior to discharge. They should be informed of the child's surgery, outcome and proposed discharge date. More detailed information should follow with the surgeon's discharge letter.

For some families, the knowledge that they can contact the surgical ward for advice is reassuring. This service should be automatically available and must be re-emphasized to the family prior to discharge.

DAY SURGERY

The advent of day surgery has provided yet another facet to paediatric surgery. Minor operations, such as the insertion of grommets, circumcision, orchidopexy, and in some instances tonsillectomies, now reduce the length of stay in hospital. These types of admissions can dovetail with the needs of the family unit. Disruption of the family unit and routine is, therefore, kept to a minimum (Glasper and Stradling, 1989). Ideally, paediatric day surgery facilities should be linked to the paediatric unit. Where this is not the case, the culture and attitude of the unit should reflect the needs of children. In mixed adult and paediatric day care units, Registered Children's Nurses should be employed to care for the paediatric patients.

Preparation for day surgery requires advanced planning from the nursing staff to ensure that high standards of family-centred care are provided. Maintaining high standards of practice ensures that the potential to develop a 'conveyor-belt' attitude to this par-

ticular type of admission does not exist. The child and parents expect to be treated as individuals, not as 'one-of-five' circumcisions to be operated on that day (Foale, 1991).

Discharge planning and follow-up appointments are equally important, if not more important, following day surgery. Advice and relevant information must be provided to enable the child to a have speedy and successful recovery at home, with minimal anxiety and stress for the parents. Discharge should occur only when the child's condition has been stable for several hours, when the child has taken and tolerated oral fluids, and when the child has passed urine. Inpatient paediatric beds should be available for children who are not deemed fit for discharge on the same day (Valman, 1988).

PLAY

Play is a highly successful vehicle for preparing children for a variety of procedures. The role and experience of the play specialist is fundamental to helping children gain insight about their impending surgery. Play therapy can be directed at a specific age range, on a group or individual basis (Save the Children, 1989).

Allowing children to express their fears and anxieties through play enables the health care team to identify potential problem areas. These can then be addressed by involving the child, the family, and all members of the health care team.

Whenever possible, play therapy should begin on admission to the ward and continue until the child is discharged. Ideally, play therapy should be integrated into pre-admission visits to the ward (Keegan, 1990). The concept of a structured 'fun day' in hospital is possibly the best method of allaying childhood apprehensions about hospitals and their functions.

It is also beneficial to instruct parents about suitable play therapy in the home prior to admission. This provides the parents with an important role in preparing their child for admission and continuing their participation in the care of their child, while having the support of trained individuals as a resource (Save The Children, 1989).

Using specific items of medical and nursing equipment (e.g., nurse's uniforms, syringes, and stethoscopes) as constructive and educational play therapy (Fig. 7.2), coupled with visits to appropriate hospital departments, can often nullify many myths and misconceptions the child may have (Jago, 1987).

Children (aged 0-18 years) comprise almost 25% of the workload in the main surgical specialities (ear, nose and throat, general surgery, trauma and orthopaedics and ophthalmology). Although paediatric surgical admissions have plateaued since the early 1970s, the average length of stay has been reduced from eight days to under three days. Nurses caring for children and families undergoing a surgical procedure must develop the necessary skills to care for the children effectively, must facilitate and coordinate the work of other members of the health care team, and must support and nurture the children and familes during this potentially stressful time. The nurse must also be aware of the need to adapt his or her care according to the demands placed on the service by the current health care environment. Although many aspects of preoperative and postoperative care are influenced by the proposed surgical procedure, the general principles to be considered remain constant. Many of the issues explored in this chapter have been identified as quality measures (Audit Commission, 1993). The goal of nursing interventions must be the provision of a quality paediatric surgical nursing service, which integrates all aspects of care into a holistic, family-centred approach.

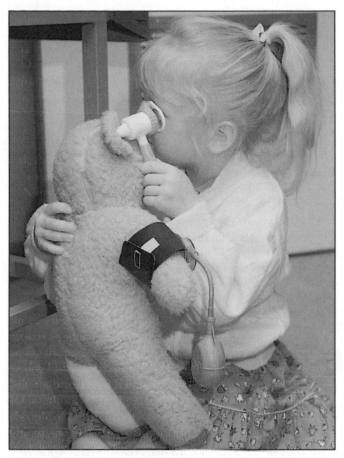

Fig. 7-2 Child using toy hospital equipment. (Courtesy of Professor E A Glasper)

KEY POINTS

- The provision of paediatric surgical care has changed dramatically over the last twenty years.
- Preoperative nursing care should focus on ensuring the child is 'fit' for the operation, or ensuring appropriate interventions are carried out if a pre-existing condition and/or underlying pathology is identified.
- Many pain assessment tools are available. They can be broadly divided into three categories: verbal response to pain, behavioural response, and physiological response.
- Parents should be encouraged to accompany their child to the anaesthetic room. Appropriate preparation for this will ensure that the parents are able to help and support their child effectively.
- Pre-emptive analgesia may diminish the hormonal response to surgery.
- Balanced analgesia blocks modify the pain pathway simultaneously at different points in the body by the use of several analgesic interventions.

- Peripheral nerve blocks using a local anaesthetic solution can provide postoperative analgesia for up to eight hours and may be particularly useful for day care surgery.
- The use of patient-controlled analgesia may be a means to empower certain groups of children in a potentially powerless situation.
- Discharge planning should begin during the admission assessment and should be a continuous process that enables the child and family to return home with few anxieties or worries, and with a comprehensive knowledge and understanding about future care or follow-up.
- Children's nurses have a crucial role to perform in coordinating and communicating with other members of the multidisciplinary team to ensure the child and family receive optimum care which is individually tailored to their needs.

REFERENCES

Adams J: Pediatric pain assessment: trends and research directions, *J Ped Oncol Nurs*, 6(30):79, 1989.

Adamson F, Hull D: *Nursing sick children*, Edinburgh, 1984, Churchill Livingstone.

Alder S: Taking children at their word, *Prof Nurs* 5(8):397, 1990.

Audit Commission: *Children first: a study of hospital services*, London, 1993, HMSO.

Baker CM, Wong DL: QUEST: a process of pain assessment in children, *Orthopaed Nurs* 6(1):11, 1987.

Barnes A: After Gillick—the implications for nursing, *Prof Nurs*, 1(3):79, 1985.

Berde C, Burrows FA: Optimal pain relief in infants and children, *BMJ* 307(6908):815, 1993.

Beyer JE *et al.*: The creation, validation and continuing development of the Oucher: a measure of pain intensity in children, *J Pediatr Nurs* 7(5):335, 1992.

Bieri D *et al*: The faces pain scale for the self-assessment of the severity of pain experienced by children: development, initial validation and preliminary investigation for ratio scale properties, *Pain* 41: 139–150, 1990.

Birch E: The key to real partnership—the importance of parent information, *Child Health* 1(1):25, 1993.

Broome M *et al*: Children's medical fear, coping behaviors, and pain perceptions during a lumbar puncture, *Oncol Nurs Forum* 17(3): 361–367, 1990.

Broome ME: Measurement of behavioural response to pain, *J Pediatr Oncol Nurs* 8(4):180, 1991.

Brykczynska G: Ethical issues in paediatric nursing, *Nurs* 3(23):862, 1987.

Campbell S, Summersgil P: Keeping it in the family—defining and developing family centred care, *Child Health* 1(1):17, 1993.

Carpenter PJ: New method for measuring young children's self-report of fear and pain, *J Pain Symptom Manage* 5(4):233, 1990.

Casey A: Development and use of the partnership model of nursing care. In Glasper EA, Tucker A, editors: *Advances in child health nursing*, London, 1993, Scutari Press.

Coulson D: A proper place for parents, *Nurs Times* 84(19):26, 1988.

Darbyshire P: Happiness is an old blanket, *Nurs Times* 81(10):40, 1985.

Day A: Can Mummy come too? *Nurs Times* 83(51):51, 1987.

Department of Health: *Welfare of children and young people in hospital*, London, 1991, HMSO.

Dilworth NM, MacKellar A: Pain relief for pediatric surgical patient, *J Pediatr Surg* 22(3):264, 1987.

Dingwell R: *Socio-legal aspects of medical practice*, London, 1989, The Royal College of Physicians.

Eland JM: Persistence in pediatric pain research: one nurse researcher's efforts, *Recent Adv Nurs* 21:43, 1988.

Foale H: Concerns in surgical paediatric nursing, *Paediatr Nurs* 3(1):9, 1991.

Gedaly-Duff V: Palmar sweat index use with children in pain research, *J Pediatr Nurs* 4(1):3, 1989.

Gillies M: Post-operative pain in children: a review of the literature, *J Clin Nurs* 2(1):5, 1993.

Glasper A, Stradling P: Preparing children for admission, *Paediatr Nurs* 1(5):18, 1989.

Glasper EA, Thompson M: Preparing children for hospital admission. In Glasper EA, Tucker A, editors: *Advances in child health nursing*, London, 1993, Scutari Press.

Gourlay GK, Boas RA: Fatal outcome with the use of rectal morphine for postoperative pain control in an infant, *BMJ* 304(6829):766, 1992.

Harris S: The role of the theatre nurse, *Paediatr Nurs* 3(1):13–14, 1991.

Hendrick J: Acting for sick children, *Nurs Times* 87(17):64, 1991.

Hester NO *et al.*: Excerpts from guidelines for the management of pain in infants, children and adolescents undergoing operative and medical procedures, *Matern Child Nurs* 17(3):146, 1992.

Jago D: Communicating with children in hospital, *Matern Child Health* 12(6):186, 1987.

Keegan S: Pre-admission visiting, *Nurs* 4(16):13, 1990.

Kuhn S *et al.*: Perceptions of pain relief after surgery, *BMJ* 300(6741):1687, 1990.

Lewer H, Robertson L: *Care of the child*, ed 2, London, 1987, Macmillan.

Lloyd-Thomas AR: Pain management in paediatric patients, *Br J Anaesthesia* 64(1):85, 1990.

McGrath PA, deVeber LL, Hearn MT: Multidimensional pain assessment in children. In Fields HL, Dubner R, Cervero F (Eds) *Advances in pain research and therapy*, vol 9, New York, 1985, Raven Press.

McGrath PJ: CHEOPS: A behavioural scale for rating postoperative pain in children, *Adv Pain Res Therapy* 9:395, 1985.

McIlvain WB: Perioperative pain management in children: a review, *J Pain Symptom Manage* 4(4):215, 1989.

McQuay HJ: Pre-emptive analgesia, *Br J Anaesthesia* 69(1):1, 1992.

Mitiguy J: A surgical liaison programme—making the waiting more bearable, *Am J Matern Child Nurs* 11(6):388, 1986.

Morton N: Balanced analgesia for children, *Nurs Stand Supple* 7(25):8, 1993.

Muller D, Harris P, Wattley L: *Nursing children—psychology, research and practice*, London, 1986, Harper & Row.

Pethen C: Involving the parents, *Nurs* 4(19):12, 1990.

Robertson J: Pediatric pain assessment: validation of a multidimensional tool, *Pediatr Nurs* 19(3):209, 1993.

Save the Children: *A deprived environment for children? The case for hospital playschemes*, London, 1989, Save the Children.

Schreiner MS. Preoperative and postoperative fasting in children, *Ped Clinics North Am* 41(1): 111–120, 1994.

Taylor D: Prepare for the best, *Nurs Times* 87(1): 64, 1991.

The Children Act, London, 1989, HMSO.

The Royal College of Surgeons of England, The College of Anaesthetists: *Report of the working party on pain after surgery*, London, 1990, RCS.

Thornes R: J*ust for the day—children admitted to hospital for day treatment*, London, 1991, NAWCH.

Valman HB: *ABC of one to seven*, London, 1988, British Medical Association.

Watt-Watson JH, Donovan MI: *Pain management nursing perspective*, St Louis, 1992, Mosby–Year Book.

Welborn LG *et al*, Effects of minimizing preoperative fasting on perioperative blood glucose hemeostasis in children, *Paed Anaesthesia*, 3, 167–171, 1993.

Whaley LF, Wong DL: *Nursing care of infants and children*, ed 3, St Louis, 1987, CV Mosby.

Willatts S: *Lecture notes on fluid and electrolyte imbalance*, Oxford, 1982, Blackwell Scientific.

Wilson PTJ, Lloyd-Thomas AR: An audit of extradural analgesia using bupivacaine and diamorphine, *Anaesthesia* 48(8):718, 1993.

Wong DL, Baker CM: Pain in Children; comparison of assessment scales, *Ped Nurs* 14(1): 9–17, 1988.

FURTHER READING

Action for Sick Children: *Children and pain,* London, 1992, Action for Sick Children.

Alderson P: *Choosing for children: parents' consent to surgery,* Oxford, 1990, Oxford University Press.

Alex MR, Ritchie JA: School-aged children's interpretation of their experience with acute surgical pain, *J Pediatr Nurs* 7(3):171, 1992.

Althea: *Going into hospital,* London, 1986, HarperCollins.

Carter B: *Child and infant pain—principles of nursing care and management,* London, 1994, Chapman & Hall.

Civardi A, Cartwright S: *First experiences going to the hospital,* London, 1986, Usbourne.

Gadish HS, Gonzalez JL, Hayes JS: Factors affecting nurses' decision to administer pediatric pain medication postoperatively, *J Pediatr Nurs* 3(6):383, 1988.

Jolly J: *The other side of paediatrics,* London, 1981, Macmillan.

Kempton D: *The hospital highway code,* London, 1994, Piccolo.

Llewellyn NE: The use of PCA for paediatric post-op pain management, *Paediatr Nurs* 5(5):12, 1993.

Schecter NL, Berde CB, Yaster M: *Pain in infants, children and adolescents,* Baltimore, 1993, Williams & Wilkins.

Thornes R: All in a day's work, *Paediatr Nurs* 3(1):7, 1991.

White R *et al.*: *A guide to the children act,* London, 1989, Butterworths.

Whiting M: Play and surgical patients, *Paediatr Nurs* 5(6):11, 1993.

Chapter 8

Paediatric Variations of Nursing Interventions

LEARNING OUTCOMES

After studying this chapter you should be able to:

◆ Discuss appropriate ways to prepare children for medical procedures.
◆ Describe how play therapy can be used to help children undergoing specific procedures.
◆ Identify the important role played by parents when their children are in hospital.
◆ Discuss ways to ensure compliance with treatment regimes.
◆ Identify adaptations required when planning nursing care for children of different ages.
◆ Describe how children can be encouraged to be involved in their care.
◆ Discuss the importance of safe administration of medicine using a variety of routes.
◆ Identify ways a child's safety can be maintained during various procedures.
◆ Define glossary terms.

GLOSSARY

antipyretic An agent that relieves or reduces fever

febrile Pertaining to fever

febrile convulsion A fit assouated with a high temperature in young children

fever Elevation in set point such that body temperature is regulated at a higher level

gastrostomy An opening in the abdominal wall through which a feeding tube is passed

HIV Human immunodeficiency virus

hyperthermia Body temperature exceeds the set point

IM Intramuscular

infant A child in the first year of life

informed consent Legal and ethical requirement that patients/parents must completely understand proposed treatments, including risks and benefits

IV Intravenous

set point Temperature around which body temperature is regulated by a thermostat-like mechanism in the hypothalamus`

hildren are not simply small adults. They differ from their older counterparts in biological, cognitive, and emotional function and response. Consequently, many standard interventions employed in nursing practice must be altered to meet the special needs of children at various developmental stages. This chapter presents an overview of psychological preparation of children for procedures; strategies to enhance compliance; application of the principles of growth and development in planning, implementing, and evaluating nursing procedures; and selected aspects of skills that require modification in caring for infants and children.

GENERAL CONCEPTS RELATED TO PAEDIATRIC PROCEDURES

Children, regardless of their age, require preparation for procedures. Family members, especially parents, also need adequate preparation. For some procedures, parents are required to give consent. This section discusses consent, general aspects of preparation for procedures, and the use of play in procedures.

CONSENT TO TREATMENT

Consent from a parent or guardian of a young child will normally be required for medical treatment and diagnostic procedures. Should the parents or guardians refuse such consent it is possible for application to be made to the court, which may grant consent in such situations. Adolescents over the age of 16 years may give their own consent to medical treatment, even if it overrides the wishes of the parents. Children under the age of 16 years who are of sufficient understanding and intelligence are considered capable, in English law, of giving consent to treatment, even if it is against the wishes of their parents. For children under the age of 18 years there is, however, no express right to refuse treatment (Korgaonkar and Tribe, 1993; McCall Smith, 1992). (See Chapter 7 for additional discussion of informed consent.)

PREPARATION FOR PROCEDURES

Although many children are now prepared for admission to hospital (see Chapter 5), some present without previous preparation or as the result of a medical emergency. These children and those who have received prior preparation can benefit greatly from preparation for specific procedures.

PSYCHOLOGICAL PREPARATION

Preparing children for procedures decreases their anxiety (Glasper and Thompson, 1993), promotes their cooperation, supports their coping skills and may teach them new ones. Most preparation strategies used by nurses are informal, focus on providing information about the experience, and are directed at stressful and/or painful procedures. Preparatory

interventions are most effective in: (1) reducing behavioural distress (crying, resisting), (2) decreasing children's rating of pain, and (3) reducing signs of physiological distress (heart rate, blood pressure, oxygen saturation) (Broome, Lillis, and Smith, 1989).

When individualizing the preparatory process, nurses should consider the child's temperament, existing coping strategies, and previous experiences. Children with previous health-related experiences still need preparation for repeat or new procedures, but the nurse must assess what they know, correct their misconceptions, supply new information, and introduce new coping skills as indicated by their previous reactions (Bates and Broome, 1986). There are general guidelines which can be followed (see Box 8-1) but nurses should also take into account the child's age and stage of development (see Box 8-2).

Some children want, and actively solicit, information about the intended procedure, whereas others characteristically avoid information. Parents can often guide nurses in deciding how much information is enough for the child. Asking older children their preferences about the amount of explanation is also important.

The exact timing of the preparation for a procedure varies with the child's age and the type of procedure. In general, the younger the child, the closer the explanation should be to the actual procedure to prevent undue fantasizing and worry. With complex procedures, more time may be needed for assimilation of information, especially with older children.

Establish trust and provide support
The nurse who has spent time with and who has established a positive relationship with a child will usually find it easier to gain cooperation. If the nurse does not know the child, it is best if the nurse is introduced by an other person whom the child trusts. The first visit with the child ideally focuses on the child first and then on explanation of the procedure only; performing the procedure should be avoided.

Children need support during procedures, and for young children the greatest source of support is the parents. The parents' preferences for assisting, observing, or waiting outside the room should be assessed, as well as the child's preference for parental presence. The child's choice should be respected (Rollins and Brantly, 1991). Parents who wish to stay need to know what will occur and how they can help. Parents who do not wish to be present or participate, should be supported in their decision and encouraged to remain close by, so they can be available to console the child immediately following the procedure. Parents should also know that someone will be with their child to provide support. This person should inform the parents after the procedure about how the child managed.

Provide an explanation
Before performing a procedure, the nurse explains to the child what is to be done and what is expected of them. The explanation should be short, simple, and appropriate to the child's level of comprehension. This is especially true regarding painful

procedures. When explaining the procedure to parents with the child present, the nurse uses language appropriate to the child. If the parents need additional preparation, this is done away from the child. Teaching sessions are planned at times most conducive to the child's learning and usual span of attention.

For young children who cannot yet think in concepts, using objects to supplement verbal explanation is important. Allowing children to handle actual items that will be used in their care, such as a stethoscope or sphygmomanometer, helps them to develop familiarity with these items and to reduce the threat often associated with their use. Hospital items, such as intravenous equipment, can be used to explain what the children can expect and permit them to safely experience situations that are unfamiliar and potentially frightening. Written and illustrated materials are also valuable aids to preparation.

PHYSICAL PREPARATION

One area of special concern is the administration of appropriate sedation and/or analgesia prior to stressful procedures. The drug is given before the procedure to allow time for the medication to reach its peak effect. Whenever possible, the intravenous (through an existing infusion), oral, transdermal, or rectal route is used rather than the intramuscular route, because children dislike injections. Some hospitals use short-acting anaesthetics (e.g., ketamine), general anaesthetics, or potent analgesics (e.g., fentanyl) to eliminate the pain and trauma associated with treatments, such as bone marrow tests, lumbar punctures, burn debridement, and suturing (Forlini, Morin, and Treacy, 1987). (See also Chapter 7.)

PERFORMANCE OF PROCEDURE

Ideally, the same nurse who explained the procedure should perform it or assist. If possible, procedures should be performed in a special treatment room rather than on the child's bed. Traumatic procedures should never be performed in 'safe' areas, such as the playroom. As the procedure is nearing completion, the nurse should inform the child that it is almost over.

Expect success
Nurses who approach children with confidence and who convey the impression that they expect to be successful, are less likely to encounter difficulty. It is best to approach a child as though cooperation is expected. Children can sense anxiety in an adult and will respond to a perceived threat by striking out or actively resisting. A firm approach with a positive attitude from the nurse tends to convey a feeling of security to most children.

Involve the child
Involving children helps to gain their cooperation. Permitting them to make choices gives them some measure of control. However, a choice is given only in situations in which one is available.

◆ BOX 8-1

General guidelines for preparing children for procedures

- Determine the details of the exact procedure to be performed.
- Review the parents' and child's present level of understanding.
- Plan the actual teaching based on the child's developmental age and existing level of knowledge.
- Incorporate parents in the teaching if they desire, and especially if they plan to participate in the care.
- Inform parents of their role during the procedure, such as standing near child's head or in child's line of vision and talking softly to the child.
- While preparing the child and family, allow for ample discussion to prevent information overload and to ensure adequate feedback.
- Use concrete, not abstract, terms and visual aids to describe the procedure. For example, use a simple line drawing of a boy or girl, and mark the body part that will be involved in the procedure.
- Emphasize that no other body part will be involved.
- If the body part is associated with a specific function, stress the change or noninvolvement of that ability (e.g., following tonsillectomy, the child can still speak).
- Use words appropriate to the child's level of understanding (a rule of thumb for number of words is the age in years plus 1).
- Avoid words/phrases with dual meanings unless the child understands such words.
- Clarify all unfamiliar words (e.g., 'Anaesthesia is a *special sleep*').
- Emphasize the sensory aspects of the procedure — what the child will feel, see, smell, and touch and what the child can do during the procedure (e.g., lie still, count out loud, squeeze a hand, hug a doll).
- Allow the child to practise those procedures that will require cooperation (e.g., turning, deep breathing, using a mask).
- Introduce anxiety-laden information last (e.g., the preoperative injection).
- Be honest with the child about the unpleasant aspects of a procedure, but avoid creating undue concern. When discussing that a procedure may be uncomfortable, state that it feels differently to different people and have the child describe how it felt.
- Emphasize the end of the procedure and any pleasurable events afterward (e.g., going home, seeing parents). Stress the positive benefits of the procedure (e.g., 'After your tonsils are fixed, you won't have as many sore throats').

◆ BOX 8-2

Age-specific guidelines for preparing children for procedures based on developmental characteristics

Infancy: Developing a Sense of Trust

Attachment to parent

- *Involve parent in procedure if desired.
- Keep parent in infant's line of vision.
- If parent is unable to be with infant, place familiar object with infant (e.g., stuffed toy).

Stranger anxiety

- *Have usual caregivers perform or assist with procedure.
- Make advances slowly and in nonthreatening manner.
- *Limit number of strangers entering room during the procedure.

Sensorimotor phase of learning

- During the procedure, use sensory soothing measures (e.g., stroking skin, talking softly, giving a dummy).
- *Use analgesics (e.g., local anaesthetic, intravenous opioid) to control discomfort.
- Cuddle and hug child after stressful procedure; encourage parent to comfort child.

Increased muscle control

- Expect older infants to resist.
- Restrain adequately.
- Keep harmful objects out of reach.

Memory for past experiences

- Realize that older infants may associate objects or persons with prior painful experiences and will cry and resist at sight of them.
- *Keep frightening objects out of view.
- *Perform painful procedures in a separate room, not in cot (or bed).

Imitation of gestures

- Model the desired behaviour (e.g., opening mouth).

Toddler: Developing a Sense of Autonomy

Use same approaches as for infant in addition to following:

Egocentric

- Explain procedure in relation to what child will see, hear, taste, smell, and feel.
- Emphasize aspects of procedure that require cooperation (e.g., lying still).
- Tell the child it's okay to cry, yell, or use other means to express discomfort verbally.

Negative behaviour

- Expect treatments to be resisted; child may try to run away.
- Use firm, direct approach.
- Ignore temper tantrums.
- Use distraction techniques (e.g., singing a song *with* a child).
- Restrain adequately.

  *Applies to any age.

  Limited language skills

- Communicate using behaviours.

- Use a few, simple terms familiar to child.
- Give one direction at a time (e.g., 'Lie down', then 'Hold my hand').
- Use small replicas of equipment; allow child to handle equipment.
- Use play; demonstrate on doll but avoid child's favourite doll since child may think doll is really 'feeling' procedure.
- Prepare parents separately to avoid child's misinterpreting words.

Limited concept of time

- Prepare child shortly or immediately before procedure.
- Keeping teaching sessions short (about 5-10 minutes).
- Have preparations completed before involving child in procedure.
- Have extra equipment nearby (e.g., alcohol swabs, new needle, plasters) to avoid delays.
- Tell child when procedure is completed.

Striving for independence

- Allow choices whenever possible, but realize that the child may still be resistant and negative.
- Allow the child to participate in care and to help whenever possible (e.g., drink medicine from a cup, hold a dressing).

Preschool Child: Developing a Sense of Initiative

Preoperational thought: egocentric

- Explain procedure in simple terms and in relation to how it affects the child (as with toddler, stress sensory aspects).
- Demonstrate use of equipment.
- Allow the child to play with miniature or actual equipment.
- Encourage 'playing out' experience on a doll both before and after procedure to clarify misconceptions.
- Use neutral words to describe the procedure.

Increased language skills

- Use verbal explanation, but avoid overestimating the child's comprehension of words.
- Encourage the child to verbalize ideas and feelings.

Concept of time and frustration tolerance still limited

- Implement same approaches as for toddler, but may plan longer teaching session (10-15 minutes); may divide information into more than one session.

Illness and hospitalization often viewed as punishment

- Clarify why each procedure is performed; a child will find it difficult to understand how medicine can make him or her feel better and can taste bad at the same time.
- Ask child thoughts regarding why a procedure is performed.
- State directly that procedures are never a form of punishment.

Fears of bodily harm, intrusion, and castration

- Point out on drawing, doll, or child where procedure is performed.

(Cont.)

◆ BOX 8-2

Age-specific guidelines for preparing children for procedures based on developmental characteristics

- Emphasize that no other body part will be involved.
- Use nonintrusive procedures whenever possible (e.g., axillary temperatures, oral medication).
- Apply a plaster over puncture site.
- Encourage parental presence.
- Realize that procedures involving genitals provoke anxiety.
- Allow child to wear underpants with gown.
- Explain unfamiliar situations, especially noises or lights.

Striving for initiative

- Involve child in care whenever possible (e.g., hold equipment, remove dressing).
- Give choices whenever possible but avoid excessive delays.
- Praise child for helping and attempting to cooperate; never shame child for lack of cooperation.

School-Aged Child: Developing a Sense of Industry

Increased language skills; interest in acquiring knowledge

- Explain procedures using correct scientific/medical terminology.
- Explain reason for procedure using simple diagrams of anatomy and physiology.
- Explain function and operation of equipment in concrete terms.
- Allow child to manipulate equipment; use doll or another person as model to practice using equipment whenever possible (doll play may be considered 'childish' by older school-aged child).
- Allow time before and after procedure for questions and discussion.

Improved concept of time

- Plan for longer teaching sessions (about 20 minutes).
- Prepare in advance of procedure.

Increased self-control

- Gain child's cooperation.
- Tell child what is expected.
- Suggest ways to maintain control (e.g., deep breathing, relaxation, counting).

Striving for industry

- Allow responsibility for simple tasks (e.g., collecting specimens).

- Include in decision making (e.g., time of day to perform procedure, preferred site).
- Encourage active participation (e.g., removing dressings, handling equipment, opening packages).

Developing relationships with peers

- May prepare two or more children for same procedure or encourage one to help prepare another peer.
- Provide privacy from peers during procedure to maintain self-esteem.

Adolescent: Developing a Sense of Identity

Increasingly capable of abstract thought and reasoning

- Supplement explanations with reasons why procedure is necessary or beneficial.
- Explain long-term consequences of procedures.
- Realize that adolescent may fear death, disability, or other potential risks.
- Encourage questioning regarding fears, options, and alternatives.

Conscious of appearance

- Provide privacy.
- Discuss how procedure may affect appearance (e.g., scar) and what can be done to minimize it.
- Emphasize any physical benefits of procedure.

Concerned more with present than future

- Realize that immediate effects of procedure are more significant than future benefits.

Striving for independence

- Involve in decision making and planning (e.g., choice of time; place; individuals present during procedure, such as parents; clothing to wear).
- Impose as few restrictions as possible.
- Suggest methods of maintaining control.
- Accept regression to more childish methods of coping.
- Realize that adolescents may have difficulty in accepting new authority figures and may resist complying with procedures.

Developing peer relationships and group identity

- Same as for school-aged child, but assumes even greater significance.

Provide distraction

A child who is occupied with an interesting activity is less likely to focus on the procedure. For example, when an injection is given, it is helpful to give the child something to do or something on which to focus attention. For example, asking the child to tightly squeeze the hands of a parent or an assistant, count aloud, sing a familiar song, or verbally express discomfort.

Allow expression of feelings

The child should be allowed to express feelings of anger, anxiety, fear, frustration, or any other emotion. It is natural for children to strike out in frustration or to try to avoid stress-provoking situations. The child needs to know that it is alright to cry. Whatever the response, the nurse must accept the behaviour for what it is.

POSTPROCEDURAL SUPPORT

After the procedure, the child continues to need reassurance that he or she performed well and is accepted and loved. If the parents did not participate, the child should be united with them as soon as possible so that they can provide comfort.

Praise the child

Children need to hear from adults that they did the best they could in the situation. It is important for children to know that their worth is not being judged on the basis of behaviour in a stressful situation.

Returning to the child a short while after the procedure helps the nurse to strengthen a supportive relationship. Relating with the child in a relaxed and nonstressful period allows him or her to see the nurse not only as someone associated with stressful situations but as someone with whom to share pleasurable experiences, as well.

USE OF PLAY IN PROCEDURES

The use of play is an integral part of relationships with children (see Chapter 5). As such, its value in specific situations is discussed throughout this book. There has been an increasing realization of the importance of play for children in hospital. The Department of Health (1991) recommends that there should be provision for play in all areas of the hospital where children are found and that play specialists should be employed. Provision, however, remains variable; the Audit Commission (HMSO, 1993) found that one-third of wards surveyed had a play specialist for only half the week. No matter what the hospital provides for children, nurses can still include play activities as part of nursing care. Play can be used to teach, for expression of feelings, or as a method to achieve a therapeutic goal. Consequently, it should be included in preparing children for and encouraging their cooperation during procedures. Suggestions for incorporating play into nursing procedures and activities for hospitalized children that facilitate learning and adjustment to a new situation are described in Box 8-3.

COMPLIANCE

One of the most significant nursing interventions concerning procedures that must be repeated in the hospital and/or continued at home is related to compliance. Compliance refers to the extent to which the patient's behaviour in terms of taking medication, following diets, or executing other life-style changes coincides with the prescribed regimen (Blum, 1984).

ASSESSMENT

In developing strategies to improve compliance, the nurse must first assess the child's level of compliance. Since many children are too young to assume partial or total responsibility for their care, parents are usually the primary caregivers in terms of

---

◆ **BOX 8-3**

Play activities for specific procedures

Fluid Intake
- Make ice lollies using child's favourite juice.
- Make game of taking sip when turning page of book or in games such as 'Simon Says'.
- Use small medicine cups; decorate the cups.
- Have tea party; pour at small table.
- Let child fill a syringe and squirt it into mouth or use it to fill small decorated cups.
- Use a 'crazy' straw.
- Make a 'progress poster'; give rewards for drinking a predetermined quantity.

Deep Breathing
- Blow bubbles with bubble blower.
- Blow on pinwheel, feathers, whistle, harmonica, balloons, toy horns.
- Have blowing contest using balloons, boats, feathers, marbles, ping-pong balls, pieces of paper; blow such objects on a tabletop over a goal line, over water, through an obstacle course, up in the air, against an opponent, or up and down a string.
- Suck paper or cloth from one container to another using a straw.
- Do straw-blowing painting.

Range of Motion and Use of Extremities
- Throw bean bags at fixed or movable target, wadded paper into wastebasket.
- Touch or kick balloons held or hung in different positions (if child is in traction, hang balloon from trapeze).
- Play 'tickle toes'; wiggle them on request.
- Play Twister game or 'Simon Says'.
- Play kick or throw ball with soft foam ball in safe area.
- Position bed so that child must turn to view television or doorway.
- Pretend to teach 'aerobic' dancing or exercises; encourage parents to participate.
- Play video games or pinball (fine motor movement).
- Play 'hide and seek' game: hide toy somewhere in bed (or room, if ambulatory) and have child find it using specified hand or foot.
- Provide clay to mould with fingers.
- Paint or draw on large sheets of paper placed on floor or wall.
  (Cont.)

---

home management. Consequently the nurse needs to assess their ability to carry out instructions.

Factors that influence compliance

Research on compliance has identified several influencing factors (Box 8-4). The first area relates to factors about the

---

◆ **BOX 8-3 continued**

Play activities for specific procedures

Injections

- Let child handle syringe, vial, alcohol swab and give an injection to doll or stuffed animal.
- Use syringes to squirt paint, or target shoot into a container.
- Draw a 'magic circle' on area before injection; draw smiling face in circle after injection.
- Allow child to have a 'collection' of syringes (without needles); make 'wild' creative objects with syringes.
- If multiple injections or venepunctures, make a 'progress poster'; give rewards for predetermined number of injections.

Ambulation

- Give child something to push.
  Toddler: push-pull toy
  School-aged child: wagon or decorated IV stand
  Adolescent: a baby in a pushchair or wheelchair
  Have a parade; make hats, drums, etc.

Extending Environment (Patients in Traction, etc.)

- Make bed into a pirate ship or aeroplane with decorations.
- Put up mirrors so patient can see around room.
- Move patient's bed frequently, especially to playroom, hallway, or outside.

◆ **BOX 8-4**

Guidelines for referral regarding communication impairment

Individual/Family Factors

- High self-esteem.
- Positive body image.
- High degree of autonomy (increased locus of control).
- Supportive and well-adjusted family.
- Effective family communication.
- Family expectation for successful completion of therapy.

Care Setting Factors

- Perceived satisfaction with care.
- Positive interactions with practitioners.
- Continuity of care.
- Individualized care.
- Minimum waiting time for appointments.
- Convenient care setting.

Treatment Factors

- Simple regimen.
- Minimum disruption in usual life-style.
- Short duration.
- Inexpensive.
- Visible benefits.
- Tolerable side effects.

---

patient. Some evidence suggests that higher levels of self-esteem and increased autonomy favourably affect adolescent compliance (Pidgeon, 1989). Family factors are important, and characteristics associated with good compliance include family support, family reminders, good communication, and expectations for successful completion of therapeutic regimen (Pidgeon, 1989).

Any aspect of the health care setting that increases the family's satisfaction with the physical setting and the relationship with the practitioner positively influences adherence to the treatment regimen. In addition, the type of care required to manage the disorder is important. The more complex, inconvenient, longer, and disruptive the treatment protocol, the less likely the family is to comply.

COMPLIANCE STRATEGIES

Strategies to improve compliance include interventions that encourage families to follow the prescribed treatment regimen. Ideally, such strategies should be implemented prior to or concurrent with the initiation of treatment, in order to avoid compliance problems. Several strategies have been identified as effective.

Organizational strategies

Organizational strategies refer to interventions concerned with the care setting and the therapeutic plan. These include manip-ulating the factors listed in Box 8-4, which are known to positively affect compliance. Depending on the individual situation, this may involve increasing the frequency of appointments, designating a primary practitioner, reducing the disruption of the treatment on the family's life-style, and using 'cues' to minimize forgetting. Many devices are available commercially or can be improvised for cueing; these include pill dispensers, watches with alarms, charts to record completed therapy; reminders, such as messages on the refrigerator; and treatment schedules that incorporate the treatment plan into the daily routine, such as physiotherapy after the evening bath.

Educational strategies

Educational strategies teach the family about the treatment plan. It is important that all members of the team follow similar guidelines, as indicated in Box 8-5. Although education is an important component in enhancing compliance and patients who are more knowledgeable about their condition are more likely to comply, education alone does not ensure compliant behaviour. Written materials are essential, especially in any regimen requiring multiple or complex treatments, and need to be readable by the average individual.

Behavioural strategies

Behavioural strategies encompass interventions designed to modify behaviour directly. Several strategies are effective in encouraging the desired behaviour and are very useful with children. Ideally, positive reinforcement should be used to strengthen the behaviour. This may consist of earning stars or tokens, which gains the child a special privilege or gift. However, at times disciplinary techniques, such as time-out for young children or withholding privileges for older children, may be needed to reduce noncompliance (Rapoff, 1986).

Contracting

Contracting is a process in which the exact elements of desired behaviour are explicitly outlined in the form of a written contract. It is very effective, especially with older children who are involved in the process of defining the rules of the agreement. Ideally, it should involve tangible rewards but may include negative consequences, such as demerits or 'checks' for failing to comply. Often, the contract includes a commitment from the parent, such as agreeing to stop nagging about taking medication.

An effective contract includes components listed in Box 8-6, although more informal arrangements can be used with

---

◆ BOX 8-5

Guidelines for effective teaching of family members

- Establish rapport; reduce anxiety and fear.
- Assess what family knows and expects to learn, especially if they have concerns, and address their concerns before beginning teaching.
- Assess family's learning style; ask if they prefer having everything explained in detail or knowing only the major facts.
- Direct teaching to family decision maker.
- Use a variety of teaching materials (lecture, demonstration, video or slide presentation, written material).
- Speak family's language, avoid jargon, and clarify all terms.
- Be specific when giving information; divide information into small steps.
- Keep information short, simple, and concrete.
- Introduce most important information first.
- Use 'verbal' headings to organize information, such as, 'There are two things you need to learn: how to give the medicine and what side effects to look for. First, how to give... Second, what side effects... '
- Stress importance of instructions and expected benefits; explain detrimental effects of inadequate treatment but avoid fear tactics.
- Evaluate teaching by eliciting feedback to ensure that family understands information.
- Repeat information as needed.
- Reward family for learning through verbal praise.
- Use 'teachable' moments — times when family is most likely to accept new information (e.g., when symptoms are present).

---

young children, such as awarding desired behaviour with stars or stickers. Once the contract is implemented, it is evaluated at the end of the time specified in the agreement and revisions are made.

PERSONAL HYGIENE AND CARE

Attention to personal hygiene is continued throughout the child's hospital stay. Certain caregiving activities present special challenges, especially feeding the sick child. In addition, children often have high fevers that require attention. Any of these activities presents excellent opportunities for family health teaching.

BATHING

Unless contraindicated, most infants and children can be bathed at the bedside, on the bed, or in a standard bath located on the ward.

Infants and small children should *never* be left unattended in a bath, and infants who are unable to sit alone should be securely held with one hand. The infant's head should be supported securely with one hand or the farther arm should be firmly grasped in the nurse's hand while the head rests comfortably on the wrist. This provides secure control of the infant while the other hand is free to wash the infant's body. Infants or children who are able to sit without assistance need only close supervision and a pad placed in the bottom of the bath to prevent slipping and loss of balance, which could result in a bumped head or submersion of the face.

Most children who feel well require little encouragement to participate in their daily care. Nurses will need to use judgement regarding the amount of supervision the child requires. Children with cognitive impairments, physical limitations such as severe anaemia or leg deformities, or suicidal or psychotic problems (who may commit bodily harm) require close supervision.

◆ BOX 8-6

Components of a contract

- The goal or desired behaviour is realistic and seems possible.
- The behaviour is measurable (e.g., agreeing to take the drug before leaving for school without reminding).
- The contract is written and signed by all those involved in any of the agreements.
- The contract is dated, and if appropriate, a date is specified when a goal should be reached (e.g., number of pounds of weight loss in two weeks).
- The identified rewards or consequences are reinforcing.
- The goal can be evaluated (e.g. counting the number of tablets, using a scale for weight measurement).

Areas that require special attention during bed baths, and for children performing their own care, are the ears, between skinfolds, the neck, the back, and the genital area. The genital area should be carefully cleansed and dried with particular care to skinfolds. Older children sometimes avoid the genitalia, therefore they may need a gentle reminder.

Children who are ill or debilitated will need more extensive assistance with bathing and other aspects of care, but they should be encouraged to perform as much as they are capable of without overtaxing their energies. Children with limited capacity for self-help but no other contraindications benefit greatly from baths. They can be transported to the bath with the aid of lifting devices and/or an appropriate number of persons to assist.

ORAL HYGIENE

Mouth care is an integral part of daily hygiene and should be continued in the hospital. Infants and debilitated children will require the nurse or a family member to perform mouth care. Although small children can manage a toothbrush and are encouraged to use it, most will need assistance to perform a satisfactory job. Older children, although capable of brushing without assistance, sometimes need to be reminded that this is a part of their care.

HAIR CARE

Brushing and combing hair are a part of the daily care for all people in hospital, including infants and children. If the child does not have a brush or comb, many hospitals provide one. If not, the parents should be asked to bring hair care equipment for the child's use. Both boys and girls are helped to comb or brush their hair, or it is done for them, at least once daily. Hair should not be cut without parental permission, although shaving hair to provide access to a scalp vein for intravenous needle insertion may be necessary.

If children are hospitalized for more than a few days, the hair may need shampooing. With infants, the hair may be washed during the daily bath or less frequently. For most children, washing the hair and scalp once or twice weekly is sufficient, unless there is an indication to wash it more frequently, such as following a high fever and profuse sweating.

Black children require special hair care, and this need is frequently neglected or inadequately managed. For the black child with kinky hair, most standard combs are inadequate and may cause hair breakage and discomfort to the child. If a special comb with widely spaced teeth is not available on the unit, parents can be reminded to bring a comb, if possible, for the child's use. It is also much easier to comb the hair after shampooing, when it is wet. This type of hair requires a special hair dressing or pomade, which usually has a coconut oil base. The preparation is rubbed on the hands and then transferred to the hair to make it more pliable and manageable. The child's parents should be consulted regarding the preparation they wish to be used on their child's hair and asked if they can provide some for use during the child's hospitalization.

FEEDING THE SICK CHILD

Loss of appetite is a symptom common to most childhood illnesses and is frequently the initial evidence of illness, preceding fever and other overt signs of infection. In most cases children can be permitted to determine their own need for food. Since an acute illness is usually short, the nutritional state is seldom compromised.

Refusing to eat may also be one way children can exert power and control in an otherwise helpless situation. For young children, loss of appetite may be related to the depression of separation from their parents. Parents' concern with eating can intensify the problem. Forcing a child to eat only meets with rebellion and reinforces the behaviour as a control mechanism. Although it is best to encourage high quality, nutritious foods, the child may desire foods and liquids that contain mostly calories. Some well-tolerated foods include diluted clear soups, carbonated drinks, dry toast, and hard-boiled sweets. Even though these substances are not nutritious, they can provide necessary fluid and calories.

Dehydration is always a hazard when children are febrile or anorexic, especially when this is accompanied by vomiting or diarrhoea. An adequate fluid intake is encouraged by offering small amounts of favoured fluids at frequent intervals and by providing salty foods, if allowed. If diarrhoea is present, high-carbohydrate liquids are avoided because they may aggravate the diarrhoea by an osmotic effect. Also, replacing abnormal losses with plain water, which may worsen the electrolyte imbalance, is not advocated. Fluids should not be forced, and the child should not be wakened from rest to take fluids. Gentle persuasion with preferred drinks will usually meet with success. Using play techniques can also be very effective (see Box 8-3).

It is better to work with preferred food choices than with selections that children rarely eat. Box 8-7 lists different ways in which children may be encouraged to eat.

An understanding of children's feeding habits can also increase food consumption. For example, if they are presented with large portions, they often push the food away because the amount overwhelms them. If young children are not supervised during mealtime, they tend to play with the food rather than eat it.

Once the child is feeling better, appetite usually begins to improve. It is best to take advantage of any hungry period by serving high quality foods and snacks. If the child still refuses to eat, nutritious fluids, such as prepared breakfast drinks, should be encouraged. Parents can be very helpful by bringing these food items from home. This is especially important if the family's cultural eating habits differ from the hospital's food services.

Regardless of the type of diet, charting the amount consumed is an important nursing responsibility. Descriptions must be detailed and accurate, such as '120 ml of orange juice, no bacon, and 240 ml of milk'. Comments such as 'ate well' or 'ate poorly' are inadequate. If parents are involved in the child's care, they should be encouraged to keep a list of everything

---

◆ BOX 8-7

Guidelines for feeding the sick child

- Take a dietary history and use information to make eating time as much like home as possible.
- Encourage parents or other family members to feed child or to be present at mealtimes.
- Have children eat at tables in groups; bring nonambulatory children to eating area.
- Use familiar eating utensils, such as a favourite plate, cup, or bottle for small children.
- Make mealtimes pleasant; avoid any procedures immediately before or after eating; make sure child is rested and pain free.
- Have a nurse present at mealtimes to offer assistance, prevent disruptions, and praise children for their eating.
- Serve small, frequent meals rather than three large meals or serve three meals and nutritious between-meal snacks.
- Bring in foods from home, especially if food preparation is very different from hospital's; consider cultural differences.
- Provide finger foods for young children.
- Involve children in food selection and preparation whenever possible.
- Serve small portions, and serve each course separately, such as soup first, followed by meat, potatoes, and vegetables, and ending with dessert; with young children camouflage size of food by cutting meat thicker so less appears on plate or by folding a cheese slice in half; offer second helpings; ensure a variety of foods, textures, and colours.
- Provide food selections that are favourites of most children, such as hamburgers, pizza, spaghetti, chicken, and fruit yoghurt.
- Avoid foods that are highly seasoned, have strong odours, are served hot, or are all mixed together, unless typical of cultural practices.
- Provide fluid selections that are favourites of most children, such as fruit juice, cola, ginger ale, sweetened tea, ice cream, milk and milkshakes, pudding, or creamed soups.
- Offer nutritious snacks, such as frozen yoghurt or pudding, ice cream, biscuits, hot cocoa, cheese slices, pieces of raw vegetable or fruit, and dried fruit or cereal.
- Make food attractive and different, for example:
  Serve a 'picnic lunch' in a paper bag.
  Pack food in a Chinese-food container; decorate container.
    Put a 'face' or a 'flower' on a hamburger or sandwich with pieces of vegetable.
  Use a pastry cutter to shape a sandwich.
  Serve pudding, yoghurt, or juice frozen as an iced lolly.
  Serve fluids through brightly coloured or unusually shaped straws.
  Make 'bowtie' sandwiches by cutting them in triangles and placing two points together.
  Slice sandwiches into 'fingers'.
  Grate mounds of cheese.
  Cut apples horizontally to make circles.
  Break uncooked spaghetti into toothpick lengths and skewer cheese, cold meat, vegetables, or fruit chunks.
- Praise children for what they do eat.
- Do *not* punish children for not eating by removing their sweet or putting them to bed.

---

eaten. Using a pre-measured cup for fluids ensures a more accurate estimate of intake. Behaviours associated with mealtime also identify possible factors influencing appetite. For example, the observation, 'Child eats well when with other children, but plays with food if left alone in room', helps the nurse plan mealtime activities that stimulate the appetite.

CONTROLLING ELEVATED TEMPERATURES

An elevated temperature is one of the most common symptoms of illness in children.

Most pyrexias in children are of viral origin, are of relatively brief duration, and have limited consequences. In addition, there is mounting evidence that fever plays a role in enhancing the development of both specific and nonspecific immunity and aiding recovery and survival from infection.

THERAPEUTIC MANAGEMENT

The principal reason for treating a pyrexia is the relief of discomfort. Relief measures include pharmacological and/or environmental intervention. The most effective intervention is the use of antipyretics. Paracetamol is the preferred drug.

The temperature is usually retaken 30 minutes after the antipyretic is given to assess its effect, but should not be repeatedly measured. The child's level of discomfort is the best indication for continued treatment.

Environmental measures to reduce pyrexia may be used if they are tolerated by the child and if they do not induce shivering, because compensatory shivering greatly increases metabolic requirements above those already caused by the pyrexia.

Traditional cooling measures, such as minimum clothing, exposing the skin to the air, reducing room temperature, increasing air circulation, and cool moist compresses to the skin (e.g., the forehead), are effective if employed approximately one hour *after* an antipyretic is given, so the set point is lowered.

Convulsions associated with a fever occur in 3-4% of all children, usually in those between three months and five years of age. Although most children never have febrile after the first occurrence, a younger age at onset and a family history of febrile convulsions seizures are associated with recurring episodes (Hardman, 1990).

FAMILY TEACHING AND HOME CARE

Nurses have a unique opportunity to teach the family about health care practices while the child is hospitalized. The daily bath, handwashing before meals and after bowel and bladder evacuation, and conscientious dental hygiene should be taught, by example, during routine care. Clean hair, nails, and clothing, as well as good grooming, should be emphasized as essential to a pleasing appearance.

While sick children's appetites may be poor and not characteristic of their home eating habits, the hospital stay provides numerous opportunities for nurses to assess the family's knowledge of good nutrition and to implement teaching as needed to improve nutritional intake.

Parents should know how to take the child's temperature, read the thermometer accurately, and have guidelines for seeking professional care. Some of the newer temperature-measuring devices, such as plastic strip or digital thermometers, may be better suited for home use. If the use of paracetamol is indicated, the parents need instruction in administering the drug. It is important to emphasize accuracy in both the amount of drug given and the time intervals at which the drug is administered. As children grow, the dosage needs to be recalculated. To ensure the correct dose, parents should be advised to read the instructions on the bottle.

SAFETY

Children have special characteristics that require great concern for safety. It is the responsibility of everyone who comes into contact with them to maintain protective measures throughout their hospital stay. A report by the Child Accident Prevention Trust and the Royal College of Nursing highlighted the fact that children in hospital have accidents, many of which are preventable (CAPT, 1992). Nurses need a good understanding of the age level at which each child is operating and must plan for safety, accordingly.

Name bands are particularly important for children in the paediatric age group. Infants and unconscious patients are unable to tell or respond to their names. Toddlers may answer to any name or to a nickname only. Older children may exchange places, give an erroneous name, or choose not to respond to their own names as a form of joke, unaware of the hazards of such practices.

INFECTION CONTROL

The need for medical asepsis and appropriate barrier precautions to reduce the risk of nosocomial (hospital associated) infections is essential in caring for children. In addition, children may not have developed good hygiene habits, such as handwashing after toileting. Young children are especially at risk for infection because of their high oral activity. Children in nappies present infection risks if caregivers do not practise meticulous cleaning techniques.

Nurses must ensure they thoroughly understand the different policies which relate to the control of infection. Units should have clear policies and continuing education programmes which address infection control for health care professionals and for visitors, such as families (RCN, 1990).

While the principles of infection control should be universal, different units may interpret them differently. Nurses who move from one area to another, such as students, should therefore receive appropriate education to ensure they maintain adequate precautions.

ENVIRONMENTAL FACTORS

All the environmental safety measures for the protection of adults apply to children as well. Electrical equipment should be maintained in good working order, used only by personnel familiar with its use, and should not be in contact with moisture or near baths. Beds of ambulatory patients should be locked in place and at a height that allows easy access to the floor. Staff members should practise proper care and disposal of small breakable items, such as thermometers and bottles, and know a well-organized fire plan.

All windows should be securely screened, and lifts and stairways made safe. Ideally, electrical outlets should be provided with covers to prevent burns in small children, whose exploratory activities may extend to inserting objects into the small openings. Bath water temperature should be carefully checked before placing the child in it, and children must never be left alone in a bath.

Furniture is safest when it is scaled to the child's proportions, is sturdy, and is well balanced to prevent its being easily tipped over. Infants and small children must be securely strapped into infant seats and feeding chairs. Infants, young children, and those who are weak, paralyzed, agitated, confused, sedated, or cognitively impaired should never be left unattended on treatment tables, on scales, or in treatment areas.

Cot sides should be kept up and fastened securely unless an adult is at the bedside. It is safer to leave cot sides up, even when the cot is unoccupied. Anyone attending an infant or small child in a cot with the sides down should never turn away without maintaining hand contact with the child (see Fig. 8-1). Banco and Powers (1988) reported that falls from cots by infants tended to occur when siderails had carelessly been left down. Children in beds, however, tended to fall, despite raised siderails, by climbing over them.

TOYS

Toys have a vital role in the everyday life of children, and they are no less important in the hospital setting. Toys should be appropriate to the child's age, condition, and treatment. Toys should be inspected to make certain they are nonallergenic, washable and unbreakable, and that they have no small, removable parts that can be aspirated or swallowed or that can otherwise inflict injury to a child.

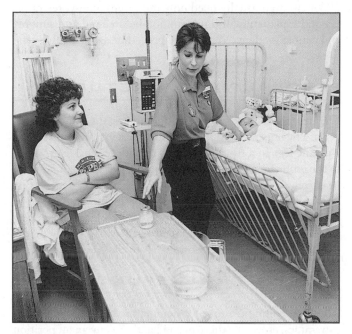

Fig. 8-1 Nurse maintains hand contact when back is turned. (Courtesy of Southampton University Hospitals Trust)

LIMIT-SETTING

Setting limits is essential to a child's safety. Children must understand where they are permitted to go and what they are permitted to do in the hospital. These limitations should be made clear to them, consistently enforced, and repeated as frequently as necessary to make certain that they are understood. Normally, active older children often become restless when their activity is restricted. Children in hospital require surveillance; appropriate tension-reducing activities can be planned and supervised by nurses and/or by the play therapist.

TRANSPORTING INFANTS AND CHILDREN

Infants and children usually need to be transported within the unit and to areas outside the paediatric unit. It is ordinarily safe to carry infants and small children for short distances within the ward. It is important that infants are well supported when being carried (Fig. 8-2). For more extended trips, the child should be securely transported in a suitable conveyance.

Infants can be transported to other areas in their bassinet or cot. Prams are sometimes used for infants who are not likely to stand up. Pushchairs and wheeled feeding chairs are also convenient transporters in some situations.

The method of transporting children is determined by their age, condition, and destination. Most older children are safe in wheelchairs. Younger children can be transported in their cot, on a trolley with raised sides, or in a wheelchair.

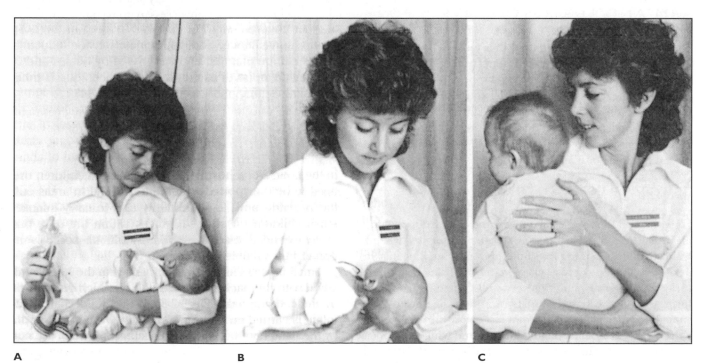

A   **B**   **C**

Fig. 8-2 Transporting infants. A, Infant's thigh firmly grasped in nurse's hand. B, Under arm hold. C, Back supported.

THE USE OF RESTRAINTS

Some method of restraint may be needed to ensure a child's safety or comfort, to facilitate examination, or to carry out procedures. Restraint can often be avoided with adequate preparation of the child, parental or staff supervision of the child, and adequate protection of a vulnerable site, such as an infusion device.

When a child must be restrained, the child and parents need a simple explanation. Alternative methods may be devised to replace the need for passive restraints. Holding children for periods is a pleasant alternative, as is restraining them in a highchair, where they can observe nearby activities. If feasible, distraction techniques, such as play and reading, can be used to gain the child's cooperation without resorting to restraints. Parental participation is always encouraged.

MUMMY RESTRAINT

When an infant or small child requires short-term restraint for examination or treatment that involves the head and neck (e.g., venepuncture, throat examination, nasogastric feeding), the mummy device effectively controls the child's movements. A blanket or sheet is opened on the bed or cot with one corner folded to the centre. The infant is placed on the blanket with shoulders at the fold and feet towards the opposite corner. Safety pins can be used to fasten the blanket in place at any step in the process.

To modify the mummy restraint for chest examination, the folded edge of the blanket is brought over each arm and under the back, after which the loose edge is folded over and secured at a point below the chest to allow visualization and access to the chest.

ARM AND LEG RESTRAINTS

Occasionally, one or more extremities must be restrained or limited in motion. When this type of restraint is used, it must be appropriate to the child's size; it must be padded to prevent undue pressure, constriction, or tissue injury; and the extremity must be observed frequently for signs of irritation or impaired circulation. The ends of the restraints are never tied to the cot rails, since lowering the rail will disturb the extremity and may hurt or injure the child.

ELBOW RESTRAINT

Sometimes, it is important to prevent the child from reaching his or her head or face; for example, after lip surgery, when a scalp vein infusion is in place, or to prevent scratching in skin disorders. For this purpose, elbow restraints, fashioned from a variety of materials, function very well. The most common form of elbow restraint consists of a piece of muslin long enough to reach comfortably from just below the axilla to the wrist, with a number of vertical pockets into which a wooden spatula inserted. The restraint is wrapped around the arm and secured with tapes or pins. It may be necessary to pin the top of the restraint to the undershirt sleeve to prevent the restraint

from slipping. Similar restraints can be made from readily available items.

POSITIONING FOR PROCEDURES

Infants and small children are unable to cooperate for many procedures; therefore, the nurse is responsible for minimizing their movement and discomfort with proper positioning. Older children usually need only minimum, if any, restraint. Careful explanation and preparation beforehand and support and simple guidance during the procedure, are usually sufficient.

FEMORAL VENEPUNCTURE

Frequently used sites for venepuncture are the large femoral veins. The nurse restrains the infant by placing the child supine with the legs in a frog position to provide extensive exposure of the groin area. Both the arms and the legs of the infant can be effectively controlled by the nurse's forearms and hands (Fig. 8-3). Only the side used for the venepuncture is uncovered so that the operator is protected should the child urinate during the procedure. Pressure is applied to the site after the withdrawal of blood to prevent oozing from the site.

EXTREMITY VENEPUNCTURE

The most common sites of venepuncture are the veins of the extremities, especially the arm and hand. A convenient position for restraint is having one person on either side of the bed. The child's outstretched arm is partially stabilized by the person taking the blood. It is rarely necessary to restrain a child for extremity venepuncture. The procedure is performed following therapeutic play intervention (Fig. 8-4).

LUMBAR PUNCTURE

Children are usually controlled best in the side-lying position, with the head flexed and the knees drawn up towards the chest. Even cooperative children need to be restrained to prevent possible trauma from unexpected, involuntary movement. They can be reassured that, although they are trusted, the restraint will serve as a reminder to maintain the desired position. It also provides a measure of support and reassurance to them (Fig. 8-5, A).

An alternative position, used with small infants and some older children, is the sitting position. The child is placed with the buttocks at the edge of the table and with the neck flexed so that the chin rests on the chest. The infant's arms and legs are immobilized by the nurse's hands (Fig. 8-5, B).

Specimens and spinal fluid pressure are obtained, measured, and sent for analysis. Vital signs are taken as ordered, and the child is observed for any changes in level of consciousness, motor activity, or other neurological signs. Postlumbar puncture headache may occur and is related to postural changes; this is

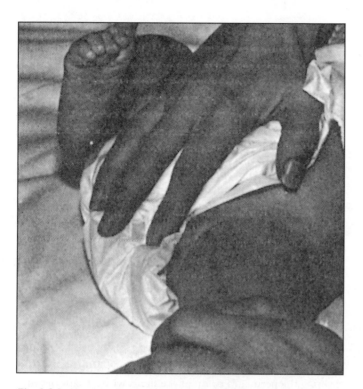

Fig. 8-3 Restraining infant for femoral venepuncture.

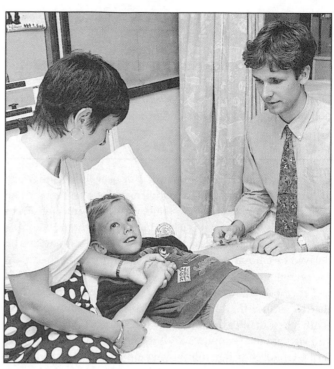

Fig. 8-4 Therapeutic play intervention for extremity venepuncture. (Courtesy of Southampton University Hospitals Trust)

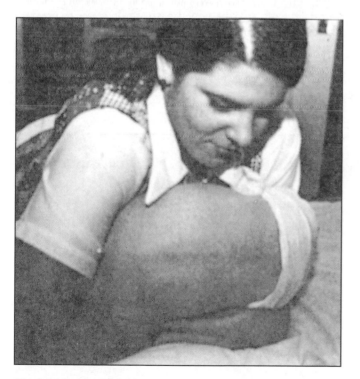

Fig. 8-5A Position for lumbar puncture, lying on side.

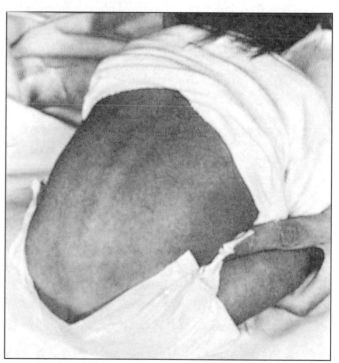

Fig. 8-5B Position for lumbar puncture, sitting.

less severe when the child lies flat. Headache is seen much less frequently in young children than in adolescents.

BONE MARROW ASPIRATION/BIOPSY

Position for a bone marrow aspiration or biopsy depends on the location of the chosen site. In children, the posterior or anterior iliac crest is most frequently used, although in infants the tibia may be selected because of easy access to the site and restraint of the child.

COLLECTION OF SPECIMENS

Older children are able to cooperate if given proper instruction regarding what is expected from them.

URINE SPECIMENS

Children admitted to the hospital or seen in a clinic may require a urine specimen as a routine diagnostic procedure. The presence of menses may be an embarrassment or a concern to teenage girls; therefore it is a good idea to ask them about this and make adjustments as necessary. The specimen can be delayed or a notation made on the laboratory slip to explain the presence of red blood cells.

Preschool children and toddlers are less cooperative, primarily because they are usually unable to void on request. It is often best to offer them water or other liquids that they enjoy and wait about 30 minutes until they are ready to void voluntarily. Children will better understand what is expected if the nurse uses familiar terms for the function, such as 'wee wee'. Some will have difficulty voiding in an unfamiliar receptacle. Potties or a bedpan placed on the toilet are usually satisfactory. Toddlers who have recently acquired bladder control may be especially reluctant. A useful approach is to enlist the help of parents; they are likely to be successful, and this helps them to feel a part of the child's care.

For infants and toddlers who are not toilet trained, special urine collection devices are used. These devices are clear plastic, single-use bags with self-adhering material around the opening at the point of attachment. To prepare the infant, the genitalia, perineum, and surrounding skin are washed and dried thoroughly. The collection bag is easiest to apply if attached first to the perineum, progressing to the symphysis (Fig. 8-6). With females, the perineum is stretched taut during application to that area to ensure a leak-proof fit. With males, the penis and scrotum are placed inside the bag. The adhesive portion of the bag must be firmly applied to the skin all around the genital area to avoid possible leakage. The nappy is carefully replaced. The bag should be checked frequently and removed as soon as the specimen is available, since the moist bag may become loosened on an active child.

CLEAN-CATCH SPECIMENS

Clean-catch specimens traditionally refer to urine samples obtained for culture after the urethral meatus is cleaned and the first few millilitres of urine are voided before the urine is collected (midstream specimen). The procedure consists of cleaning the perineum or tip of the penis with a soap- or antiseptic-soaked sterile pad, and in females wiping from front to back only once with each pad. This is repeated at least two times. The area may be wiped with sterile water to prevent accidental contamination of the urine with a solution that may destroy the pathogens.

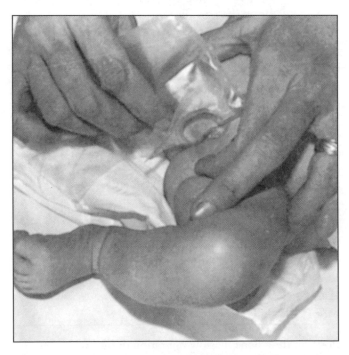

Fig. 8-6A Application of urine collection bag. For female infants, adhesive portion is applied to exposed and dried perineum first.

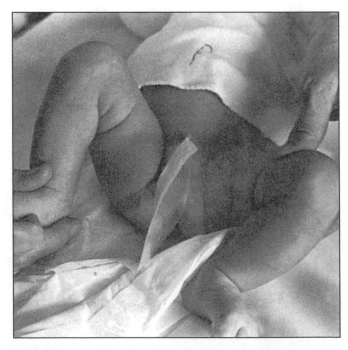

Fig. 8-6B Application of urine collection bag. Bag adheres firmly around perineal area to prevent urine leakage.

TWENTY-FOUR-HOUR COLLECTION

The need to collect urine voided over a 24-hour period creates a special challenge in infants and children. Collection bags are required in infants and small children. Older children require special instruction about notifying someone when they need to void or have a bowel movement so that urine can be collected separately and not discarded. Some older school-aged children and adolescents can be trusted to take responsibility for collection of their own 24-hour specimens.

Infants and small children who are bagged for 24-hour urine collection require a special collection bag; frequent removal and replacement of adhesive collection devices can produce skin irritation. Plastic collection bags with collection tubes attached are ideal when the container must be left in place for a time. These can be connected to a collecting device or emptied periodically by aspiration with a syringe.

SPECIAL TECHNIQUES

Catheterization or *suprapubic aspiration* are employed when a specimen is urgently needed or when the child is unable to void or otherwise provide an adequate specimen. Catheterization is most often used when urethral obstruction or anuria caused by renal failure is believed to be the cause of the child's failure to void. Suprapubic aspiration is useful in clarifying the diagnosis of suspected urinary tract infection in acutely ill infants.

Most children are frightened of catheterization, and few small children are entirely cooperative; therefore even when the procedure is adequately explained, an assistant is needed to help restrain and reassure the child. Special care must be exercised when catheterizing young males to avoid trauma to the ductal and glandular openings into the urethra, which might result in sterility.

Suprapubic aspiration, which is performed by a doctor, involves aspirating bladder contents by inserting a needle in the midline approximately 1 cm above the symphysis and directed vertically downwards. The bladder should contain an adequate volume of urine. This can be assumed if the infant has not voided for at least 1 hour or the bladder can be palpated above the symphysis. This technique is especially useful for obtaining sterile specimens from young infants.

STOOL SPECIMENS

Stool specimens are frequently collected in children to identify parasites and other organisms that cause diarrhoea, to assess gastrointestinal function, and to check for occult (hidden) blood. Ideally, the stool should be collected without contamination with urine. An ample amount of stool is collected and placed in the appropriate container, which is covered and labelled. If several specimens are needed, the containers are marked with the date and time and kept in a specimen refrigerator. Special care is exercised in handling the specimen because of the risk of contamination.

BLOOD SPECIMENS

Most blood specimens are obtained by the laboratory staff or doctors. However, whether the specimen is collected by the nurse or others, the nurse is responsible for ensuring that specimens, such as serial examinations and fasting specimens, are collected on time and that the proper equipment is available, such as correct collection tubes and ice for blood gas samples.

The best method for taking peripheral blood samples from infants is by a heel prick. Before the blood sample is taken, the heel is warmed to dilate the vessels in the area. The area is cleansed with alcohol and, with the infant's foot firmly restrained with the free hand, the heel is punctured with a disposable blood lancet.

The most serious complication of infant heel puncture is necrotizing osteochondritis from lancet penetration of the underlying calcaneus bone. To avoid this, the puncture should be no deeper than 2.4 mm and should be made at the outer aspect of the heel. The boundaries of the calcaneus can be marked by an imaginary line extending posteriorly from a point between the fourth and fifth toes and running parallel to the lateral aspect of the heel and another line extending posteriorly from the middle of the great toe and running parallel to the medial aspect of the heel (Fig. 8-7).

The needed specimens are quickly collected, and pressure is applied to the puncture site with a dry gauze square until bleeding stops. The site is then covered with a plaster. In young children, 'spot' plasters pose an aspiration hazard; their use should be avoided, or the plaster should be removed as soon as the bleeding stops.

No matter how or by whom the specimen is collected, children, even some older ones, fear the loss of their blood. Explaining to them that their blood is continually being produced by their bodies provides them with a measure of reassurance regarding this aspect of the stress-provoking procedure.

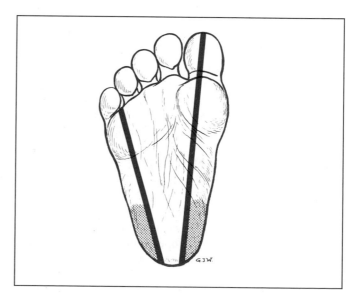

Fig. 8-7 Puncture site (red stippled area) on sole of infant's foot.

When the blood is drawn, a simple comment such as, 'Just look how red it is. You're really making a lot of nice red blood', confirms this information and gives them an opportunity to express their concern. A plaster gives them added assurance that the vital fluids will not leak out through the puncture site.

Children also dislike the discomfort associated with venous, arterial, or capillary punctures. In fact, children have identified these procedures as the ones most frequently causing pain during hospitalization and arterial punctures as being one of the most painful of all procedures experienced (Wong and Baker, 1988). Younger children are more distressed by venepuncture than are older children (Fradet *et al.,* 1990).

RESPIRATORY SECRETION SPECIMENS

Collection of sputum or nasal discharge is sometimes required for diagnosis of respiratory infections. Older children and adolescents are able to cough as directed and supply sputum specimens when given proper directions. It must be made clear to them that a coughed specimen, not mucus cleared from the throat, is needed. Infants and small children are unable to follow directions to cough; therefore gastric washings (lavage) may be used to collect a specimen. Sometimes a satisfactory specimen can be obtained by using a suction device such as a mucous trap if the catheter is inserted into the trachea and the cough reflex elicited. Other respiratory secretion collection methods include nasopharyngeal swabs (to diagnose *Bordetella pertussis*) and throat cultures.

ADMINISTRATION OF MEDICATION

Children vary widely in age, weight, surface area, and the ability to absorb, metabolize, and excrete medications. Nurses must be particularly alert when computing and administering drugs to infants and children.

DETERMINING DRUG DOSAGE

It is the doctor's responsibility to prescribe drugs in the correct dosage to achieve the desired effect without endangering the child's health. However, nurses must understand the safe dosage of medications they administer to children as well as the expected action, possible side effects, and signs of toxicity (UKCC, 1989).

PREPARATION FOR SAFE ADMINISTRATION

The ability to calculate fractional doses from larger dosages is absolutely essential. In addition, measuring doses, identifying patients, and gaining cooperation create problems not usually encountered in giving medications to adults.

CHECKING DOSAGE

Administering the correct dosage of a drug is a shared responsibility between the doctor who orders the drug and the nurse who carries out that order. Children react with unexpected severity to some drugs, and ill children may be especially sensitive to drugs. Therefore, checking the dose if there is any doubt about its accuracy is a professional duty. When a dose is ordered that is outside the usual range, or if there is some question regarding the preparation or the route of administration, the nurse should always check with the doctor before proceeding with the administration, since the nurse is legally liable for any drug administered (UKCC, 1989).

Many hospitals where medications are given to children have regulations requiring that drugs be double-checked.

IDENTIFICATION

Before the administration of any medication, the child must be correctly identified. Parents may be present to identify their child, but the only safe method for identifying children is to check their hospital identification bands with the medication card.

PARENTS

Parents can be useful sources of information regarding the child and his or her capabilities. Nearly all parents have given some type of medication to their child and can describe the approaches they have found to be successful. They can also provide information regarding the child's reaction to similar experiences. In some cases it is less traumatic for the child if a parent gives the medication, provided the nurse prepares the medication and supervises its administration and the practice is consistent with hospital or ward policy.

CHILD

Every child requires psychological preparation for parenteral administration of medication and supportive care during the procedure. Even if children have received several injections, they rarely become accustomed to the discomfort and have as much right to understanding and patience from those involved in giving the injection as any other child.

ORAL ADMINISTRATION

The oral route is preferred for administering medications to children whenever possible. Because of the ease of administration of oral medications – most are dissolved or suspended in liquid preparations. There is danger of aspiration in any oral preparation, but solid forms (pills, tablets, capsules) are especially hazardous if their administration causes extreme resistance or crying.

Most paediatric medications come in palatable and colourful preparations for added ease of administration. Some have a slightly unpleasant aftertaste, but the majority of children will swallow these liquids with little if any resistance. The nurse should taste a very small amount of an oral preparation to ascertain if it is palatable or bitter. In this way, legitimate complaints of dislike from the child can be accepted and the taste camouflaged whenever possible.

PREPARATION

The devices available to measure medicines are not always sufficiently accurate for measuring the small amounts needed in children's nursing practice. Many medications are supplied with caps or droppers designed to measure each specific preparation. These are accurate when used to measure that specific medication, but are not reliable for measuring other liquids. Emptying dropper contents into a medicine cup invites additional error. Since some of the liquid clings to the sides of the cup, a significant amount of the drug can be lost.

The most accurate means for measuring small amounts of medication is the plastic disposable syringe. Not only does the syringe provide a reliable measure, but it also serves as a convenient means for transporting and administering the medication. The medication can be placed directly into the child's mouth from the syringe.

Young children, and some older children, have difficulty swallowing tablets or pills. Since several drugs are not available in paediatric preparations, the tablet will need to be crushed before it can be given to these children. However, not all drugs can be crushed; for example, medication with an enteric or protective coating or formulated for slow release.

Since paediatric doses often require dividing adult preparations of medication, the nurse may be faced with the dilemma of accurate dosage. With tablets, only those that are scored can be halved or quartered accurately.

ADMINISTRATION

While administering liquids to infants is relatively easy, care must be observed to prevent aspiration. With the infant held in a semireclining position, the medication is placed in the mouth from a spoon, plastic cup, plastic dropper, or plastic syringe (without needle). The dropper or syringe is best placed along the side of the infant's tongue and administered slowly in small amounts, waiting for the child to swallow.

Medicine cups can be used effectively for older infants who are able to drink from a cup. Because of the natural outward tongue thrust in infancy, medications may need to be retrieved from lips or chin and readministered. Medication should not be added to the infant's formula feeding.

The young child who refuses to cooperate or resists consistently despite explanation and encouragement, may require mild physical coercion. This should be carried out quickly and carefully. Every effort should be made to determine why the child resists, and the reasons for this alternative should be explained in such a way that the child will know it is being carried out for his or her well-being and is not a form of punishment. There is always a risk in using even mild forceful techniques. A crying child can aspirate a medication, particularly when lying on his or her back. If the nurse holds the child in the lap with the child's right arm behind the nurse, the left hand firmly grasped by the nurse's left hand, and the head securely restrained between the nurse's arm and body, the medication can be slowly poured into the child's mouth (Fig. 8-8).

INTRAMUSCULAR ADMINISTRATION

Injections, including intramuscular (IM), intradermal, subcutaneous, and intravenous (IV), constitute some of the most traumatic health-related experiences for children. No one likes an injection, especially young children, who may associate the procedure with other meanings such as fear of body mutilation and punishment. Consequently, injections are given only when the drug cannot be given by any other route.

SELECTING SYRINGE AND NEEDLE

The volume of medication prescribed for small children and the small amount of tissue for injection require that a syringe be selected that can measure very small amounts of solution. For volumes less than 1 ml, a syringe, calibrated in one-hundredth increments, is appropriate.

The needle length must be sufficient to penetrate the subcutaneous tissue and deposit the medication into the body of the muscle. Needle gauge should be as small as possible to deliver the fluid safely. Small gauges (25 to 30) cause the least discomfort, but larger sizes are needed for viscous medication and when longer length needles are used (to prevent accidental bending).

DETERMINING SITE

Factors that are considered when selecting a site for an IM injection on an infant or child include:
- The amount and character of the medication to be injected.
- The amount and general condition of the muscle mass.
- The frequency or number of injections to be given during the course of treatment.
- The type of medication being given.
- Factors that may impede access to or cause contamination of the site.
- The ability of the child to assume the required position safely.

Older children and adolescents usually pose few problems in selecting a suitable site for IM injections, but infants, with their small and underdeveloped muscles, have fewer available sites. It is sometimes difficult to assess the amount of fluid that can be injected safely into a single site. Usually 1 ml is the maximum volume that should be administered in a single site to small children and older infants. The muscles of small infants may not tolerate more than 0.5 ml. The larger the amount of solution, the larger the muscle into which it must be injected.

Injections must be placed in muscles large enough to accommodate the medication, but major nerves and blood vessels must be avoided. There is no universal agreement regarding the best IM injection site for children. Nurses should follow the current policy for the unit they are working in.

ADMINISTRATION

Although injections that are executed with care seldom produce trauma to the child, there have been reports of serious disability related to IM injections in children. Repeated use of a single site has been associated with fibrosis of the muscle with subsequent muscle contracture. Injections close to large nerves, such as the sciatic nerve, have been responsible for permanent disability, especially when potentially neurotoxic drugs are administered. One of the difficulties in administering the opaque preparations is that aspirated blood cannot be detected at the bottom of the syringe, thus increasing the risk of injecting into a blood vessel. When such drugs are injected, great care must be used in locating the correct site.

Most children are unpredictable and few are totally cooperative when receiving an injection. Even children who appear to be relaxed and constrained can lose control under the stress of the procedure. It is advisable to have someone available to help restrain the child, if needed. Since children often jerk or pull away unexpectedly, it is a good idea to carry an extra capped needle to exchange for a contaminated one so that delay is minimized. The child, even a small one, is told that he or she is receiving an injection, and then the procedure is carried out as quickly and skilfully as possible to avoid prolonging the stressful experience. Delay caused by lengthy explanations, attempts to hide the syringe from sight, or efforts to soothe the child will only increase anxiety.

Small infants offer little resistance to injections. Although they squirm and may be difficult to hold in position, they can usually be restrained without assistance. The muscle mass of the thigh to be injected is firmly grasped in one hand to stabilize the limb and compress the muscle mass for injection with the other hand. The body of a larger infant can be securely restrained between the nurse's arm and body.

If medication is given around the clock, the nurse must be careful to wake the child before giving the injection. Although it may seem easier to surprise the sleeping child and do it as quickly as possible, performing the procedure in this way can cause the child to fear going back to sleep. If awakened first, children will know that nothing will be done to them unless forewarned.

INTRAVENOUS ADMINISTRATION

The IV route for administering medications is frequently used. For some important drugs it is the only effective route of administration. This method is used for giving drugs to children who have poor absorption as a result of diarrhoea, dehydration, or peripheral vascular collapse; children who need a high serum concentration of a drug; children who have resistant infections that require parenteral medication over an extended time; children who need continuous pain relief; and children who require emergency treatment.

Several factors need to be considered in relation to IV medication. When a drug is administered intravenously, the effect is almost instantaneous and further control is limited. Most drugs for IV administration require a specified minimum dilution and/or rate of flow, and many are highly irritating or toxic to tissues outside the vascular system. In addition to the precautions and nursing observations related to IV therapy, factors to consider when preparing and administering drugs to infants and children by the IV route include:

- Amount of drug to be administered.
- Minimum dilution of drug and whether child is fluid restricted.
- Type of solution in which drug can be diluted.
- Length of time over which drug can be safely administered.
- Rate of infusion that child and vessels can tolerate.
- IV tubing volume capacity.
- Time that this or another drug is to be administered.
- Compatibility of all drugs that child is receiving intravenously and compatibility with infusion fluids.

Before any IV infusion, the site of insertion is checked for patency. Medications are never administered with blood products. Only one antibiotic should be administered at a time.

When a drug is to be administered within a specific time, such as one hour, the infusion rate should take into account the volume of fluid in the tubing from the injection point that must infuse before the drug reaches the bloodstream. Therefore, the rate must always be considered to ensure that the entire dose is administered over the desired time.

For the very small infant or fluid-restricted child who is not able to tolerate the increased rate or fluids, the direct technique can be used. Although the medication must still be minimally diluted as recommended, the dose is administered closer to the child's vein, avoiding the need to infuse also the tubing volume.

For the *direct technique*, appropriately diluted medication is injected into the tubing at the site of the Y connection or through a stopcock in the direction of the child. A syringe pump may be used for a controlled rate. As syringe pumps become increasingly available, this method is being used more often for children because of convenience, greater control over administration time, and the need to flush with less fluid when administering medications.

NASOGASTRIC OR GASTROSTOMY ADMINISTRATION

When a child has an indwelling feeding tube or a gastrostomy, oral medications are usually given via that route. This should only be done with medicine which is in a liquid form or safe to crush (Box 8-8). An advantage of this method is the ability to administer oral medications around the clock without disturbing the child. A disadvantage is the risk of occluding or 'clogging' the tube, especially when giving viscous solutions through small-bore feeding tubes. The most important preventive measure is adequate flushing after the medication is instilled (Williams, 1989).

RECTAL ADMINISTRATION

The rectal route for administration is less reliable, but sometimes used when the oral route is difficult or contraindicated. Some of the drugs available in suppository form are sedatives, analgesics (morphine), and anti-emetics. The difficulty in using the rectal route is that, unless the rectal ampulla is empty at the time of insertion, the absorption of the drug may be delayed, diminished, or prevented by the presence of faeces. However, the rectal route can be used in children who are unable to take anything by mouth and are unlikely to have large amounts of stool. It is also used when oral preparations are unsuitable to control vomiting.

The suppository is lubricated with water-soluble jelly or warm water. Using a glove or finger cot, the suppository is quickly but gently inserted into the rectum, making certain that it is placed beyond both the rectal sphincters. The buttocks are then held together firmly to relieve pressure on the anal sphincter until the urge to expel the suppository has passed — five to ten minutes.

If medication is administered via a retention enema, the same procedure is used. Drugs given by enema are diluted in the smallest amount of solution possible, to minimize the likelihood of being evacuated.

OPTIC, OTIC, AND NASAL ADMINISTRATION

The major difficulty is in gaining children's cooperation or employing restraining techniques. The infant's or young child's head is immobilized. Older children need only explanation and direction. Although the administration of optic, otic, and nasal medication is not painful, these drugs can cause unpleasant sensations.

To instil eye medication, the child is placed supine or sitting with the head extended and is asked to look up. One hand is used to pull the lower lid downwards; the hand that holds the dropper rests on the head so that it may move synchronously with the child's head, thus reducing the possibility of trauma to a struggling child or dropping medication on the face (Fig. 8-8). As the lower lid is pulled down, a small conjunctival sac is formed; the solution or ointment is applied to this area, never directly on the eyeball. Another effective technique is to pull the lower lid down and out to form a cup effect, into which the medication is dropped.

The lids are gently closed to prevent expression of the medication, and the child is asked to look in all directions to enhance even distribution of the preparation. Excess medication is wiped from the inner canthus outward to prevent contamination to the contralateral eye.

Instilling eye drops in infants can be difficult because they often clench the lids tightly closed. One approach is to place the drops in the nasal corner where the lids meet. The medication pools in this area, and when the child opens the lids,

---

◆ **BOX 8-8**

Guidelines for nasogastric or gastrostomy medication administration in children

- Use elixir or suspension (rather than syrup) preparations of medication whenever possible.
- If administering tablets, crush tablet to a very fine powder and dissolve drug in a small amount of warm water. Never crush enteric-coated or sustained-release tablets or capsules.
- Avoid oily medications because they tend to cling to side of tube.
- Dilute viscous medication if possible.
- Do not mix medication with enteral formula unless fluid is restricted. If adding a drug:
  Check with pharmacist for compatibility.
  Shake formula well and observe for any physical reaction (e.g., separation, precipitation).
  Label formula container with name of medication, dosage, date, and time infusion started.
- Have medication at room temperature.
- Measure medication in calibrated cup.
- Check for correct placement of nasogastric tube.
- Attach syringe (with adaptable tip but without plunger) to tube.
- Pour medication into syringe.
- Unclamp tube and allow medication to flow by gravity.
- Adjust height of container to achieve desired flow rate (e.g., increase height for faster flow).
- As soon as syringe is empty, pour in water to flush tubing. Amount of water depends on length and gauge of tubing. Determine amount before administering any medication by using a syringe to completely fill an unused nasogastric tube with water. The amount of flush solution is usually 1 5 times this volume. With certain drug preparations (e.g., suspensions) more fluid may be needed.
- If administering more than one drug at the same time, flush the tube between each medication with clear water.
- Clamp tube after flushing, unless tube is left open.

the medication flows onto the conjunctiva. For young children, playing a game can be helpful, such as instructing the child to keep the eyes closed until the count of three, then to open them, at which time the drops are quickly instilled.

Ear drops are instilled with the child restrained in the supine position and the head turned to the appropriate side. For children younger than three years of age, the external auditory canal is straightened by gently pulling the pinna downwards and straight back. The pinna is pulled upwards and back in children older than three years of age. After instillation, the child should remain lying on side for a few minutes. Gentle massage of the area immediately anterior to the ear facilitates the entry of drops into the ear canal. The use of cotton pledgets prevents medication from flowing out of the external canal. However, they should be loose enough to allow any discharge to exit from the ear. Premoistening the cotton with a few drops of medication prevents the wicking action from absorbing the medication instilled in the ear.

Unpleasant sensations associated with medicated nose drops are minimized when care is taken to position the child with the head extended well over the edge of the bed or a pillow. Depending on their size, infants can be positioned in the nurse's arm with the head extended and stabilized between the nurse's body and elbow, and the arms and hands immobilized with the nurse's hands, or with the head extended over the edge of the bed or a pillow. Following instillation of the drops, the child should remain in position for one minute to allow the drops to come in contact with the nasal surfaces.

FAMILY TEACHING

The nurse usually assumes the responsibility for preparing families to administer medications at home. The family should have an understanding of why the child is receiving the medication and the effects that might be expected, as well as the amount, frequency, and length of time the drug is to be administered. Instruction should be carried out in an unhurried, relaxed manner, preferably in an area away from busy ward or office routine.

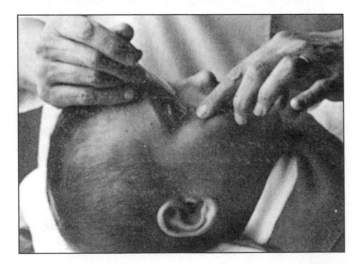

Fig. 8-8 Administering eye drops.

The caregiver is carefully instructed regarding the correct dosage, and the nurse is responsible for preparing parents for the specifics of the task. It is important to ascertain if they have acceptable devices for measuring the drug. If the drug is packaged with a dropper, syringe, or plastic cup, the nurse should show the point on the device that indicates the prescribed dose and demonstrate how the dose is drawn up into a dropper or syringe and measured, and how to eliminate bubbles. Ample time for instruction and practice must be allotted.

Home modifications are often necessary, because the availability of equipment or assistance can differ from the hospital setting. For example, restraint is often required when giving medications to children, and the parent may need guidance in devising methods that allow one person to restrain the child and safely give the drug.

The time that the drug is to be administered is clarified with the parent. When a drug is to be given several times during the day, together the nurse and parents can work out a schedule that accommodates the family routine. This is particularly significant if the drug must be given at equal intervals throughout a 24-hour period. For example, telling parents that the child needs one teaspoon of medicine four times a day is subject to misinterpretation, since parents may routinely schedule the doses at incorrect times. Instead, a preplanned schedule based on six-hour intervals should be set up with the number of days required for therapeutic dosage listed.

GASTRIC FEEDING TECHNIQUES

Some children are unable to take nourishment by mouth because of conditions such as anomalies of the throat, oesophagus, or bowel; impaired swallowing capacity; severe debilitation; respiratory distress; or unconsciousness. These children are frequently fed by way of a tube inserted nasally to the stomach or duodenum/jejunum, or by a tube inserted directly into the stomach (gastrostomy) or jejunum (jejunostomy). Such feedings may be intermittent or by continuous drip. During non-oral feedings, infants are given a dummy. Non-nutritive sucking has been shown to have several advantages, such as increased weight gain and decreased crying (Anderson, 1986). However, only dummies with a safe design must be used to prevent the possibility of aspiration.

When a child is concurrently receiving continuous-drip gastric or enteral feedings and parenteral (intravenous) therapy, the potential exists for inadvertent administration of the enteral formula through the circulatory system. The possibility for error increases when the parenteral solution is a fat emulsion, a milky appearing substance. Safeguards to prevent this potentially serious error include (Garvin and Franck, 1990):

- Using a separate, specifically designed enteral feeding pump mounted on a separate pole for continuous-feeding solutions.
- Labelling all tubing for continuous enteral feeding with brightly coloured tape or labels.
- Using specifically designed continuous-feeding bags to contain the solutions instead of parenteral equipment, such as a burette.

NASOGASTRIC FEEDING

Infants and children can be fed simply and safely by a tube passed into the stomach through either the nares or the mouth. The tube can be left in place or inserted and removed with each feeding. In older children, it is usually less traumatic to tape the tube securely in place between feedings. When this alternative is used, the tube should be removed and replaced with a new tube according to hospital policy and according to the type of tube used. Meticulous handwashing is practised during the procedure to prevent bacterial contamination of the feeding, especially during continuous-drip feedings.

PREPARATION

The equipment needed for gavage feeding includes:
- A suitable tube selected according to the size of the child and the viscosity of the solution being fed. Feeding tubes are available in silicone rubber, polyurethane, polyethylene, or polyvinylchloride. Polyurethane and silicone rubber tubes are smaller in diameter and more flexible than the others. These are often referred to as *small-bore tubes*.
- A receptacle for the fluid; for small amounts a 10-30 ml syringe barrel is satisfactory; for larger amounts a 50 ml syringe with a catheter tip is more convenient.
- A syringe to aspirate stomach contents and/or to inject air after the tube has been placed.
- Water or water-soluble lubricant to lubricate the tube; sterile water is used for infants.
- Paper or nonallergenic tape to mark the tube and to attach the tube to the infant's or child's cheek.
- A stethoscope to determine the correct placement in the stomach.
- The solution for feeding.

Not all feeding tubes are the same. Polyethylene and polyvinylchloride types lose their flexibility and need to be replaced frequently. The polyurethane and silicone rubber tubes are indwelling and remain flexible, so they can remain in place longer and are more comfortable. Use of these small-bore tubes for continuous feeding has greatly reduced the incidence of complications, such as pharyngitis, otitis media, and incompetence of the lower oesophageal sphincter. While the increased softness and flexibility of the tubes are advantages, they also cause disadvantages, such as difficult insertion, collapse of the tube during aspiration of gastric contents to test for correct placement, dislodgement during forceful coughing, and unsuitability for thick feedings (Moore and Green, 1985). Traditional methods for verifying placement are less reliable with the small-bore tubes (Metheny, 1988).

PROCEDURE

Infants will be easier to control if they are first wrapped in a mummy restraint. Care must be taken so that breathing is not compromised.

Whenever possible, the infant should be held during the procedure to associate the comfort of physical contact with the feeding. When this is not possible, feeding is carried out with the infant or child on the back or towards the right side, and the head and chest elevated. Feeding the child in a sitting position helps maintain the placement of the tube in the lowest position, thus increasing the likelihood of correct placement in the stomach.

The feeding tube can be passed through either the nose or the mouth. An indwelling tube is almost always placed through the nose; the tube is alternated between nares with each insertion to minimize irritation, chance of infection, and possible breakdown of mucous membranes from pressure that occurs over time.

Two important issues remain unresolved regarding gavage feeding: measuring the insertion distance and checking the tube placement. Two standard methods of measuring tube length for insertion are: (1) measuring from the nose to the bottom of the earlobe and then to the end of the xiphoid process or (2) measuring from the nose to the earlobe and then to a point midway between the xiphoid process and umbilicus (Fig. 8-9). However, research on using these methods in premature infants has found both placements to be too high. Until more definitive data are available, no method that results in a shorter distance than these methods should be used.

Unfortunately, 'bedside' methods used to verify the placement of the tube have serious shortcomings (Box 8-9). The only accurate method for testing tube placement is radiography, but this practice is not feasible before each feeding (Metheny, 1988). One method that appears promising is pH testing of aspirated fluid, since respiratory, gastric, and intestinal fluid have different pH (Metheny *et al.*, 1989). Until pH is studied further, especially in children, nurses need to use the traditional methods with an awareness of their limitations. If doubt exists regarding correct placement, the doctor should be consulted.

GASTROSTOMY FEEDING

Feeding by way of gastrostomy tube is a variation of tube feeding often used for children in whom passage of a tube through the mouth, pharynx, oesophagus, and cardiac sphincter of the stomach is contraindicated or impossible. It is also used to avoid the constant irritation of a nasogastric tube in children who require tube feeding over an extended period. The tube is inserted through the abdominal wall into the stomach about midway along the greater curvature and secured by a purse-string suture. The stomach is anchored to the peritoneum at the operative site. The tube used can be a Foley, wing-tip, or mushroom catheter. Immediately after surgery the catheter is left open and attached to gravity drainage for 24 hours or more.

Postoperative care of the wound site is directed towards prevention of infection and irritation. The area is cleansed and covered with a sterile dressing daily or as often as needed to keep the area dry. After healing occurs, meticulous care is needed to keep the area surrounding the tube clean and dry to prevent excoriation and infection. Care is exercised to prevent excessive pull on the catheter that might cause widening of the opening and subsequent leakage of highly irritating gastric juices.

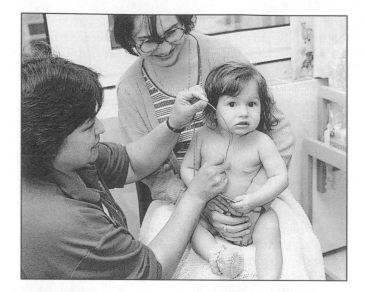

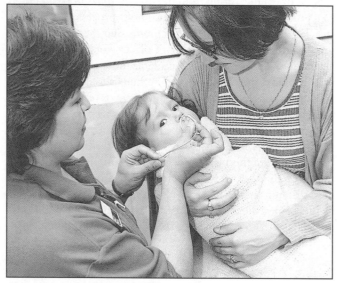

Fig. 8-9 Gavage feeding. Measuring tube for orogastric feeding from tip of nose to earlobe and to midpoint between end of xiphoid process and umbilicus (above). Inserting the tube (below). (Courtesy of Southampton University Hospitals Trust)

For children on long-term gastrostomy feeding, the recently developed skin level device (Button) offers several advantages. The small, flexible silicone device protrudes slightly from the abdomen, is cosmetically pleasing in appearance, affords increased comfort and mobility to the child, is easy to care for, and is fully immersible in water.

After feedings, the infant or child is positioned on the right side or in the Fowler position, and the tube may be left open and suspended, or clamped between feedings, depending on the child's condition (Fig. 8-10). A clamped tube allows more mobility but is only appropriate if the child can tolerate intermittent feedings without vomiting or prolonged backup of feeding into the tube. When the gastrostomy tube is no longer needed, it is removed; the skin opening usually closes spontaneously by contracture.

FAMILY TEACHING

When gastric tube feedings are needed for an extended period, the child may be discharged home before the tube is removed. The family will require appropriate instruction and preparation for performing the skill.

PROCEDURES RELATED TO ELIMINATION

Children seldom have problems with elimination, but in cases of severe constipation, or when an empty rectum is needed before surgery or diagnostic procedures, an enema may be administered to stimulate rectal emptying. Various conditions in the newborn and childhood period also require formation of an ostomy for purposes of elimination.

ENEMA

The prescribed isotonic solution is used in children. Plain water is not used because, being hypotonic, it can cause rapid fluid shift and fluid overload.

Since infants and young children are unable to retain the solution after it is administered, the buttocks must be held together for a short time to retain the fluid. The enema is administered and expelled while the child is lying with the buttocks over the bedpan and with the head and back supported by pillows. Older children are ordinarily able to hold the solution if they understand what to do and if they are not expected to hold it for too long. The nurse should have the bedpan handy or, for the ambulatory child, ensure that the

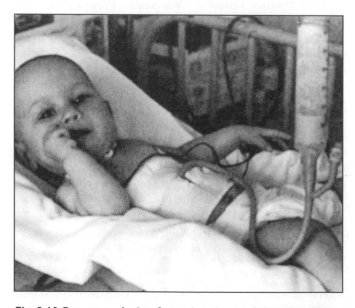

Fig. 8-10 Gastrostomy feeding. Syringe barrel suspended to allow thick formula to enter stomach by gravity. Note child sucking on thumb for oral gratification.

◆ BOX 8-9

Guidelines for nasogastric tube feedings in children

- Place the child supine with head slightly hyperflexed or in a sniffing position (nose pointed towards ceiling).
- Measure the tube for approximate length of insertion, and mark the point with a small piece of tape.
- Insert the tube that has been lubricated with sterile water or water-soluble lubricant through either the mouth or one of the nares to the predetermined mark. Since most young infants are obligatory nose breathers, insertion through the mouth causes less distress and helps to stimulate sucking. In older infants and children, the tube is passed through the nose and alternated between nostrils. An indwelling tube is almost always placed through the nose.

When using the nose, slip the tube along the base of the nose and direct it straight back toward the occiput.

When entering through the mouth, direct the tube toward the back of the throat (Fig. 8-15, *B*).

If the child is able to swallow on command, synchronize passing the tube with swallowing.

- Check the position of the tube by using *both* of the following:

Attach the syringe to the feeding tube and apply negative pressure. Aspiration of stomach contents indicates proper placement, but aspiration of respiratory secretions may be mistaken for stomach contents. However, absence of fluid is not necessarily evidence of improper placement. The stomach may be empty, or the tube may not be in contact with stomach contents. Note the amount and character of any fluid aspirated and return the fluid to the stomach.

With the syringe, inject a small amount of air (0.5 to 1 ml in premature or very small infants to 5 ml in larger children) into the tube while simultaneously listening with a stethoscope over the stomach area. Sounds of gurgling or growling will be heard if the tube is properly situated in the stomach, although it is possible to hear the air entering the stomach even when the tube is positioned above the gastroesophageal sphincter.

- Stabilize the tube by holding or taping it to the cheek, not to the forehead, because of possible damage to the nostril. To maintain correct placement, measure and record the amount of tubing extending from the nose or mouth to the distal port when the tube is first positioned. Recheck this measurement before each feeding.
- Warm the formula to room temperature. Pour formula into the barrel of the syringe attached to the feeding tube. To start the flow, give a gentle push with the plunger, but then remove the plunger and allow the fluid to flow into the stomach by gravity. The rate of flow should not exceed 5 ml every 5-10 minutes in premature and very small infants and 10 ml/minute in older infants and children to prevent nausea and regurgitation. The rate is determined by the diameter of the tubing and the height of the reservoir containing the feeding and is regulated by adjusting the height of the syringe. A usual feeding may take from 15-30 minutes to complete.
- Flush the tube with sterile water (1 or 2 ml for small tubes to 5 ml or more for large ones, or see discussion of flushing for administering medication through nasogastric tubes in Box 8-8 to clear it of formula.
- Cap or clamp indwelling tubes to prevent loss of feeding.

If the tube is to be removed, first pinch it firmly to prevent escape of fluid as the tube is withdrawn. Withdraw the tube quickly.

- Position the child on the right side or abdomen for at least 1 hour in the same manner as following any infant feeding to minimize the possibility of regurgitation and aspiration. If the child's condition permits, bubble the youngster after the feeding.
- Record the feeding, including the type and amount of residual, the type and amount of formula, and how it was tolerated. For most infant feedings, any amount of residual fluid aspirated from the stomach is refed to prevent electrolyte imbalance, and the amount is subtracted from the prescribed amount of feeding. For example, if the infant is to receive 30 ml and 10 ml is aspirated from the stomach before the feeding, the 10 ml of aspirated stomach contents is refed plus 20 ml of feeding.

---

bathroom is readily available before beginning the procedure. An enema is an intrusive procedure and thus threatening to the preschool child; therefore, a careful explanation is especially important to ease possible fear.

STOMAS

Children may require stomas for various health problems. The most frequent causes are necrotizing enterocolitis and imperforate anus in the infant, less often Hirschsprung disease. In the older child the most frequent causes are inflammatory bowel disease, especially Crohn's disease (regional enteritis),

and ureterostomies for distal ureter or bladder defects.

The major emphasis in paediatric care is the preparation of the child for the procedure and teaching care of the stoma to the child and family. Simple, straightforward language is most effective, together with the use of illustrations and a replica model; for example, drawing a picture of a child with a stoma on the abdomen and explaining it as 'another opening where bowel movements [or any other term the child uses] will come out.' At another time the nurse can draw a pouch over the opening to demonstrate how the contents are collected. Using a doll to demonstrate the process is an excellent teaching strategy.

Except in infants, an appliance is usually fitted immediately after surgery. Once an appliance is in place, drainage is directly measured from the collecting pouch. To measure colostomy drainage accurately before a collecting appliance is in place, the nurse weighs the dry dressing and reweighs it when wet. The difference in weight is calculated as fluid because 1 g equals 1 ml. If formed stool is passed, it is not weighed and calculated as part of fluid loss.

FAMILY TEACHING AND HOME CARE

Since these children are almost always discharged with a functioning colostomy, preparation of the family should begin as early as possible in the hospital. The family is instructed in the application of the device, care of the skin, and instructions regarding appropriate action in case skin problems develop. Early evidence of skin breakdown or stomal complications, such as ribbon-like stools, excessive diarrhoea, bleeding, prolapse, or failure to pass flatus or stool, is brought to the attention of the doctor, the nurse, or the stoma specialist.

KEY POINTS

◆ Most parents and children want to be together during stressful procedures and should be offered this opportunity, with guidance on how the parent can comfort the child.

◆ In giving postprocedural support, the nurse should encourage children to express their feelings and praise them for completion of the procedure.

◆ Assessment of compliance entails measuring factors that affect compliance (through clinical judgement, self-reporting, and direct observation), monitoring therapeutic response, taking pill counts, and performing chemical assay.

◆ Knowledge of the sick child's eating habits and favourite foods can help in maintaining adequate nutrition.

◆ Control of elevated temperatures may be accomplished, depending on cause, by pharmacological means (administration of antipyretics) and environmental means (minimum clothing, increased air circulation, cool compresses).

◆ Ensuring safety in the hospital setting is a major concern and can be achieved through environmental measures, infection control measures, limit-setting, and safe transportation.

◆ Family teaching regarding medication administration includes telling parents why the child is receiving the drug, its possible effects, and the amount, frequency, and length of time the drug is to be administered.

REFERENCES

Anderson GC: Pacifiers: the positive side, *MCN* 11(2):122, 1986.

Banco L, Powers A: Hospitals: unsafe environments for children, *Pediatr* 82(5):794, 1988.

Bates T, Broome M: Preparation of children for hospitalization and surgery: a review of the literature, *J Pediatr Nurs* 1(4):230, 1986.

Blum RW: Compliance with therapeutic regimens among children and youths. In Blum R, editor: *Chronic illness and disabilities in childhood and adolescence*, New York, 1984, Grune & Stratton.

Broome M, Lillis P, Smith M: Pain interventions in children: a meta-analysis of the research, *Nurs Res* 38(3):154, 1989.

Child Accident Prevention Trust: *Accidents to children on hospital wards*, London, 1992, CAPT.

Department of Health: *Children and young people in hospital*, London, 1991, HMSO.

Forlini J, Morin DM, Treacy S.: Painless peds procedures, *AJN* 87(3):321, 1987.

Fradet C *et al.*: A prospective survey of reactions to blood tests by children and adolescents, *Pain* 49(1):53, 1990.

Garvin G, Franck L: Preventing delivery of enteral formula via parenteral route, *Pediatr Nurs* 15(1):17, 1990.

Glasper A: Patients in the anaesthetic room: a blessing or a curse? In Glasper A, editor: *Child care: some nursing perspectives*, London, 1991, Wolfe.

Glasper EA, Thompson M: Preparing children for hospital admission. In Glasper EA, Tucker A, editors: *Advances in child health nursing*, London, 1993, Scutari Press.

Ghrishan FK: The transport of electrolytes in the gut and the use of oral rehydrating solutions, *Pediatr Clin North Am* 35(1):35, 1988.

Hardman M: Febrile convulsions, *J Paed Nurs* 2(4):12, 1990.

Children first: a study of hospital services, London, 1993, HMSO.

Korgaonkar G, Tribe D: Children and consent to medical treatment, *BMJ* 2(7):383, 1993.

McCall Smith A: Consent to treatment in childhood, *Arch Dis Child* 67(11):1247, 1992.

Metheny N: Measures to test placement of nasogastric and nasointestinal feeding tubes: a review, *Nurs Res* 37(6):324, 1988.

Metheny N *et al.*: Effectiveness of pH measurements in predicting feeding tube placement, *Nurs Res* 38(5):280, 1989.

Moore MC, Green HL: Tube feedings of infants and children, *Pediatr Clin North Am* 32(2):401, 1985.

Pidgeon V: Compliance with chronic illness regimens: school-aged children and adolescents, *J Pediatr Nurs* 4(1):36, 1989.

Rapoff MA: Helping parents to help their children comply with treatment regimens for chronic diseases, *Issues Compr Pediatr Nurs* 9(3):147, 1986.

Rollins J, Brantly D: Preparing the child for procedures. In Smith, DP et al, editors: *Comprehensive child and family nursing skills,* St Louis, 1991, Mosby–Year Book.

Royal College of Nursing *Standards of Care*: *Paediatric nursing,* London, 1990, Scutari.

United Kingdom Central Council: *Exercising accountability,* London, 1989, UKCC.

Williams PJ: How do you keep medicines from clogging feeding tubes? *Am J Nurs* 89(2):181, 1989.

Wong DL, Baker CM: Pain in children: comparison of assessment scales, *Pediatr Nurs* 14(1):9, 1988.

FURTHER READIING

Preparing for Procedures/Use of Play

Bates TA, Broome M: Preparation of children for hospitalization and surgery: a review of the literature, *J Pediatr Nurs* 1(4):230, 1986.

Collier J, Mackinley D: Play at work, *Child Health* 3(3):123, 1993.

Petrillo M, Sanger S: *Emotional care of hospitalized children,* ed 2, Philadelphia, 1980, JB Lippincott.

Price S: Preparing children for admission to hospital, *Nurs Times* 87(9):46, 1991.

Pridham KF, Adelson F, Hansen MF: Helping children deal with procedures in a clinic setting: a developmental approach, *J Pediatr Nurs* 2(1):13, 1987.

Waidley EK. Show and tell: preparing children for invasive procedures, *Am J Nurs* 85(7):811, 1985.

Surgical Procedures

Berde CB: Pediatric postoperative pain management, *Pediatr Clin North Am* 36(4):921, 1989.

Carter JH, Hancock J: Caring for children: how to ease them through surgery, *Nurs '88* 18(10):46, 1988.

Demarest DS, Hooke JF, Erickson MT: Preoperative intervention for the reduction of anxiety in pediatric surgery patients, *Child Health Care* 12(4):179, 1984.

Moushey R, Sinacore M, Diomede B: A perioperative teaching program: a collaborative process, *J Pediatr Nurs* 3(1):40, 1988.

Rushton CH: The surgical neonate: principles of nursing management, *Pediatr Nurs* 14(2):141, 1988.

Zeltzer LK, Jay SM, Fisher DM: The management of pain associated with pediatric procedures, *Pediatr Clin North Am* 36(4):941, 1989.

Compliance

Austin JK: Predicting parental anticonvulsant medication compliance using the theory of reasoned action, *J Pediatr Nurs* 4(2):88, 1989.

McHatton M: A theory for timely teaching, *Am J Nurs* 85(7):798, 1985.

Melnyk K: Barriers to care: operationalizing the variable, *Nurs Res* 39(2):108, 1990.

Miller A: When is the time ripe for teaching? *Am J Nurs* 85(7):801, 1985.

Russell FF, Mills BC, Zucconi T: Relationship of parental attitudes and knowledge to treatment adherence in children with PKU, *Pediatr Nurs* 14(6):514, 523, 1988.

Sallis JF: Improving adherence to pediatric therapeutic regimens, *Pediatr Nurs* 11(2):118, 1985.

Spicher CM, Yund C: Effects of preadmission preparation on compliance with home care instructions, *J Pediatr Nurs* 4(4):255, 1989.

Yoos L: Factors influencing maternal compliance to antibiotic regimens, *Pediatr Nurs* 10(2):141, 1984.

General Care and Hygiene/Fever

Burson JZ, Brannigan CN: The use of play in the nutritional support of hospitalized children, *Issues Compr Pediatr Nurs* 7(4-5):283, 1984.

Irwin M: Encourage oral intake—yes, but how? *Am J Nurs* 87(1):100, 1989.

Kilmon CA: Home management of children's fevers, *J Pediatr Nurs* 2(6):400, 1987.

Younger JB, Brown BS: Fever management: rational or ritual? *Pediatr Nurs* 11(1):26, 1985.

Safety/Collection of Specimens

Jackson MM et al.: Why not treat all body substances as infectious? *Am J Nurs* 87(9):1137, 1987.

Rutledge JC: Pediatric specimen collection for chemical analysis, *Pediatr Clin North Am* 36(1):37, 1989.

Administration of Medication

Beecroft PC, Redick S: Possible complications of intramuscular injections on the pediatric unit, *Pediatr Nurs* 15(4):333, 1989.

Birdsall C, Uretsky S: How do I administer medication by NG? *Am J Nurs* 84(10):1259, 1984.

Frank T, Fischer RG: What are some of the most common reasons for medication errors? *Pediatr Nurs* 10(4):294, 1984.

Raju TN et al.: Medication errors in neonatal and paediatric intensive-care units, *Lancet* 2(8659):374, 1989.

Rettig FM, Southby JR: Using different body positions to reduce discomfort during dorsogluteal injection, *Nurs Res* 31(4):219, 1982.

Royal College of Nursing: *Drug administration—a nursing responsibility,* London, 1987, RCN.

Gastric Feeding Techniques/Elimination

Paarlberg J, Balint JP: Gastrostomy tubes: practical guidelines for home care, *Pediatr Nurs* 11(2):99, 1985.

Smith DB: The ostomy: how is it managed? *Am J Nurs* 85(11):1246, 1985.

Wink DM: The physical and emotional care of infants with gastrostomy tubes, *Compr Pediatr Nurs* 6:195, 1983.

Chapter 9

Nursing Assessment and Communication

LEARNING OUTCOMES

After studying this chapter you should be able to:

◆ Describe the relationship between nursing assessment, intervention and evaluation.
◆ List the components of holistic paediatric nursing assessment.
◆ Identify the reasons for, and appreciate the importance of, recording nursing assessments.
◆ Define communication.
◆ Distinguish between verbal communication and the different kinds of nonverbal communication.
◆ Identify impediments to effective communication with children and parents.
◆ Identify strategies for conducting successful interviews with children and parents.
◆ Describe the development of language and thought processes in children and how this knowledge helps you to communicate with them.

GLOSSARY

assessment data Subjective or objective findings which are used to make inferences about the health and circumstances of an individual

confidentiality Trust or duty to keep information secret or limited to specified individuals

evaluation The process of reassessing an individual/family to identify the effects of interventions

euphemism Substitution of a mild or vague expression for a harsh or direct one

facilitation Supporting and enabling another

nursing assessment The process of collecting and interpreting data about the physical and psychosocial effects of health problems on individuals and their families

nursing diagnosis A term which is synonymous with the patient problem or need identified as a result of nursing assessment

observation The processing of watching and noting signs, behaviours and events as part of clinical asssessment

outcome A judgement about the effects and effectiveness of interventions

ommunication consists of the behaviours by which one person, consciously or unconsciously, affects another. All behaviour transmits a message; even the attempt not to communicate creates a particular impression. Communication is essential to the nursing of children. It is fundamental to forming a trusting relationship with the child and family, and to developing a caring partnership with them. Along with skilled observation, communication is the main source of information for assessing the nursing needs of children and families, and their responses to nursing interventions.

This chapter is concerned primarily with the communication process as it relates to assessment of the child and family. A brief overview of assessment in children's nursing is presented, followed by a review of strategies for communication and interviewing. The use of communication to help the child and family express their emotions and manage the child's care is also explored.

NURSING ASSESSMENT

Assessment is an activity which includes gathering data, interpreting the significance of the data, and deciding whether there is a need for further action. One kind of action may be to collect more data, another to remedy any problem identified, another to pass information to another person. If remedial action is taken, data are collected afterwards to evaluate the effectiveness of that action.

In nursing, the activity of assessment produces data which are used to identify the child's and family's needs for, and responses to, nursing care. The results of nursing assessment may be expressed as a problem, a need, or a nursing diagnosis. Reassessment after taking action is expressed as an evaluation or an outcome.

For example, a nurse observing a child with a flushed face might interpret the flushing as a sign of pyrexia. To confirm this first impression, the nurse will collect more data by touching the child or measuring the child's temperature. Finding that the child is pyrexial, the nurse will take action to attempt to remedy the problem; for example, recommending removal of excess clothing and getting the child to drink fluids. The nurse may also notify a doctor, if the situation requires medical intervention.

Having taken some nursing action and perhaps, in response to a medical prescription, administered an anti-pyretic, the nurse again measures the child's temperature. This reassessment determines whether the actions have been effective (Fig. 9-1).

Nurses use *observation*, *measurement* and *interview* to gather data about a child's physical and psychosocial state, and the family's needs and concerns. Historical data, for example about the child's response to recent hospitalization, are an essential part of assessment. Information is also obtained from other health care professionals, verbally or through written communications, such as records and referral letters.

Conversely, data collected by nurses are relevant to the activities of other carers, especially medical staff. Many of the observations that nurses make will be directly related to the medical problem and its treatment, rather than to the nursing problem.

LEVELS OF ASSESSMENT

Assessment occurs at different levels, ranging from formal, structured data collection to informal, virtually subconscious observation. Formal assessment, often according to a structured assessment protocol, is carried out upon first contact with the child, and needs to be repeated at significant times, such as admission to hospital, transfer into another ward, and discharge to the care of a community nurse. The child who is being cared for over a long period will need to be reassessed at regular intervals so that care is appropriate to his or her changing needs.

At the first contact with the child and family, nursing assessment is as thorough as possible to establish baseline information and to develop a plan of care. The timing of the assessment and the kind of information required will depend on the particular context. A child and family facing treatment for malignant disease will be assessed differently from the well child admitted for minor elective surgery. A balance must be found between assessment which is too narrow and misses problems, and assessment which obtains irrelevant information.

A structured assessment guide based on a model of care, such as Activities of Living (Roper *et al.*, 1983), helps ensure an holistic approach is taken and that no areas are missed. Assessment of relevant psychosocial, developmental and physical parameters enables the nurse to identify the child's response to the health problem and its management. A more family-centred model (Casey, 1993) guides holistic assessment of the child, as well as assessment of the family's need for support, information and teaching (Box 9-1).

Ongoing assessment, both formal and informal, identifies changes over time, or as result of care and treatment. Informal assessment occurs continually, almost subconsciously, throughout the time the nurse is in contact with the child and family. This is especially true during communication, because participants in an interaction constantly monitor each other's verbal

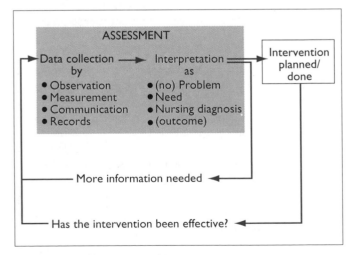

Fig. 9-1 Nursing Assessment and Intervention.

and nonverbal cues. Experienced nurses observe and listen *continuously*. The nature of the infant's crying, the tension in the mother's hands, the withdrawal of the child from company, are all data which need to be interpreted.

RECORDING ASSESSMENT

Assessment is used to make decisions about what care is needed and who should give that care. The record of assessment communicates to all concerned the basis for those decisions. Assessment data are recorded in the nursing record and also on observation charts, fluid balance charts, growth charts - any part of the complete patient record may contain information which is used to make decisions about care and treatment.

Information in the record must be able to be retrieved easily when needed. In the hospital setting, a 24-hour diary format for recording the child's usual pattern of care or routines helps the nurse to find this information quickly when a parent is not present. This format also provides a plan of care which is the basis for maintaining or restoring the child's customary routines while in hospital.

Deciding what to record is a professional skill based on a judgement of what is significant (UKCC, 1993) and what is useful. Recording too much data wastes time and clutters the record, making it hard to find relevant facts. Recording too little, including omission of some normal findings, may leave

out data which become significant or useful for another purpose, such as retrospective audit.

Guidance on record keeping is available (NHSTD, 1993) and most units have local guidelines or standards. The move towards computerized record keeping and multidisciplinary or patient-held records provides an opportunity to explore what is important to record about patient care and how best to record, and use, such information (Information Management Group, 1992).

It is particularly difficult to decide what to record about the child and family's psychosocial state and needs. One way to help with such decisions is to bear in mind the use of assessment information. Who needs it and for what purpose? If the record is shared with the family, it may not be appropriate to have recorded the nursing assessment of their inability to cope or their concerns about money. Such information, however, may have been the basis for arranging frequent visits by the community nursing service, or for referral to social services.

Education and experience equip the children's nurse with the skills required to assess the child's and family's needs for, and responses to, care and treatment. Most difficult to acquire is the skill that is central not only to assessment, but to the whole of nursing — communication.

COMMUNICATION

Communication may be verbal, nonverbal, or abstract. *Verbal* communication involves language and its expression, such as vocalizations in the form of laughs, moans, and sobs, or the implications of what is not said in light of what has been said. *Nonverbal* communication is often called 'body language' and includes gestures, movements, facial expressions, postures, and reactions. *Abstract* communication includes play, artistic expression, symbols, photographs, and choice of clothing. Because it is possible to exert greater conscious control over verbal communication, it is a less reliable indicator of true feelings, especially in relationships with children.

Many factors influence the communication process. To be successful, communication must be appropriate to the situation, properly timed, and clearly delivered. This implies that nurses understand and use techniques of effective communication. Verbal and nonverbal messages must be congruous; that is, two or more messages sent via different means must not be contradictory.

Nurses need to recognize their own feelings and must attempt to recognize the feelings of people with whom the communicative interchange takes place. Biases and judgements interfere with all aspects of this process. The tendency to approve or disapprove of another's statements inhibits positive reactions. In addition, the transmission and reception of messages may be altered by influences of intimacy or distance, trust and mistrust, security and insecurity, or caring and not caring on the part of the participants. Most human biases and judgements are based on recognition of differences between ourselves and others. Nurses in our multicultural society need to be particularly aware of cultural differences and

---

◆ **BOX 9-1**

Paediatric nursing assessment

Where relevant, assessment identifies:

1. The nature of the health problem (actual or potential) and its management, and the child's and family's understanding of it.

2. The physical, psychosocial and developmental effects (actual and potential) on the child of the health problem and its management.

3. The family's situation, its responses to the child's health problem and the nature and effectiveness of its coping strategies.

4. The family's wishes and educational needs related to participation in care.

5. The child's usual routines and self-care abilities and how these are affected by the health problem.

6. The child's and family's expectations related to care, treatment, and discharge.

must be open to other ways of doing or expressing things. It is not only language that blocks communication between people of different cultures. Lack of awareness of one's own responses and lack of understanding of another's culture can be difficult to overcome (Dobson, 1991). The value of effective communication is an increased understanding between the nurse, child, and family. Since nursing of infants and children always involves the inclusion of a caregiver, nurses must be able to communicate not only with children of all ages, but also with the adults in their lives.

VERBAL COMMUNICATION — THE POWER OF WORDS

Words shape reality and thus hold tremendous power. Use of particular words in place of others can affect more than just understanding. For example, if the diagnosis of cancer is always referred to as a tumour, cyst, malignancy, or carcinoma, patients may never really know that they have cancer. Consequently, they may assume less responsibility for their care than if they were aware of the seriousness of the condition. By learning to recognize how patients and health professionals use language to manipulate reality, one can also learn how to change perceptions and communicate more effectively.

AVOIDANCE LANGUAGE

Probably the most common way people try to alter reality is by avoiding words that truly describe it. For example, euphemisms such as 'passed on' are used instead of the word 'death'. Avoidance language usually indicates that a person wants to hide something, especially feelings. As a rule, accepting a person's use of euphemisms only perpetuates the fears and never helps the person deal with them. In contrast, use of straightforward, precise, descriptive language lends perspective to the situation and allows the person to discuss the fears. Most often, imagined fears are far greater than the actual reality. For a discussion of explaining death to children, see Chapter 21.

DISTANCING LANGUAGE

Sometimes people use impersonal words to shield themselves from the painful reality of a situation. For example, parents may state that they know *someone* with a child who is slow, but are actually talking about personal fears regarding *their* child. By realizing that parents need to talk about this difficult subject, the nurse can provide sensitive statements that ease them into discussing their situation.

One of the dangers in supporting distancing language is that the parent may effectively deny that a problem exists. To return to the previous example, if the issue of retardation is never approached directly but is allowed to be 'someone else's problem', the parents may not be able to make decisions for special schools or individualized training.

Sometimes distancing is desirable because the topic may be too painful to discuss directly. Using the third-person tech-

nique ('them' rather than 'us') may be very therapeutic in allowing an individual the opportunity to indirectly approach a subject and receive feedback, but still remain in control.

NONVERBAL COMMUNICATION — PARALANGUAGE

In addition to the spoken word, messages are relayed through nonverbal means, or paralanguage, which involves pitch, timing, tone, rate, volume, and accent in speech (Burnard, 1992). Young children become very adept at understanding paralanguage; long before they know the meaning of words, they sense anxiety or fear by the rise in pitch or the accelerated rate of the parent's voice. By careful attention to the spoken word, nurses can better understand the meaning of another's verbal message and more accurately control their own paralanguage.

Because most people do not exert conscious control over paralanguage, it is a valuable clue to such things as feelings and concerns. For example, *pausing* may signify a need to formulate thoughts, recall information, or sometimes fabricate a story. Frequent pauses, however, often make the speaker sound insecure. Long pauses may mean that the individual needs more information.

Rate also sends unspoken messages. Talking too fast usually makes the speaker sound glib and insensitive. Talking slowly with a firm tone and appropriate pauses conveys authority. Therefore, a person is much more likely to 'hear' instructions if the latter approach is used. Children, in particular, respond attentively to a slow, even, steady voice.

CONFIRMING AND DISCONFIRMING BEHAVIOURS

People respond to each other through *confirming behaviours*, such as nodding the head, using direct eye contact, repeating or requesting clarification, and making appropriate comments, or through *disconfirming behaviours*, such as tapping fingers or a foot, turning away from the speaker, avoiding eye contact, and interrupting (Heineken and Roberts, 1983). Since there is a reciprocal relationship between such behaviours, nurses need to use confirming behaviours to receive confirmation in return. This 'mirroring' effect is particularly evident in children because of their sensitivity to nonverbal cues.

GUIDELINES FOR COMMUNICATION AND INTERVIEWING

The most widely used method of communicating with parents on a professional basis is the interview process. Interviewing, unlike social conversation, is a specific form of goal-directed communication. As nurses converse with children and adults, they focus on the individuals to determine the kind of persons they are, their usual ways of handling problems, whether help is needed, and the way in which they react to their situation. Developing interviewing skills requires time and patience, but adherence to some guiding principles and avoiding some obstacles facilitate this process.

ESTABLISHING A SETTING FOR COMMUNICATION

Part of the success in interviewing depends on the type of physical and psychological setting the interviewer constructs. Appropriate introduction, role clarification, explanation of the reason for the interview, preliminary acquaintance with the family, and assurance of privacy and confidentiality are prerequisites for establishing a setting conducive to communication.

APPROPRIATE INTRODUCTION

Nurses should introduce themselves to, and ask the name of, each family member who is present. During the interview, each person is addressed by name, after asking them their preference regarding form of address. Using the person's preferred name conveys respect and communicates a personal interest in each family member. The preferred name should be recorded on the medical record and communicated to other staff members (Elizabeth, 1989).

At the beginning of the visit, children are included in the interaction by asking them their name, age, and other information. Nurses often direct all questions to adults, even when children are old enough to speak for themselves. However, this terminates one extremely valuable source of information - the patient.

ROLE CLARIFICATION AND EXPLANATION OF THE INTERVIEW

During the introduction, it is also necessary to clarify the nurse's particular role in the health setting. For example, nurses performing interviews may be paediatric nurse specialists, inpatient staff nurses, community paediatric nurses, health visitors, or school nurses. A parent is much more likely to reveal personal information about the child and family if the relevance and importance of the interview are stressed. If this is not done, parents may refuse to elaborate about certain areas because they feel it has no bearing on the 'problem'. In addition, since more than one member of the health team may take a history during the course of a hospital admission, it is important to clarify the reason for each interview.

PRELIMINARY ACQUAINTANCE

Because of the personal and private nature of an in-depth interview, the person being interviewed must trust the interviewer in order to reveal sensitive information. Therefore, it is best to begin with some general conversation. Comments such as, 'How have things been since your last visit?' 'Tell me about Johnny', or (to the child) 'What do you think is going to

happen today?' allow the parent or child to express their concerns in a casual, relaxed atmosphere.

The preliminary acquaintance conversation also reveals how responsive the informant may be to questions. For example, using open-ended statements may lead the person into a lengthy detailed discussion. In this case, it is more beneficial to direct questions towards specific answers to avoid tangential remarks. At other times a person may respond to open-ended questions with only minimal information, in which case the continued use of open-ended questions probably will reveal more data than 'yes' or 'no' type questions.

ASSURANCE OF PRIVACY AND CONFIDENTIALITY

The place where the interview is conducted is almost as important as the interview itself. The physical environment should allow for as much privacy as possible with distractions, such as interruptions, background noise, or other visible activity, kept to a minimum. At times it is necessary to turn off a television or radio. The environment should also have some play provision for young children to keep them occupied during the parent-nurse interview (Fig. 9-2). Parents who are constantly interrupted by their children are unable to concentrate fully and tend to give short, brief answers to terminate the interview as quickly as possible.

Confidentiality is also an essential component of the initial phase of the interview. Since information is usually shared with other members of the health team, it is the interviewer's responsibility and obligation to inform the family of the confidential limits of the conversation. If there is concern regarding confidentiality in a situation, such as talking to a parent suspected of child abuse or a teenager contemplating suicide, the nurse must deal with this directly and inform the person that in such instances confidentiality cannot be ensured.

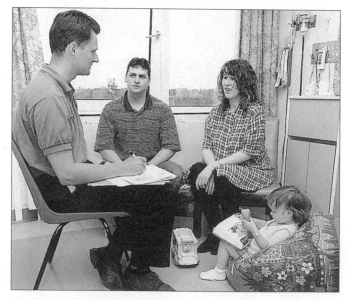

Fig. 9-2 Child plays while nurse interviews parents. (Courtesy of Southampton University Hospitals Trust)

COMMUNICATING WITH FAMILIES

Communicating with the family is a triangular process involving the nurse, parents, and child. Although the following discussion focuses primarily on this triad, in many circumstances significant others, for example, siblings, relatives, or other caregivers, may be part of the communication process.

COMMUNICATING WITH PARENTS

Although the parent and child are separate and distinct entities, relationships with the child are frequently mediated via the parent, particularly in the case of younger children. For the most part, information about the child is acquired by direct observation or communicated to the nurse by the parents. Usually, it can be assumed that, because of the close contact with the child, the information imparted by the parent is reliable. Making an assessment of the child requires input from the child (verbal and nonverbal), information from the parent, and the nurse's own observations of the child and interpretation of the relationship between the child and the parent.

ENCOURAGING THE PARENT TO TALK

Interviewing parents not only offers the nurse an opportunity to determine the health and developmental status of the child, but also offers information about all factors that influence the child's life. Whatever the *parent* sees as a problem should also be a concern of the nurse. These problems are not always easy to identify. Nurses need to be alert for clues and signals by which a parent communicates worries and anxieties. Careful phrasing with broad open-ended questions such as 'What is Jimmy eating now?' provides more information than several single-answer questions such as 'Is Jimmy eating what the rest of the family eats?' that can be answered with 'yes' or 'no'.

Sometimes the parent will take the lead without stimulation. At other times it may be necessary for the nurse to direct another question on the basis of an observation such as 'Connie seems unhappy today', or 'How do you feel when David cries?' If the parent appears to be tired or distraught, the nurse might ask, 'What do you do to relax?' or 'What help do you have with the children?' A comment such as 'You handle the baby very well. What kinds of experience have you had with babies?' to new mothers who appear comfortable with their first child gives them positive reinforcement and provides an opening for any questions they might have regarding the care of the infant. Often, all that is required to keep the parent talking is a nod and saying 'yes'.

When attempting to elicit feelings and covert problems, it is best to avoid closed-ended questions that begin with 'Does... ', 'Did... ' or 'Is... ', which usually require only a single response. In addition, asking questions such as, 'Does your son have any problems at school?' subtly implies a lack of parental skills and evokes defensiveness. Instead, it is helpful to say 'What... ', 'How... ', 'Tell me about... ', and encourage elaboration with 'You were saying... ', 'You say that... ', or reflecting back key words or phrases, such as 'He was depressed?'. Open-ended questions are nonthreatening and encourage description.

Another useful approach is to elicit information about a topic and compare the answer to the person's perception of what 'things' should be. For example, after the parent describes what the child is eating, it is helpful to ask, 'What do you think your child should be eating?' If there is a discrepancy between the two answers, it is important to ask the parent to comment on how important the difference is. This approach allows the parent to discuss areas of concern that may not be disclosed otherwise.

DIRECTING THE FOCUS

Ability to direct the focus of the interview while allowing for maximum freedom of expression is one of the most difficult goals in effective communication. One approach is the use of open-ended or broad questions, followed by guiding statements. For example, if the parent proceeds to list the other children by name, the nurse can also say: 'Tell me their ages, too'. If the parent continues to describe each child in depth, which is not the purpose of the interview, the nurse can redirect the focus by stating, 'Let's talk about the other children later. You were beginning to tell me about Paul's activities at school.' This approach conveys interest in the other children, but focuses the data collection on the patient.

In the event that the parent has suggested that a problem exists with one of the other children, the nurse should reintroduce this subject at the end of the interview to assess the need for further family follow-up. Saying to the parent, 'Earlier, you mentioned that your older son is having trouble in school. Tell me what you see as the problem', reintroduces this subject but only in terms of the possible problem.

LISTENING

Listening is the most important component for effective communication. When listening is truly aimed at understanding the other person, it is an active process that requires concentration and attention to all aspects of the conversation — verbal, nonverbal, and abstract. Two of the greatest impediments to listening are environmental distraction and premature judgement.

The attitudes and feelings of the nurse are easily injected into an interview. Often, nurses' perceptions of a parent's behaviour are influenced by their own perceptions, prejudices, and assumptions, which may include racial, religious, and cultural stereotypes. What may be interpreted as passive hostility or disinterest in a parent may be shyness or an expression of anxiety. For example, in Western cultures eye contact and directness are signs of paying attention. However, in many non-Western cultures, directness, such as looking someone in the eye, is considered rude. Children are taught to avert their gaze and to look down when being addressed by an adult, especially one with authority (Petrie, 1989). Therefore, judgements about 'listening' need to be made with an appreciation of cultural differences.

Although it is necessary to make some preliminary judgements, the nurse must attempt to listen with as much objectivity as possible, by clarifying meanings and attempting to see the situation from the parent's point of view. Effective interviewers use conscious control over their reactions, responses, and the techniques they use.

Use of minimal verbal activity with active listening facilitates parent involvement. It is tempting to spend time explaining, describing, and interpreting health information when the opportunity presents itself. However, it is possible to provide effective health education by properly timing the information and presenting only as much as is necessary at the moment.

Careful listening facilitates the use of cues, verbal leads, or signals from the interviewer to move the interview along. Frequent references to an area of concern, repetition of certain key words, or a special emphasis on something or someone serve as cues to the interviewer for the direction of inquiry. Concerns and anxieties are often mentioned in a casual, offhand manner. Even though they are casual, they are important and deserve more careful scrutiny to identify problem areas. For example, a parent who is concerned about a child's habit of bed-wetting may casually mention that the child's bed was 'wet this morning'.

Because the interview is almost always triangular — nurse, child, and parent — the parent may wish to convey information in such a way as to prevent the child from hearing it. This requires active listening on the part of the nurse to hear the *unspoken* message.

Listening is also helpful in assessing reliability. For example, the answers elicited at the beginning of the interview may differ from those at the end, when the parent feels more confident in revealing problems. It is important to identify any discrepancies and to reintroduce those topics for further investigation.

USING SILENCE

Silence, as a response, is often one of the most difficult interviewing techniques to learn. It requires a sense of confidence and comfort on the part of the interviewer to allow the interviewee space in which to think uninterrupted. Silence permits the interviewee to sort out thoughts and feelings, search for responses to questions, and to share feelings in which two or more people absorb the emotion to its depth.

Sometimes it is necessary to break silence and reopen communication. This should be done in such a way that the person is given a choice to continue talking about what is considered important. Breaking a silence by introducing a new topic or by prolonged talking essentially terminates the interviewee's opportunity to use the silence. Suggestions for breaking the silence include statements such as, 'Is there anything else you

wish to say?' 'I see you find it difficult to continue; how may I help?' or 'I don't know what this silence means. Perhaps there is something you would like to put into words but find difficult to say.'

BEING EMPATHIC

Empathy means feeling and participating in the inner feelings of another, while remaining objective. The empathic interviewer attempts to see the world from the interviewee's perspective with as much understanding as possible. Empathy differs from sympathy, which is subjectively thinking or feeling like the other person. Although important and necessary at times, sympathy is not always therapeutic in the helping relationship. Empathy, however, is a very beneficial supportive technique.

Some individuals are naturally empathic and easily 'feel' with another person. However, empathy can be learned by attending to the verbal and nonverbal language of the interviewee. Empathy building exercises, reflection and other experiential learning methods are a vital part of nursing education (Burnard, 1985).

DEFINING THE PROBLEM

To arrive at a solution to a problem or concern, the nurse and the parent must agree that a problem exists. If neither believes that there is a problem, there is certainly no need to create one. Sometimes the parent may believe there is a problem the nurse is unable to see. For example, a mother was overly concerned about every small cold, sneeze, or cough in her baby who had been carefully examined and found to be healthy with no evidence of a respiratory problem. On careful questioning, the nurse discovered that a previous child had died of pneumonia in infancy. Consequently, the nurse was able to better understand the mother's concern. Once the nurse acknowledges the mother's fear, she can help the mother deal with her special anxieties about her baby and teach her how to recognize when there is need for concern.

Occasionally, the nurse identifies a problem that the parent denies exists. In this case the nurse should pursue the situation and either find a way to deal with it or enlist the aid of other health team members. For example, the parents of a child with Down syndrome may refuse to believe that their child is different from any other child of the same age. They may say, 'He is just a little slow', and 'All she needs to do is to try harder'. A child with an obvious behaviour problem may be described by the parents as 'just stubborn' or 'just behaving that way to spite us'. Such statements may be clues that the parents have not progressed past the stage of denial in adjusting to the problem.

SOLVING THE PROBLEM

Once the problem is identified and agreed on by parent and nurse, they can begin to arrive at a solution. A parent who is included in the problem-solving process is more likely to follow through with a course of action. Questions such as, 'What have you tried so far?' or 'What have you thought about doing?' provide leads for exploration and enable parents to believe that their ideas and solutions are worthwhile. These can be followed by, 'What prevents you from trying that?', 'That sounds like a good plan', and 'Have you considered trying this?' Such approaches encourage participation and reinforce, rather than belittle, parents' efforts to solve problems.

Sometimes a parent arrives at a solution that the nurse does not consider to be the best alternative. If it can be ascertained that it will do no harm and the parents are convinced of its merits, it is usually best to allow them to continue with the plan. A course of action is more likely to be carried out when parents can reach their own conclusions. However, when parental decisions are inappropriate, nurses will need to discuss the risks with the family and try to reach an agreed solution. Whenever possible, decisions should be theirs, with the nurse serving as a *facilitator* in problem solving.

AVOIDING IMPEDIMENTS TO COMMUNICATION

Many impediments to communication can adversely affect the quality of the relationship between nurse and family. Many of these blocks are initiated by the interviewer, such as giving unrestricted advice or forming prejudged conclusions. Another type of block occurs primarily with the interviewees and deals with information overload. When individuals are presented with too much information or information that is overwhelming, they will often demonstrate signals of increasing anxiety or decreasing attention. Such signals should alert the interviewer to give less information or to clarify what has been said. Some common impediments to communication are listed in Box 9-2.

Impediments to communication can be corrected by careful analysis of the interview process. One of the best methods for improving interviewing skills is audiotape and/or videotape feedback in a classroom situation. With supervision and

guidance, the interviewer can recognize the impediments and consciously avoid them.

COMMUNICATING WITH FAMILIES THROUGH AN INTERPRETER

Sometimes, verbal communication is impossible because two people speak different languages. In this case, it is necessary to exchange information through a third party, the interpreter. Specific guidelines for using an adult interpreter are listed in Box 9-3. In many families, the school-aged children may speak good English but should not be used to interpret, as this could cause distress and might be culturally inappropriate.

Communicating with families through an interpreter requires sensitivity to cultural, legal, and ethical considerations. In some cultures, class and gender differences between the interpreter and the family may cause the family to feel intimidated and less inclined to offer information. Therefore, care should be exercised in choosing someone to translate, and time should be provided for the interpreter and family to establish rapport (Slater, 1993).

Legal and ethical issues may also arise. For example, in obtaining informed consent through an interpreter, it is important that the family be fully informed of all the aspects of the particular procedure to which they are consenting. Issues of confidentiali-

---

◆ **BOX 9-2**

• Some impediments to communication

- Giving unrestricted and sometimes unasked-for advice.
- Offering premature or inappropriate reassurance.
- Giving overready encouragement.
- Defending a situation or opinion.
- Using stereotyped comments or cliches.
- Limiting expression of emotion by asking directed, closed-
- ended questions.
- Interrupting and finishing the person's sentence.
- Talking more than the interviewee.
- Forming prejudged conclusions.
- Deliberately changing the focus of the discussion.

◆ **BOX 9-3**

Guidelines for using an interpreter

- Explain to the interpreter the reason for the interview and the type of questions that will be asked.
- Clarify whether a detailed or brief answer is required and whether the translated response can be general or literal.
- Introduce the interpreter to the family and allow some time before actual interview so that they can become acquainted.
- Communicate directly with family members when asking questions to reinforce interest in them and to observe nonverbal expressions.
- Refrain from interrupting the family member and interpreter while they are conversing.
- Avoid commenting to interpreter about family members since they may understand some English.
- Respect cultural differences; it is often best to pose questions about sex, marriage, or pregnancy indirectly—ask about a child's 'father' rather than mother's 'husband'.
- Allow time following interview for the interpreter to share something that he or she felt could not be said earlier; ask about the interpreter's impression of nonverbal clues to communication and family members' reliability or ease in revealing information.
- Arrange for family to speak with the same interpreter on subsequent visits whenever possible.

ty may arise if family members related to another patient are asked to interpret for the family, thus revealing sensitive information that may be shared with other families on the unit. It is, of course, important for nursing staff to ascertain who has 'parental responsibility' as defined within the *Children Act* published in 1989.

COMMUNICATING WITH CHILDREN

Although the greatest amount of verbal communication may be carried out with the parent, the child should not be excluded during the interview. Periodic attention to infants and younger children through play or by occasionally directing questions or remarks to them makes children participants in the interview. Older children can be actively included as informants.

In communication with children of all ages, the nonverbal components of the communication process convey the most significant messages. It is difficult to disguise feelings, attitudes, and anxiety when relating to children. They are very alert to surroundings and attach meaning to every gesture and move that is made. This is particularly true with very young children.

Active attempts to make friends with children before they have had an opportunity to evaluate an unfamiliar person tend to increase their anxiety. A helpful tactic is to continue to talk to the child and parent, but go about activities that do not involve the child directly, thus allowing the child to observe from a safe position. If the child has a special toy or doll, it is helpful to 'talk' to the doll first (Fig. 9-3). Asking simple questions such as, 'Does your teddy bear have a name?' may ease the child into conversation. Other guidelines for communicating with children are listed in Box 9-4.

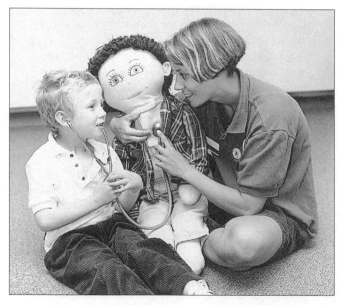

Fig.9-3 Nurse talks to child using puppets and assumes position at child's level. (Courtesy of Southampton University Hospitals Trust)

COMMUNICATION RELATED TO DEVELOPMENT OF THOUGHT PROCESSES

The normal development of language and thought offers a frame of reference in knowing how to communicate with children. Thought processes progress from concrete to functional and finally to abstract, formal operations.

Infancy

Because they are unable to use words, infants primarily use and understand nonverbal communication. Infants communicate their needs and feelings through nonverbal behaviours and vocalizations that can be interpreted by someone who is around them for a sufficient amount of time. Infants smile and gurgle when content and cry when distressed. Crying is provoked by unpleasant stimuli from inside or outside, such as hunger, pain, body restraint, or loneliness. Adults interpret this to mean that an infant needs something and consequently try to alleviate the discomfort and reduce tension. Crying (or the desire to cry) persists as a part of everyone's communication repertoire.

Infants respond to adults' nonverbal behaviours. They become quiet when they are cuddled, patted, or receive other forms of gentle, physical contact. They derive comfort from the sound of a voice, even though they do not understand the words that are spoken. Until infants reach the age at which they experience 'stranger anxiety', they readily respond to any firm, gentle

---

◆ **BOX 9-2**

Guidelines for communicating with children

- Allow children time to feel comfortable and settled.
- Avoid sudden or rapid advances, broad smiles, extended eye contact, or other gestures that may be seen as threatening.
- Talk to the parent if child is initially shy.
- Communicate through transition objects such as dolls, puppets, or stuffed animals before questioning a young child directly.
- Give older children the opportunity to talk without the parents present.
- Assume a position that is at eye level with the child.
- Speak in a quiet, unhurried, and confident voice.
- Speak clearly, be specific, use simple words, and short sentences.
- State directions and suggestions positively.
- Offer choices only when one exists.
- Be honest with children.
- Allow them to express their concerns and fears.
- Use a variety of communication techniques.

handling and quiet, calm speech. Loud, harsh sounds and sudden movements are frightening.

Older infants' attentions are centred on themselves and their parents; therefore, any stranger is a potential threat until proved otherwise. Holding out the hands and asking the child to 'come' is seldom successful, especially if the infant is with the parent. If infants must be handled, the best approach is simply to pick them up firmly without gestures. It is helpful to observe the position in which the parent holds the infant. Most infants have learned to prefer a particular position and manner of handling. In general, infants are more at ease upright than horizontal. It is also best to hold infants in such a way that they can keep their parents in view. Until they have developed the understanding that an object (in this case the parent) removed from sight can still be present, they have no way of knowing that the object is still there.

Early childhood

Children under five years of age are almost completely egocentric. They see things only in relation to themselves and from their point of view. Therefore, any communication to them should be focused on *them*. They need to be told what they can do or how they will feel. Experiences of others are of no interest to them. It is futile to use another child's experience as an attempt to gain the cooperation of very small children. Although they have not yet acquired sufficient language skills to express their feelings and wants, toddlers are able to communicate effectively with their hands to transmit ideas without words. They push an unwanted object away, pull another person to show them something, point, and cover the mouth that is saying something they do not wish to hear.

Everything is direct and concrete to small children. They are unable to work with abstractions and base all deductions on literal formulations. Analogies escape them because they are unable to separate fact from fantasy. For example, they attach literal meaning to such common phrases as 'two-faced', 'sticky fingers', or 'coughing your head off'. Children who are told they will get 'a little stick in the arm' may not be able to envision an injection. Nurses must be aware of inadvertently using a phrase that might be misinterpreted by a small child.

Language should be used that is consistent with the child's developmental level. For example, in talking with a toddler, it is best to use simple, *short* sentences, repeat words that are *familiar* to the child, and limit descriptions to *concrete* explanations.

Children in this age category assign human attributes to inanimate objects. They endow mechanical devices and instruments with living characteristics. Consequently they fear that these objects may jump, bite, cut, or pinch all by themselves. Children do not know that these devices are unable to perform without human direction. They should be allowed to touch, examine, and familiarize themselves with articles that will come in contact with them. A stethoscope will feel cold; a blood pressure cuff squeezes.

School-aged years

Children aged five to eight years rely less on what they see and more on what they know when faced with new problems. They want explanations and reasons for everything, but require no verification beyond that. They are interested in the functional aspect of all procedures, objects, and activities. They want to know why an object exists, why it is used, how it works, and the intent and purpose of its user. They need to know what is going to take place and why it is being done to *them* specifically. For example, to explain a procedure such as taking a blood pressure, the nurse might show the child how squeezing the bulb pushes air into the cuff and makes the 'silver' in the tube go up. The child should be permitted to operate the bulb. An explanation for the reason might be as simple as, 'I want to see how far the silver goes up when the cuff squeezes your arm.' Consequently the child becomes an enthusiastic participant. Allowing children to ask questions about what is happening to them and maintaining a permissive atmosphere are conducive to open communication.

Children at this age have a heightened concern about body integrity. Because of the special importance and value they place on their body, they are overly sensitive to anything that constitutes a threat or suggestion of injury to it. This concern extends to their possessions also, so that they may appear to overreact to loss or threatened loss of treasured objects. Helping children to voice their concerns enables the nurse to provide reassurance and to implement activities that reduce their anxiety. For example, if a reticent child fears being the single object of probing inquiry, the nurse can ignore that particular child by talking and relating to other children in the family or group. When children no longer feel like single targets, they will usually interject personal ideas, feelings, and interpretations of events.

Older children have an adequate and satisfactory use of language. They still require relatively simple explanations, but their ability to think concretely can facilitate communication and explanation. They may have previous experience of health care to draw on in understanding what is expected of them.

Adolescence

As children move into adolescence, they fluctuate between child and adult thinking and behaviour. They are riding a current that is moving them rapidly towards a maturity that may be beyond their coping ability. Therefore, when tensions rise, they may seek the security of the more familiar and comfortable expectations of childhood. Anticipating these shifts in identity allows the nurse to adjust the course of interaction to meet the needs of the moment. No single approach can be relied on consistently, and one can expect to encounter cooperation, hostility, anger, bravado, and a variety of other behaviours and attitudes. It is as much a mistake to regard the adolescent as an adult with an adult's wisdom and control, as it is to confine to the teenager the concerns and expectations of a child.

Frequently, adolescents are more willing to discuss their concerns with an adult outside the family. They are extremely susceptible to the advances of anyone who displays a genuine interest in them. However, adolescents are quick to reject persons who attempt to impose their values on them, whose interest is feigned, or who appear to have little respect for who they are and what they think or say.

As with children, adolescents need to express their feelings. Generally they talk quite freely when given an opportunity. However, what adolescents say cannot always be taken at face value. When emotional factors are involved, the feelings that are interjected into words are as significant as the words that are used. The best way to give support is to be attentive, try not to interrupt, and avoid comments or expressions that convey disapproval or surprise. Prying and asking embarrassing questions should be avoided, and any impulse to give advice should be resisted. Frequently, adolescents reveal their feelings or a source of concern, or ask a question when they are involved in routine matters such as a physical assessment.

Teenagers characteristically have a language and culture all their own that further sets them apart from others. To avoid misinterpretation, frequent clarification of terms is advisable. Occasionally adolescents are reticent and answer only in monosyllables. Usually this happens when they are unwilling patients or do not yet feel safe enough to reveal themselves. In this instance the best approach is to confine discussions to irrelevant topics to reduce the element of threat until such time as they feel more secure. The nurse must be alert for signals that indicate they are ready to talk. The major sources of concern for adolescents are attitudes and feelings towards sex, relationships with parents, peer group acceptance, and developing a sense of identity.

Assessing the adolescent presents some questions for the nurse. The first may be whether to talk to the adolescent alone, with the parents, or to each individually. Of course, if the adolescent is alone, there is no question, except that the nurse might want to suggest to the teenager that she may talk with the parents at another time. If parents and teenager are together, talking with the adolescent first has the advantage of immediately identifying with the young person, thus fostering the interpersonal relationship. However, talking with the parents initially may provide insight into the family relationship. Whichever decision is made, both parties need an opportunity to be included in the interview. If time constraints are important, such as during history-taking, these need to be clarified at the onset to avoid appearing to 'take sides' by talking more with one person than the other.

Confidentiality is very important when interviewing adolescents. Parents and teenagers need to know the limits of confidentiality - specifically that young persons' disclosures will be kept between them and the nurse. However, exceptions also must be clarified, such as breaking confidence if it is necessary for the welfare of adolescents, as in the case of suicidal behaviour.

Another dilemma in interviewing adolescents is that two views of a problem frequently exist — the teenager's and the parents'. Clarification of the problem is a major task. However, providing both parties with an opportunity to discuss their perceptions in an open and unbiased atmosphere can, by itself, be therapeutic. By demonstrating positive communication skills, the nurse can help families communicate more effectively.

COMMUNICATION TECHNIQUES

In addition to conventional interviewing methods such as reflection and open-ended questions, several techniques encourage family members to express their thoughts and feelings in a less directive and confrontational manner.

VERBAL TECHNIQUES

Various verbal techniques can be used to encourage communication. The interviewer can use some of these techniques to pose questions or explore concerns in a less threatening manner. Others can be presented as 'word games' that are often well received by children.

Third-person technique
The third-person technique involves expressing a feeling in terms of a third person (he, she, they). This technique is less threatening than directly asking individuals how they feel, because it gives them the opportunity to agree or disagree without being defensive. For example, the nurse may comment, 'Sometimes when people are sick they feel angry and sad because they cannot do what others can' and either wait silently for a response or encourage a reply with a statement such as, 'Did you ever feel that way?'. This approach allows three choices: (1) to agree and, hopefully, express how they feel, (2) to disagree, or (3) to remain silent, in which case they may have such feelings but are unable to express them at that time. Demonstrating to parents how useful such techniques are also helps them learn new ways of communicating with the child.

Another variation of the third-person technique is to ask about friends, for example, 'Do any of your friends smoke or drink alcohol?'. Since peer group activity often reflects the children's activity, this may introduce the topic in such a way that young persons are able to talk about their habits or concerns.

Facilitative responding
Facilitative responding is the careful listening and reflecting back to patients the feelings and content of their statements. Such responses are empathetic and nonjudgemental, and legitimize the person's feelings. The formula for facilitative responses is, 'You feel ___ because ___' (Henrich and Bernheim, 1981). For example, if a child states, 'I hate coming to the hospital and getting jabs', a facilitative response is, 'You feel unhappy because of all the things that are done to you.'

Storytelling

Storytelling uses the language of children to probe into areas of their thinking while bypassing conscious inhibitions or fears. Children respond to a variety of storytelling techniques. The simplest is asking them to relate a story about an event, such as 'being in the hospital'. Another approach involves showing children a picture of a particular event, such as a child in a hospital with other people in the room, and asking them to describe the scene. Comic strips cut from a newspaper with the words removed or originally drawn to depict a particular scenario are excellent vehicles when children ascribe their own statements to each comic scene (Walker, 1988). There are also many other techniques for encouraging expression of emotions and concerns. These range from word association through to guided imagery, and require special training to be used safely.

NONVERBAL TECHNIQUES

Many children and adults find talking about their feelings difficult. For them, verbal communication may be more stressful than supportive. Several nonverbal techniques can be used to encourage communication.

Touch

Touch is one of the most meaningful forms of communication, particularly when communicating feelings and attitudes. Children are particularly sensitive to messages conveyed by touch, and the nurse can use touch in a most therapeutic manner. Numerous types of touch can be used, such as massaging, stroking, and swaddling.

Regardless of the particular method of touch that is used to communicate to the child or adult, nurses must assess what is considered positive touch. For example, a child may be frightened by premature touching that may be perceived as an aggressive attack, whereas another child might be comforted by light stroking or rubbing. When using touch, the duration, location, intensity, and sensation must be altered to find the correct balance for the child, especially the neonate. A parent will be able to describe the kind of touch the child finds comforting.

Writing

Writing is an alternative communication approach for older children and adults. Specific suggestions include: (1) keeping a journal or diary, (2) writing feelings or thoughts that are difficult to express, (3) writing 'letters' that are never mailed (a variation is making up a 'pen pal' to write to), or (4) keeping an account of the child's progress from both a physical and an emotional viewpoint.

To encourage writing about feelings, it is helpful to give some instruction while keeping the format as open-ended as possible. For example, rather than asking children to write about things that worry them, it is better to request them to complete the specific statement, 'These are the things that upset me today:... '. Any form of writing can also be supplemented with drawings. To initiate a conversation, the nurse can inquire about the writing, possibly even asking to read some of it. Frequently, as

one writes down ideas, thoughts, or feelings, there is also an urge to discuss them. Once they are written, they are more real and tangible but often less frightening than when kept locked inside one's mind.

Writing can also have a long-term benefit. After the experience, there can be growth in rereading about it. One mother used her journal to help her teenage daughter understand a serious childhood illness that had threatened the youngster's life. The adolescent had become resentful of comments about 'when she was ill', but after reading the journal with the mother, she realized what a stressful time those earlier years had been and gained a deeper appreciation of her parents' continuing concern for her health.

Drawing

Drawing is one of the most valuable forms of communication — both nonverbal, from looking at the drawing, and verbal, from the child's story of the picture. Children's drawings are usually of themselves, their experiences, or those who are significant to them. Besides communicating about themselves, art also provides children with a natural activity that helps them deal with both conscious and unconscious feelings.

Drawing can be spontaneous or directed. *Spontaneous drawings* involve giving children a variety of art supplies (older children like felt-tipped pens) and providing the opportunity to draw. The only encouragement may be the statement, 'Draw something for me.' *Directed drawing* involves a more specific direction, such as 'draw a person'. Interpretation of children's drawing requires special training, but nurses can use drawings to help children communicate both their concern and their understanding of what is happening to them.

Play

Play is a universal language of children. It is one of the most important forms of communication and can be an effective technique in relating to them. Clues about physical, intellectual, and social developmental progress can often be gleaned from the form and complexity of a child's play behaviours. Play requires a minimum of equipment or none at all. Therapeutic play is often used to reduce the trauma of illness and hospitalization (see Chapter 5) and to prepare children for therapeutic procedures (see Chapter 8).

Because their ability to perceive precedes their ability to transmit, small infants respond to activities that register on their senses. Patting, stroking, and other skin play convey messages. Repetitive actions, such as stretching infants' arms out to the side while they are lying on the back and then folding them across the chest or raising and revolving the legs in a bicycling motion, will elicit pleasurable sounds. Colourful items to catch the eye or interesting sounds such as a ticking clock, chimes, bells, or singing can be used to attract children's attention.

Older infants respond to simple games. The old game of peekaboo is an excellent way to initiate communication with infants while maintaining a 'safe', nonthreatening distance. After this intermittent eye-to-eye contact, the nurse is no longer viewed as a stranger, but as someone who is a friend. This can be followed by touch games. Clapping an infant's hands together for pat-a-cake or wiggling the toes for 'this little piggy' delights an infant or small child. Much of the nursing assessment can be carried out with the use of games and simple play equipment while the infant remains in the safety of the parent's arms or lap. Talking to a foot or other part of the child's body is an effective tactic.

The nurse can capitalize on the natural curiosity of small children by playing games such as 'Which hand do you take?' and 'Guess what I have in my hand' or by manipulating items such as a flashlight or stethoscope. Finger games are very useful. More elaborate materials, such as puppets and replicas of familiar or unfamiliar items, serve as excellent means to communicate with small children. The variety and extent are limited only by the nurse's imagination.

Through play, children reveal their perceptions of interpersonal relationships with their family, friends, or hospital personnel. Children may also reveal the wide scope of knowledge they have acquired from listening to others around them. For example, through needle play, children may disclose how

carefully they have watched each procedure by precisely duplicating the technical skills. They may also reveal how well they remember those who performed procedures. One child who painstakingly re-enacted every detail of a tedious medical procedure also played the role of the doctor who had repeatedly shouted at her to be still for the long ordeal. Her anger at him was most evident during the play session and revealed the cause for her abrupt withdrawal and passive hostility towards the medical and nursing staff following the test.

Play sessions serve not only as assessment tools for determining children's awareness and perception of their illness, but also as methods of intervention and evaluation. In the previous example, when the child revealed anger towards the doctor, the nurse acted the part of the patient, but this time did not accept the doctor's harsh commands to stay still. Instead the nurse said to the doctor all the things the child had wished she could say.

Subsequent play sessions can also be used for evaluation of the child's progress. A change in the type of drawing or the theme of the play may indicate progression towards or away from ability to deal with anxiety.

KEY POINTS

◆ Assessment includes collection and interpretation of data, as well as identification of the child's and family's need for, and reponse to, nursing care.

◆ Nurses use observation, measurement, interviewing and existing records to gather data about the child and family.

◆ A structured assessment guide, based on a family-centred model of nursing, ensures that a holistic approach is taken for both initial and ongoing assessment.

◆ The record of a nursing assessment communicates to all concerned the basis for decisions about what care is needed and who should give that care.

◆ Communication, the most important skill nurses must possess in the care of children, has verbal, nonverbal, and abstract components.

◆ To effectively establish a setting for communication, nurses must make an appropriate introduction, clarify their role and the purpose of the interview, and ensure privacy and confidentiality.

◆ When communicating with parents, nurses need to encourage parental involvement, listen carefully, use silence, and be empathic.

◆ Communication with children must reflect their developmental stage.

REFERENCES

Burnard P: *Communicate!—a communication skills guide for healthcare workers*, London, 1992, Edward Arnold.

Burnard P: *Learning human skills: a guide for nurses*, London, 1985, Heinemann.

Casey A: Developing a model of paediatric nursing practice. In Glasper A, Tucker A: *Advances in child health nursing*, London, 1993, Scutari.

Dobson S: *Transcultural nursing*, London, 1991, Scutari.

Elizabeth J: Form of address: an addition to history taking? *BMJ* 298(6669):257, 1989.

Heineken J, Roberts FB: Confirming, not disconfirming: communicating in a more positive manner, *MCN* 8(1):78, 1983.

Henrich AP, Bernheim KF: Responding to patients' concerns, *Nurs Outlook* 29(7):428, 1981.

Information Management Group: *Information management and technology strategy overview*, London, 1992, Department of Health.

National Health Service Training Directorate: *Keeping the record straight*, Bristol, 1993, NHSTD.

Petrie P: *Communicating with children and infants*, London, 1989, Edward Arnold.

Roper N, Logan W, Tierney A: *Using a model for nursing*, Edinburgh, 1983, Churchill Livingstone.

Slater M: *Health for all our children: achieving appropriate healthcare for black and ethnic minority children and their families,* London, 1993, Action for Sick Children.

United Kingdom Central Council for Nursing, Midwifery and Health Visiting: *Standards for records and record keeping,* London, 1993, UKCC.

Walker C: Stress and coping in siblings of childhood cancer patients, *Nurs Res* 37(4):208, 1988.

FURTHER READING

Cluroe S: Educate to communicate, *Paediatr Nurs* 4(6):26, 1992.

Denehy J: Communicating with children through drawings. In Craft M, Denehy J, editors: *Nursing interventions for infants and children,* Philadelphia, 1990, WB Saunders.

Eiser C, Eiser JR, Hunt J: Developmental changes in analogies used to describe parts of the body: implications for communicating with sick children, *Child Care Health Devel* 12(5):277, 1986.

Hahn K: Therapeutic storytelling: helping children learn and cope, *Pediatr Nurs* 13(3):175, 1987.

Jolly J: Communicating with children. In Glasper A: *Child care: some nursing perspectives,* London, 1991, Wolfe.

Jolly J: *The other side of paediatrics: a guide to the everyday care of sick children,* London, 1981, Macmillan.

Kitzinger S, Kitzinger C: *Talking with children about things that matter,* London, 1989, Pandora.

Morrison P, Burnard P: *Caring and communicating: the interpersonal relationship in nursing,* Basingstoke, 1991, Macmillan.

Pederson CJ, Anderson JM: Factors that impact data collection from children, *Cancer Nurs* 3(6):439, 1980.

Perry J: Commmunicating with toddlers in hospital, *Paediatr Nurs* 6(5):14, 1994.

Petrie P: *Communicating with children and adults: interpersonal skills for those working with babies and children,* London, 1989, Edward Arnold.

Phillips T: Communication in the health care of children. In Lindsay B, editor: *The child and family: comtempory nursing issues in child health and care,* London, 1994, Baillière Tindall.

Smith DP, editor: *Comprehensive child and family nursing skills,* St Louis, 1991, Mosby.

Chapter 10

Growth and Development of Children

LEARNING OUTCOMES

After studying this chapter you should be able to:

◆ Describe the foundations for healthy growth and development.
◆ Outline the stages of growth and development.
◆ Identify some of the conditions that threaten normal growth and development.
◆ Define the glossary terms.
◆ Describe the stages of language development.
◆ Outline the importance of play and its charactetistics.

GLOSSARY

cephalocaudal Head-to-tail direction of growth

cross-sectional Method of study that measures a group at the same point in time

development A gradual change and expansion; advancement from lower to more advanced stages of complexity; the emerging and expanding of an individual's capacities through growth, maturation and learning

developmental task A set of skills and competencies, peculiar to each developmental stage, that children must accomplish or master in order to deal effectively with their environment

differentiation Processes by which early cells and structures are systematically modified and altered to achieve specific and characteristic physical and chemical properties

growth An increase in number and size of cells as they divide and synthesize new proteins; results in increased size and weight of the whole or any of its parts

longitudinal A method of study that compares the same individual at different points in time

maturation An increase in competence and adaptability; ageing; usually used to describe a qualitative change; a change in the complexity of a structure that makes it possible for that structure to begin functioning; to function at a higher level

proximodistal near-to-far direction of growth

rowth and development are complex processes involving numerous components that are subject to a wide variety of influences. All facets of the child's body, mind and personality develop simultaneously (although not independently), and emerge at varying rates and sequences. Infants depend totally on adults for satisfaction of the most basic needs (with the exception of limited reflex responses). As development proceeds, children begin to communicate their needs verbally and nonverbally, and to assume increasing responsibility for their basic need gratification.

Those who care for children come to understand the physical changes that take place during the process of development and the special needs generated by these changes; for example, the nature and quantity of food intake, the method and frequency of feeding, and the amount of sleep and activity that change during childhood. Health and safety hazards associated with every phase of development require provisions for the child's physical safety (including prevention of injuries and disease) and education of children, families and communities regarding these potential threats to health and well-being.

This chapter introduces the general progression and flow of developmental changes that take place throughout childhood.

GROWTH AND DEVELOPMENT

All children are basically alike. They follow the same pattern of development and maturation, although their genetic, cultural and experiential backgrounds make each child unique. However, individual children differ in their rate of growth, their ultimate size and capabilities, and the way in which they respond to their environment.

FOUNDATIONS OF GROWTH AND DEVELOPMENT

'Growth and development' includes the numerous changes that occur during the lifetime of an individual. It is a dynamic process that encompasses several related dimensions: growth, development, maturation and differentiation (see Glossary).

All of these processes are inter-related. Although they are simultaneous, ongoing processes, none normally occurs without the others. For example, the child's body becomes

larger and the personality simultaneously expands in scope and complexity. Very simply, growth can be viewed as a *quantitative* change, and development as a *qualitative* change.

STAGES OF GROWTH AND DEVELOPMENT

Many authorities in the field of child development conveniently categorize child growth and behaviour into approximate age stages or in terms that describe the features of an age group. Since the age ranges of these stages are broad and do not account for individual differences, they cannot be applied to all children with any degree of precision. However, this categorization is a convenient way to describe characteristics associated with the majority of children at periods when distinctive developmental changes appear and when specific developmental tasks are accomplished. The sequence of descriptive age periods and sub-periods used here is listed in Box 10-1.

PATTERNS OF GROWTH AND DEVELOPMENT

There are definite and predictable patterns in growth and development that are continuous, orderly and progressive. These patterns are universal and basic to all human beings. Although they are more apparent with respect to physical growth, most of these patterns also apply to psychological and social skills development. They follow predetermined trends in direction, sequence and pace. However, each human being accomplishes these with a unique manner and time-frame.

Directional trends
Growth and development proceed in regular, related directions, or gradients, and reflect the physical development and maturation of neuromuscular functions (Fig. 10-1). The first pattern is the *cephalocaudal*, or head-to-tail, direction. The head end of the organism develops first, whereas the lower end takes shape at a later period. The physical evidence of this trend is most apparent during the period before birth, but also applies to postnatal development. Infants achieve structural control of the head before the trunk and extremities, hold their back erect before they stand, use their eyes before their hands, and gain control of their hands before they have control of their feet.

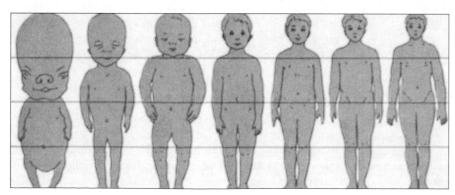

Fig. 10-1 Changes in body proportions from before birth to adulthood. (From Crouch JE, McClintic JR: Human anatomy and physiology, ed 2, New York, 1976, John Wiley & Sons.)

♦ **BOX 10-1**

Developmental Age Periods

Prenatal period: Conception to birth
GERMINAL: conception to approximately two weeks
EMBRYONIC: 2-8 weeks
FETAL: 8-40 weeks (birth)
A rapid growth rate and total dependency make this one of the most critical periods in the developmental process. The relationship between maternal health and certain manifestations in the newborn emphasizes the importance of adequate antenatal care to the health and well-being of the infant.

Infancy period: Birth to 12 or 18 months
NEONATAL: Birth to 28 days
INFANCY: 1 to approximately 12 months
The infancy period is one of rapid motor, cognitive and social development. Through mutuality with the care-giver (parent/ guardian), the infant establishes a basic trust in the world and establishes the foundation for future interpersonal relationships. The crucial first month of life, although part of the infancy period, is often differentiated from the remainder, because of the major physical adjustments to extrauterine existence and the psychological adjustment of the parent.

Early childhood: 1-5 years
TODDLER: 1-3 years
PRESCHOOL: 3-5 years
This period, which extends from the time the children attain upright locomotion until they enter school, is characterized by intense activity and discovery. It is a time of marked physical and personality development. Motor development advances steadily. Children at this age acquire language and wider social relationships, learn role standards, gain self-control and mastery, develop increasing awareness of dependence and independence, and begin to develop a self-concept.

Middle childhood: 5-11 or 12 years
Frequently referred to as the 'school age', this period of development is one in which the child is directed away from the family group and is centred around the wider world of peer relationships. There is steady advancement in physical, mental and social development with emphasis on developing skill competencies. Social cooperation and early moral development take on more importance with relevance for later life stages. This is a significant period in the development of a self-concept.

Later childhood: 11-19 years
PREPUBERTAL: 10-13 years
ADOLESCENCE: 13 to approximately 18 years
The tumultuous period of rapid maturation and change known as adolescence is considered to be a transitional period that begins at the onset of puberty and extends to the point of entry into the adult world. Biological and personality maturation are accompanied by physical and emotional turmoil, and there is redefining of the self-concept. In the late adolescent period, the child begins to internalize all previously learned values and to focus on an individual, rather than a group, identity.

The *proximodistal* (near-to-far) trend applies to the midline-to-peripheral concept. A conspicuous illustration is the early embryonic development of limb buds, followed by rudimentary fingers and toes. In the infant, shoulder control precedes mastery of hands (the whole hand is used as a unit before the fingers can be manipulated), and the central nervous system develops more rapidly than the peripheral nervous system.

These trends or patterns are bilateral, and appear to be symmetrical: each side develops in the same direction and at the same rate as the other.

The third trend in directional growth, *mass-to-specific* (sometimes referred to as 'differentiation'), describes development from simple operations to more complex activities and functions. From very broad patterns of behaviour, more specific, refined patterns emerge. Through the processes of development and differentiation, early embryonal cells with vague, undifferentiated functions progress to an immensely complex organism composed of highly specialized and diversified cells, tissues and organs. Generalized development will precede specific or specialized development; gross, random muscle movements take place before fine muscle control. The child will initially run and jump for the sake of motion, but eventually these activities take the more complex form of a race, hopscotch, or similar game.

Sequential trends

In all aspects of growth and development there is a definite, predictable sequence. It is orderly and continuous, and children normally passes through every stage. Each stage is affected by those preceding it and affects those that follow. Sequential patterns have been described for motor skills such as locomotion and use of hands, and types of behaviour such as language and social skills. Children crawl before they stand, and stand before they walk. Children first play alone, then with others in increasing numbers and increasingly complex activities.

New biological parts and behaviours arise from and build upon those already established. This continuity with the past (*epigenesis*) serves as a foundation for the future and requires interaction with a suitable environment at the proper time.

Developmental pace

Although there is a fixed, precise order to development, it does not progress at the same rate or pace in all children. There are periods of accelerated growth and periods of decelerated growth in both total body growth and growth of subsystems. The rapid growth rate before and after birth gradually levels off throughout early childhood. It is relatively slow during middle childhood, increases markedly at the beginning of adolescence, and levels off in early adulthood.

Research suggests that normal growth, in particular height in infants, may occur in brief (possibly even 24-hour) bursts that punctuate long periods in which no measurable growth takes place (Lampl, 1992). Further, findings indicate a stuttering or *saltatory* pattern of growth that follows no regular cycle and can occur after 'quiet' periods that last as long as four weeks. Mothers reported that their children were usually fussy and voraciously hungry a day or two before the growth spurt.

Sensitive periods

There are limited times during the process of growth when children interact with a particular environment in a specific manner. The terms *critical periods*, *sensitive periods* and *vulnerable periods* describe those times in an organism's lifetime when it is more susceptible to positive or negative influences. Colombo (1982) describes a 'critical' period as one when the developing organism is more sensitive to beneficial stimulation or more susceptible to detrimental influences. Touwen (1989) suggests that 'critical' period implies the need for specific stimulation, while 'sensitive' and 'vulnerable' periods of maturation are those during which external conditions may be particularly harmful to specific tissues, organs or systems.

The quality of interactions during these sensitive periods determines whether the effects on the children will be beneficial or harmful. The character and extent of the interaction's consequences depend upon the nature of the environmental influences and upon the child's stage of development. For example, physiological maturation of the central nervous system is influenced by adequacy and timing of contributions from the environment, such as stimulation and nutrition.

Psychological development also appears to have sensitive periods when an environmental event has maximum influence on the developing personality. Observers have identified periods in development when behaviour patterns are most readily acquired. For example, primary socialization occurs during the first year, when infants make their initial social attachments and establish a basic trust in the world. At this time, a warm relationship with the caregiver is fundamental to a healthy parent-child relationship (Mitchell and Mills, 1983). The sensitive period concept might also be applied to readiness for learning skills, such as toilet training or reading. In these instances there appears to be an opportune time when the skill is best learned. However, if the skill is not learned at this time, acquisition at a later time is still possible.

BIOLOGICAL GROWTH AND DEVELOPMENT

As children grow, their external dimensions change. These changes are accompanied by corresponding alterations in structure and function of internal organs and tissues. Although these alterations are progressive and interdependent, they are not a uniform process: they are characterized by cycles of accelerated and slow development that vary from organ to organ and system to system.

EXTERNAL PROPORTIONS

Variations in the growth rate of different tissues and organ systems produce significant changes in body proportions during childhood. The cephalocaudal trend of development is most evident in total body growth as indicated by these changes

(Fig. 10-1). During fetal development, the head is the fastest growing part. At two months of gestation, the head comprises 50% of total body length. During infancy, growth of the trunk predominates. During childhood, the legs are the most rapidly growing part. During adolescence, the trunk once again elongates. In newborns, the lower limbs are one-third of total body length, but only 15% of total body weight. In adults, the lower limbs comprise one-half of total body height and 30% of total body weight. As growth proceeds, the midpoint in head–to-toe measurements gradually descends from a level even with the umbilicus at birth, to the level of the symphysis pubis at maturity.

The first year is a period of rapid growth, dominated by lengthening of the trunk and accumulation of subcutaneous fat. When infants begin to walk, their large head, heavy trunk and protuberant abdomen atop short legs force them to walk with a wide stance, outward rotation of the hips, and everted feet. The high centre of gravity created by such disproportion causes infants to walk unsteadily and contributes to frequent stumbling and falls.

After the first year and until puberty, the legs grow more rapidly than any other part. The bowlegged appearance disappears with locomotion, the abdomen is held in, and the body becomes slender and elongated. Until puberty, this slender, long-legged build is characteristic of both sexes.

With the onset of puberty, there is marked alteration in body proportion, when all structures show the effects of the pubertal growth spurt. The feet and hands are first to increase in rate of growth, therefore, during this transient period they appear large and ungainly in relation to the rest of the body (this is often embarrassing to adolescents). The trunk again grows faster than the legs, so that a large portion of the increase in height at adolescence is a result of trunk growth.

One of the more outstanding features of changing body proportion is the breadth of shoulders and hips resulting from hormone secretion of maturing gonads. Shoulder and hip growth increase in both sexes, but the shoulder width in boys is considerably greater than in girls. The anteroposterior hip diameter increases in girls, and the female pelvis becomes wider, shallower and roomier than the male pelvis. The differences in deposition of fat produce the distinctive feminine contours in girls and loss of subcutaneous fat in boys.

Facial proportions

Facial proportions show characteristic changes during childhood. In infancy and early childhood, the face is small in relation to the skull (Fig. 10-2). The size of the cranial vault reflects the advanced development of the human brain. The brain has achieved 25% of its adult size at birth and 50% at the end of one year. More than 90% of the growth of the brain cavity has been reached by the end of the fifth year, and 98% has been achieved at age 15 years.

After the first year, the facial skeleton grows more rapidly than the brain case. The principal growth occurs in the jaws, as they enlarge to accommodate the teeth, and in the muscles of mastication as they develop. The face grows first in width

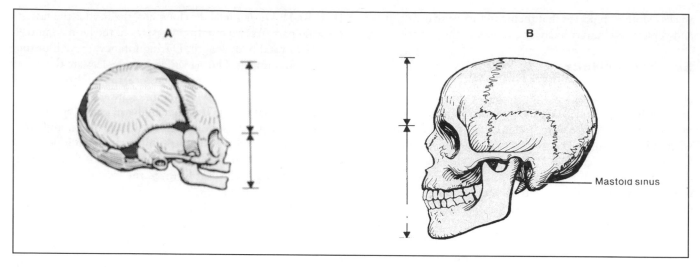

Fig. 10-2 Comparison of face and cranial proportions in A, infant, and B, adult, skulls. Note differences in relative size of face and angle of mandible, absence of mastoid sinus in infant and absence of fontanels (red) in adult.

and then in length, so that the child's face appears to emerge from underneath the skull, particularly during adolescence.

The size of the face relative to the skull has implications for health in the infant and young child. The large, heavy cranium is the primary site of injury in falls. The changing dimensions of the face alter the diameter and angle of ear structures, particularly the external auditory meatus and the eustachian tube. The latter contributes significantly to the incidence of middle ear infection.

BIOLOGICAL DETERMINANTS OF GROWTH AND DEVELOPMENT

A prominent feature of childhood and adolescence is physical growth. In some tissues, growth is continuous (e.g., bone growth and dentition); in others, significant alterations occur at specific stages (e.g., appearance of secondary sex characteristics). Satisfactory growth achievement is most commonly judged in terms of increase in body weight, height and skeletal growth. Serial measurements taken over time and compared with standardized norms can predict a child's developmental progress with a high degree of confidence. Table 10-1 and Fig. 10-3 indicate the general trends in height and weight gain during childhood.

Height

Linear growth (height) occurs almost entirely as a result of skeletal growth, and is considered to be a stable measure of general growth. It is not uniform throughout life, but when maturation of the skeleton is complete, linear growth ceases. By two years of age, children normally have achieved 50% of their adult height. By four years of age, birth length (height) has usually doubled.

At approximately three years of age, children begin a relatively stable and steady growth rate of 5-6 cm per year that continues for the next nine years. This long midgrowth period

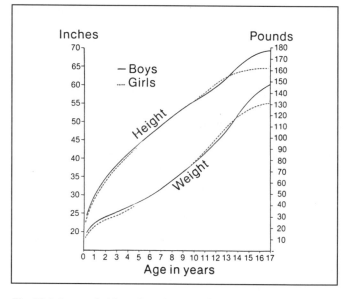

Fig. 10-3 Average height and weight curves for boys and girls. The earlier increase for girls at adolescence is clearly shown. Most girls are larger than boys between ages 11 and 13, probably a result of earlier influence of sex hormones on physical growth. (From Lowrey GH: *Growth and development of children*, ed 8, St Louis, 1986, Mosby–Year Book.)

ends with a sudden and marked acceleration — the adolescent growth spurt. Although there is wide variation, this increase, which begins about ages 10.5-11 in girls and 12.5 in boys, lasts approximately 2-2.5 years. During this time, boys may add 20 cm to their height and girls may add 16 cm. Usually, 98% of the terminal height is reached by age 16.5 in girls, but not until age 17 in boys (Table 10-2).

From analysis of data derived from longitudinal studies, it is possible to state the percentage of terminal height that has been achieved at any given age, and to predict the future height

AGE	WEIGHT*	HEIGHT*
Infants		
Birth–6 months	Weekly gain: 140-200 g (5-7 oz) Birth weight doubles by end of first 4-7 months†	Monthly gain: 2.5 cm(1 inch)
6–12 months	Weight gain: 85-140 g (3-5 oz) Birth weight triples by end of first year	Monthly gain: 1.25 cm(0.5 inch) Birth length increases by approximately 50% by end of first year
Toddlers	Birth weight triples by 14-17 months† Birth weight quadruples by age 2.5 Yearly gain: 2-3 kg (4.5-6.5 lb)	Height at age 2 is approximately 50% of eventual adult height Gain during second year: about 12 cm (4.75 inches) Gain during third year: about 6-8 cm (2.375-3.25 inches)
Preschool Children	Yearly gain: 2-3kg (4.5-6.5 lb) Yearly gain: 5-7.5cm (2-3 inches)	Birth length doubles by age 4
School-Aged Children	Yearly gain: 2-3kg (4.5-6.5 lb)	Yearly gain after age 7: 5 cm (2 inches) Birth length triples by about age 13
Pubertal Growth Spurt		
Females – 10-14 years	Weight gain: 7-25 kg (15-55 lb) Mean: 17.5kg (38.125lb)	Height gain: 5-25 cm (2-10 inches); approximately 95% of mature height achieved by onset of menarche or skeletal age of 13 Mean: 20.5 cm (8.25 inches)
Males – 11-16 years	Weight gain: 7-30 kg (15-65 lb) Mean: 23.7kg (52.125 lb)	Height gain: 10-30 cm (4-12 inches); approximately 95% of mature height achieved by skeletal age of 15 years Mean: 27.5 cm (11 inches)

*Yearly height and weight gains for each age-group represent averaged estimates from a variety of sources.
†Jung and Czajka-Narins, 1985.

Table 10-1 General trends in height and weight gain during childhood.

CHRONOLOGICAL AGE	PERCENT OF EVENTUAL HEIGHT	
Years	**Boys**	**Girls**
1	42.2	44.7
2	49.5	52.8
3	53.8	57.0
4	58.0	61.8
5	61.8	66.2
6	65.2	70.3
7	69.0	74.0
8	72.0	77.5
9	75.0	80.7
10	78.0	84.4
11	81.1	88.4
12	84.2	92.9
13	87.3	96.5
14	91.5	98.3
15	96.1	99.1
16	98.3	99.6
17	99.3	100.0
18	99.8	100.0

From Bayley, 1956.

Table 10-2 Percentage of mature height attained at different ages.

of an individual from measurements taken in childhood. Predictions are of little value until the second year of life. By this time, the child has frequently compensated for any deviations related to prematurity or other prenatal influences. However, children with lower birth weights are likely to remain shorter and lighter throughout childhood (Binkin *et al.*, 1988). Variability in the onset of puberty may also alter the predictive value in this age group.

Weight

At birth, weight is more variable than height and, to a greater extent, is a reflection of the intrauterine environment. After an initial loss of weight in the days following birth, the rate of weight gain increases rapidly, but soon slows. After the second year, the 'normal' rate of weight gain, just like the growth rate in height, assumes a steady annual increase (approximately 2-2.75 kg per year), until the adolescent growth spurt.

Weight gain is usually considered to be an indication of satisfactory growth progress in a child. However, it may be difficult to determine if this increase in weight is caused by healthy tissue development or by an unhealthy deposition of fat.

SKELETAL GROWTH AND MATURATION

Growth of the skeleton follows a genetically programmed plan. It provides evidence for the best estimate of biological age. Skeletal age has been shown to correlate more closely with other measures of physiological maturity (e.g., onset of menarche) than with chronological age or height. This 'bone age' is determined by comparing the mineralization of ossification centres and advancing bony form to age-related standards. Skeletal maturation begins with the appearance of centres of ossification in the embryo and ends when the last epiphysis is firmly fused to the shaft of its bone.

In a healthy child, skeletal growth and development consist of two concurrent processes: (1) creation of new cells and tissues (growth), and (2) consolidation of these tissues into a permanent form (maturation). Early in fetal life, closely packed connective tissue forms cartilage, which enlarges within the forming structures and builds successive layers onto the surface of the mass. Bone formation begins during the second month of fetal life, when calcium salts are deposited in the intercellular substance (matrix) to form calcified cartilage first, and then true bone.

NEUROLOGICAL MATURATION

In contrast to other body tissues, which grow rapidly after birth, the nervous system grows proportionately more rapidly before birth. Two periods of rapid brain cell growth occur during fetal life: (1) a dramatic increase in the number of neurons between 15-20 weeks of gestation, and (2) another increase at 30 weeks, which extends to one year of age. The rapid growth of infancy continues during early childhood, then slows to a more gradual rate during later childhood and adolescence. It is believed that no new nerve cells appear after the sixth month of fetal life.

Brain

Brain volume is reflected in head circumference, which increases six times as much during the first year as it does in the second year of life. One-half of post-natal brain growth is achieved by one year of age, 75% by age three and 90% by age six. The brain comprises 12% of the body weight at birth, doubles in weight in the first year, and has tripled by age five or six. Thereafter, growth slows until the brain is only about 2% of total body weight in adulthood.

LYMPHOID TISSUES

Lymphoid tissues contained in the lymph nodes, thymus, spleen, tonsils, adenoids and blood lymphocytes follow a distinctive growth pattern unlike that of other body tissues. These tissues are small in relation to total body size, but they are well developed at birth. They increase rapidly to reach adult dimensions by six years of age and continue to grow. At 10-12 years, the tissues reach maximum development (approximately twice their adult size), followed by a rapid decline to stable adult dimensions by the end of adolescence.

Lymph nodes are large, and the superficially located nodes are often palpable. The tonsils, massive during early childhood, become inconspicuous in adults. The thymus gland beneath the sternum, a prominent feature in infancy, will probably be impossible to detect in an adult. The growth pattern of lymphatic tissues parallels the development of immunity, and probably reflects the repeated exposure to new infectious agents.

DENTITION

The course of dentition is sometimes divided into four major stages: growth, calcification, eruption and attrition. The primary teeth arise as outgrowths of the oral epithelium during the sixth week of embryonic life and begin to calcify during the fourth to sixth months. Tooth buds form at ten different points in each arch and eventually become the enamel organs for the 20 primary (deciduous) teeth. All the buds are present at birth, but the amount of enamel laid down varies with each set of teeth.

Teeth are divided into quadrants of the mandible and maxilla, and are named for their location in each quadrant of the dental arch, such as central incisor, lateral incisor, and first and second molars. Teeth are also named after their specific function in the mastication of food. The knife-like or scissors-like, central and lateral incisors cut the food. The single-pointed cuspids, also called *canines,* tear the food. The two premolars, called *bicuspids* because of their two-pointed crown, crush the food. The permanent molars, which have four or five cusps, grind the food.

Dental maturation does not correlate well with bone age and is unreliable as an index of biological age. Delayed eruption is more common than accelerated eruption, and may be caused by heredity or may, rarely, indicate health problems such as endocrine disturbance, nutritional factors or malposition of teeth.

SLEEP AND REST

Sleep, a protective function in all organisms, allows for repair and recovery of tissues following activity. As in most aspects of development, a wide variation exists among individual children, and ages of children, in the amount and distribution of sleep. As the child matures, the quantity and quality of sleep changes. Family influences, social expectations and cultural variations in sleep patterns must be considered when analyzing sleep problems.

TIME AND QUALITY OF SLEEP

The length of time spent in sleep decreases throughout childhood. New-borns sleep much of the time not occupied with feeding and other aspects of their care. Larger new-borns sleep for longer periods than smaller ones, because of their larger stomach capacity. As infants mature, total time spent in sleep gradually decreases, and they remain awake for longer periods

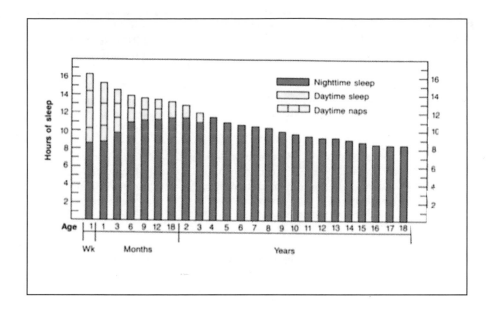

Fig. 10-4 Changes in number of hours of sleep with increasing age. (Modified from Ferber R: *Solve your child's sleep problems*, New York, 1985, Simon & Schuster.)

and sleep longer at night. During the later part of the first year, most children sleep through the night and take one or two naps during the day. By the time they are one-and-one-half years old, most children have eliminated the second nap. After age three, children have usually given up daytime naps, except in cultures in which an afternoon nap or siesta is customary. From ages 4-10, sleep time declines slightly, then increases somewhat during the pubertal growth spurt. The changes in length of sleep in relation to age are illustrated in Fig. 10-4.

DEVELOPMENT OF COGNITIVE FUNCTION AND PERSONALITY

Personality and cognitive skills develop in much the same manner as biological growth — new accomplishments, building on previously mastered skills. Table 10-3 summarizes some of the developmental theories.

THEORETICAL FOUNDATIONS OF LANGUAGE DEVELOPMENT

Children learn the complex symbol system of language with astonishing speed. They can express hundreds of different messages by age two, and know and use most of the syntactic structures of their native tongue by age five. However, at all stages of language development, children's comprehension vocabulary is greater than their expressed vocabulary, and the acquisition of vocabulary and language keeps pace with cognitive advancement (see Box 10-2).

THEORIES OF LANGUAGE DEVELOPMENT

There are three major theories of language acquisition: learning theory, nativism, and the interactional approach. *Learning theorists* believe language is acquired as children hear and respond to the speech of their companions. However, some disagreement exists regarding how children learn to speak. One faction believes that language is learned through operant conditioning as adults reinforce children for their attempts to produce grammatical speech. Others argue that children acquire language by listening to and imitating the speech of their older companions.

Nativists propose that humans have an inborn linguistic processor, or language acquisition mechanism, that is specialized for language learning. They also believe there is a

---

◆ BOX 10-2

Stages in Development of Language

Prelinguistic stage — the period before children utter their first meaningful words; develops in step-like fashion over first 10-12 months, from crying through cooing to babbling.

Holophrastic stage — the period when children's speech consists of one-word utterances, some of which are thought to be holophrases (single-word utterances that represent the meaning of an entire sentence); begins at about one year of age.

Telegraphic stage — the period when children's speech consists solely of content words, omitting the less meaningful parts of speech (such as articles, prepositions, and auxiliary verbs); begins at about 18-24 months of age.

Preschool period — when children begin to produce some very lengthy sentences and speech increases in complexity; ages 30 months to five years.

Middle childhood period — when children refine their language skills and increase linguistic competence; ages 6-14 years. They use bigger words, produce longer and more complex utterances, and learn subtle exceptions to grammatical rules. They begin to understand even the most complex syntactic structures of their native language.

STAGE/age	RADIUS OF SIGNIFICANT RELATION- SHIPS	PSYCHO- SEXUAL STAGES*	PSYCHO- SOCIAL STAGES+	COGNITIVE STAGES §	MORAL JUDGEMENT STAGES¶
I Infancy Birth to I year	Maternal person (unipolar-bipolar)	Oral sensory	Trust vs mistrust	Sensorimotor (birth to 18 months)	
II Toddlerhood 1-3 years	Parental persons (tripolar)	Anal-urethral	Autonomy vs shame and doubt	Preoperational thought, preconceptual phase (transductive reasoning) (e.g., specific to specific) (2-4 years)	Preconventional (prehmoral) level Punishment and obedience orientation
III Early childhood 3-5 years	Basic family	Phallic- locomotion	Initiative vs guilt	Preoperational thought, intuitive phase (transductive reasoning) (4-7 years)	Preconventional (pre-moral) level Naive instrumental orientation
IV Middle childhood 5-12 years	Neighbourhood, school	Latency	Industry vs inferiority	Concrete operations (inductive reasoning and beginning logic)	Conventional level Good-boy, nice-girl orientation Law-and-order orientation
V Adolescence 13-19 years	Peer group and outgoups Models of leadership Partners in frienship, sex, competition, cooperation	Genitality	Identity and repudiation vs identity confusion	Formal operations (deductive and abstract reasoning)	Postconventional or principled level Social-contract orientation Universal ethical principle orientation (no longer included in revised theory)
VI Early adulthood	Divided labour and shared household		Intimacy and solidarity vs isolation		
VII Young and middle adulthood	Mankind 'my kind'		Generativity vs self-absorption		
VII Later adulthood			Ego integrity vs despair		

Table 10-3 Summary of personality, moral and cognitive development theories. (According to *Freud, +Erikson, §Piaget and ¶Kohlberg.)

critical period for language development and that humans are most proficient at language learning between two years of age and puberty.

The *interactional* proponents acknowledge that children are biologically prepared to acquire language, but suggest that what may be innate is the development and maturation of the nervous system, rather than a special linguistic processor. They also recognize the crucial role of environment in language learning, because children must hear simplified versions of adult speech in order to acquire the needed linguistic concepts.

FACTORS AFFECTING LANGUAGE ACQUISITION

Girls are more advanced in language development than boys. First-born children develop language earlier than do later-born children, and children of multiple births (twins, triplets, etc.) develop language later than children of single births. Delayed, lack of, or impaired speech can result from several sources, including congenital structural defects of the mouth and nasopharynx, a hearing deficit, neurological dysfunction (including learning disability), maternal deprivation and other emotional factors.

THEORETICAL FOUNDATIONS OF SOCIAL LEARNING

Learning occurs when behaviour changes as a result of experience. Learning theories attempt to explain the ways in which controlled changes in the environment produce predictable changes in behaviour. Basically, children acquire new behaviours and produce alterations in existing behaviours through: (1) forming associations through conditioning and (2) observing models.

CONDITIONING (SKINNER)

Conditioning is learning by association, that is, establishing a connection between a stimulus and a response. In *classical* (Pavlovian) conditioning, two events which occur simultaneously or close together in time come to have similar meanings to the child, and thus evoke the same response. For example, infants learn very early to associate the sight of the mother's face and the sound of her voice with feeding and other pleasant sensations. Consequently, an infant will cease crying or somehow indicate pleasure when the mother speaks or enters the infant's visual field. This type of learning appears to be the predominant form that occurs during infancy (particularly in the first six months), before the development of motor control.

Operant (*instrumental*) conditioning uses rewards or reinforcements to encourage performance of specific behaviours. Reinforcing desired responses, whenever they occur, increases the likelihood that they will be repeated. Behaviour that is not in some way reinforced or rewarded will be extinguished. The principles of instrumental conditioning are especially applicable to learning that occurs naturally in toddlers and preschool children. These children can appreciate the significance of rewards and punishments, even though they may not be able to conceptualize the context or framework in which they are operating.

Avoidance conditioning discourages undesired behaviours through the use of punishment and fear of punishment. The effectiveness of rewards and punishments depends on the child's subjective assessment of the reward or punishment.

Operant conditioning is the basis of behaviour-modification procedures that have achieved varying degrees of success in speech therapy and in behaviour modification in children who are overly aggressive and/or children who have learning disabilities. Behaviour is shaped by reinforcing closer approximations to the behaviour being taught.

MODELLING OR OBSERVATIONAL LEARNING (BANDURA)

Much of childhood learning takes place because of children's innate tendency to observe and imitate the behaviour of people who are significant in their lives. Children learn by observing parents, siblings and peers, and through audio-visual sources such as video and television programmes. Learning is immediate, and children can often correctly imitate a behaviour on the first attempt. They are more likely to imitate those whom they believe to be prestigious and those whom they see being rewarded for their behaviour.

As children gain more complex cognitive skills and the use of language, learning assumes broader dimensions, involving creativity, problem solving and abstract conceptualization. Modelling requires no reinforcement, although in most situations children imitate a behaviour because they are in some way reinforced for doing so. A child may proudly proclaim to be doing something 'just like mummy and daddy'. Apparently, modelling is its own reward (Fig. 10-5).

ROLE LEARNING IN CHILDREN

A role is a set of duties, rights, obligations and expected behaviours that accompanies a given position in a social structure. Children are expected to play a variety of roles such as son or

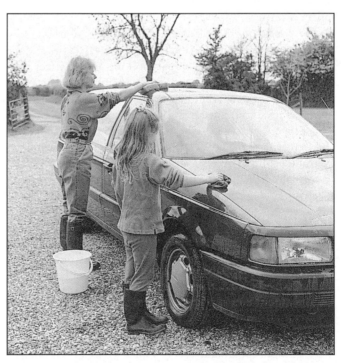

Fig. 10-5 Children learn by imitating the behaviour of others. (Courtesy of Southampton University Hospitals Trust)

daughter, sister or brother, student, classmate and playmate. They learn and practise these roles, and learn something of the characteristics of other roles, through play and through inter-action with others. Children will behave in patterned and pre-dictable ways, because they learn roles that define mutual expectations in typical and recurring social relationships.

The ability to interact successfully with other people is closely related to role-taking skills. Relationships change as children recognize that other people have different motives and intentions. For example, in Selman's Stage 1, a friend is someone who not only lives nearby, but also does nice things; at Stage 2 the term *friend* implies a reciprocal relationship with mutual respect, kindness and affection (Furman and Bierman, 1983). In adolescence, friendship becomes a relationship of common interests and values with a reasonably well-coordi-nated outlook on life, and a 'friend' becomes someone with whom intimate information can be shared (Berndt, 1982). It has also been found that children who are adept in role-taking abilities are better able to establish intimate friendships (McGuire and Weisz, 1982) and are more popular with class-mates (Kurdek and Krile, 1982).

DEVELOPMENT OF SELF-CONCEPT

'Self-concept' encompasses all the notions, beliefs, and con-victions that constitute children's knowledge of themselves and that influence their relationships with others. It is not present at birth, but develops gradually as a result of each child's unique experiences within the self, with significant others and with the realities of the world (Stuart and Sundeen, 1995). However, the self-concept is subjective and therefore may or may not reflect reality.

The content of the self-concept differs at various stages of development and results from the cognitive capacities and the dominant motives of individuals coming into contact with stage-related cultural expectations. In infancy, self-concept is primarily an awareness of one's independent existence learned, in part, from social contacts and experiences with other people. The process becomes more active during toddlerhood as children explore the limits of their capacities and the nature of their impact upon others (Newman and Newman, 1984).

School-aged children are more aware of differences in per-spectives among people, social norms and moral imperatives. They are sensitive to social pressures and become preoccupied with issues of self-criticism and self-evaluation. Because school-aged children depend upon adults for material and emo-tional resources, their self-concept is likely to be most vulner-able during this time. Little change in self-concept occurs during early adolescence, when children anxiously focus on their physical and emotional changes and peer acceptance. Self-concept crystallizes during later adolescence, as young people review and evaluate their childhood experiences and organize their self-concept around a set of values, goals and competen-cies (Newman and Newman, 1984).

BODY IMAGE

Body image, a vital component of the self-concept, is the sub-jective concepts and attitudes individuals have towards their own bodies. Central to the concept of self, body image is the picture of the body formed in the mind, including feelings about size, function, appearance and potential. The picture appears to be a learned phenomenon that may be conscious or unconscious, and may be cognitive and/or emotional. Body image has physical, psychological and social components, and includes present and past perceptions. It changes with advanc-ing development, and is continually modified by new percep-tions and experiences.

The 'significant others' in children's lives exert the most important and meaningful impact on children's body image. Labels that are attached to a child (such as 'skinny', 'pretty' or 'fat') or body parts are frequently incorporated into the child's body image.

Development during growth
Infants receive input about their bodies through self-exploration and sensory stimulation from others. As they begin to manip-ulate their environment, they become aware of their bodies as separate from others. Toddlers learn to identify various parts of their bodies and are able to use symbols to represent objects. Preschool children become aware of the wholeness of their bodies, and discover their genitals. Exploration of the genitals and the discovery of differences between the sexes become important. There is only a vague concept of internal organs and function (Selekman, 1983; Stuart and Sundeen, 1995).

School-aged children begin to learn about internal body structure and function, and become aware of differences in the body size and configurations of others. They are highly influ-enced by the cultural norms of society and the fads of the times. Children whose bodies deviate from the norm are often subject to criticism and ridicule.

Adolescence is the stage when children become most con-cerned about the physical self. The familiar body changes and the new physical self must be integrated into the self-concept. Adolescents face conflicts over what they see and what they visualize as the ideal body structure. Body image formation during adolescence is a crucial element in shaping their identity, and results in the 'psychosocial crisis' of adolescence.

SELF-ESTEEM

Self-esteem is the affective component of the self, and self-concept is the cognitive component; however, the two are almost indistinguishable, and the terms are often used inter-changeably (Stanwyck, 1983). Self-esteem is a personal, sub-jective judgement of one's worth derived from and influenced by the social groups in the immediate environment, and by the individual's perceptions of how he or she is valued by others. Self-esteem is primarily a function of being loved and of gaining the respect of others.

Self-esteem is a product of both competence and social acceptance that changes with development. Throughout childhood, children experience an increased ability to differentiate components of competence, an increased concern with a variety of significant others who may give or withhold approval, and an increased capacity to experience guilt when internal norms for either competence or social acceptance are violated (Newman and Newman, 1984). *High self-esteem* is described as a feeling based on unconditional acceptance of oneself as a worthy and important being (Stuart and Sundeen, 1995).

Highly egocentric toddlers are unaware of any difference between competence and social approval. They are the centre of their world, and to them all positive experiences are evidence of their importance and value. Preschool and early school-aged children, on the other hand, are increasingly aware of the discrepancy between their competencies and the abilities of more advanced children. As their competencies increase and they develop meaningful relationships, their self-esteem rises. Their self-esteem is again at risk during early adolescence when they are defining an identity and sense of self in the context of their peer group.

Children who experience warm, affectionate relationships with their family and who are aware of their parents' acceptance and positive attitudes towards them, are more accepting of themselves. Children who have a strong sense of their own worth are confident, able to initiate activities, explore their environment and take risks in their behaviour when confronted with new or novel situations. They approach tasks and relationships with the expectation that they will be well received and successful.

DEVELOPMENT OF SEXUALITY

From the moment of birth, children are treated differently by their families, based on their biological sex. Almost immediately, infants are placed in male or female categories with given names that clearly indicate a sex, dressed in pink if girls or blue if boys, and referred to as either 'he' or 'she'. Thus, information regarding a sexual identity is conveyed to children and to the world. Along with these overt messages, a set of sex-related attitudes towards them emerge. The outcome of the identification process depends on the characteristics of the parents and other role models, the innate capacities and preferences of the child, and the cultural and family values placed on the child's sex.

Families recognize the importance of sex differences and even in infancy treat boys differently from girls. Parental attitudes and expectations regarding sex-appropriate behaviours, generally acquired from the parents' own upbringing, influence how they react to their children. These attitudes and expectations are transmitted to infants first in subtle, then in more obvious, ways. For example, family members relate to infants differently: girls are handled more tenderly; boys are stimulated with boisterous activity and vigorous motor play. Families provide sex-appropriate toys and encourage play consistent with the sex-role expectations of the children, such as dolls for girls and cars for boys.

GENDER LABEL

The gender label is achieved early and subtly through imitation of the parents' expressions as they refer to children's gender, for example, 'That's a good girl' or 'That's a good boy'. Gender orientation has more effect on development than does chromosomal determination of sex.

However, with the increasing number of nontraditional gender roles portrayed on television, children's stereotypical perceptions of men and women may be changing. Children who are familiar with shows that depict men performing traditionally feminine tasks such as cooking, cleaning, and caring for children and women employed outside the home have a more flexible view of sex-related roles (Rosenwasser, Lingenfelter, and Harrington, 1989).

SEX-ROLE STANDARDS

Beginning when children are toddlers, sex-role standards are differentiated and continuously developed throughout childhood. By the time children are three years old, they know whether they are boys or girls, and they have acquired considerable knowledge of and a preference for sex-appropriate behaviours. They can differentiate one sex from the other even before they learn anatomical differences; two-year-old children can identify others as girls or boys, based on external appearances.

Preschool children have definite impressions of masculinity and femininity, and these are reflected in overt play. Most children in this age group engage in stereotyped sex-appropriate play activities. Girls are more likely to play at housekeeping, taking care of dolls, dressing up and cooking; boys choose cars, blocks, and more physically active play. Boys are generally more aggressive in their play, and in disagreements with peers they are more likely to react with shouting or fighting. Girls tend to be more dependent and introverted in their play (Maccoby and Jacklin, 1974).

Families expect children to learn appropriate sex-role behaviour early and to deviate little from it. Each family has its own concept of what constitutes male or female attributes and the types of sex-linked behaviour they wish to cultivate in their children. These beliefs are conveyed to the children by a variety of means, and parents exert special efforts to gain compliance with their expectations.

Observing siblings' interaction at play can provide insight into sex-role relationships. Sibling relationships mirror parent relationships, whether divorced or intact. For example, older boys from discordant families have been observed to bully their younger sisters (MacKinnon, 1989).

ROLE OF PLAY IN DEVELOPMENT

Play is claimed to be the work of the child (Eaton, 1993). Through the universal medium of play, children learn what no one can teach them. They learn about their world and how to deal with this environment of objects, time, space, structure and people. They learn about themselves operating within that environment — what they can do, how to relate to things and situations, and how to adapt themselves to the demands society makes on them. It has been said that play is the *work* of the child. In play, children continually practise the complicated, stressful processes of living, communicating and achieving satisfactory relationships with other people. In addition, while promoting and advancing development and relationships, play is an intrinsically motivated, often purposeless, and satisfying activity — something children do for the sheer fun of it.

CLASSIFICATION OF PLAY

From a developmental point of view, patterns of children's play can be categorized according to *content* and *social character*. In both, there is an additive effect; each builds on past accomplishments, and some element of each is maintained throughout life. At each stage in development, the new predominates.

CONTENT OF PLAY

The content of play involves primarily the physical aspects of play, although social relationships cannot be ignored. The content of play follows the directional trend, from simple to complex.

Social-affective play
Play begins with social-affective play, wherein infants take pleasure in relationships with people. As adults talk, cuddle, nuzzle, and in various ways elicit a response from an infant, the infant soon learns to provoke parental emotions and responses with such behaviours as smiling, cooing or initiating games and activities. The type and intensity of the adult behaviour with children vary among cultures.

Sense-pleasure play
Sense-pleasure play is a nonsocial stimulating experience that originates from without. Objects in the environment (light and colour, tastes and odours, textures and consistencies) attract children's attention, stimulate their senses and give pleasure. Pleasurable experiences are derived from handling raw materials (water, sand, food), from body motion (swinging, bouncing, rocking), and from other uses of senses and abilities (smelling, humming) (Fig. 10-6).

Skill play
Once infants have developed the ability to grasp and manipulate, they persistently demonstrate and exercise their newly acquired abilities through skill play, repeating an action over and over again. The element of sense-pleasure play is often evident in the practising of a new ability, but all too frequently the determination to conquer the elusive skill produces pain and frustration (e.g., learning to ride a bicycle).

Unoccupied behaviour
In unoccupied behaviour, children are not playful, but focus their attention momentarily on anything that strikes their interest. Children daydream, fiddle with clothes or other objects, or walk aimlessly. This role differs from that of onlookers, who actively observe the activity of others.

Dramatic, or pretend, play
One of the vital elements in children's process of identification is dramatic play, also known as *symbolic* or *pretend play*. It begins in late infancy (11-13 months) as children engage in simple pretending with familiar activities, such as eating, sleeping, or drinking from a cup. In toddlerhood, the activities are still primarily those that are familiar. As children enter the preschool stage, their play becomes further removed from everyday activities and becomes much more complex. Dramatic play is the predominant form of play in the preschool child.

Once children begin to invest situations and people with meanings, and to attribute affective significance to the world, they can pretend and fantasize almost anything. By acting out events of daily life, children learn and practise the roles and identities modelled by members of their family and society. Pretend play provides a framework within which mature behaviours are tested and assimilated (Connolly, Doyle, and Reznick, 1988).

Children's toys, replicas of the tools of society, provide a medium for learning about adult roles and activities that may be puzzling and frustrating to them. Interacting with the world is one way children get to know it. The simple, imitative, dramatic play of the toddler, such as using the telephone, driving a car, or rocking a doll, evolves into more complex, sustained dramas of the preschool child, which extend beyond

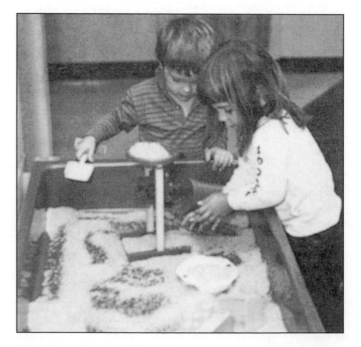

Fig. 10-6 Children derive pleasure from handling raw materials.

common domestic matters to wider aspects of the world and society, such as playing policeman, shopkeeper, teacher, or nurse. Older children work out elaborate themes, act out stories and compose plays.

Games

Children in all cultures engage in games alone and with others. Solitary activity involving games begins as very small children participate in repetitive activities and progress to more complicated games that challenge their independent skills, such as puzzle-solving and playing computer or video games.

Preschool children learn and enjoy *formal games* that begin with ritualistic, self-sustaining games, such as ring-around-a-rosy and London Bridge. With the exception of some simple board games, preschool children do not engage in *competitive games*. They do play competitively, but find it difficult not to take competition seriously. Preschool children hate to lose and will try to cheat, want to change rules, or demand exceptions and opportunities to change their moves. Competitive games are the province of school-aged children and adolescents, who enjoy a variety of physically active games such as football or netball.

SOCIAL CHARACTER OF PLAY

The play interactions of infancy are mainly between a child and an adult. Children continue to enjoy the company of an adult, but are increasingly able to play alone. As age advances, interaction with age-mates increases in importance and becomes an essential part of the socialization process (Fig. 10-7). Through interaction, highly egocentric infants, unable to tolerate delay or interference, ultimately acquire concern for others and the ability to delay gratification or even to reject gratification at the expense of others. A pair of toddlers engage in considerable combat, because their personal needs cannot tolerate delay or compromise. By the time they reach age five or six, children are able to compromise or arbitrate, usually after individual children have attempted, but failed, to gain their own way. Through continued interaction with peers, and the growth of conceptual abilities and social skills, children are able to increase participation with others.

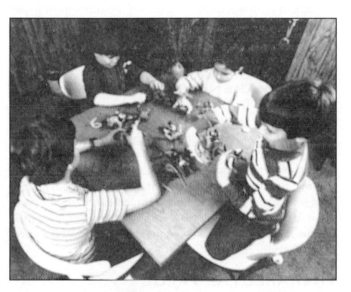

Fig. 10-7 Children show interest and pleasure in the company of others.

Associative play

When children play together and are engaged in a similar or even identical activity, but there is no organization, division of labour, leadership assignment, or mutual goal, the play is associative. Children borrow and lend play materials, follow each other with ride-on cars and tricycles, and sometimes attempt to control who may or may not play in the group. Each child acts according to his or her own wishes; there is no group goal (Fig. 10-8). For example, two children play with dolls, borrowing articles of clothing from each other and engaging in similar conversation, but neither directs the other's actions nor establishes rules regarding the limits of the play session. There is a great deal of behavioural contagion: when one child initiates an activity, the entire group follows the example.

Cooperative play

Cooperative play is organized, and the children play in a group *with* other children. The children discuss and plan activities for the purposes of accomplishing an end — to make something, to attain a competitive goal, to dramatize situations of adult or group life, or to play formal games. The group is loosely formed, but there is a marked sense of belonging or not belonging. The goal and its attainment require organization of activities, division of labour, and playing roles. The leader-follower relationship is definitely established, and the activity is controlled by one or two members who assign roles and direct the activity of the others. The activity is organized to allow one child to supplement another's function in order to complete the goal.

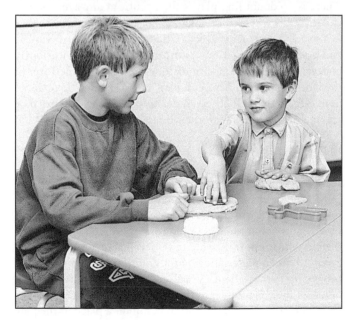

Fig. 10-8 Associative play.

FUNCTIONS OF PLAY

The specific values of play (the functions it serves throughout childhood) include sensorimotor development, intellectual development, socialization, creativity, self-awareness, and therapeutic and moral value.

SENSORIMOTOR DEVELOPMENT

Sensorimotor activity is a major component of play at all ages and is the predominant form of play in infancy. Active play is essential for muscle development and serves a useful purpose as a release for surplus energy. Through sensorimotor play, children explore the nature of the physical world. Infants gain impressions of themselves and their world through tactile, auditory, visual and kinaesthetic stimulation. Toddlers and preschool children revel in body movement and exploration of things in space. Older children also engage in sensorimotor play, although with increasing maturity, the play becomes more differentiated and involved. Whereas very young children run for the sheer joy of body movement, older children incorporate or modify the motions into increasingly complex and coordinated activities such as races, games, roller skating and bicycle riding.

INTELLECTUAL DEVELOPMENT

Through exploration and manipulation, children learn colours, shapes, sizes, textures and the significance of objects. They learn the significance of numbers and how to use them, they learn to associate words with objects, and they develop an understanding of abstract concepts and spatial relationships, such as up, down, under and over. Activities such as puzzles and games help them develop problem-solving skills. Play provides a means to practise and expand language skills.

SOCIALIZATION

From very early infancy, children show interest and pleasure in the company of others. Their initial social contact is with the mothering person, but through play with other children, they learn to establish social relationships and solve the problems associated with these relationships.

Children pass through four distinct phases in developing social competence in play during their first five years. Infants under one year of age investigate other infants in much the same manner as they investigate other objects in their environment. Children between ages two and three generally engage in considerable pretend play with mutually dependent roles such as mother and baby, doctor and patient, grocer and customer. Their social circle expands to include both short- and long-term friends. When they reach the preschool years, children become increasingly aware of a peer group and can identify stable characteristics of individual playmates. They have one or two favourite playmates with whom they play almost exclusively. They can verbalize judgements about each

other and sense a distinction between good friends and mere acquaintances (Howes, 1987).

In play, children learn to give and take, which is more readily learned from critical peers than from more tolerant adults. They learn the sex role that society expects them to fulfill, as well as approved patterns of behaviour. Closely associated with socialization is development of moral values and ethics. Children learn right from wrong, the standards of the society, and to assume responsibility for their actions.

CREATIVITY

In no other situation is there more opportunity to be creative than in play. Children can experiment and test their ideas in play through every medium at their disposal, including raw materials, fantasy and exploration. Creativity is stifled by pressure to conform; therefore, striving for peer approval may inhibit creative endeavours in the school-aged or adolescent child. Creativity is primarily a product of solitary, as opposed to group, activity.

SELF-AWARENESS

Beginning with active exploration of their bodies and awareness of themselves as separate from the caregiver, the process of self-identity is facilitated through play activities. Children learn who they are and what their place is in the world. They become increasingly able to regulate their own behaviour, to learn what their abilities are and to compare their abilities with those of others. Through play, children are able to test their abilities, assume and try out various roles, and learn the effect their behaviour has on others.

THERAPEUTIC VALUE

There is no doubt that play is therapeutic at any age. In play, children can express emotions and release unacceptable impulses in a socially acceptable fashion. Children are able to experiment and test fearful situations and can assume, and vicariously master, the roles and positions they are unable to perform in the world of reality. Through play, children are able to communicate, to the alert observer, the needs, fears and desires they are unable to express with their limited language skills.

MORAL VALUE

Although children learn at home and at school the behaviours considered right and wrong in the culture, their interaction with peers during play contributes significantly to their moral training. Nowhere is the enforcement of moral standards so rigid as in the play situation. If they are to be acceptable members of the group, children must adhere to the culturally accepted codes of behaviour: fairness, honesty, self-control and consideration for others. Children soon learn that their peers are less tolerant of violations than are adults, and to maintain a place in the play group they must conform to the standards of the group.

CHARACTERISTICS OF PLAY

There are several aspects of play that display developmental changes and that differentiate children's play from adult play.

TRADITION

In general, the play of small children varies little from generation to generation within a culture. Each generation of children imitates the play of the preceding generation. In this way, the more satisfying forms of play are perpetuated. Many types of play are characteristic of all cultures; for example, playing with balls, some form of doll, or some type of walking toy to help children, who are just beginning to walk, to maintain balance.

TIME AND AGE

The amount of time children spend in play decreases with age. Older children have less time available for play, because of an increase in schoolwork and other responsibilities. The number of playmates decreases with age as children progress from play with anyone available, to play with a few selected friends of the same age.

Children's play can be divided into the following four categories: (1) imitative, (2) exploratory, (3) testing, and (4) model building. At all ages, each type is evident in children's play, but one type will predominate over the others at specific ages. For example, imitative play is seen in infants who mimic the actions of other people (pat-a-cake), but it reaches its peak in the dramatic play of preschool children who play 'house', 'astronaut', or 'school'.

As children grow older, play activities become less spontaneous, more formal and structured, and increasingly sex appropriate.

PATTERNS OF DEVELOPMENT

Throughout childhood, certain play activities are popular at one age and not at another (Box 10-3). These activities are so consistent and predictable that childhood is sometimes divided into age stages according to the types of play characteristic of each particular phase of development.

As they grow older, children also use materials in more meaningful ways.

TOYS

Toys are the inanimate objects with which children interact. Cognitive development appears to be related to the variety and accessibility of objects for children to explore, experiment with, and come to know. Access to playthings, particularly during the earlier years, correlates with the accessibility of caregivers who make objects available, react to children's response to the objects, encourage further exploration and talk about what is happening. Consequently, although they can be significant in themselves, playthings assume an important aspect as a medium of social interchange.

SELECTING TOYS

The type of toys chosen by and/or provided for children can facilitate learning and development in the areas just described. Toys that are small replicas of the culture and its tools help children assimilate their culture and learn sex and occupational roles. Toys that require pushing, pulling, rolling and manipulating teach children about physical properties of the items and help to develop muscles and coordination. Rules and the basic elements of cooperation and organization are learned through board games.

Because they can be employed in a variety of ways, raw materials or multidimensional toys are best for enhancing skills and stimulating the imagination. Through manipulation, playthings such as boxes, clay and blocks can assume a multitude of symbolic objects and can inspire creative impulses. For example, building blocks can be used to construct a variety of things, to count, and to learn shapes and sizes. 'Educational' toys are less flexible. There are several ways in which families can encourage children's toy play.

Play materials need not be expensive or elaborate. Infants and small children derive enjoyment from simple kitchen utensils, such as wooden spoons and small plastic plates to bang, pot lids to clang together, and a nest of measuring spoons to rattle. Empty cartons, especially oversized ones used to pack furniture for shipping, can assume the function of a clubroom, a study or another private area. A waist-high mound of impacted dirt can become a place for small children to roll toy cars and balls, to dig holes during summer and a place for

---

◆ **BOX 10-3**

Age Characteristics of Play

Exploratory Stage

Age: Approximately 3-12 months

Activities: Grasping, holding, and examining articles

Exploration via crawling

Toy Stage

Age: 1-7 or 8 years

Activities: Imitating adult behaviour with replicas of adult tools

Play Stage

Age: 8-12 years

Activities: Interest in toys diminishes

Interest in games, sports, and hobbies increases

Daydreaming Stage

Age: Characteristic of older children and pubescents

Activities: Playing the martyr misunderstood and mistreated by everyone, or the hero or beauty admired by everyone

sliding in winter. Paper is a fascinating and versatile raw material for children of any age, and most books about toy materials include recipes for play dough and finger paint.

TOY SAFETY

Selection of toys and play equipment is a joint effort between parents and children, but evaluation of their safety is the responsibility of the adult. Although there are safety standards for most toys, age-specific safety depends on the parents (Avery and Jackson, 1993).

FACTORS THAT INFLUENCE DEVELOPMENT

Children are engaged in a continuous, dynamic, and reciprocal relationship with their environment in order to achieve and maintain an equilibrium. This equilibrium, or balance, is continually upset and regained through numerous and varied complex interactions. It is impossible to include a discussion of all the complex and interrelated factors that influence the development of children as unique individuals. However, some of the major areas of importance are presented.

PHYSICAL ENVIRONMENT

Some physical conditions have been shown to effect growth, although their influence is less evident than factors such as heredity, nutrition, or hormonal excesses or deficiencies.

SEASON, CLIMATE AND OXYGEN CONCENTRATION

There is some evidence that season and climate may have an influence on growth. Growth in height appears to be faster in the spring and summer months, whereas growth in weight proceeds more rapidly during the autumn and winter. These observations have not been satisfactorily explained. This phenomenon may have a hormonal basis, or it may be related to seasonal differences in activity levels.

There seems to be some evidence regarding the effects of hypoxia on growth. Children with disorders that produce chronic hypoxia are characteristically small when compared with children of the same chronological age. In addition, children native to high altitudes are smaller than those living at lower altitudes (Yip, Binkin, and Trowbridge, 1988).

NUTRITION

Probably the single most important influence on growth is nutrition. Dietary factors regulate growth at *all* stages of development, and their effects are exerted in numerous and complex ways (Horne and Ibbotson, 1991). Adequate nutrition provides the essential nutrients in the amount and balance necessary to sustain the needs of growing children. These needs vary widely according to age, level of activity and environmental conditions. Inadequacies in any or all of these essential nutrients will alter growth.

The nutritional requirements of childhood are directly related to the rate and direction of growth. During the rapid prenatal growth period, faulty nutrition may negatively influence development from the time of implantation of the ovum until birth. The nutritional needs are met entirely through the maternal system; as a result, maternal deficiencies or abnormalities in the supplementary intrauterine structures will be manifest in fetal development. Although the fetus is usually able to obtain adequate nutrition for prenatal growth unless the mother's nutrition is very poor, severe maternal malnutrition during the period of most rapid brain growth is associated with permanent reduction in the total number of fetal brain cells and can have a critical effect on the child's intellectual functioning.

During infancy and childhood, the demand for calories is relatively great, as evidenced by the rapid increase in both height and weight. Protein and calorific requirements are higher at this time than at almost any period of postnatal development. As the growth rate slows with its concomitant decrease in metabolism, a corresponding reduction in calorific and protein requirement occurs. Growth is uneven during the periods between infancy and adolescence, when there are plateaus and small growth spurts. The child's appetite fluctuates in response to these variations until the turbulent growth spurt of adolescence, when adequate nutrition is extremely important, but may be subject to numerous emotional influences. Children's calorific intake must equal their energy output plus that needed for growth. It is estimated that the average child (e.g., the 6- to -10-year-old child) expends 55% of the energy for metabolic maintenance, 25% for physical activity, 8% in faecal loss and 12% for growth.

Adequate nutrition is closely related to good health throughout life, and an overall improvement in nourishment is evidenced by the gradual increase in size and early maturation of children in this century. Furthermore, recent findings suggest that the pathogenesis of fatal coronary heart disease begins in fetal life and infancy, with the strongest relationship being identified between weight at one year and subsequent increased risk of mortality in adulthood (Fall *et al.*, 1995; Osmond *et al.*, 1993; Lucas, 1991). In the growing child, inadequate nutrition is dangerous, particularly during periods critical for growth. Inadequate nutrition has the greatest impact during the critical periods of rapid cell division. For example, normal development of the central nervous system depends on adequate nutrition during fetal life and throughout the first two years of postnatal life.

MALNUTRITION

The term *malnutrition* in its strictest sense is usually used to describe undernutrition, primarily that resulting from insufficient calorie intake. However, malnutrition may result from the following: (1) a dietary intake that is quantitatively or qualitatively inadequate, or both, including overnutrition; (2)

disease that interferes with appetite, digestion or absorption while increasing nutritional requirements; (3) excessive physical activity or inadequate rest; or (4) disturbed interpersonal relationships and other environmental or psychological factors. Severe malnutrition during the critical periods of development, particularly the first six months of life, is positively correlated with diminished height, weight, and intelligence scores. The importance of nutrition as a vital aspect of health promotion during all phases of the illness-wellness continuum is included as it relates to developmental phases and specific health problems.

INTERPERSONAL RELATIONSHIPS

Warm interpersonal relationships are essential to psychological well-being. Relationships with significant others play an important role in development, particularly in emotional, intellectual and personality development. Not only do the quality and quantity of contacts with other persons exert an influence on growing children, but the widening range of contacts is essential to learning and to the development of a healthy personality. During the formative years, culturally determined, age-appropriate behaviours are reinforced and consequently repeated. Thus, patterns of reward, punishment and modelling continually modify children's individuality of character and temperament. Children behave in a manner that elicits rewards from the persons most significant in their lives.

SIGNIFICANT OTHERS

Normal children routinely turn to parents, teachers and friends for comfort, protection, education, acceptance and material needs. Parents and care-giving persons are unquestionably the most influential persons during early infancy. They meet the infants' basic needs of food, warmth, comfort and love; provide stimulation for their senses; and facilitate their expanding capacities. Through these individuals, children learn to trust the world and feel secure to venture in increasingly wide relationships. Through constant reinforcement, children learn and incorporate the behaviours that bring satisfaction to the nurturing persons. Eventually, these behaviours become self-motivating.

As they get older, children seek approval from a widening sphere of persons, including other members of their family, their peers and, to a lesser degree other authority figures (e.g., teachers). The increasing importance of the peer group in determining the behaviour of school-aged children and adolescents is well documented. However, it is the quality of the parent-child relationship that determines, to a large extent, the impact of peer influence on a child.

Generally, parents are most influential in helping children to assume sex-role identification. Parents define and reinforce acceptable sex-role behaviour and provide sex-appropriate role models for the children. In the absence of a suitable sex-role model in the family, children may adopt some characteristics of the opposite-sex parent or sibling. Frequently, children identify with a teacher or other significant person of the same sex.

Siblings are children's first peers, and the way they learn to relate to each other can affect later interactions with peers outside the family group. For example, first-born children who are accustomed to a position of leadership with siblings tend to assume the same position with peers; younger children are more often followers. Ease in relationships with peers of the same or opposite sex is frequently associated with similar associations in the home.

Pets can also serve as an object for love and affection and play an important role in the lives of many young children. They provide close, nonjudgemental companionship, are on call 24 hours per day, and can be an excellent tool for helping build children's self-esteem. By assuming responsibility for the care of a pet, children can develop confidence in their abilities and gain respect for a job well done (Pets are Wonderful Council, 1985). Pets can also help children learn to develop a concern for other people.

LOVE AND AFFECTION

The most important emotional need of children is to be loved and to feel secure in that love. Children strive, above all else, to gain the love and acceptance of those who are significant in their lives. When they feel secure in this love, they are able to withstand the normal crises associated with growing up, as well as the unexpected crises (e.g., illness or loss) that are superimposed on the anticipated course of development.

Children cannot receive too much love. However, this love must be communicated to them through words and actions that tell them they are loved, not for their actions or achievement, but for what they are or simply *because they are*. Although love is closely associated with discipline, independence and other factors that influence the child's self-concept, it should be an undemanding, accepting love that is indispensable to the development of a healthy personality. Unconditional love, freely bestowed, helps establish a sense of security and a positive sense of self within children that will persist throughout their lifetime (Fig. 10-9). Children must know they are loved and that whatever happens, they can depend on this love. Without the security of loving relationships, children may become tense and insecure, and may develop undesirable behaviour patterns as they attempt to obtain that love or try to compensate for its loss.

SECURITY

Closely allied to the need for love, is the need for a sense of security. As they grow and develop in a complex world, children encounter many threats to their sense of security. Indeed, many childhood behaviour problems are associated with an element of insecurity. Every change in themselves or their environment creates a feeling of uncertainty. Faced with confusing, conflicting adjustments, young children need the security provided by relatively stable situations and dependable

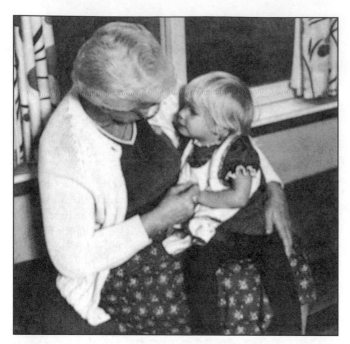

Fig. 10-9 A grandmother is a primary source of unconditional love and comfort.

human relationships. The degree to which they can cope with these stresses depends on the patience and support they receive from those most closely involved in their care.

DISCIPLINE AND AUTHORITY

Because children live in an organized society, they must be prepared to accept boundaries to their behaviour. Discipline is not punishment. Rather, it is the teaching of desirable behaviour. Children need to learn the rules governing behaviour in the home, neighbourhood, school and community at large. To learn acceptable behaviour that permits them to live enjoyably with themselves and others, children need the steady, firm guidance of loving parents and others in authority roles. Good discipline provides children with protection from dangers within and without, relieves them of the burden of decisions they are not prepared to make, but allows them to develop independence of thought and action within a secure framework.

DEPENDENCE AND INDEPENDENCE

As children grow and mature, they are increasingly able to direct their own activities and to make more independent decisions. However, there are great fluctuations in their ability to function independently. Even with a compelling inner drive to master and achieve, they are not always able to cope with difficult and frustrating problems or conflicts. Independence should be permitted to grow at its own rate.

Periods of regression and dependence not only are normal, but are often necessary and helpful. If children feel sufficiently comfortable and content in a situation or relationship, and

reasonably certain that they can return to this safety and security, they will venture into the untried and untested on their own. If they feel doubtful concerning their abilities to cope, regression to a more comfortable level of competence allows them to replenish their inner resources and move ahead once again. Independence grows out of dependence; one cannot be considered as distinct from the other.

EMOTIONAL DEPRIVATION

The most prominent feature of emotional deprivation, particularly during the first year, is developmental delay. Much of the information regarding the adverse effects of interpersonal influences on development has been acquired through retrospective studies of gross deprivation and trauma. The most notable instances involved homeless infants who were placed in institutions for care. These infants, who did not receive consistent care-giving, failed to gain weight even with an adequate diet. They were pale, listless and immobile, and unresponsive to stimuli that usually elicit a response (such as a smile or cooing) in normal infants. If the emotional deprivation continues for a sufficient length of time, the child does not survive.

Harlow's classic experiments with infant monkeys illustrate the extensive effects of emotional and social deprivation in infancy (Harlow and Harlow, 1962). In these experiments, the monkeys were raised by substitute, inanimate 'mothers', made of cloth-covered wire, from whom they derived nourishment and a measure of comfort, but no mothering. These monkeys developed abnormal play and sex behaviour. The few who bore offspring were unable to 'mother' them. However, those who were allowed peer associations developed normal play and social-sex behaviour. By correlating these findings with retrospective studies of human infants in comparable age-groups, attempts have been made to explain some of the behaviours observed in these children in later interpersonal relationships.

STRESS IN CHILDHOOD

Stress has been defined and described by numerous authorities from both a physiological and an emotional point of view. Most discussions centre on adult responses, but children are frequently among the most affected victims of a variety of threatening events. Essentially, stress is 'an imbalance between environmental demands and a person's coping resources that... disrupts the equilibrium of the person' (Masten, 1988).

Most research related to children has been restricted to specific stressors and stress-provoking experiences, such as hospitalization, separation and loss, and pain. Studies indicate a support for an association between the occurrence of stressful life events and physical and psychological problems in children (Grey, 1993). A description of all the stressors to which children are exposed is beyond the scope of this chapter; however, some common manifestations and stressful events are discussed briefly.

Although children are not strangers to stress, some children appear to be more vulnerable than others. Children's age, temperament, life situation and state of health affect their vulnerability, reactions and ability to handle stress. It is impossible, unrealistic, and undesirable to protect children from stress, but providing them with interpersonal security helps them develop coping strategies for dealing with stress. The concept of an emotional bank can help parents and caregivers maintain a proper perspective regarding the effects of stress and coping. According to Usdin (1988), children have an emotional bank in which deposits, as well as withdrawals, can be made. 'If the child has a good positive balance in the account, he or she can tolerate significant withdrawal experiences. If the child has a low balance, then even a minor withdrawal may bankrupt the account, causing it to be overdrawn.'

Parents and other caregivers can try to recognize signs of stress (Box 10-4) in order to help children manage stresses before they become overwhelming. If several stresses are imposed on children at the same time, the children are more vulnerable. When a succession of stresses produces an excessive stress load, children may experience a serious change in health and/or behaviour.

COPING

Coping is defined as 'flexible strategies for dealing with environmental challenges' (Murphy and Moriarity, 1976). It refers to a special class of individual reactions to stressors: specifically, a reaction to a stressor that resolves, reduces or replaces the affect state classified as stressful. Children, like adults, respond to everyday stress by trying to change the circumstances (primary control coping) or trying to adjust to circumstances the way they are (secondary control coping) (Band and Weisz, 1988). An example of primary control are tantrums or aggressive behaviour; withdrawal and submission are examples of secondary control.

Any strategy that provides relaxation is effective in reducing stress. Most children have their own natural methods; for example, withdrawal, physical activity, reading, listening to music, working on a project or taking a nap. The list is endless. Some turn to parents to solve their problems, or they may develop socially unacceptable strategies such as cheating, stealing or lying (Kuczen, 1982).

Children can be taught stress-reduction techniques. First, they must be helped to recognize signs of tension in themselves and then taught appropriate strategies, such as special exercises, relaxation and breathing, mental imagery and many other simple activities. Parents and other caregivers can anticipate possible stress-provoking events and can prepare children for coping by role playing a scenario or 'talking it through' beforehand.

Probably the most useful tool that children can learn is how to solve problems. When children can view any new situation as a problem to be solved and an opportunity to learn, they are not vulnerable to the control of others. It provides them with a sense of mastery over their own lives and reinforces the fact that they have within themselves the ability and information to handle whatever comes their way. Problem-solving skill

---

◆ **BOX 10-4**

Warning Signs: Childhood Stress

Bed-wetting in older children
Boasts of superiority
Complaints of feeling afraid or upset without being able to identify the source
Complaints of neck or back pains
Complaints of pounding heart
Complaints of stomach upset, nausea or vomiting
Compulsive cleanliness
Compulsive ear tugging, hair pulling or eyebrow plucking
Cruel behaviour towards people or pets
Decline in school achievement
Defiance
Demand for constant perfection
Depression
Dislike of school
Downgrading of self
Easily startled by unexpected sounds
Encopresis
Explosive crying
Extreme nervousness
Frequent daydreaming and retreats from reality
Frequent urination or diarrhoea
Headaches
Hyperactivity, or excessive tension or alertness
Increased number of minor falls, and other accidents
Irritability
Listlessness or lack of enthusiasm
Loss of interest in activities usually approached with vigour
Lying
Nightmares or night terror
Nervous laughter
Nervous tics, twitches or muscle spasms
Obvious attention-seeking
Overeating
Poor concentration
Poor eating
Poor sleep
Psychosomatic illnesses
Stealing
Stuttering
Teeth grinding (sometimes during sleep)
Thumb-sucking
Uncontrollable urge to run and hide
Unusual difficulty in getting along with friends
Unusual jealousy of close friends and siblings
Unusual sexual behaviour, such as spying or exhibitionism
Unusual shyness
Use of alcohol, drugs or cigarettes
Withdrawal from usual social activities

From Kuczen B, 1982.

gives them the confidence to know where and how to seek help when they need it.

CHILDHOOD FEARS

Fear is a normal function. It is a self-preservation signal that mobilizes the physiological resources of the organism. *Fear* and *anxiety* are often used interchangeably, and the physical reactions to both are almost identical. *Fear* is an emotional reaction to a specific real or unreal threat or danger; *anxiety* refers to a general uneasiness, apprehension or feeling of impending doom. Fear is a momentary reaction to danger based on a low estimate of one's own power. Fearful children perceive a threat (person, animal or situation) as being stronger than themselves and thus capable of harming them. When the balance of power is altered, the fear disappears. For example, children's fears can be alleviated by the presence of an adult whom they perceive as a source of protection; or fear can be overcome by familiarity with the source of the threat, such as a dark room. Anxiety is general, lasting, internally generated, and reflects overall feelings of weakness, ineptitude and helplessness (Wolman, 1978).

In childhood, the distinction between fear and anxiety is important, because childhood fears are specific and, except for the specific fear (or fears), children are happy and active. Childhood fears are limited problems and most are alleviated with growth and children's increased self-confidence. Unrealistic fears are abandoned with maturation and learning, to be replaced by realistic fears. As with other stresses, there are individual differences in susceptibility to fear, and certain fears are age related. Fears that are likely to persist into adulthood are fear of physical danger, death, sickness, bodily injury, physical assault, car accidents, aeroplane crashes and war. Nurses can help parents learn to recognize fear in their children by explaining that not all children express fear in the same way. Although some children cry and look afraid, other may make 'smart' remarks, act silly, bite their nails, suck their thumb, pretend they are not afraid, and/or change their playing, eating, or sleeping patterns.

Coping with fears is the same as coping with other stresses. To help children overcome their fears, parents and others should not shame or show disapproval for their fears, encourage their unreasonable fears, overprotect them, or force them into a situation they fear. For example, throwing a fearful child into deep water will probably increase a fear of water to the point of a lasting phobia. Parents can serve as models by demonstrating strength, decisiveness and self-confidence. For instance, parents can take their children by the hand and gently guide them into shallow water or around a dark room. Desensitization by gradually facing the fearsome object or situation is effective with most children. Parents can allow their children to express their fears and encourage them to cope with certain dangers. Most of all, parents need to make their children feel that they will always be loved and will be protected whenever necessary.

RESILIENCE

Some children manage to achieve stable personalities and a sense of competence despite adverse conditions and a series of stressful events in their childhood, such as biological insults, a pathological family environment, or the negative effects of poverty. This ego-resiliency has been observed in several studies (Anthony and Cohler, 1987; Garmezy and Rutter, 1989; Sroufe, 1983; Werner and Smith, 1982). The findings of these observations have determined that resilient children share several common characteristics: they were active, alert, responsive and sociable as infants, with the ability to elicit positive responses from other people, and acquired a strong sense of autonomy. As children, they enjoyed school, often using it as a refuge from a disordered home, and are well liked by peers. Although a more recent study of high-risk adolescents found similar results, findings also revealed that children labelled as resiliant were significantly more depressed and anxious than were competent children from low-stress backgrounds (Luthar, 1991).

Ego-resilient children use a wide variety of coping strategies, have hobbies and interests that give them a sense of mastery and pride, and have problem-solving and communication skills that they use effectively (Green, 1991). Central in the histories of all these children, regardless of the type and extent of their adversity, is that they had the opportunity to establish a secure relationship with at least one stable person who accepted them uncritically.

INFLUENCE OF THE MASS MEDIA

There is no doubt that communications media provide children with a means for extending their knowledge about the world. However, there is growing concern regarding the enormous influence the media can have on the developing child. Linkages have been established between mass media use and risk-taking behaviours in adolescents (Klein *et al.*, 1993). The images of risky behaviour presented by the media may serve to establish or reinforce teenagers' perceptions of their social environment.

READING MATERIALS

The oldest form of mass media (books, newspapers and magazines) contributes to children's competence in almost every direction, and provides enjoyment. Recognition of the influence of reading matter used in schools on children's value system and socialization processes prompted re-evaluation of textbook content regarding the biased presentation of male and female role models, the sugar-coated view of life situations, and the unrealistic, biased history of minority groups.

Fairy tales, for generations the mainstay of young children's literature, were once condemned as being sexist, overly violent in content, and riddled with unfavourable stereotypes, such as the wicked stepmother and physical unattractiveness associated with evil. These stories are now believed to provide an excellent medium for explaining puzzling and important topics such as death, step-parents, and inner feelings and turmoils. To a young child, the world is peopled by giants — adults who control their lives and threaten their autonomy, who want children to do something against their will. Children can see these giants overcome. The split view of parents is also portrayed in fairy tales: the 'good' parents who give children whatever they want and the 'mean' parents who deprive their children of things. Although they do not provide solutions, fairy tales confront children with emotional predicaments and offer suggestions for dealing with them.

Comic books have been popular in every generation, usually at the expense of literature provided by schools, libraries and parents. Many children have nothing else to read. The easy reading, quick action and adventure in brief episodes seem to fulfil a need for children who are striving to understand both aggression in others and their own impulses. Reading ability, intelligence and school adjustment apparently have no relationship to the number and type of comics read. Most comics appear to be relatively harmless to most children and are in some ways even beneficial. Comic books seem to have only a minor influence on acquisition of beliefs, values and behaviours. The popularity of this medium has prompted some educators to encourage translations of literature into comic book form in order to stimulate students' interest in the classics.

TELEVISION, FILMS AND VIDEOS

Many children watch two to three hours' television daily from the age of three or earlier, and during school age they average more time in front of the television than in the classroom (Gunter and McAleen, 1990). Although watching television is believed to provide benefits in terms of portraying an assortment of socially approved behaviours (Buckingham, 1993) by far the most attention has been given to the negative aspects. It has been reported in over 1000 studies that there is an association in some children and young people between screen violence and an increased level of aggression (Newson, 1994; Black and Newman, 1995). Increased aggression is not the only reported negative effect. The content of films, videos and television has changed markedly during the past few years with increasing amounts of violence being a major feature. Children who are unable to distinguish between reality and fantasy may find these images frightening and as a result develop night-time fears, short-term sleeplessness and other problems (Melville-Thomas and Sims, 1985; Schmitt, 1989).

Children need adults to be aware of the content of films, videos and television and to screen out unsuitable programmes. In some cases, they need the adult to sit and be with them, just as today's adults needed adults to reduce their fears of the wolf in Red Riding Hood. The medium may be different, but the need for adult supervision and support is, if anything, greater today.

KEY POINTS

- Growth and development of children are strongly influenced by genetic and environmental factors.
- The major development phases are the prenatal, infancy, early childhood, middle childhood and later childhood, or adolescent, phases.
- Growth and development follow predictable patterns in direction, sequence and pace.
- Biological growth is determined by height, weight, bone age and dentition.
- External proportions and organ systems change with advancing age.
- Critical periods in development are those times when the child is more sensitive to beneficial stimulation or more susceptible to detrimental influences.
- According to social learning theory, children learn appropriate behaviour through conditioning and observation of role models.
- In the context of the family, children learn to apply appropriate sex labels to themselves, acquire sex-appropriate behaviours, develop a preference for their biological sex, and identify with the parent of the same sex.
- To develop a positive self-concept, children need recognition for their achievements and the approval of others.
- Play provides a means of development in the areas of sensorimotor and intellectual progress, socialization, creativity, self-awareness and moral behaviour; it serves as a means for release of tension and expression of emotions.
- Growth and development are affected by a variety of conditions and circumstances, including heredity, physiological function, sex of the child, disease, physical environment, nutrition and interpersonal relationships.
- Children's vulnerability and reaction to stress depend to a large extent on their age, coping behaviours and support systems.
- The mass media can be influential in children's learning and behaviour.
- Growth and development are affected by a variety of conditions and circumstances, including heredity, physiological function, sex of the child, disease, physical environment, nutrition and interpersonal relationships.
- Children's vulnerability and reaction to stress depend to a large extent on their age, coping behaviours and support systems.
- The mass media can be influential in children's learning and behaviour.

REFERENCES

Anthony EJ, Cohler B, editors: *The invulnerable child*, New York, 1987, Guilford Press.

Avery and Jackson, RH; *Children and their accidents*, London, 1993. Edward Arnold.

Bayley N; *Growth curves of height and weight for boys and girls, scaled according to physical maturity*, J Paedicatr 48:187, 1956.

Band EB, Weisz JR: How to feel better when it feels bad: children's perspectives on coping with everyday stress, *Dev Psychol* 24:247, 1988.

Berndt TJ: The features and effects of friendship in early adolescence, *Child Dev* 53:1447, 1982.

Binkin NJ, et al: Birth weight and childhood growth, *Pediatr* 82:828, 1988.

Black D, Newman M: Television violence and children, *BMJ* 310:273, 1995.

Colombo J: The critical period concept: research, methodology and theoretical issues, *Psychol Bull* 81:260, 1982.

Connolly JA, Doyle AB, Reznick E: Social pretend play and social interaction in preschoolers, *J Appl Dev Psychol* 9:301, 1988.

Eaton N: A play progamme. In Glasper A, Tucker A, editors: *Advances in child health nursing*, London, 1993, Edward Arnold.

Fall et al: Weight in infancy and prevalence of coronary heart disease in adult life, *BMJ* 310:17, 1995..

Furman W, Bierman KL: Developmental changes in young children's conception of friendship, *Child Dev* 54:549, 1983.

Garmezy N, Rutter M, editors: *Stress, coping, and development in children*, New York, 1989, McGraw-Hill.

Green C: *Toddler taming: a parent's guide to the first four years*, London, 1991, Century.

Grey M: Stressors and children's health, *J Pediatr Nurs* 8(2):85, 1993.

Gunter B, McAleen JL: *Children and television: one eyed monster?* London, 1990, Routledge.

Harlow HF, Harlow MK: Social deprivation in monkeys, *Sci Am* 203:136, Nov. 1962.

Horne E, Ibbotson M: Weaning: a first step to independence. In Glasper A, editor: *Child care: some nursing perspective*, London, 1991, Wolfe.

Howes C: Social competence with peers in young children: developmental sequences, *Dev Rev* 7:252, 1987.

Jung FE, Czajka-Nairns DM: Birth weight doubling and tripling times: an updated look at the effects of birth weight, sex, race and type of feeding, *Am J Clin Nutr* 42:1820,1985.

Klein et al.: Adolescents' risky behavior and massmedia use, Pediatrics 92(1):24, 1993.

Kuczen B: *Childhood stress: don't let your child be a victim*, New York, 1982, Delacorte Press.

Kurdek LA, Krile D: A developmental analysis of the relation between peer acceptance and both interpersonal understanding and perceived social self-competence, *Child Dev* 53:1485, 1982.

Lampl M: Saltation and stasis: a moldel of human growth, *Science* 258(5083):801, 1992.

Liebert RM, Sprafkin JN, Davidson ES: *The early window: effects of television on children and youth*, New York, 1982, Pergamon Press

Lucas, A: Programming by early nutrition in man. In Bock GR, Whelan J, editors: *The childhood environment and adult disease*, Chichester, 1991, Wiley.1991.

Luthar SS: Vulnerability and resiliance: a study of high-risk adolescents, *Child Dev* 62(3):600, 1991.

Maccoby EE, Jacklin CN: *The psychology of sex differences*, Stanford, CA, 1974, Stanford University Press.

MacKinnon CE: An observational investigation of sibling interactions in married and divorced families, *Dev Psychol* 25:36, 1989.

Masten A et al: Competence and stress in school children: moderating effects of individual and family qualities, *J Child Psychol Psychiatr* 29:747, 1988.

McGuire KD, Weisz JR: Social cognition and behavioral correlates of preadolescent chumship, *Child Dev* 53:1478, 1982.

Melville-Thomas G, Sims A: Psychiatrists' case studies. In Barlow G, Hill A, editors: *Video violence and children*, London, 1985, Hodder & Stoughton.

Mitchell K, Mills NM: Is the sensitive period in parent-infant bonding overrated? *Pediatr Nurs* 9(2):91, 1983.

Murphy LB, Moriarity AE: *Vulnerability, coping and growth*, New Haven, CT, 1976, Yale University Press.

Murray JP: *Television and youth: 25 years of research and controversy*, Boys Town, NE, 1980, Boys Town Center for the Study of Youth Development.

Newson E: Video violence and the protection of children, *Psychologist* 7:272, 1994.

Newson, 1994; Newman BM, Newman PR: *Development through life: a psychosocial approach*, ed 3, Homewood, IL, 1984, The Dorsey Press.

Osmond et al.: Early growth and death from cardiovascular disease in women, *BMJ* 307:1517, 1993.

Pets Are Wonderful Council in consultation with Dr Lee Salk: *Raising better children: how a pet can help*, Chicago, 1985, Pets Are Wonderful Council.

Rosenwasser SM, Lingenfelter AF, Harrington AF: Nontraditional gender role portrayals on television and children's gender role perceptions, *J Appl Dev Psychol* 10:97, 1989.

Schmitt BD: Nightmares on main street, *Am J Dis Child* 143:649 (editorial), 1989.

Selekman J: The development of body image in the child: a learned response, *Top Clin Nurs* 5(1):13, 1983.

Sroufe LA: Infant-caregiving attachment and patterns of adaptation and competence. In Perlmutter M, editor: *Minnesota symposia in child psychology*, vol 16, Hillsdale, NJ, 1983, Lawrence Erlbaum Associates.

Stanwyck DJ: Self-esteem through the life span, *Top Clin Nurs* 6(2):11, 1983.

Stuart GW, Sundeen SJ: *Principles and practice of psychiatric nursing*, ed 5, St Louis, 1995, Mosby–Year Book.

Touwen BCL.: Perspective: critical periods of early brain development, *Inf Young Child* 1:vii, 1989.

Usdin G: Investing in the 'emotional bank' concept, *Child Teens Today* 8(6):7, 1988.

Werner EE: The roots of resiliency, *Early Childhood Update* 3(4):1, 1987.

Werner EE, Smith RS: *Vulnerable but invincible: a longitudinal study of children and youth*, New York, 1982, McGraw-Hill.

Wolman BB: *Children's fears*, New York, 1978, Grosset and Dunlop.

Yip R, Binkin NJ, Trowbridge FL: Altitude and childhood growth, *J Pediatr* 113:486, 1988.

FURTHER READING

General

Brazelton TB: Forces for development in infants and parents, *Early Childhood Update* 2:1, 1986.

Brown MS *et al*: Type A behavior in children: what a pediatric nurse practitioner needs to know, *J Pediatr Health Care* 3:131, 1989.

Ferber R: *Solve your child's sleep problems*, New York, 1985, Simon & Schuster.

Ferber R: The sleepless child. In Guilleminault C, editor: *Sleep and its disorders in children*, New York, 1987, Raven Press.

Harlow HF, Harlow MK: Learning to love, *Am Sci* 54:244, 1966.

Honig AS: Development of academically competent children, *Early Childhood Update* (3)1:2, 1987.

Howes C: Pressuring children to learn versus developmentally appropriate education, *J Pediatr Health Care* 3:181, 1989.

Lewis CE, Siegel JM, Lewis MA: Feeling bad: exploring sources of distress among pre-adolescent children, *Am J Public Health* 74:117, 1984.

Messer DJ *et al*: Relation between mastery behavior in infancy and competence in early childhood, *Dev Psychol* 22:366, 1986.

Parker S, Greer S, Zuckerman B: Double jeopardy: the impact of poverty on early child development, *Pediatr Clin North Am* 35:1227, 1988.

Phillips JL: *The origins of intellect: Piaget's theory*, San Francisco, 1969, WH Freeman.

Power TG, Parke RD: Patterns of early socialization: mother- and father-infant interaction in the home, *Int J Behav Dev* 9:331, 1986.

Seidner B, Stipek DJ, Feshbach ND: A developmental analysis of elementary school-aged children's concepts of pride and embarrassment, *Child Dev* 59:367, 1988.

Sherwen LN: *Separation: the forgotten phenomenon of child development*, Top Clin Nurs 5:1, 1983.

Stone LJ, Church J: *Childhood and adolescence*, ed 5, New York, 1984, Random House.

Thomas RM: *Comparing theories of child development*, ed 2, Belmont, CA, 1985, Wadsworth.

Withrow C, Fleming JW: Pediatric social illness: a challenge to nurses, *Issues Compr Pediatr Nurs* 6:261, 1983.

Language

Bonvillian JD, Orlansky MD, Novack LL: Developmental milestones: sign language acquisition and motor development, *Child Dev* 54:1435, 1983.

Castiglia PT: Speech-language development, *J Pediatr Health Care* 1:165, 1987.

LeNormand MT: A developmental exploration of language used to accompany symbolic play in young, normal children, Child Care Health Dev 12:121, 1986.

McCabe AE: Differential language learning styles in young children: the importance of context, *Dev Rev* 9:1, 1989.

Rosenthal MK: Vocal dialogues in the neonatal period, *Dev Psychol* 18:17, 1982.

Sande DR, Billingsley CS: Language development in infants and toddlers, *Nurse Pract* 10(9):39, 1985.

Play

Axelsson A, Jerson T: Noisy toys: a possible source of sensorineural hearing loss, *Pediatr* 76:574, 1985.

Bellack JP, Fleming JW: Theoretical practical aspects of play: a universal need. In Fore C, Poster EC, editors: *Meeting psychosocial needs of children and families in health care*, Washington, DC, 1985, Association of Care of Children's Health.

Betz CL, Poster EC: Incorporating play into the care of the hospitalized child, *Issues Compr Pediatr Nurs* 7:343, 1984.

Cohen D: *The development of play*, New York, 1987, New York University Press.

Lee J, Fowler MD: Merely child's play? Developmental work and playthings, *J Pediatr Nurs* 1:260, 1986.

Marino BL: Assessments of infant play: applications to research and practice, *Issues Compr Pediatr Nurs* 11:227, 1988.

Nutrition

American Academy of Pediatrics, Committee on Nutrition: Toward a prudent diet of children, *Pediatr* 71:78, 1983.

Barness LA *et al*: Straight talk about feeding young children, *Contemp Pediatr* 5(6):22, 1988.

Dwyer J: Promoting good nutrition for today and the year 2000, *Pediatr Clin North Am* 33:799, 1986.

Endres JB, Rockwell RE: Food, nutrition, and the young child, ed 2, St Louis, 1985, Mosby–Year Book.

Pipes PL: *Nutrition in infancy and childhood*, ed 4, St Louis, 1989, Mosby–Year Book.

Williams SR: *Nutrition and diet therapy*, ed 5, St Louis, 1985, Mosby–Year Book.

Stress and Fear

Berman BD, Boyce WT: Environmental stresses and protective factors in child health and development, *Curr Opin Pediatr* 1:172, 1989.

Colton JA: Childhood stress: perceptions of children and professionals, *J Psychopathol Behav Assess* 7(2):155, 1985.

Compas BE: Coping with stress during childhood and adolescence, *Psychol Bull* 101:393, 1987.

Grey M, Hayman LL: Assessing stress in children: research and clinical implications, *J Pediatr Nurs* 2:316, 1987.

Kagan J: Stress and coping in early development. In Garmezy N, Rutter M, editors: *Stress, coping, and development in children*, New York, 1983, McGraw-Hill.

Langbaum T: What are children worrying about? *Clin Pediatr* 3(12):79, 1986.

Lewis CE, Siegel JM, Lewis MA: Feeling bad: exploring sources of distress among pre-adolescent children, *Am J Public Health* 74:117, 1984.

Witmer D, Crouthamel CS: Overcoming the common fears of childhood, *Contemp Pediatr* 3(9):76, 1986.

Mass Media

Comstock GA: Influences of mass media on child health behavior, *Health Educ Q* 8(1):32, 1981.

Dail PW, Way WL: What do parents observe about parenting from prime time television, *Fam Rel* 34:491, 1985.

Eron LD *et al*: Age trends in the development of aggression, sex-typing, and related television habits, *Dev Psychol* 19:71, 1983.

Pearl D, Bouthilet L, Lazar J: *Television and behavior: ten years of scientific progress and implications for the eighties*, vols. 1 and 2, Washington, DC, 1982, US Department of Health and Human Services.

Rothenberg MB: In my opinion... role of television in shaping the attitudes of children, *Child Health Care* 13:148, 1985.

Singer DG: Does violent television produce aggressive children? *Pediatr Ann* 14:804, 1985.

Strasburger VC: When parents ask about... the influence of TV on their kids, *Contemp Pediatr* 2:18, 1985.

Unit Two

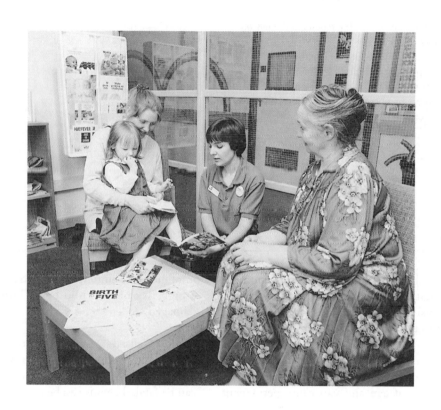

Health Problems
and Health Promotion

Chapter 11

Principles of Health Promotion in Childhood

LEARNING OUTCOMES

After studying this chapter you should be able to:

♦ Define the key terms listed.
♦ Understand what health education means.
♦ Define three stages of prevention.
♦ Describe the main causes of death for infants and children.
♦ State the main causes of accidents.
♦ Describe the immunization schedule for children.
♦ Identify measures to prevent dental decay.
♦ Describe how infants should be placed for sleeping.
♦ Describe the main ways to ensure a healthy diet.
♦ Define the glossary terms.

GLOSSARY

measles Common and highly infectious, measles can cause encephalitis (inflammation of the brain), which can lead to brain damage, convulsions, ear infections, bronchitis, and pneumonia, sometimes resulting in lasting lung damage.

mumps Usually a mild illness, but serious complications can occur. It is the most common cause of viral meningitis among children under 15 years of age and can cause permanent deafness.

polio A disease which attacks the nervous system and can cause muscle paralysis. Can affect any muscle in the body. A child can be protected for life by immunization.

rubella A mild disease, but if a pregnant woman who is not immune comes into contact with an infected person, there is a high risk of the child being born blind, deaf, or brain-damaged.

tetanus Caused by organisms from soil getting into an open wound and producing a poison which attacks the nervous system, causing painful muscle cramps. Tetanus is rare, but can be fatal. Tetanus can be avoided by immunization.

whooping cough Causes long, distressing bouts of coughing and choking, and can last from between 3–4 weeks to up to 12 weeks. Can cause convulsions, pneumonia, collapsed lungs, ear infections, and occasionally brain damage. Immunization can reduce the severity of the illness.

Nurses working with children and parents have a major role to play in health education. The World Health Organization (1985) defines the goals of health education as: (1) to persuade people to adopt and sustain healthful life practices, (2) to use health services wisely, and (3) to make their own decisions (individually and collectively) to improve their health status and environment.

PRINCIPLES OF HEALTH PROMOTION IN CHILDHOOD

Ewles and Simnett (1985) describe seven dimensions of health education:

1. Health, and therefore health education, is concerned with the whole person, and encompasses physical, mental, social, emotional, spiritual, and societal aspects.
2. Health education is a life-long process from birth to death, helping people to change and adapt at all stages.
3. Health education is concerned with people at all points of health and illness, from the completely healthy to the chronically sick and handicapped, to maximize each person's potential for healthy living.
4. Health education is directed towards individuals, families, groups, and whole communities.
5. Health education is concerned with helping people to help themselves and with helping people to work towards creating healthier conditions for everybody, making healthy choices easier choices.
6. Health education involves formal and informal teaching and learning using a range of methods.
7. Health education is concerned with a range of goals, including giving information, attitude change, behaviour change and social change.

They also emphasize that health education is often given a narrow interpretation (e.g., primary prevention, patient education, or education aimed at changing behaviour) which limits its comprehensive nature; consequently, other health education activities, such as improving the environment or informal learning from television, friends and family are often forgotten.

There is frequently confusion about the difference between *health education* and *health promotion*, and the terms are often used imprecisely. Nurses must be able to differentiate between these terms. Health promotion is defined by Green *et al.* (1979) as 'any combination of health education and related organisational, economic and legislative supports for behaviour conducive to individual or community health'.

Parents need teaching, support, and guidance from nursing staff in order to promote health and wellness. Nurses will need to offer a range of health education approaches to meet parental and children's needs. These may include:

- Assessing parents' knowledge through verbal or observational feedback.
- Providing parents with written and verbal guidance on a range of health issues.
- Providing classes for parents in child care and management.
- Demonstrating appropriate care giving to children, e.g., role modelling.
- Referring parents to a support group or other professional worker who can offer help.
- Providing anticipatory guidance at appropriate times, e.g., to ensure parents understand the importance of accident prevention for toddlers.
- Ensuring that the hospital environment fosters an awareness of health education.

This is reinforced by Coutts and Hardy (1985) who emphasize that in teaching for health, the nurse may help to identify and solve health-related problems by:

- Informing.
- Advising.
- Helping with the acquisition of skills.
- Assisting with the process of clarifying beliefs, feelings and values.
- Enabling the adaptation of life-style.
- Promoting change in the structures and organizations which influence health status.
- Providing a model of values and behaviour related to health.

Nurses must also be aware of what is meant by 'prevention' in order to identify topics and approaches in health education.

PREVENTION

There are three levels of prevention: primary, secondary, and tertiary.

PRIMARY PREVENTION

Primary prevention is implemented before the disease process or disability has started. A potential problem or illness is anticipated and action is taken to avoid the condition. An example is the immunization programmes which protect a population from diseases, such as polio, measles, and rubella. Another example would be giving advice to parents on how to make their homes safe and thus reduce the risk of accidents in the home.

SECONDARY PREVENTION

Secondary prevention is undertaken when an illness or disability may still be alleviated or arrested. This includes the early detection (e.g., screening), diagnosis, and treatment of health problems. An example is motivating a patient with dental caries to apply for dental treatment.

TERTIARY PREVENTION

This occurs following illness or disability. The goal of this type of prevention is maintenance and rehabilitation. The damage resulting from a previous mental or physical illness, or any chronic condition, must be alleviated as much as possible. An example is helping a family cope with a child who has a disability that requires long-term care. In tertiary prevention, the emphasis is often on rehabilitation.

All nurses should be involved in prevention, but this varies according to the area of work; for example, in the community the health visitor is the nurse most involved in primary prevention, with some focus on secondary, and less on tertiary prevention.

POLICY FOR HEALTH

A discussion of the government focus on the prevention of ill health and the main causes of death in infants and children will enable us to identify the focus for health education.

The *Health of the Nation* (Department of Health, 1991) establishes the agenda for preventive health care in the future. One of these areas is the health of pregnant women and children. The document states that 'it has long been recognised that the health status of pregnant women, infants and children are important indicators of the general state of health of any population. The WHO Health for All by the Year 2000 programme and the recent United Nations World Summit for Children in which the UK participated, have both set objectives for these groups. The health of pregnant women influences the health of their babies, and fetal and infant health is one of the main determinants of health in childhood and later in life.'

The report notes that the infant mortality rate is 8.4 per 1000 live births and is at its lowest level ever; it does go on to say that better rates have been achieved overseas, and there are significant variations nationally within the UK.

The distribution of causes of death in newborn infants, other infants, and children aged 1–4 or 5–14 years, is given in Box 11-1.

TARGETS FOR HEALTH

Health of the Nation identifies several targets for improving health:

(a) Young children:
- Immunization against childhood diseases.
- Early detection of congenital and acquired abnormalities including impairments in hearing, vision, growth and development.

(b) Older children:
- Promotion of healthy life-styles.
- Prevention (particularly through education) of smoking and misuse of alcohol and drugs.

(c) All children:
- Accident prevention and safety education.
- Improvements in the quality of the environment, particularly housing.
- Avoidance of smoking in the household.
- Prevention, identification, and treatment of emotional and behavioural problems.
- Prevention of dental decay.

◆ **BOX 11-1**

Guidelines for referral regarding communication impairment

Neonatal Deaths
(0–27 days)

Congenital anomalies	32%
Hypoxia, birth asphyxia and other respiratory conditions	32%
Low birth weight or short gestation	10%
Obstetric complications	6%
Fetal/neonatal haematological causes	5%
Other	16%
	(Total = 3531)

Other Infant Deaths, 1989
(28 days to under 1 year)

Sudden infant death syndrome	46%
Congenital anomalies	17%
Respiratory diseases	9%
Conditions originating in the perinatal period	8%
Other	19%
	(Total = 2536)

Deaths Age 1–4 Years, 1989

Accidents	21%
Congenital anomalies	21%
Neoplasms	13%
Diseases of nervous and sense organs	10%
Respiratory diseases	9%
Other	26%
	(Total = 1078)

Deaths Age 5–14 Years, 1989

Accidents	36%
Neoplasms	18%
Congenital anomalies	11%
Diseases of nervous and sense organs	10%
Other	24%
	(Total = 1175)

(Department of Health, 1991)

168

The report also establishes the following targets:

(a) Breast-feeding:
- To increase the proportion nationally of infants who are breast-fed at birth from 64% in 1985 to 75% by the year 2000.
- To increase the proportion of infants aged six weeks being wholly or partly breast-fed from 39% in 1985 to 50% by 2000.

(b) Child health:
- Prevention and reduction of ill-health caused by respiratory diseases (including asthma).
- The early diagnosis of impairments of hearing, vision, growth, and development.
- Improved sexual health, e.g., reduction in pregnancies below the age of 16.
- The prevention of behavioural disorders in children.

(c) Dental caries:
- Despite recent improvements in the dental health of children, dental decay remains one of the most common childhood diseases, causes pain and discomfort, affects well-being and appearance, and is a prime example of preventable morbidity — there is no clinical reason why dental decay in children could not virtually be eliminated.

TOPICS FOR HEALTH

Although several health education topics are identified, this section will concentrate on the key areas of accident prevention, dental health, immunization, nutrition, and sleep.

ACCIDENT PREVENTION

When the potential environmental dangers to which infants are vulnerable are considered, the task of preventing these injuries only begins to be appreciated. Nurses must be aware of the possible causes of injury in each age group in order for anticipatory preventive health teaching to occur.

Injury prevention requires protection of the child and education of the parents or caregiver. Nurses in hospitals and the community are in a favourable position to educate others about injury prevention.

One approach to teaching injury prevention is to discuss why children in various age groups are prone to specific types of injuries. Stressing prevention is just as important as emphasizing the way injuries occur. However, injury prevention must also be practical. Asking parents for their ideas leads to realistic suggestions that can be followed.

Injuries do not always indicate neglect. It is a difficult task to watch children carefully without overprotecting or unnecessarily confining them. Allowing children to explore while maintaining consistent, age-appropriate limits is sound advice.

An additional factor must be stressed concerning injury prevention and education. Children are imitators; they copy what they see and hear. *Practising safety teaches safety.* This applies to parents and their children and to nurses and their patients. Saying one thing but doing another confuses children and can lead to difficulties as the child grows older.

Every year, one in five children has an accident which is serious enough to require medical attention. Most accidents occur between the time children begin to crawl, at about nine months, and the age of four years (Child Accident Prevention Trust, 1990).

Constant vigilance, awareness, and supervision are essential as the child gains increased locomotor and manipulative skills that are coupled with an insatiable curiosity about the environment. Injuries can be grouped into the following categories: (1) aspiration of foreign objects, (2) suffocation, (3) motor vehicle injuries, (4) falls, (5) poisoning, (6) burns, and (7) bodily damage.

Aspiration of foreign objects

Asphyxiation by foreign material in the respiratory tract, combined with mechanical suffocation, may cause fatal injury in children younger than one year of age. The size, shape, and consistency of foods or objects are important determinants of fatal obstruction. For example, small objects (less than 3.2 cm) are more likely to completely obstruct the airway. A spherical or cylindrical object plugs the airway more completely than any other shaped object. Pliable objects are less likely to be expelled than rigid ones. Unfortunately, common household items can be deadly to infants.

All toys must be carefully inspected for potential danger. An active child can grab a low-hanging mobile and quickly chew off a small piece. As soon as the infant crawls or plays on the floor, the floor must be kept free of any small articles that can be picked up and swallowed, such as coins.

Food is the second most common cause of aspiration. Foods which should be avoided include hard sweets, fruits with seeds, or foods containing nuts. Snack foods such as peanuts should be kept away from young children. Dummies can also be dangerous because the entire object may be aspirated if it is small, or the teat and shield may become detached from the handle and become lodged in the pharynx.

Another commonly aspirated substance is baby powder. Talcum powder containers often become favourite playthings and are placed in the mouth (Mofenson *et al.*, 1981). The improper use of powder, by sprinkling it directly on the skin, creates a cloud of talc dust that is easily inhaled. Parents are advised of the danger of baby powder.

Whenever a powder is used, it should be placed in the hand and then applied to the skin — never shaken directly from the container to the skin. The container should be kept closed and stored immediately in a safe place, especially away from curious toddlers who often imitate caregiving activities and may accidentally shake it on the infant.

Suffocation

Mechanical suffocation is another important cause of death by asphyxiation and includes asphyxiation by covering the mouth and nose, by pressure on the throat and chest, and by exclusion of air, such as by refrigerator entrapment.

An infant who is placed in a bed under blankets and sheets that are tucked in can be caught under them and be unable to wriggle free. Pillows and duvets are not safe for babies less than one year old because of the risk of suffocation. Duvets can also cause overheating. Baby nests and quilted sleeping bags are not suitable for unattended babies to sleep in (at any time) because of the danger of suffocation. The mattress on a cot should fit snugly without leaving spaces around the edges in which the baby could trap his or her head and suffocate (Child Accident Prevention Trust, 1990).

Plastic bags also cause suffocation. Large plastic bags used over garments are very lightweight and can easily and quickly be wrapped around the head of an active infant or pressed against the infants face. Pillows and mattresses should not be covered with plastic for this reason. Older infants may play with a plastic bag and accidentally pull it over their heads. Because plastic is non-porous, suffocation takes place in a matter of minutes.

Anything tied around an infant's neck can potentially cause strangulation. Bibs should be removed at bedtime, and objects such as soothers should never be hung on a string around the infant's neck.

Toys that have strings attached, such as a telephone, or toys that are tied to cots or playpens can be hazards. Cot toys should be hung high enough that the infant cannot become entangled in them or should no longer be used once the child is able to reach them.

Restraining straps, if applied too loosely or left unfastened, can be a hazard. For example, a child may slide off a high chair beneath the tray and become strangled on the loose strap. All straps should be fastened securely.

Motor vehicle injuries

Approximately 300 babies are killed or injured in cars each year (Child Accident Prevention Trust, 1988). Some are disabled or disfigured for the rest of their lives. By using a proper safety system, the risk of child injury in a crash can be reduced. For a very young baby, a baby seat or a carrycot with restraints can be used. Both are much safer and more convenient than carrycots. A baby seat or carrycot with restraints should be used on every trip, including the first ride home from hospital. Parents should never put a seat belt around both themselves and their child, as this could cause the baby to be crushed in the event of an accident.

Child car seats can be secured with an adult seat belt or with two anchorage straps. It is vitally important to secure the child car seat according to the manufacturer's instructions. Ensure the child keeps the harness correctly fastened at all times.

Falls

Infants are at risk of falling or rolling off raised surfaces; for example, a bed or changing unit. Always stay with the baby while it is on a raised surface. Care is necessary when using high chairs, as serious accidents can occur when the child is not firmly strapped in. The use of baby walkers is not recommended by the Child Accident Prevention Trust and the Royal Society for the Prevention of Accidents. Baby walkers cause more accidents among young children than any other single item of equipment. Every year there are serious accidents when babies

in walkers get close to hazardous objects such as a fire, or trip and fall down stairs (Child Accident Prevention Trust, 1990).

Once infants are mobile, they should not be allowed to crawl unsupervised on any raised surface, near stairs, or near any water reservoir. Gates should be used at the bottom and top of stairs, because both present dangers to the crawling and climbing infant.

Sometimes, even when the environment is made safe, infants may literally trip over their own feet. Slippery socks; hard, slick soles on shoes or rubber soles that can catch, especially on a carpet; and long trousers or pyjama bottoms can easily upset a child's balance. Such dangers need to be pointed out to parents, especially when infants are taking their first steps.

During this age playground injuries become common, and many of the injuries are related to playground equipment and occur at home or at nursery. Children need to be taught safety at play areas, such as no horseplay on high slides or jungle gyms, sitting on swings, and staying away from moving swings.

The climbing and running activity of the typical toddler is complicated by total neglect for and lack of appreciation of danger combined with immature coordination and a high centre of gravity. Falling from stairs is a major cause of injury, with more children in this age-group sustaining head injury than older children (Joffe and Ludwig, 1988). Accessible windows that are left open during warm weather must be screened or guarded with a rail.

Poisoning

Poisoning is almost always the result of inadequate supervision, but it does not always represent neglect. Children are very fast, and it takes only seconds to eat a bar of soap or a handful of cleanser or detergent. Although infants usually do not possess the manipulative skill to open closed jars, they are amazingly persistent and inventive.

Plants are another source of poisoning for infants. Plants are frequently placed on the floor, and the leaves or flowers are attractive and easy to pull off. More than 700 species of plants are known to have caused illness or death.

Another danger is ingestion of button-sized batteries that are used in devices such as hearing aids, calculators, watches, and cameras. Because they are bright and shiny, they are attractive to children. However, they can cause severe morbidity, even death, if lodged in the oesophagus. The strong alkali in a battery can leak and cause a severe caustic burn. As a precaution, small batteries should be safely stored and discarded where young children cannot easily retrieve them.

The only sure way to prevent poisoning is to remove toxic agents, which means placing them out of the infant's reach. However, because crawling infants soon become climbing toddlers, it is best to keep all toxic agents, especially medicines, in a locked cabinet. Special plastic hooks can be attached to the inside of cabinet doors to keep them securely closed. Firm thumb pressure is required to unlatch the hook, and small children are usually unable to manipulate them. Locks are best, but for cleaning agents frequently used, such as under the kitchen sink, hooks are a practical alternative.

No potentially hazardous substance should be stored in any type of food container. Soft drink bottles are sometimes used for the storage of toxic liquids, putting a child who is unaware of the dangerous contents at great risk from poisoning.

If a parent suspects that a child has swallowed medicine or other substances, the child should be taken to the local hospital or the family GP immediately, depending on proximity. If possible, the container or a sample of the substance swallowed should also be brought. Attempts to make the child sick with salt and water should be avoided, as this can be very dangerous in case the substance causes further damage to the throat and mouth when the child is vomiting.

Drowning

With well-developed skills of locomotion, toddlers are able to reach potentially dangerous areas, such as baths, swimming pools, and lakes. Even unlikely sources of water, such as toilets and buckets, are dangerous. As inquisitive toddlers lean over the rim of the receptacle, their high centre of gravity and poor coordination make it difficult for them to extricate themselves (Jumbelic and Chambliss, 1990). Their intense drive for exploration and investigation, combined with an unawareness of the danger of water and their helplessness in water, makes drowning always a viable threat. It is also one category of injuries that results in death within minutes, diminishing the chance for rescue and survival. Supervising children when near any source of water is essential; teaching swimming and water safety can be helpful, but cannot be regarded as sufficient protection.

Burns

Children's ability to climb, stretch, and reach objects above their head makes any hot surface a potential source of danger. Scalds from pulling pots on top of themselves are a major source of burns. As a precaution, pot handles should be turned towards the back of the stove. Ideally, the knobs for controlling the hob should be out of reach, not on the front panel where nimble fingers can turn them on and accidentally touch the hotplates. Oven doors should be closed whenever the oven is turned on or when it is cooling. The outside of doors of automatic self-cleaning ovens may become hot and, if touched, could cause a burn. Other sources of heat, such as radiators, fireplaces, and gas or electric heaters are also potentially hazardous.

Scald burns are the most common type of heat injury in children. Among young children, a significant type of scalding burn is caused by high temperature tap water, which children come in contact with either as a result of turning on the hot water tap, falling into a bath of hot water, or deliberate abuse. Besides the obvious prevention of always supervising young children when they are near tap water and checking bathwater temperatures, a recommended passive prevention is to limit household water temperatures to less than 49°C. At this temperature, it takes only 10 minutes for exposure to the water to cause a full-thickness burn.

DENTAL HEALTH

The Committee on Medical Aspects of Food Policy (COMA, 1989) states that dental caries can occur at any age. 'Bottle caries' are found in infants who use a feeding bottle over prolonged periods and/or at night. While lactose, the sugar naturally occurring in milk, is not considered to be the main cause of dental caries (COMA, 1991), it will cause decay when allowed to remain in contact with teeth for long periods. Bottle caries are also associated with the prolonged use of sweetened soothers. Good dental hygiene is important from birth, as even newborn babies have unseen developing teeth which need to be protected.

The importance of oral hygiene in preserving the teeth and maintaining healthy gums cannot be overemphasized or begun too early. Nurses are in an optimum position to promote dental hygiene in their care of both well children and ill children during hospitalization. It is also important for health visitors and school nurses working in the community to emphasize the importance of oral hygiene.

Parents should start brushing their child's teeth at an early age, so that it becomes habitual. It is necessary to help with toothbrushing, at least until the child starts school and perhaps for longer. Even when children take over their own brushing, parents should check to ensure it is effective. Every surface of every tooth should be well brushed on both sides, and the chewing surface should be well brushed. A child's teeth can be cleaned more successfully using a toothbrush with a small head.

Children should be taken to the dentist regularly so they become used to going. This also means decay can be detected in its early stages and treated appropriately.

Attention to the child's diet is also recommended to ensure that the frequency of sugary snacks is reduced and that healthy eating patterns are promoted (Health Education Authority, 1980).

By the beginning of the preschool period, the eruption of the primary teeth is complete. Dental care is essential to preserve these temporary teeth and to teach good dental habits. Although children's fine motor control is improved, they still require assistance and supervision with brushing, and flossing should be done by parents.

Nurses can give the following advice to parents:
* Start brushing your child's teeth at an early age.
* Help with toothbrushing, at least until your child starts school. Even when your child takes over brushing, check to see that it is done correctly.
* Take your child to the dentist regularly, so that any decay can be treated before it causes trouble.
* Avoid feeding with sugary foods or drinks right from the start, so your child does not get a taste for sweet things.
* The more often sweet things are eaten, the worse it is for teeth. Decrease the frequency that sweet foods are consumed each day.
* When shopping, avoid buying foods and drinks with sugar in them.

IMMUNIZATION

One of the most dramatic advances in paediatrics has been the decline of infectious diseases over the past 50 years because of the widespread use of immunization for preventable diseases.

Childhood immunization is available against diphtheria, whooping cough, tetanus, polio, measles, mumps, and rubella. In addition, immunization has recently been introduced against haemophilus influenzae type B.

Diphtheria

Diphtheria is a disease which begins with a simple sore throat and develops into a serious illness which can last for weeks. It blocks the nose and throat making it difficult for the child to breathe. It also produces a poison which, when in the child's bloodstream, can attack the heart and nervous system. Though very rare, diphtheria can be fatal.

Whooping cough (pertussis)

Whooping cough is a serious disease which is transmitted by direct contact or droplet infection. It has an incubation period of approximately 10 days. It begins with symptoms of upper respiratory infection for one or two weeks, and then the child develops a dry, hacking cough which can be very severe. The cough most often occurs at night, and consists of short, rapid coughs followed by sudden inspiration associated with a high-pitched crowing sound or 'whoop'. The complications are pneumonia, convulsions, and otitis media.

Haemophilus influenzae type B

Haemophilus influenzae type B affects children in the first five years of life. It is a leading cause of bacterial meningitis, and can also cause pneumonia, joint or bone infections, and throat inflammation.

Measles

Measles is an acute viral illness transmitted via droplet infection. Clinical features include Koplik spots, coryza, conjunctivitis, bronchitis, rash, and fever. The incubation period is about 10 days, with a further two to four days before the rash appears. It is highly infectious from the beginning of the prodromal period to four days after the appearance of the rash. Complications have been reported in one in 15 notified cases, and include otitis media, bronchitis, pneumonia, convulsions, and encephalitis, which has an incidence of one in 5000 cases, has a mortality of about 15%, and 20–40% of survivors have residual neurological effects. Complications are more common, and are severe in poorly nourished and chronically ill children; **it is therefore particularly important that such children should be immunized against measles.**

Mumps

Mumps is an acute viral illness characterized by parotid swelling which may be unilateral or bilateral; some cases are asymptomatic. The incubation period is 14–21 days, and mumps is transmissible from several days before to several days

AGE	DISEASE	IMMUNIZATION
2 months	Diphtheria	1st dose
	Whooping cough	Triple vaccine
	Tetanus	One injection
	Haemophilus influenzae type B	One injection
	Polio	Polio drops
3 months	Diphtheria	2nd dose
	Whooping cough	One injection
	Tetanus	
	Haemophilus influenzae type B	One injection
	Polio	Polio drops
4 months	Diphtheria	Final dose
	Whooping cough	One injection
	Tetanus	
	Haemophilus influenzae type B	One injection
	Polio	Polio drops
15 months	Measles	MMR
	Mumps	One injection
	Rubella (German measles)	
4–5 years	Diphtheria	Booster
	Tetanus	Injection
	Polio	Booster (Drops)

Table 11-1 Childhood immunizations.

after the parotid swelling appears. Complications include pancreatitis, oophoritis, and orchitis; even when orchitis is bilateral, there is no firm evidence that it causes sterility. Neurological complications, including meningitis and encephalitis, may precede or folllow parotitis and can occur in its abscence. Before the introduction of mumps, measles, and rubella (MMR) vaccine, mumps was the cause of about 1200 hospital admissions each year in England and Wales. In the under 15 age group, it was a common cause of viral meningitis; it can also cause permanent unilateral deafness at any age.

Rubella

Rubella is a mild infectious disease, most common among children aged four to nine years. It causes a transient erythmatous rash, lymphadenopathy involving post-auricular and suboccipital glands, and, occasionally in adults, arthritis and arthralgia. Clinical diagnosis is unreliable, since the symptoms are often fleeting and can be caused by other viruses; in particular, the rash is not diagnostic of rubella. A history of 'rubella' should never be accepted without serological evidence of previous infection. The incubation period is 14–21 days, and the period of infectivity from one week before until four days after the onset of the rash.

Maternal rubella infections in the first eight to ten weeks of pregnancy result in fetal damage in up to 90% of infants, and multiple defects are common. The risk of damage declines to about 10–20% by 16 weeks and, after this stage of pregnancy, fetal damage is rare. Fetal defects include mental handicap, cataract, deafness, cardiac abnormalities, retardation of intra-uterine growth, and inflammatory lesions of brain, liver, lungs, and bone marrow. Any combination of these may occur; the only defects which commonly occur alone are perceptive deafness and pigmentary retinopathy following infection after the first eight weeks of pregnancy. Some infected infants may appear normal at birth, but perceptive deafness may be detected later.

Rubella immunization was introduced in the UK in 1970 for pre-pubertal girls and immune women with the aim of pro-tecting women of childbearing age from the risks of rubella in pregnancy. This policy was not intended to prevent the circula-tion of rubella, but to increase the proportion of women with antibody to rubella. This increased from 85–90% before 1970 to 97–98% by 1987.

Tetanus

Tetanus is an acute disease characterized by muscular rigidity with superimposed agonizing contractions. It is induced by the toxin of tetanus bacilli which grow anaerobically at the site of an injury. The incubation period is between 4 and 21 days, commonly about 10. Tetanus spores are present in soil, and may be introduced into the body during injury, often through a puncture wound, but also through burns or trivial, unnoticed wounds. Tetanus is not spread from person to preson.

Effective protection against tetanus is provided by active immunization, introduced in some localities as part of the primary immunization of infants from the mid-1950s and nationally from 1961. In 1970 it was recommended that active immunization in the UK should be routinely provided in the treatment of wounds, when immunization against tetanus should be initiated and subsequently completed.

Side-effects of immunization

Diphtheria, tetanus, and whooping cough are combined into one triple vaccine which protects against all three diseases. The vaccine is given by injection. Polio vaccine is given by drops in the mouth and is administered in three doses. Side-effects from the triple vaccine, if any, are almost always very mild. The child may become irritable and slightly feverish in the 24 hours fol-lowing the injection. Infant paracetamol can be used to lower a raised temperature. If used, the nurse should follow recom-mended dosage instructions carefully. Sometimes the skin becomes red, sore, or swollen around the injection site. This is usually not a cause for worry, but a health visitor or family doctor should be consulted if in doubt.

The MMR vaccine protects children from measles, mumps, and rubella. Most children experience no adverse side effects following immunization. Some children, however, may

develop a mild fever and rash one week to ten days later, which should only last for 2–3 days. A few children develop swollen faces, similar in appearance to mumps, approximately three weeks after the injection. This will gradually disappear. None of these reactions are infectious. If the child appears hot and irritable during the first week or so following the injection, infant paracetamol may be given. The risk of a child having any serious side effects is extremely slight and is far outweighed by the risks of the diseases (Health Education Authority, 1988). A summary of the childhood immunization schedule is provided in Table 11-1.

Reinforcing doses in children

A booster dose of adsorbed diptheria /tetanus should be given prior to school entry, preferably with an interval of at least three years from the last dose of the primary course. If the primary course is only completed at school entry, then the booster dose should be given three years later. A further reinforcing dose of tetanus vaccine alone is recommended for those aged 15–19 years or before leaving school.

Contraindications

- Children with acute febrile illness when they present for immunization; this should be deferred.
- Children with untreated malignant disease or altered immunity, those receiving immunosuppressive or x-ray therapy or high-dose steroids.
- Children who have received another live vaccine — includ-ing BGS — within three weeks.
- Children with allergies to neomycin or kanamycin.
- If MMR vaccine is given to adult women, pregnancy should be avoided for one month, as for rubella vaccine.
- MMR vaccine should not be given within three months of an injection of immunoglobulin (Salisbury and Begg, 1992).

Contraindications for pertussis

Pertussis immunization is contraindicated for children in which there is a family history of idiopathic epilepsy or if the child has had convulsions. In addition, pertussis is con-traindicated in children who have suffered cerebral damage.

There is some recent work which suggests that children with histories of neurological problems can be safely immunized against pertussis, but this is not yet policy. In all such cases, the risks should be discussed fully with parents (Baxter, 1994).

NUTRITION

From birth to four months of age, a baby's nutritional require-ments are met by either breast-feeding or bottle feeding with formula milk. After this time, milk alone may not meet these needs, so it is necessary to introduce semi-solid foods to ensure the baby receives adequate nourishment for healthy growth and development. As all babies are different, there is no fixed time to start weaning; but this should begin between four and six months of age.

In the early stages of weaning, the baby should be offered only a small amount of food in addition to breast or bottle milk. A few drops or a tiny piece of mashed food is enough in the initial stages. Food should be bland with a smooth texture and no added salt or sugar. Finely mashed or sieved foods should be mixed to a sloppy consistency with a little milk. It is best to avoid spiced or highly flavoured foods and it is important to ensure an adequate fluid intake during weaning.

The key to healthy eating is variety. By the age of one year, the infant's diet should include fruit, vegetables, wholemeal bread, cereals, milk, cheese, poultry, fish, pulses, and potatoes (Early Childhood Development Unit, 1988). The Department of Health *Guidelines on the Weaning Diet* (Department of Health, 1994a) say that 'fat is the major contributor to the total energy intake of infants in the first months of life, but by six months, fat contributes proportionately less than carbohydrate. The high-energy density of fat allows infants and young children to obtain their energy requirements from a manageable volume of food' (p. 21).

Growth in infancy and young children must be safeguarded because poor growth has been associated with increased risk of ill health in adult life. The *Report* goes on to say that fat intake should be moderated for children over five years of age in line with the Department of Health recommendations of 1994 on the nutritional aspects of cardiovascular disease (Department of Health, 1994b).

Never introduce more than one new food at a time. This will make it easier to identify which foods the child likes and dislikes.

Parents of infants with special dietary requirements; for example, children who have diabetes, who belong to some ethnic groups, or who are brought up as either vegetarian or vegan, need specific advice and guidance. Information should be sought from the hospital or community dietitian. Eating habits established in the first 2–3 years of life tend to have lasting effects on subsequent years.

For some young children, sitting at the table may be more disruptive than functional. Frequent nutritious snacks can replace a meal. Grazing — nibbling and snacking — is a good way to ensure proper nutrition, if appropriate foods are provided.

The method of serving food is also important. Toddlers need to feel control and achievement in their abilities. Giving them large portions contributes to their feeling overwhelmed. In general, *what* is eaten is much more significant than *how much* is consumed. Small amounts of meat and vegetables supply greater food value than a large consumption of bread or potato. Serving sizes need to be appropriate for age. Substitutions should be provided for foods that they do not enjoy, but this practice should be used sparingly to avoid catering to all toddlers' eating requests.

Toddlers often like the same dish, cup, or spoon every time they eat. For some children, a regular mealtime schedule also contributes to their desire and need for predictability and ritualism.

Appetite and food preferences are sporadic during these years. A child may enjoy one food for three days in a row and then suddenly refuse to eat it again for days. It is preferable to accept such extremes and to offer other foods in small portions. Generally, the child will choose another favourite food that may compensate for the nutritional inadequacy. Introducing at least three items from the basic four food groups at each meal helps develop a variety of taste preferences and well-balanced habits. When offering snacks, several small pieces of food (carrot sticks, cheese blocks, raisins, or sliced cold meat, bread, or apple) are appropriate.

Developmentally, most children by 12 months of age are eating the same food as the rest of the family. Some may have mastered using a cup with occasional spilling, although most cannot adeptly use a spoon until 18 months of age or later, and generally prefer using their fingers.

Some preschool children still have food habits that are typical of toddlers, such as food fads and strong taste preferences. When children reach four years of age, they seem to enter another period of finicky eating, which is generally characteristic of the more rebellious and rowdy behaviour of children in this age group. By the age of five years, children are more agreeable to trying new foods, especially if encouraged by an adult who allows the child to help with food preparation or experiments with new tastes or different dishes. Mealtimes can become battlegrounds if parents expect impeccable table manners. Usually, the five-year-old child is ready for the social side of eating, but the three- or four-year-old child still has difficulty sitting quietly through a long family meal.

Parents sometimes worry about the quantity of food preschool children consume. In general, the quality is much more important than the quantity. Young children often consume more food than parents realize.

SLEEP

Guidelines regarding sleeping position, particularly in relation to reducing the risk of cot death, have been developed by the Department of Health (1992). Cot death, also known as sudden infant death syndrome (SIDS), usually affects babies between one and five months of age. It happens while the baby is asleep and is always sudden and unexpected. Cot death is comparatively rare and the causes are not yet known. Although there is no method of prevention, studies have shown that some simple precautions can reduce the risk. However, parents should be reassured that cot deaths are rare, in order to prevent undue anxiety during the baby's first few months of life.

Recent research shows that cot death is more common in babies who sleep face downwards. By ensuring a baby goes to sleep in the right position, the risk of cot death can be greatly reduced. There is no evidence to suggest that babies might be sick and choke if laid on their backs.

Some babies who require special treatment, or who have particular medical problems, need to be nursed on their fronts. The nurse, midwife, or doctor should explain the need for this to the parents.

The right sleeping position is important only until the infant is able to roll over in its sleep. Once able to do this, it is safe to let the infant adopt its preferred position.

Babies should be laid down to sleep either 1) on their backs or 2) on their sides, with the lower arm forward to stop them rolling over.

The infant should be kept warm, but must not be allowed to get too hot. Lightweight blankets should be used, as these can be added and taken away according to room temperature. The Department of Health (1992) do not recommend the use of a duvet or baby nest, as these can be too warm and can easily cover the baby's head. Feverish babies should have few blankets, if any. The baby should be cared for in a smoke-free zone. Smoking should not be permitted anywhere near the baby.

If a baby seems unwell, medical advice should be sought immediately.

As babies spend many hours alone in cots, it is vital that it is safe. The mattress must fit snugly, leaving no spaces in which a baby's head could become stuck. The bars of the cot must be smooth and securely fixed, and the distance between each bar should not be less than 25 mm and not more than 60 mm, to prevent the baby's head from becoming trapped. The cot should be sturdy, and moving parts should work smoothly and not permit fingers or clothing to become trapped. Check that there are not footholds in the sides, or cutouts in the ends which could help the baby climb out, or trap its head, arms, or legs. Cots with transfers on the inside should be avoided, as the baby may chew them off. New cots should carry the British Standard Mark BS1753 (Child Accident Prevention Trust, 1990). Avoid situating the cot near curtains or anything that might help a baby climb out, or near blinds where cords could strangle an infant.

Sleep and activity

Sleep patterns vary among infants, and active infants typically sleep less than placid children. Generally, by 3–4 months of age most infants have developed a nocturnal pattern of sleep lasting from 9–11 months. The total daily sleep is about 15 hours. The number of naps per day varies, but by the end of one year infants may take one or two naps. Breast-fed infants usually sleep for less prolonged periods, with more frequent waking, especially during the night, than do bottle-fed infants.

Sleep disturbances

Concerns regarding sleep are common during the child's infancy. Sometimes they are as basic as parents questioning if the infant needs additional sleep. In this case, it is best to investigate the reason for their concern, stressing the individual needs of each child. Infants who are active during wakeful periods and who are growing normally are sleeping a sufficient amount of time.

However, there are many more serious concerns that require intervention. Sleep disturbances caused by organic dysfunction are rare, with the exception of colic. The more common sleep disturbances are a learned pattern or developmental characteristic of some infants. Although many families may report sleep problems that are typical of these patterns, interventions are offered only when the pattern is disruptive to the family.

However, when a sleeping problem is presented, a careful assessment is essential. Charting sleep habits, both before and after interventions, is also an important strategy. Questions regarding the frequency and duration of waking, the usual bedtime routine, the number of night-time feedings, the perceived problem (e.g., how much disruption the behaviour generates), and the attempted interventions are important in planning effective approaches designed for the specific sleep problem. An equally effective, but more practical approach, for trained night crying is to let the child cry for progressively longer times between brief parental interventions that consist only of reassurance, not rocking, holding, or using the bottle or soother. For example, the parents may check on the child every five minutes during the first night and progressively extend this interval by five minutes on successive nights (Green, 1989).

The best way to prevent sleep problems is to encourage parents to establish bedtime rituals that do not foster problematic patterns. One of the most constructive is placing infants in their own cot while still awake.

KEY POINTS

◆ Nurses need to offer a range of health education approaches which are sensitive to parents' and children's needs. It is vital to assess parents' knowledge before undertaking health education.

◆ Every year one in five children has an accident which is serious enough to need medical attention. Most accidents occur between nine months and four years of age.

◆ Approximately 300 babies are killed or injured in cars each year.

◆ Childhood immunization is available against diphtheria, whooping cough, tetanus, polio, measles, mumps, and rubella. In addition, immunization has recently been introduced against *Haemophilus influenzae* type B.

◆ Dental decay is one of the most common childhood diseases. Good dental hygiene is important from birth, as even newborn babies have unseen developing teeth which need to be protected.

◆ Attention to a child's diet is recommended to ensure that the frequency of sugary snacks is reduced and that healthy eating patterns are promoted.

◆ Children need an adequate intake of fat in their diet up to the age of five.

◆ Parents should be more concerned about the quality of food that children eat rather than the quantity.

◆ Cot death, also known as sudden infant death syndrome (SIDS), usually affects babies between one and five months of age.

◆ Babies should be laid down to sleep on their backs or on their sides, with the lower arm forwards to stop them rolling over.

◆ Babies should be cared for in a smoke-free zone.

REFERENCES

Baxter DN: Pertussis immunization of children with histories of neurological problems, *BMJ*, Dec. 17; 309 (6969) 1619, 1994.

Child Accident Prevention Trust: *First ride safe ride — keeping your baby safe in the car*, London, 1988, Child Accident Prevention Trust.

Child Accident Prevention Trust: *Keep your baby safe – a guide to safe nursery equipment*, London, 1990, Child Accident Prevention Trust.

COMA (Committee on Medical Aspects of Food): *Dietary reference values for food energy and nutrients for the United Kingdom: report of the Panel on Dietary Sugars of the Committee on Medical Aspects of Food Policy*, London, 1991, HMSO.

Coutts L, Hardy L: *Teaching for health*, Edinburgh, 1985, Churchill Livingstone.

Department of Health: *Back to sleep — reducing the risk of cot death*, London, 1992, HMSO.

Department of Health: *The Health of the Nation - a consultative document for health in England*, London, 1991, HMSO.

Department of Health: *Guidelines on the weaning diet*, London, 1994a, HMSO.

Department of Health: *Nutritional aspects of cardiovascular disease*, London, 1994b, HMSO.

Early Childhood Development Unit: *Nutritional and weaning ideas for parents of infants*, 1988, Bristol University.

Ewles L, Simnett I: *Promoting Health. A practical guide to health education*, Chichester, 1985, John Wiley & Sons.

Green C: *Babies! A parents guide to surviving (and enjoying!) baby's first year*, London, 1989, Simon & Schuster.

Green L *et al*: *Health education planning: a diagnostic approach*, Palo Alto, 1979, Mayfield.

Health Education Authority: *The MMR vaccination*, London, 1988, Health Education Authority.

Health Education Authority: *Your children's teeth*, London, 1980, Health Education Authority.

Joffe M, Ludwig S: Stairway injuries in children, *Pediatr* 82(3, pt 2):457, 1988.

Jumbelic MI, Chambliss M: Accidental toddler drowning in 5-gallon buckets, *JAMA* 263:1952, 1990.

Mofenson HC *et al*: Baby powder — a hazard! *Paediatr* 68(2):265, 1981.

Salisbury D and Begg A (Eds): *Immunization against infectious diseases*, Department of Health Welsh Office, Scottish Office Home and Health Department, DHSS Northern Ireland, London, 1992, HMSO.

World Health Organization: *Targets for health for all*, Copenhagen, 1985, WHO.

FURTHER READING

Armstrong N: Promoting physical activity in schools, *Health Visitor* 66(10):362, 1993.

Baillie L: Health promotion. Childhood accidents; the A&E nurse's role, *Nursing Standard* 8(39):30, 1994.

Brodt J: A crying need for immunisation, *American Nurse* 25(1):3, 1993.

Brooks L *et al*: Group child health assessments, *Health Visitor* 66(8):287, 1993.

Bryar R, Frisk L: Setting up a community health house, *Health Visitor* 67(6):203, 1994.

Bunton R, MacDonald G, editors: *Health promotion: disciplines and diversity*, London, 1992, Routledge.

Campbell A, Edgar S: Teenage screening in a general practice setting, *Health Visitor* 66(10):365, 1993.

Draper P, ed: *Health through public policy*, London, 1991, Greenprint.

Gott M, O'Brien M: Health promotion: practice and the prospect for change, *Nursing Standard* 5(3):30, 1990.

Igoe J: Health promotion, health protection and disease prevention in childhood, *Pediatric Nurse* 18(3):291, 1992.

Jacobson B, Smith A, Whitehead M, eds: *The nation's health. A strategy for the 1990s*, London, 1991, Kings Fund.

Jones S: Fluoride: spanning the health divide, *Nursing Standard*, 7(10):36, 1992.

Whelan C: Promoting positive parenting, *Health Visitor*, 67(6):207, 1994.

Wilson-Barnett J, Clark JM: *Research in health promotion and nursing*, London, 1993, Macmillan.

Chapter 12

Genetics and the Family

LEARNING OUTCOMES

After studying this chapter you should be able to:

◆ Appreciate the influence of genetic factors on health and disease.
◆ Define patterns of inheritance.
◆ Discuss the impact of hereditary disorders on families.
◆ Describe the process of genetic counselling.
◆ Identify situations that necessitate referral to specialist genetic services.
◆ Define the glossary terms.

GLOSSARY

autosome A chromosome other than a sex (X or Y) chromosome

carrier An individual who possesses and can transmit the gene for a given trait, but does not exhibit the trait

chromosomal aberration The addition, loss, or structural alteration of a chromosome

congenital A condition present at birth; causes may be genetic, nongenetic, or both

dominant Refers to a gene that produces an effect (is expressed) whenever it is present

familial A trait or disorder that 'runs in families' or is present in more members of a family than would be expected by chance

genetic Caused by a single gene, several genes, or a deviation in chromosome number or structure; may or may not be apparent at birth

genotype The genetic constitution that determines the physical and chemical characteristics of an individual

heterozygous Having dissimilar genes at a given position (locus) on a pair of chromosomes

homozygous Having the same genes at a given position (locus) on a pair of chromosomes

inherited (heritable, hereditary) Describes traits or disorders appearing in parent and offspring over several generations

monogenic Caused by a single gene

multifactorial A complex interaction of both genetic and environmental factors

mutation A permanent, heritable change in the sequence of DNA in a gene

phenotype The physical or chemical characteristics of an individual; produced by interaction of the environment on the genotype

polygenic Inheritance involving many genes at separate loci whose combined, additive effects produce a given phenotype

recessive Refers to a gene that produces its effect (is expressed) only when it is present in the homozygous or monozygous state

translocation The transfer of all or part of a chromosome to another location on the same chromosome or to a different chromosome following chromosome breakage

X-linked Refers to a gene located on the X chromosome, and thus always transmitted by the X chromosome

Child development begins before birth and is directed by the action of many genetic mechanisms controlled by a strict chronology. But no less significant are the influences of environment, particularly during the time of critical differentiation. The physical, biochemical, and mental characteristics of the child include not only traits that create the individuality of each child, but also characteristics that produce unpleasant symptoms or undesirable physical abnormalities that are interpreted as disease.

Numerous defects and diseases seen frequently in the population show an increased incidence in some families or under certain environmental conditions. Parents and health workers alike are concerned with the probability that a specific disease or disorder will recur in a family. To better counsel families and to anticipate probable problems, the nurse needs a fundamental understanding of the principles of genetics and the importance of heredity as an aetiological factor in diseases and disorders of childhood. This chapter is concerned with some genetic factors that play a role in growth and development, and with counselling the family about problems related to hereditary disorders.

GENETIC INFLUENCES ON HEALTH

Hereditary influences on health and disease are assuming increasing importance to persons in the health professions. Medical science has made rapid advances in the control of infectious diseases and nutritional disorders that formerly accounted for the major share of deaths in infancy. At the same time, contributions from the fields of biochemistry, cytogenetics and molecular genetics have established a genetic basis and the means for identifying an increasing number of diseases and defects. Consequently, there has been a corresponding increase in the proportion of conditions in which genetic factors are prominent, especially in the paediatric population.

HEREDITY IN HEALTH PROBLEMS

There is probably a genetic component in all disease processes. In some disorders, the genetic defect is known; in others the precise nature of the genetic component is more obscure. In some, the disorder is apparent at birth; in others the manifestations do not appear for weeks, months, or years. Some diseases and disorders, such as muscular dystrophy, Marfan's syndrome, and Down's syndrome, are determined by the genetic constitution of the individual. Other diseases, although genetically determined, do not become clinically apparent until environmental factors precipitate the onset of symptoms. For instance, an infant with phenylketonuria (a disorder caused by lack of an enzyme essential for the metabolism of the protein phenylalanine) does not display any symptoms until a sufficient amount of milk containing the protein is ingested; and the serious effects of sickle cell anaemia develop under conditions of lowered oxygen tension.

Genetic diseases can usually be classified into one of three broad categories according to the hereditary factors that produce the observed effect: (1) cytogenetic, (2) monogenic and (3) multifactorial.

CYTOGENETIC DISORDERS

Chromosomal abnormalities, or cytogenetic disorders, are deviations in either structure or number of a chromosome. The consequences in either situation can usually be readily observed in the affected individual. Although the types of cytogenetic disorders are not as varied as those caused by a single gene, the incidence for many of the specific abnormalities is significantly higher than that for any of the single-gene (monogenic) disorders.

A structural abnormality involves loss, addition, rearrangement, or exchange of part of a chromosome. If there is sufficient remaining genetic material to render the organism viable, structural alterations can produce an endless variety of clinical manifestations.

The addition of one chromosome to a normal pair of chromosomes is called *trisomy*. Several deviations that are compatible with life occur in humans, especially those involving the sex chromosomes, but the more serious outcomes are related to abnormalities of the autosomes. Trisomies are the chromosomal aberrations encountered most commonly by health workers.

The clinical consequences that attend variations in chromosome number frequently consist of discrete, identifiable syndromes, particularly with regard to the trisomies. The chromosomal structural anomalies form a more diverse group of reported physical deviations with few recognized syndromes. Some of the chromosomal disorders, such as Down's syndrome, can be identified on the basis of physical characteristics; all require chromosomal analysis to establish a chromosomal abnormality as a causative factor.

CAUSES OF CHROMOSOME DEFECTS

There is considerable speculation regarding the precise cause of chromosome errors.

Most of the information regarding factors that cause chromosome errors is related to parental age. The incidence of trisomic births corresponds strongly with increasing maternal age, regardless of the number of pregnancies. For example, the risk for trisomy 21, or Down's syndrome, increases dramatically for mothers more than 35 years of age (see Down's Syndrome, Chapter 22, for further discussion). There is no positive explanation for this observation.

Nondisjunction
The mechanism considered to be responsible for maldistribution of chromosomes in the majority of cases is nondisjunction during meiosis. Nondisjunction is failure of the chromosomes

to separate and migrate during cell division. The consequence of this prolonged attachment during division is an unequal distribution of chromosomes between the two resulting cells. Nondisjunction can take place during ova formation or sperm formation and can involve autosomes or sex chromosomes.

Translocation

A *translocation* occurs when two chromosomes exchange material. A balanced translocation involves a reciprocal exchange with no loss or gain of material. This normally has no phenotypic effect, but there is the possibility of an unbalanced chromosome constitution being passed on to offspring, resulting in abnormality or early fetal loss.

Recognizing autosomal anomalies

The best known viable trisomies (21, 18, 13) are easily identified, and the diagnosis can nearly always be made early, based on physical characteristics alone — usually in the delivery room or newborn nursery. Often, nurses in the newborn nursery see infants who have a facial appearance that sets them apart from other infants. The infant may have no obvious congenital malformation, but on closer inspection, may evidence other variations, the sum of which disclose the specific features of known syndromes.

It need not be appearance only that suggests more careful scrutiny of such infants. They may exhibit hypotonia and other neurological manifestations such as an unusual cry, poor feeding behaviour or abnormal reflex responses.

ABNORMALITIES OF SEX CHROMOSOMES

An increase in the number of sex chromosomes does not produce the profound effects that are associated with the autosomal trisomies.

Many sex chromosome abnormalities have been described. The more common of these, Klinefelter's and Turner's syndromes, are discussed further in Chapter 18 in relation to developmental problems of later childhood. Some general characteristics of chromosomal abnormalities of sex chromosome numbers are listed in Box 12-1.

Fragile X syndrome (see Chapter 22) is attributed to a fragile (unstable) site on the X chromosome. This disorder is now known to be caused by a previously undescribed gene mutation.

MONOGENIC (SINGLE-GENE) DISORDERS

Disorders for which a simple, definite inheritance pattern can be identified are rare individually, but collectively they constitute a significant portion of health problems seen in infants and children. They can involve any system in the body. They can be of minor importance and have little effect on the child, or they can cause serious disability or can be incompatible with life.

Conditions that can be directly attributed to a single gene

mutation are often distributed in families in characteristic patterns according to basic Mendelian principles. Genes are either dominant or recessive in their effect, and most disorders caused by a single mutation gene can be recognized readily by the simple family patterns that they display. Nontraditional patterns of interference such as new mutations, mosaicism, and uniparental disomy are increasingly being recognized as responsible for disorders in a family not exhibiting Mendelian inheritance.

AUTOSOMAL INHERITANCE PATTERNS

The characteristic major inheritance patterns are described and accompanied by sample pedigree charts.

Autosomal dominant inheritance

The first case in a family may appear suddenly as the result of a fresh mutation and, depending on the degree of disability the condition imposes on the individual, will either die out or continue to be passed on through several generations (Fig. 12-1). There is wide variability in expression and later onset may occur. Examples of autosomal-dominant disorders include achondroplasia, Huntington's disease, and Marfan's syndrome.

Autosomal recessive inheritance

Children who display an autosomal recessive disorder will always be homozygous for that trait. Carriers will be heterozygous and unaffected. It is estimated that each person carries from three to eight recessive genes (Fig. 12-2). However, the probability of mating between two persons who carry the same deleterious gene is highly unlikely. If they are blood relatives, the likelihood is increased. Examples of autosomal recessive disorders include cystic fibrosis, phenylketonuria (PKU), and galactosaemia.

◆ BOX 12-1

Characteristics of Sex Chromosome Abnormalities

There is a direct relationship between the male or female phenotype and the presence or absence of a Y chromosome. The Y chromosome is essential for development of male characteristics.

The severity of defects is not related to the number of extra X chromosomes, except for mental retardation, which increases proportionally with each X chromosome.

The presence of more than one Y chromosome appears to have variable but as yet not well-defined effects on the phenotype.

X-LINKED INHERITANCE PATTERNS

Genes on the X chromosome differ from those on the Y chromosome; therefore, the transmission of traits caused by these genes will vary according to the sex of the individual who carries the gene. The two X chromosomes in the female are alike in gene constitution, with two genes for each trait. Genes on the X chromosome have no counterpart on the Y chromosome; therefore a characteristic determined by a gene on the X chromosome is *always* expressed in the male. One of the most significant aspects of X-linked inheritance is the absence of father-to-son transmission. The Y chromosome carries only a few known genes, mostly related to the development of the male phenotypes.

X-linked dominant inheritance

Superficially, this pattern resembles an autosomal dominant inheritance pattern. This type of inheritance is relatively uncommon, and because severe effects in the male may be fatal prenatally, transmission of the gene takes place primarily in the female. An example of an X-linked dominant disorder is hypophosphataemic vitamin D–resistant rickets.

X-linked recessive inheritance

The abnormal gene behaves as any recessive gene; that is, its effect will be hidden by a normal dominant gene. Examples of X-linked recessive disorder include haemophilia and Duchenne muscular dystrophy.

MULTIFACTORIAL DISORDERS

Several diseases and defects encountered frequently in the population show an increased incidence in some families, that is, higher than expected by chance, but show no specific mode of inheritance. In some, environmental factors appear to play an important role. These are the conditions classified as *multifactorial* — disorders in which a genetic susceptibility, combined with the appropriate environmental agents, interact to produce a disease state. Disorders that are considered to be multifactorial include many congenital defects such as spinabifida and a number of common chronic diseases such as hypertension and non-insulin-dependent diabetes mellitus.

		Affected parent	
	Gametes	A	a
Normal parent	a	A a Affected	a a Normal
	a	A a Affected	a a Normal

Characteristics of autosomal dominant inheritance

Males and females are affected with equal frequency.
Affected individuals will have an affected parent (unless the condition is caused by a fresh mutation).
Half the children of a heterozygous affected parent will have the probability of possessing the defective gene, although it may be nonpenetrant.
Unaffected children of affected parents will have unaffected children (unless the gene is nonpenetrant).
Traits can be traced vertically through previous generations—a positive family history.

Fig. 12-1 Possible offspring of mating between normal parent and one with autosomal dominant trait.

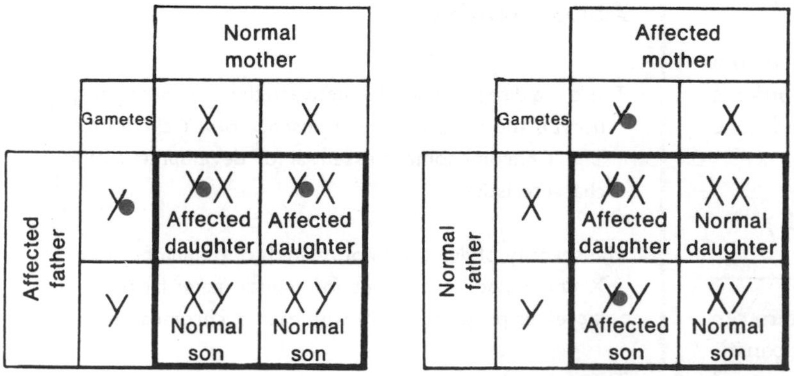

Characteristics of X-linked dominant inheritance

Affected individuals will have an affected parent.
All the daughters but none of the sons of an affected male have the probability of being affected.
Half the sons and half the daughters of an affected female will be affected.
Normal children of an affected parent will have normal offspring.
There are no carriers.
The inheritance pattern shows a positive family history.

Fig. 12-2 Possible offspring of mating between two parents with recessive gene on an autosome.

CONGENITAL ANOMALIES

The development of an organism, especially during embryogenesis, is an intricate process in which all parts must be properly integrated to ensure a coordinated whole. The rate must be such that one part is ready when needed by another part; otherwise, either part may cease to grow or may deviate from its normal path. Congenital anomalies, or birth defects, can arise at any stage of development and show wide variability in determining factors as well as in type, extent, and frequency of defects. Some defects result when a state, present in one phase of development as a normal condition, persists into another phase, becoming abnormal. For example, cleft lip is normal in a young embryo, and patent ductus arteriosus is essential during fetal life. Any agent that interferes with these complex processes will produce a defect in development ranging in severity from an insignificant local anomaly to complete degeneration.

A few congenital defects are clearly caused by a single gene; some are associated with chromosomal abnormalities, and others are produced by known intrauterine environment risk factors. In many cases an aetiological factor cannot be identified.

Because of the steady decline in infant mortality from other causes, congenital anomalies are responsible for an increasing proportion of all deaths in infancy and constitute an increasing proportion of infants requiring intensive newborn care. Some defects are of minor significance and have little or no effect on survival or the quality of life; others are severe and are incompatible with life or are a serious threat to survival.

THERAPEUTIC MANAGEMENT OF GENETIC DISEASE

No cures are available for most genetic diseases at present, although preventive and corrective therapy is helping to reduce the harmful effects in an increasing number of conditions. Genetic research is making progress in methods of altering the genetic material directly known as 'gene therapy'. Meanwhile, the major goal of therapy is modification of the internal or external environment to correct or minimize the effects of the genetic defect.

GENETICS AND SOCIETY

There is no doubt that genetic diseases constitute a significant portion of world health problems, and the advantages of improving the human race are seldom questioned. Controversy exists, however, between those who advocate improvement in the species by selective breeding and those who recommend providing a better environment.

Eugenics is essentially planned breeding designed to alter future generations. Such practice has been used successfully for many years by animal and plant breeders to develop superior food products. For many persons, any discussion of controlling heredity creates visions of Hitler's interpretation and misuse of directed evolution - some racial groups view it as the code word for genocide, and religious groups protest that it is tampering with God's creation. Further discussion of this issue is beyond the scope of this chapter. It is important, however, to learn from the abuses of the past when formulating future health policy.

IMPACT OF HEREDITARY DISORDERS ON THE FAMILY

The presence of a genetic disorder presents multiple problems and concerns to the family and to health workers. The disorder may have been present in a family for generations, or it may appear suddenly in a family. In either situation the family is faced with decisions regarding their reproductive future.

GENETIC SCREENING

Tests to determine the presence of a defective gene are rapidly assuming greater importance in management of genetic disorders as more defects are identified and techniques are developed for easy detection. It is probable that with improved technology, mass screening for numerous defects may eventually be a routine procedure. However, to be truly effective, screening programmes depend on education of health professionals and the public regarding the programmes. The religious, moral, and ethical issues associated with screening and prenatal diagnosis are extensive and beyond the scope of this discussion; therefore, only a few are mentioned, and the reader is encouraged to investigate these issues further in other resources.

PURPOSES OF SCREENING

Genetic screening is presumptive identification of an unrecognized genotype in individuals or populations. There are several purposes for this screening: (1) to detect the carrier state or presence of disease, incipient or overt, (2) to provide reproductive information, and (3) to gain information concerning the incidence of a disorder in the population.

Screening for disease
The rationale for screening for disease is to discover people who: (1) have the disease, either manifest or incipient, or (2) may, in time or under special circumstances, develop the disease. The purpose of this knowledge is to anticipate serious consequences and provide the individual with treatment and management that will prevent, reverse, or diminish the adverse effects of the disorder. An example is the generalized, systematic screening of newborn infants for PKU.

Screening for reproductive information
Screening for heterozygotes (carriers) can detect unaffected people with certain genes who, when they mate with an individual who carries a similar gene, are at high risk of producing an affected offspring. These individuals are thus provided with

the knowledge they need for use in decisions about family planning. Carriers of a number of diseases can be detected by laboratory tests, but because of the rarity of these diseases, mass screening is not feasible except in persons or populations known to be at risk. People at risk include close relatives of persons with an inborn error of metabolism or other detectable disorder, or certain ethnic populations known to have a high incidence of a specific disease, such as sickle cell anaemia in blacks, Tay-Sachs disease in Ashkenazi Jews, thalassaemia in people of Mediterranean ancestry and cystic fibrosis in people originating from North West Europe.

PRENATAL DIAGNOSIS

A variety of techniques are available for diagnosing several diseases and defects in the fetus. As more diseases can be diagnosed prenatally, and parents at risk are recognized early, these procedures provide the means to detect defects that are best corrected soon after delivery, conditions that may require preterm delivery for early correction, conditions that may require Caesarean delivery, conditions that may require medical or surgical treatment before birth, and conditions on which a decision may be based to terminate a pregnancy.

SIGNIFICANCE OF SCREENING TO FAMILIES

Mass screening programmes have not been enthusiastically endorsed and carried out by all members of the health professions or wholeheartedly accepted by the public — especially compulsory screening. The reasons for this resistance are justified in many instances. Many practitioners are unfamiliar with the techniques required for genetic screening, and some of the tests have limitations to accuracy. The perceived stigma attached to carriers of a disease is also a prohibiting factor. Much of family concern about screening focuses on the issues of informed consent and the use to be made of the information from the screening.

Release of information to persons other than the family is also subject to debate. At present, the reporting of genetic findings is not mandatory, as it is for certain contagious diseases, and it is questionable whether this would be desirable. A family may not wish for other family members, or even the family practitioner, to receive the results of screening. Third parties who may make use of such information detrimentally are insurance companies and employers. All of these possibilities should be made clear to families in order to provide them with some selective control.

The social stigma, however unfounded, attached to the carrier of a defective gene may be a negative effect of screening. In some families, such knowledge is a source of embarrassment and damaging to the self-esteem of its members. Teenagers are especially vulnerable to the effects of knowing they carry a specific defective gene at a time when identity formation and peer approval are extremely important. Cultural views regarding this knowledge can have profound effects on the members of some

ethnic groups. In some cases, social status within the cultural group can be impaired.

Probably the most important area for nursing practice is teaching. Families need to understand why the screening is proposed, what the results mean, and how the family can interpret false positive and false negative results. Parents are concerned, and their anxiety is greater when they have not received sufficient information about the screening or testing process and its significance for the health of their infant (Sorenson and Mangione, 1984). The nurse is a valuable resource person in making families aware of alternatives and in helping them select the one that best suits their particular situation.

GENETIC COUNSELLING

In recent years, the significance of heredity as an aetiological agent in disease and disability has assumed a more prominent place in children's nursing. With the expanded recognition of genetic diseases and defects, an increasingly well-informed public is assuming more responsibility for the quality of future populations and creating a justified demand for accurate information regarding risks to present and future generations. The actual number of people who need advice is relatively small compared with those who have many other health problems,

Questions & Controversies

Should routine genetic screening be performed for a disease with no known adverse clinical consequences? Also, should incidental but unexpected findings of genetic screening be disclosed? To whom?

Some argue that screening for a disease with no known clinical repercussions is desirable because it allows follow-up that may reveal subtle consequences unrecognized before (Cohen, 1984). However, there is no reason to subject children and families to the stress of screening procedures if there is no visible evidence of disease and no untoward symptoms.

Sometimes screening information alters family relationships. Disruption of parent-child bonding can occur in the newborn period. The common consequences of detecting a genetic disease in a child are blaming, overprotectiveness of the child resulting in impaired psychological development, and guilt feelings in the family. Knowledge that they have a disease can seriously alter identity information in adolescents. It makes them 'different' from their peers, and persons who are carriers of a genetic disease often exhibit an altered self-concept.

Unexpected information that might seriously alter family relationships includes nonpaternity and discovery of a disorder other than the one for which the individual was screened (Korsch, 1984).

but their need is great. When expert counselling is not accessible, these people may become victims of well-meaning but uninformed quasi-professionals or misguided relatives and acquaintances.

It is estimated that only a small proportion of people who need counselling are seen by clinical genetics services. Many families who might benefit from genetic counselling do not recognize the need, or this special need is not apparent to those who supervise their care. Children's nurses continually encounter genetic diseases and families in which there is a risk that a disorder may be transmitted to an offspring. It is a responsibility of nurses to be alert to situations in which families could benefit from genetic counselling, to become familiar with facilities in their areas where genetic counselling is available, and to learn the basic principles of heredity. In this way, they will be able to direct individuals and families to take advantage of counselling services and to be active participants in the counselling process. Nurses should also be knowledgeable regarding special services that are available to help in management and support of affected children.

A comprehensive definition of genetic counselling prepared by a group of eminent medical geneticists states that genetic counselling is a communication process that deals with the human problems associated with the occurrence, or risk of occurrence, of a genetic disorder in a family. This process involves an attempt by one or more appropriately trained persons to help the individual or family (Fraser, 1974):

* Comprehend the medical facts, including the diagnosis, the probable course of the disorder, and the available management
* Appreciate the way heredity contributes to the disorder, and the risk of recurrence in specified relatives
* Understand the options for dealing with the risk of recurrence
* Choose the course of action that seems appropriate to them in view of their risk and their family goals and act in accordance with that decision
* Make the best possible adjustment to the disorder in an affected family member and/or to the risk of recurrence of that disorder

CLIENTS

Clients may or may not be affected themselves, but may request genetic counselling about the heritability of a trait that may be deleterious, beneficial, or merely troublesome. Clients might be a young couple contemplating marriage or childbearing, who are concerned about a disorder in one of their families, no matter how remote the relationship, or who may seek advice because they are related. A couple who are both members of a population at risk for certain diseases may wish to determine whether they carry the harmful gene (e.g., blacks and sickle cell anaemia, Ashkenazi Jews and Tay-Sachs disease, or persons of Mediterranean ancestry and thalassaemia).

More often, persons who inquire about the possibility of recurrence of a disease or disorder are parents of a child with a specific disease or defect that significantly impairs fitness who are concerned that they might produce another similarly affected child. This advice may be sought before the couple

initiates another pregnancy, after the mother is already pregnant, or after the birth of another child. There is often concern regarding the risk to unaffected siblings of the affected child or to the affected child's future children.

More than ever before, parents plan and feel responsible for their children. They need to know the risk in *their particular situation* and how it relates to the random risk for <u>any</u> prospective parents.

Some families may need counselling regarding the advisability of sterilization, artificial insemination, prenatal diagnosis, or termination of a pregnancy. Infertility or recurrent abortion in a family may also indicate a need for counselling.

Special risk situations

When health personnel are alerted to the possibility of an inherited disease in a family, this knowledge makes possible the early detection and subsequent treatment of the disorder. This early detection is increasingly important, as treatments are becoming available for more genetically determined diseases. This is especially true in situations where treatment is effective only when initiated early. The history of a condition in an older sibling, such as PKU or galactosaemia, provides a clue for specific and thorough testing for the condition in a newborn. In this way, early therapy can be initiated when indicated, thus minimizing or eliminating the effects of the disease or defect.

INFORMATION ESSENTIAL FOR GENETIC COUNSELLING

Unlike a medical prognosis that predicts the outcome of a disease, a genetic prognosis directly involves other persons: the affected child, members of the immediate family, relatives, and future offspring. Effective genetic counselling requires a

---

Questions & Controversies

*S*hould parents be permitted prenatal diagnosis for sex determination unrelated to X-linked disease?

Prenatal ultrasonography and chromosome analysis from amniotic fluid or chorionic villus sample allow determination of sex before birth. It has long been employed for detecting sex in carrier mothers at risk of passing a sex-linked disorder to a male offspring. Parents may also be informed of the sex of the fetus when amniocentesis is performed to rule out a chromosomal anomaly or some other undesirable disorder. The technique could easily be employed for sex determination alone. To date, the long-term effects on society if parents are allowed to selectively terminate a pregnancy with a fetus of the 'wrong sex' are unknown. However, it is well-known that a male is the preferred firstborn (Fletcher, 1979).

thorough evaluation of each situation. Information from which the counsellor derives risks of recurrence is acquired from several sources: an accurate diagnosis, a thorough family history, and an extensive knowledge of genetics.

Accurate diagnosis

The first and most important component in the counselling process is an accurate diagnosis. There are more than 3,000 known inherited disorders, many of which have similar clinical manifestations but may have different modes of inheritance. For example, symptoms in the early stages of severe X-linked muscular dystrophy appear much like those of the milder autosomal recessive and autosomal dominant varieties, autosomal recessive neurogenic muscular atrophies, and nongenetic poliomyelitis. The significance of the risks related to each type of disorder is readily apparent. It is especially difficult to assign a cause to deafness or mental retardation.

Family history

A careful, detailed family history is necessary to the counselling process. Not only does it provide a picture of the *proband* (the affected person, or *index case*) in relation to other family members, but it may also serve to identify other persons who are similarly affected or who might be at risk of producing affected children. Analysing the pattern of affected members of the family can assist in confirming a tentative diagnosis or in determining the level of risk in multifactorial inheritance.

Knowledge of genetics

In order to counsel families regarding their particular problem, a counsellor must have a thorough understanding of genetic principles, a knowledge of the risks related to multifactorial inheritance, and up-to-date information on genetic diseases.

ESTIMATION OF RISKS

The mode of inheritance determines the degree of risk in the major categories of genetic disorders. In general, the more definite and clear-cut the genetics, the greater the risks; as the causative factors become more obscure, recurrence risks are usually lower.

INTERPRETATION OF RISKS

When explaining risk estimates, the counsellor does not attempt to make recommendations or decisions for consultants. The counsellor provides appropriate and accurate information about the nature of the disorder, the extent of the risk involved, the probable consequences, and alternative solutions but remains nondirective, leaving the final decision to the persons concerned.

Families may misunderstand probabilities, even when they are fully explained. It is important to impress on them that *each pregnancy is an independent event*. It is not uncommon for parents who are told that a recessive disorder carries a 1:4 risk of recurrence to feel secure with one affected child. They incorrectly reason that because they already have one affected child

the next three will be unaffected. However, chance has no memory; the risk is 1:4 for each and every pregnancy.

NURSES AND GENETIC COUNSELLING

Nurses skilled in counselling techniques are in a unique position to help meet the counselling needs of families in which there is a genetic disease or disorder. Genetics nurse specialists, with advanced preparation in genetic theory, are assuming a prominent position on counselling teams; and practitioners in the specialty areas of midwifery and children's nursing are constantly involved with families in which there is a genetic defect. Nurses are frequently the persons who recognize clues that indicate a genetics-related problem, who assist the family in obtaining the needed services for diagnosis and treatment, and who provide follow-up care.

GENETIC COUNSELLING SERVICES

The most efficient service consists of a group of specialists that may include geneticists, psychologists, biochemists, cytogeneticists, molecular geneticists, nurses, social workers, and other auxiliary personnel.

ROLE OF THE NURSE IN GENETIC COUNSELLING

It is a nurse who is frequently the family's initial contact with a counselling service. Families who have a relaxed and nonstressful initial discussion are able to gain more from a counselling session.

Taking a family history

The family history is recorded in the form of a pedigree chart or family tree using standard symbols to indicate persons, relationships, and significant details related to them.

It is important to include information about previous pregnancies and family history. Sometimes the place of birth and ethnic background are significant. For example, the incidence of Tay-Sachs disease is higher in Ashkenazi Jews from eastern Europe than in Jews from other geographic origins. Also, when a pedigree chart is being evaluated, the fact that a sister died in infancy as a 'blue baby' might be genetically significant, whereas a healthy sibling who drowned at age one year would not. Information concerning first-degree relatives is most important and should be complete.

Follow-up care

The success of counselling is measured by the way in which the family uses the information presented to them. Maintaining contact with the family or referral to an agency that can provide a sustained relationship is one of the most important aspects of the counselling process. Some families do not choose to have follow-up visits, but in most instances these visits make the family feel that they have not been abandoned and facilitate the process of adjustment to the problem.

Follow-up visits to the counselling service or in the home provide the family with the opportunity to ask questions that they did not ask on previous visits. Often the family members have not really 'heard' the information presented to them or have misinterpreted what they have heard, so that it may be necessary to repeat and reinforce counselling. In some disorders, a diagnosis in one family member places relatives at risk and is an indication for further screening. Follow-up counselling letters, summarizing the information provided to the family, are an excellent documentation tool and provide future reference.

Nurses should be prepared to help families arrive at tentative decisions regarding the future. Initial and ongoing assessments of the family's coping abilities, resources, and support systems are vital in order to determine their need for additional assistance and support. Locating agencies and clinics specializing in a specific disorder or its consequences that can provide services (e.g., equipment, medication, and rehabilitation), educational programmes, and parent groups is part of the nurse's resources.

SUPPORTIVE COUNSELLING

It requires time and understanding to deal with the emotional tension and anxiety generated in families who are faced with the prospect of a genetic disorder. Knowledge of and the ability to deal with the range of psychological responses and all their ramifications (e.g., the grief reaction, guilt, anger, and coping mechanisms) are essential components of the nursing role in genetic counselling. Many of these factors determine the degree to which a counsellor's message is understood and influence the family's attitudes and the use they make of counselling information. Awareness and understanding of these feelings make the difference between a genetic informant and a genetic counsellor.

Timing of the counselling requires careful evaluation. Some families may not be ready to listen immediately after a diagnosis is made; many do not listen effectively the first time information is presented to them. Families who seek genetic counselling, spontaneously or by referral, are apprehensive and know that decisions made on the basis of the information they receive may alter their lives significantly and may even alter their view of themselves. There may be numerous impediments to getting information across to families. Often, they are so angry or frightened that they do not hear what is being said to them; they may feel guilty, embarrassed, or somehow inferior or inadequate.

It is important early in counselling to get a clear understanding of the family's initial concerns, their state of knowledge about the disease, their attitudes and beliefs concerning the condition, and to determine the kind and amount of information they need or want. Some are not sure they should be at a counselling service. Whether the people needing help are parents who have given birth to an affected child, relatives of an affected individual, or persons who have been identified

as carriers of a deleterious gene, their feelings, attitudes, and fears must be dealt with.

Guilt and self-blame are very natural and universal reactions. Nurses must deal with parents' feelings of guilt about carrying 'bad genes' or having 'made my child sick'. For example, the young father of a child with translation Down's syndrome refused to submit to chromosome analysis for fear he might be identified as the carrier of the translocation and thought he could not endure the guilt this knowledge would generate. Often, the counsellor is in a position to absolve the parents of guilt by explaining the random nature of segregation during both gamete formation and fertilization. Sometimes there is comfort in knowing that everyone carries defective genes and that it is mere chance that a particular couple happen to carry the same abnormal gene. Reactions may be different in situations where one member can pinpoint the 'blame' (dominant or X-linked disorders), whereas there is some reassurance in recessive disorders for the couple to know that it is not just one of them who carries the defective gene. Anxieties generated by old wives' tales, superstitions, and misconceptions can be dispelled. A large and vital part of the nurse's role in genetic counselling is that of sympathetic and supportive listener.

Burden of genetic defect

The way in which members of a family respond to the probability of a genetic disorder will depend a great deal on the nature of the condition and the burden, actual or perceived, that it may place on them. A burden is considered to be the total amount of distress, economic and emotional, that is placed on persons, their families, and society by the birth of an affected child — the anticipated burden as well as the threat of disability. Various factors associated with disorders produce a burden in different ways to determine the total impact on a family. These include severity, chronicity, age of onset, mor-

Questions & Controversies

Should society allow a couple to have children when one or both have a severely disabling condition known to be hereditary that inhibits or impairs their ability to function?

In order to solve such a dilemma, several issues must be addressed. How is the competence or incompetence of the involved family to be determined (Kilpack, 1986)? Do persons with a disability have the same right to procreate as persons without a physical or mental disability? If society is to have a voice in such decisions, society will need to determine what constitutes a 'disabling condition'. Who will determine whether a condition is disabling (doctors, lawyers, politicians)? How will such a decision be enforced?

tality, morbidity, presence or absence of chronic pain, mental retardation and cosmetic disfigurement.

There is a great deal of variability in the ability of individuals and families to withstand stress, and people respond differently to probabilities. A degree of risk that is reassuring to one may be threatening or intolerable to another. Also, two individuals will respond differently to a hazard that both perceive as threatening. Some parents will choose to have children even in the face of high risk; others believe that even a moderate risk is too much to take. Some may risk having a child with a disorder that produces a minor defect or even one that causes early death, but elect not to risk having a child with

a lifelong disability. The longer the duration of the disability, the greater the financial and emotional burden.

All of these matters confront a family when they must make a decision about whether to risk a pregnancy that might result in a child with a disability, and nurses should be prepared to explore these probabilities with them. Decisions are often irrevocable; therefore, the choice must be mutually achieved. Parents who elect to have children despite a fairly high risk of recurrence will need education and emotional support. By learning about the disorder, they will be alert to signs of the disease so that early treatment can be initiated to minimize the ill effects of the disorder.

KEY POINTS

◆ There is a probably a genetic component in all disease processes.

◆ Genetic diseases are usually classified as those produced by chromosomal aberrations, those caused by a single mutant gene, or those resulting from interaction of genetic and environmental factors (multifactorial).

◆ Chromosomal aberrations are caused by deviations in either chromosome structure or number.

◆ Disorders caused by a single gene are distributed in families according to predictable Mendelian principles of inheritance.

◆ Although no cure for genetic disease is presently available, various therapeutic measures are used to modify or correct the basic defect.

◆ The objectives of genetic screening are to detect the presence of disease in individuals, detect unaffected carriers of a disease, and monitor the incidence of disease and/or malformations in a population.

◆ Genetic counselling is directed towards providing individuals and families with information needed to make decisions about a course of action appropriate to them.

REFERENCES

Cohen FL: *Clinical genetics in nursing practice,* Philadelphia, 1984, JB Lippincott.

Fletcher JC: Ethics and amniocentesis for fetal sex identification, *N Engl J Med* 301:550, 1979.

Fraser FC: Genetic counseling, *Am J Hum Genet* 26:636, 1974.

Kilpack V: Ethical issues in procedural dilemmas in measuring patient competence. In Chinn PL, editor: *Ethical issues in nursing,* Rockville, MD, 1986, Aspen Systems.

Korsch BM: What do patients and parents want to know? What do they need to know? *Pediatr* (suppl), pp. 917, 1984.

Sorenson JR, Mangione TW: Parental response to repeat testing of infants with 'false-positive' results in a newborn screening program, *Pediatr* 73(2):183, 1984.

FURTHER READING

Clarke A, editor: *Genetic counselling: practice and principles,* London, 1994, Routledge.

Conner JM, Ferguson Smith MA: *Essential medical genetics,* Oxford, 1991, Blackwell Scientific.

Evers-Kiebooms G *et al,* editors: *Psychosocial aspects of genetic counselling,* New York, 1992, Wiley/Liss.

Harper PS: *Practical genetic counselling,* ed 4, Oxford, 1993, Butterworth-Heinemann.

Jones KL: *Smiths recognisable patterns of human malformation,* ed 4, Philadelphia, WB Saunders.

Kingston H: *ABC of clinical genetics,* ed 2, London, 1989, *British Medical Association.*

McKusick VA: Mendelian inheritance in man, ed 10, London, 1992, The John Hopkins University Press.

Nuffield Council on Bioethics: *Genetic screening—ethical issues,* London, 1993, Nuffield Council on Bioethics.

Ratcliffe S, Paul N, editors: *Prospective studies on children with sex chromosome aneuploidy,* New York, 1986, Alan R Liss.

Chapter 13

Health Problems of the Newborn and the Family

LEARNING OUTCOMES

After studying this chapter you should be able to:

◆ Identify problems newborn infants may experience immediately or shortly after birth.
◆ Describe the three most common types of extracranial haemorrhagic injury in the newborn.
◆ Identify disorders related to the immature physiological system of the newborn.
◆ Identify the causes of increased erythrocyte destruction.
◆ Discuss the reason for blood incompatability.
◆ Discuss the care of infants and children with congenital hypothyroidism, phenylketonuria, and galactosaemia.
◆ Discuss the management and care of high-risk newborns.
◆ Describe how high risk newborns are classified.
◆ Identify the characteristics of premature infants.
◆ Discuss the high risk conditions associated with prematurity.
◆ Define the glossary terms.

GLOSSARY

birth injuries Injuries suffered by the infant during the birth process

birth marks Discolouration of the skin found in newborn infants

jaundice Yellowish discolouration of the skin, mucous membranes and sclerae of the eyes

necrotizing enterocolitis A severe and acute inflammatory disease of the bowel

seizure Fit or convulsion

The newborn may experience a number of problems immediately or shortly after birth. Examples include birth injuries, inborn errors of metabolism, and disorders related to the immature physiological system of the newborn. If identified early, these can be successfully managed to prevent deleterious effects.

BIRTH INJURIES

Birth injuries are injuries that occur during the birth process. The forces of labour and delivery may result in trauma, especially when the infant is large, the presentation is breech, following forceps delivery, or if inexperienced practitioners are in attendance. Birth trauma is a leading cause of neonatal mortality.

Many birth injuries are minor and resolve spontaneously in a few days. Birth injuries can be classified according to the type of body structure involved (Box 13-1).

SOFT TISSUE INJURY

Various types of soft tissue injury may be sustained during the birth process. Soft tissue injury usually occurs when there is some degree of disproportion between the presenting part and the maternal pelvis (cephalopelvic disproportion). Common types of soft tissue injury are listed in Box 13-2. These traumatic lesions generally fade spontaneously within a few days without treatment.

IMPLICATIONS FOR NURSING

Nursing care is primarily directed towards identifying and assessing the injury, maintaining asepsis of the area to prevent breakdown and infection, and providing parents with explanation and reassurance.

Regardless of how benign the injury, parents are concerned. Explanations of the cause and treatment, if any, need to be thorough and repeated frequently. Even if the injuries are temporary, the bonding process can be affected by the parents' initial feelings of shock, grief, and disappointment.

HEAD TRAUMA

Trauma to the head that occurs during the birth process is usually benign, but occasionally results in more serious injury. Injuries that produce serious trauma are intraventricular haemorrhage and subdural haematoma. The three most common types of extracranial haemorrhagic injury are caput succedaneum, subgaleal haemorrhage and cephalhaematoma.

CAPUT SUCCEDANEUM

The most commonly observed scalp lesion is caput succedaneum, a vaguely outlined area of oedematous tissue situated over the portion of the scalp that presents in a vertex delivery. The swelling consists of serum and/or blood, which accumulate in the tissues above the bone. Typically, the swelling extends

---

◆ BOX 13-1

Types of physical injuries at birth

Soft Tissue Injury
Erythema
Abrasion
Petechiae
Ecchymoses
Subcutaneous fat necrosis
Subconjunctival (scleral) haemorrhage
Retinal haemorrhage
Haemorrhage into abdominal organ(s)
Head Injury
Skull moulding
Caput succedaneum
Subgaleal haemorrhage
Cephalhaematoma
Fracture (depressed or linear)
Intracranial haemorrhage
Subdural or epidural haematoma
Neurological Injury
Facial paralysis
Brachial palsy (Erb-Duchenne paralysis, Klumpke palsy)
Phrenic nerve palsy (diaphragmatic paralysis)
Spinal cord injury

◆ BOX 13-2

Common types of soft tissue injury

Erythema and abrasions — usually the result of the application of forceps; discolouration is in the same configuration as the instrument.
Petechiae — nonraised, pinpoint haemorrhages caused by a sudden increase and then release of pressure during passage through the birth canal; may be seen on the chest, face, and head.
Ecchymoses — small haemorrhagic areas (larger than petechiae) that may occur after traumatic, rapid (or 'precipitate'), or breech delivery.
Subcutaneous fat necrosis — clearly outlined masses located in the subcutaneous tissues that are firm to the overlying skin but movable over the underlying tissue; most likely caused by traumatic manipulation during delivery.
Subconjunctival (scleral) haemorrhages — the result of rupture of capillaries in the sclera from pressure on the fetal head during delivery; most common location is the limbus of the iris.
Retinal haemorrhages — flame-shaped, irregular, or round areas of bleeding in the retina from excessive pressure on the fetal head during delivery; extensive areas may indicate subdural haematoma or brain trauma.

beyond the bone margins and may be associated with overlying petechiae or ecchymosis (Thomas and Harvey, 1992). It is present at or shortly after birth. No specific treatment is needed, and the swelling subsides within a few days.

SUBGALEAL HAEMORRHAGE

Subgaleal haemorrhage is bleeding into the subgaleal compartment. The subgaleal compartment is a potential space that contains loosely arranged connective tissue; it is located beneath the galea aponeurosis, which is the tendinous sheath that connects the frontal and occipital muscles and forms the inner surface of the scalp. The injury occurs as a result of forces that compress and then drag the head through the pelvic outlet (Minarcik and Beachy, 1989). The bleeding extends beyond the bone and can continue after birth, with potential complications. Treatment is usually not needed, but may be required for blood loss and shock. Resolution of the bleeding may cause hyperbilirubinaemia.

CEPHALHAEMATOMA

Infrequently, a cephalhaematoma is formed when blood vessels rupture during labour or delivery to produce bleeding into the area between the bone and its periosteum. The injury occurs most often with primiparous women, and it is often associated with forceps delivery. Unlike caput succedaneum, the boundaries of the cephalhaematoma are sharply demarcated and do not extend beyond the limits of the bone. The cephalhaematoma may involve one or both parietal bones. Less commonly, the occipital and rarely the frontal bones are affected. The swelling is usually minimal at birth and increases in size on the second or third day. Blood loss is not significant.

No treatment is indicated for uncomplicated cephalhaematoma. Most lesions are absorbed within two weeks to three months. Lesions that result in severe blood loss to the area or that involve an underlying fracture require further evaluation. Hyperbilirubinaemia may result during resolution of the haematoma.

IMPLICATIONS FOR NURSING

Nursing care is directed towards assessment and observation of the common scalp injuries, and vigilance in observing for possible complications such as infection, subdural haematoma, or intraventricular haemorrhage. Because these visible injuries resolve spontaneously, parents need to be reassured that the injuries are usually benign.

FRACTURES

Fracture of the clavicle (collarbone) is the most common birth injury. It is associated with difficult vertex or breech delivery of infants of above average weight. The fracture may be

detected during delivery by an audible 'click' or 'snap', although the newborn may be asymptomatic. The problem should be suspected in infants who demonstrate limited use of the affected arm, a malposition of the arm, asymmetric Moro reflex, local swelling or tenderness, or who cry in pain when the arm is moved. Crepitus (the crackling sound produced by the rubbing together of fractured bone fragments) is often heard and/or felt on further examination, and X-rays usually reveal a complete fracture with overriding of the fragments.

Fractures of long bones, such as the femur or humerus, may be undetected because the epiphysis is mostly cartilage, which is usually not dense enough to show clearly on an X-ray. Presence of fracture(s), especially in the absence of difficulty at birth, may be an indication to evaluate the infant for osteogenesis imperfecta.

Fractures of the neonatal skull are uncommon. Skull fractures usually follow prolonged, difficult delivery or forceps extraction. Most fractures are linear, but some may be visible as depressed indentations resembling a table tennis ball.

IMPLICATIONS FOR NURSING

No intervention may be prescribed other than proper body alignment, careful dressing and undressing of the infant, and handling and carrying that support the affected bone. Occasionally, for immobilization and relief of pain, the arm on the side of the fractured clavicle is stabilized by pinning the sleeve to the shirt or by using a triangular sling or a figure-8 bandage.

Skull fractures usually require no treatment, although a fracture of the 'ping-pong' type (resembling a ping-pong ball) may be decompressed by nonsurgical methods. The infant is carefully observed for neurological signs and evidence of cerebral complications.

PARALYSES

Pressure exerted on nerves during a difficult labour can cause injury and paralysis of muscles that the nerves supply. The most frequently observed nerve injuries are those involving the facial nerve and the brachial plexus.

FACIAL PARALYSIS

Pressure on the facial nerve during delivery may result in injury to cranial nerve VII. Clinical manifestations are primarily loss of movement on the affected side (such as inability to completely close the eye), drooping of the corner of the mouth, and absence of wrinkling of the forehead and nasolabial fold. Paralysis is most noticeable when the infant cries. The mouth is drawn to the unaffected side, the wrinkles are deeper on the normal side, and the eye on the involved side remains open.

No medical intervention is necessary. The paralysis usually disappears spontaneously in a few days, but may take up to six months.

BRACHIAL PALSY

Plexus injury results from forces that alter the normal position and relationship of the arm, shoulder, and neck. *Erb palsy* (Erb-Duchenne paralysis), caused by damage to the upper plexus, is usually a result of stretching or pulling away of the shoulder from the head. The less common lower plexus palsy, or *Klumpke palsy*, results from severe stretching of the upper extremity while the trunk is relatively less mobile (Thomas and Harvey, 1992).

The clinical manifestations of Erb palsy are related to the paralysis of the affected extremity and muscles. The arm hangs limp alongside the body and is internally rotated, and the wrist is pronated. The muscles of the hand are paralysed in lower plexus palsy with consequent wrist drop and relaxed fingers. In severe forms of brachial palsy, the entire arm is paralysed and hangs limp and motionless at the side.

Treatment of an affected arm is aimed at preventing contractures of the paralysed muscles and maintaining correct placement of the humeral head within the glenoid fossa of the scapula. Complete recovery from stretched nerves usually takes three to six months. Avulsion of the nerves may result in permanent damage, requiring surgical and orthopaedic intervention.

IMPLICATIONS FOR NURSING

Nursing care of the infant with facial nerve paralysis involves aiding the infant in sucking and helping the mother with feeding techniques. Sometimes the infant needs to be tube fed to prevent aspiration. Breast-feeding is not contraindicated, but the mother will need additional assistance in helping the infant to grasp and compress the areolar area.

If the lid of the eye on the affected side does not close completely, artificial tears can be instilled daily to prevent drying of the conjunctiva, sclera, and cornea. The lid is often taped shut to prevent accidental injury.

Nursing care of the newborn with brachial palsy is concerned primarily with proper positioning of the affected arm. The position may be maintained with intermittent splinting. The arm should be put through complete passive range of exercises to maintain muscle tone and function.

DERMATOLOGICAL PROBLEMS IN THE NEWBORN

Numerous dermatological problems may be encountered in the newborn period. Many are innocuous conditions that are of concern only to the parents; others require intervention to prevent complications.

ERYTHEMA TOXICUM NEONATORUM

Erythema toxicum neonatorum, also known as *newborn rash*, is a benign, self-limiting eruption that usually appears within the first two days of life. The lesions are firm, 1-3 mm, pale yellow or white papules, or pustules on an erythematous base (Thomas and Harvey, 1992). The rash appears most commonly on the face, proximal extremities, trunk, and buttocks, but it may be located anywhere on the body except the palms and soles.

The aetiology is unknown. However, a smear of the pustule shows numerous eosinophils, which may be related to mechanical or thermal stimulation (Berg and Solomon, 1987). Although no treatment is necessary, parents are usually concerned about the rash and need to be reassured of its benign and transient nature.

CANDIDIASIS

Candida infections, also known as *moniliasis*, are not uncommon in the newborn. *Candida albicans*, the organism usually responsible, may cause disease in any organ system. It is a yeastlike fungus that can be acquired from a maternal vaginal infection during delivery, by person-to-person transmission, or from contaminated hands, bottles, nipples, or other articles. It is usually a benign disorder in the neonate, often confined to the oral and nappy regions.

CANDIDAL NAPPY DERMATITIS

The warm, moist atmosphere created in the nappy area provides an optimal environment for candidal growth. The dermatitis appears in the perianal area, inguinal folds and lower abdomen. The usual source of infection is through the gastrointestinal tract when organisms are swallowed from the birth canal during delivery. It may also appear two to three days after an oral infection.

Therapy consists of applications of an anticandidal ointment, such as nystatin. Sometimes the infant is given an oral antifungal preparation to eliminate any gastrointestinal source of infection (Greenough *et al*, 1992).

ORAL CANDIDIASIS

Oral candidiasis (*thrush*) is characterized by white adherent patches on the tongue, palate and inner aspects of the cheeks. It is often difficult to distinguish from coagulated milk that may remain in these areas after feeding (Thomas and Harvey, 1992).

The condition tends to be acute in the newborn, chronic in infants and young children, and to appear when the oral flora are altered as a result of antibiotic therapy. Although the disorder is usually self-limiting, spontaneous resolution may take as long as two months. The disease is treated with good hygiene, application of a fungicide and correction of any underlying disturbance.

Topical application of 1 ml nystatin over the surfaces of the oral cavity is usually sufficient to prevent spread of the disease or prolongation of its course.

IMPLICATIONS FOR NURSING

Nursing care is directed towards preventing spread of the infection and towards correct application of the prescribed topical medication. Good hygiene is essential to prevent the spread of infection. For candidiasis in the nappy area, the caregiver is taught to keep the nappy area as clean and dry as possible, and to apply the medication to affected areas as prescribed.

Oral nystatin is applied after feedings. The medication is distributed over the surface of the oral mucosa and tongue.

Mothers are encouraged to sterilize all bottles and dummies prior to use. Breast-feeding mothers are taught to care for their breasts correctly.

BULLOUS IMPETIGO

Bullous impetigo (impetigo neonatorum) is an infectious skin condition caused by various strains of group A beta-haemolytic streptococci or coagulase-positive *Staphylococcus aureus*. It is characterized by the eruption of bullous vesicular lesions on previously untraumatized skin (Thomas and Harvey, 1992). The lesions may appear on any body surface and sometimes become widespread, but the usual distribution involves the buttocks, perineum, trunk, and face. They vary in size from a few millimetres to several centimetres, contain turbid fluid, and are easily ruptured. The bullae rupture in one to two days, leaving a superficial red, moist, denuded area with very little crusting.

IMPLICATIONS FOR NURSING

Once the diagnosis is suspected, appropriate precautionary measures are instituted to prevent spread of the infection to other infants. Persons who have come in contact with the infant are investigated to determine a possible source of the infecting organism. Other infants in the nursery should be scrutinized for early detection of any evidence of infection. Parents and other visitors are instructed regarding precautions for prevention of infection.

'BIRTHMARKS'

Discolourations of the skin are common findings in the newborn infant (Thomas and Harvey, 1992). Most, such as mongolian spots or telangiectatic nevi, involve no therapy other than reassurance to parents of the benign nature of these discolourations. Some can be a manifestation of a disease that suggests further examination of the child and other family members (e.g., the multiple flat, light brown *café au lait spots* that often characterize the autosomal-dominant hereditary disorder neurofibromatosis and are common findings in Albright syndrome).

Darker and/or more extensive lesions demand further scrutiny, and excision of the lesion is recommended when feasible or when excisional biopsy is performed.

Strawberry haemangiomas, which appear as red, rubbery nodules with a rough surface, may not be present at birth but may appear at two to four weeks of age. The parents can be reassured that the lesions (even very large ones) resolve spontaneously during childhood and usually require no treatment. If there is evidence of ulceration on the surface of the lesion

(because of poor blood supply), the child should receive systemic antibiotics to prevent infection and subsequent scar formation.

IMPLICATIONS FOR NURSING

Although most birthmarks are benign, they can cause parents considerable anxiety if they are located on highly visible areas, such as the face. A complete explanation of the type of birthmark and treatment options is given.

PROBLEMS RELATED TO PHYSIOLOGICAL FACTORS

Neonates are susceptible to several problems related to pathological variations of certain physiological peculiarities. Examples include hyperbilirubinaemia, neonatal hypocalcaemia, and neonatal hypoglycaemia.

HYPERBILIRUBINAEMIA

The term *hyperbilirubinaemia* refers to an excessive accumulation of bilirubin in the blood and is characterized by *jaundice*, or *icterus*, a yellowish discolouration of the skin and other organs. Hyperbilirubinaemia is a common finding in the newborn and in most instances is relatively benign. However, it can also indicate a pathological state. For causes of hyperbilirubinaemia in the newborn, see Box 13-3.

CLASSIFICATION

Hyperbilirubinaemia is classified according to the types of bilirubin responsible: *unconjugated* (indirect reacting) and *conjugated* (direct reacting). Special tests distinguish between the direct-reacting and indirect-reacting pigments. Hyperbilirubi-

---

◆ **BOX 13-3**

Causes of hyperbilirubinaemia in the newborn

Excess production of bilirubin (e.g., haemolytic disease, biochemical defects, bruises)
Disturbed capacity of the liver to secrete conjugated bilirubin (e.g., enzyme deficiency, bile duct obstruction)
Combined overproduction and undersecretion (e.g., sepsis)
Physiological (developmental) factors (prematurity)
Association with breast-feeding or breast milk
Some disease states (e.g., hypothyroidism, galactosaemia, infant of a diabetic mother)
Genetic predisposition to increased production (e.g., Asians)

naemia that is characterized by elevation of unconjugated bilirubin is the type most commonly seen in newborns. Hyperbilirubinaemia caused by increased levels of conjugated bilirubin (rare in newborns) implies a functioning liver but signifies serious hepatic problems, such as biliary atresia (Levene *et al,* 1987).

Complications.

The signs of kernicterus are those of central nervous system depression or excitation. Generally, the clinical symptoms appear after the peak plasma bilirubin level has been established for several hours. Prodromal symptoms consist of decreased activity, lethargy, irritability, and a loss of interest in feeding. Within several hours, these subtle findings are followed by rigid extension of all four extremities, opisthotonos, irritable cry, seizures, and gastric or pulmonary haemorrhage. Those who survive may eventually show evidence of neurological damage, such as mental retardation.

PHYSIOLOGICAL JAUNDICE

Physiological or developmental jaundice *(icterus neonatorum)* results from the functional immaturity of the newborn liver combined with an increased bilirubin load from haemolysis of RBCs. It is not associated with any pathological process, as is haemolytic disease of the newborn. Although almost all newborns experience elevated bilirubin levels, only about half demonstrate observable signs of jaundice.

The severity of physiological jaundice differs among races. For example, infants of Oriental descent have mean bilirubin levels higher than white infants and black infants.

JAUNDICE IN BREAST-FEEDING INFANTS

Breast-feeding is associated with an increased incidence of jaundice. Two types have been identified: early-onset breast-feeding jaundice (or 'jaundice associated with breast-feeding') and late-onset jaundice (or 'breast-milk jaundice'). In late-onset jaundice, increasing levels of bilirubin peak during the third week, then gradually diminish. Despite high levels of bilirubin that may persist for three to 12 weeks, these infants are well. The reason for the jaundice is unknown, although it has been observed that infants with good functional nursing stimulate an earlier adequate supply of breast milk (Osborn, 1986). Early and frequent breast-feeding appears to reduce the likelihood of breast-feeding jaundice (RCM, 1991).

CLINICAL MANIFESTATIONS

Almost all newborns experience elevated bilirubin levels. However, about half demonstrate observable signs of jaundice - a yellowish discolouration observable principally in the sclera, nails, or skin. Jaundice caused by unconjugated bilirubin is bright yellow or orange; jaundice produced by conjugated bilirubin is a greenish, muddy yellow. As a rule, jaundice that appears within the first 24 hours is caused by haemolytic disease of the newborn, sepsis, or one of the maternally derived diseases, such as diabetes mellitus or infections. Jaundice that appears on the second or third day, peaks on the second to fourth days, and decreases between the fifth and seventh days is usually the result of physiological jaundice. Jaundice appearing after the third day but within the first week, suggests sepsis.

THERAPEUTIC MANAGEMENT

The aims of therapy for hyperbilirubinaemia are to prevent kernicterus and, in any blood group incompatibility, to reverse the haemolytic process. The main forms of treatment involve phototherapy.

Phototherapy

Phototherapy consists of the application of fluorescent light on the infant's exposed skin. Light promotes excretion by photo-oxidation, or photoisomerization, a process that alters the structure of bilirubin to a soluble form for easier excretion. Sunlight also acts in the same way as fluorescent light. It is well documented that phototherapy effectively reduces or prevents increasing bilirubin levels, but the long-term effects are unclear.

The effectiveness of phototherapy is determined by a decrease in bilirubin. Concurrently, the infant's total physical status is assessed because the suppression of jaundice may mask signs of sepsis, haemolytic disease, or hepatitis.

IMPLICATIONS FOR NURSING

The primary implications for nursing is recognition of jaundice and helping to distinguish between a benign disorder and a life-threatening one.

Part of the routine physical assessment includes observing for evidence of jaundice at regular intervals. Jaundice is most reliably assessed by observing the infant's skin colour from head to toe and colour of sclera and mucous membranes. For dark-skinned infants, the colour of gums is the most reliable indicator (Kelnar and Harvey, 1985; Jenkins, 1991).

When jaundice is observed, blood levels of bilirubin must be determined and monitored as necessary to establish the pattern of increase.

When blood samples are taken for bilirubin measurement, the phototherapy unit should be turned off and the blood sample tube should be covered for transport to prevent a false reading from bilirubin destruction by exposure to sunlight.

Other considerations in assessment include the ethnic origin of the family (e.g., higher incidence in Asian infants), type of delivery (e.g., induction of labour), and infant characteristics such as weight loss after birth, gestational age, gender, presence of bruising, and method and frequency of feeding. The blood types of both infant and mother are reviewed and any medications being given to the infant (e.g., cephalosporins) are noted.

Side effects of phototherapy

Presently, the long-term risks from phototherapy are not known. Although some minor side effects occur, there appears to be no increased mortality in infants treated with phototherapy (Lipsitz, Gartner and Bryla, 1985). Minor side effects for which the nurse should be alert include loose, greenish stools; hyperthermia; increased metabolic rate; increased water loss (especially from increased bowel motility); and electrolyte disturbances, such as hypocalcaemia. Although the effect of phototherapy on the eyes is uncertain, animal studies indicate that retinal degeneration may occur after several days of continuous exposure (Fig. 13-1).

Family support

Parents need constant reassurance concerning their infant's progress. All the procedures are explained to familiarize them with the benefits and risks. To facilitate bonding, eyeshields may be removed when the parents are visiting.

One of the most important nursing interventions is recognition of breast-feeding jaundice. Lack of familiarity among health professionals has caused many newborns prolonged hospitalization, termination of breast-feeding, and unnecessary phototherapy. Supportive care of the new mother can encourage successful and frequent breast-feeding. Parents also need reassurance of the benign nature of the jaundice and encouragement to resume breast-feeding if temporary cessation is prescribed.

Discharge planning and home care

Discharge planning and home care depend on the type of jaundice and the treatment instituted. In jaundice associated with breast-feeding, follow-up blood studies are usually

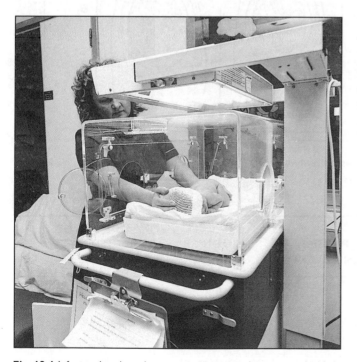

Fig. 13-1 Infant under phototherapy unit. Note that the eyes are shielded and the skin is exposed for maximum safety and therapeutic effect. (Courtesy of Southampton University Hospitals Trust)

required to assess the progress of the jaundice. Families requiring continued surveillance in the home are referred to the family care sister, midwife, health visitor, or GP.

HAEMOLYTIC DISEASE OF THE NEWBORN

Hyperbilirubinaemia in the first 24 hours of life is most often the result of haemolytic disease of the newborn (HDN) *(erythroblastosis fetalis)*, an abnormally rapid rate of red cell destruction. Anaemia caused by this destruction stimulates the production of red blood cells, which, in turn, provides increasing numbers of cells for haemolysis. Major causes of increased erythrocyte destruction are isoimmunization (primarily Rh) and ABO incompatibility (Levene *et al*, 1987).

BLOOD INCOMPATIBILITY

The membranes of human blood cells contain a variety of antigens, also known as *agglutinogens,* which are substances capable of producing an immune response if recognized by the body as a foreign substance (Bowman, 1986). It is the reciprocal relationship between antigens on red blood cells and antibodies in the plasma that causes agglutination (clumping) to take place. In other words, antibodies in the plasma of one blood group (except the AB group, which contains no antibodies) will produce agglutination when mixed with antigens of a different blood group. In the ABO blood group system, the antibodies occur naturally. In the Rh system, the person must be exposed to the Rh antigen before significant antibody formation takes place to cause a sensitivity response.

Rh incompatibility (isoimmunization)

The Rh blood group consists of several antigens, but for simplicity, only the terms *Rh-positive* (presence of antigen) and *Rh-negative* (absence of the antigen) are used in this discussion. The presence or absence of the naturally occurring Rh factor determines the blood type. Ordinarily, no problems are anticipated when the Rh blood types are the same in both mother and fetus or if the mother is Rh-positive and the infant Rh-negative. Difficulty may arise when the blood of the mother is Rh-negative and that of the infant is Rh-positive.

Although the maternal and fetal circulations are separate and distinct, sometimes fetal red blood cells (with antigens foreign to the mother) gain access to the maternal circulation through minute breaks in the placental vessels. The mother's natural defence mechanism responds to these alien cells by producing anti-Rh antibodies (isoimmunization).

Under normal circumstances, this process of isoimmunization has no effect on the fetus during the first pregnancy with an Rh-positive fetus, because the initial sensitization to Rh antigens rarely occurs before the onset of labour. However, as larger amounts of fetal blood are transferred to the maternal circulation during placental separation, maternal antibody production is stimulated. During a subsequent pregnancy with an Rh-positive fetus, these previously formed maternal antibodies to Rh-positive blood cells enter the fetal circulation, where they attack and destroy fetal erythrocytes (Fig. 13-2). Because the disease begins in utero, the fetus attempts to compensate for the progressive haemolysis by accelerating the rate of erythropoiesis. As a result, immature red blood cells (erythroblasts) appear in the fetal circulation; hence the term *erythroblastosis fetalis.*

There is wide variability in the development of maternal sensitization to Rh-positive antigens. Sensitization may occur during the first pregnancy if the woman had previously received an Rh-positive blood transfusion. In the most severe form of erythroblastosis fetalis, *hydrops fetalis,* the progressive haemolysis causes fetal hypoxia, cardiac failure and generalized oedema (anasarca).

ABO incompatibility

Haemolytic disease can also occur when the major blood group antigens of the fetus are different from those of the mother. The major blood groups are A, B, AB, and O. The incidence of these blood groups varies according to race and geographical location. The presence or absence of antibodies and antigens determines whether agglutination will occur (Table 13-1).

The most common blood group incompatibility in the neonate is between a mother with O blood group and an infant with A or B blood group (see Table 13-2 for possible ABO incompatibilities). Naturally occurring anti-A or anti-B antibodies already present in the maternal circulation cross the placenta and attack the fetal red blood cells, causing haemolysis. Usually the haemolytic reaction is less severe than in Rh incompatibility.

CLINICAL MANIFESTATIONS

Jaundice appears during the first 24 hours and serum levels of unconjugated bilirubin rise rapidly. Anaemia results from the haemolysis of large numbers of erythrocytes, and hyperbilirubinaemia and jaundice from the liver's inability to conjugate and excrete the excess bilirubin. Most newborns with HDN are not jaundiced at birth. However, hepatosplenomegaly may be evident. If the infant is severely affected, signs of anaemia (notably, marked pallor) and hypovolaemic shock are apparent.

PROCESS OF DIAGNOSIS

Maternal blood group and Rh typing is routine prenatally so that health professionals can be alert to the possibility of incompatibility at birth. The maternal blood group is compared with the

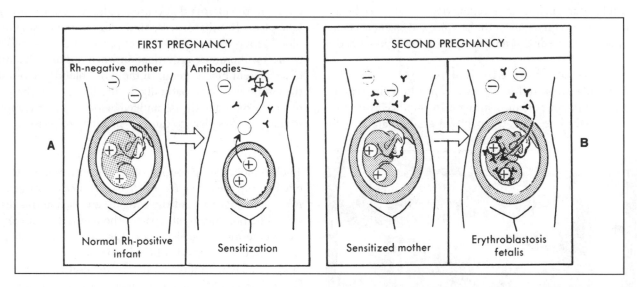

Fig. 13-2 Development of maternal sensitization to Rh antigens. A, Fetal Rh-positive erythrocytes enter maternal system. Maternal anti-Rh antibodies are formed. B, Anti-Rh antibodies cross placental barrier and attack fetal erythrocytes.

BLOOD GROUP (PHENOTYPE)	GENOTYPE	RED CELL ANTIGENS	PLASMA ANTIBODIES	RED CELL COMPATIBILITY	
				AS DONOR TO TYPE	AS RECIPIENT FROM TYPE
A	AA,AO	A	B	AB,A	O,A
B	BB,BO	B	A	AB,B	O,B
AB	AB	A and B	None	AB	O,A,B,AB
O	OO	None	A and B	AB,A,B,O	O

Table 13-1 ABO relationships of antigens/antibodies and donor-recipient compatibility.

MATERNAL BLOOD GROUP	INCOMPATIBLE FETAL BLOOD GROUP
O	A or B
B	A or AB
A	B or AB

Table 13-2 Potential maternal - fetal ABO incompatibilities

infant's blood group and Rh type immediately after birth, and a direct Coombs test is performed on cord blood to rule out the possibility of the infant developing HDN (Swanwick, 1989).

Antibody titre levels are measured periodically during pregnancy in Rh-negative mothers. Rising antibody titres (indirect Coombs test) indicate incompatibility. The disease can be confirmed postnatally by detecting antibodies attached to the circulating erythrocytes of affected infants (direct Coombs test).

THERAPEUTIC MANAGEMENT

The primary aim of therapeutic management of isoimmunization is prevention. Postnatal therapy is usually exchange transfusion. Although phototherapy may control bilirubin levels in mild cases, the haemolytic disease can continue, causing severe anaemia.

Prevention

The administration of Rh_o immunoglobulin (RhoGAM) to all unsensitized Rh-negative mothers after delivery or abortion of an Rh-positive infant or fetus prevents the development of maternal sensitization to the Rh factor. Rh_o immunoglobulin must be administered after the first delivery and repeated after subsequent ones. RhoGAM is not effective against existing Rh-positive antibodies in the maternal circulation.

Exchange transfusion

Exchange transfusion, in which the infant's blood is removed in small amounts (usually 10-20 ml at a time) and replaced with compatible blood (such as Rh-negative blood), is a standard therapy for treatment of severe hyperbilirubinaemia. It is the treatment of choice for hyperbilirubinaemia caused by Rh incompatibility. Exchange transfusion removes the sensitized erythrocytes, lowers the serum bilirubin level to prevent kernicterus, corrects the anaemia, and prevents cardiac failure.

Intrauterine transfusion

Infants of mothers already sensitized are sometimes treated by intrauterine transfusion, which consists of infusing blood into the peritoneal cavity or the umbilical vein of the fetus.

IMPLICATIONS FOR NURSING

The possibility of HDN can be anticipated from the prenatal and perinatal history. Prenatal evidence of incompatibility and the laboratory results of the Coombs test are cause for increased vigilance for early signs of jaundice in an infant.

Exchange transfusions

In addition to assisting the doctor during the initial stages of this procedure, the nurse keeps accurate records of blood volumes exchanged, including amounts of blood withdrawn and infused, time of each procedure and cumulative record of the total volume exchanged. Vital signs that are monitored electronically are evaluated frequently and correlated with removal and infusion of blood. If signs of restlessness or cardiac arrhythmias occur, rate of infusion is decreased. Throughout the procedure, the infant requires attention to thermoregulation.

After the procedure is completed, the nurse inspects the umbilical site for evidence of bleeding. A sterile dressing is applied and checked periodically for evidence of bleeding or infection.

Unless kernicterus develops, most infants recover satisfactorily after HDN. If kernicterus has occurred, the family is apprised of the need for periodic assessments to detect sensorineural hearing loss, cerebral damage or developmental delay in the child.

HYPOGLYCAEMIA

Hypoglycaemia is said to be present when the infant's blood glucose concentration is significantly lower than that of the majority of infants of the same age and weight (Levene *et al*, 1987). In the full-term newborn, hypoglycaemia is defined as plasma glucose concentrations of less than 1.7 mmol/l (30 mg/100 ml) in the first 72 hours and 2.2 mmol/l (40 mg/100 ml) thereafter; in low-birth-weight infants it is less than 1.1 mmol/l (20 mg/100 ml) (Pildes and Lilien, 1983). For causes of hypoglycaemia, see Box 13-4.

CLINICAL MANIFESTATIONS

The signs of hypoglycaemia are usually vague and often indistinguishable from those observed in other conditions, such as hypocalcaemia, septicaemia, central nervous system disorders, or cardiorespiratory problems. Because the brain depends on glucose for energy, cerebral signs such as jitteriness, tremors, twitching, weak or high-pitched cry, lethargy, limpness, apathy and convulsions are prominent. Other clinical manifestations are cyanosis, apnoea, rapid and irregular respirations, sweating, eye rolling, and refusal to feed. Frequently, the symptoms are transient but recurrent.

◆ BOX 13-4

Causes of Hypoglycaemia in the newborn

Decreased substrate availability

Some infants exhibit hypoglycaemia as a result of diminished glycogen and fat stores that are unable to provide sufficient energy to maintain glucose homeostasis until gluconeogenesis reaches adequate levels; e.g., preterm infants, infants with intrauterine growth retardation. Other infants are unable to use stored glycogen as a result of enzyme deficiencies; e.g., those with glycogen storage disease or other inborn errors of metabolism.

Endocrine disturbances

Hyperinsulinism is the most common endocrinological disturbance resulting in hypoglycaemia; it most commonly (15%-75%) occurs in the infant of the diabetic mother. Other infants with hyperinsulinism include those with Beckwith-Wiedemann syndrome, erythroblastosis fetalis, islet cell dysplasia, those who have just had exchange transfusion, and those whose mothers have had tocolytic (labour-inhibiting) agents.

Increased use

Infants with normal energy stores at birth may be stressed by perinatal events such as asphyxia or hypothermia to the extent that available supplies are unable to meet the energy requirements of the neonate.

Miscellaneous and multiple mechanisms

Hypoglycaemia caused by stimulation of glucose use by circulating endotoxins has been observed in infants with sepsis. Adrenal failure and hypoglycaemia can occur as a result of adrenal haemorrhage in association with sepsis. Increased metabolism and a resultant need for increased caloric intake result from congestive heart failure secondary to congenital heart disease, which is compounded by feeding difficulties.

THERAPEUTIC MANAGEMENT

Intravenous infusion of glucose is the treatment for hypoglycaemia. Infants who are at increased risk of developing hypoglycaemia should have their blood glucose measured within one hour after birth using blood glucose testing equipment. The procedure should be repeated every one to two hours for the first six to eight hours, then every four to six hours for two days.

Hypoglycaemia can be prevented in most instances by initiating early feeding in normoglycaemic newborns. Breast-fed infants should be put to breast as soon as possible after delivery. Feeding by tube may be necessary. If feeds are poorly tolerated, intravenous glucose may be administered to these infants if they develop hypoglycaemia.

IMPLICATIONS FOR NURSING

Major nursing objectives include preventing, anticipating, and recognizing potential dangers of concentrated dextrose infusion. Infusing the hypertonic solution too rapidly can cause circulatory overload, hyperglycaemia, and intracellular dehydration.

Because hypoglycaemia may be a symptom of some other underlying pathophysiological process, parents are usually very concerned about their infant's progress, particularly since these infants do not feed well or behave responsively.

HYPERGLYCAEMIA

Hyperglycaemia in the newborn is usually defined as a blood glucose concentration greater than 125mg/dl in the term infant or greater than 150mg/dl in the preterm infant. Affected infants are usually low-birth-weight infants who are unable to tolerate intravenous glucose infusions at the usual rate. Increased blood glucose levels may also occur in infants with sepsis or decreased insulin sensitivity.

Hyperglycaemia is usually asymptomatic, but is detected on routine screening. It is usually treated by reducing the infant's glucose intake. Insulin infusion is sometimes administered to very low-birth-weight infants who are unable to tolerate glucose solutions with concentrations greater than 5 g/dl.

IMPLICATIONS FOR NURSING

Blood glucose is monitored frequently, especially in infants receiving insulin. This requires numerous heel sticks, and sites should be rotated to minimize tissue damage. Urine output is carefully measured to detect any evidence of osmotic diuresis.

As in care of all infants, parents are given a careful explanation of the therapy and provided with frequent progress reports as well as support to reduce anxiety.

HYPOCALCAEMIA

Like many conditions in the neonate, hypocalcaemia is difficult to differentiate from other disorders and the aetiology is ill defined (Kelnar and Harvey, 1985).

THERAPEUTIC MANAGEMENT

In most instances, onset of hypocalcaemia is temporary and reverses itself in one to three days. Restoration of a normal calcium level is facilitated by early feedings, physiological correction of the hypoparathyroidism, and sometimes administration of calcium supplements.

If treatment is required, this may involve intravenous or oral administration of 10% calcium gluconate.

IMPLICATIONS FOR NURSING

The nurse observes for signs of acute hypercalcaemia (vomiting, bradycardia). If such symptoms occur, the injection or infusion of calcium gluconate is discontinued and the doctor is notified. During the acute phase, the infant should have maximal rest and minimal activity.

The restlessness, irritability, and convulsive activity of the infant are of much concern to the parents. The nurse should emphasize that the condition will subside rapidly with no subsequent ill effects. During the acute phase, parents are advised not to disturb the infant.

HAEMORRHAGIC DISEASE OF THE NEWBORN

Haemorrhagic disease of the newborn is a bleeding disorder that may appear within one to five days of life as a result of a deficiency of vitamin K. Newborn vitamin K stores are virtually absent. Breast-fed infants are particularly at risk because human milk is a poor source of vitamin K. Haemorrhagic manifestations rarely occur in infants fed fortified cow's milk formula from the first day of life, because this formula is an adequate source of the vitamin.

Signs and symptoms of haemorrhagic disease typically appear 24-72 hours after birth and can include oozing from the umbilicus or circumcision site, bloody or black stools, haematuria, ecchymoses on skin and scalp, epistaxis, or bleeding from punctures. Diagnosis can be confirmed in the presence of prolonged prothrombin time (PT) and partial thromboplastin time (PTT) accompanied by normal platelet count and fibrinogen levels.

A late form (late-onset haemorrhagic disease) appears at about four to seven weeks of age. This late-onset disease occurs in totally or predominantly breast-fed infants. It appears to be related to a factor in breast milk that inhibits vitamin K synthesis by the infant's bacterial flora. Manifestations of late-onset disease are evidence of intracranial haemorrhage, deep ecchymoses, bleeding from the gastrointestinal tract, and/or bleeding from mucous membranes and skin punctures.

THERAPEUTIC MANAGEMENT

The goal of management is prevention of haemorrhagic disease of the newborn with prophylactic administration of vitamin K.

INBORN ERRORS OF METABOLISM

Inborn error(s) of metabolism (IEM) is a term applied to inherited diseases caused by the absence or deficiency of a substance essential to cellular metabolism, usually an enzyme. Most IEMs are characterized by abnormal protein, carbohydrate, or fat metabolism (Danks and Brown, 1986).

Prenatal diagnosis enables special care of the infant immediately after birth. Neonatal screening is useful in detecting some disorders after a few days of life, but is less helpful in detecting symptoms early in the neonatal period.

Although there are innumerable IEMs only two are selected for discussion.

CONGENITAL HYPOTHYROIDISM

Congenital hypothyroidism (CH) (sometimes called by the undesirable term, *cretinism*) is a deficiency of thyroid hormones believed to be present at birth. Results of screening tests in the United Kingdom indicate that CH occurs in one of every 3,500 newborns.

A number of aetiological factors are implicated in hypothyroidism and the condition may be permanent or transient. Permanent CH can result from defective thyroid gland development, an enzymatic defect in thyroxine synthesis or (rarely) pituitary dysfunction. Transient hypothyroidism results from intrauterine transfer of goitre-inducing substances (such as the antithyroid drugs), which inhibit thyroid secretion. Although self-limiting, this type is potentially fatal because, once the maternal supply is terminated, the infant's thyroid is unable to produce its own hormones. In addition, regardless of aetiology, a large goitre in a neonate may cause total obstruction of the airway.

CLINICAL MANIFESTATIONS

The severity of the disorder depends on the amount of thyroid tissue present. Usually the newborn does not exhibit obvious signs of hypothyroidism, probably because of the exogenous source of prenatal thyroid hormone supplied by the maternal circulation. Clinical manifestations may be delayed in infants with a functional remnant of thyroid gland, infants with some types of familial hypothyroidism, and breast-fed infants, who may not display symptoms until weaned. Bone age is greatly retarded from birth. Reports of intellectual capacity are varied.

Classic features of untreated CH usually appear after about six weeks of life and include typical facial features (depressed nasal bridge, short forehead, puffy eyelids, and large tongue); thick, dry, mottled skin that feels cold to the touch; coarse, dry, lacklustre hair; abdominal distention, umbilical hernia, hyporeflexia, bradycardia, hypothermia, hypotension with narrow pulse pressure, anaemia, and widely patent cranial sutures. The infant displays difficulty feeding, decreased gastric motility, minimal crying, and excessive sleepiness. The most serious consequence is delayed development of the nervous system, which leads to severe mental retardation. The severity of the intellectual deficit is related to the degree of hypothyroidism and the duration of the condition before treatment. Other nervous system manifestations include slow, awkward movements and abnormal deep tendon reflexes.

PROCESS OF DIAGNOSIS

Diagnosis is aimed at early identification of the disorder to prevent the serious effects on mental development resulting from delayed treatment. Neonatal screening consists of initial thyrosurie (T_4) measurement followed by measurement of thyroid-stimulating hormone (TSH) in specimens with low

T_4 values (American Academy of Pediatrics and American Thyroid Association, 1987). Specimens are usually taken after six days of feeds on the Guthrie card.

Screening results that show a low level of T_4 and a high level of TSH indicate CH and the need for further tests.

THERAPEUTIC MANAGEMENT

Treatment involves thyroid hormone replacement therapy, as soon as possible after diagnosis, to abolish all signs of hypothyroidism and re-establish normal physical and mental development. To prevent the risk of overdosage of thyroid hormones, thyroxine and triiodothyronine levels are measured regularly. Bone age surveys are also performed to ensure optimum growth. If adequate thyroid hormone replacement is begun shortly after birth, the chance for normal growth and intelligence appears to be excellent (Glorieux *et al*, 1985).

IMPLICATIONS FOR NURSING

Nurses caring for neonates must be certain that screening is performed.

If CH is diagnosed, parents need an explanation of the disorder and the necessity of life-long treatment. The importance of compliance with the drug regimen must be stressed. Parents also need to be aware of signs indicating overdose, such as rapid pulse, dyspnoea, irritability, insomnia, fever, sweating, and weight loss. Signs of inadequate treatment are fatigue, sleepiness, decreased appetite, and constipation.

Genetic counselling is important, especially if the disorder is caused by an inborn error of thyroid hormone synthesis, which is autosomal recessive.

PHENYLKETONURIA

Phenylketonuria (PKU) is a disease of protein metabolism, inherited as an autosomal recessive trait, characterized by the inability to metabolize the essential amino acid phenylalanine. The disorder is detected in 1:10,000-15,000 live births.

In recent years it has become apparent that severe, classic PKU is at one end of a spectrum of conditions now known as *hyperphenylalaninaemia*. Rarer forms, or *variants*, are the result of a deficiency of other enzymes, such as *dihydropteridine reductase* (DHPR) or *dihydrobiopterin synthetase* (DHBS) and are diagnosed and treated differently from classic PKU.

CLINICAL MANIFESTATIONS

Clinical manifestations of PKU include failure to thrive, frequent vomiting, irritability, hyperactivity, and unpredictable, erratic behaviour. Bizarre or schizoid behaviour patterns are common in older children, such as fright reactions, screaming episodes, head banging, arm biting, disorientation, failure to respond to strong stimuli, and catatonia-like positions.

PROCESS OF DIAGNOSIS

The objective in diagnosing or treating the disorder is to prevent mental retardation. The most commonly used test for screening newborns is the *Guthrie blood test,* which is mandatory for all newborns. If properly done, it detects serum phenylalanine levels greater than 4 mg/dl (normal value is 2 mg/dl). Only fresh heel blood, not cord blood, can be used for the test.

The screening test is most reliable if the blood sample is taken after the infant has ingested a source of protein.

THERAPEUTIC MANAGEMENT

Treatment of PKU is dietary. Since the genetic enzyme is intracellular, systemic administration of phenylalanine hydroxylase is of no value. Phenylalanine cannot be eliminated because it is an essential amino acid in tissue growth. Therefore, dietary management must do the following:

1. Meet the child's nutritional need for optimum growth.
2. Maintain phenylalanine levels within a safe range.

The diet is calculated to maintain serum phenylalanine levels between 2 and 8 mg/dl. Significant brain damage usually occurs when levels are greater than 10 to 15 mg/dl. At levels less than 2 mg/dl the body begins to catabolize its protein stores, resulting in growth retardation.

Since all natural food proteins contain about 15% phenylalanine, specially prepared milk substitutes, such as Lofenalac or PKU-1, are prescribed for the infant. Total or partial breast-feeding, because of the low phenylalanine content of breast milk, may be possible with close monitoring of phenylalanine levels (Lawrence, 1990).

The low-phenylalanine diet is implemented as soon as possible after birth. It is not yet known for how long the diet therapy must be continued. Presently, many centres discontinue the diet when the child is six to eight years old. However, there is evidence that increased phenylalanine levels beyond this age have neuropsychological sequelae, such as lowered intelligence quotient, attentional and academic difficulties (especially in arithmetic) and visual-spatial problems (Brunner, Jordan, and Berry, 1983; Seashore *et al*, 1985). There is also the difficulty of compliance in resuming the diet, such as during pregnancy (Michals *et al*, 1985).

Since there is a strong correlation between maternal blood phenylalanine levels and improved fetal outcome, the low-phenylalanine diet should be resumed *prior* to pregnancy (Drogari *et al*, 1987; Rohr *et al*, 1987).

IMPLICATIONS FOR NURSING

The principal nursing consideration is teaching the family the dietary restrictions. The task of maintaining such a strict dietary regimen is very demanding. Foods with low phenylalanine levels, such as vegetables, fruits, juices, and some cereals, breads, and starches, must be measured to provide the prescribed amount of phenylalanine. Most high-protein foods, such as meat and dairy products, are either eliminated or restricted to small amounts.

During infancy, maintaining the diet presents few problems. Solid foods, such as cereal, fruits, and vegetables, are introduced as usual to the infant. Difficulties arise as the child gets older. The child's increasing independence may inhibit absolute control of what he or she eats. Either factor can result in decreased or increased phenylalanine levels. During the school years, peer pressure becomes a major force in deterring the child from eating the prescribed foods or abstaining from high-protein foods, such as milkshakes or ice cream. Illness and growth spurts also increase the body's need for this essential amino acid.

Family support

In addition to the problems related to a child with a chronic disorder, the parents have the burden of knowing that they are carriers of the defect and must make serious decisions regarding future children. Prenatal testing is now available to detect the presence of the defective gene in heterozygotes. Genetic counselling is especially important for an affected child, who theoretically has a 50% chance of bearing an affected offspring.

GENERAL MANAGEMENT OF HIGH-RISK NEWBORNS

High-risk neonates can be defined as newborns, regardless of gestational age or birth weight, who have a greater than average chance of morbidity or mortality because of conditions or circumstances that are superimposed on the normal course of events associated with birth and the adjustment to extrauterine existence.

In recent years, there has been an increase in the survival rate of newborns that has coincided with the establishment of programmes to improve the health of mothers, the timing of their pregnancies, and the introduction of new techniques in neonatal care. Birth weight is the most important predictor of infant survival. Survival increases exponentially as birth weight increases to its optimum level (Mutch, 1986). When problems are anticipated, preparations can be made for intensive care during the periods of greatest threat; through this care the incidence of fetal and neonatal mortality can be significantly reduced.

IDENTIFICATION OF HIGH-RISK NEWBORNS

In the prenatal period, the most important aspect in anticipating or averting problems is early and consistent prenatal care. Midwives and health visitors are in a position to detect families in need and to arrange opportunities for ongoing antenatal observation. During labour and delivery, the midwife should be alert to signs of fetal distress and maternal condi-

tions that contribute to neonatal morbidity, in order to avert numerous problems. Assessment and prompt intervention in life-threatening emergencies often make the difference between a favourable outcome and a lifetime of disability. The neonatal nurse is familiar with the characteristics of neonates and recognizes the significance of serious deviations from expected observations.

CLASSIFICATION OF HIGH-RISK NEWBORNS

High-risk infants are most often classified according to size, gestational age, and predominant pathophysiological problems. The more common problems related to physiological status are closely associated with the state of maturity of the infant and usually involve chemical disturbances (e.g., hypoglycaemia, hypocalcaemia) and consequences of immature functioning organs and systems (e.g., hyperbilirubinaemia, respiratory distress, hypothermia). Since high-risk factors are common to several specialty areas, particularly obstetrics, paediatrics, and neonatology, specific terminology is needed to describe the developmental status of the newborn (Box 13-5).

NURSING CARE OF HIGH-RISK NEWBORNS

Neonatal intensive care nursing is a highly specialized area of knowledge and practice that requires lengthy supervised experience to reach a level of competence that permits independent nursing care (Townshend, 1987).

Nurses working in NICUs are subject to stresses not found in most nursing units. The critical nature of their patients' conditions generates a stressful atmosphere (Thornton, 1984).

Since the majority of infants admitted to intensive care facilities are born before the estimated date of delivery, the major discussion of problems related to the high-risk neonate will be directed towards the preterm infant. Low birth weight (LBW) is generally accepted as the single largest factor contributing to infant mortality. The incidence of neonatal complications (e.g., hyperbilirubinaemia and hyaline membrane disease) is highest in this group.

ASSESSMENT

At birth, the newborn is given an assessment to determine any apparent problems and identify those that demand immediate attention. This examination is primarily concerned with the evaluation of cardiopulmonary and neurological functions. The assessment includes the assignment of an Apgar score and an evaluation for pallor, cyanosis, prematurity, any obvious congenital anomalies, or evidence of disease.

SYSTEMATIC ASSESSMENT

The assessment of the infant should proceed in a systematic manner. An observational assessment is usually performed hourly. However, any assessment procedures that require that the infant be disturbed should be timed to allow for sufficient rest between assessments.

To conserve the infant's energy, the position changing and periodical treatments should be timed to coincide with an assessment. Much of the assessment can be accomplished without moving the child, but necessary handling is minimum and as atraumatic as possible. During all activities, a prime consideration is the conservation of body heat.

MONITORING PHYSIOLOGICAL DATA

Most neonates under intensive observation are placed in a controlled thermal environment and monitored for heart rate, respiratory activity, and temperature (see Fig. 13-3). Respiratory activity is monitored, because the heart rate does not always drop with apnoea, although bradycardia frequently follows an apnoeic spell.

Blood pressure is monitored routinely in the sick neonate by either internal or external means. Direct recording with arterial catheters is often employed.

Weighing the nappy is the simplest and least traumatic means of measuring urine output. Plastic collecting devices can be used when it is necessary to collect urine for laboratory examination. Specific gravity is often measured as a screening for renal function and adequacy of hydration.

Blood examinations are a necessary part of the ongoing assessment and monitoring of the sick neonate's progress. The tests performed most often are blood glucose, bilirubin, calcium, haematocrit, blood gases, and electrolytes. Samples may be obtained by taking blood from the heel, by venepuncture, or by an indwelling catheter in an umbilical vein, umbilical artery or peripheral artery. The indwelling catheter is usually maintained at a slow rate with heparin infusion in order to prevent clotting of blood in the system.

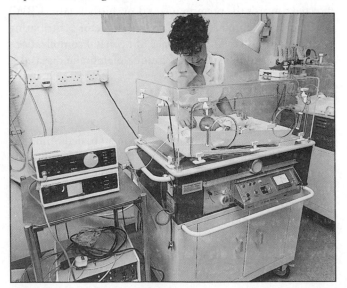

Fig. 13-3 Infant in incubator. (Courtesy of Southhampton University Hospitals Trust)

◆ **BOX 13-5**

Classification of high-risk infants

CLASSIFICATION ACCORDING TO SIZE

Low-birth-weight (LBW) infant — an infant whose birth weight is less than 2500 g regardless of gestational age

Very-low-birth-weight (VLBW) infant — an infant whose weight is less than 1500 g

Appropriate-for-gestational-age (AGA) infant — an infant whose weight falls between the 10th and 90th percentiles on intrauterine growth curves

Small-for-date (SFD) or small-for-gestational-age (SGA) infant — an infant whose rate of intrauterine growth was slowed and whose birth weight falls below the 10th percentile on intrauterine growth curves

Intrauterine growth retardation (IUGR) — found in infants whose intrauterine growth is retarded (sometimes used as a more descriptive term for the SGA infant)

Large-for-gestational-age (LGA) infant — an infant whose birth weight falls above the 90th percentile on intrauterine growth curves

CLASSIFICATION ACCORDING TO GESTATIONAL AGE

Premature (preterm) infant — an infant born before completion of 37 weeks of gestation, regardless of birth weight

Term infant — an infant born between the beginning of the 38 weeks and the completion of the 42 weeks of gestation, regardless of birth weight

Postmature (post-term) infant — an infant born after 42 weeks of gestational age, regardless of birth weight

CLASSIFICATION ACCORDING TO MORTALITY

Live birth — birth in which the neonate manifests any heartbeat, breathes, or displays voluntary movement, regardless of gestational age

Fetal death — death of the fetus after 20 weeks of gestation and before delivery, with absence of any signs of life after birth

Neonatal death — death that occurs in the first 28 days of life; early neonatal death occurs in the first week of life; late neonatal death occurs at 7-27 days

Perinatal mortality — describes the total number of fetal and early neonatal deaths per 1,000 live births

Postnatal death — death that occurs at 28 days to 1 year

Capillary samples are usually collected from the heel after the foot has been warmed to approximately 45.5°C, which takes 5-10 minutes. This is a stressful procedure for the infant.

Invasive and noninvasive methods are available for monitoring acid-base and oxygenation status. Arterial blood gas samples may be obtained from indwelling lines or from intermittent arterial punctures. Noninvasive techniques include transcutaneous monitors and pulse oximeters. Transcutaneous monitors provide continuous readings of oxygen (PaO_2) and carbon dioxide ($PaCO_2$) levels from sensors secured to the skin by electrodes. Pulse oximeters provide continuous oxygen saturation (SaO_2) measurements from a sensor taped to an extremity (hand, foot, big toe). The nurse must note any changes in oxygenation associated with handling the infant and adjust care accordingly. Hourly readings are recorded with vital signs.

RESPIRATORY SUPPORT

The primary objective in the care of high-risk infants is to establish and maintain respiration. Many infants require supplemental oxygen and assisted ventilation.

THERMOREGULATION

After the establishment of respiration, the most crucial need of the LBW infant is application of external warmth. Prevention of heat loss in the distressed infant is absolutely essential for survival, and maintaining a neutral thermal environment is a challenging aspect of neonatal intensive nursing care. Heat production is a complicated process that involves the cardiovascular, neurological, and metabolic systems, and the immature neonate has all the problems related to heat production that are faced by the full-term infant (Stewart, 1990). However, LBW infants are placed at further disadvantage by a number of additional problems. They have a smaller muscle mass and deposits of brown fat for producing heat, they lack insulating subcutaneous fat, and they have poor reflex control of skin capillaries.

Maintaining thermoneutrality
To prevent the effects of cold stress, newborns at risk are placed in a heated environment. This balances heat production, and promotes heat conservation and dissipation. Since overheating produces an increase in oxygen and calorie consumption, the infant is also jeopardized in a hyperthermic environment. A *neutral thermal environment* is one that permits the infant to maintain a normal core temperature with minimum oxygen consumption and calorie expenditure. This means a deep body temperature that stays within a normal range of 36.5-37.5°C.

The VLBW infant, with thin skin and almost no subcutaneous fat, can control body heat loss or gain only within a very limited range of environmental temperature.

The three methods for maintaining a neutral thermal environment are: (1) use of a radiant warming panel, (2) an incubator and (3) an open bassinet with cotton blankets. The dressed infant under blankets can maintain a temperature within a wider range of environmental temperatures; however, the close observations required by a high-risk infant are best accomplished if the infant remains unclothed. The incubator should always be prewarmed before placing an infant in it (Greer, 1988).

The most effective means for maintaining the desired range of temperature in the naked infant is by way of a manually adjusted or automatically controlled (servocontrolled) heat panel incubator. The latter mechanism, when set at the upper and lower limits of the desired circulating air temperature range, adjusts automatically in response to signals from a thermal sensor attached to the abdominal skin. If the infant's temperature drops, the warming device is triggered to increase heat output. The servocontrol is set to a desired skin temperature between 36 and 36.5°C.

Oxygen, or any source of air, such as an oxygen mask or tube, should not blow directly on the infant's face. Oxygen concentrated around the head, such as that supplied to a headbox, must be warmed.

The skin, followed by the axillary temperature, provides the best indication of an infant's core temperature. Rectal temperature, in addition to the possibility of producing injury and vagal stimulation, is often misleading, since it reflects a drop in core temperature, a late response to cold stress. Heat production is activated by a lowered skin temperature; therefore core temperature drops only after body heat cannot be maintained by increased metabolic activity. Nursing interventions to alleviate cold stress should be initiated with a drop in skin temperature (36.5°C) rather than when core temperature decreases.

Radiant heat loss is one of the greatest threats to temperature regulation in the incubator, since the temperature of circulating air within has no influence on heat loss to cooler surfaces without, such as windows, walls, or a lower nursery temperature.

A high-humidity atmosphere contributes to body temperature maintenance by reducing *evaporative* heat loss. Humidity is provided in some incubators by air circulating over a heated water reservoir, which has the additional advantage of decreasing heat loss by convection as the air flows over the infant. Since stagnant, warm water provides an excellent breeding medium for microorganisms, the reservoir is emptied every 24 hours and replaced with sterile distilled water.

Conductive heat loss can be reduced by warming all items that come in direct contact with the infant, such as scales, x-ray plates, blankets, and the hands of caregivers. Warming the items before use can reduce this source of heat loss (Topper and Stewart, 1984).

Two simple methods have been employed to reduce oxygen consumption, insensible water loss, and radiant heat demand, especially in VLBW infants under open radiant warmers. A heat shield of plastic food wrap stretched across the open cot produces a micro-environment around the infant that reduces evaporative, convective, and radiant heat loss). Use of a plastic heat shield, clothing, blankets, or incubating devices (e.g., bubble wrap) should NOT be used under radiant warmers, since these interfere with radiant heat delivery.

PROTECTION FROM INFECTION

Protection from infection is an integral part of all newborn care, but preterm and sick neonates are particularly susceptible. The protective environment of a regularly cleaned and changed incubator provides effective isolation from airborne infective agents. However, thorough, meticulous, and frequent handwashing is the foundation of a preventive programme. This includes *all* persons who come in contact with the infants and their equipment. After handling another infant or equipment, never touch an infant without washing hands first.

The sources of infection rise in direct relationship to the number of persons and pieces of equipment coming in contact with the infants. Protocol is established by each institution. Since organisms thrive best in water, plumbing and humidifying equipment are particularly hazardous. Disposable equipment used for water-related therapies, such as nebulizers and tubing, should be changed regularly.

HYDRATION

It is not uncommon for high-risk infants to receive supplemental parenteral fluids to supply additional calories, electrolytes, or water. Adequate hydration is particularly important in premature infants, because extracellular water content is higher than that of a full-term infant, and the capacity for osmotic diuresis is limited in premature infants' underdeveloped kidneys. Consequently, preterm infants are highly vulnerable to water depletion, especially when there are increased losses through the gastrointestinal tract, lungs, and skin.

Peripheral IV sites allow for maximal infant mobility, except for the restrained IV site. If these sites are exhausted by long-term therapy, then percutaneous central venous lines, Broviac catheters, or a venous cutdown (usually inserted in the saphenous or antecubital vein) may be employed.

IVs must always be delivered by continuous infusion pumps that deliver minute volumes at a preset flow rate. Since very small infants are highly vulnerable to fluid shifts, the rates are very slow, carefully regulated, and checked hourly to prevent dehydration and to detect inadvertent fluid overload that could cause congestive heart failure, pulmonary oedema, or intraventricular haemorrhage.

Observations are especially important when using hypertonic solutions and IV drugs, which can cause severe tissue damage. Restraints should be assessed frequently for tightness and to ascertain that they are accomplishing their purpose.

Infants who are tachypnoeic, receiving phototherapy, or under a radiant warmer have increased insensible water losses, which require appropriate fluid adjustments. Nurses must observe fluid status by accurate intake and output, specific gravity, dipstick measurements of urine, and evaluation of serum electrolyte levels.

NUTRITION

Optimal nutrition is critical in the management of LBW preterm infants, but there are difficulties in providing for their nutritional needs. The various mechanisms for ingestion and digestion of foods are not fully developed, and the younger the infant, the greater the problem. In addition, the nutritional requirements for this group of infants are not known with certainty. It is known that all preterm infants are at risk because of poor nutritional stores and because of several physical and developmental characteristics.

Nutritional needs

The demand for nutrients in LBW infants is much higher than in larger infants, and individual infants vary in activity level, ease of achieving basal energy expenditure, thermoneutrality, physical condition, and efficacy of nutrient absorption (Lucas, 1986). Since most of the nutritional stores are accumulated in the final months of gestation, preterm infants are also hampered by low stores of calcium, iron, phosphorus, proteins, and vitamins A and C.

The amount and method of feeding are determined by the size and condition of the infant. Nutrition can be provided by either the parenteral or the enteral routes, or by a combination of the two. Very small or ill infants are fed by the parenteral route until their condition is stabilized and their neurological and physical state permits enteral feedings. Often, enteral feedings must be supplemented by parenteral infusions to ensure an adequate intake of carbohydrates and water.

There is still some controversy regarding the type of enteral feeding that best meets the nutritional needs of LBW infants. In one study, infants fed with their own mother's milk displayed a more rapid rate of growth in all parameters and a shorter length of time to regain birth weight (Gross, Oehler, and Eckerman, 1983). Human milk supplements are available for infants on breast milk who require additional calories and nutrients. The anti-infectious attributes of human milk provide additional advantages for preterm infants. Secretory immunoglobulin A (IgA) concentration is higher in the milk from mothers of preterm infants than in the milk from mothers of full-term infants. Immunoglobulin A is important in the control of bacteria in the intestinal tract, where it inhibits adherence and proliferation of bacteria at epithelial surfaces (Gross *et al*, 1981). Finally, the psychological advantages of using the milk from an infant's own mother cannot be overlooked.

Although the timing of the first feeding has been a matter of controversy, most authorities now believe that early feeding, usually within 3-6 hours after birth, reduces the incidence of complicating factors such as hypoglycaemia, dehydration, and the degree of hyperbilirubinaemia. The feeding regimen employed varies in different units. However, the initial enteral feeding is not attempted until infants have adapted to extrauterine existence as evidenced by temperature neutrality, normal breathing, and good colour, tone and cry (Sani, 1988).

Bottle feeding

Vigorous infants can be fed from a bottle with little difficulty, whereas weaker infants require alternative methods. The amount to be fed is determined largely by the infant's weight and is gradually and cautiously increased.

The rate of increase that is well tolerated varies from one infant to another, and determining this rate is often a nursing responsibility. Preterm infants require more time and patience to feed compared with full-term infants (Shaker, 1990). It is important not to tire the infants or overtax their capacity to retain the feedings. When infants require more than 30 minutes to complete a feed, the next one should be given by tube. When infants are unable to tolerate bottle-feeds, intermittent feeds by tube are instituted until they gain enough strength and coordination to use the bottle.

The teat used should be relatively firm and stable. A high-flow pliable teat, although it requires less energy to use, provides a flow rate too rapid for most preterm infants to manage without risk of aspiration.

Stroking the infant's lips, cheeks, and tongue before feeding helps promote oral sensitivity (Kimble, 1992). Inward and upward support to the infant's cheeks and a slightly upward lift to the chin are provided by the fingers to assist teat compression during feeding (Shaker, 1990).

Bottle feedings are continued if infants are able to tolerate the feeds and take the required amount. The infant is best fed when fully alert. Drowsy infants feed more slowly, and liquid is more likely to fill the relaxed pharynx before the infant swallows, causing choking (Shaker, 1990).

The complications of aspiration make it important that infants are not overfed. If infants take very little and appear to be tired, their feeds may have to be repeated in a short while and then at more frequent intervals. Preterm infants are often slow feeders and require periods of rest and frequent 'winding'.

Breast-feeding

Studies indicate that even small preterm infants are able to breast-feed if the infant has adequate sucking and swallowing reflexes and if there are no other contraindications, such as facial defects, respiratory complications or concurrent illness (Jones, 1994). Mothers who wish to breast-feed their preterm infants are encouraged to express their breasts until their infants are sufficiently stable to tolerate breast-feeding.

Time, patience, and dedication on the part of the mother and the nursing staff are needed to help infants with breast-feeding. The process is begun slowly — beginning with once daily feeds and gradually increasing the feeds as the infant tolerates them. Infants should not be placed on an empty breast to feed, since the infant will become exhausted. The infant will become frustrated and refuse to feed without the reward of milk. Supplementary bottle feeding is inefficient, since the baby expends energy and calories to feed twice. Feeding more often, supplementing by tube feeding is more energy and calorie efficient (Gardner, O'Donnell, and Weisman, 1989).

Tube feeding

Tube feeding is one of the safest means of meeting the nutritional requirements of infants who are less than 32 weeks of gestation or infants who weigh less than 1,650 g. These infants are usually too weak to suck effectively, are unable to coordinate swallowing, and lack a gag reflex. Tube feeds may be provided continuously via an infusion pump or by intermittent bolus feeds. For infants learning to bottle feed and who become excessively tired, are listless, or become cyanotic, intermittent tube feeding is used as an energy-conserving technique.

The stomach is aspirated, the contents measured, and the aspirant returned as part of the feeding. The amount of the aspirant depends on the length of time since the previous feeding or concurrent illness. Whether or not the amount of the aspirant is deducted from the total feeding varies among units.

The formula is allowed to flow by gravity, and the length of time should approximate the time required for a bottle feed. This procedure is not used as a time-saving method for the nurse. Complications of indwelling tubes include obstructed nares, mucous plugs, purulent rhinitis, epistaxis, and possible stomach perforations that sometimes occur with indwelling catheters.

The nurse needs to observe premature infants closely for behaviours that indicate readiness for bottle feeds. These include: (1) a strong, vigorous suck; (2) coordination of sucking and swallowing; (3) a gag reflex; (4) sucking on the nasogastric tube, hands, or dummy; and (5) rooting and wakefulness before and sleeping after feeds. When these behaviours are noted, infants can be challenged with bottle feeds.

Oxygen is supplied via either nasal cannula or through the oxygen source held in the vicinity of the nose (Fig. 13-4). Also, sucking on a dummy helps infants associate the sucking with

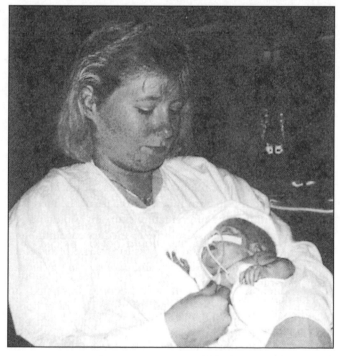

Fig. 13-4 Infant held during tube feeding. Note oxygen source held in the vicinity of the face.

the feeling of satiety. When compared with other LBW infants, those who are allowed to suck are ready for bottle feeding earlier, require fewer tube feeds, demonstrate better weight gain, are discharged earlier, and have fewer complications (Bernbaum *et al*, 1983; Field *et al*, 1982; Paludetto *et al*, 1984).

FEEDING RESISTANCE

Any feeding technique that bypasses the mouth precludes the opportunity for the affected child to 'practice sucking and swallowing, or the opportunity to experience normal hunger and satiation cycles' (Orr and Allen, 1986). Infants may demonstrate aversion to oral feedings by such behaviours as averting the head to the presentation of the teat, extruding the teat by tongue thrust, gagging, or even vomiting (Geertsma *et al*, 1985).

The longer the period of nonoral feeding, the more severe are the feeding problems, especially if this period occurs during the time when the infant progresses from reflexive to learned and voluntary feeding actions (Orr and Allen, 1986). Infancy is the period during which the mouth is the primary instrument for reception of stimulation and pleasure.

ENERGY CONSERVATION

One of the major goals of care for the high-risk infant is conservation of energy. For example, disturbing the infant as little as possible, maintaining a neutral thermal environment and providing tube feeding. When the infant is not required to expend energy to cope with efforts to breathe, eat and alter body temperature, this energy can be used for growth and development. Diminishing environmental noise levels and shading the infant from bright lights also promote rest.

The prone position is optimum for most preterm infants and results in improved oxygenation, better-tolerated feedings, and more organized sleep-rest patterns (Masterson, Zucker, and Schulze, 1987). Infants exhibit less physical activity and energy expenditure when they are placed in the prone position (Fox and Molesky, 1990; Masterson, Zucker, and Schulze, 1987).

SKIN CARE

The skin of premature infants is characteristically immature relative to that of full-term infants. Because of the increased sensitivity and fragility of premature skin, any topical preparation (including creams, lotions, or medicated ointments) should be carefully assessed for possible toxic effects before application. The increased permeability of the skin facilitates absorption of ingredients.

The skin is easily excoriated and denuded; therefore, care must be taken to avoid damage to the delicate structure. The total thickness of the skin is less than that of full-term infants, has fewer elastic fibres, and has less cohesion between the thinner skin layers. Adhesives used after heel pricks, or to secure monitoring equipment or intravenous infusions, may excoriate the skin or adhere to the skin surface so well that the skin can be separated from understructures and pulled away with the tape (Sparshott, 1991). Transpore tape is a safe tape to apply directly to the skin of small infants. It is best to use as little tape as possible (Lund *et al*, 1986).

FAMILY INVOLVEMENT

Often, professional health workers are so absorbed in the life-saving physical aspects of care that the emotional needs of infants and their families are ignored. The significance of early parent-child interaction and infant stimulation has been documented by reliable research, and nurses, aware of these infant and family needs, must incorporate activities that facilitate family interaction into the nursing care plan (Archdeacon, 1989; Stewart, 1991; McHaffie, 1987; Whitby, 1988).

The birth of a preterm infant is an unexpected and stressful event for which families are emotionally unprepared. They find themselves simultaneously coping with their own needs, the needs of their infant, and the needs of their families (especially when there are other children). To compound the situation, the precarious nature of their infant's condition engenders an atmosphere of apprehension and uncertainty. They are faced with multiple crises and overwhelming feelings of responsibility, expense, and frustration.

All parents have some anxieties about the outcome of a pregnancy, but following a premature birth, the concern is heightened about both the viability and the intactness of their infant. Parents see their infant only briefly before the newborn is removed to the intensive care unit or even to another hospital, leaving them with just the recollection of the infant's very small size and unusual appearance. They usually feel alone or lost in the maternity ward, belonging neither with parents who have lost their infants nor with those who delivered healthy, full-term infants. The staff and doctors are often guarded in discussing the infant's condition; parents are continually expecting to hear that their infant has died, and they are sensitive to the anxieties of other parents and staff members. Leaving their infant and going home empty-handed only compounds their feelings of disappointment, failure, and deprivation.

When an infant is to be transported from the hospital, the parents need a description of the unit where the infant is going. They need to know the location of the facility and the care that the infant is expected to receive. The name of the infant's doctor and the telephone number of the nursery should be given to them, and unfamiliar terms explained to them, such as *neonatologist, ventilator, infusion,* and *incubator.* Explanations should be simple, and parents should be given the opportunity to ask questions. If booklets are available that describe the facility, they should be given to the family.

Perhaps most importantly, the parents, especially the mother, should have some contact with the infant before the transport. To be able to see, touch, and (if possible) hold their infant facilitates the attachment process. Often a photograph, or even a videotape, of their infant can serve as a bond until the parents are able to travel to the regional facility. When possible, it is often advisable to transfer the mother to the same institution as her infant.

Parents need to be informed of their infant's progress and reassured that the infant is receiving proper care. They need to understand the smallest aspects of the infant's condition and treatment. Parents need a realistic assessment of the situation that is honest and direct. Using nonmedical terminology, moving at a pace that is comfortable for parents to assimilate the information, and avoiding lengthy technical explanations facilitate communication with family members (Klaus and Faranoff, 1989).

FACILITATING PARENT–INFANT RELATIONSHIPS

Because of their physiological instability, infants are separated from their mothers immediately and surrounded by a complex, impenetrable barrier of glass windows, mechanical equipment, and special caregivers. There is increasing evidence that the emotional separation that accompanies the physical separation of mothers and infants interferes with the normal maternal-infant attachment process. Maternal attachment is a cumulative process that begins before conception, is strengthened by significant events during pregnancy, and matures through maternal-infant contact during the neonatal period.

Before the first visit, the parents should be prepared for their infant's appearance, the equipment that is attached to the child, and some indication of the general atmosphere of the unit. The initial encounter with the intensive care unit is a stressful experience, and the frightening array of people, equipment, and activity is likely to be overwhelming. A book of photographs or pamphlets describing the NICU environment (infants in incubators or under radiant warmers, monitors, mechanical ventilators, and intravenous equipment) provides a useful and nonthreatening introduction to the NICU.

Parents should be encouraged to visit their infant as soon as possible. Even if they saw the infant at the time of transport or shortly after birth, the infant may have changed considerably, especially if there are many medical and equipment requirements associated with the infant's hospitalization. At the bedside, the nurse should explain the function of each piece of equipment and the role it plays in facilitating recovery.

Parents appreciate the support of a nurse during the initial visit with their infant, but they may also appreciate some time alone with the infant for a short while. It is important during the early visits to emphasize positive aspects of their infant's behaviour and development so that parents can focus on their infant as an individual rather than on the equipment that surrounds the child.

Parents vary greatly in the degree to which they are able to interact with their infant. Some may wish to touch or hold their infant during the first visit, whereas others may not feel comfortable enough even to enter the nursery. It is essential to recognize that the individualized pacing and quality of the interactions are more important than early onset of these inter-

actions. Parents may not be receptive to early and extended infant contact, since they need time to adjust to the impact of an infant with birth problems, and must be helped to grieve before acceptance of their infant can take place.

Most parents feel shaky and insecure about initiating interaction with their infant. Nurses can sense parents' level of readiness and can offer encouragement in these initial efforts. Parents of premature infants follow the same acquaintance process as do parents of term infants. They may quickly proceed through the process or may require several days or even weeks to complete the process. Parents begin by touching their infant's extremities with their fingertips and poking the infant tenderly, then proceed to caresses and fondling. Touching is the first act of communication between parents and their child.

Eventually, parents begin to endow their infant with an identity — a part of the family. When an infant no longer appears as a foreign object and begins to take on aspects of family members, such as the father's chin or the sister's nose, nurses can facilitate this incorporation. Parents are encouraged to bring in clothes and toys for their infant, and the nurse can help parents set goals for themselves and for the infant. Feeding schedules are discussed, and parents should be encouraged to visit at times when they can become involved in the care of their infant (Fig. 13-5).

Nurses must encourage and reinforce parents during their caregiving activities and interactions with their infant in order to promote healthy parent-child relationships.

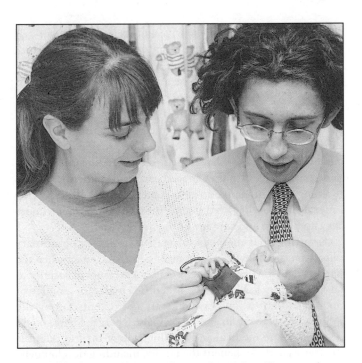

Fig. 13-5 Mother and father visit their newborn infant. (Courtesy of Southampton University Hospitals Trust)

Siblings

In the past, concerns about sibling visitation in the NICU focused on fear of infection and disruption of nursing routines. These fears have not been substantiated (Kowba and Schwirian, 1985; Doll-Speck *et al*, 1993), and sibling visits are now part of the normal operation of most NICUs.

Birth of a preterm infant is a difficult time for siblings, who rely on the support of understanding parents. When the happy anticipation is changed to sadness, worry, and altered routines, siblings are bewildered and deprived of their parents' attention. They know something is wrong, but they have only a dim understanding of what it is. Concern about negative effects of seeing the ill newborn on visiting siblings has not been confirmed. Children have not hesitated to approach or touch the infant, and children less than five years of age have been less reluctant than older children (Schwab *et al*, 1983); in addition, there have been no measurable differences between previsit and postvisit behaviours (Trause *et al*, 1981).

Support groups

Parents need to feel that they are not alone. Parent support groups have been valuable to families of infants in the NICU. Some groups consist of parents who have infants in hospital who share the same anxieties and concerns. Other groups include parents who have had infants in the NICU and who have dealt with the crisis effectively. The groups are usually under the leadership of a staff person and involve doctors, nurses, and social workers; but it is the parents who can offer other parents something that no one else can provide.

DISCHARGE PLANNING AND HOME CARE

Parents become very apprehensive and excited as time for discharge approaches. They have many concerns and insecurities regarding the care of their infant. They fear the child may still be in danger, that they will be unable to recognize signs of distress or illness in their infant, and that the infant may not yet be ready for discharge. Nurses need to begin early to assist parents in acquiring or increasing their skills in the care of their infant. Appropriate instruction must be provided and sufficient time allowed for the family to assimilate the information and learn the continuing special care requirements. Where rooming-in or other live-in arrangements are available, parents can stay for a few days and assume the care of their infant under the supervision and support of the nursery staff.

Knowing that members of staff (especially the primary nurse) are available for telephone or personal contact when the parents take the infant home provides a measure of security to anxious parents. Most NICU facilities maintain a policy of open communication between staff and parents during the infant's hospitalization and following discharge. There should be appropriate medical and nursing follow-up and referrals to services that can benefit the family, including developmental follow-up.

DEVELOPMENTAL OUTCOME

Some physiological systems in preterm infants mature earlier than they would have if the infant had remained within the uterus; for example, the function of some enzyme and immunological systems and organs, such as the kidneys and gastrointestinal system efficiency. Others slow down, such as growth in height and weight. Others keep pace with the development of fetuses still in utero; for example, reflex behaviours.

Longitudinal studies of infants born prematurely indicate there are differences in many aspects of development that may be a consequence of the immaturity at birth and related perinatal problems. Preterm infants remain in a lower percentile range for height, weight, and head circumference, although they follow the same general growth pattern as infants born at term (Ross, Lipper, and Auld, 1985; Westwood *et al*, 1983). There is a rapid increase in growth during the first six months, and growth remains somewhat accelerated until the normal growth curve is reached by age two to three years.

Neurological impairment (such as intraventricular haemorrhage) and serious sequelae correlate with the size and gestational age of infants at birth and with the severity of neonatal complications (Hack *et al*, 1984). The greater the degree of immaturity, the greater the degree of disability. A greater incidence of cerebral palsy, attention deficit disorder, visual-motor deficits, and altered intellectual functioning is observed in preterm than in full-term infants. However, behavioural development can be enhanced when families are provided with support and infants are referred to appropriate services for neurological and developmental interventions (Slater *et al*, 1988). Parental interest and involvement are very important variables in developmental progress of infants.

All infants at risk seem to benefit from special care, since undesirable sequelae appear to be decreased in infants who receive intensive medical and nursing care as opposed to those whose care is delayed or less than intensive. Although the risk of perinatal complications is highest in VLBW infants and the mortality is higher, a positive outcome is believed to be possible even for these survivors of extremely low birth weight (Bennett, Robinson, and Sells, 1983).

A concern of personnel in NICUs is the incidence of sensory impairment in surviving premature infants, such as retinopathy of prematurity (a complication of oxygen therapy). More difficult to anticipate and detect is a hearing deficit. Because LBW infants show significant visual-motor deficits compared with full-term infants at a later time, many NICUs routinely screen infants for hearing acuity.

NEONATAL LOSS

The precarious nature of many high-risk infants makes death a very real and ever-present possibility. Although infant mortality has been reduced sharply with improved technology, the mortality rate is still greatest in the neonatal period of life. Nurses in the NICU are the persons who must prepare the parents for an inevitable death and facilitate a family's grieving process after an expected or an unexpected death (Tom-Johnson, 1990).

The loss of an infant has special meaning for the grieving parents. It represents a loss of a part of themselves (especially for mothers), a loss of the potential for immortality that offspring represent, and the loss of the dream child that has been fantasized throughout the pregnancy. There is a sense of emptiness and failure. In addition, when an infant has lived for such a short time, there are few, if any, pleasant memories to serve as a basis for identification and idealization that are part of the resolution of a loss (Newman, 1984).

To help the parents understand that the death is a reality, it is important to encourage them to hold their infant before death and, if possible, be present at the time of death so that their infant can die in their arms if they choose. Many who deny the need to hold the infant later regret the decision (Null, 1989). Parents should be provided with an opportunity to see, touch, hold, caress, examine, and talk to their infant privately after death and to bathe their infant if they desire as a final act of caring. If parents are hesitant about seeing their dead infant, it is advisable to keep the body in the unit for a few hours, since many parents change their minds after the initial shock of the death (Symes, 1991; Thomas, 1990).

Parents may need to see and hold the infant more than once: the first time to say 'hello' and the last time to say 'goodbye'. If parents wish to see the infant after the body has been taken to the mortuary, the infant should be retrieved, wrapped in a blanket, and taken to the mother's room or other private place. The nurse should stay with the parents and provide them with an opportunity for private time alone with their dead infant (Marriott, 1988).

Some units have implemented a hospice approach for families with infants for whom the decision has been made not to prolong life and who are receiving only palliative care. A special 'family' room is set aside that contains all supportive equipment needed for the care of the infant and also provides a homelike atmosphere for the family (Landon-Malone, Kirkpatrick, and Stull, 1987). All hospice services are available to the family, and the infant remains under the care and supervision of a primary nurse on the NICU staff (Hill, 1994).

A photograph of the infant, taken before or after death, is highly desirable. The parents may not wish to see the photograph at the time of death, but the chance to refer to it later will help make their infant seem more real, which is a part of the normal grief process. A photograph of their infant being held by the hand or touched by an adult offers a more positive image than a morgue type of photograph. Other tangible remembrances of the child can be provided, such as name tags, armbands, and locks of hair shaved for intravenous insertion or other procedures. If the parents have not done so, they should be encouraged to name their infant.

At least one nurse who is familiar to the family should be present during the discussion about a dead or dying infant. The nurse should talk with parents openly and honestly about funeral arrangements, since few of them have had experience with this aspect of death. Someone from the NICU should take the responsibility for acquiring this type of information.

Families need to be informed of options available, but it is preferable to encourage a funeral because the ritual provides an opportunity for parents to feel the support of friends and relatives. Clergy of the appropriate faith may be notified if the parents wish.

Before the parents leave the hospital, they should be given the telephone number of the unit (if they do not have it) and invited to call any time they have any further questions. Several organizations are available to offer support and understanding to families who have lost a newborn, including the Stillbirth and Neonatal Death Society (SANDS). (For useful professional guidelines, see SANDS, 1991.)

HIGH-RISK CONDITIONS RELATED TO DYSMATURITY

A dysmature baby is born outside of the normal parameters of the 'term' baby (a baby delivered at between 37-42 weeks gestation). Postmature babies have defined problems; after 42 weeks gestation the placenta starts to degenerate, and the fetus may not withstand the stress of labour. Consequently, these babies are prone to birth asphyxia, birth injuries, and expiration.

Preterm infants have several distinctive characteristics. The mature systems of these infants are designed to cope with the transition to extrauterine life. This can cause a number of difficulties for the infant, such as respiratory distress, jaundice, and thermoregulation.

PRETERM INFANTS

Prematurity accounts for the largest number of admissions to an NICU. Not only does the immaturity of these infants place them at risk for neonatal complications (e.g., hyperbilirubinaemia and respiratory distress syndrome, which is highest in the preterm infant), but also other high-risk factors (e.g., congenital abnormalities in association with prematurity).

CHARACTERISTICS

Preterm infants have several characteristics that are distinctive at various stages of development. Identification of these characteristics provides valuable clues to the gestational age and hence to the physiological capabilities of infants. The general, outward physical appearance changes as the fetus progresses to maturity. Characteristics of skin, general attitude (or posture) when supine, appearance of hair, and amount of subcutaneous fat provide clues to a newborn's physical development. Observation of spontaneous, active movements and response to stimulation and passive movement contributes to the assessment of neurological status.

On inspection, premature infants are very small and appear scrawny because they lack or have only minimum subcutaneous fat deposits, with a proportionately large head in relation to the body, which reflects the cephalocaudal direction of growth. Of all the body measurements, the head is reduced least, and sucking pads in the cheeks are strikingly prominent. The skin is bright pink, smooth, and shiny (may be oedematous), with small blood vessels clearly visible underneath the thin, transparent epidermis. The fine lanugo hair is abundant over the body but is sparse, fine, and fuzzy on the head. The ear cartilage is soft and pliable, and the soles and palms have minimum creases, resulting in a smooth appearance. The bones of the skull and the ribs feel soft, and the prominent eyes may be closed. Male infants have few scrotal rugae, and the testes are undescended; the labia and clitoris are prominent in females.

Premature infants are inactive and torpid. The extremities maintain an attitude of extension and remain in any position in which they are placed. Reflex activity is only partially developed — sucking is absent, weak, or ineffectual; swallowing, gag, and cough reflexes are weak; and other neurological signs are absent or diminished. Physiologically immature, preterm infants are unable to maintain body temperature, have limited ability to excrete solutes in the urine, and have increased susceptibility to infection. A pliable thorax along with immature lung tissue and regulatory centre lead to periodic breathing, hypoventilation, and frequent periods of apnoea. Preterm infants are more susceptible to biochemical alterations, such as hyperbilirubinaemia and hypoglycaemia. They have a higher extracellular water content that renders them more vulnerable to fluid and electrolyte derangements.

The soft cranium is subject to characteristic nonintentional deformation, or 'premature head', caused by positioning from one side to the other on a mattress. The head looks disproportionately longer from front to back, is flattened on both sides, and lacks the usual convexity seen at the temporal and parietal areas (Budreau, 1987). This positional moulding is frequently a concern to parents and may influence the parents' perception of the infant's attractiveness and their responsiveness to the infant.

POSTMATURE INFANTS

Infants born of a gestation that extends beyond 42 weeks as calculated from the mother's last menstrual period are considered to be postmature or post-term, regardless of birth weight. This constitutes approximately 12% of all births. Some infants are appropriate for gestational age, but many show the characteristics of progressive placental dysfunction. Frequently the skin is cracked, parchment-like, and desquamating. A common finding in postmature infants is a wasted physical appearance that reflects intrauterine deprivation. Depletion of subcutaneous fat gives them a thin, long appearance. The little vernix caseosa that remains in the skin folds is usually stained a deep yellow or green.

There is a significant increase in fetal and neonatal mortality in post-term infants compared with those born at term. They are especially prone to intrauterine hypoxia associated with the decreasing efficiency of the placenta and to the meconium aspiration syndrome. The greatest risk occurs during the stresses of labour and delivery, particularly in infants of *primigravidas*, women delivering their first child.

HIGH RISK RELATED TO DISTURBED RESPIRATORY FUNCTION

Respiratory distress in a newborn baby may be caused by many conditions. The baby with respiratory distress will be tachypnoeic with a respiratory rate greater than 60/min. Intercostal recession may be present. Central cyanosis may also be present, but should be differentiated from peripheral cyanosis, which is normal in the first 24 hours of extrauterine life.

APNOEA OF PREMATURITY

Apnoea of prematurity (AOP) is a common phenomenon in the preterm infant. Rarely observed in full-term infants, the prevalence of apnoeic spells increases the younger the gestational age. Approximately one-third of infants less than 32 weeks of gestation and almost all apparently healthy infants less than 30 weeks of gestation have apnoeic spells. Characteristically, premature infants are periodic breathers; they have periods of rapid respiration separated by periods of very slow breathing and often short periods during which there are no visible or audible respirations. Apnoea is primarily an extension of this periodic breathing and can be defined as a lapse of spontaneous breathing for 20 or more seconds, which may or may not be followed by bradycardia and colour change (Vyas and Milner, 1986). Apnoea of prematurity should not be confused with apnoea of infancy (see Chapter 15).

CLINICAL MANIFESTATIONS

Several factors that appear to promote the incidence of apnoea in preterm neonates can be treated. Conversely, one of these disorders may be suspected in infants with persistent apnoeic spells. Although apnoea is an expected event in preterm neonates, it should not be designated as such until all other causes are ruled out.

THERAPEUTIC MANAGEMENT

It has been found that oral administration of theophylline is often effective in reducing the frequency of primary apnoea-bradycardia spells in newborns. Theophylline and caffeine act as central nervous system (CNS) stimulants to breathing. Neonates who receive these drugs have serum theophylline levels measured regularly and must be closely observed for symptoms of toxicity.

IMPLICATIONS FOR NURSING

Management of periodic apnoea consists of monitoring respiration and heart rate routinely in all small preterm infants and of prevention of conditions that might precipitate it. Without close observation, even of monitored infants, many unidentified episodes of prolonged apnoea and severe bradycardia occur (Southall *et al*, 1983). Nursing observation combined with monitoring is the most effective means of identifying neonatal apnoea (Muttitt *et al*, 1988).

If it is begun early, gentle tactile stimulation, such as rubbing the back or chest gently or turning the infant over, will stop most apnoeic spells. If stimulation fails to reinstitute respiration, the nose and oropharynx are suctioned, and if breathing does not begin, the chin is raised gently and sufficient pressure is applied with mask and bag to lift the rib cage. The infant is never shaken. It is important for nurses to document episodes of apnoea. A careful record is maintained of the number of apnoeic spells, the appearance of the infant during and after attacks, and whether the infant self-stimulates or if exogenous stimulation is needed to restore breathing. Persistent and repeated periods of apnoea are treated by mechanical ventilation with the respirator set at low pressure and rate.

IDIOPATHIC RESPIRATORY DISTRESS SYNDROME

Respiratory distress is a name applied to respiratory dysfunction in neonates and is primarily a disease related to developmental delay in lung maturation. The terms *respiratory distress syndrome* (RDS) and *hyaline membrane disease* (HMD) are most often applied to the severe lung disorder that is not only responsible for more infant deaths than any other disease but also carries the highest risk in terms of long-term respiratory and neurological complications. It is seen almost exclusively in preterm infants. The disorder is rare in infants of narcotic-addicted mothers or infants who have been subjected to intrauterine stress (e.g., maternal pre-eclampsia or hypertension).

PATHOPHYSIOLOGY

Preterm infants are born before the lungs are fully prepared to serve as efficient organs for gas exchange. This appears to be a critical factor in the development of RDS.

Before birth, there is evidence of fetal respiratory activity. The lungs make feeble respiratory movements, and fluid is excreted through the alveoli. Since the final unfolding of the alveolar septa, which increases the surface area of the lungs, takes place during the last trimester of pregnancy, premature infants are born with numerous underdeveloped and many uninflatable alveoli. Because of the increased pulmonary vascular resistance, the major portion of fetal blood is shunted from the lungs by way of the ductus arteriosus and foramen ovale (see Chapter 28).

At the time of birth, infants must initiate breathing and then keep the previously fluid-filled lungs inflated with air. At the same time the pulmonary capillary blood flow must be increased approximately tenfold to provide for adequate lung perfusion and to alter the intracardiac pressure that closes the fetal cardiac structures. Most full-term infants successfully accomplish these adjustments; preterm infants with respiratory distress are unable to do so (Morley, 1986).

Surfactant is a surface-active phospholipid secreted by the alveolar epithelium. Acting much like a detergent, this sub-stance reduces surface tension of fluids that line the alveoli and respiratory passages, resulting in uniform expansion and maintenance of lung expansion at low intra-alveolar pressure. Immature development of these functions produces consequences that seriously compromise respiratory efficiency. Deficient surfactant production causes unequal inflation of alveoli on inspiration and collapse of alveoli on end expiration. Without surfactant, infants are unable to keep their lungs inflated and therefore exert a great deal of effort to re-expand the alveoli with each breath. Infants use more oxygen to expend this energy than they take in, which rapidly leads to exhaustion. With increasing exhaustion, they are able to open fewer and fewer alveoli. This inability to maintain lung expansion produces widespread atelectasis.

In the absence of alveolar stability (normal functional residual capacity) and with progressive atelectasis, the pulmonary vascular resistance (PVR) increases, whereas with normal lung expansion it would decrease. Consequently there is hypoperfusion to the lung tissue with a decrease in effective pulmonary blood flow.

Inadequate pulmonary perfusion and ventilation produce hypoxaemia and hypercapnia. Thus a decrease in oxygen tension causes vasospasm in the pulmonary arterioles that is further enhanced by a decrease in blood pH. This vasoconstriction contributes to a marked increase in PVR. In normal ventilation with increased oxygen concentration, the ductus arteriosus constricts and the pulmonary vessels dilate to decrease PVR.

Pulmonary oedema observed in the early stages of RDS also contributes to impaired gas exchange. Factors believed to facilitate this fluid accumulation in the lungs include renal immaturity or insufficiency resulting from hypoxaemia, high fluid intake and patent ductus arteriosus, left ventricular dysfunction associated with papillary muscle necrosis, low serum protein concentration and low colloid osmotic pressure, increased alveolar surface tension that enhances the shift of interstitial fluid to alveolar spaces, oxygen toxicity, and high plasma vasopressin (summarized by Yeh *et al*, 1982).

Deficiencies in other systems contribute to respiratory distress. For example, a high threshold of the respiratory centre to afferent stimuli and weak gag and cough reflexes reflect the immaturity of the nervous system. In addition, the persistence of fetal haemoglobin, so beneficial in prenatal existence, may place the infant at a disadvantage during respiratory distress. Although the binding power of fetal haemoglobin for oxygen is much greater than in adult haemoglobin, this increased affinity also causes less oxygen to be released to the tissues at normal oxygen tension.

Affected lungs are stiffer and require far more pressure than do normal lungs to achieve an equal amount of expansion. The major factors that produce respiratory distress in immature infants are summarized in Table 13-3.

RDS is a self-limiting disease, and following a period of deterioration (approximately 48 hours) and in the absence of complications, affected infants begin to improve by 72 hours. Often heralded by the onset of diuresis, this improvement has

CAUSE	EFFECT
Increased surface tension of alveoli (surface deficiency)	Alveolar collapse; atelectasis; increased difficulty of breathing
Impaired gas exchange	Hypoxaemia and hypercapnia with respiratory acidosis
Increased pulmonary vascular resistance	Hypoperfusion of pulmonary circulation
Hypoperfusion (with hypoxaemia)	Tissue hypoxia and metabolic acidosis
Increased transudation of fluid into lungs	Hyaline membrane formation; impaired gas exchange

Table 13.3 Major factors in respiratory distress.

been attributed primarily to increased production and greater availability of surface-active material.

CLINICAL MANIFESTATIONS

Infants with RDS can develop respiratory insufficiency either acutely or over a period of hours. Usually the observable signs produced by the pulmonary changes begin to appear in infants who apparently achieve normal breathing and colour soon after birth. In 30 minutes to two hours breathing gradually becomes more rapid (greater than 60 breaths per minute). Infants may display recession — suprasternal or substernal; supracostal, subcostal, or intercostal — which result from a compliant chest wall. Weak chest wall muscles and the highly cartilaginous nature of the rib structure produce an abnormally elastic rib cage. During this early period, the infant's colour remains satisfactory and auscultation reveals good air entry.

Within a few hours, respiratory distress becomes more obvious. The respiratory rate continues to increase (to 80 to 120 breaths per minute), and breathing becomes more laboured. It is significant to note that infants will increase the *rate* rather than the *depth* of respiration when in distress. Substernal recession becomes more pronounced as the diaphragm works hard in an attempt to fill collapsed air sacs, and there is an audible expiratory grunt. This grunt, a useful mechanism observed in the earlier stages of RDS, serves to increase end-expiratory pressure in the lungs. Flaring of the nares is also a sign that accompanies tachypnoea, grunting, and recession in respiratory distress. Central cyanosis (a bluish discolouration of oral mucous membranes and generalized body cyanosis) is a late and serious sign of respiratory distress. Initially, cyanosis may be abolished by supplemental oxygen.

At this point, the respiratory distress may gradually decrease over 12 to 24 hours with eventual recovery, or it may increase in severity. In distressed infants cyanosis becomes more marked despite increases in ambient oxygen concentration. The infants become flaccid and unresponsive, and begin to display frequent apnoeic episodes. Severe RDS is often manifested by diminished cardiac inflow and low arterial blood pressure.

Infants with RDS who survive the first 96 hours have a reasonable chance of recovery. Complications of IRDS include those described as complications of oxygen therapy (see Chapter 26), patent ductus arteriosus and congestive heart failure, persistent pulmonary hypertension, intraventricular haemorrhage, bronchopulmonary hyperplasia, retinopathy of prematurity, necrotizing enterocolitis, and neurological sequelae.

PROCESS OF DIAGNOSIS

X-ray findings characteristic of RDS include: (1) a diffuse granular pattern over both lung fields closely resembling ground glass that represents alveolar atelectasis, and (2) dark streaks, or bronchograms, within the ground glass areas that represent dilated air-filled bronchioles. It is important to distinguish between RDS and pneumonia in infants with respiratory distress.

Prenatal diagnosis
Fetal lung maturity depends on gestational age, except in some specific instances that may not be known until the time of labour or delivery.

THERAPEUTIC MANAGEMENT

The treatment of RDS is largely supportive and includes all the general measures required for any premature infant, as well as those instituted to correct imbalances. The supportive measures that are most crucial to a favourable outcome are: (1) maintain a neutral thermal environment to conserve utilization of oxygen, (2) provide additional fraction of inspired oxygen (FiO_2) content by increasing ambient oxygen concentration or by assisted ventilation, (3) prevent hypotension and hypovolaemia, (4) correct respiratory acidosis by assisted ventilatory support, and (5) correct metabolic acidosis by intravenous administration of sodium bicarbonate, which also dilates pulmonary vessels and reduces the constriction response. Bottle and tube feeds are contraindicated in any situation that creates a marked increase in respiratory rate, because of the greater hazards of aspiration. Nutrition may be provided by parenteral therapy during the acute stage of the disease.

Oxygen therapy
The goals of oxygen therapy are to provide adequate oxygen to the tissues, prevent lactic acid accumulation resulting from hypoxia, and at the same time avoid the toxic effects of oxygen. All methods require that the gas be warmed and humidified before entering the respiratory tract. If the infant does not require mechanical ventilation, oxygen can be supplied to a plastic hood placed over the infant's head to supply variable concentrations of humidified oxygen (see Chapter 26). If oxygen saturation of the blood cannot be maintained at a sat-

isfactory level and the carbon dioxide level (PaCO$_2$) rises, infants will require ventilatory assistance (see Table 13-4).

Continuous positive airway pressure (CPAP) or *continuous positive pressure breathing* (CPPB), the application of 3-10 cm of water (positive) pressure to the airway, uses the infant's spontaneous respiration to improve oxygenation by helping prevent alveolar collapse and increasing diffusion time. If oxygenation is not improved, or if infants require assisted ventilation to decrease PaCO$_2$ levels, *intermittent mandatory ventilation* (IMV) or *continuous positive pressure ventilation (CPPV)* is used with *positive end–expiratory pressure (PEEP).* This allows infants to breathe at their own rate but provides positive pressure at regular preset intervals and end-expiratory pressure to prevent alveolar collapse and overcome tube resistance.

Complications of oxygen therapy

Although it can save lives, oxygen therapy is not without hazards. Positive pressure introduced by mechanical apparatus has caused an increased incidence of air leaks that produce complications, such as *pneumothorax* and *pneumomediastinum.* Other complications directly related to oxygen therapy include *retinopathy of prematurity, bronchopulmonary dysplasia,* and various problems associated with intubation.

Medical therapies

In addition to the establishment of one or more intravenous lines to maintain hydration and nutrition, infants with respiratory distress syndrome receive a variety of medications (see Table 13-5).

METHOD	DESCRIPTION	HOW PROVIDED
• Common methods		
Continuous positive airway pressure (CPAP) or continuous distending pressure (CDP)	Provides constant distending pressure to airway in spontaneously breathing infant	Nasal prongs Nasopharyngeal tubes Endotracheal tube
Positive end-expiratory pressure (PEEP)	Provides increased end-expiratory pressure that prevents alveolar collapse during controlled ventilation	Endotracheal intubation
Continuous positive-pressure ventilation (CPPV)	Maintains continuous positive pressure to airways in infant attached to ventilator	Endotracheal intubation and either volume- or pressure-controlled ventilators
Intermittent mandatory ventilation (IMV)	Allows the infant to breathe spontaneously at own rate but provides mechanical cycled respirations and pressure at regular preset intervals	Endotracheal intubation and venitilator
• Alternative methods		
High frequency ventilation (HFV):		
High-frequency positive-pressure ventilation (HFPPV)	Low-compliant circuit provides high gas flow through the circuit; operates at rates between 60 and 150 breaths/minute	Conventional infant ventilators: endotracheal tube
High-frequency oscillation (HFO)	Application of high-frequency, low-volume, sine-wave flow oscillations to the airway at rates between 480 to 1200 breaths/minute	Variable-speed piston pump (or loudspeaker, fluidic oscillator); endotracheal tube
High-frequency jet ventilation (HFJV)	Uses a separate, parallel, low-compliant circuit and injector port to deliver small pulses or jets of fresh gas deep into airway at rates between 250 and 900 breaths/minute	May be used alone or with low-rate IMV with endotracheal tube

Table 13-4 Common methods for assisted and controlled ventilation in respiratory distress syndrome.

A relatively recent addition to the medical therapies for RDS is the administration of artificial surfactant. The surfactant is given on diagnosis of RDS at 16-24 hours of age. Treatment prevents atelectasis and contributes to fluid clearance from alveoli, thereby increasing compliance and decreasing the work of breathing. Treated infants exhibit fewer respiratory complications (Collaborative European Multicenter Study Group, 1988; Lang et al, 1990).

Prevention

Since RDS is a maturational disorder primarily related to the production of pulmonary surfactant, one approach to prevention is through stimulation of surfactant production. Some experiments with administration of corticosteroids to mothers from 24 hours to seven days before delivery have demonstrated a significant reduction in the incidence of RDS in their infants (Kling, 1986).

The most successful approach to prevention of RDS is prevention of premature delivery, especially in elective early delivery and caesarean section. An aggressive approach using tocolysis (ritadine administration) to delay delivery and maternal administration of corticosteroids to induce surfactant production appears to reduce the incidence of RDS in preterm infants (Kwong and Egan, 1986; Papageorgiou *et al*, 1989).

IMPLICATIONS FOR NURSING

Care of infants with RDS involves all the observations and interventions described for high-risk infants. In addition, the nurse is concerned with the complex problems related to respiratory therapy and the constant threat of hypoxaemia and acidosis that complicates the care of patients in respiratory difficulty.

The most essential nursing function is to observe and assess the infant's response to therapy. Since oxygen concentration and ventilation parameters are prescribed according to the infant's blood gas measurements and transcutaneous oxygen ($TcPO_2$) and pulse oximeter readings and because an infant's status can change rapidly, continuous monitoring and close observation are mandatory.

Changes in oxygen concentration are based on these observations. The amount of oxygen administered, expressed as the

MEDICATION	PURPOSE	COMMENTS
Antibiotics	Treat pneumonia and/or septicaemia Pneumonia prophylaxis	Observe for adverse response Check serum blood levels for selected medications
Aminoglycosides	Therapy for sepsis	Nephrotoxic; observe urine output and electrolytes Ototoxic; test for possible hearing impairment Check serum drug levels
Pancuronium	Muscle paralysis to prevent additive pressures generated when infant is breathing spontaneously during mechanical ventilation, to prevent air leaks, to provide better oxygenation and ventilation	Close observation of infant for muscle involvement and need for repeat dose Causes relaxed arterioles and pooling of blood Ventilator alarms in 'on' position in case of accidental disconnection; infant unable to make any respiratory effort Eye taped closed; eye drops to prevent corneal irritation
Frusemide	Facilitates renal excretion of fluid; reduces pulmonary oedema Especially valuable when spontaneous diuresis does not occur	Observe for onset of diuresis Requires observation and fluid regulation to prevent dehydration Assess electrolyte status; K+ replacement may be necessary Long-term use may result in calculi and hydronephrosis
Vitamin E	Decreases oxygen-derived free radical production Given prophylactically to infants on oxygen therapy to prevent or reduce the severity of retinopathy of prematurity, intraventricular haemorrhage, and bronchopulmonary dysplasia	Oxygen-free radicals believed to cause oxidative damage to tissues Use of drug is experimental

Table 13-5 Medications used in the treatment of respiratory distress syndrome.

fraction of inspired air (FiO_2), is determined on an individual basis according to pulse oximeter and/or direct or indirect measurement of arterial oxygen concentration. Capillary samples, collected from the heel, are useful for pH and $PaCO_2$ determinations but not for oxygenation status. Pulse oximetry readings are recorded at least hourly. Blood sampling is necessary 15-30 minutes after ventilator changes for the acutely ill infant and every two to four hours for sick infants (Foss, 1988).

Thick, tenacious mucous may form in the respiratory tract as a result of the infant's pulmonary condition, including the endotracheal (ET) tube. Suctioning should be performed as often as necessary based on individual infant assessment, which includes auscultation of the chest, evidence of decreased oxygenation, excess moisture in the ET tube, or increased infant irritability. Instillation of 0.25-0.5 ml of sterile normal saline in the ET tube before insertion of the suction catheter aids in loosening mucus and removing secretions. Removal of secretions can be further facilitated by positioning and application of percussion and vibration to the thoracic wall.

The FiO_2 should be increased by 10% before suctioning to compensate for a decrease in (FiO_2) during the procedure (see Chapter 26).

Mouth care is especially important when infants are receiving nothing by mouth, and the problem is often aggravated by the drying effect of oxygen therapy. Drying and cracking can be prevented by good oral hygiene using saline swabs.

MECONIUM ASPIRATION SYNDROME

Meconium aspiration is a serious condition that accounts for a substantial number of neonatal fatalities. It occurs when fetuses have been subjected to fetal asphyxia or other intrauterine stress that causes increasing peristalsis, relaxing of the anal sphincter, and passage of meconium into the amniotic fluid. The majority of meconium aspiration takes place with the first breath. However, a severely compromised fetus may aspirate in utero. At delivery of the chest and initiation of the first breath, infants inhale fluid and meconium in the naso-oropharynx.

CLINICAL MANIFESTATIONS

Infants who have been stressed for some time are stained from passage of green meconium stools (those with more recent meconium passage are not stained), tachypnoeic, hypoxic, and depressed at birth. They develop expiratory grunting and retractions similar to those experienced by infants with RDS. The infants are often stressed, hypothermic, hypoglycaemic, and hypocalcaemic. Severe meconium aspiration progresses to respiratory failure.

PROCESS OF DIAGNOSIS

At birth, meconium can often be visualized in the respiratory passages and vocal cords. Chest x-rays show uneven distribution of patchy infiltrates, air trapping, and hyperexpansion.

THERAPEUTIC MANAGEMENT

Prevention of meconium aspiration includes vigorous suctioning of the hypopharynx before delivery of the shoulders. Resuscitation is initiated and maintained until the infant is breathing spontaneously and has good colour.

Infants with respiratory distress are admitted to the NICU. Management of chemical pneumonitis consists of ventilatory support, intravenous fluids, and chest percussion and postural drainage. Since these infants are prone to develop persistent pulmonary hypertension, they are maintained somewhat hyperoxic as a precautionary measure and may be candidates for extracorporeal membrane oxygneation therapy.

BRONCHOPULMONARY DYSPLASIA

Bronchopulmonary dysplasia (BPD), also known as *chronic* or *respirator lung disease,* is a pathological process that may develop in the lungs of infants, primarily VLBW infants, with lung disorders (e.g., RDS, meconium aspiration, and persistent pulmonary hypertension) (Vyas and Milner, 1986). BPD is an iatrogenic disease caused by therapies used to treat lung disease: exposure to high oxygen concentrations, use of positive-pressure ventilation (CPAP or PEEP), endotracheal intubation; prolonged use of these therapies; fluid overload; and patent ductus arteriosus (PDA). The reported incidence of the disorder in survivors of RDS is between 20% and 30% (Koops, Abman, and Accurso, 1984), and the incidence of infants surviving with milder forms of chronic lung disease is much higher (Bancalari and Gerhardt, 1986). The infants who survive are at risk for frequent hospitalization because of their borderline respiratory reserve, hyperactive airway, and increased susceptibility to respiratory infection.

THERAPEUTIC MANAGEMENT

The first approach to management is prevention of the disorder in susceptible infants. To reduce the risk of barotrauma when mechanical ventilation is being used, the lowest peak inspiratory pressure (PIP) necessary to obtain adequate ventilation is maintained and the lowest level of inspired oxygen is used to maintain adequate oxygenation. Fluid administration is carefully controlled and restricted. Drug or surgical intervention is indicated when there is a PDA.

There is no specific treatment for BPD, except to maintain adequate arterial blood gases with the administration of oxygen and avoid progression of the disease. Some have reported improvement in infants administered dexamethasone (Gladstone, Ehrenkranz, and Jacobs, 1989; Harkavy *et al*, 1989), although the infants exhibited significant delay in weight gain. Weaning infants from the ventilator is difficult and must be accomplished gradually.

Oral diuretics are used to control interstitial fluid. Bronchodilators may be effective and promote improvement in infants with chronic lung disease. Theophylline improves lung compliance and reduces expiratory resistance in BPD ventilated infants.

Growth and development are delayed in some infants with BPD, related in part to the difficulties in providing adequate nutrition and in part to the lack of normal sensory stimulation due to prolonged hospitalization. Children with BPD have metabolic needs far greater than those of the average child. This can create a problem for the caregiver who must meet the goals of adequate nutrition while avoiding overhydration, especially if the child is ill, eats poorly, or has cardiopulmonary instability (Goldson, 1990). The infant may be further compromised by gastroesophageal reflux, a frequent complication in premature infants (see Chapter 27).

Prognosis

Reports vary regarding the mortality rate for this disorder. The hospital stay is frequently long because of the infant's need for supplemental oxygen, although home oxygen therapy provides selected infants the opportunity for discharge. However, a significant proportion of deaths occur after discharge from hospital. Use of nasal cannulas provides an acceptable way to administer oxygen for the dependent infant to promote development of motor and social skills. A large percentage of survivors have significant disabilities, such as cerebral palsy, mental retardation, deafness and blindness, which are consistent with the VLBW infant population and probably unrelated to the BPD.

IMPLICATIONS FOR NURSING

Infants with BPD expend considerable energy in their efforts to breathe; therefore it is important that they receive plenty of opportunities for rest and additional calories. Growth records provide clues to the need for change in their diets, and some infants require nutritional supplements. Since they tire easily and large quantities of feed compromise respiration, small frequent feedings are better tolerated.

Parents are extremely anxious regarding the prognosis when their infant has BPD. In addition, the lengthy hospitalization interferes with parent-child relationships and deprives the infant of parental stimulation. Nurses should encourage the parents to visit the infant and become involved in the routine care. The parents need to be informed regarding medical care, equipment, and procedures related to their infant and taught procedures, such as suctioning and chest physiotherapy.

Home care

Since the availability of home cardiac/apnoea monitors and home oxygen therapy has increased, many of these infants can be discharged when they are gaining weight and oxygen need is low (less than 1 l/min). Home care is desirable to promote parent-infant bonding, minimize health care costs, and prevent nosocomial infections. Preparation for home care requires education and considerable reassurance (see Chapter 5). Management of home monitoring equipment and home oxygen therapy is stressful, but most families become comfortable with the machinery while their infant is still in the hospital. Families must be reminded about their infant's increased risk of infection and cautioned regarding contact with persons who have respiratory infections. Because of their minimum respiratory reserve, these infants can be threatened by even a minor illness.

HIGH RISK RELATED TO INFECTIOUS PROCESSES

Newborns are highly susceptible to infection. Their immature immune systems and their inability to localize infection render them especially vulnerable to infectious organisms. Prevention of infection in neonates, particularly in infants who are already compromised by physiological or structural disorders, is a primary nursing function. The nurse must be aware of potential sources of transmission and recognize those infants who are at risk (Pearse and Robertson, 1986).

SEPSIS

Sepsis, or *septicaemia*, refers to a generalized bacterial infection in the bloodstream. Neonates are highly susceptible to infection as a result of diminished non-specific (inflammatory) and specific (humoral) immunity, such as impaired phagocytosis, delayed chemotactic response, minimum or absent IgA and IgM, and decreased complement levels. Because of the infant's poor response to pathogenic agents, there is usually no local inflammatory reaction at the portal of entry to signal an infection and the resulting symptoms tend to be vague and non-specific. Consequently, diagnosis and treatment may be delayed.

Although the mortality from sepsis has diminished, the incidence of septicaemia has not diminished. The high-risk infant has a four times greater chance of developing septicaemia than does the normal neonate. The frequency of infection is almost twice as great in male infants as in females and carries a higher mortality for males as well. Other factors increasing the risk of infection are prematurity, bottle feeding, and use of steroids for treating lung disease.

Breast-feeding has a protective benefit against infection. Colostrum contains agglutinins that are effective against gram-negative bacteria. Human milk contains large quantities of IgA and iron-binding protein that exert a bacteriostatic effect on *Escherichia coli*. Human milk also contains macrophages and lymphocytes that promote a local inflammatory reaction.

SOURCES OF INFECTION

Sepsis in the neonatal period can be acquired prenatally across the placenta from the maternal bloodstream or during labour from ingestion or aspiration of infected amniotic fluid. Prolonged rupture of the membranes always presents a risk of this type from maternal-fetal transfer of pathogenic organisms. *In utero* transplacental transfer of organisms can occur, such as cytomegalovirus, *Toxoplasma,* and *Treponema pallidum* (syphilis), which cross the placental barrier during the latter half of pregnancy.

Early sepsis (less than three days) is acquired at birth; infection can occur from direct contact with organisms from the maternal gastrointestinal and genitourinary tracts. The most common infecting organisms are Streptococcus agalactiae and Escherichia coli, which may be present in the vagina from fecal contamination. E. coli accounts for about two-thirds of all cases of sepsis caused by gram-negative organisms. Proper hygiene of the perineum is one method of preventing this mode of transmission. Other pathogens that are harboured in the vagina and that may infect the infant include gonococci, Candida albicans, herpes simplex virus (type II), Listeria organisms, chlamydia, and ß-haemolytic streptococci.

Late sepsis (1-3 weeks following birth) is primarily nosocomial, and the offending organisms are usually the staphylococci, *Klebsiella*, enterococci, and sometimes *Pseudomonas*. The infant is at risk for self-infection because of the proximity of the umbilical wound to the perineum. Bacterial invasion can also occur through sites other than the umbilical stump, such as the skin; mucous membranes of the eye, nose, pharynx, and ear; and internal systems such as the respiratory, nervous, urinary, and gastrointestinal systems.

Postnatal infection is acquired by cross-contamination from other infants, personnel, or objects in the environment. Neonatal sepsis is most common in the infant at risk, particularly the preterm infant or the infant born following a difficult or traumatic labour and delivery, who is least capable of resisting such bacterial invasion.

PROCESS OF DIAGNOSIS

Because sepsis is so easily confused with other neonatal disorders, the definitive diagnosis is established by laboratory and radiographic examination. Isolation of the specific organism is always attempted through cultures of blood, urine, and cerebrospinal fluid. Direct (conjugated) hyperbilirubinaemia often occurs in infants with sepsis, particularly sepsis of gram-negative origin. Blood studies may show signs of anaemia, leukocytosis, or leukopenia. Leukopenia is usually an ominous sign because of its frequent association with high mortality. See Box 13-6 for manifestions observed in neonatal sepsis.

THERAPEUTIC MANAGEMENT

Early recognition and diagnosis with institution of vigorous therapeutic measures are essential to increase the infant's chance for survival and reduce the likelihood of permanent neurological damage. Often diagnosis of sepsis is based on suspicion, and antibiotic therapy is initiated before laboratory results are available for confirmation and identification of the exact organism. Treatment consists of circulatory support, respiratory support, aggressive administration of antibiotics, and immunotherapy.

Supportive therapy usually involves administration of oxygen if respiratory distress or cyanosis is evident, careful regulation of fluids and correction of electrolyte or acid-base imbalance, and temporary discontinuation of oral feedings. Blood transfusions may be needed to correct anaemia and

shock, and electronic monitoring of vital signs and regulation of the thermal environment are mandatory.

Antibiotic therapy is continued for 7-10 days if cultures are positive, discontinued in three days if cultures are negative, and most often administered via intravenous infusion. This has proved to be highly effective in lowering mortality from this disease. Intravenous gammaglobulin has also proved effective as a prophylactic measure against nosocomial infections (Chirico *et al*, 1987; Clapp *et al*, 1989).

◆ **BOX 13-6**

Manifestations observed in neonatal sepsis

General Signs
Infant generally 'not doing well'
Poor temperature control — hypothermia, hyperthermia (rare)

Circulatory System
Pallor, cyanosis, or mottling
Cold, clammy skin
Hypotension
Oedema
Abnormal heartbeat — bradycardia, tachycardia, arrhythmia

Respiratory System
Irregular respirations, apnoea, or tachypnoea
Cyanosis
Grunting
Dyspnoea
Retractions

Central Nervous System
Diminished activity — lethargy, hyporeflexia, coma
Increased activity — irritability, tremors, seizures
Full fontanelle
Increased or decreased tone
Abnormal eye movements

Gastrointestinal System
Poor feeding
Vomiting, increased stomach residual after feeding
Diarrhoea or decreased stool
Abdominal distention
Hepatomegaly

Haematopoietic System
Jaundice
Pallor
Purpura, petechiae, ecchymosis
Splenomegaly
Bleeding

Prognosis is variable. Before the discovery of antibiotics the mortality from bacterial sepsis was 95% to 100%, but early recognition, antibiotics, and supportive therapy have reduced mortality to less than 50% (Bruhn and Jones, 1985). However, mental retardation can occur with late diagnosis of meningitis or inadequate length of treatment.

IMPLICATIONS FOR NURSING

Nursing care of the infant with sepsis involves observation and assessment as outlined for any high-risk infant. Recognition of the existing problem is of paramount importance; it is usually the nurse who observes and assesses infants and who identifies that 'something is wrong' with them. Much of the care of infants with sepsis involves the medical treatment of the illness. Knowledge of the side effects of the specific antibiotic and proper regulation and administration of the drug are vital.

Prolonged antibiotic therapy poses additional hazards for affected infants. Oral antibiotics destroy intestinal flora responsible for synthesis of vitamin K, which can reduce blood coagulability. In addition, they predispose the infants to growth of resistant organisms and superinfection from fungal or mycotic agents, such as *Candida albicans*. Nurses must be alert for evidence of such complications.

Part of the total care of infants with sepsis is to decrease any additional physiological or environmental stress. This includes providing an optimum thermoregulated environment and anticipating potential problems, such as dehydration or hypoxia. Precautions are implemented to prevent spread of infection to other newborns, but to be effective, activities must be carried out by all caregivers. Proper handwashing, use of disposable equipment (e.g., linens, catheters, feeding utensils, and intravenous equipment), disposing of excretions (e.g., vomitus and stool), and adequate housekeeping of the environment and equipment are essential. Since nurses are the most consistent caregivers involved with sick infants, it is usually their responsibility to oversee that all phases of isolation are maintained by everyone.

Another aspect of caring for infants with sepsis involves observation for signs of complications including meningitis and shock, a severe complication caused by the release of toxins into the bloodstream.

Other complications of sepsis include pyarthrosis (which may affect any joint, but most commonly localizes in the hip) and osteomyelitis. Local inflammation of the involved area is again uncommon, so identification is difficult. Limited movement of the affected joint and/or extremity may be one of the few indications of infection.

NECROTIZING ENTEROCOLITIS

Necrotizing enterocolitis (NEC) is an acute inflammatory disease of the bowel with increased incidence in preterm and other high-risk infants, but it is most common in those who weigh less than 2,000 g. Three factors appear to play an important role in its development: intestinal ischaemia, colonization by pathogenic bacteria, and excess substrate (artificial formula feeding) in the intestinal lumen.

CLINICAL MANIFESTATIONS

The prominent clinical signs of NEC are a distended (often shining) abdomen, gastric retention, and blood in the stools or gastric contents. Nonspecific signs include lethargy, poor feeding, hypotension, apnoea, vomiting (often bile-stained), decreased urine output, and unstable temperature. The onset is usually between four and ten days, but signs may be evident as early as four hours and as late as 30 days. NEC in full-term infants almost always occurs in the first ten days when the gut is least mature; late-onset NEC is confined primarily to preterm infants (Wilson *et al*, 1982).

PROCESS OF DIAGNOSIS

Radiographic studies show a sausage-shaped dilation of the intestine that progresses to marked distention and the characteristic pneumatosis intestinales — 'soapsuds' or bubbly appearance of thickened bowel wall and ultralumina. There may be air in the portal circulation or free air observed in the abdomen, indicating perforation. Laboratory findings may include anaemia, leucopenia, leucocytosis, and electrolyte imbalance. In severe cases, coagulopathy and/or thrombocytopenia may be evident. Organisms are often cultured from blood, although bacteraemia or septicaemia may not be prominent early in the course of the disease. Breath hydrogen measurements are suggested as an aid to diagnosis of NEC and have proved to be 99% effective in detecting absence of the disease, thereby preventing prolonged withholding of feedings from these infants (Kenner *et al*, 1988).

THERAPEUTIC MANAGEMENT

Treatment of NEC begins with prevention. Breast milk is the preferred enteral nutrient because it confers some passive immunity (IgA), macrophages, and lysozymes.

Treatment of confirmed NEC consists of discontinuation of all oral feedings, institution of abdominal decompression via nasogastric suction, administration of intravenous antibiotics, and correction of extravascular volume depletion, electrolyte abnormalities, acid-base imbalances, and hypoxia. Replacing oral feedings with parenteral fluids decreases the need for oxygen and circulation to the bowel.

Prognosis

With early recognition and treatment, medical management is increasingly successful. If there is progressive deterioration under medical management or evidence of perforation, surgical resection and anastomosis are carried out. Extensive involvement may necessitate establishment of an ileostomy, jejunostomy, or colostomy. Sequelae in surviving infants include short-gut syndrome (see Chapter 27), colonic stricture with obstruction, fat malabsorption, and failure to thrive secondary to intestinal dysfunction.

IMPLICATIONS FOR NURSING

Nursing responsibilities begin with early recognition. Because the signs are similar to those observed in many other disorders of the newborn, nurses must constantly be aware of the possibility of this disease.

When the disease is suspected, the nurse assists with diagnostic procedures and implements the therapeutic regimen. Vital signs, including blood pressure, are monitored for changes that might indicate impending sepsis or cardiovascular shock. It is especially important to avoid rectal temperatures, because of the increased danger of perforation. To avoid pressure on the distended abdomen and to facilitate continuous observation, infants are frequently left naked and positioned supine or on the side.

Conscientious attention to nutritional and hydration needs is essential, and antibiotics are administered as prescribed. The time at which oral feedings are reinstituted varies considerably but is usually at least 7-10 days following diagnosis and treatment.

The infant who requires surgery requires the same careful attention and observation as any infant with abdominal surgery, including stoma care. This disorder is one of the most frequent reasons for performing ileostomies on newborns. Throughout the medical and surgical management of infants with NEC, the nurse is continually alert to signs of complications, such as sepsis, disseminated intravascular coagulation, hypoglycaemia, and other metabolic derangements.

HIGH RISK RELATED TO CARDIOVASCULAR COMPLICATIONS

LBW infants and those who are otherwise physically compromised are subject to complications in all major systems. This segment is not concerned with congenital cardiac anomalies or the complications that result from these lesions (see Chapter 28). The disorders described here are observed in the neonatal period, usually as complications of pulmonary dysfunction and respiratory therapy.

PERSISTENT PATENT DUCTUS ARTERIOSUS

A common complication of severe respiratory disease in preterm infants is persistent patent ductus arteriosus (PDA) (Wilkinson and Cooke, 1986). It occurs in the majority of preterm infants under 1,200 g, and the incidence diminishes in direct relationship to increasing birth weight. During fetal life the ductus remains patent through the vasodilatory action of prostaglandins within its tissues. Postnatally the increase in oxygen tension has a constricting effect on the ductus, but it may reopen in these small infants in response to the lowered oxygen tension associated with respiratory impairment. It is

still unknown whether PDA is a contributing factor in the development of respiratory distress or whether respiratory distress contributes to the development of PDA.

IMPLICATIONS FOR NURSING

Nursing observations are important in the recognition and management of PDA. Assisting in early detection, assessing cardiovascular status carefully, and monitoring for complications following implementation of therapy are nursing responsibilities (Cohen, 1983).

Other nursing observations and management are the same as for the high-risk infant and the infant with PDA (see Chapter 28).

PERSISTENT PULMONARY HYPERTENSION OF THE NEWBORN

Persistent pulmonary hypertension of the newborn (PPHN), or *persistent pulmonary hypertension* (PPH), formerly known as *persistent fetal circulation* (PFC), is a condition in which affected infants display severe pulmonary hypertension, with pulmonary artery pressure levels equal to or greater than systemic pressure, and large right-to-left shunts through both the foramen ovale and the ductus arteriosus. Since full development of pulmonary arterial musculature occurs late in gestation, PPHN is primarily a condition of full-term or postterm infants, many of whom were products of complicated pregnancies or deliveries. The condition is often associated with massive aspiration (especially meconium aspiration), cold stress, and/or respiratory distress (e.g., IRDS or pneumonia) and is believed to be precipitated by perinatal factors, such as perinatal asphyxia, that cause or contribute to vasospasm.

PPHN can be either primary or secondary: primary PPHN occurs when the pulmonary vascular system fails to open with the initial respiration at birth; secondary PPHN results from stress that increases pulmonary vascular resistance and causes a return to fetal cardiopulmonary circulation. PPHN is most frequently observed in infants at 35-44 weeks of gestation who have a history of perinatal asphyxia, polycythaemia, acidosis, or sepsis and respiratory distress within the first 24 hours. The infants become hypoxic when agitated and display marked cyanosis, tachypnoea with grunting and recession, and decreased peripheral perfusion. Mild cases may display only minimum tachypnoea and cyanosis during stressful episodes, such as crying or feeding.

Diagnosis is established from clinical signs and diagnostic tests including chest radiography.

IMPLICATIONS FOR NURSING

The nursing care is the same as for infants with respiratory difficulties and infants supported by mechanical respirators.

ANAEMIA

Preterm infants tend to develop anaemia that is more severe and appears earlier than in more mature infants. It may be the result of haemorrhage during the course of labour and delivery (into brain, liver, spleen, or kidneys), blood disorders (haemolytic disease, thrombocytopenia), conditions that produce swelling or distention of abdominal organs, or iatrogenic from blood withdrawn in the NICU for laboratory tests. Physiological characteristics of prematurity tend to contribute to development of anaemia, that is, a drop in the production of fetal haemoglobin and shortened survival time of the red blood cells.

IMPLICATIONS FOR NURSING

One of the most common causes of anaemia in preterm infants is blood loss associated with frequent sampling for blood gas and metabolic analyses. Therefore, an important nursing responsibility is careful monitoring and recording of all blood drawn for tests. It is surprising how easily and rapidly the small total blood volume of premature infants is depleted by repeated withdrawals.

Observation for signs of anaemia is a vital nursing function. The traditional signs of anaemia in the child are often observed in the preterm infant: feeding difficulties, dyspnoea, tachycardia, tachypnoea, diminished activity, and pallor. However, some infants may not display all of these signs. Poor weight gain may be an indication of a lowered haemoglobin level. Nursing precautions and observations during blood transfusion for the preterm infant are similar to those for any child.

RETINOPATHY OF PREMATURITY

Although often discussed in relation to respiratory dysfunction, *retinopathy of prematurity* (ROP) is a disorder involving blood vessels. ROP is a term used to describe all phases of retinal changes in the eye observed in preterm infants. The older term, *retrolental fibroplasia* (RLF), describes the cicatricial changes that characterize the later stages in the most severely affected infants. The incidence of the disease correlates with the degree of the infant's maturity — the younger the gestational age, the greater the likelihood of the development of ROP (Levene *et al*, 1987).

Numerous factors have been implicated in the cause of ROP in addition to immaturity, including hyperoxaemia and hypoxaemia, hypercarbia and hypocarbia, patent ductus arteriosus, prostaglandin synthetase inhibitors, apnoea, intraventricular haemorrhage, infection, vitamin E deficiency, lactic acidosis, maternal diabetes, prenatal complications, and genetic factors. Previously considered to be an iatrogenic disease related to hyperoxia, ROP is now believed to be a complex disease of prematurity with multiple causes and therefore difficult to prevent and manage.

IMPLICATIONS FOR NURSING

Adherence to the principles of oxygen administration and careful monitoring of oxygenation status are the first lines of defence against development of ROP (Gracey *et al*, 1991). Constant assessment and vigilance are necessary just as for any high-risk neonate. When the infant suffers partial or complete visual impairment, the parents will need a considerable amount of support and assistance in meeting the special developmental needs of the infant (see Chapter 23).

HIGH RISK RELATED TO NEUROLOGICAL DISTURBANCE

Neurological complications are observed with increased frequency in preterm infants and in infants born following a difficult labour and delivery (Levene, 1986). A disproportionately high incidence of perinatal encephalopathy, or cerebral palsy, and psychomotor retardation is found in the high-risk infant population, especially VLBW infants. Preterm infants are also more vulnerable to cerebral insults, such as hypoxia and chemical alterations. In addition, fragility and increased permeability of capillaries and prolonged prothrombin time predispose the brain of the preterm infant to trauma when delicate structures are subjected to increased pressure, such as the forces of labour, high mechanical ventilatory pressures, and seizure activity. All of these factors contribute to intracranial insults, including traumatic bleeding in the newborn, which consists of four major types: intraventricular, subdural, primary subarachnoid, and intracerebellar. (See Box 13-7 for causes of perinatal hypoxaemia and cerebral ischaemia.)

◆ BOX 13-7

Primary causes of perinatal hypoxaemia and cerebral ischaemia

Perinatal Hypoxaemia
1. Intrauterine asphyxia with respiratory failure at the time of birth
2. Postnatal respiratory insufficiency secondary to severe IRDS or recurrent apnoea
3. Severe cyanotic heart defects (right-to-left shunts) or persistent pulmonary hypertension

Primary Cerebral Ischaemia
1. Intrauterine asphyxia with cardiac insufficiency
2. Postnatal cardiac insufficiency secondary to severe congenital heart disease or recurrent apnoea
3. Postnatal cardiovascular collapse secondary to sepsis

Data from Hill, 1981.

PERINATAL HYPOXIC-ISCHAEMIC BRAIN INJURY

IMPLICATIONS FOR NURSING

Nursing care is primarily the same as for any high-risk infant: careful assessment and observation for signs that might indicate cerebral hypoxia or ischaemia, monitoring of ventilatory and intravenous therapy, observation and management of seizures, and general supportive care to infants and parents, including guidelines for management in the event of learning disabilities (see Chapter 22). These infants are usually on intravenous alimentation.

PERIVENTRICULAR-INTRAVENTRICULAR HAEMORRHAGE

Most authorities use the term IVH to describe this disorder, which is responsible for a significant percentage of seriously ill infants and neonatal mortality. Intraventricular haemorrhage is extremely common in preterm infants, especially VLBW infants less than 32 weeks of gestation and less than 1500 g (Minarcik and Beachy, 1989). Classification data are given in Box 13-8.

IMPLICATIONS FOR NURSING

In addition to the routine observations and management, nursing care is directed towards prevention of increased cerebral blood pressure. Some nursing procedures (e.g., suctioning) increase intercranial pressure (ICP).

Interventions that may reduce the risk of increased ICP include avoiding interventions that cause crying (such as painful procedures). Crying can impede venous return, increase cerebral blood volume, and compromise cerebral oxygenation in LBW infants. These consequences must be considered when nursing care includes activities that precipitate crying. Care includes evaluating manipulations and handling, and administering analgesics to reduce discomfort. 'Each intervention should be preceded by the questions, "How stressful will this be for the infant?" and "Is it necessary?"' (Kling, 1989).

◆ BOX 13-8

Classification of brain haemorrhage

0 no bleeding

1 germinal matrix only

2 germinal matrix with blood in the ventricles

3 germinal matrix with blood in the ventricles and ventricular dilatation

4 intraventricular and parenchymal bleeding (other than

INTRACRANIAL HAEMORRHAGE

Intracranial haemorrhage (ICH) in neonates, although manifested in the same ways as those described in older children, occurs with different frequencies and different degrees of severity.

SUBDURAL HAEMATOMAS

Subdural haematomas, life-threatening collections of blood in the subdural space, are most often produced by the stretching and tearing of the large veins in the *tentorium cerebelli*, the dural membrane that separates the cerebrum from the cerebellum. With improved obstetric care these have become relatively uncommon; however, they are especially serious because of the inaccessibility of the haematoma to aspiration by subdural tap. Less frequently, haemorrhage occurs when veins in the subdural space over the surface of the brain are torn (see Chapter 31).

SUBARACHNOID HAEMORRHAGE

Subarachnoid haemorrhage, the most common type of intracranial haemorrhage, occurs in term infants as a result of trauma and in preterm infants as a result of hypoxia. Small haemorrhages are the most common. Bleeding is of venous origin, and underlying contusion may also occur.

INTRACEREBELLAR HAEMORRHAGE

Intracerebellar haemorrhage is a common finding on postmortem examination of the premature infant and can be a primary haemorrhage in the cerebellum associated with skull compression during abrupt, precipitous delivery, or it may occur secondary to extravasation of blood into the cerebellum from a ventricular haemorrhage. In the full-term infant the bleeding may follow a difficult delivery.

IMPLICATIONS FOR NURSING

Nursing care is the same as care of the infant with periventricular-intraventricular haemorrhage or with perinatal hypoxic-ischaemic brain injury.

NEONATAL SEIZURES

Seizures in the neonatal period are usually the clinical manifestation of a serious underlying disease. Although not life-threatening as an isolated entity, seizures constitute a medical emergency because they signal a disease process that may produce irreversible brain damage. Consequently, it is imperative to recognize a seizure and its significance so that the cause as well as the seizure, can be treated (Box 13-9).

◆ **BOX 13-9**

Causes of neonatal seizures

Metabolic
Hypoglycaemia; hyperglycaemia
Hypocalcaemia
Hypomagnesaemia
Pyridoxine deficiency
Aminoacidurias (e.g., phenylketonuria, maple syrup urine disease)

Toxic and Electrolyte
Hypernatraemia
Hyponatraemia
Narcotic withdrawal
Uraemia
Bilirubin encephalopathy (kernicterus)

Prenatal Infections
Toxoplasmosis
Syphilis
Cytomegalic inclusion disease
Herpes simplex
Hepatitis

Postnatal Infections
Bacterial meningitis
Viral meningoencephalitis
Sepsis
Brain abscess

Trauma at Birth
Hypoxic encephalopathy
Intracranial haemorrhage
Subarachnoid, epidural haemorrhage
Intraventricular haemorrhage of prematurity

Malformations
Central nervous system agenesis
Hydroencephalopathy
Parencephalopathy
Tuberous sclerosis

Miscellaneous

IMPLICATIONS FOR NURSING

The major nursing responsibilities in the care of infants with seizures are to recognize when the infant is having a seizure so that therapy can be instituted, to carry out the therapeutic regimen, and to observe the response to the therapy and any further evidence of seizures or other symptomatology. Assessment and other aspects of care are the same as for all high-risk infants. Parents need to be informed of their infant's status, and the nurse should reinforce and clarify the explanations of the practitioner. The infant's behaviours need to be interpreted for the parents, and the infant's responses to the treatment

must be anticipated and their significance explained. Parents are encouraged to visit their infant and perform the parenting activities consistent with the plan of care. Seizures are a frightening phenomenon and generate a great deal of anxiety and fear, which is easily compounded by the justifiable concern of the staff. Providing support and guidance is an important nursing function.

HIGH RISK RELATED TO MATERNAL CONDITIONS

Conditions in the maternal system can have a significant effect on the fetus that extends into the postnatal period. Many of these conditions are congenital malformations and disorders and can cause permanent disability. Maternal diabetes is presented in the following section.

Many maternal infections are detrimental to both the mother and the fetus. Some produce permanent physical or mental defects; others cause illness in the newborn period. It is important to be aware of a possible infection in the mother, in order to be alert for evidence of the illness in the newborn, and to be aware of signs in the newborn that indicate intrauterine exposure to a maternal infection.

INFANTS OF DIABETIC MOTHERS

Effective control of maternal diabetes and an increased understanding of fetal disorders has resulted in significant reduction in the morbidity and mortality of infants.

Severity of maternal diabetes is determined by the duration of the disease before pregnancy, the age of onset, the extent of vascular complications, and abnormalities of the current pregnancy, such as pyelonephritis, diabetic ketoacidosis, pregnancy-induced hypertension, and noncompliance. The single most important factor influencing fetal well-being is the euglycaemic status of the mother. It has been found that reasonable metabolic control started before conception and continued during the first weeks of pregnancy can prevent malformations in infants of diabetic mothers (IDMs). (Aynsley-Green and Soltesz, 1986).

EFFECTS OF DIABETES ON THE FETUS

It is generally agreed that during fetal life high maternal blood sugar levels provide a continual stimulus to the fetal islet cells for insulin production. This sustained state of hyperglycaemia promotes fetal insulin secretion that ultimately leads to excessive growth and deposition of fat, which probably accounts for the infants who are large for gestational age (LGA). When the glucose supply is removed abruptly at the time of birth, the continued production of insulin soon depletes the blood of circulating glucose, creating a state of hyperinsulinism and hypoglycaemia (Aynsley-Green and Soltesz, 1986a). Precipitous drops in blood glucose levels can cause serious neurological damage or death.

Tests of fetal well-being are performed routinely on the expectant mother with diabetes during pregnancy. Ultrasonography is performed at 18-20 weeks to determine fetal size and to rule out the presence of fetal anomalies. It may be repeated periodically during the course of fetal development.

THERAPEUTIC MANAGEMENT

The most effective management appears to be careful observation of all IDMs. The infants are examined for the presence of any anomalies or birth injuries, and blood studies for initial determinations of glucose, calcium, haematocrit, and bilirubin are obtained on a regular basis.

Feeding with breast milk or formula feeds is begun within the

first hour after birth. Approximately half of these infants do very well and adjust without complications. Critically ill infants require IV infusions. Oral and intravenous intake may be titrated to maintain adequate blood sugar levels. Frequent blood glucose determinations are needed for the first two days of life to assess the degree of hypoglycaemia present at any given time.

IMPLICATIONS FOR NURSING

Because some IDMs are born prematurely, they are subject to the problems discussed in relation to the preterm infant. In addition to the routine care of the newborn, the infants require observation for signs of complications.

KEY POINTS

- Parental involvement in the care of high-risk infants is important, and nurses should help to facilitate parent-infant relationships by guiding them to support groups and home health teaching.
- Several severe respiratory conditions place the infant at high risk: apnoea of prematurity, IRDS, meconium aspiration syndrome, extraneous air syndromes, and BPD. Therapeutic management of IRDS includes oxygen therapy and assisted ventilation.
- Cardiovascular complications in the high-risk infant may include persistent patent ductus arteriosus, persistent pulmonary hypertension, anaemia, and polycythaemia/hyperviscosity syndrome.
- Neurological disturbances in the high-risk newborn may include perinatal hypoxic-ischaemic brain injury, periventricular-intraventricular haemorrhage, intracranial haemorrhage, and neonatal seizures.
- Diabetes is one of several maternal conditions that poses a threat to the newborn.

- The most common forms of paralysis in the newborn are facial nerve, brachial plexus, and phrenic nerve palsies.
- Hyperbilirubinaemia is classified according to the two types of bilirubin: unconjugated and conjugated. In the newborn it may result from excess production of bilirubin, disturbed capacity of the liver to conjugate bilirubin, or bile duct obstruction resulting from biliary atresia.
- Haemolytic disease of the newborn is characterized by abnormally rapid destruction of red blood cells as a result of blood incompatibility between mother and fetus.
- Categories of hypoglycaemia are: (1) decreased substrate availability, (2) endocrine disturbances, (3) increased utilization, and (4) other mechanisms.
- Haemorrhagic disease of the newborn is characterized by oozing from the umbilicus or circumcision site, bloody or black stools, haematuria, ecchymoses on skin and scalp, and epistaxis.
- The most significant inborn errors of metabolism are congenital hypothyroidism, phenylketonuria, and galactosaemia.

REFERENCES

American Academy of Pediatrics and American Thyroid Association: Newborn screening for congenital hypothyroidism: recommended guidelines, *Pediatrics* 80:745-747, 1987.

Archdeacon H: Somebody's baby, *Nurs Times* 85(21):44, 1989.

Aynsley-Green A, Soltesz G: Disorders of blood glucose homeostasis in the neonate. In Robertson NRC, editor: *Textbook of neonatology,* London, 1986a, Churchill Livingstone.

Aynsley-Green A, Soltesz G: Metabolic and endocrine disorders. In Robertson NRC, editor: *Textbook of neonatology,* London, 1986b, Churchill Livingstone.

Bancalari E, Gerhardt T: Bronchopulmonary dysplasia, *Pediatr Clin North Am* 33:1, 1986.

Bennett FC, Robinson NM, Sells CJ: Growth and development of infants weighing less than 800 grams at birth, *Pediatr* 71:319, 1983.

Berg FJ, Solomon LM: Erythema neonatorum toxicum, *Arch Dis Child* 62:327, 1987.

Bernbaum JC *et al*: Nonnutritive sucking during gavage feeding enhances growth and maturation in premature infants, *Pediatr* 71:41, 1983.

Bowman JM: Haemolytic disease of the newborn. In Robertson NRC, editor: *Textbook of neonatology,* London, 1986, Churchill Livingstone.

Bruhn FW, Jones B: Infection in the neonate. In Merenstein GB, Gardner SL: *Handbook of neonatal intensive care,* St Louis, 1985, Mosby–Year Book.

Brunner RL, Jordan MK, Berry HK: Early-treated phenylketonuria: neuropsychologic consequences, *J Pediatr* 102(6):831, 1983.

Budreau GK: Postnatal cranial modeling and infant attractiveness: implications for nursing, *Neonatal Network* 5(5):13, 1987.

Chirico G *et al*: Intravenous gammaglobulin therapy for prophylaxis of infection in high-risk neonates, *J Pediatr* 110:437, 1987.

Clapp DW *et al*: Use of intravenously administered immune globlulin to prevent nosocomial sepsis in low birth weight infants: report of a pilot study, *J Pediatr* 115:973, 1989.

Cohen MA: The use of prostaglandins and prostaglandin inhibitors in critically ill neonates, *MCN* 8:194, 1983.

Collaborative European Multicenter Study Group: Surfactant replacement therapy for severe neonatal respiratory distress syndrome: an international clinical trial, *Pediatr* 82:683, 1988.

Danks DM, Brown G: Inborn errors of metabolism in the neonate. In Robertson NRC, editor: *Textbook of neonatology,* London, 1986, Churchill Livingstone.

Doll-Speck L, Miller B, Rohrs K: Sibling education: implementing a programme for the NICU unit, *Neonatal Network* 12(4):49, 1993.

Drogari E *et al*: Timing of strict diet in relation to fetal damage in maternal phenylketonuria, *Lancet* 2:927, 1987.

Field T *et al*: Nonnutritive sucking during tube feedings: effects on preterm neonates in an intensive care unit, *Pediatr* 70:381, 1982.

Foss M: Acid base balance, *Prof Nurs* :509, 1988.

Fox MD, Molesky MG: The effects of prone and supine positioning on arterial oxygen pressure, *Neonatal Network* 8:25, 1990.

Gardner SL, O'Donnell JP, Weisman LE: Breastfeeding the sick neonate. In Merenstein GB, Gardner SL: *Handbook of neonatal intensive care,* ed 2, St Louis, 1989, Mosby–Year Book.

Geertsma, M.A., *et al*: Feeding resistance after parenteral hyperalimentation, *Am J Dis Child* 139:255-256, 1985.

Gladstone IM, Ehrenkranz RA, Jacobs HC: Pulmonary function tests and fluid balance in neonates with chronic lung disease during dexamethasone treatment, *Pediatr* 84:1072, 1989.

Glorieux J *et al*: Follow-up at ages 5 and 7 years on mental development in children with hypothyroidism detected by Quebec Screening Program, *J Pediatr* 107:913, 1985.

Goldson E: Bronchopulmonary dysplasia, *Pediatr Ann* 19:13, 1990.

Gracey KM *et al*: Caring for the infant with retinopathy of prematurity undergoing cryotherapy, *Neonatal Network* :7, 1991.

Greenough A, Osborne J, Sutherland S: *Congential, perinatal and neonatal infections,* Edinburgh, 1992, Churchill Livingstone.

Greer PS: Head coverings for newborns under radiant warmers, *JOGNN* 17(4):265, 1988.

Gross SJ *et al*: Elevated IgA concentration in milk produced by mothers delivered of preterm infants, *J Pediatr* 99:389, 1981.

Gross SJ, Oehler JM, Eckerman CO: Head growth and developmental outcome in very low-birth-weight infants, *Pediatr* 71:70, 1983.

Hack, M. *et al*: Catch-up growth in very-low-birth-weight infants, *Am J Dis Child* 138:370-375, 1984.

Harkavy KL *et al*: Dexamethasone therapy for chronic lung disease in ventilator- and oxygen-dependent infants: a controlled trial, *J Pediatr* 115:979, 1989.

Hill L: *Caring for dying children and their families,* London, 1994, Chapman & Hall.

Hill A, Volpe JJ: Seizures, hypoxic-ishemic brain injury, and intraventricular haemorrhage in the newborn, *Ann Neurol* 10:109, 1981.

Jenkins HR: Care of the jaundiced infant, *Update* :289, 1991.

Jones E: Breast feeding preterm infant, *Modern Midwife* :22, 1994.

Kelnar CJH, Harvey D: *The sick newborn baby,* ed 2, London, 1985, Baillière Tindall.

Kenner C *et al*: *Neonatal surgery—a nursing perpective,* Orlando, 1988, Grune & Stratton.

Kimble C: Nonnutritive sucking: adoptation and health for the neonate, *Neonatal Network* 2(2):29, 1992.

Klaus MH, Faranoff AA: *Care of the high risk neonate,* ed 2, London, 1989, WB Saunders.

Kling P: Nursing interventions to decrease the risk of periventricular-intraventricular hemorrhage, *JOGNN* 18:457, 1989.

Kling P: Respiratory distress syndrome in the tiny baby, *Neonatal Network* vol(issue):19, 1986.

Koops B, Abman S, Accurso F: Outpatient management and followup of BPD, *Clin Perinatol* 11:101, 1984.

Kowba MD, Schwirian PM: Direct sibling contact and bacterial colonization in newborns, *JOGNN* 14:412, 1985.

Kwong MS, Egan EA: Reduced incidence of hyaline membrane disease in extremely premature infants following delay of delivery in mother with preterm labor: use of ritodrine and betamethasone, *Pediatr* 78:767, 1986.

Landon-Malone KA, Kirkpatrick JM, Stull SP: Incorporating hospice care in a community hospital NICU, *Neonatal Network* 6(1):13, 1987.

Lang MJ *et al*: A controlled trial of human surfactant replacement therapy for severe respiratory distress syndrome in very low birth weight infants, *J Pediatr* 116:295, 1990.

Lawrence RA: *Breastfeeding: a guide for the medical profession,* ed 3, St Louis, 1990, Mosby–Year Book.

Levene MI: *Current reviews in neonatal neurology,* Edinburgh, 1986, Churchill Livingstone.

Lipsitz PJ, Gartner LM, Bryla DA: Neonatal and infant mortality in relation to phototherapy, *Pediatr* 75(suppl):422, 1985.

Lucas A: Nutritional psychology: dietary requirements of term and preterm infants. In Robertson NRC, editor: *Textbook of neonatology,* London, 1986, Churchill Livingstone.

Lund C *et al*: Evaluation of a pectin-based barrier under tape to protect neonatal skin, *JOGNN* 15:39, 1986.

Marriott S: The long goodbye, *Nurs Times* 84(6):45, 1988.

Masterson J, Zucker C, Schulze K: Prone and supine positioning effects on energy expenditure and behavior of low birth weight neonates, *Pediatr* 80:689, 1987.

McHaffie H: Isolated but not alone, *Nurs Times* 83(28):73, 1987.

Michals K *et al*: Return to diet therapy in patients with phenylketonuria, *J Pediatr* 106:933, 1985.

Minarcik CJ, Beachy P: Neurologic disorders. In Merenstein GB, Gardner SL: *Handbook of neonatal intensive care,* ed 2, St Louis, 1989, Mosby–Year Book.

Morley C: The respiratory distress syndrome. In Robertson NRC, editor: *Textbook of neonatology,* London, 1986, Churchill Livingstone.

Mutch CM: Epidemiology, perinatal mortality, and morbidity. In Robertson NRC, editor: *Textbook of neonatology,* London, 1986, Churchill Livingstone.

Muttitt SC *et al*: Neonatal apnea: diagnosis by nurse versus computer, *Pediatr* 82:713, 1988.

Newman A: Coping with grief, *Nurs Times* :32, 1984.

Null, S.: Nursing care to ease parents' grief, *MCN* 14:84-89, 1989.

Orr, M.J. and Allen, S.S.: Optimal oral experiences for infants on long term total parenteral nutrition, *Nutr Clin Pract,* 9:288-295, 1986.

Osborn LM: Management of neonatal jaundice, *Nurse Pract* 11(4):41 1986.

Paludetto R *et al*: Transcutaneous oxygen tension during nonnutritive sucking in preterm infants, *Pediatr* 74:539, 1984.

Papageorgiou AN *et al*: Reduction of mortality, morbidity, and respiratory distress syndrome in infants weighing less than 1,000 grams by treatment with betamethasone and ritodrine, *Pediatr* 83:493, 1989.

Pearse RWI, Robertson NRC: Infection in the newborn. In Robertson NRC, editor: *Textbook of neonatology,* London, 1986, Churchill Livingstone.

Pildes RS, Lilien LD: Carbohydrate metabolism in the fetus and neonate. In Fanaroff A, Martin R, editors: *Behrman's neonatal-perinatal medicine,* ed 4, St Louis, 1987, Mosby–Year Book.

Rohr FJ *et al*: New England maternal PKU project: prospective study of untreated and treated pregnancies and their outcomes, *J Pediatr* 110:391, 1987.

Ross G, Lipper EG, Auld PAM: Physical growth and developmental outcome in very low birth weight premature infants at 3 years of age, *J Pediatr* 107:284, 1985.

Royal College of Midwives: *Successful breastfeeding,* Edinburgh, 1991, Churchill Livingstone.

SANDS (Stillbirth and Neonatal Death Society): *Stillbirth and neonatal death: guideline for professionals,* London, 1991, SANDS.

Sani J: Infant feeding: best for baby, *Nurs Times* 84(15):65, 1988.

Schwab F *et al*: Sibling visiting in a neonatal intensive care unit, *Pediatr* 71:835, 1983.

Seashore MR *et al*: Loss of intellectual function in children with phenylketonuria after relaxation of dietary phenylalanine restriction, *Pediatr* 75(2):226, 1985.

Shaker CS: Nipple feeding premature infants: a different perspective, *Neonatal Network* 8(5):9, 1990.

Slater, M.A. *et al*: Neurodevelopment of monitored versus non-monitored very low birth weight infants: the importance of family influences, *J Dev Behav Pediatr* 8(5):278-285, 1988.

Southall DP *et al*: Undetected episodes of prolonged apnea and severe bradycardia in preterm infants, *Pediatr* 72:541, 1983.

Sparshott M: Maintaining skin integrity, *Paediatr Nurs* :12, 1991.

Stewart A: Carers or outsiders, *Midwives Chronicle Nurs Notes* :118, 1991.

Stewart A: SCBU — Maintaining the ideal body temperature, *Prof Nurs* :544, 1990.

Swanwick T: The cases of neonatal jaundice, *Nurs* 13(39):3, 1989.

Symes J: What comfort for this grief, *Prof Nurs* **vol(issue)**:437, 1991.

Thomas J: Supporting parents when their baby dies, *Nurs Stand* 5(**issue**):52, 1990.

Thomas R, Harvey D: *Neonatology,* ed 2, Edinburgh, 1992, Churchill Livingstone.

Thornton S: Stress in the neonatal unit, *Nurs Times* **vol(issue)**:35, 1984.

Tom-Johnson C: Talking through grief, *Nurs Times* 86(1):44, 1990.

Topper WH, Stewart TP: Thermal support for the very-low-birth-weight infant: role of supplemental conductive heat, *J Pediatr* 105:810, 1984.

Townshend P: Impact of intensive care, *Midwives Chronicle Nurs Notes* :194, 1987.

Trause, M.A. *et al*:Separation for childbirth: the effect on the sibling, *Child Psychiatry Hum Dev* 12:94-104, 1983.

Vyas H, Milner AD: Respiratory diseases of the neonate. In Robertson NRC, editor: *Textbook of neonatology,* London, 1986, Churchill Livingstone.

Westwood M *et al*: Growth and development of full-term nonasphyxiated small-for-gestational-age newborns: follow-up through adolescence, *Pediatr* 71:376, 1983.

Whitby C: Caring for patients with a baby receiving intensive care, *Care Crit Ill* 4(2):24, 1988.

Wilkinson J, Cooke RWI: Cardiovascular disorders. In Robertson NRC, editor: *Textbook of neonatology,* London, 1986, Churchill Livingstone.

Wilson, R. *et al*: Age onset of necrotizing enterocolitis: an epidemiologic analysis, *Pediatr Res* 12:82-84, 1982.

Yeh TF *et al*: Furosemide prevents the renal side effects of indomethacin therapy in premature infants with patent ductus arteriosus, *J Pediatr* 101:433, 1982.

FURTHER READING

General

Bethea SW: Primary nursing in the infant special care unit, *JOGNN* 14:202, 1985.

Cunningham N, Hutchinson S: Neonatal nurses and issues in research ethics, *Neonatal Network* 8(5):29, 1990.

Grassi LC: Life, money, quality: the impact of regionalization on perinatal/neonatal intensive care, *Neonatal Network* 6(4):53, 1988.

Harpin VA, Rutter N: Barrier properties of the newborn infant's skin, *J Pediatr* 102:419, 1983.

27, 1989.

Oehler JM, Peter MA, Seyler S: Support groups: are they really helpful in dealing with NICU stress? *Neonatal Network* 8(2):21, 1989.

Tribotti S: Admission to the neonatal intensive care unit: reducing the risks, *Neonatal Network* 8(4):17, 1990.

Birth Injuries

Greenwald AG *et al*: Brachial plexus birth palsy: a ten year report on incidence and prognosis, *J Pediatr Orthop* 4:689, 1984.

Ingardia CJ, Cetrulo CL: Forceps—use and abuse, *Clin Perinatol* 8:163, 1981.

Joseph PR, Rosenfeld W: Clavicular fractures in neonates, *Am J Dis Child* 144:165, 1990.

Dermatological Problems

Abramovits W: Resistant oral candidiasis in an infant due to pacifier contamination, *Clin Pediatr* 20:393, 1981.

Finn MC, Glowacki J, Mulliken JB: Congenital vascular lesions: clinical application of a new classification, *J Pediatr Surg* 18(6):894, 1983.

Hyperbilirubinaemia

Costarino AT *et al*: Bilirubin photoisomerization in premature neonates under low- and high-dose phototherapy, *Pediatr* 75(3):519, 1985.

Dortch E, Spottiswoode P: New light on phototherapy: home use, *Neonatal Network* 4(4):30, 1986.

Hill AS, Cochran CK, Dickerson C: Nursing care of the infant with erythroblastosis fetalis, *J Pediatr Nurs* 4:395, 1989.

Mauer HM *et al*: Phototherapy for hyperbilirubinemia of hemolytic disease of the newborn, *Pediatr* 75(suppl 2):407, 1985.

Metabolic Problems

Shannon LF: Insulin usage in the neonate, *Neonatal Network* 6(5):31, 1988.

Inborn Errors of Metabolism

Aronson R *et al*: Growth in children with congenital hypothyroidism detected by neonatal screening, *J Pediatr* 116:33, 1990.

Berger LR: When should one discourage breast-feeding? *Pediatr* 67:300, 1981.

Burton BK: Inborn errors of metabolism: the clinical diagnosis in early infancy, *Pediatr* 79:359, 1987.

Coody D: Congenital hypothyroidism, *Pediatr Nurs* 10:342, 1984.

Kotzer AM, McCabe ERB: Newborn screening for inherited metabolic disease: principles and practice, *Neonatal Network* 6(4):15, 1988.

Rovet JF: Does breast-feeding protect the hypothyroid infant whose condition is diagnosed by newborn screening? *Am J Dis Child* 144:319, 1990.

60, 1989.

Phenylketonuria

Barnico LM, Cullinane MM: Maternal phenylketonuria: an unexpected challenge, *MCN* 10:108, 1985.

Lott JW: PKU: a nursing update, *J Pediatr Nurs* 3:29, 1988.

Russell FF, Mills BC, Zucconi T: Relationship of parental attitudes and knowledge to treatment adherence in children with PKU, *Pediatr Nurs* 14:514, 1988.

Schor DP: Phenylketonuria and temperament in middle childhood, *Child Health Care* 14(3):163, 1986.

Thermoregulation

Haddock BJ, Merrow DL, Vincent PA: Comparisons of axillary and rectal temperatures in the preterm infant, *Neonatal Network* 6(5):67, 1988.

Mayfield SR *et al*: Temperature measurement in term and preterm neonates, *J Pediatr* 104:271, 1984.

Vaughlans B: Early maternal-infant contact and neonatal thermoregulation, *Neonatal Network* 8(5):19, 1990.

Feeding and Nutrition

Churella HR, Bachhuber WL, MacLean WC: Survey: methods of feeding low-birth-weight infants, *Pediatr* 76:243, 1985.

Moore AC: Total parenteral nutrition for infants, *Neonatal Network* 6(2):33, 1987.

2, 1983.

Tietjen SD: Starting an infant's IV, *AJN* 90(5):44, 1990.

Developmental Outcome

Bauchner H, Brown E, Peskin J: Premature graduates of the newborn intensive care unit: a guide to follow-up, *Pediatr Clin North Am* 35:1207, 1988.

Termini L *et al*: Reasons for acute care visits and rehospitalization in very low-birthweight infants, *Neonatal Network* 8(5):23, 1990.

Developmental Intervention

Barb SA, Lemons PK: The premature infant: toward improving neurodevelopmental outcome, *Neonatal Network* 7(6):7, 1989.

Lott JW: Developmental care of the preterm infant, *Neonatal Network* 7(4):21, 1989.

Rushton CH: Promoting normal growth and development in the hospital environment, *Neonatal Network* 4(6):21, 1986.

Family Support

Arenson J: Discharge teaching in the NICU: the changing needs of NICU graduates and their families, *Neonatal Network* 6(4):29, 47, 1988.

Censullo M: Home care of the high-risk newborn, *JOGNN* 15:146, 1986.

Edwards KA, Allen ME: Nursing management of the human response to the premature birth experience, *Neonatal Network* 6(5):82, 1988.

Harrison LL, Twardosz S: Teaching mothers about their preterm infants, *JOGNN* 15:165, 1986.

Johnson SH: The premature infant. In Johnson SH, editor: *Nursing assessment and strategies for the family at risk,* ed 2, Philadelphia, 1986, JB Lippincott.

Kelting S: Supporting parents in the NICU, *Neonatal Network* 4(6):14, 1986.

McCain GC: Family functionng 2 to 4 years after preterm birth, *J Pediatr Nurs* 5:97, 1990.

Mussell G *et al*: Use of live video transmission in the NICU, *Neonatal Network* 8(4):37, 1990.

Oehler JM: The very low-birthweight infant as an early social partner: exploring maternal reactions, expectations, and attitudes, *Neonatal Network* 9(2):79, 1990.

Smith SM: Primary nursing in the NICU: a parent's perspective, *Neonatal Network* 5(4):25, 1987.

Respiratory Conditions

Kleiber C, Hummel PA: Factors related to spontaneous endotracheal extubation in the neonate, *Pediatr Nurs* 15:347, 1989.

Perehudoff B: Newborn resuscitation in the delivery room, *J Perinat Neonatal Nurs* 3(2):81, 1989.

Turnage CS: Meconium aspiration syndrome, *J Perinat Neonatal Nurs* 3(2):69, 1989.

Bronchopulmonary Dysplasia

Adams D: Kasey's story, *Neonatal Network* 7(3):19, 1988.

Jackson DF: Nursing care plan: home management of children with BPD, *Pediatr Nurs* 12:342, 1986.

McElheny JE: Parental adaptation to a child with bronchopulmonary dysplasia, *J Pediatr Nurs* 4:346, 1989.

Perry MA, Hayes NM: Bronchopulmonary dysplasia: discharge planning and complex home care, *Neonatal Network* 7(3):13, 1988.

Sepsis

Amspacher KA: Necrotizing enterocolitis: the never-ending challenge, *J Perinat Neonatal Nurs* 3(2):58, 1989.

Larson E: Trends in neonatal infections, *JOGNN* 16(6):404, 1987.

Walsh M, Kliegman RM: Necrotizing enterocolitis: treatment based on staging criteria, *Pediatr Clin North Am* 33:179, 1986.

Cardiovascular Conditions

Dooley KJ: Management of the premature infant with a patent ductus arteriosus, *Pediatr Clin North Am* 31:1159, 1984.

Dudell GG, Gersony WM: Patent ductus arteriosus in neonates with severe respiratory disease, *J Pediatr* 104:915, 1984.

Lawson M: Persistent pulmonary hypertension of the newborn: current trends in classification and diagnosis, *Neonatal Network* 6(1):27, 1987.

Stockman JA: Anemia of prematurity, *Pediatr Clin North Am* 33:111, 1986.

Retinopathy of Prematurity

An international classification of retinopathy of prematurity. II. The classification of retinal detachment, *Pediatr* 82:37, 1988.

Noerr B: Vitamin E (alpha-tocopherol), *Neonatal Network* 9(2):85, 1990.

Neurological Disturbances

Guzzetta F *et al*: Periventricular intraparenchymal echodensities in the premature newborn: critical determinant of neurologic outcome, *Pediatr* 78:995, 1986.

Kuban K, Teele RL: Rationale for grading intracranial hemorrhage in premature infants, *Pediatr* 74:358, 1984.

Painter MJ, Bergman I, Crumrine P: Neonatal seizures, *Pediatr Clin North Am* 33:91, 1986.

Conditions Related to Maternal Conditions

Kennard MJ: Cocaine use during pregnancy: fetal and neonatal effects, *J Perinat Neonatal Nurs* 3(4):53, 1990.

Chapter 14

Conditions Caused by Defects in Physical Development

LEARNING OUTCOMES

After studying this chapter you should be able to:

◆ Understand the importance of adequate analgesia in the neonate.
◆ Offer appropriate support to parents of an infant born with a physical defect and understand the differing reactions they may have.
◆ Discuss the different types of neural tube defect and their long-term treatment.
◆ Discuss the team approach to care of the child with cleft lip and palate.
◆ Understand the anatomy and physiology of congenital diaphragmatic hernia and why this condition has a high mortality.
◆ Discuss pre- and post-operative care of the child with oesophageal atresia.
◆ Define the glossary terms.

GLOSSARY

agenesis Absence of a body part caused by lack of primordial tissue

anomaly Marked deviation from the normal; anything structurally unusual, irregular, or contrary to a general rule

aplasia Absence of a body part caused by failure of the normal primordial tissue to develop

association A nonrandom occurrence of multiple malformations for which no specific or common aetiology has been identified

atrophy Decreased development of a mass of tissue or an organ as a result of a decrease in cell size or number

deformity Abnormal form, shape, or position of a part caused by mechanical forces

differentiation Process whereby embryonic cells acquire individual characteristics and function

dysplasia Abnormal organization of cells into tissue(s) and its morphologic result(s)

hyperplasia, hypoplasia Overdevelopment or underdevelopment of an organ or tissue that results from an increase or decrease in the number of cells

hypertrophy Increase in the size of organs, tissues, or cells

malformation Morphogenic defect of an organ, part of an organ, or larger region of the body resulting from an intrinsically abnormal developmental process

nociception Perception by nerve endings of traumatic or painful stimuli

pathogenesis Mechanisms leading to an abnormal structure, form, or function

syndrome A recognized pattern of malformations with a single, specific aetiology

teratogen A substance, agent, or process that interferes with normal prenatal development, producing one or more developmental abnormalities in the fetus

ongenital malformations constitute a large percentage of the health problems of infants and children. Although many severe disorders of childhood can be prevented or effectively treated, very little progress has been achieved in the prevention of congenital defects. Birth defects are detected in 20.5% of reported infant deaths, making birth defects the leading cause of infant mortality (OPCS, 1990).

DEFECTS IN PHYSICAL DEVELOPMENT

Congenital malformations may be caused by genetic or environmental factors. Not all congenital defects are considered to be malformations; for example, inborn errors of metabolism and mental disability. However, this chapter is primarily concerned with structural abnormalities (most of which are apparent at birth) and with their impact on the child and family.

BIRTH OF A CHILD WITH A PHYSICAL DEFECT

Parents are the most significant influence in the life of the child. The initial parent–infant attachment is the relationship on which future interactions are based. The birth of any child is considered by some to constitute a crisis situation, but when the newborn suffers from a physical or mental defect, the parents' need for understanding and supportive care from health professionals is magnified. The manner in which nurses and other health personnel work with the parents immediately after the birth profoundly influences this situation.

PARENTAL RESPONSES

Parents may experience shock, frustration, or anger at what has happened to them and may ask themselves, 'Why me?'. Despite reassurance that the cause of many congenital defects is unknown, the mother may still believe that something she has done or omitted to do during pregnancy has caused her baby's abnormality.

Parental reactions may be varied and may include guilt, anger, anxiety, and sadness, which often extend for years and which depend to a large extent on the type and severity of the defect. A gross, visible anomaly, especially one involving the face, usually elicits a more intense emotional response than one that is less apparent, such as a heart defect. The extent of the impairment cannot be used as a criterion to determine the degree of parental depressive reactions. Because of their limited contact with congenital defects, parents' perception of the abnormality and its implications may be distorted, and much depends on previous feelings they may have experienced with a similar abnormality. Therefore, their reactions may seem out of proportion to the actual extent and severity of the impairment as viewed by health professionals.

Supplying information
Parents need to have accurate, up-to-date information given to them early and in language they can understand. Since they do not hear all that is said the first time it is told to them, they want careful explanations about the child's defect, the treatments, and what will be expected of them. Parents often misinterpret information and therefore require repeated explanations. Often the nurse's responsibility is to explain, interpret, and clarify information that has been given by the doctor, and to answer questions. Following the basic concepts of interviewing, the nurse determines what the parents know and proceeds from that point. One cannot assume that the parents' failure to ask questions means they understand. Most parents have little or no knowledge of basic anatomy or physiology; therefore, pictures and other visual aids can be used effectively to explain both normal and deviant structures.

Numerous agencies and organizations offer services to families of children with congenital defects. Some provide services for a variety of defects; others are devoted to specific disorders. They help families with ongoing problems and with anticipating problems they will encounter in raising a child with a defect, including financial burdens. Many have local support groups. All have unique and specialized services to help support the family and to aid parents in solving problems.

NURSING CARE OF THE SURGICAL NEONATES

Advances in early detection of defects (including prenatal diagnosis), surgical techniques, and anaesthesia have made it possible for correction or amelioration of many physical defects in the newborn. Approximately 0.5–1% of newborn infants have anomalies that require surgery during the neonatal period, often as emergencies. Fortunately most are correctable with a high degree of success, even those that are dramatic in their presentation.

PREOPERATIVE CARE

Most of the problems encountered in infants undergoing surgery have been discussed in relation to the high-risk infant (e.g., airway maintenance, cardiovascular support, thermoregulation, fluid and electrolyte balance, and nutritional needs). Electronic monitoring of cardiovascular and respiratory status is implemented and maintained, as well as regular comprehensive assessments. Some congenital defects are often associated with other anomalies; therefore, assessment should include careful observation for evidence of these.

Fluid and electrolyte disturbances are corrected and the infant is stabilized before surgery. Prophylactic antibiotic administration may begin before surgery, and the infant is observed for any evidence of infection. In addition to routine care, special attention is directed to specific needs, such as abdominal decompression, management of open lesions, and specific measurements (e.g., abdominal girth, head dimensions).

POSTOPERATIVE CARE

Surgery imposes significant stresses on the neonate, especially the preterm or ill infant. The assessment and observations remain much the same as for preoperative care, with the additional problems related to surgery, such as anaesthesia and pain. It is essential to maintain physiological stability to avoid undesirable consequences (Rushton, 1988). Because the neonate is subject to many adverse effects of stress in all physiological parameters, continual vigilance is mandatory.

Because of the respiratory characteristics of the newborn, some compromising responses may be anticipated. The newborn's poor chest wall stability, smaller and more reactive airways, fewer and smaller alveoli, and poorly developed accessory muscles contribute to respiratory dysfunction. Compression by intrapleural fluid, air, or blood, or a distended abdomen can further compromise pulmonary efforts. Respiratory distress is a common problem in preterm infants. Many postoperative neonates require mechanical ventilation, which may be further influenced by the type, duration, and urgency of the surgery. Neonates are highly subject to acidosis and hypoxia, and require continuous monitoring of oxygen levels.

Cardiovascular support is of particular importance because the immature sympathetic innervation of the myocardium makes the neonate particularly sensitive to vagal stimulation induced by many postoperative procedures, such as nasogastric (NG) tubes, endotracheal (ET) tubes, and suctioning (Rushton, 1988). The infant may be given atropine preoperatively to block these responses. Any evidence of early compensation for diminished cardiac output is noted and interventions are implemented before decompensation occurs.

Careful management of fluid and electrolyte status is vital to surgical care. The natural tendency for rapid fluid shifts related to characteristics of the neonate may be aggravated by stress and any abnormal losses associated with some surgical procedures.

NEONATAL PAIN

It had previously been believed that the nerve pathways of newborn infants were not sufficiently myelinated to transmit painful stimuli, that the infant did not possess sufficiently integrated cortical function to interpret or recall pain experiences, and that the risk of anaesthesia was too great to justify any possible benefit of pain relief (Anand and Hickey, 1987; Shapiro, 1989). Consequently, invasive procedures (including some types of surgery) were performed on infants without anaesthesia. This traditional view has been refuted by several research studies which indicate that infants, both preterm and full term, perceive and react to pain in much the same manner as children and adults. Evidence indicates that pain pathways, cortical and subcortical centres needed for pain perception, and neurochemical systems associated with pain transmission and modulation are intact and functional in the neonate. Slower conduction speed is offset by shorter interneuron distances travelled by the impulse (Anand and Hickey, 1987).

Pain perception has both physiological and psychological components, and it is accepted that newborns recognize and respond to painful stimuli. However, because pain is a sensation with strong emotional associations, it is difficult to differentiate between pain perception and nociceptive activity

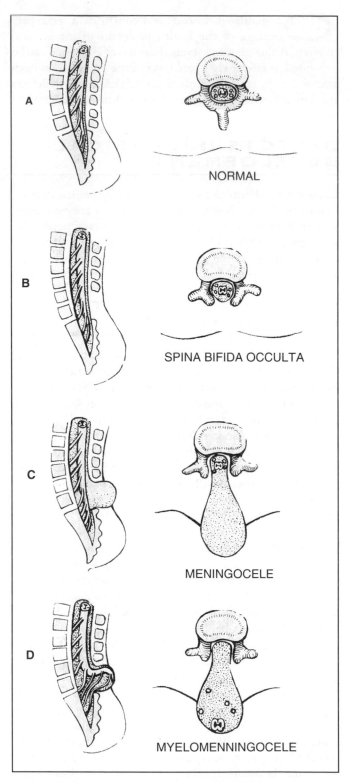

Fig. 14-1 Midline defects of osseous spine with varying degrees of neural herniations. **A**, Normal. **B**, Spina bifida occulta. **C**, Meningocele. **D**, Myelommeningocele.

in neonates. Consequently, the term *nociception* (the perception by nerves of injurious influences or painful stimuli) is frequently used to discuss pain in the neonate.

It has also been found that neonates release endorphins in response to stress and that the supply may become depleted (Hindmarsh, Sankaran, and Watson, 1984). It is now recommended that infants receive appropriate analgesia or anaesthesia for potentially painful procedures. Relatively safe local or systemic pharmacological agents are available to permit anaesthesia or analgesia to neonates and are indicated for those undergoing surgical procedures. Local anaesthetic techniques can suppress stress responses better than opioids by blocking the nerves carrying nonreceptive impulses.

Other effects of pain may include increased wakefulness and irritability, as well as alterations in feeding, vomiting, loss of appetite, and loss of interest in or energy for sucking. Interruptions in sleep–wake patterns, behavioural states, and parent–infant interactions also occur and may interfere with recovery from surgery (Shapiro, 1989).

PAIN ASSESSMENT

Assessment of pain in the preverbal child is difficult, especially in the neonate, because evaluative tools and verbal responses do not apply. Evaluation must be based on physiological changes and behavioural observations. Although behaviours including vocalisations, facial expressions, body movements, and general state are common to all infants, they vary with different situations. Crying associated with pain is more intense and sustained. Facial expression is the most consistent characteristic, and most infants respond with increased body movements. However, the infant may be experiencing pain even when lying quietly with eyes closed (Shapiro, 1989). Nursing assessment for evidence of pain is indicated any time the infant suffers tissue damage.

PAIN MANAGEMENT

Nonpharmacological measures may be used to alleviate pain and are essentially comforting measures. They are not a substitute for analgesia, but can be used to calm a distressed neonate. These include repositioning, swaddling, containment, cuddling, rocking, music, reducing environmental stimulation, tactile comfort measures, and non-nutritive sucking.

Morphine is the most widely used narcotic analgesic for pharmacological management of neonatal pain, with fentanyl as an effective alternative (Maguire and Maloney, 1988). Fentanyl is also used as an anaesthetic during surgery, especially in the preterm, low-birth-weight infant (Anand, Sippell, and Aynsley-Green, 1987; Collins *et al.*, 1985).

FAMILY SUPPORT

Parents are universally concerned that their infants are suffering pain during procedures. Nurses need to address these concerns and encourage the parents to speak with the professionals involved. It is important that parents are aware that nurses are sensitive to the infant's pain and are reassured that the infant will not suffer unduly (Shapiro, 1989).

MALFORMATIONS OF THE CENTRAL NERVOUS SYSTEM

Defects of the central nervous system (CNS) are usually the result of embryological developmental failures. Some can be attributed to genetic factors; others may be a result of postnatal infections. However, in most cases the aetiology is obscure. The defects discussed in this section are abnormalities of neural tube closure and hydrocephalus, which is characterized by an increase of free fluid in the cranial cavity.

DEFECTS OF NEURAL TUBE CLOSURE

Abnormalities that are derived from the embryonic neural tube (neural tube defects [NTDs]) constitute the largest group of congenital anomalies that is consistent with multifactorial inheritance. Normally the spinal cord and cauda equina are encased in a protective sheath of bone and meninges (Fig. 14-1A). Failure of neural tube closure produces defects of varying degrees. They may involve the entire length of the neural tube or may be restricted to a small area.

SPINA BIFIDA OCCULTA

Noncystic SB is failure of the spinous processes to join posteriorly in the lumbosacral area (L5 and S1). Routine radiographic examinations indicate that the disorder is quite common, but it may not be apparent unless there are associated cutaneous manifestations or neuromuscular disturbances. The incidence is estimated to occur in up to 25% of younger children, in whom there is eventual fusion of the vertebral arches, and in approximately 5–10% of the US population (Scarff and Fronczak, 1981).

Superficial indications include a skin depression or dimple, port-wine angiomatous naevi, dark tufts of hair, or soft, subcutaneous lipomas. These signs may be absent, appear singly, or be present in combination.

Neuromuscular disturbances are not uncommon in children with SB occulta and usually consist of progressive disturbance of gait with foot weakness and/or bowel and bladder sphincter disturbances. The usual cause is abnormal adhesion, or *tethering*, to a bony or fixed structure, resulting in traction on the spinal cord and cauda equina. Manifestations may not be evident during periods of slow growth, but tend to arise during periods of rapid growth, especially during the adolescent growth spurt at the end of the first decade and beginning of the second decade of life (Anderson, 1989). Therefore, the progress of these children is followed by the paediatrician.

Plain radiography is employed to disclose the precise bony defect in the symptomatic lesion and to establish the diagnosis in the suspected, nonsymptomatic occult variety.

MYELOMENINGOCELE (MENINGOMYELOCELE)

The cystic defect myelomeningocele affects about 1.7 of every 1000 live births (OPCS, 1990), but the incidence varies throughout the country. It accounts for 90% of spinal cord lesions, and may be located at any point along the spinal column. Usually, the sac is encased in a fine membrane that is prone to tears through which cerebrospinal fluid leaks. In other instances the sac may be covered by dura, meninges, or skin, in which instances there is rapid and spontaneous epithelialization. Since the lumbar segment is the last portion of the neural tube to close, the largest number of myelomeningoceles is found in the lumbar or lumbosacral area (Fig. 14-2).

The anomaly most frequently associated with myelomeningocele is hydrocephalus; and 90–95% of children with SB have hydrocephalus (Anderson, 1989). In myelomeningocele, obstruction to cerebrospinal fluid (CSF) is caused by downward displacement of the brainstem and cerebellum through the foramen magnum secondary to a defect known as the *Arnold-Chiari malformation (ACM)*, usually type II. In most cases hydrocephalus is apparent at birth; in other children it appears shortly thereafter.

CLINICAL MANIFESTATIONS

The manifestations of SB vary widely according to the degree of the spinal defect. The degree of neurological dysfunction is directly related to the anatomic level of the defect and thus the nerves involved. Sensory disturbances usually parallel motor dysfunction.

Defective nerve supply to the bladder affects both sphincter and detrusor tone, which often causes constant dribbling of urine or produces overflow incontinence in childhood. However, some infants void in a stream. Frequently, there is poor anal sphincter tone and poor anal skin reflex, which result in lack of bowel control and sometimes rectal prolapse. If the defect is located below the third sacral vertebra, there is no motor impairment, but there may be saddle anaesthesia with bladder and anal sphincter paralysis.

Sometimes the denervation to the muscles of the lower extremities will produce joint deformities *in utero*. These are primarily flexion or extension contractures, talipes valgus or varus contractures, kyphosis, lumbosacral scoliosis, and hip dislocations. The extent and severity of these associated deformities again depend on the degree of nerve involvement. Most flexion deformities result from the pull of stronger, fully innervated muscles acting without the counterpull of their nonfunctioning paralysed antagonists.

Antenatal diagnosis

It is possible to determine the presence of some major open NTDs prenatally. Ultrasonic scanning of the uterus and elevated concentrations of alpha-fetoprotein (AFP), a fetal-specific gamma-1 globulin, in amniotic fluid may indicate the presence of anencephaly or myelomeningocele. The optimum time for performing these diagnostic tests is between 16 and 18 weeks of gestation before AFP concentrations normally diminish. Testing is offered to all pregnant women.

THERAPEUTIC MANAGEMENT

Management of the child who has a myelomeningocele requires a multidisciplinary approach involving the specialities of neurology, neurosurgery, paediatrics, urology, orthopaedics, occu-

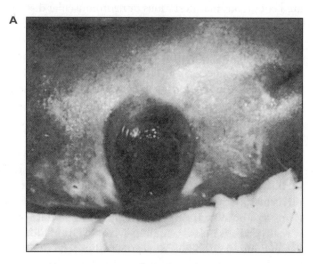
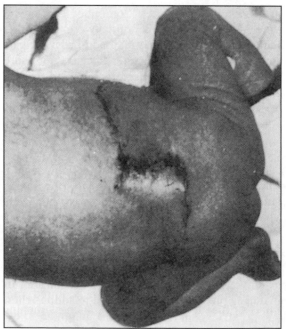

Fig. 14-2 A, Meningomyelocele before surgery. (An antibacterial dressing was used.) **B**, Repair of same patient. (Courtesy of MC Gleason, MD, San Diego, CA. From Ingallus AJ, Salerno MC: *Maternal and child health nursing*, ed 6 St Louis, 1987, Mosby–Year Book, Inc.)

pational therapy, and physiotherapy, as well as intensive nursing care in a variety of specialty areas. The collaborative efforts of these specialists are focused on: (1) the myelomeningocele and the problems associated with the defect, including hydrocephalus, paralysis, orthopaedic deformities, and genitourinary abnormalities; (2) possible acquired problems that may or may not be associated, such as meningitis, hypoxia, and haemorrhage; and (3) other abnormalities, such as cardiac or gastrointestinal malformations.

Infancy

Initial care involves prevention of infection, neurological assessment, including observation for associated anomalies, and dealing with the impact of the anomaly on the parents. Although meningoceles are repaired early, especially if there is danger of rupture of the sac, the philosophy regarding skin closure of myelomeningocele varies radically. Most authorities believe that early closure, within the first 24–48 hours, offers the most favourable outcome, especially with regard to morbidity and mortality from serious infection. Delay is thought to be beneficial by some because early closure contributes to the development of hydrocephalus by reducing the absorptive surface provided by the meningocele (Linder *et al.*, 1984).

The objective of the surgical procedure is satisfactory skin coverage of the lesion and meticulous closure. Wide excision of the large membranous covering may damage functioning neural tissue. Where the skin over the defect is intact, as often occurs with meningocele, surgical intervention may be performed to prevent tethering of the spinal cord.

Associated problems are assessed and managed by appropriate surgical and supportive measures. Shunt procedures provide relief from imminent or progressive hydrocephalus. Meningitis, urinary tract infection, and pneumonia are treated with vigorous antibiotic therapy and supportive measures.

Outcome

The early prognosis for the child with myelomeningocele depends on the neurological deficit present at birth, including motor ability and bladder innervation, and the presence of associated cerebral anomalies. Early surgical repair of the spinal defect, antibiotic therapy to reduce the incidence of meningitis and ventriculitis, and correction of hydrocephalus have significantly increased the survival rate.

Improved surgical techniques do not alter the major physical disability and deformity, or chronic urinary tract and pulmonary infections, that affect the quality of life for these children. Superimposed on these physical problems are the effects that the disorder has on family life and finances, and on schooling because of frequent hospital attendances.

Orthopaedic considerations

Musculoskeletal problems that will affect later locomotion are evaluated, and treatment, where indicated, is instituted in coordination with the activities of the surgeon. Casting, bracing, traction, and surgical techniques for correction of hip, knee, and foot deformities are employed when they may aid later ambulation. The minimum degree of future disability can usually be ascertained, although the maximum degree of disability is impossible to predict.

Management of genitourinary function

Myelomeningocele is one of the most common causes of neuropathic (or neurogenic) bladder impairment in childhood, and the prognosis for children who survive the early hazards of meningitis and hydrocephalus ultimately depends on the severity of their renal disease. Not only does renal failure pose a threat to life, but the lack of bladder control is important to the development of self-image and the social acceptability of the child. Since the majority of these children suffer from incontinence and are subject to recurrent or persistent pyuria, prevention and treatment of renal complications are a constant goal.

In children with myelomeningocele, decreased bladder tone produces the *flaccid* bladder with incomplete emptying. Increased tone causes a *spastic* bladder in which there are uninhibited bladder contractions. When coordination is faulty, high intravesical pressure may be created, predisposing the bladder to vesicoureteric reflux and incomplete emptying. The residual urine predisposes to infection, and the vesicoureteric reflux can lead to hydronephrosis. This combination can cause progressive renal damage and eventual renal failure.

Treatment of renal problems includes regular follow up with periodic imaging studies of the kidneys and bladder, with prompt and vigorous treatment of infections. Regular emptying of the bladder is established by a variety of means. Clean intermittent catheterization (CIC) can be performed easily by parents and self-catheterization can be taught successfully to children as young as four to six years of age. Although many children achieve dryness for two hours or more with CIC, the technique is not successful for others.

Medications are often used to improve bladder storage and continence.

When continence cannot be attained by CIC and medication, surgical intervention may be necessary. Surgical procedures include implantation of an artificial urinary sphincter, bladder augmentation, creating a continent ileal reservoir (Kropp procedure), or creating a urinary diversion, such as ureteroileostomy, ureterostomy, or cystostomy.

Bowel control

Some degree of faecal continence can usually be achieved in most children with myelomeningocele through diet modification, regular toilet habits, and prevention of constipation and impaction. It is frequently a lengthy process. Medications that increase stool firmness and decrease peristalsis often help when used in conjunction with other methods. Degree of continence varies, but in one study only 24% were reliably clean and dry (Malone *et al.*, 1994).

IMPLICATIONS FOR NURSING

Care of the infant or child with myelomeningocele requires both immediate and long-term nursing and medical supervision. Long-term management involves an interdisciplinary team effort to help the child and family with the multitude of problems associated with this disability. The following discussion is limited to care of the infant.

Implementation

The basic needs of the infant with a myelomeningocele are essentially the same as for any newborn infant. Special needs related to the defect and potential complications are discussed in the following section.

Care of myelomeningocele sac

The infant is usually placed in an incubator or warmer so that temperature can be maintained without clothing or covers that might irritate the delicate lesion.

Before surgical closure, the myelomeningocele is prevented from drying by the application of a sterile, moist, nonadherent dressing over the defect. The moistening solution is usually sterile normal saline or Vaseline gauze. Dressings are changed frequently (every 2-4 hours), and the sac is closely inspected for leaks, abrasions, irritation, or any signs of infection. It must be carefully cleansed if it becomes soiled or contaminated. Most sacs rupture during delivery or transport, and any opening in the sac greatly increases the risk of infection to the CNS. If early surgical closure is not anticipated, special measures to toughen the skin or membrane may be indicated, but care must be taken to prevent a dressing from adhering to and damaging the sac.

The infant should be nursed in the prone position to minimize tension on the sac and the risk of trauma. Keeping the infant's head higher than his or her buttocks will help prevent contamination of the sac from urine or faeces. Soft rolls or sandbags can be used to keep the hips slightly flexed to decrease tension on the sac. A pad should be placed between the knees to counteract hip subluxation, and a small roll under the ankles to prevent aggravation of foot deformities.

General care

The use of nappies is contraindicated until the defect has been repaired and healing is well advanced or epithelialization has taken place. The padding beneath the nappy area is changed as needed to keep the skin dry and free of irritation. The majority of these infants dribble urine constantly. Those who do develop retention have an indwelling catheter placed or have gentle bladder expression. Since the bowel sphincter is frequently affected, there is continual passage of stool, often misinterpreted as diarrhoea, which is a constant irritant to the skin and a source of infection to the spinal lesion. A protective drape is applied to minimize stool contamination of the lesion.

Areas of sensory and motor impairment are subject to skin breakdown and therefore require meticulous care. Placing the infant on a soft foam or fleece pad reduces pressure on the knees and ankles. Changing linen is best accomplished by two persons — one changes the linen while the other holds the infant, ensuring that the spine is maintained in good alignment without tension in the area of the defect.

Gentle range of motion exercises are sometimes carried out to prevent contractures, and stretching of contractures is performed when indicated. However, these exercises may be restricted to the foot, ankle, and knee joint. Where the hip joints are unstable, stretching against tight hip flexors or adductor muscles, which act much like bowstrings, may aggravate a tendency towards subluxation. A physiotherapist will advise on appropriate care.

With careful positioning, infants can be held for feeding and cuddles. Parents may be anxious that they are hurting the baby, but should be reassured that they and the baby will benefit from the contact.

Postoperative care

Postoperative care of the infant with myelomeningocele involves the same basic care as that of any postsurgical infant- monitoring vital signs, monitoring intake and output, nourishment, and observation for signs of infection, such as elevated temperature (axillary), irritability, lethargy, and nuchal rigidity. Wound management is carried out according to the directions of the surgeon, and general care is continued as preoperatively.

The prone position is maintained after operative closure, although many surgeons allow a side-lying or partial side-lying position unless it aggravates a coexisting hip dysplasia or permits undesirable hip flexion.

Over the next week, sensory and motor charting is repeated by a physiotherapist. The head circumference is measured daily, the fontanelles are examined for signs of tension or bulging, and skull ultrasound is repeated to check for increasing hydrocephalus. The infant is also assessed for urine retention. Although it may not have been a problem preoperatively, swelling around the operative site may cause transient urine retention, which resolves in 1–2 days.

Family support and home care

As soon as the parents are able to cope with the infant's condition, they are encouraged to become involved in care. They need to learn how to continue at home the care that has been initiated in the hospital — positioning, feeding, skin care, and range of motion exercises when appropriate. The family needs to know the signs of complications and how to reach assistance when needed. In cases in which the defect has not been repaired, they are taught to care for the lesion.

It is important for the family to understand the level and nature of sensory deficit in a child with a spinal defect. The child will be insensitive to pressure or other sources of tissue injury. Therefore, the family must be alert to hot or cold items that could cause thermal injury to tissues and to inspect the skin regularly for signs of pressure, especially over bony prominences. Because of sensory impairment, the child is unaware of bladder discomfort; therefore, signs of urinary tract infections may be easily overlooked. Urinary tract infection is often considered when the child becomes ill.

Prognosis

Long-range planning with, and support of, the parents and

child begin in the hospital and extend throughout childhood and beyond. The child may need numerous hospitalizations over the years, and each one will be a source of stress to which the younger child is especially vulnerable.

The Association for Spina Bifida and Hydrocephalus (ASBAH, see Useful Addresses) is organized to provide services and support for families of children with spinal lesions. Special reading materials are also available from them.

ANENCEPHALY

Anencephaly, the most serious NTD, is a congenital malformation in which both cerebral hemispheres are absent. The condition is incompatible with life, and most affected infants are stillborn. For those who survive, no specific treatment is available. The infants have intact brainstems and are able to maintain vital functions (such as temperature regulation and cardiac and respiratory function) for a few hours to several days, but eventually die of respiratory failure (Erlen and Holzman, 1988). Traditionally, these infants have been provided comfort measures, but with no effort at resuscitation.

HYDROCEPHALUS

Hydrocephalus is a condition caused by an imbalance in the production and absorption of CSF in the ventricular system. When production is greater than absorption, CSF accumulates within the ventricular system, usually under increased pressure, producing passive dilation of the ventricles. The disorder occurs in association with a number of anomalies.

Arnold–Chiari malformation is a brain defect involving posterior fossa contents. The type II malformation, seen almost exclusively with myelomeningocele, is characterized by caudal displacement of a small cerebellum, medulla, pons, and fourth ventricle into the cervical spinal canal through an enlarged foramen magnum. The resulting obstruction of CSF flow causes the hydrocephalus.

CLINICAL MANIFESTATIONS

The two factors that influence the clinical picture in hydrocephalus are the acuity of onset and the presence of pre-existing structural lesions. In infancy, before closure of the cranial sutures, head enlargement is the predominant sign, whereas in older infants and children the lesions responsible for hydrocephalus produce other neurological signs through pressure on adjacent structures.

Infancy

In infants, the head grows at an abnormal rate, although the first signs may be bulging fontanelles without head enlargement. The anterior fontanelle is tense, often bulging, and nonpulsatile. Scalp veins are dilated and markedly so when the infant cries. With the increase in intracranial volume, the bones of the skull become thin and the sutures become palpably separated to produce the 'cracked-pot' sound (MacEwen sign) on percussion

of the skull. There may be frontal enlargement or 'bossing' with depressed eyes and a 'setting-sun' sign, in which the sclera is visible above the iris because of pressure on a thinned orbital roof or the third ventricle on the tectum of the mesencephalon. Pupils are sluggish with unequal response to light.

The infant is irritable and lethargic, and may display changes in level of consciousness, opisthotonos (often extreme), and lower extremity spasticity. The infant will cry when picked up or rocked and quieten when allowed to lie still. Early infantile reflex acts may persist, and normally expected responses fail to appear, indicating failure in the development of normal cortical inhibition. However, these severe symptoms are seldom seen, as hydrocephalus rarely progresses to this stage without detection.

If hydrocephalus is allowed to progress, development of lower brainstem functions is disrupted, as manifested by difficulty in sucking and feeding, and a shrill, brief, high-pitched cry. Even if the infant's long-term prognosis is poor, a shunt is inserted as a palliative measure to facilitate care.

Childhood

The signs and symptoms in early to late childhood are caused by increased intracranial pressure(ICP), and specific manifestations are related to the focal lesion. Most commonly resulting from posterior fossa neoplasms and aqueduct stenosis, the clinical manifestations are primarily those associated with space-occupying lesions; that is, headache on awakening with improvement following emesis or upright posture; papilloedema; strabismus; and extrapyramidal tract signs such as ataxia (see Chapter 31). As with infants, the child will be irritable, lethargic, apathetic, confused, and often incoherent. In one of the congenital defects with later onset, the Dandy–Walker syndrome, characteristic manifestations are bulging occiput, nystagmus, ataxia, and cranial nerve palsies.

PROCESS OF DIAGNOSIS

In infancy, the diagnosis of hydrocephalus is based on increasing head circumference and on associated neurological signs that are present and progressive. Routine daily head circumference measurements are carried out in infants with myelomeningocele and intracranial infections. In the evaluation of a premature infant, specially adapted head circumference charts are consulted to distinguish abnormal head growth from rapid head growth that takes place normally.

The primary diagnostic tools for detecting hydrocephalus are skull ultrasound, computed tomography (CT), and magnetic resonance imaging (MRI). In older children sedation is required, since the child must remain absolutely still for an accurate picture. Diagnostic evaluation of children who have symptoms of hydrocephalus after infancy is similar to that employed in those with a suspected intracranial tumour. Sometimes isotope ventriculograms are used to assess the flow and patency of existing shunts and to check the size of the ventricles.

Problems in differential diagnosis are related to the child whose head circumference is greater than the 97th percentile, but whose head growth parallels the normal growth curve. It is sometimes valuable to measure parental occipitofrontal circumference (OFC) to detect a possible normal familial characteristic (benign familial megalencephaly).

THERAPEUTIC MANAGEMENT

The treatment of hydrocephalus is directed towards: (1) relief of the hydrocephalus, (2) treatment of complications, and (3) management of problems related to the effect of the disorder on psychomotor development. The treatment is, with few exceptions, surgical.

Medical therapy has been largely disappointing. Many newborn infants with progressive cranial enlargement secondary to intracranial haemorrhage demonstrate spontaneous stabilization and resolution. Serial lumbar punctures and medications have been used with varying success. The administration of acetazolamide and isosorbide has proved beneficial in decreasing the production of CSF in selected cases of slowly progressive disease. The medication reduces the ICP until spontaneous arrest of hydrocephalus takes place or as a temporizing measure when surgery is contraindicated.

Surgical treatment

Improved techniques have established surgical treatment as the therapy of choice in almost all cases of hydrocephalus. This is accomplished by direct removal of an obstruction, for example, resection of a neoplasm, cyst, or haematoma or, in rare instances of fluid overproduction, by choroid plexus extirpation (plexectomy or electric coagulation). However, most children require a shunt procedure that provides primary drainage of the CSF from the ventricles to an extracranial compartment, usually the peritoneum.

Most shunt systems consist of a ventricular catheter, a flush pump, a unidirectional flow valve, and a distal catheter. All are radiopaque for easy visualization after placement, and all are tested for accuracy before insertion. A reservoir is frequently added to allow direct access to the ventricular system for administration of medications and removal of fluid. In all models, the valves are designed to open at a predetermined intraventricular pressure and close when the pressure falls below that level, thus preventing backflow of secretions. High-pressure valves are used to prevent complications from rapid decompression of the ventricles. Medium-pressure valves are used in most children, especially those with long-standing hydrocephalus. Low-pressure valves are used in small infants. Some models also have an on/off mechanism.

The preferred procedure is the ventriculoperitoneal (VP) shunt, especially in neonates and young infants (Fig. 14-3). There is greater allowance for excess tubing, which minimizes the number of revisions needed as the child grows. Since it requires repeated lengthening, the ventriculoatrial (VA) shunt (ventricle to right atrium) is reserved for older children who have attained most of their somatic growth and for children with abdominal pathology. The VA shunt is contraindicated in children with cardiopulmonary disease or elevated CSF protein.

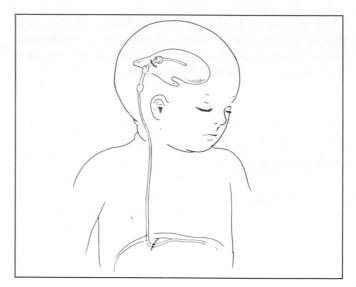

Fig. 14-3 Ventriculoperitoneal shunt. Catheter is threaded beneath the skin.

The initial shunt is placed when indicated on the basis of individual assessment. There is wide variation in the time of revisions. In most instances, revisions are performed when physical signs indicate shunt malfunction. Sometimes revisions are planned for specific times during development. In all mechanisms, the initial success rate is relatively high; however, shunts are associated with complications that interfere with continued shunt function or that threaten the life of the child.

Complications

The major complications of VP shunts are infection and malfunction. All shunts are subject to mechanical difficulties, such as kinking, plugging, or separation and migration of tubing. Malfunction is most often caused by mechanical obstruction either within the ventricles from particulate matter (tissue or exudate) or at the distal end from thrombosis or displacement as a result of growth. The child with a shunt obstruction often presents as an emergency with clinical manifestations of increased ICP, frequently accompanied by worsening neurological status.

The most serious complication, shunt infection, can occur at any time, but the period of greatest risk is 1-2 months following placement. The infection is generally the result of intercurrent infections at the time of shunt placement. Infections include septicaemia, bacterial endocarditis, wound infection, shunt nephritis, meningitis, and ventriculitis. Meningitis and ventriculitis are of greatest concern, since any complicating CNS infection is a significant predictor of intellectual outcome. Infection is treated with massive doses of antibiotics administered by the intravenous route. A persistent infection requires removal of the shunt until the infection is controlled. External ventricular drainage (EVD) is used until the CSF is sterile.

Prognosis

The prognosis of children with treated hydrocephalus depends largely on the rate at which hydrocephalus develops, the duration of raised ICP, the frequency of complications, and the cause of the hydrocephalus. For example, malignant tumours may have a high mortality regardless of other complicating factors.

IMPLICATIONS FOR NURSING

General nursing care of the infant with hydrocephalus may present special problems. Maintaining adequate nutrition often requires flexible feeding schedules to accommodate diagnostic procedures, since feeding before or after handling can precipitate an episode of vomiting. Small feedings at more frequent intervals are often better tolerated than larger ones spaced farther apart. These infants are often difficult to feed and require extra time and innovation.

The nurse is responsible for preparation of the child for diagnostic tests, such as tomography, and for assisting the doctor with procedures such as a ventricular tap (often performed to relieve excessive pressure during the preoperative period) and CSF examination. If surgery is anticipated, intravenous infusions should not be placed in a scalp vein.

Fortunately, almost all children with hydrocephalus are recognized, and treatment is begun early. For children with significant head enlargement, care must be exercised to see that the head is well supported when the infant is fed or moved, to prevent extra strain on the infant's neck, and measures must be taken to prevent development of pressure areas.

Postoperative care

In addition to routine postoperative care and observation, the infant or child is positioned carefully on the unoperated side to prevent pressure on the shunt valve and pressure areas. The child is kept flat to help avert complications resulting from too rapid a reduction of intracranial fluid. When the ventricular size is reduced too rapidly, the cerebral cortex may pull away from the dura and tear the small interlacing veins, producing a subdural haematoma. This is not a problem in children with elective shunt revision, since their intraventricular size and pressure have been normal. The surgeon indicates the position to be maintained and the extent of activity allowed. If there is increased ICP, the surgeon will prescribe the head of the bed to be elevated and/or allow the child to sit up to enhance gravity flow through the shunt. Sedation is avoided because the level of consciousness is an important observation.

Intake and output are carefully monitored. The intravenous infusion is closely monitored to prevent fluid overload. Routine feeding is resumed after the prescribed nil by mouth period, but the presence of bowel sounds is determined before feeding children with VP shunts.

Since infection is the greatest hazard of the postoperative period, nurses are continually on the alert for the usual manifestations of CSF infection, which may include elevated vital signs, poor feeding, vomiting, decreased responsiveness, and seizure activity. There may be signs of local inflammation at the operative sites and along the shunt tract. Antibiotics are administered by the intravenous route as ordered, and the nurse may also need to assist the doctor with intraventricular instillation. The incision site is inspected for leakage, and any suspected drainage is tested for glucose, an indication of CSF.

Meticulous skin care is continued postoperatively, with extra care taken to prevent tissue damage from pressure. A sheepskin pad/watermattress underneath the child helps prevent pressure on prominent areas. Skin is inspected regularly for any signs of pressure, irritation, or infection.

Family support

Often, parents have very little understanding of anatomy; therefore, they need further explanation and reinforcement of information that was given to them by the doctor and surgeon, as well as information about what they can expect. They are especially frightened of any procedure that involves the brain, and the fear of retardation or brain damage is very real and pervasive.

To prepare for the child's discharge and home care, the parents are instructed on how to recognize signs that indicate shunt malfunction or infection and how to pump the shunt and switch it off, if necessary. Active children may have accidents, such as a fall, that can damage the shunt, and the tubing may pull out of the distal insertion site or become disconnected during normal growth.

The management of hydrocephalus in a child is a demanding task for both family and health professionals, and helping a family cope with the child is an important nursing responsibility. Families can be referred to community agencies for support and guidance. ASBAH provides information, leaflets and local support for families.

CRANIAL DEFORMITIES

In the normal newborn, the cranial sutures are separated by membranous seams several millimetres wide. For the first few hours to 1–2 days after birth, the cranial bones are highly mobile, which allows them to mould and slide over one another, adjusting the circumference of the head to accommodate to the changing shape and character of the birth canal. The principal sutures in the infant's skull are the sagittal, coronal, and lambdoidal sutures, and the major soft areas at the juncture of these sutures are the anterior and posterior fontanelles.

Following birth, growth of the skull bones occurs in a direction *perpendicular* to the line of the suture, and normal closure occurs in a regular and predictable order. Although there are wide variations in the age at which closure takes place in individual children, solid union of all sutures is not completed until very late childhood. Normally, sutures and fontanelles are ossified by the following ages:

- 8 weeks — posterior fontanelle closed.
- 6 months — fibrous union of suture lines and interlocking of serrated edges.
- 18 months — anterior fontanelle closed.
- 12 years — sutures unable to be separated by ICP.

Closure of a suture before the expected time inhibits the perpendicular growth. Since normal increase in brain volume requires expansion, the skull is forced to grow in a direction *parallel* to the fused suture. This alteration in skull growth always produces a distortion of the head shape when the underlying brain growth is normal. The small head with closed and normal shape is the result of deficient brain growth; the suture closure is secondary to this brain growth failure. Failure of brain growth is not secondary to suture closure.

Various types of cranial deformities are encountered in early infancy. These include the enlarged head with frontal protrusion, or bossing, characteristic of hydrocephalus, the parietal bossing that is seen in chronic subdural haematoma, the small head, and a variety of skull deformities. Some occur during prenatal development; in others, head circumference is usually within normal limits at birth and the deviation from normal development becomes apparent with advancing age.

MICROCEPHALY

Primary microcephaly reflects a small brain and may be caused by an autosomal-recessive disorder, a chromosomal abnormality, or irradiation (especially between 4–20 weeks of gestation), maternal infection (notably toxoplasmosis, rubella, or cytomegalovirus), or chemical agents. *Secondary microcephaly* can result from a variety of insults that occur during the third trimester of pregnancy, the perinatal period, or early infancy. Infection, trauma, metabolic disorders, and anoxia are all capable of causing decreased brain growth and early closure of cranial sutures.

In both types, there appears to be a decided relationship between microcephaly and mental disability of varying degrees.

CRANIOSYNOSTOSIS (CRANIOSTENOSIS)

In craniosynostosis, suture closure is the primary defect. As a consequence, brain growth continues, and the clinical picture depends on which sutures close, the duration of the closure process, and the success or failure of the other sutures to compensate by expansion. The most common form is premature closure of the sagittal suture with resulting elongation of the skull in the anteroposterior direction. (A similar head shape is seen as a result of post-natal position maintenance in some premature infants.) Craniosynostosis causes some increase in ICP, and if uncorrected may or may not cause mental disability but can result in progressive papilloedema, optic atrophy, and eventual blindness.

THERAPEUTIC MANAGEMENT

Treatment, if any, involves surgical excision of long bars of bone along or parallel to the fused suture. Various surgical procedures are employed in an effort to release the fused suture and direct growth. Lining the bony margins of the suture with silicone, to delay closure, is infrequently used. Surgery is performed to achieve the best possible cosmetic effect and, in severe cases, to relieve cerebral pressure symptoms and complications. The advised timing of suture release is before six months of age for best cosmetic results.

IMPLICATIONS FOR NURSING

Nursing care is primarily observation for signs of haemorrhage or infection. Following cranial surgery, pressure bandages are applied and carefully maintained to reduce swelling. Providing emotional support to families is an important nursing function.

CRANIOFACIAL ABNORMALITIES

Craniofacial abnormalities are deformities involving the skull and facial bones. They have a low incidence rate in the population, but their effects can be psychologically devastating to affected children and their families. The disorders are compatible with life; therefore, unless they are corrected or modified, affected children go through their growing period under the burden of a grotesque, freak-like appearance often so severe that parents keep their children away from school, playmates, and sometimes even siblings (Koop, 1981).

THERAPEUTIC MANAGEMENT

Surgical correction of defects involves peeling the patient's face away from the skull and remoulding the understructures. Parts can be brought together, the skull reshaped, and pieces removed. The procedures are performed at various ages, depending on the anomaly, in centres specializing in this paediatric problem. The timing of surgery is determined on an individual basis to ensure normal growth and to occur before school entry. Depending on the abnormality, other surgeries are performed, such as mandibular and digit correction. Following surgery, continued growth conforming to the inborn abnormality is unlikely.

IMPLICATIONS FOR NURSING

A helmet is worn to protect the operative site and bone grafts for varying lengths of time, from six months to two years. Follow-up care is very important.

PLAGIOCEPHALY

Plagiocephaly is a rhomboid-shaped deformity that occurs in at least one of 300 live births and is rarely caused by brain malformation or unilateral suture stenosis (Clarren, 1981). The rapidly growing infant head is easily moulded by continued pressure against a surface, such as the uterine wall or a mattress. As a result, the skull is progressively flattened. There is usually a history of the infant lying on the flattened aspect of the head with limited head movement when lying down.

THERAPEUTIC MANAGEMENT

Surgical correction of cosmetically disfiguring plagiocephaly is performed according to the nature and extent of the deformity. A recent innovation involves application of a helmet constructed of polypropylene shaped normally but large enough to fit the largest diameter of the head. Treatment is begun at 4–10 months of age, and the helmet is worn until the head conforms to the shape of the helmet.

SKELETAL DEFECTS

The types and variations of deformity in developmental skeletal defects are numerous and display an equally diverse spectrum of physical disability. Some skeletal deformities constitute one or more of the manifestations associated with a syndrome; for example, the short extremities of the various forms of dwarfism, the long, thin extremities and sternal deformities of arachnodactyly (Marfan syndrome), and somatic defects in chromosomal aberrations. Many are isolated defects with hereditary (clawhand, polydactyly), environmental (thalidomide phocomelia or amelia), or multifactorial (congenital hip dysplasia) aetiology. This discussion is limited to defects in development that are most common, that are amenable to therapy, and that involve nurses to a considerable extent.

CONGENITAL HIP DYSPLASIA

The broad term *congenital hip dysplasia* describes imperfect development of the hip that can affect the femoral head, the acetabulum, or both. More commonly known as congenital hip dislocation (CHD) or congenital dislocated hip (CDH), the disorder is apparent at birth and displays various degrees of deformity. The condition is reversible with early treatment, but can rapidly progress to dislocation as the child begins to walk. The cause of hip dysplasia is unknown, but it is one of the most common congenital defects, with an incidence of about 5:1000 births (OPCS, 1990).

The disorder occurs more frequently in females than in males (5:2) and occurs 25–30 times more often in first-degree relatives than in the general population. The concordance in monozygotic twins is 40%, but only 3% in dizygotic twins, which suggests that genetic factors play a role in the aetiology. One-quarter of cases involve both hips, and when only one hip is involved, the left hip is affected three times more often than the right. Congenital diaphragmatic hernia is frequently associated with other conditions, such as SB.

CLINICAL MANIFESTATIONS

The diagnosis of congenital diaphragmatic hernia should be made in the newborn period if possible, since treatment initiated before two months of age achieves the highest rate of success. In the newborn period, dysplasia usually appears as hip joint laxity rather than as outright dislocation. Subluxation and the tendency to dislocate can be demonstrated by the Ortolani

(Fig. 14-4*D*) or Barlow tests. Barlow observed that 60% of unstable hips will be clinically normal by 1 week of age (Barlow, 1962), therefore immediate treatment may be postponed. Ultrasound is now a diagnostic aid and can also assess improvement once splinting is commenced (Clarke, 1994).

These tests are most reliable from birth to two months of age and must be performed by experienced operators to prevent fracture or other damage to the hip. For example, when these tests are performed too vigorously in the first two days of life, when the hip subluxates freely, persistent dislocation may occur (Cheetham *et al.*, 1983). Adduction contractures develop at about 6–10 weeks, and the Ortolani sign disappears. After this time, the most sensitive test is limited abduction (Fig. 14-4B). Other signs are shortening of the limb on the affected side *(Galleazzi sign, Allis sign)* (Fig. 14-4C), asymmetric thigh, and gluteal folds (Fig. 14-4A), and broadening of the perineum (in bilateral dislocation). Weight bearing may precipitate a transition from subluxation to dislocation in unrecognized cases. Often the disorder is not apparent at birth.

In the older infant and child the affected leg will be shorter than the other with telescoping or piston mobility, that is, the head of the femur can be felt to move up and down in the buttock when the extended thigh is pushed first toward the child's head and then pulled distally. Instability of the hip on weight bearing delays walking and produces a characteristic limp. When the child stands first on one foot and then on the other (holding onto a chair, rail, or someone's hands), bearing weight on the affected hip, the pelvis tilts downwards on the normal side instead of upwards as it would with normal stability. (*Trendelenburg sign*) (Fig. 14-4E). The practitioner should test the child for at least 30 seconds. In both unilateral and bilateral dislocations the greater trochanter is prominent and appears above a line from the anterosuperior iliac spine to the tuberosity of the ischium. The child with bilateral dislocations has marked lordosis and a peculiar waddling gait.

THERAPEUTIC MANAGEMENT

Treatment is begun as soon as the condition is recognized, since early intervention is more favourable to the restoration of normal bony architecture and function. The longer treatment is delayed, the more severe the deformity, the more difficult the treatment, and the less favourable the prognosis. The treatment varies with the age of the child and the extent of the dysplasia.

Newborn to six months

The hip joint is maintained by dynamic splinting in a safe position with the proximal femur centred in the acetabulum in an attitude of flexion. A variety of abduction devices are available for maintaining the femur in the acetabulum. Of these, the Pavlik harness is the most widely used device, and with time, motion, and gravity the hip works into a more abducted, reduced position (Fig. 14-5). The device is worn continuously until the hip is clinically and radiographically stable, usually about 3–6 months. It is highly effective when the device is well constructed, follow-up care is adequate, and the parents follow instructions in its use.

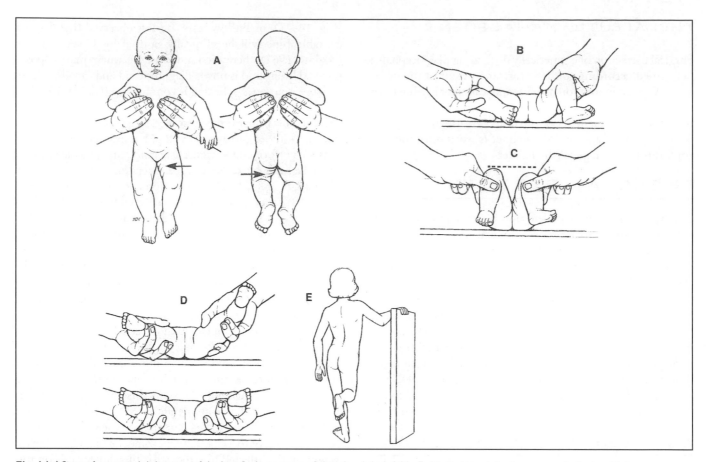

Fig. 14-4 Signs of congenital dislocation of the hip. **A**, Asymmetry of gluteal and thigh folds. **B**, Limited hip abduction, as seen in flexion. **C**, Apparent shortening of the femur, as indicated by the level of the knees in flexion. **D**, Ortolari click (if infant is under 4 weeks of age). **E**, Positive Trendelenburg sign or gait (if child is weight bearing).

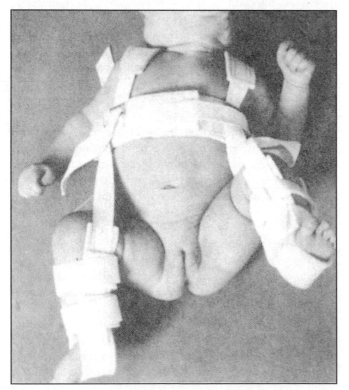

Fig. 14-5 Child in Pavlik harness.

When adduction contracture is present, other devices (such as skin traction) are employed to slowly and gently stretch the hip to full abduction, after which wide abduction is maintained until stability is attained. When there is difficulty in maintaining stable reduction, a hip spica cast is applied and changed periodically to accommodate the child's growth. After 3–6 months, sufficient stability is acquired to allow transfer to a removable protective abduction brace. The duration of treatment depends on development of the acetabulum, but is usually accomplished within the first year.

Six to eighteen months

In this age group, the dislocation is not recognized until the child begins to stand and walk, when attendant shortening of the limb and contractures of hip adductor and flexor muscles become apparent. Gradual reduction by traction is followed by plaster cast immobilization, which is maintained until radiographic examination confirms a stable joint. Often, soft tissue may obstruct and complicate reduction and subsequent joint development. In this case open reduction is performed to remove the obstruction, followed by postoperative spica cast immobilization and, later, replacement with an abduction splint.

Older child

Correction of the hip deformity in the older child is inherently more difficult than in the preceding age groups, because secondary adaptive changes and other aetiologic factors (such as juvenile rheumatoid arthritis or nonambulatory cerebral palsy) complicate the condition. Operative reduction, which may involve preoperative traction, tenotomy of contracted muscles, and any one of several innominate osteotomy procedures designed to construct an acetabular roof, is usually required. After cast removal and before weight bearing is permitted, range of motion exercises help restore movement. Next, rehabilitative measures are instituted. Successful reduction and reconstruction become increasingly difficult after the age of four years and are usually impossible or inadvisable after age six because of severe shortening and contracture of muscles, and deformity of the femoral and acetabular structures.

Family support, home care and nursing care

Casts and braces offer more challenging nursing problems, since they cannot be removed for routine care; however, sometimes the doctor allows a brace to be removed for bathing. Care of an infant or small child with a cast requires nursing innovation to reduce irritation and to maintain cleanliness of both the child and the cast, particularly in the nappy area. Parents are taught the proper care of the cast (or brace) and are helped to devise means for maintaining cleanliness and positioning the child for feeding, playing, and transport.

Generally, treatment and follow-up care of these children are carried out in a clinic or outpatient unit. Hospitalization may be necessary for cast application or brace fitting but seldom exceeds 24-48 hours. Longer hospitalization is required for open reduction or if the child is hospitalized for a concurrent illness.

CONGENITAL CLUBFOOT

Clubfoot is a general term used to describe a common deformity in which the foot is twisted out of its normal shape or position. Any foot deformity involving the ankle is called *talipes*, derived from *talus*, meaning ankle, and *pes*, meaning foot. Deformities of the foot and ankle are described according to the position of the ankle and foot.

The most frequently occurring type of clubfoot (approximately 95%) is the composite deformity talipes equinovarus (TEV), in which the foot is pointed downwards and inwards in varying degrees of severity (Fig. 14-6). Unilateral clubfoot is somewhat more common than bilateral clubfoot and may occur as an isolated defect or in association with other disorders or syndromes, such as chromosomal aberrations, arthrogryposis (a generalized immobility of the joints), or spina bifida.

The frequency of clubfoot in the general population is 1:1000 live births, with boys affected twice as often as girls. There is a 35% concordance in monozygotic twins as opposed to a 3% concordance in dizygotic twins, which indicates a hereditary component.

PROCESS OF DIAGNOSIS

The deformity is readily apparent and easily detected at birth. However, it must be differentiated from some positional deformities that can be passively corrected or overcorrected. The true clubfoot is fixed, whereas paralytic changes in the lower extremities of children with neuromuscular involvement often produce equinovarus deformity.

THERAPEUTIC MANAGEMENT

Treatment is begun as soon as the deformity is recognized and involves three stages: (1) correction of the deformity, (2) maintenance of the correction until normal muscle balance is regained, and (3) follow-up observation to avert possible recurrence of the deformity. Some feet respond to treatment readily, some respond only to prolonged, vigorous, and sustained efforts, and the improvement in others remains disappointing even with maximum effort on the part of all concerned.

Correction of TEV is most reliably accomplished by manipulation and the application of a series of casts or Denis Browne splints, begun immediately or shortly after birth and continued until marked overcorrection is reached (Fig. 14-7). Gradual stretching of tight structures on the medial side and gradual contraction of lax structures on the lateral side of the foot is achieved by manipulation and casting, or restrapping frequently (every few days for 1–2 weeks, then at 1- to 2-week intervals) in order to accommodate the rapid growth of early infancy. Because of

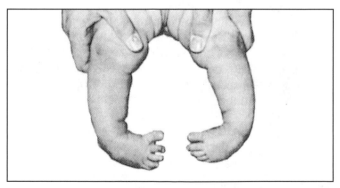

Fig. 14-6 Bilaterral *congenital talipes equinovarus* (congenital clubfoot) in 2-month-old infant. (From Broshearst Raney 1986.

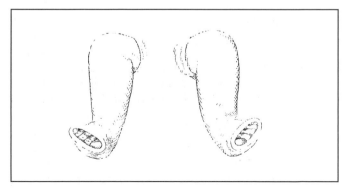

Fig. 14-7 Feet casted for correction of bilateral congenital talyses equinovarus. (From Brashear Raney 1986.

strong, thickened ligaments, cartilaginous anlages of the bone may become distorted. If manipulation is ineffective, surgical correction is performed to correct bony deformity, release tight ligaments, or lengthen or transplant tendons. The extremity or extremities are casted until the desired result is achieved.

IMPLICATIONS FOR NURSING

Parents need to understand the overall treatment programme, the importance of regular cast changes, and the role they play in the long-term effectiveness of the therapy. Reinforcing and clarifying the doctor's explanations and instructions, teaching parents about care of the cast or appliance, including vigilant observation for potential problems, and encouraging parents to facilitate normal development within the limitations imposed by the deformity or therapy are all part of nursing responsibilities.

SKELETAL LIMB DEFICIENCY

Congenital limb deficiencies, or reduction malformations, are manifest by a variety of degree of loss of functional capacity. They are characterized by underdevelopment of skeletal elements of the extremities. The range of malformation can extend from minor defects of the digits to serious abnormalities, such as *amelia*, absence of an entire extremity, or *meromelia*, partial absence of an extremity, which includes *phocomelia* (seal limbs), an intercalary deficiency of long bones with relatively good development of hands and feet attached at or near the shoulder or the hips.

In rare instances, prenatal destruction of limbs has been reported, but most reduction deformities are primary defects of development (agenesis, aplasia). Therefore, congenital 'amputations', in the literal sense, are not amputations, since nonexistent limbs cannot be amputated.

THERAPEUTIC MANAGEMENT

It is generally agreed that children with congenital limb deficiencies should be fitted with prosthetic devices whenever possible and that such a functional replacement should be applied at the earliest possible stage of development in an attempt to match the motor readiness of the infant. This favours natural progression of prosthetic use. For example, an infant with an upper extremity deficiency is fitted with a simple passive device, such as a mitten prosthesis, between three and six months of age when limb exploration is active, sitting is beginning with the extremities needed for support, and bilateral hand activities are to be encouraged. Lower limb prostheses are applied when the infant is ready to pull to a standing position. In preparation for prosthetic devices, surgical modification is often necessary to ensure the most favourable use of the device, since severe deformity can interfere with its effective use. Phocomelic digits are preserved for controlling switches of externally powered appliances in upper extremities. Digits (in both upper and lower extremities) provide the child

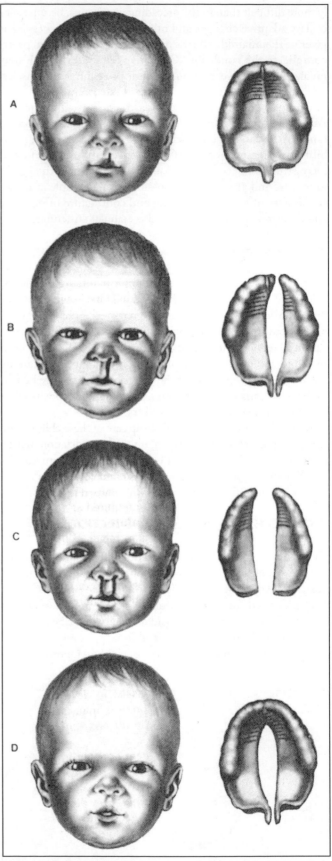

Fig. 14-8 Variations in clefts of lips and palate at birth. **A,** Notch in vermilion border. **B,** Unilateral cleft lip and palate. **C,** Bilateral cleft lip and cleft palate. **D,** Cleft palate.

with surfaces for tactile exploration and stimulation. Prostheses are replaced to accommodate growth and increasing capabilities of the child. REACH, the association for children with artificial arms, offers leaflets and support to parents and raises funds to promote research into new technology and discovering the causes of congenital limb deficiencies.

DISORDERS OF THE GASTROINTESTINAL TRACT

Congenital defects of the gastrointestinal (GI) tract can involve any portion from the mouth to the anus. Most are apparent at birth, or shortly after, and are anomalies in which normal growth ceased at a crucial stage of embryonic development, leaving the structure in an embryonic form or only partially completed.

Atresia is absence or closure of a normal body orifice. Closure at any point along the length of the GI tract creates an obstruction to the normal progress of nutrients and secretions. Most common anomalies are atresias of the oesophagus, intestine, and anus, requiring surgical intervention.

Other defects of development include *annular pancreas,* in which the head of the pancreas surrounds and constricts the second segment of the duodenum, and *malrotation of the colon,* in which associated structures remain in abnormal positions. For example, the caecum remains in the upper right quadrant and the posterior fixation of the mesentery is inadequate and allows twisting of the small intestine, or *volvulus,* to create an obstruction.

Obstruction can also be caused by *peritoneal bands* or *folds* that cross the duodenum as they attach the abnormally placed caecum to the right peritoneum. Thus, the duodenum is partially obstructed by the external pressure of the bands. In *meconium ileus* the intestine becomes obstructed by thick, inspissated, impacted meconium — the earliest manifestation of cystic fibrosis. *Congenital megacolon (Hirschsprung disease)* is caused by the absence or deficiency of innervation to the musculature of the rectum and distal colon, which inhibits propulsive peristalsis and creates a functional obstruction.

The diagnosis and management of most intestinal atresias and obstructions are similar to the diagnosis and management of intestinal obstruction from other factors, most of which are discussed in Chapter 27. The congenital defects considered in this chapter include abnormalities of the lip and palate, oesophagus, anus, and biliary tree. Biliary atresia is also considered here, because the liver is part of the digestive system, although the condition does not interfere with the passage of food.

CLEFT LIP AND/OR PALATE

Clefts of the lip and palate are facial malformations that are common to all human populations and constitute a severe handicap to the affected individual. The defects are classified into two major groups. The first includes those clefts that involve the lip and anterior maxilla, regardless of whether the defect involves the remaining portions of the hard and soft

---

◆ **BOX 14-1**

Cleft lip and /or palate

CL — clefts that involve the lip
CLP — clefts that involve the lip and palate
CL(P) — clefts that involve the lip with or without cleft palate
CP — clefts that involve the hard and soft palate only
CL/P — all types of clefts that involve the lip and/or palate

---

palate. The second group consists of clefts that involve only the hard and soft palate. Although there are differences in the severity and extent of deformities within each category, the terms and the abbreviations associated with these groups are defined in Box 14-1. The term *complete cleft* indicates the maximum degree of clefting.

Isolated CP is rarer than CL(P) and affects more females than males. The incidence of some form of clefting in the United Kingdom is 1:700 births.

PROCESS OF DIAGNOSIS

A cleft that involves the lip with or without cleft palate is readily apparent at birth and is one of the defects that elicit the most severe emotional reactions in parents. Incomplete fusion of the primary palate produces a variation in the degree of malformation (Fig. 14-8). Clefts of the lip may be unilateral or bilateral and may range from a notch in the vermilion border of the lip to complete separation extending to the floor of the nose.

Clefts of the palate may occur as an isolated defect or in association with cleft lip. Less obvious than cleft lip, the defect may not be detected without a thorough assessment of the mouth. The deformity can be identified by placing the examiner's fingers directly on the palate. Without a proper evaluation, the defect may not be detected until the infant has difficulty with initial feedings. As with cleft lip, the degree of deformity varies and may involve only the uvula or may extend through both the soft and hard palates to the incisive foramen. The isolated cleft palate occurs in the midline, but, when associated with cleft lip, the defect may involve the midline of the soft palate and extend into the hard palate on the side of the lip cleft or on both sides in bilateral clefts. Clefts of the hard palate form a continuous opening between the mouth and the nasal cavity. This creates special feeding problems. The infant is unable to develop suction because of the defect and has difficulty in swallowing. The open pathway must be closed in order to provide sufficient pressure for the swallowing sequence.

THERAPEUTIC MANAGEMENT

Treatment of the child with clefts involving the lip and palate involves the cooperative efforts of several specialists — paediatrician, nurses, plastic surgeon, orthodontist, prosthodontist, otolaryngologist, speech and language therapist, dietitian, and sometimes a psychiatrist. Treatment continues over a long time, but even after completion of a programme of health care, the child will probably retain defects of speech, facial appearance, or other problems related to the cleft. Management is directed towards closure of the cleft(s), prevention of complications, rehabilitation, and facilitation of normal growth and development of the child.

Surgical correction: cleft lip

Closure of the lip defect precedes that of the palate, although the optimum times for surgery are still being debated. Those who favour immediate repair of the lip argue that it makes the infant more acceptable to the parents before discharge from the hospital, thereby improving establishment of satisfactory parent–child relationships. Others prefer to wait until the infant shows a steady weight gain and a satisfactory haemoglobin level.

Improved surgical techniques have minimized deformity related to scar retraction, but good cosmetic results are difficult to obtain in defects that are more severe initially. In the absence of infection or trauma, healing takes place with little scar formation; however, in some instances the results are less than satisfactory from the parents' (and, later, the child's) viewpoint. Undesirable physical characteristics of the older child are residual nasal deformity, mildly protruding lower lip, and a somewhat flattened lower third of the upper lip, usually with an abnormally shaped red lip margin. Not infrequently, revisions may be required at a later age.

Surgical correction: cleft palate

Cleft palate repair is generally postponed until a later age than repair of the CL in order to take advantage of palatal changes that occur with normal growth. Since clefts vary considerably in size, shape, and degree of deformity, the timing of repair is individualized but is usually performed between one and two years of age, before the child develops faulty speech habits.

Implementation

The immediate nursing problems in the care of an infant with CL/P deformities are related to feeding the infant and dealing with the severe parental reaction to the defect. Facial deformities are particularly disturbing to parents, and parent–infant attachment may be negatively affected. A CL is the most disfiguring of the visible defects and generates strong negative responses in both nurses and parents. It is especially important for nurses to emphasize the positive aspects of the infant's physical appearance and to express optimism regarding surgical correction. Many surgeons have an album of 'before and after' photographs.

Feeding

Feeding the infant offers a special challenge to nurses. Clefts of lip or palate reduce the infant's ability to generate the suction required to compress the areola or teat and often renders both breast and bottle feeding difficult. Small, frequent feeds will prevent the baby becoming exhausted.

Contrary to previous thought, breastfeeding is possible if the mother perseveres and experiments with different positions. This is best accomplished with the child in the upright position with the nipple stabilized well back in the oral cavity so that the tongue action facilitates milk expression. As the suction required to stimulate the let down reflex may initially be absent, expressing by hand or with a breast pump before feeds may help.

Expressed breast milk or formula may also be given using a variety of teats and feeding devices. If these prove unsuccessful, spoon feeding or nasogastric feeding may be necessary to ensure good weight gain. Feeding devices have the advantage of helping to meet the infant's sucking needs and encouraging use of the sucking muscles. Muscle development is especially important for later speech development.

The parents should begin to feed the infant as soon as possible. In this way they are able to help determine the method best suited to them and the infant, and to become adept in the technique before the infant is discharged from hospital.

Preoperative care

In preparation for surgical repair, the parents are frequently instructed to accustom the infant to some of the needs of the early postoperative period, particularly if surgery is delayed several months. If they are to be used, it is also helpful to place the infant or child in arm restraints periodically before admission and, after admission, to feed the infant in the manner to be used postoperatively. No special formula is required, and the infant is usually allowed to eat up to about six hours preoperatively. Preoperative preparation, including medication, is determined by the surgeon and anaesthetist, and may include naseptin cream applied to the nostrils.

Postoperative care: cleft lip

The major efforts in the postoperative period are directed towards protecting the operative site. Before the infant leaves the operating room, the lip protective device (if used) or the butterfly closure is taped securely to the cheeks to relax the operative site and prevent tension on the suture line caused by crying or other facial movement. Arm restraints may be applied to prevent the infant from rubbing or otherwise disturbing the suture line. However, in many units the child is supervised for 24 hours and arms are left unrestrained, as experience has shown that an infant who is restrained will become agitated and difficult to console.

Feeding is essentially the same as before surgery. It is safe to offer clear liquids when the infant has fully recovered from the anaesthesia, and formula feeding is usually resumed when tolerated. The surgeon will specify any preferences or restrictions in feeding method. The mouth should be rinsed with water before and after each feeding. The method of care of the suture line is also determined by the surgeon and may vary.

A side-lying or partial side-lying position is helpful for the infant in the immediate postoperative period and for one who has difficulty in handling secretions. As with any infant, the child with cleft lip repair is placed on the right side after feedings to reduce the chance of aspirating regurgitated formula.

Preparation for discharge and home care

Parents are encouraged to participate in the care of the infant as soon as feasible following surgery. They can resume the pre-operative feeding method with the infant in a sitting position. The infant should be fed slowly and carefully and winded at frequent intervals.

Postoperative care: cleft palate

The child who has undergone an operation to repair CP is constantly supervised for 24 hours postoperatively. The child may be fed with a wide-bowl spoon (such as a soup spoon) or from the side of the spoon, with the nurse or parent taking care not to insert the spoon into the mouth where it might damage the suture line. Fluids are best taken from a cup.

Sometimes the child will have difficulty breathing following surgery, since it is often necessary to alter an established pattern of breathing and adjust to breathing through the nose. This is frustrating, but seldom requires more than positioning and support. Sometimes the infant or child is placed in a mist tent for a short period after surgery. Some surgeons place a single suture at the end of the tongue to facilitate extending the tongue if the airway should become obstructed. It is usually removed after the first 24 hours.

The child is usually discharged on a soft diet, which parents are instructed to continue until the surgeon directs them otherwise. They should be cautioned against allowing the child to eat hard items, such as toast, hard biscuits, or crisps, which could damage the newly repaired palate. The nurse might suggest that the parents not offer the child any food harder than mashed potatoes. The Cleft Lip and Palate Association (CLAPA, see Useful Addresses) offers support to parents and raises funds for research into the causes and treatment of CL and CLP.

OESOPHAGEAL ATRESIA WITH TRACHEO-OESOPHAGEAL FISTULA

Congenital oesophageal atresia (OA) and tracheo-oesophageal fistula (TOF) are rare malformations that represent a failure of the oesophagus to develop as a continuous passage and of the trachea and oesophagus to separate into distinct structures. These defects may occur as separate entities or in combination, and without early diagnosis and treatment they are rapidly fatal.

The incidence of OA and TOF is not known. Authorities in the United Kingdom have estimated the incidence to be 1:3000 live births. There appear to be no sex differences, but the birth weight of most affected infants is significantly lower than average and there is an unusually high percentage of prematurity. A history of maternal polyhydramnios is common, and approximately half the infants with oesophageal defects have associated anomalies, especially congenital heart disease, anorectal malformations, and genitourinary (GU) anomalies. The possibility of VACTER, an association of congenital defects (vertebral anomalies, anus-imperforate, cardiac anomalies, tracheo-oesophageal fistula, oesophageal atresia, renal/radial anomalies), should be considered in infants with OA and TOF.

There is little evidence to implicate heredity as a factor.

CLINICAL MANIFESTATIONS

The presence of OA is suspected in an infant with excessive salivation that is frequently accompanied by choking, coughing and sneezing. If fed, the infant swallows normally but suddenly coughs and struggles, and the fluid returns through the nose and mouth. The infant becomes cyanotic and may stop breathing as the overflow of fluid from the blind pouch is aspirated into the trachea or bronchus. The cyanosis is the result of laryngospasm, the protective mechanism that operates to prevent aspiration into the trachea, and, over time, respiratory distress develops.

In the infant with OA with a distal TOF (type III) the stomach becomes distended with air, and thoracic and abdominal compression (especially during crying) cause the gastric contents to be regurgitated through the fistula into the trachea, producing a chemical pneumonitis. When the upper segment of the oesophagus opens directly into the trachea (types II and IV), the infant is in danger of aspirating any swallowed material. Cyanosis or choking during feeding may be the only early symptom of type V (known as H type) fistula.

PROCESS OF DIAGNOSIS

To establish a diagnosis of OA, a catheter is gently passed into the oesophagus. It will meet with resistance if the lumen is blocked, but will pass unobstructed if the lumen is patent. A moderately stiff catheter is used to avoid coiling in the oesophageal pouch. Aspiration of stomach contents or auscultation over the stomach as air is introduced through the catheter confirms a patent oesophagus. Gastric lavage immediately after delivery, although not a universal practice, offers earlier diagnosis of OA.

Diagnosis is confirmed by radiographic studies. A radiopaque catheter is inserted into the hypopharynx and advanced until it encounters an obstruction. Chest films are taken to ascertain whether the tube reaches the stomach. Films that show air in the stomach indicate a connection between the trachea and the distal oesophagus in types III and IV. No gas is observed in the bowel in types I and II. Occasionally, the fistula is not patent, which makes their presence more difficult to diagnose. H type fistula (V) is suspected in an infant who has recurrent respiratory tract infection (especially right upper lobe pneumonia), tachypnoea, and abdominal distension (due to the passage of air through the fistula into the alimentary tract). Diagnosis is confirmed by barium swallow or bronchoscopy.

The presence of polyhydramnios prenatally is a clue to the possibility of OA in the unborn infant. Amniotic fluid, normally swallowed by the fetus, is unable to reach the GI tract.

THERAPEUTIC MANAGEMENT

The treatment of OA and TOF includes prevention of pneumonia, supportive therapy, and surgical repair of the anomaly.

Since type III is the most common, the discussion is directed primarily towards that anomaly.

When OA with a TOF is suspected, the infant is immediately deprived of oral intake, and intravenous fluids are begun. Humidified oxygen is given if indicated.

The infant is nursed in an incubator tilted to 30° so that his or her head is elevated. Secretions which gather in the oesophageal pouch are removed by intermittent nasopharyngeal suctioning or an indwelling sump tube attached to continuous low pressure suction. The second lumen of this tube allows air to be drawn in, preventing blockage by secretions or the mucous membrane of the pouch. Frequent installation of 1 ml normal saline will ensure patency. The tube should be changed every 24 hours, or more often if necessary. This position will also help reduce the risk of reflux of gastric contents.

Surgical correction

Most malformations can be corrected surgically in one operation or staged with two or more procedures. The success depends on early diagnosis, skilled nursing care, and the technical skill and judgement of the surgeon. With measures instituted to prevent aspiration pneumonia and to ensure adequate hydration and nutrition, surgery can be postponed to allow an opportunity for further evaluation and assessment in order to rule out any associated anomalies, optimize respiratory support, and treat problems associated with prematurity.

The surgery consists of a thoracotomy with division and ligation of the TOF and an end-to-end anastomosis of the oesophagus. This is known as primary repair. A chest tube is inserted to drain chest fluid. For infants who are premature, have multiple anomalies, or are in very poor condition, a staged operation is preferred that involves palliative measures, including gastrostomy, ligation of the TOF, and provision of constant drainage of the oesophageal pouch. Further surgery to correct anomalies is done when the infant's condition allows.

There are rare instances in which a primary anastomosis cannot be accomplished because of insufficient length of the two segments of oesophagus. In these cases, one of a variety of procedures may be considered. An oesophageal replacement procedure using bowel or gastric tube oesophagostomy may be necessary to bridge the missing oesophageal segment. When the stomach is used, a tube is fashioned from the greater curvature of the stomach, tunnelled into the chest, and anastomosed to the oesophagus. Alternatively, a segment of either the right or the transverse colon is dissected and transplanted, along with its undisturbed blood and nerve supply, through a surgical opening in the diaphragm and ligated to the oesophageal pouches, maintaining the proximodistal orientation. In both types of repair, peristalsis is largely ineffective and food is conducted to the stomach by gravity. Another alternative is a gastric pull-up, where the oesophagus and stomach are mobilized and 'pulled-up' and oesophageal anastamosis performed. This means the stomach is now within the thoracic cavity, but with gradual introduction of feeds, respiratory compromise is prevented.

Prognosis

In all surgical procedures involving the oesophagus there may be problems with stricture caused by scar tissue contraction that require evaluation by barium x-ray studies, oesophagoscopy, and mechanical dilation. Many surgeons routinely perform dilation at regularly scheduled intervals for some time after surgery. The procedure may need to be repeated several times during growth. Strictures that do not respond to dilation require surgical intervention.

Postoperative care

Postoperative care for these infants is essentially the same as for any high-risk newborn. Some paediatric surgeons elect to leave the infant intubated and ventilated for several days postoperatively, especially if the anastasmosis is tight. Muscle relaxants and analgesia are given intravenously (Davies and Beale, 1991). The infant is returned to the warm atmosphere of the incubator, the chest tube is attached to an underwater drainage bottle, and nutrition is supplied by hyperalimentation. A transanastamotic nasogastric tube is placed during the operative procedure and this must be guarded carefully postoperatively. Drainage from the nasogastric tube is inspected and measured, since saliva in the collection container is evidence of a patent oesophagus. Saliva in the chest drain indicates breakdown of anastasmosis and refistulation.

Enteral feeds are gradually introduced and parenteral nutrition withdrawn. The initial attempt at oral feeding (7–10 days postoperatively) must be carefully observed to make certain that the infant is able to swallow without choking. Contrast studies to assess anastamosis are usually done prior to this. Chest drains are removed when advised by surgeon.

Special problems

In the infant awaiting oesophageal replacement surgery, the sump tube is removed and the upper oesophageal segment is drained by means of an artificial opening in the neck (cervical oesophagostomy), which allows escape of the swallowed saliva. This is a source of annoyance, since the skin may become irritated by moisture from the continual discharge of saliva. Frequent removal of drainage and application of a thin layer of protective ointment are usually sufficient treatment. Non-nutritive sucking is provided by a pacifier and small amounts of water or milk are given orally. In this case, the fluid drains from the oesophagostomy but allows the infant to develop mature sucking patterns. This is known as sham feeding. Children who must remain nil orally for an extended period have not been able to go through the processes of eating in the normal manner. They frequently have difficulty with this new task and may become extremely resistant to learning it. Some paediatric hospitals have multidisciplinary teams to assist these children.

Family support, discharge planning, and home care

Preparing parents for discharge of their infant involves teaching the techniques that will be continued in home care, such as careful suctioning, gastrostomy feeding, and skin care. The parents are taught child or infant behaviours that might be expected after corrective surgery, such as those that indicate that the child needs to be suctioned, signs of respiratory difficulty, and signs that indicate constriction of the oesophagus (poor feeding, dysphagia, drooling, or regurgitating small amounts).

Parents are reminded that it is particularly important to guard against the child swallowing foreign objects. They are instructed to cut solid food into small pieces, teach the child to chew thoroughly, and avoid foods such as whole hot dogs or large pieces of meat that may become lodged in the oesophagus. With a child in any of the stages of locomotion, this is no simple problem.

Most infants will have some tracheomalacia; therefore, parents should be reassured that their infant's 'barky' cough is normal and will gradually diminish as the infant grows and the trachea becomes stronger. Since over one-half of the infants with OA/TOF will develop gastro-oesophageal reflux, precautions should be initiated (see Chapter 27). Parents may also need help in acquiring needed equipment, such as a suction machine. Most hospitals have a supply which can be lent to parents for home use.

ANORECTAL MALFORMATIONS

Malformations in the anorectal region of the GI tract are manifested in several variations, often termed *imperforate anus*. The incidence is approximately 1:5000 and seems to more common in males. The incidence of associated anomalies is high.

Clinically, anorectal malformations are classified in three ways (Box 14-2). A distinction between these categories is important for planning therapy and determining a prognosis (Seashore, 1986).

PROCESS OF DIAGNOSIS

Checking for patency of the anus and rectum is a routine part of the newborn assessment and includes observation or inquiries regarding the passage of meconium. Inspection of the perineal area reveals absence of an anal opening or a thin, translucent membrane. The appearance of the perineum alone does not accurately predict the level of the lesion. However, complete absence of anal features, a flat perineum, and absence of external sphincter contraction when stimulated generally indicate an intermediate or high lesion. TOF and cardiac anomalies are common findings in association with anorectal malformations and should be considered in the assessment when an anorectal anomaly is noted.

Digital and endoscopic examination identify constriction or the blind pouch of rectal atresia. Stenosis may not become apparent until 1 year of age or older when the child has a history of difficult defecation, abdominal distention, and ribbon-like stools. Fistulae may not be apparent at birth, but as peristalsis gradually forces the meconium through the fistula, they can be identified by careful examination. A rectourinary fistula is suspected on the basis of meconium in the urine and

---

◆ **BOX 14-2**

Classification of anorectal malformations

Low anomalies — rectum has descended normally through the puborectalis muscle, the internal and external sphincters are present and well developed with normal function, and there is no connection to the genitourinary tract. These may be anal stenosis with or without an obstructive membrane, frequently with an external fistula to the perineum or vestibule through which meconium is passed.

Intermediate anomalies — rectum is at or below the level of the puborectalis muscle, the anal dimple and external sphincter are positioned normally, but the anal opening is located anteriorly in the perineum. There may be a persistent connection to the genitourinary tract.

High anomalies — rectum ends above the puborectalis muscle. There is absence of internal and external sphincters, and the puborectalis muscle is relatively ineffectual. These anomalies occur almost exclusively in males, where there is usually a rectourethral fistula; a rectovaginal communication is found in females. Wide variations are found in high anomalies; these are often associated with maldevelopment of the sacrum, which interferes with innervation to anal and urethral musculature.

---

confirmed by radiographs of contrast media injected through a tiny catheter into the fistula.

Definitive diagnosis of the extent and location of the high lesion is made by radiographic examination. Abdominal and perineal ultrasound may be performed to verify the infant's anatomy. Renal ultrasound and voiding cystourethrography are recommended for the infant with a high lesion to identify or rule out the possibility of associated anomalies of the urinary tract. Further examination is also indicated if there is evidence of urinary tract infection or other symptoms. In addition, cardiac evaluation and skeletal films may be done to rule out other anomalies.

THERAPEUTIC MANAGEMENT

Successful treatment for anal stenosis is generally accomplished by manual dilations. The procedure, begun by the doctor, is repeated on a regular basis by the nurses in the hospital and continued at home by the parents, after they are carefully instructed in the technique. An imperforate anal membrane is excised and followed by daily anal dilations.

Reconstruction of an anus in the proper position is the goal of surgical treatment of intermediate anorectal malformations. The most important consideration in the probable success of reconstruction is the level at which the rectum terminates, especially in its relationship to the puborectalis sling of the levator ani muscle. Where the bowel has come through this structure, surgical correction often can be accomplished in the neonatal period by way of an abdominal–perineal pull-through procedure and/or anoplasty.

Infants with high anomalies require a divided sigmoid colostomy in the newborn period. This allows time for the infant to gain weight, for a more leisurely evaluation of the anomaly, and for protection of the GU tract from faecal contamination if a fistula is present. Antibiotics are usually administered prophylactically. Final correction of higher defects is usually postponed for a year. The most common procedure is the posterior sagittal anorectoplasty. When children, after a pull-through procedure, fail to achieve bowel control at a reasonable age, a permanent colostomy may be necessary.

IMPLICATIONS FOR NURSING

Postoperative nursing care ordinarily presents few problems and is primarily directed towards healing of the anoplasty without infection or other complications. There may or may not be a temporary dressing and drain, but when the infant is passing stool, dressings are of little value. The preferred placement is a side-lying prone position with the hips elevated or a supine position with the legs suspended at a 90° angle to the trunk to prevent pressure on perineal sutures. Frequent perineal cleansing in a tub and measures to reduce friction on skin are initiated. If skin irritation becomes problematic, a stoma therapist should be consulted.

The infant is given regular enteral feeds as soon as peristalsis returns. In the meantime, there may be intravenous feeding and a nasogastric tube for abdominal decompression. Care of the infant with a colostomy involves frequent dressing changes, meticulous skin care, and correct application of a collection device.

Nursing care of children with permanent colostomies is the same as for any child with a colostomy.

Family support, discharge planning, and home care

Long-term follow-up is essential for children with high lesions. Following a definitive pull-through procedure, toilet training is delayed. Complete continence is seldom achieved at the usual age of three to four years. Bowel habit training, diet modification, and administration of stool softeners help children slowly improve bowel management, but optimum results may not be achieved until later childhood or adolescence. Support and reassurance during the slow progression to normal function are essential, and any type of coercive toilet training is discouraged. Approximately 80% will ultimately achieve normal or at least socially acceptable continence (Seashore, 1986).

Parents are instructed in perineal and wound care or care of the colostomy. Anal dilations may be necessary for some infants. Parents are advised to observe bowel habit and for signs of anal stricture or complications. Information on dietary modifications and/or administration of medications is included in counselling. For infants with high lesions, plans for corrective surgery should be discussed.

BILIARY ATRESIA

Biliary atresia is the obstruction or absence of a portion of the bile ducts. Blockage may be either *intrahepatic*, the absence of bile ducts within the liver, or *extrahepatic*, in which there is absence or obstruction of the main bile passages outside the liver. Numerous variations are encountered, but the most common abnormality is complete atresia of the extrahepatic structures. The cause is unknown. It is generally considered to be a developmental anomaly, but recent evidence implicates a viral infection before or shortly after birth (Glaser, Balistreri and Morecki, 1984). The predictable course of the disease terminates in irreversible obliteration of the extrahepatic bile ducts.

CLINICAL MANIFESTATIONS

Jaundice is usually the earliest evidence of biliary atresia and is the most striking feature of the disorder. It is first observed in the sclera. It may be present at birth, but is not usually apparent until the child is two to three weeks of age, when normal physiological jaundice has resolved. Any baby with persistent jaundice should be investigated. Early diagnosis of biliary atresia is critical, as surgical procedures performed after three months of age are uniformly unsuccessful (Hussein *et al.*, 1991; Nelson, 1989). The urine becomes dark and stains the nappy, and the stools are lighter than expected. Hepatomegaly and abdominal distention are common, and splenomegaly occurs later. Poor fat metabolism results in poor weight gain and general failure to thrive. As the disease progresses, the child becomes irritable and difficult to comfort.

PROCESS OF DIAGNOSIS

No single test or combination of tests is diagnostic. The disease is suspected on the basis of clinical signs, including a steady increase in *conjugated* hyperbilirubinaemia. Percutaneous or open surgical liver biopsy with cholangiogram is performed to identify the presence or absence of intrahepatic bile ducts. Presence of intrahepatic bile ducts indicates that the atresia is of extrahepatic origin and amenable to surgical exploration. Hepatobiliary scans and a complete work-up for other causes of neonatal jaundice, such as hepatitis, may be undertaken.

THERAPEUTIC MANAGEMENT

The major hope in care of these children is that the condition will benefit from surgery. Surgical reconstruction is possible in about 10% of cases of extrahepatic atresia when the lesion is either a distal atresia with patent proximal hepatic duct or a cystic dilation of ducts adjacent to the hilum of the liver. Surgery is most successful when performed early; therefore, diagnosis is urgent.

In the more common atresias there are no patent extrahepatic ducts. In these cases a hepatic portoenterostomy (Kasai procedure) is employed, in which a substitute duct is formed from a segment of jejunum if there are any hepatic duct remnants. The procedure provides effective palliation for some patients; for others complications of progressive liver disease occur despite initially satisfactory bile secretion (Lally *et al.*, 1989).

Liver transplantation has become a more realistic solution for children who, despite portoenterostomy, subsequently develop progressive failure or portal hypertensive complications (Ryckman *et al.*, 1993). The recent success with partial liver transplants and those from living donors offers an encouraging alternative to scarce cadaver donors.

Medical management is primarily supportive. It is the method of choice for intrahepatic atresia and supplemental to surgical therapy in extrahepatic atresia. Medical management consists of a high-calorie formula containing fats that can be digested without bile (Pregestimil, Generaid Plus, Portagen) and water-miscible vitamins. The bile–acid-binding drug cholestyramine is sometimes useful to prevent reabsorption of bile from the intestines. However, it is not effective where bile is not excreted into the intestines. Phenobarbital helps reduce irritability and enhances bile flow. A low-salt diet and diuretics may reduce ascites formation.

HERNIAS

A hernia is a protrusion of a portion of an organ or organs through an abnormal opening. The danger from herniation arises when the organ protruding through the opening is constricted to the extent that circulation is impaired or when the protruding organs encroach on and impair the function of other structures. The herniations of concern here are those that protrude through the diaphragm, the abdominal wall, or the inguinal canal. Because they involve the GU tract, inguinal and femoral hernias are discussed in the next section.

UMBILICAL HERNIA

Ordinarily, the umbilical ring, through which the umbilical blood vessels provide essential elements to the developing fetus, undergoes spontaneous, gradual closure after birth. Incomplete closure of this fascial ring results in the protrusion of portions of omentum and intestine through the opening. The size of the defect varies from less than 1 cm to 4 or 5 cm. The hernias are seen as soft swellings or protrusions covered by skin that are readily reducible with the finger, and small defects usually close spontaneously by three to four years of age. However, very large hernias often persist. Those that have not disappeared by school age require surgical closure. Strangulation or incarceration of herniated bowel is rare but requires immediate surgical intervention.

IMPLICATIONS FOR NURSING

Because the sight of an umbilical hernia is very disconcerting to parents, they need reassurance regarding the innocuous nature of the defect. Taping or strapping appears to be of no value in expediting closure and may even retard it. The application can also cause troublesome skin irritation; when done improperly, it may cause strangulation.

DIAPHRAGMATIC HERNIA

In congenital diaphragmatic hernia the abdominal contents herniate through the diaphragm into the pleural cavity, seriously compromising respiration. The defect is associated with an exceptionally high mortality.

PATHOPHYSIOLOGY

The herniation represents failure of the pleuroperitoneal canal to close completely during embryonic development, which allows various degrees of protrusion of abdominal viscera through the defect into the thoracic cavity. The defect can vary from a minimal opening to complete absence of the diaphragm. It is not unusual to find most of the abdominal organs (stomach, small intestine, spleen, left lobe of liver, left kidney, and all but the descending colon) in the thorax. The more severe defects occur with herniation through the foramen of Bochdalek on the left side (80%); less severe are herniations on the right side (20%), which are often blocked by the liver, preventing other organs from entering the thoracic cavity.

Respiration is compromised by hypoplasia and compression of the lung, airways, and blood vessels on the affected side. Ineffective motion of the leaf of the diaphragm on the affected side interferes with the normal diaphragmatic breathing of the neonate. Respiration is further compromised when the stomach and intestine (generally found within the chest) rapidly become distended with swallowed air as the result of crying. Negative thoracic pressure from crying tends to pull the intestines into the chest and further distends those already there. This increased volume in the chest cavity displaces the mediastinum to the unaffected side to produce a partial collapse of the opposite lung.

The high mortality associated with congenital diaphragmatic hernia was previously attributed to pulmonary hypoplasia, resulting in ventilatory insufficiency. However, recent studies have shown that persistent pulmonary hypertension with increased pulmonary vascular resistance, right to left shunting, and progressive hypoxaemia is a major problem (Kinsella and Abman, 1992).

PROCESS OF DIAGNOSIS

Prenatal diagnosis is becoming more common and delivery at a regional centre with surgical facilities is recommended. The diagnosis is usually established by radiographic examination, which shows fluid- and air-filled loops of intestine in the affected side of the chest (80% are present on the left side). The mediastinum is shifted to the unaffected side, causing a similar shift in the point of maximum intensity on auscultation. Auscultation also reveals absence of breath sounds on the affected side of the thorax, and bowel sounds may be present. Blood gas and pH determinations are made to assess the status of oxygenation and acidosis. Heart beat will be heard deviated to the right side.

CLINICAL MANIFESTATIONS

Clinical manifestations include severe respiratory distress, often present at birth, with dyspnoea and cyanosis. The infant has the typical appearance of a barrel-shaped chest and a markedly scaphoid (sunken) abdomen. Distress will increase as air is swallowed.

There are many prognostic indicators which may help predict the outcome for infants with diaphragmatic hernia. The following indicate poor prognosis:

- Polyhydramnios during pregnancy — survival rate is 55% when not present and 11% when present.
- Onset of symptoms — infants diagnosed within six hours of life carry a mortality risk of over 50%, decreasing to 40% within 24 hours. Mortality approaches 0% when signs appear after 24 hours. Right-sided defects may be asymptomatic and discovered later during radiograph examination for other reasons.
- Prematurity.
- Associated anomalies — infants with congenital diaphragmatic hernia who are still-born or die soon after birth have a high incidence of associated anomalies.

THERAPEUTIC MANAGEMENT

The affected infant will require immediate respiratory support of varying degree, depending on time of onset and severity of respiratory distress. If diaphragmatic hernia is suspected, positive pressure ventilation using a bag or mask is avoided as this increases distension of the stomach and bowel, further compromising respiratory function. Facial oxygen is provided and, if necessary, the child is intubated and ventilated using low pressures and high rates. Pneumothorax is a constant danger because of the uneven distribution of intrapulmonary pressures in the hypoplastic, atelectic, and compressed lung tissue.

The infant is positioned with the head and thorax higher than the abdomen and feet. This facilitates downwards displacement of the abdominal organs. A wide bore (10 French guage) tube is passed into the stomach to allow decompression.

Intravenous fluids are begun by way of an umbilical artery catheter, metabolic and respiratory acidosis is corrected, and antibiotics may be administered prophylactically. Traditional management has previously been early surgical repair of the defect; however, increased survival rates have been reported with surgery delayed following a period of preoperative stabilization (Cartlidge, Mann and Kapilar, 1986; Sakai *et al*, 1987). If the infant is to be transported to a special facility, stabilization and transport are accomplished as quickly as possible. The infant may be electively intubated and ventilated prior to transfer to ensure optimum oxygenation.

Preoperative care includes many modes of ventilation (e.g., high rate, low pressure IPPV, high frequency oscillatory). The use of muscle relaxants and opioids may increase ventilatory efficiency. Pre- and post-ductal arterial lines or saturation monitoring will assist in the assessment of pulmonary hypertension and shunting through patent ductus arteriosus and foramen ovale. If necessary, vasodilators, such as tolazoline, enoximone, and inhaled nitric oxide may be given to reduce pulmonary vascular resistance and reverse shunting. Inotropic support (e.g., dopamine) may be required if associated peripheral vasodilatation leads to hypotension.

Timing of surgery varies from centre to centre. If the diaphragmatic defect is large, various techniques, such as muscle flaps or insertion of prosthetic materials, may be used to facilitate closure. A chest drain is placed in the pleural cavity on the affected side and connected to an underwater seal.

Postoperative care continues as preoperative care, with a gradual reduction of ventilation and medication as the infant's condition improves. However, despite maximum intervention, many of these infants do not improve.

IMPLICATIONS FOR NURSING

The degree of care required for an infant with diaphragmatic hernia can vary greatly, but in severe cases will be at the highest level seen in a neonatal surgical unit. Despite this, mortality rates remain high.

Extracorporeal membrane oxygenation (ECMO) is a technique which may provide support to the infant until pulmonary hypertension decreases. It can be used pre- and/or post-operatively, but should be instituted early and not seen as 'rescue therapy'.

Future therapy may include fetal surgery to repair the defect, allowing the lung on the affected side to grow and mature normally (Scott *et al*, 1994). Partial fetal tracheal occlusion results in fluid collecting in the lung, preventing it from being compressed and allowing normal or increased growth (Wilson *et al*, 1993).

HIATUS HERNIA

Congenital herniations through the normal oesophageal hiatus in the newborn are usually of the sliding type. Because the muscular ring of the hiatus is not snug, it permits the cardiac end of the stomach to slide above the diaphragm and back into the abdomen. This produces the symptoms seen with associated incompetent or relaxed cardiac sphincter *(chalasia)*, that is, reflux of gastric contents into the oesophagus with subsequent regurgitation.

Therapeutic management is directed towards treatment of the oesophageal reflux. When conservative management, such as upright posture and feeding modification, is disappointing, the defect is repaired surgically.

ABDOMINAL WALL DEFECTS

Omphalocele and gastroschisis, the most common abdominal wall defects, have been considered for some time to be embryologically distinct disorders. The distinction at birth has been that an omphalocele is a covered defect of the umbilical ring with a sac into which intra-abdominal contents may herniate. Gastroschisis is a defect in the anterior abdominal wall, uncovered, and with a normally inserted umbilical cord.

OMPHALOCELE

Omphalocele is a serious congenital malformation in which a variable amount of the abdominal contents protrudes into the base of the umbilical cord. As the embryonic midgut grows and elongates, it projects from the abdomen, which is too small to contain it, into the umbilical cord. This migration takes place from the sixth to the tenth week of fetal life. Normally, the intestines return rapidly into the abdomen by the eleventh week of gestation; failure to return produces an omphalocele.

In contrast to an umbilical hernia, the omphalocele is covered only by a translucent sac of amnion to which the umbilical cord inserts. The sac may contain only a small loop of bowel or most of the bowel and other abdominal viscera. If the sac ruptures, the abdominal contents eviscerate through the opening in the abdominal wall. The abdomen is smaller than usual, making replacement of the bowel more difficult. Omphalocele is often associated with other anomalies, such as trisomy 18, cardiac defects, imperforate anus, and meningocele. Antenatal diagnosis may include amniocentesis for chromosome analysis. Termination of pregnancy may be considered.

Since the advent of prenatal ultrasonography, an increasing number of these defects are detected before birth. This has created a debate regarding the optimum mode of delivery — vaginal versus surgical; term versus preterm. Where possible, delivery in a regional surgical facility is preferred.

The omphalocele is covered immediately with moist gauze and kept moist until the infant is taken to the operating room. The moist dressing is covered with plastic wrap to avoid loss of heat and moisture. Small lesions are repaired as soon as possible to prevent infection or tissue damage. Larger lesions may require gradual reduction by way of plastic material (Silastic or Gortex) sewn to the margins of the defect and pulled together at the top to form a chimney, with steady pressure applied to the protruding mass over a course of days to gradually enlarge the intra-abdominal space to accommodate the intestinal contents. A second operation is then performed to close the wound.

Management of ruptured omphalocele is similar to that for gastroschisis. Complications include infection, rupture, and intestinal obstruction. Blood glucose level is closely monitored, as Beckwith-Wiedemann's syndrome with hypoglycaemia may be associated.

GASTROSCHISIS

Gastroschisis is herniation through a defect of the abdominal wall that permits extrusion of abdominal contents without involving the umbilical cord. The defect is usually located to the right of the intact umbilicus and is not encased in a protective sac. Herniation through the defect can take place pre-

natally or perinatally. If the evisceration is of long standing, the abdominal cavity will be small and the protruding bowel thickened as a result of poor blood return and irritation from amniotic fluid. The bowel is almost normal and the abdominal cavity adequate in eviscerations that take place just before birth. Major anomalies outside the GI tract are uncommon in children with gastroschisis.

Therapy is directed towards prevention of infection, nutrition, and surgical closure of the defect. A primary closure is preferred but is not always possible. When the abdomen is too small to accommodate the extruded contents, a Silastic, Gortex, or collagen-coated Vicryl mesh pouch is placed over the herniated viscera to contain the bowel and to aid in reduction until surgical closure is attempted (Fig. 14-9). As with exompholos, the pouch is reduced each day until the opening is surgically closed. The return may take a few hours to a few days, depending on the size of the abdominal cavity relative to the amount of viscera.

Some of the problems that may be encountered postsurgically when the abdomen is unable to accommodate the viscera are respiratory compromise caused by the increased pressure on the diaphragm, decreased venous return to the heart because of pressure on the vena cava, and possible bowel necrosis from excessive crowding and prolonged ileus. If the infant develops respiratory distress, the sutures may need to be released and the pouch replaced until adequate respiratory function can be reinstated. Postoperatively, many surgeons prefer elective intubation and ventilation with muscle relaxants and analgesia to prevent respiratory compromise and tension on the suture line.

IMPLICATIONS FOR NURSING

Nursing care is the same as for any high-risk infant. Infection is a constant threat before surgery, and careful positioning and handling are needed to prevent rupture of the intact omphalocele sac or disturbance of the Silastic bag used for gradual reduction. Viscera should be protected with plastic wrap (cling film) wrapped around the defect. Heat and fluid losses from the exposed viscera are major concerns in the pre-

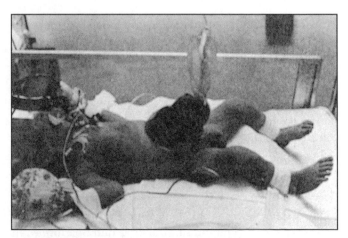

Fig. 14-9 Gastroschisis enclosed in a silastic pouch.

operative period; therefore thermoregulation is critical, and fluid resuscitation may be massive to compensate for losses. The gastrointestinal tract is decompressed via a nasogastric tube before surgery to aid in reduction. It may take several weeks for bowel function to begin, so parenteral nutrition is necessary. Enteral feeds are introduced gradually, and many centres advocate the use of expressed breast milk or modified formula milk. Postsurgical care includes particular attention to observation for signs of complications and indications that the replaced bowel is functioning.

DEFECTS OF THE GENITOURINARY TRACT

External defects of the genitourinary (GU) tract are usually obvious at birth. Several, such as hypospadias, epispadias, and undescended testes (cryptorchidism), do not necessitate immediate repair but may require one or more staged repairs during early childhood. Others, such as extrophy of the bladder, require initial intervention at birth with repeated medical and surgical treatment for several years. The anatomical location of these defects frequently causes more psychological concern to children and parents than does the actual condition or treatment. Hernias are common in young children and are usually repaired as soon as diagnosis is established.

PHIMOSIS

Phimosis is a narrowing or stenosis of the preputial opening of the foreskin that prevents retraction of the foreskin over the glans penis. It is a normal finding in infants and very young boys and usually disappears as the child grows and the distal prepuce dilates. Occasionally, the narrowing obstructs the flow of urine, resulting in a dribbling stream or even ballooning of the foreskin with accumulated urine during voiding.

Inflammation or infection of the phimotic foreskin occurs occasionally and is managed as any other inflammation or infection. Severe phimosis is treated surgically by circumcision.

IMPLICATIONS FOR NURSING

Proper hygiene of the phimotic foreskin in infants and young boys consists of external cleansing during routine bathing. The foreskin should not be forcibly retracted, because this may create scarring, which can prevent future retraction. Furthermore, retraction of the tight foreskin can result in paraphimosis, a condition in which the retracted foreskin cannot be replaced in its normal position over the glans. This causes oedema and venous congestion created by constriction by the tight band of foreskin -a urologic emergency that requires immediate evaluation.

INGUINAL HERNIA

Inguinal hernias account for approximately 80% of all hernias and are the most common surgical procedures performed in infancy (with the possible exception of circumcision).

CLINICAL MANIFESTATIONS

This very common defect is asymptomatic unless the abdominal contents are forced into the patent sac. Most often it appears as a painless inguinal swelling that varies in size. It disappears during periods of rest or is reducible by gentle compression; it appears when the infant cries or strains, or when the older child strains, coughs, or stands for a long period. The defect can be palpated as a thickening of the cord in the groin, and the 'silk glove' sign can be elicited by rubbing together the sides of the empty hernial sac.

Sometimes the herniated loop of intestine becomes partially obstructed, producing variable symptoms that may include fretfulness and irritability, tenderness, anorexia, abdominal distention, and difficulty in defecating. Occasionally, the loop of bowel becomes incarcerated (irreducible), with symptoms of complete intestinal obstruction that, left untreated, will progress to strangulation and gangrene. Incarceration occurs more often in infants under ten months of age and is more common in girls.

THERAPEUTIC MANAGEMENT

The treatment for hernias is prompt, elective surgical repair in healthy infants and children as soon as the defect is diagnosed. Since there is a significant incidence of bilateral involvement, many doctors advocate exploration of both sides. This practice of exploration remains controversial, however. It is preferable to attempt reduction of a recently incarcerated hernia in order that surgery can be delayed to allow the injured tissues to recover somewhat, but irreducible or strangulated hernias are treated as emergencies.

IMPLICATIONS FOR NURSING

Preterm infants usually have surgery delayed until they are fit and ready for discharge from the special care unit. Apnoea is not uncommon after general anaesthesia; therefore, regional anaesthetic techniques are often used. Full-term infants and children tolerate surgery very well. There is usually no restriction placed on their activities, and it is not uncommon for the child to be discharged from hospital on the day of surgery. Every attempt is made to keep the wound clean and reasonably dry. With infants and small children who are not yet toilet trained, the wound may be left without a dressing, or airstrips may be applied. Changing nappies as soon as they become damp helps reduce the chance of irritation or infection of the incision, or the child may be left without a nappy. It is unnecessary to apply a urine-collecting device.

Parents are instructed to give the child sponge baths instead of conventional baths for 2-5 days and to change nappies more frequently than usual during the day and once or twice during the night. There are no restrictions placed on the infant's or toddler's activity, but older children are cautioned against lifting, pushing, wrestling and fighting, bicycle riding, and athletics for about three weeks (Gans and Austin, 1986). School children are permitted to attend classes as soon as they are comfortable but are excused from physical education activities for the same length of time as specified for restricting physical activity.

If surgery is postponed, the parents need to be taught the signs of incarcerated hernia and where to call for assistance.

FEMORAL HERNIA

Femoral hernias are rare in children. When they occur, there is a higher incidence in girls than in boys. The disorder is suspected from a swelling in the groin area associated with severe pain. Treatment and management are the same as for inguinal hernia. Strangulation is a frequent complication.

HYDROCELE

Hydrocele is the presence of fluid in the persistent processus vaginalis and is the result of the same developmental process as inguinal hernia. When the upper segment of the processus vaginalis has been obliterated but the tunica vaginalis still contains peritoneal fluid, this is called a *noncommunicating hydrocele*. This type of hydrocele is common in newborns and often subsides spontaneously as fluid is gradually absorbed.

A *communicating hydrocele* is one in which the processus vaginalis remains open and into which peritoneal fluid may be forced by intra-abdominal pressure and gravity. The length of the hydrocele depends on the length of the processus vaginalis and may extend into the tunica vaginalis within the scrotum. The hydrocele is asymptomatic except for a palpable bulge in the inguinal or scrotal areas. Unlike a hernia, the hydrocele may not be reducible and may not be produced by a sudden increase in intra-abdominal pressure (such as straining). The scrotum appears to be larger after an active day and smaller in the morning. Since a communicating hydrocele represents a patent processus vaginalis, it can predispose to herniation; therefore, surgical repair is indicated if spontaneous resolution does not take place by one year of age.

CRYPTORCHIDISM (CRYPTORCHISM)

Cryptorchidism is failure of one or both testes to descend normally through the inguinal canal into the scrotum. Absence of testes within the scrotum can be the result of: (1) *undescended (cryptorchid)* testes, (2) *retractile* testes, or (3) *anorchia* (absence of testes). Undescended testes can be categorized further according to location (Box 14-3). The incidence of cryptorchidism is 3-4% of full-term infants and falls to approximately 1% at age one year. The rate does not change in the years that follow (reported in Saggese *et al.*, 1989).

CLINICAL MANIFESTATIONS

Undescended testes are rarely a cause of discomfort. The entire scrotum, or one side of it, appears smaller than normal and incompletely developed, an observation made by concerned parents who often bring the child for medical evaluation.

THERAPEUTIC MANAGEMENT

A retractile testis that can be manipulated into the scrotum will eventually assume a satisfactory scrotal position without medical or surgical intervention. The diagnosis is not made at a single examination, and parents are asked if they have observed the testes in the scrotum at some time. If so, the anomaly probably represents the retractile variety and the parents can be reassured. By one year of age, the cryptorchid testes will descend spontaneously in approximately 75% of cases in both term and preterm infants (Penny, 1986). In contrast true undescended testes rarely descend spontaneously after one year of age.

If the testes do not descend spontaneously, orchidopexy is performed preferably between one and two years of age. Surgical repair is done to: (1) prevent damage to the undescended testicle by exposure to the higher degree of body heat in the undescended location, (2) decrease the incidence of tumour formation, which is higher in undescended testicles, (3) avoid trauma and torsion, (4) close the processus vaginalis, and (5) prevent the cosmetic and psychological handicap of an empty scrotum. Because of increased propensity toward neoplastic changes (even after orchidopexy), cryptorchid testes are better observed in the scrotal position.

In the routine procedure for undescended testes, the testes are brought down into the scrotum and secured in that position without tension or torsion. A simple orchidopexy for a palpable testis can usually be performed in an outpatient surgical unit without the need for overnight hospitalization. Intra-abdominal testes require considerable surgical skill because of technical problems resulting from variations in the length of the spermatic cord, and overnight hospitalization may be necessary.

In most cases, the family can be reassured of normal function in adulthood; however, untreated children are at high risk for developing testicular cancer eventually.

IMPLICATIONS FOR NURSING

The postoperative nursing care is directed towards prevention of infection and instructing parents in home care of the child. Infection is prevented by carefully cleansing the operative site

---

◆ **BOX 14-3**

Classification of Cryptorchid testes

Abdominal—located proximal to the internal inguinal ring

Canalicular—located between the internal and external inguinal rings

Ectopic—located outside the normal pathways of descent between the abdominal cavity and the scrotum

of stool and urine. Observation of the wound for complications and activity restrictions are discussed.

HYPOSPADIAS

Hypospadias refers to a condition in which the urethral opening is located below the glans penis or anywhere along the ventral surface of the penile shaft. In very mild cases, the meatus is just below the tip of the penis. In the most severe malformations the meatus is located on the perineum between the halves of the scrotum. Chordee, or ventral curvature of the penis, results from the replacement of normal skin with a fibrous band of tissue and usually accompanies more severe forms of hypospadias. In addition, the foreskin is usually absent ventrally and, when combined with chordee, gives the organ a hooded and crooked appearance. In severe cases, the altered appearance may leave the gender in doubt at birth, since the perineal position of the meatus may be mistaken for a female urethra. Since undescended testes may also be present, the small penis may appear to be an enlarged clitoris. In any case of ambiguous genitalia, further study, such as chromosomal analysis, is essential.

SURGICAL CORRECTION

The principal objectives in surgical correction are: (1) to enable the child to void in the standing position by voluntarily directing the stream in the usual manner, (2) to improve the physical appearance of the genitalia for psychological reasons, and (3) to produce a sexually adequate organ. The procedure involves releasing the chordee (when present), extending the length of the urethra, and constructing a new meatal opening. Since the prepuce is valuable skin for the reconstructive surgery, circumcision should not be done on these infants.

The preferred time for surgical repair is 6-18 months, before the child has developed body image and castration anxiety. Occasionally, a short course of testosterone is administered preoperatively to achieve additional penile size to facilitate the surgery. Microscopic optical magnification and delicate instruments are used during surgery. Sometimes repairs for more severe cases of hypospadias may result in fistulae and strictures, necessitating additional surgical intervention.

Hypospadias repair may require some type of urinary diversion (e.g., suprapubic catheterization) to promote optimum healing and to maintain the position and patency of the newly formed urethra. Following repair of more severe hypospadias the child is often placed under a bed cradle and on bed rest. Sedation may be required for the excessively irritable or restless child, and pain is controlled with analgesics. It is recommended that one parent should be resident with the child to reduce separation anxiety.

Parents are taught to care for the indwelling catheter or stent and irrigation technique if indicated. They need to know how to empty the urine bag and how to avoid kinking, twisting, or blockage of the catheter or stent. Often the child is discharged with a catheter or stent dripping directly into the nappy. In older children a urine collection device can be used. Parents are taught how to tape the drainage bag to the leg to allow the child to be mobile. An extra bag is sent home with the family in case of tears or leakage. The family is advised to encourage the child to increase fluid intake. Twice-daily bathing is recommended, as is loose clothing. Straddle toys, sandboxes, swimming, and rough activities are avoided until allowed by the surgeon.

EPISPADIAS

Epispadias is a rare defect in which the meatal opening is located on the dorsal surface of the penis. As in hypospadias, the defect can occur in differing degrees of severity. The treatment is surgical and usually includes penile and urethral lengthening plus bladder neck reconstruction for continence when necessary. The nursing considerations are similar to those discussed for hypospadias.

EXSTROPHY OF BLADDER

Exstrophy of the bladder is an obvious and serious congenital defect that occurs three times more frequently in males than in females (Fig. 14-10). Although the mode of inheritance is unclear, there is an increased risk of recurrence in a given family.

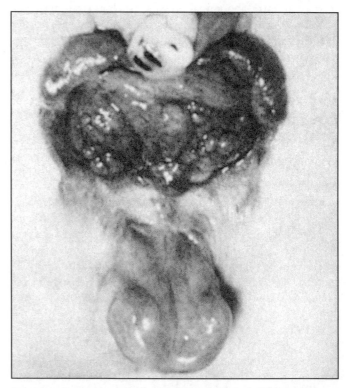

Fig. 14-10 Exstrophy of bladder. (Courtesy of BS Tant, MD, Division of Urology, University of Oregon Health Services Center, Portland, OR.)

PATHOPHYSIOLOGY

Exstrophy results from failure of the abdominal wall and underlying structures, including the ventral wall of the bladder, to fuse *in utero*. As a result the lower urinary tract is exposed and the everted bladder appears bright red through the abdominal opening. This is accompanied by a constant seepage of urine from the exposed ureteral orifices, making the area malodorous and susceptible to infection. The constant accumulation of urine on the surrounding skin produces tissue ulceration and further infection. Progressive renal damage from infection and obstruction may terminate in renal failure if left untreated.

In males, the defect is almost always associated with epispadias and may include other problems, such as undescended testes, a short penis, or inguinal hernia. The sexual handicap in males may be severe because the penis protrudes inadequately. In females, the genitalia may be affected, with a cleft or bifid clitoris, completely separated labia, and absent vagina. In either sex, separation of the pubic bones causes difficulty in walking, such as a waddling gait.

THERAPEUTIC MANAGEMENT

The objectives of treatment include: (1) preservation of renal function, (2) attainment of urinary control, (3) adequate reconstructive repair for psychological benefit, and (4) improvement of sexual function, particularly in males. Closure of the bladder is ideally accomplished within the first 48 hours of life when the circulating maternal hormones allow the pelvis to be approximated anteriorly without the need for iliac osteotomies. If this is not done, repair may be staged: (1) iliacosteotomies (postoperative Gallows traction), (2) closure of bladder. To promote optimum healing, the infant is usually maintained in traction or elastic external compression for a few weeks until adequate union of the separated pubis takes place.

Final repair is completed before school age. Essentially, all patients with exstrophy have vesicoureteral reflux that requires antireflux surgery, usually accompanied by bladder neck reconstruction in an attempt to produce urinary continence. These initial procedures are ordinarily performed at 2.5-3 years of age, and penile lengthening, release of dorsal chordee, and urethral construction with advancement of the urinary meatus at about 4-6 years of age.

In females, the urethroplasty and other reconstruction are performed at the same time as the anti-incontinence procedure, but vaginoplasty is delayed until puberty. Both boys and girls in whom surgery is delayed may require a temporary urinary diversion procedure. Those with complications or continued problems with continence are candidates for an artificial genitourinary sphincter or antirefluxing intestinal diversion, such as ureteral sigmoid implant, bilateral ureterostomy, or ileal conduit.

IMPLICATIONS FOR NURSING

Physical care of the unrepaired defect includes meticulous hygiene of the bladder area to prevent infection and excoriation of the surrounding tissue. A sterile nonadherent dressing or vaseline gauze is placed over the exposed bladder area to prevent infection and to keep the nappy from adhering to the mucosa. A barrier cream may be prescribed for the surrounding skin to protect it from the constantly draining urine.

Other aspects of preoperative care are similar to those for any major abdominal surgery. Since a routine urinalysis is part of most admission procedures, a urine specimen can be obtained by allowing urine to drip into a container by holding the child prone over a basin or by aspirating some urine directly from the bladder area into a medicine dropper or syringe. If a sterile specimen is needed for evaluation of existing infection, the former procedure is preferable, but a sterile container must be used.

Postoperative nursing care following bladder neck reconstruction and antireflux surgery (ureteral reimplantation) includes routine wound care and careful monitoring of urine output from the bladder and/or ureteric drainage tubes. Care following a penile lengthening, chordee release, and urethral reconstruction is similar to care following hypospadias repair.

In addition to routine postsurgical care, nursing following a continent diversion includes wound care, observation of nasogastric suction (surgery requires bowel resection), and measurement and observation of urinary output. In most cases, a continent urinary diversion can be created. Regular emptying of the urinary reservoir by clean intermittent catheterization is needed but preferable to permanent urinary conduits, which require a drainage appliance. Therefore, permanent urinary conduits are rarely performed.

Family support and prognosis
When the infant is discharged with an unrepaired defect, ordinarily nappies are placed over the defect in the usual manner. Nappies are changed frequently to prevent infection, ulceration and odour, and after a bowel movement to prevent contamination of the exposed area. General infant care remains unchanged except for sponge baths rather than immersion in water.

Even with improved reconstructive surgery for these patients, substantial psychologtc support and guidance are needed to help them adjust to their fears of inadequaate penile size, appearance of the genitalia, potential inability to procreate, and rejection by peers, especially the opposite sex. Ongoing discussion groups for parents and children are particularly useful in promoting resolution of these fears and allowing for optimum psychologic adjustment, particularly durtng adolescence.

OBSTRUCTIVE UROPATHY

Structural or functional abnormalities of the urinary system that obstruct the normal flow of urine can produce renal disorders. When there is interference with urine flow, the collecting system above the obstruction causes *hydronephrosis* (the collection of urine in the renal pelvis to the point of cyst formation from the distension) with eventual pressure destruction to renal parenchyma, although the dilating ureters form a reservoir that reduces the effect on the kidneys for a long time.

Obstruction may be congenital or acquired, unilateral or bilateral, complete or incomplete, and the manifestations acute or chronic. The obstruction can occur at any level of the upper or lower urinary tract. Partial obstruction may not be symptomatic unless there is a water or solute diuresis. Boys are affected more commonly than girls, and malformations should be suspected when patients have some other congenital defects (e.g., prune belly syndrome, chromosome anomalies, hypospadias, anorectal malformations, and aural defects). The severity of damage at birth depends on duration, type and severity of obstruction.

CLINICAL MANIFESTATIONS

The clinical manifestations depend on the type of obstruction and the extent of complications (e.g., infection). There may be pain or strangury (slow and painful urination, drop by drop) and haematuria (if caused by calculi). The type and location of pain are related to the area of obstruction (e.g., abdominal, flank, suprapubic, or radiating to the testicle or inguinal region).

Chronic obstruction may cause polyuria and polydipsia as a result of the inability to concentrate urine, anaemia caused by renal damage that impairs the secretion of erythropoietin, failure to thrive, unexplained febrile episodes caused by urinary infection, frequent voiding, weak or forceful urinary stream, and daytime and nocturnal enuresis. A full bladder and/or enlarged kidney may be evident on examination of the abdomen (Kaplan, 1983). Hydronephrosis is often an antenatal diagnosis after routine scans (Greig *et al.*, 1989).

PROCESS OF DIAGNOSIS

Laboratory examination reveals findings of acute or chronic renal failure. A voiding cystoureterogram may demonstrate the presence of posterior ureteral valves or vesicoureteral reflux, and ultrasonography may help identify and localize the site of obstruction. Radio-isotope scans can estimate the degree of function. Early identification of affected infants permits early management of abnormalities that otherwise may not be recognized until later in life after irreversible renal damage.

THERAPEUTIC MANAGEMENT

Early diagnosis and surgical correction or bypass procedures, such as ileal conduit or cutaneous ureterostomy, that divert the flow of urine are essential in order to prevent progressive renal damage. Often, a percutaneous nephrostomy tube or tubes are inserted through the skin and underlying tissues into the renal pelvis to relieve intrarenal pressure until an alternative diversion is established. Medical complications of acute or chronic renal failure and/or infection are managed as described for those disorders. In future, urinary tract decompression before birth may be routine treatment, but at present many problems are encountered (Adzick and Harrison, 1994).

Prognosis

The prognosis depends on the type of obstruction, the degree of irreversible renal damage, presence of renal dysplasia, the age at which the diagnosis was established, and the severity of complications. Despite the improvements in corrective surgery, some patients develop renal failure, which may evolve over a highly variable period of time that can extend into adulthood. Renal failure can result from hypoplasia-dysplasia, pyelonephritic scarring, and other proposed mechanisms that cause progressive nephron loss (Warshaw, Hymes and Woodard, 1982). Careful follow-up of children should extend throughout childhood and adolescence, especially when any degree of renal insufficiency is present.

ABERRANT SEXUAL DEVELOPMENT

The birth of a child with ambiguous genitalia is a situation that constitutes a crisis quite different from that of many other congenital anomalies. Uncertain gender is a potential lifetime social tragedy for the child and family. Furthermore, the electrolyte disturbances that accompany conditions in which gender is doubtful can be life-threatening. Thus, the problem of appropriate gender must be solved quickly and accurately and requires no less speed and skill than life-threatening anomalies such as tracheo-oesophageal fistula. There are studies that can be carried out during the first few days of life that help guide those involved in making a correct gender choice. Even a brief delay in gender assignment can generate rumours that can be a source of distress to a child and family for years.

TYPES OF ABNORMALITIES

Some disorders with abnormal sexual development are not characterized by ambiguous genitalia in the newborn period. For example, the most common sex chromosomal disorders do not become apparent until later childhood, adolescence, or even young adulthood when the individual seeks medical attention because of problems of delayed development or infertility. The four conditions producing ambiguous genitalia in the newborn that require prompt and accurate evaluation are the masculinized female (female pseudohermaphrodite), the incompletely masculinized male (male pseudohermaphrodite), the true hermaphrodite, and mixed gonadal dysgenesis.

Ambiguous genitalia in the newborn is most often the result of virilization in the female by adrenal androgens after the time of early gonadal differentiation. The most common type, congenital adrenal hyperplasia (CAH), is an inherited deficiency of adrenal corticoid hormones (see Chapter 32). The resulting decrease in cortisol stimulates pituitary secretion of corticotropin (ACTH), which causes the adrenal cortex to increase production of adrenal hormones, including the androgens. Since the adrenal gland differentiates later than the gonadal duct systems but before differentiation of the external genitalia, the masculinization of the external genitalia is the predominant feature. Internal female anatomy is normal.

Congenital adrenal hyperplasia is the only intersex problem that is life-threatening and should be considered in any situation where sex is doubtful.

External genitalia in the incompletely masculinized male may be incompletely male, ambiguous, or completely female. The complex nature of virilization offers numerous opportunities for disturbance in the process. Defects may be the result of deficient production of fetal androgen, deficiency in any of the enzymes needed for testosterone biosynthesis, or unresponsiveness or subresponsiveness of genital structures to testosterone. True hermaphrodites are rare and may be either genetic males or females with *both* ovarian and testicular tissues, with an ovary on one side and a testis on the other, or a combination of ovotestis. The external genitalia may be male, usually cryptorchid, or normal female, but in the majority of cases are ambiguous.

Mixed gonadal dysgenesis is the second most common disorder, in which affected infants are sex chromosomal mosaics. Genitalia vary greatly, but in those who appear predominantly female, the dysplastic testis may cause masculinization at puberty.

THERAPEUTIC MANAGEMENT

The assignment of a gender sex to the infant whose sex is doubtful constitutes a social emergency. The long-term implications are such that a hasty decision based on appearance alone may be disastrous, and the optimum sex of rearing may not be the same as the genetic or gonadal sex. The infant's anatomy rather than genetic sex is the primary criterion on which the choice of gender should be based. An incomplete female is better able to adjust than is an inadequate male. A functional vagina can be constructed surgically, and with appropriate administration of hormones the anatomically incomplete female can lead a relatively normal life, but it is as yet impossible to construct a satisfactory penis from an inadequate phallus for an equally satisfactory adjustment of the incomplete male.

In most instances of ambiguous genitalia it is recommended that the infant be reared as a female. Genetic males with a phallus of adequate size that will respond to testosterone at the time of puberty can be considered for male rearing. Adequate studies should be carried out early to assist in gender selection, even though they may delay final sex assignment for several days or even weeks. Supportive measures, such as appropriate surgical reconstruction techniques, that provide normal-appearing external structures are carried out. Removal of inappropriate internal structures and dysgenic gonads is recommended.

CONGENITAL DEFECTS CAUSED BY PRENATAL FACTORS

Before birth, the maternal host determines the well-being of the fetus by the manner in which she protects, favours, or deprives it. An unfavourable maternally imposed environment may produce effects on the fetus that are of a transient nature with few, if any, deleterious consequences or effects serious enough to cause long-range health problems in the infant or child. Several syndromes involving a variety of malformations have been attributed to an adverse prenatal environment.

FETAL ALCOHOL SYNDROME

The term *fetal alcohol syndrome (FAS)* is now widely used to describe infants with characteristic facial and associated features attributed to excessive ingestion of alcohol by the mother during pregnancy. It is now known that alcohol (ethanol) definitely interferes with normal pregnancy, that the effects on the fetus are permanent, and that even moderate use of alcohol during pregnancy may impair the mother-child bonding process. Observers have concluded that there is no safe level of alcohol consumption in pregnancy (Davis, Partridge and Storrs, 1982) and that women who plan to become pregnant are advised to stop consuming alcohol at least three months before they plan to become pregnant.

It is unclear to what extent the defects of FAS are related to the amount of alcohol consumed. It is not the degree of alcoholism in the mother that is related to the presence of abnormalities in the fetus; rather, it is the amount consumed in excess of the liver's ability to detoxify that places the fetus at risk. The liver's capacity to detoxify is limited and inflexible — when the liver receives more alcohol than it is able to handle, the excess is continually recirculated until the organ is able to reduce it to carbon dioxide and water. This circulating alcohol has a special affinity for brain tissue. Other factors that contribute to the teratogenic effects include toxic acetyl aldehyde (a degradation by-product of ethanol) and other substances that may be added to the alcohol. The poor nutritional state of the alcoholic mother further compromises the fetus.

The effects on the fetal brain are reflected in the central nervous system manifestations of fetal alcohol syndrome. mental disability, hearing disorders, and a variety of defects in craniofacial development are prominent features. Affected infants display the physical features of the syndrome and the characteristic behaviours beginning in the first 24 hours of life (Lemons, 1983). These include difficulty in establishing respirations, irritability, lethargy, seizure activity, tremulousness, opisthotonos, poor suck reflex, and abdominal distention. Affected infants frequently develop metabolic problems.

The initial difficulties in the newborn period are managed by preventing stimulation that might precipitate seizures, sedation and/or anticonvulsant therapy, and general supportive measures. The defects and their effects are irreversible, so the major emphasis must be aimed at prevention.

RADIATION

Ionizing radiation in large doses has been shown to be both mutagenic and teratogenic in humans. Pelvic irradiation of pregnant women — from natural background radiation that is present everywhere in varying degrees, from occupational exposure, or from diagnostic or therapeutic procedures — is believed to be hazardous to the embryo, although the extent of teratogenicity and the exact dosage required to induce somatic change are still under consideration. Radiation may damage the conceptus at any time during its prenatal existence, and it is known that rapidly dividing and differentiating cells, such as those of the embryo, have increased radiosensitivity. As with other teratogens, the type of effect produced is closely correlated with the stage of development at which the radiation exposure occurs.

NUTRITION

The human conceptus has no store of nutrients to sustain vital functions during the prenatal period; therefore it must rely on the mother as its single source of nutrition. Several related factors, acting alone or in combination, influence fetal access to nutrients. These include reduction of maternal intake of specific nutrients and the general nutritional state of the mother. The chronically malnourished mother has few nutritional reserves available for fetal use, and the accumulated effects of lifetime nutritional deficiency may produce physiological and anatomical structural defects that impair the mother's ability to support pregnancy and contribute to difficulties during labour. The teenage mother who has special nutritional requirements for meeting her own growth needs may compete with the fetus for available nutrients.

KEY POINTS

◆ Surgery initiates a number of physiological responses, including cardiovascular, respiratory, endocrine, renal, gastrointestinal, immune, neuralgic, and fluid and electrolyte.

◆ Nurses must be sensitive to pain in the neonate, be alert for signs of pain, and intervene appropriately.

◆ Care of the infant and child with myelomeningocele requires both immediate and long-term professional supervision. Associated problems include infection, neurological damage, impaired renal function, and musculoskeletal impairment.

◆ Therapeutic management of hydrocephalus focuses on relief of intracranial pressure, treatment of complications, and management of problems related to the effect of the disorder on psychomotor development.

◆ Three degrees of congenital hip dysplasia are acetabular dysplasia, subluxation and dislocation.

◆ Treatment of clubfoot involves manual overcorrection of the deformity, maintenance of the correction until normal muscle balance is gained, and follow-up observation to detect possible recurrence of the deformity.

◆ Management of cleft lip and/or palate involves a multidisciplinary approach to care involving professionals from surgery, medicine, nursing, dentistry and speech therapy.

◆ Tracheo-oesophageal fistula consists of an abnormal connection between the oesophagus and the trachea, placing the untreated infant at risk for life-threatening aspiration.

◆ Anorectal defects are often associated with other congenital anomalies, such as those involving the gastrointestinal tract and heart.

◆ Defects involving herniation through the abdominal wall range from a simple umbilical hernia to complex gastroschisis.

◆ Obstructive uropathy can result in significant renal damage unless it is recognized and managed early.

◆ Ambiguous genitalia constitute a *social* emergency; therefore, an appropriate gender should be established as early as possible.

REFERENCES

Adzick NS, Harrison MR: Fetal surgical therapy, *Lancet* 343:897, 1994.

Anand KJ: Hormonal and metabolic functions of neonates and infants undergoing surgery, *Curr Opin Cardiol* 1:681, 1986.

Anand KJ, Aynsley-Green A: Measuring the severity of surgical stress in newborn infants, *J Pediatr Surg* 23:297, 1988.

Anand KJ, Hickey P: Pain and its effects in the human neonate and fetus, *N Engl J Med* 317:1321, 1987.

Anand KJ, Sippell WG, Aynsley-Green A: Randomized trial of fentanyl anaesthesia in preterm babies undergoing surgery: effects on the stress response, *Lancet* 31:243, 1987.

Anderson, S.M.: Secondary neurologic disability in myelomeningocele, *Inf Young Child* 1(4):9-21, 1989.

Barlow TG: Early diagnosis and treatment of CDH, *J Bone Joint Surg Br* 44:292, 1962.

Broshearst HR, Raney RB: *Handbook of orthopedic surgery*, ed. 10, St Louis, 1986, Mosby-Year Book, Inc.

Cartlidge PH, Mann NP, Kapilar L: Preoperative stabilization in congenital diaphragmatic hernia, *Arch Dis Child* 61:1226, 1986.

Cheetham CH *et al*: Congenital dislocation of the hip (letter), *BMJ* 286:277, 1983.

Clarke NMO: Role of ultrasound in congenital hip displasia, *Arch Dis Child* 70(5):362, 1994.

Clarren SK: Plagiocephaly and torticollis: etiology, natural history, and helmet treatment, *J Pediatr* 98:92, 1981.

Collins C *et al*: Fentanyl pharmacokinetics and hemodynamic effects in preterm infants during ligation of patent ductus arteriosus, *Anesth Analg* 64:1078, 1985.

Davies MRQ, Beale PG: Protection of oesophageal anastamosis following uncomplicated repair of common-type oes atresia by non-reversal of anaesthesia and guarded withdrawal of respiratory support, *Pediatr Surg Int* 6:98, 1991.

Davis PJM, Partridge JW, Storrs CN: Alcohol consumption in pregnancy: how much is safe? *Arch Dis Child* 57:940, 1982.

Dixon AG: Jeff's story: a unique approach to the care of an infant with esophageal atresia and a cervical esophagostomy, *Neonatal Network* 4(6):7, 1986.

Erlen, J.A., Holzman, I.R.: Anencephalic infants: should they be organ donors? *Pediatr Nurs* 14:6-64, 1988.

Gans SL, Austin E: Hernias and hydroceles. In Gennis SS, Kagan BM: *Current pediatric therapy 12*, Philadelphia, 1986, WB Saunders.

Glaser JH, Balistreri WF, Morecki R: Role of reovirus type 3 in persistent infantile cholestasis, *J Pediatr* 105:912, 1984.

Greig JD *et al.*: Value of antenatal diagnosis of abnormalities of the urinary tract, *BMJ* 298:1417, 1989.

Hindmarsh KW, Sankaran K, Watson VG: Plasma beta-endorphin concentrations in neonates associated with acute stress, *Dev Pharmacol Ther* 7:198, 1984.

Hussein M *et al*: Jaundice at 14 days of age: exclude biliary atresia, *Arch Dis Child* 66:1177, 1991.

Kaplan MR: Hematuria in childhood, *Pediatr Rev* 5:99, 1983.

Kinsella, Abman, *Pediatrics* 91(5):997, 1992.

Koop CE: The most important advances of the last 10 years, *Pediatr Consult* 12(1):1, 1981.

Lally KP *et al*: Preoperative factors affecting the outcome following repair of biliary atresia, *Pediatr* 83.723, 1989.

Lemons PKM: The sequelae to addiction, *Crit Care Update* 10(6):7, 1983.

Linder, M. *et al*: Effects of meningomyelocele closure on the intracranial pulse pressure, *Child's Brain* 11:176-182, 1984.

Maguire DP, Maloney P: A comparison of fentanyl and morphine use in neonates, *Neonatal Network* 7(1):27, 1988.

Malone P, Wheeler R and Williams J: Continence in patients with spinabifida: long-term results, *Arch Dis Child* 70(2):107, 1994.

Nelson R: Managing biliary atresia—referral before 6 weeks is vital, *BMJ* 298:1471, 1989.

Office of Population Censuses and Surveys England and Wales, London, 1990, HMSO Publications.

Penny R: Undescended testes. In Gellis SS, Kagan BM: *Current pediatric therapy 12*, Philadelphia, 1986, WB Saunders.

Rushton CH: The surgical neonate: principles of nursing management, *Pediatr Nurs* 14:141, 1988.

Ryckman F *et al*: Improved survival in bilary atresia patients in the present era of liver transplantation, *J Ped Surg* 28(3):382, 1993.

Saggese G *et al*: Hormonal therapy for cryptorchidism with a combination of human chorionic gonadotropin and follicle-stimulating hormone, *Am J Dis Child* 143:980, 1989.

Sakai H *et al*: Effect of surgical repair on respiratory mechanics in congenital diaphragmatic hernia, *J Pediatr* 111:432, 1987.

Scarff TB, Fronczak S: Myelomeningocele: a review and update, *Rehab Lit* 42(5-6):143, 1981.

Scott Adzick N, Harrison MR: Fetal surgical therapy, *Lancet* 343, April, pp 897, 1994.

Seashore JH: Disorders of the anus and rectum. In Gellis, SS, Kagan BM: *Current pediatric therapy 12*, Philadelphia, 1986, WB Saunders.

Shapiro C: Pain in the neonate: assessment and intervention, *Neonatal Network* 8(1):7, 1989.

Warshaw BL, Hymes LC, Woodard JR: Long-term outcome of patients with obstructive uropathy, *Pediatr Clin North Am* 29:815, 1982.

Wilson JM *et al*: Experimental fetal tracheal ligation—possible application for CDH, *J Ped Surg* 28(11):1433, 1993.

FURTHER READING

The Child with a Physical Defect

Heller A *et al.*: Birth defects and psychosocial adjustment, *Am J Dis Child* 139:257, 1985.

Jackson PL: When the baby isn't 'perfect', *AJN* 85:396, 1985.

Lemons PM: Beyond the birth of a defective child, *Neonatal Network* 5(3):13, 1986.

Porter FL: Pain in the newborn, *Clin Perinatol* 16:549, 1989.

Shaw N: Common surgical problems in the newborn, *J Perinat Neonatal Nurs* 3:50, 1990.

Surgery and Pain

Anand KJS, Aynsley-Green A: Measuring the severity of surgical stress in newborn infants, *J Pediatr Surg* 23(4):297, 1988.

Beaver PK: Premature infants' response to touch and pain: can nurses make a difference? *Neonatal Network* 6(3):13, 1987.

Butler NB: More on neonatal pain, *Perinatal Press* 11(2):19, 1988.

Jones MA: Identifying signs that nurses interpret as indicating pain in newborns, *Pediatr Nurs* 15:76, 1989.

Marshall RE: Neonatal pain associated with caregiving procedures, *Pediatr Clin North Am* 36:885, 1989.

Paxton JM: Transport of the surgical neonate, *J Perinat Neonatal Nurs* 3(3):43, 1990.

Shaw N: Common surgical problems in the newborn, *J Perinat Neonatal Nurs* 3(3):50, 1990.

Wise BV, Lawrence-Nolan L: A risk of blood transfusions for premature infants, *MCN* 15:86, 1990.

Neurological Defect

Bernardo ML: Craniosynostosis: the child's care from detection through correction, *MCN* 4:234, 1979.

Burton BK: Maternal serum a-fetoprotein screening, *Pediatr Ann* 18:687, 1989.

Charney EB: Parental attitudes toward management of newborns with myelomeningocele, *Dev Med Child Neurol* 32:14, 1990.

Cohen FL: Neural tube defects: epidemiology, detection, and prevention, *JOGNN* 16(2):105, 1987.

Graham JM: Craniostenosis: a new approach to management, *Pediatr Ann* 10:258, 1981.

Guertin SR: Cerebrospinal fluid shunts, evaluation, complications, and crisis management, *Pediatr Clin North Am* 34:203, 1987.

Jeffries JS, Killam PE, Varni JW: Behavioral management of fecal incontinence in a child with myelomeningocele, *Pediatr Nurs* 8:267, 1982.

Joseph DB *et al.*: Clean, intermittent catheterization of infants with neurogenic bladder, *Pediatr* 84:78, 1989.

Scheinblum DT, Hammond M: The treatment of children with shunt infections: extraventricular drainage system care, *Pediatr Nurs* 16:139, 1990.

Skeletal Defects

Aiello DH: Congenital dysplasia of the hip, diagnosis, treatment, nursing care, *AORN J* 49:1566, 1989.

Hall JG: When a child is born with congenital anomalies, *Contemp Pediatr* 5(8):78, 1988.

Gastrointestinal Defects

Alberly EH *et al.*, editors: *Cleft lip and palate—a team approach*, Bristol, 1986, Wright.

Curtin G: The infant with cleft lip or palate: more than a surgical problem, *J Perinat Neonatal Nurs* 3(3):80, 1990.

Fentner S: Abdominal wall defects: omphalocele and gastroschisis, *Neonatal Network* 6(3):29, 1987.

Oellrich RG, Cusumano MM: Biliary atresia, *Neonatal Network* 5(5):25, 1987.

Theorell CJ: Congenital diaphragmatic hernia: a physiologic approach to management, *J Perinat Neonatal Nurs* 3(3):66, 1990.

Torfs C, Curry C, Roeper P: Gastroschisis, *J Pediatr* 116:1, 1990.

Genitourinary Defects

Bernhardt J: Percutaneous nephrostomy tubes in the neonate with obstructive uropathy, *Neonatal Network* 4:51, 1986.

Jeffs RD: Extrophy, epispadias, and cloacal and urogenital sinus abnormalities, *Pediatr Clin North Am* 34:1233, 1987.

Mitchell ME, Rink RC: Pediatric urinary diversion and undiversion, *Pediatr Clin North Am* 34:1319, 1987.

Page J: The newborn with ambiguous genitalia, *Neonatal Network* 13(5):15, 1994.

Peevy KJ, Speed FA, Hoff CJ: Epidemiology of inguinal hernia in preterm neonates, *Pediatr* 77:246, 1986.

Stevens MS, Reinitz M: Nursing a child through exstrophic bladder reconstruction surgery, *MCN* 5:265, 1980.

Prenatal Influences: General

Rhodes AM: Legal alternatives for fetal injury, *MCN* 15:111, 1990.

Vande Perre P *et al.*: Postnatal transmission of human immunodeficiency virus type I from mother to infant, *N Engl J Med* 325:593-8, 1991.

Prenatal Influences: Infectious Agents

Kaplan KM *et al.*: A profile of mothers giving birth to infants with congenital rubella syndrome, *Am J Dis Child* 1144:118, 1990.

Prenatal Influences: AIDS

Prenatal Influences: Chemical Agents

Eliason MJ, Williams JK: Fetal alcohol syndrome and the neonate, *J Perinat Neonatal Nurs* 3(4):64, 1990.

Gastroschisis

Stoodley N *et al.*: Influence of place of delivery in babies with gastroschisis, *Arch Dis Childhood* 68(31):321, 1993.

Yeo H: Expert care at a critical time: surgical repair of gastroschisis in neonates, *Child Health* 1(2):74, 1993.

Nichols *et al.*: Is specialist centre delivery of gastroschisis beneficial, *Arch Dis Childhood* 69(1):71, 1993.

Spina bifida

Malone P, Wheeler R, Williams J: Continence in patients with spina bifida: Long-term results, *Arch Dis Child* 70(2):107, 1994.

Hydronephrosis

Scott A N, Harrison MR: Fetal surgical therapy, Lancet 343, April, pp 897, 1994.

Diaphragmatic

Department of Health: *Folic acid in the prevention of neural tube defects*, letter from the Chief Medical and Nursing Officers PL/CMO(91):6, London, Aug 12, 1991.

MRC Vitamin Study Group: Prevention of neural tube defects, *Lancet* 238: 131, 1991.

Office of Population Censuses and Surveys England and Wales, London, 1990, HMSO Publications.

USEFUL ADDRESSES

The Association for Spina Bifida and Hydrocephalus, 22 Upper Woburn Place, London WC1H 0EP.

The Cleft Lip and Palate Association, 1 Eastwood Gdns, Kenton, Newcastle-upon-Tyne NE3 3DQ

Chapter 15

Health Problems During Infancy

LEARNING OUTCOMES

After studying this chapter you should be able to:

◆ Describe assessment techniques for identifying unmet needs using Maslow's hierarchy of needs.
◆ Describe the basic nursing implications concerning unmet needs.
◆ Describe the relationships among different levels of needs.
◆ Identify actual or potential conditions that threaten fulfilment of patient needs.
◆ State factors that influence the individual need priorities.
◆ Identify techniques used in guiding caregivers on the correct procedures for handling any feeding or diet problems.
◆ Assess ways to ensure caregiver/child will comply with medical or nursing advice.
◆ Identify ways to define outcomes of care/advice.
◆ Define the glossary terms.

GLOSSARY

allergens or **allergic antigens** Usually proteins that are capable of inducing IgE antibody formation ('sensitization') when ingested, injected, or inhaled

apnoea (pathological) Respiratory pause of more than 20 seconds or shorter pause associated with cyanosis, marked pallor, hypotonia, or bradycardia

atopy Allergy with tendency to be inherited

deficiency Inadequate intake of a nutrient that causes adverse clinical effects

fat-soluble vitamins Vitamins A, D, E, and K

food allergy or **hypersensitivity** Adverse reactions involving immunological mechanisms, usually IgE

food intolerance Adverse reactions involving known or unknown nonimmunological mechanisms

food sensitivity Any type of adverse reaction to food or food additives

hypervitaminosis Excessive intake of a vitamin that causes adverse clinical effects

kwashiorkor Protein deficiency with low or adequate energy sources

macrominerals Minerals that have a daily requirement greater than 100 mg

marasmus State of semistarvation from inadequate protein and energy

microminerals (trace elements) Minerals that have daily requirements less than 100 mg

sensitization Initial exposure of an individual to allergen, resulting in an immune response; subsequent exposure induces a much stronger response

vegan General term referring to individuals who exclude all animal products from the diet

vegetarian General term referring to individuals who exclude meat from the diet, but may include dairy products

water-soluble vitamins B complex and C vitamins

An infant's immaturity predisposes several potential health problems during the first year. This chapter deals primarily with health problems that are influenced by environmental factors affecting the physical or psychological development of the child. Some of the problems, such as nutritional disturbances, have special implications for nurses, because they are preventable. Others, such as sudden infant death syndrome (SIDS), are uncontrollable and unpredictable, but the intervention needed after the death of the child is crucial for the family. Although several of the topics discussed here can occur in age groups other than infancy, the greatest significance of these disorders is evident during the early months and years of life. Prompt awareness and identification of health problems hopefully will avert complications in later life. Prevention whenever possible, rather than treatment, should be every health professional's goal in the care of children.

NUTRITIONAL DISTURBANCES

Poor nutrition is a general term that refers to inadequate nutrition. Although it is generally thought of in terms of undernutrition, it also includes overnutrition, which may be manifested as obesity or hypervitaminosis. Inadequate nutrition is most commonly seen as iron deficiency anaemia (see Chapter 29), vitamin deficiencies, or failure to thrive. Each of these is related to a wide variety of factors — economic, social, and cultural. While poverty is the economic precursor of malnutrition, it is usually when certain cultural and social factors coincide with poverty that malnutrition becomes a threat. Culture influences food selection and may limit certain nutritious foods because of preference, not availability.

Since all of these nutritional disturbances are amenable to some degree of alteration through intervention, the nutritional disturbances to be discussed could potentially be eliminated. However, adequate food supplies alone are not the answer, especially when sociocultural factors that affect food consumption are considered. Therefore, nutritional counselling becomes a complex process that must take into account all the variables affecting the physical and psychological make-up of the family.

VITAMIN DEFICIENCIES

Vitamins are an essential food element and function in small quantities by regulating specific metabolic activity, usually by acting as *coenzymes*. When vitamin coenzymes enter the body, they are combined with a protein *apoenzyme* that has been synthesized within the cell to form a *holoenzyme*. The quantity of apoenzymes any cell can produce limits the body's ability to make use of excessive vitamins (Jarvis, 1984). A deficiency of the vitamin directly affects the metabolic activity it regulates. However, regular ingestion of excessive amounts of vitamins may produce a toxic effect.

True vitamin disturbances are rare in the United Kingdom, but subclinical deficiencies are commonly seen, especially in lower socioeconomic groups where proper dietary intake may be imbalanced. Vitamin D deficient rickets, once rarely seen

because of vitamin D fortified milk, has increased. Populations at risk include: (1) children born of mothers who are vitamin D deficient, (2) individuals who are exposed to minimal sunlight because of distinctive clothing, housing in areas of high pollution, or dark skin pigmentation, (3) adherence to vegetarian diets that are low in sources of vitamin D.

Children may also be at risk of vitamin deficiency due to disorders or their treatment. For example, vitamin deficiencies of the fat-soluble vitamins A and D may occur in malabsorptive disorders. Children on high doses of salicylates, such as for rheumatoid arthritis, may have impaired vitamin C storage (Olness, 1985).

Of equal, if not greater concern, is the overuse of vitamins. An excessive dose of a vitamin is generally defined as 10 or more times the recommended dietary allowance (RDA), although the fat-soluble vitamins, especially A and D, tend to cause toxic reactions at lower doses (Council on Scientific Affairs, 1987). With the addition of vitamins to commercially prepared foods, the potential for hypervitaminosis has increased, especially when combined with the injudicious use of vitamin supplements. Hypervitaminosis of A and D presents the greatest problems, because these fat-soluble vitamins are stored in the body. Vitamin D is the most likely of all vitamins to cause toxic reactions in relatively small overdoses. However, there appears to be variance in the tolerance to different vitamin intakes. For example, two children ingesting excessive amounts of vitamin A may not both demonstrate clinical features of intoxication (Carpenter *et al*, 1987).

MINERAL DEFICIENCIES

Several minerals are essential nutrients. The *macrominerals* refer to those with daily requirements greater than 100 mg and include calcium, phosphorus, magnesium, sodium, potassium, chloride, and sulphur. *Trace elements* have daily requirements less than 100 mg and include several essential minerals and those whose exact role in nutrition is still unclear. The greatest concern with minerals is deficiency, especially iron deficiency anaemia (see Chapter 29). However, other minerals that may be inadequate in children's diets, even with supplementation, include calcium, phosphorus, magnesium, and zinc (Moss *et al.*, 1989). Low levels of zinc can cause nutritional failure to thrive (Walravens, Hambidge and Koepfer, 1989).

VEGETARIAN DIETS

The importance of vegan or certain vegetarian diets and their relationship to potential nutritional deficiencies in children cannot be overemphasized. The stricter the vegetarian diet, the more difficult it becomes to ensure adequate nutrition for infants and children. The major types of vegetarianism are described in Box 15-1.

Many individuals who are concerned about healthy diets subscribe to vegetarian diets that are not typified by the categories in Box 15-1. Therefore, during nutritional assessment, it is necessary to clearly list exactly what the diet includes and excludes.

The lacto-ovovegetarian diet is associated with the least deficiencies, although protein intake needs to be monitored. The lactovegetarian diet may be low in protein, as well as iron. The major deficiencies in the stricter vegetarian diets are inadequate protein for growth, inadequate calories for energy and growth, poor digestibility of many of the natural, unprocessed foods, especially for infants, and deficiencies of vitamin B_{12}, niacin, thiamine, riboflavin, vitamin D, iron, calcium, and zinc.

Because vegetarian diets eliminate the major sources of complete proteins, protein deficiency can occur. Fortunately, this problem is easily remedied by selecting foods with complementary amino acids and consuming them at the same meal (Box 15-2).

Achieving a nutritionally adequate vegetarian diet is not difficult, but it requires careful planning and knowledge of nutrient sources. For children, the lacto-ovovegetarian diet is nutritionally adequate; however, the vegan diet requires supplementation with vitamins D and B_{12}, particularly for children ages 2-12 years. Infants on a vegan diet should be breast-fed for the first six months and preferably for one year, fed solid foods after about four months, and receive iron-fortified cereal for at least 18 months. The use of vitamin C juices with foods high in iron will further improve iron absorption. If cow's or human milk is not given, fortified soy milk is recommended.

IMPLICATIONS FOR NURSING

Since one of the best assurances of nutritional adequacy is eating a variety of foods, families need guidelines for selecting foods that provide essential nutrients without exceeding energy requirements. The health adviser is the ideal professional to advise and counsel families on the importance of a nutritionally adequate diet.

OBESITY

Obesity is a complex condition that may or may not be related to the chronic ingestion of more calories than are needed to supply the body's energy requirement. Genetic factors play a significant role, since there is a strong correlation of obesity among family members that is not evident among parents and adopted children (Stunkard *et al*, 1986, 1990).

Firm evidence links obesity in infancy and adolescence to obesity in adulthood (see Obesity, Chapter 19); the evidence for obesity in infancy remaining a risk factor for adult obesity is controversial. Although recent studies have examined the role of infant feeding methods and subsequent overweight, these results are also conflicting. One study found that infants who were breast-fed beyond six months of age had slower growth rates than bottle-fed infants during the second half of the first year (Dewey *et al*, 1989).

Despite the conflicting data on exactly what causes infant obesity, all authorities agree that *prevention* holds greater promise than treatment. Besides the physiological component of increased numbers of fat cells, there are also the psychological disadvantages of firmly entrenched food habits and dependency on food. Consequently, evaluation of overnutrition *early* in life is essential, with attention to factors that may prevent obesity.

IMPLICATIONS FOR NURSING

The principal nursing goal is prevention of obesity. If infants are overweight for their height, the goal is to slow weight gain, not cause weight loss. During infancy, the development of obesity is influenced by parental practices. Education on prevention of obesity can be obtained from the health visitor for young children, and from the school nurse for school-aged children. Intervention involves helping the parent establish appropriate feeding habits for the infant or to change inappropriate habits. This involves much more than dietary counselling. Psychological factors play an important role, particularly the philosophy that a fat baby is a healthy baby, or, more subconsciously, that a fat 'healthy' baby is a sign of good mothering (Sherman and Alexander, 1990). Such beliefs are difficult to dispel, and counselling may need to include other family members (such as grandmothers), especially in ethnic groups, who can greatly influence the mother's practices.

Although the exact role breast-feeding has on the development of subsequent obesity is unclear, its protective effect may be related to self-regulation of intake. With bottle feeding, parents may encourage the infant to finish all of the bottle, establishing a habit of eating beyond the initial feeling of

---

◆ **BOX 15-1**

Types of vegetarian diets

Lacto-ovovegetarians exclude meat from their diet, but eat milk, eggs and sometimes fish.
Lactovegetarians exclude meat and eggs, but drink milk.
Pure vegetarians (vegans) eliminate any food of animal origin, including milk and eggs.
Macrobiotics are more restrictive than pure vegetarians; cereals, especially brown or polished rice, are the mainstay of the diet.

◆ **BOX 15-2**

Food combinations for complementary amino acids

Grains (cereal, rice, pasta) and **legumes** (beans, peas, lentils, peanuts)

Grains and **milk products** (milk, cheese, yoghurt)

Seeds (sesame, sunflower) and **legumes**

satiety. During nutritional counselling, the health visitor should discuss with parents appropriate feeding habits, such as allowing the child to regulate the need for formula and solid food. With proper education, parents can come to understand that a 'good eater' is not a big eater but one who eats moderately without necessarily 'cleaning the plate'.

Weaning foods are another important aspect of nutritional counselling. When solid foods are added, the quantity of milk should be decreased to less than 1 litre to maintain the proper caloric balance. Water can be substituted for a bottle of formula milk. Substituting skimmed or low-fat milk for whole milk or formula is unacceptable. Semi-skimmed milk can only be given after the age of two years. Although they contain a significant reduction in calories, they are not nutritionally sound for infants. Their low fat content deprives the infant of essential fatty acids, their significantly increased amounts of solids and electrolytes elevate the renal solute load and water demands, and their vitamin A content is reduced.

The selection of solid foods should also be considered. Approximately 20% of commercial baby foods contain less than 50 kcal/100 g, whereas another 20% contain more than 100 kcal/100 g. Choosing low calorie foods can significantly lower the daily calorie intake without actually decreasing the total quantity of food. Parents should be encouraged to read food labels. Sweet foods should be kept to a minimum. This includes not adding additional sugar to the formula or cereal and avoiding finger foods such as biscuits. Other foods rich in calories that should be restricted in serving size rather than eliminated include butter, cream, ice cream, and chocolate.

Parents should also be encouraged to interpret the infant's signals of discomfort and to intervene in ways other than through feeding. Crying, fussiness, or sucking does not necessarily indicate hunger. Rocking, stroking, holding, and offering a pacifier may be more appropriate than automatically responding with food (Wishon and Kinnick, 1986).

Since activity is also an important factor in maintaining appropriate weight, parents should be encouraged to promote exercise in their child. Although infants are naturally active, placing them in confined areas, such as cots or playpens, and in front of televisions, establishes poor habits. There is a direct relationship between time spent viewing television and the tendency towards obesity.

FOOD SENSITIVITY

Food sensitivity is a general term that includes any type of adverse reaction to food or food additives. Food sensitivities can be divided into two broad categories (Anderson, 1986):
- **Food allergy** or **hypersensitivity,** which refers to reactions involving immunological mechanisms, usually immunoglobulin E (IgE); the reactions may be immediate or delayed and mild or severe, such as an anaphylactic reaction.
- **Food intolerance,** which refers to reactions involving known or unknown nonimmunological mechanisms; lactose intolerance is an example of a reaction that looks like allergy, but is due to deficiency of the enzyme lactase.

However, this classification is not universally accepted; therefore, the terms *food sensitivity, hypersensitivity, allergy,* and *intolerance* are often used interchangeably.

Food allergy is caused by exposure to *allergens,* also called *allergic antigens.* They are usually proteins (but not the smaller amino acids) that are capable of inducing IgE antibody formation ('sensitization') when ingested. Sensitization refers to the initial exposure of an individual to an allergen, resulting in an immune response; subsequent exposure induces a much stronger response that is clinically apparent. Consequently, food hypersensitivity typically occurs after the food has been ingested one or more times. In infants, an allergic response can occur with the first ingestion because of transplacental sensitization *in utero* or because of sensitization to the substance passed through breast milk (Wilson, Self and Hamburger, 1990). Allergens can also produce an allergic response when inhaled or injected, but these routes rarely apply to food allergens (see also discussion of asthma in Chapter 26). The most common food allergens are eggs, cow's milk, peanuts, wheat, corn, and fish.

Food allergies can occur at any time, but are common during infancy because the immature intestinal tract is more permeable to proteins than the mature intestinal tract, thus increasing the likelihood of an immune response. Allergies in general demonstrate a genetic component: children who have one parent with allergy have a 50-58% risk of developing allergy; children who have both parents with allergy have up to a 100% risk of developing allergy. Allergy with a hereditary tendency is referred to as *atopy.*

Although the reason is unknown, many children 'outgrow' their food allergies. Children who are allergic to more than one food may develop tolerance to each food at different times. The most common allergens are outgrown less readily than other food allergens. Because of the tendency to lose the hypersensitivity, allergenic foods should be reintroduced into the diet after a period of abstinence (usually one year or more) to evaluate if the food can be safely added to the diet (Sampson and Scanlon, 1989).

There is evidence that food allergies and asthma can be prevented by excluding from the mother's diet all milk, fish and egg products. The child is breast fed as normal and introduced to these foods gradually at a later than usual age (e.g., 4–6 years) (National Childbirth Trust).

COW'S MILK INTOLERANCE

Cow's milk intolerance is a multifaceted disorder representing adverse systemic and local gastrointestinal reactions to cow's milk protein. The hypersensitivity may be manifest through a variety of signs and symptoms (Box 15-3) that may appear within 45 minutes of milk ingestion or after a period of several days (Hill *et al.,* 1986, 1989). The diagnosis is initially made from careful history taking. For example, cow's milk allergy may be manifest as colic or sleeplessness in an otherwise healthy infant.

Process of diagnosis

Several diagnostic tests may be performed, including stool analysis for blood (both frank and occult bleeding can occur from the colitis), serum IgE levels and skin-prick testing.

The most definitive diagnostic strategy is elimination of milk, followed by challenge testing after improvement of symptoms. A good history is also essential.

Therapeutic management

Treatment of cow's milk allergy is elimination of all dairy products. For infants fed cow's milk formula, this primarily involves changing the formula to a casein or whey hydrolysate milk formula, in which the protein has been broken down (or 'predigested') into its amino acids through enzymatic hydrolysis. Soya-based formula is not recommended, because as many as 20% of these infants are also allergic to soya. Goat's milk is not an acceptable substitute, since it cross-reacts with cow's milk protein and is deficient in folic acid. Infants who are breast-fed but have symptoms of cow's milk hypersensitivity are treated by eliminating all dairy products from the lactating mother's diet. These women need vitamin D and calcium supplementation to prevent deficiency. Infants are maintained on the dairy-free diet for one or two years, at which time very small quantities of milk are reintroduced.

IMPLICATIONS FOR NURSING

The principal nursing objectives are identification of potential milk allergy and appropriate counselling of parents regarding substitute formulas. The protein hydrolysate formulas are less palatable than milk-based formulas. Consequently, reluctance to accept the new formula may be a problem. This can be overcome by introducing the formula gradually over a few days using 1 ounce of new formula to 7 ounces of old formula, then 2 to 6 ounces, 3 to 4, and as needed. Parents also need to be reassured that the infant will receive complete nutrition from the new formula and will suffer no ill effects from the absence of cow's milk.

Once solid foods are started, parents need guidance in avoiding all associated milk products during weaning. This requires carefully reading all food labels to avoid potential addition of milk products to the prepared food.

LACTOSE INTOLERANCE

Lactose intolerance refers to at least two different entities that involve a deficiency of the enzyme lactase, which is needed for the digestion of lactose. *Congenital lactose intolerance* appears soon after birth when the diet contains lactose from milk. *Late-onset lactose intolerance* is similar to the congenital type, but manifests later in life. The principal manifestations include diarrhoea, abdominal pain, distension, and flatus shortly after ingesting milk products.

In older children, lactose intolerance may be diagnosed on the basis of the history and improvement following a lactose-free diet.

◆ **BOX 15-3**

Clinical manifestations of cow's milk sensitivity

Gastrointestinal
- Diarrhoea*
- Vomiting*
- Colic*
- Abdominal pain*
- Haematochezia (bloody stools)
- Malabsorption
- Enteropathy
- Constipation
- Anorexia
- Colitis

Respiratory
- Rhinitis*
- Bronchitis*
- Asthma*
- Sneezing*
- Coughing*
- Chronic nasal discharge*
- Recurrent croup
- Serous otitis media

Dermatological
- Eczema*
- Urticaria
- Hives

Central Nervous and Behavioural
- Excessive crying*
- Excessive night waking; sleeplessness
- Excessive sweating
- Headache
- Hyperirritability
- Hyperactivity
- Lethargy

Vascular
- Facial pallor
- Infraorbital oedema (swelling under eyes)

Constitutional
- Failure to thrive
- Retarded growth
- Malnutrition

*Most common.

Treatment of lactose intolerance is elimination of many dairy products. In infants, soya-based formula can be substituted for cow's milk formula or human milk. Some children are able to tolerate small amounts of lactose. Since dairy products are a major source of calcium and vitamin D, supplementation of these nutrients is needed to prevent deficiency.

Implications for nursing

Nursing care is similar to the interventions discussed for cow's milk allergy: explaining the dietary restrictions to the family; identifying alternative sources of calcium, such as yoghurt and green leafy vegetables, and the need for supplementation; and discussing sources of lactose, especially hidden sources, such as its use as a bulk agent in certain medications. Parents are advised to check with the pharmacist regarding this possibility when obtaining medication.

FEEDING DIFFICULTIES

Several feeding difficulties can occur during the infant's first year. Minor breast-feeding problems are common and often cause mothers considerable concern and discomfort. Some, such as posseting, require little more than parental reassurance. Others, such as colic, can tremendously disrupt a family, although the problem resolves spontaneously.

BREAST-FEEDING PROBLEMS

Many mothers have concerns regarding breast-feeding and, with earlier discharge from maternity units, common problems, such as engorgement and painful nipples, may occur once the mother is at home. New mothers are often concerned about their milk supply, and excessive anxiety can affect successful lactation. There is increasing evidence that some exclusively breast-fed infants gain weight more slowly than bottle-fed infants, especially after the first 4-6 months, but that their growth is adequate (Dewey *et al,* 1989).

Most of the common breast-feeding problems are easily remedied, provided the mother receives the attention needed to identify the concern (Box 15-4). Many problems respond rapidly to simple interventions, such as correcting the infant's feeding position. However, the mother needs continual reassurance of success and support that allow her the needed rest and relaxation to nurse her infant. Referral to supportive agencies, such as local groups of La Leche League (see useful addresses), the National Childbirth Trust (see useful addresses), or a breast-feeding counsellor, may be beneficial.

REGURGITATION AND POSSETING

The return of small amounts of food after a feeding is a common occurrence during infancy. It should not be confused with actual vomiting, which can be associated with a number of disturbances that may be insignificant or serious. It is usually benign, although persistent regurgitation necessitates medical evaluation to rule out gastro-oesophageal reflux.

PAROXYSMAL ABDOMINAL PAIN (COLIC)

Colic is generally described as paroxysmal abdominal pain or cramping that is manifested by loud crying and drawing the legs up to the abdomen. Other definitions include variables such as duration of cry greater than three hours a day and parental dissatisfaction with the child's behaviour. It is more common in young infants under the age of three months than in older infants, and infants with 'difficult' temperaments are more likely to be colicky (Barr *et al,* 1989). Despite the obvious behavioural indications of pain, the child tolerates the formula well, gains weight, and thrives.

Many theories have been investigated as to potential causative factors, but currently no one theory is supported universally. In fact, much controversy exists over the aetiology of the condition, and some authorities question if colic merely represents a maturational stage.

While colic is considered a minor ailment, the presence of a colicky, crying, irritable infant can have an intense emotional impact on parent–child attachment and family relationships. Parents, especially mothers, often relate histories of a daily routine that is laden with feelings of frustration, anger, despair, and helplessness. A vicious cycle ensues in which the parent's own anxiety may be transferred to the infant, further increasing the tension, irritability, and crying.

IMPLICATIONS FOR NURSING

The initial step in managing colic is to take a thorough, detailed history of the usual daily events. Areas that should be stressed include: (1) diet of the breast-feeding mother, (2) time of day when attacks occur, (3) relationship of the attacks to feeding time, (4) presence of specific family members and habits, such as smoking, during attacks (5) activity of the mother or usual caregiver before, during, and after the crying, (6) characteristics of the cry (duration, intensity), and (7) measures used to relieve the crying and their effectiveness. Of special emphasis is a careful assessment of the feeding process via *demonstration* by the parent.

◆ **BOX 15-4**

Guidelines for observing the breast-feeding couple

Position of mother, her body language, and tension

Position of infant: child should be next to mother with the face directly in front of the breast; the infant cannot swallow if the head has to turn to the breast

Position of mother's hand on breast: using two fingers to compress areola and support breast facilitates infant's ability to grasp areola properly

Position of infant's lips on areola: lips should gently clamp the *entire* areola; lower lip should not be folded in so infant sucks lip

Use of alternate breasts and feeding time on each breast

Technique to break suction: should release suction using fingers between areola and lips; should not pull infant from the breast

---

If milk sensitivity is suspected, breast-feeding mothers may be asked to follow a milk-free diet for a minimum of five days in an attempt to reduce symptoms in the infant. If this approach is helpful, lactating mothers may need calcium supplements to meet the body's requirement. Bottle-fed infants may improve with the same dietary modifications as for the child with cow's milk allergy.

More often than not, no change is required in feeding practices. When no cause can be identified, it is preferable to determine the time of the onset of crying and attempt to manipulate the circumstances associated with it. For example, some infants have episodes of colic around the family's dinner time, when all household members are home and the mother is preoccupied with cooking. The overstimulating, more tense atmosphere may upset the infant. Encouraging someone else to prepare dinner or the mother to prepare dinner earlier in the day and feed the infant in a more quiet area of the house may help reverse the environmental conditions that may have provoked the attack of colic. The carrying method illustrated in Figure. 15-1 has been found to be helpful in the relief of infant colic.

One of the most important areas of nursing concern is the support of parents during the colic period. It should be stressed that despite the crying and obvious pain, the infant is doing well. Colic disappears spontaneously, usually by three months of age, although guarantees should never be given because it may continue for much longer. The disappearance of colic is as an indication of weight gain. The parent, especially the mother, should be encouraged to leave the house and arrange for some free time. Most important, it should be emphasized that colic does not indicate poor or inadequate parenting.

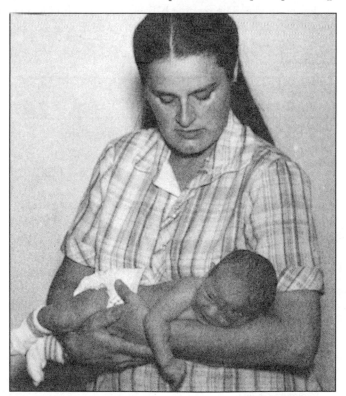

Fig. 15-1 The 'colic carry' may be comforting to an infant with colic.

Parents' negative feelings towards the infant and insecurities regarding their parenting abilities are normal. Parents are encouraged to talk about such feelings, since active listening may do more to relieve the colic syndrome than offering stereotyped advice and remedies.

FAILURE TO THRIVE

The term *failure to thrive* refers to a state of inadequate growth from inability to obtain and/or use calories required for growth. It is a symptom, not a disease, but regardless of the aetiology, all such children have malnutrition. Failure to thrive has no universal definition, although one of the more common parameters is weight and sometimes height. Percentile charts should be used for all infants. If the weight and height measurements fall off the percentile as indicated by the birthweight for that percentile, then FTT should be considered. Growth measurements alone are not used to diagnose children with FTT. Rather, the finding of a persistent deviation from an established growth curve is cause for concern.

Two general categories of failure to thrive have been defined:

- **Organic failure to thrive,** which is the result of a physical cause, such as congenital heart defects, neurological lesions, microcephaly, chronic urinary tract infection, gastro-oesophageal reflux, renal insufficiency, malabsorption syndrome, endocrine dysfunction, or cystic fibrosis. This category accounts for less than half of all FTT.
- **Nonorganic failure to thrive,** which has a definable cause that is unrelated to disease. NFTT is most often the result of psychosocial factors, such as inadequate nutritional information by the parent; deficiency in maternal care or a disturbance in maternal-child attachment; or a disturbance in the child's ability to separate from the parent, leading to food refusal in order to maintain attention (Chatoor *et al*, 1985). NFTT has been described under a variety of less acceptable names, including maternal deprivation, environmental deprivation, and deprivation dwarfism.

Traditionally, the category of nonorganic failure to thrive has implied a disturbance in the parent-child interaction. However, this is not always the case. Many other factors can lead to inadequate feeding of the infant (Box 15-5). In these instances, parent education and provision of necessary support (financial or psychosocial) are successful in correcting the reason for the malnutrition. Dealing with families in which a child has nonorganic failure to thrive because of a parent-child disturbance is much more difficult and is the focus of the nursing care discussion on the next page.

PROCESS OF DIAGNOSIS

Diagnosis is initially made on anthropomorphic findings documenting growth retardation. If FTT is recent, the weight, but not the height, is below accepted standards; if FTT is long-standing, both weight and height are depressed, indicating chronic malnutrition.

◆ BOX 15-5

Selected causes of failure to thrive usually unrelated to disturbed parent-child interactions

Poverty — lack of funds to buy sufficient food; may dilute formula to extend available supply

Health beliefs — use of fad diets; excessive concern with preventing conditions such as obesity, hypercholesterolaemia, or nursing caries

Inadequate nutritional knowledge — cultural confusion of newly arrived immigrants who are unaware of appropriate food selections in food stores; parents with cognitive impairment

Family stress — overwhelming involvement with another chronically ill child; lack of energy to deal with feeding problems in addition to other needs of child with OFTT; other stresses (financial, marital, excessive parenting and employment responsibilities, depression, drug abuse, alcohol misuse, acute grief)

Feeding resistance — result of non-oral nutritional therapy early in life (see Feeding Resistance, Chapter 13)

Insufficient breast milk — result of many different causes (fatigue, illness, poor release of milk, insufficient glandular tissue, lack of confidence)

Additional diagnostic procedures include a dietary history; a complete history and physical examination for signs of serious chronic illness or other conditions known to cause growth retardation; developmental assessment; and a family assessment. Other tests are selected only as indicated to rule out organic problems. Unfortunately, many of these children undergo exhausting, traumatic, and expensive diagnostic procedures that are unnecessary. To prevent the overuse of diagnostic procedures, NFTT should be considered *early* in the differential diagnosis.

THERAPEUTIC MANAGEMENT

Regardless of the cause of FTT, the treatment is directed at reversing the malnutrition. The goal is to provide sufficient calories to support 'catch-up' growth—a rate of growth greater than the expected rate for age.

In cases of NFTT due to a disturbed parent-child relationship, a multidisciplinary team of doctor, nurse, dietitian, health visitor, and social worker or mental health professional is needed to deal with the multiple psychological problems and to provide family-centred care.

PROGNOSIS

The prognosis for NFTT is related to the cause. If the parents have simply been ignorant of the infant's needs, teaching may remedy the child's limited caloric intake and permanently reverse the growth failure. However, when the family dys-

function is extensive, the prognosis is uncertain. Intensive health visiting may be required. Factors related to poor prognosis are severe feeding resistance, lack of awareness in and cooperation from the parent(s), low family income, low maternal educational level, and early age of onset of NFTT (Ayoub and Milner, 1985). Many of these children are below normal in intellectual development, have poorer language development and less well-developed reading skills, attain lower social maturity, and have a higher incidence of behavioural disturbances (Oates, Peacock and Forrest, 1985). Such findings indicate that a long-term plan is needed for the optimum development of these children. Admission to a hospital or family centre may be necessary.

IMPLICATIONS FOR NURSING

Caring for the child with NFTT presents many nursing challenges, whether treatment takes place in hospital or at home. Providing a positive feeding environment, teaching the parent successful feeding strategies, and supporting the child and family are essential components of care.

Assessment

Nurses and health visitors play a critical role in the diagnosis of NFTT through their assessment of the child, parents, and family interaction. Knowledge of the characteristics of children with NFTT and their families is essential in helping identify these children and hastening the confirmation of a correct diagnosis (Box 15-6). Accurate assessment of initial weight and height and daily weight is mandatory, as well as recording of all food intake. The feeding behaviour of the child is documented, as well as the parent-child interaction during feeding, other caregiving activities, and play (Box 15-7).

◆ BOX 15-6

Clinical manifestations of nonorganic failure to thrive

Growth failure — below 5th percentile in weight only or in weight and height

Developmental retardation — social, motor, adaptive, language

Apathy

Poor hygiene

Withdrawn behaviour

Feeding or eating disorders, such as vomiting, anorexia, pica, rumination

No fear of strangers (at age when stranger anxiety is normal)

Avoidance of eye-to-eye contact

Wide-eyed gaze and continual scan of the environment ('radar gaze')

Stiff and unyielding or flaccid and unresponsive

Minimum smiling

The approximate developmental age should be assessed on admission by administering an appropriate developmental test. Only after objective measurements are available is a plan of care for stimulation outlined.

Planning

Planning should begin as soon as possible on admission. The priority nursing goal is providing the infant with sufficient nutrients for growth. More specific nursing care depends on the identified cause of FTT. If an organic aetiology is confirmed, care is related primarily to management of the disorder. If the problem is one of inadequate knowledge regarding child feeding, parental education is required. When serious psychosocial factors are involved, hospitalization is needed and additional interventions are required to meet the needs of both the child and family. The following are goals for the hospitalized child with NFTT:

◆ **BOX 15-7**

Parental maladaptive behaviours towards infant

Persistent ambivalence or negative feelings about the fetus and the pregnancy during the prenatal period

Makes no plans for obtaining basic infant supplies

Appears indifferent to infant at time of delivery; may appear sad or angry; is expressionless

Makes no effort to establish eye-to-eye contact with infant

Handles infant only when necessary

Makes few or no spontaneous movements with infant

Asks few questions about care

Sees infant as ugly, fat, or unattractive

Displays disgust with infant's drooling and sucking sounds; is revolted by infant's body fluids

Annoyed with nappy changing

Holds infant with little support to head and body

Holds infant away from body during feeding or props bottle for feeding; seldom cuddles infant

Refers to infant in an impersonal manner

Develops inappropriate responses to infant's needs, such as leaving infant in one place for long periods, leaving child alone in room, overfeeding or underfeeding, overstimulating or understimulating infant, forcing or refusing eye contact, bouncing or tickling infant when child is tired

Cannot discriminate between infant's signals for hunger, comfort, rest, body contact

Is convinced the infant has a defect or disease even when reassured to the contrary

Makes negative statements regarding parenting role

Believes the infant is judging him/her and efforts as an adult

Believes the infant does not love him/her

Develops paradoxical attitudes and behaviours towards the infant

---

1. Structure a feeding environment that encourages the child to consume adequate calories; provide age-appropriate foods.
2. Provide appropriate developmental stimulation for the child.
3. Teach parents feeding techniques and other caregiving activities, such as suitable play, that are successful in the hospital.
4. Provide a nurturing environment for the parent; make appropriate referrals for supportive services.

Implementation

The effectiveness of nursing and health visiting interventions is determined by continual reassessment and evaluation of care based on the following observational guidelines and expected outcomes:

1. Record weight and calorie intake daily; document child's reaction to feeding environment; review notes to see if changes were made as necessary to improve eating and if consistent group of nurses fed child.
2. Perform periodic developmental screening tests.
3. Document parents' relationship with staff or other supportive individuals. Note length of time parents visit with these people, appointments kept with referral services, and any requests for help.
4. Keep a record of all teaching and compare taught skills with parent's actual skills.

SKIN DISORDERS

Several skin problems manifest themselves during infancy. The most common is nappy rash; others that occur during infancy are seborrhoeic dermatitis and atopic dermatitis. While these conditions can be benign, they are often of considerable concern to parents. The nurse is in an advantageous position to counsel parents regarding care of these common skin problems.

NAPPY RASH

Dermatitis in the nappy area is encountered frequently by nurses in all paediatric settings. Approximately 50% of young children demonstrate some degree of nappy rash, and about 5% have severe rash (intense erythema, scaling, papules, and ulcerations). The peak age for nappy rash is 9–12 months and may be associated with decreased frequency of nappy changes and modifications in diet, such as change from breast milk to formula and introduction of solids. The incidence is generally reported as greater in bottle-fed than in breast-fed infants.

PATHOPHYSIOLOGY AND CLINICAL MANIFESTATIONS

Nappy rash is caused by prolonged and repetitive contact with an irritant, principally urine, faeces, soaps, detergents, ointments and friction. Although the obvious irritant in the majority of incidences is urine and faeces, the specific components that contribute to irritation include a combination of factors.

THERAPEUTIC MANAGEMENT

Treatment is primarily related to the measures discussed under Implications for Nursing. For stubborn inflammations that do not respond to these interventions, topical glucocorticoid preparations are sometimes required. If steroids are prescribed, their use is generally limited to low-potency preparations such as 1% hydrocortisone cream.

Candida infections are treated with nystatin ointment. Where *Candida* is the causative agent, oral administration of a fungicide is advised because the gastrointestinal tract is usually the source of infection (see Candidiasis, Chapter 13).

IMPLICATIONS FOR NURSING

Nursing interventions are aimed at altering the three factors considered to produce dermatitis — wetness, pH, and faecal irritants. The most significant factor amenable to intervention is the moist environment created in the nappy area. Changing the nappy as soon as it becomes wet eliminates a large part of the problem, and removing the nappy entirely for extended periods, to expose the area to light and air, facilitates drying and healing. Occlusive nappy coverings, such as plastic pants, prevent evaporation and should not be used except for brief social occasions. During the night, the nappy should be changed at least once, such as before the parents retire. The use of two cotton or disposable nappies *without* the plastic lining, or the use of disposable nappies with absorbent gelling material increases absorbency, and nappies with linings draw wetness away from the skin.

After soiling, the perineal area should be cleansed, preferably with plain water and, if needed, a mild soap. Wiping with a wet cloth is usually sufficient to remove urine. However, after defecation, the area, especially the skin folds, needs to be thoroughly cleansed, rinsed, and dried. In some instances, especially with diarrhoeal stools and irritated skin, a sponge bath may be given. Exposing the skin to warm, dry air for a few minutes before applying the nappy is helpful.

Occasionally applying an occlusive ointment, such as zinc oxide or petrolatum, to noninflamed skin can prevent the development of nappy dermatitis, provided good hygiene is also practised. During cleansing, the ointment is removed and then reapplied. Zinc oxide is most easily removed with mineral oil. The use of talcum powder is of questionable benefit. Despite the known risks of talc, it is a common baby care product. The majority of parents are likely to receive a free sample of the product in the maternity ward and to continue using that brand. While no known research exists to substantiate whether the practice of free talc samples influences the incidence of inhalation injury, nurses have a responsibility to inform parents of the risks and to instruct them in the correct application and safe storage of powders.

The selection and care of nappies are very important aspects in preventing inflammation or further irritation. There is also evidence that the type of nappy can influence the development of dermatitis. If nondisposable nappies are used and washed at home, they should be soaked in a quaternary ammonium compound or dilute hypochlorite (bleach), washed in hot water with a simple laundry soap, and run through the rinse cycle twice.

SEBORRHOEIC DERMATITIS

Seborrhoeic dermatitis is a chronic, recurrent, inflammatory reaction of the skin that occurs most commonly on the scalp (cradle cap), but may involve the eyelids (blepharitis), external ear canal (otitis externa), nasolabial folds, and inguinal region. The cause is unknown, although it is more common in early infancy when sebum production is increased. The lesions are characteristically thick, adherent, yellowish, scaly, oily patches that may or may not be mildly pruritic. If pruritus is present, the infant may be irritable. Unlike atopic dermatitis, seborrhoeic dermatitis is not associated with a positive family history for allergy and is very common in infants shortly after birth and in children after puberty. Diagnosis is made primarily by the appearance and location of the crusts or scales.

IMPLICATIONS FOR NURSING

Cradle cap may be prevented with adequate scalp hygiene. Not infrequently, parents omit shampooing the infant's hair from fear of damaging the 'soft spots' or fontanels. The midwife or health visitor should discuss how to shampoo the infant's hair and emphasize that the fontanel is like skin anywhere else on the body — it does not puncture or tear with mild pressure.

When seborrhoeic lesions are present, the treatment is mainly directed at removing the crusts. Shampooing should be done daily with a mild soap or commercial baby shampoo; medicated shampoos are not needed. The shampoo is applied to the scalp and allowed to remain on until the crusts are softened, and then the scalp is thoroughly rinsed (Morelli and Weston, 1987). Using a fine-tooth comb or a soft facial brush after shampooing helps remove the loosened crusts from the strands of hair.

ATOPIC DERMATITIS (ECZEMA)

Eczema or eczematous inflammation of the skin refers to a descriptive category of dermatological diseases and not to a specific aetiology. Atopic dermatitis (AD) is a type of pruritic eczema that usually begins during infancy and is associated with allergy with a hereditary tendency (atopy). AD presents in three forms based on the age of the child and the distribution of lesions:

1. **Infantile (infantile eczema)** — usually begins between two and six months of age and generally undergoes spontaneous remission by three years of age.

2. **Childhood** — may follow the infantile form; it occurs at two to three years of age, and 90% of the children will manifest the disease by the age five years.
3. **Preadolescent and adolescent** — begins at about 12 years of age and may continue into the early adult years or indefinitely.

Because the disease occurs predominantly in infancy, this discussion is restricted to the infantile form of atopic dermatitis.

The diagnosis of eczema is based on a combination of history and morphological findings (Box 15-8). The majority of children with infantile eczema have a family history of atopy (eczema, asthma, or allergic rhinitis), which strongly supports a genetic predisposition. The cause is unknown, but appears to be related to abnormal function of the skin, including alterations in sweating, peripheral vascular function, and heat tolerance. The disease is better in humid climates and worse in autumn and winter, when homes are heated and environmental humidity is lower. The disorder can be controlled, but not cured.

THERAPEUTIC MANAGEMENT

The major goals of management are to (1) relieve pruritus, (2) hydrate the skin (moistening and softening it), (3) reduce inflammation, and (4) prevent or control secondary infection. Most of the general measures for managing AD serve to reduce pruritus as well as other aspects of the disease. General management includes avoiding exposure to skin irritants, avoiding overheating, improving skin hydration, and administration of medications such as antihistamines (topical steroids) and (sometimes) mild sedatives as indicated such as piriton (to be used with caution). Use of medications should be limited as they can cause, or can irritate, fragile skin. There is some evidence that increased doses of vitamin C reduce the severity of eczema.

Differing philosophies regarding cleansing and hydrating the skin of the child with eczema generally embrace two methods — the wet and the dry methods. In the dry method baths are infrequent, and skin is cleansed with a nonlipid, hydrophilic agent. The wet method consists of frequent baths (up to four times per day) followed immediately by the application of a lubricant (while the skin is still damp) to trap moisture in the skin. No soap or a very mild, nonperfumed soap should be used. Some advocate oil or oilated oatmeal baths with light drying so that a protective, oily film remains on the skin. Showers should be avoided because of their drying effect.

Enhancing skin hydration can be accomplished by application of preparations that occlude the skin to prevent evaporation and retain moisture in the upper skin layers and/or by replacement of natural moisturizing substances in the skin. A variety of emollients containing petrolatum or lanolin have occlusive properties and are prescribed according to the degree of occlusion desired. For the majority of infants, lotions applied twice or three times daily maintain satisfactory hydration. The frequency may be increased if greater hydration is required.

Creams or ointments provide more occlusion, and those that contain urea or lactic acid improve the binding of water in the skin as well as prevent evaporation of moisture.

Moderate or severe pruritus is usually relieved by administration of oral antihistamine drugs (hydroxyzine or diphenhydramine), and the amount is tailored to the individual child. Since pruritus increases at night, a mild sedative may be needed.

Occasional flare-ups require the use of topical steroids to diminish inflammation. Low-, moderate-, or high-potency topical corticosteroids are prescribed, depending on the degree of involvement, the area of the body to be treated, the age of the child, and the type of vehicle to be used (e.g., cream, lotion, ointment). Avoid using these preparations on the face. Secondary infection is managed with appropriate antibiotic therapy.

IMPLICATIONS FOR NURSING

Long-term treatment of eczema is usually established on an outpatient basis. As a result, the major burden of responsibility and physical care rests on the parents in the home. A vicious cycle of exacerbations – scratching, infection, irritability, frustration – is the usual course unless the initial phase can be altered.

Assessment of the child with eczema includes a family history for evidence of atopy, a history of previous involvement, and any environmental or dietary factors associated with the present and previous exacerbations. The skin lesions are examined for type, distribution, and evidence of secondary infection. The parents are interviewed regarding the child's behaviour, especially in relation to the child's scratching, irritability, and sleeping patterns. The interview should also include exploration of the family's feelings and methods of coping with the situation.

The objectives for nursing care of the child with eczema are similar to those for medical management as follows:
1. Relieve pruritus.
2. Improve skin hydration.
3. Prevent secondary infection.
4. Support child and family.

The child with AD presents a nursing challenge. Controlling the intense pruritus is imperative if the disorder is to be successfully managed, since scratching leads to the formation of new lesions and may cause secondary infection. In addition to the medical regimen, other measures can be taken to prevent or minimize the scratching. Fingernails and toenails are cut short, kept clean, and filed frequently to prevent sharp edges. Gloves or cotton stockings may have to be placed over the hands and pinned to shirtsleeves. To prevent any contact with the skin, elbow restraints are sometimes necessary. One-piece cotton outfits with long sleeves and long trousers also decrease direct contact with the skin. Whether gloves or elbow restraints are used, the child needs time to be free from such restrictions. An excellent time to remove any protective devices is during the bath or after receiving sedative or antipruritic medication.

Conditions that increase itching are eliminated when possible. Woollen clothes or blankets, rough fabrics, and furry

◆ **BOX 15-8**

Clinical manifestations of atopic dermatitis

Distribution of Lesions

Infantile form — generalized, especially cheeks, scalp, trunk, and extensor surfaces of extremities

Childhood form — flexural areas (antecubital and popliteal fossae, neck), wrists, ankles, and feet

Preadolescent and adolescent form — face, sides of neck, hands, feet, and antecubital and popliteal fossae (to a lesser extent)

Appearance of Lesions

Infantile form
  Erythema
  Vesicles
  Papules
  Weeping
  Oozing
  Crusting
  Scaling
  Often symmetric
Childhood form
  Symmetric involvement
  Clusters of small erythematous or flesh-coloured papules or minimally scaling patches
  Dry and may be hyperpigmented
  Lichenification (thickened skin with accentuation of creases)
  Keratosis pilaris (follicular hyperkeratosis) common
Adolescent/adult form
  Same as childhood manifestations
  Dry, thick lesions (lichenified plaques) common
  Confluent papules

Other Manifestations

Intense itching
Unaffected skin dry and rough
Black children likely to exhibit more papular and/or follicular lesions than white children
May exhibit one or more of the following:
  Lymphadenopathy, especially near affected sites
  Increased palmar creases (many cases)
  Atopic pleats (extra line or groove of lower eyelid)
  Prone to cold hands
  Pityriasis alba (small, poorly defined areas of hypopigmentation)
  Facial pallor (especially around nose, mouth, and ears)
  Bluish discolouration beneath eyes ('allergic shiners')
  Increased susceptibility to unusual cutaneous infections (especially viral)

stuffed animals are removed. Cotton clothing is encouraged, as is a cool environment. Pruritus is often precipitated by exposure to the irritant effects of certain components of common products such as soaps, detergents, fabric softeners, perfumes, and powders. Most children experience less itching when soft cotton fabrics are worn next to the skin. During cold months, synthetic fabrics (not wool) should be used for overcoats, hats, gloves, and snowsuits.

Clothes and sheets should be laundered in a mild detergent and rinsed thoroughly in clear water (without fabric softeners and antistatic chemicals). Putting the clothes through a second complete wash cycle without using detergent minimizes the amount of residue remaining in the fabric.

Preventing infection is usually secondary to preventing scratching. Baths should be given as prescribed, the water kept tepid, and soaps (except as indicated) and bubble baths, oils and powders should be avoided. Skinfolds and nappy areas need frequent cleansing with plain water. A room humidifier or vaporizer may benefit children with extremely dry skin. The lesions should be examined for signs of infection, usually the presence of honey-coloured crusts with surrounding erythema.

If the child is being treated with frequent baths for hydration, it is imperative that the emollient preparation be applied immediately following bathing (while the skin is still slightly moist) to prevent drying.

Wet wrap dressings are applied and medications for pruritus or infection are administered as directed. The family should be given *explicit written* instructions on the preparation and use of soaks, special baths, and topical medications, including the order of application if more than one is prescribed. Directions are worded in language the family understands. For example, if a solution is to be diluted in the ratio of 1:20 parts of water, it is preferable to express the ratio concretely, such as 1 cup of solution mixed with 20 cups of water. It is important to emphasize that one thick application of a topical medication is *not* equivalent to several thin applications, and that excessive use of an agent, particularly steroids, can be hazardous. If children have difficulty remaining still for a 10- or 15-minute soak, bath, or dressing application, these can be carried out at bedtime or when the child is engrossed in television or a story.

Since adequate rest is also important for these children, who are usually fretful and irritable, planning meals, baths, medications, and treatments during awake periods is paramount. Sleepy, tired children are normally cranky, and such behaviour only intensifies the urge to scratch.

Diet modification is another source of frustration to parents. When a hypoallergenic diet is prescribed, parents need help in understanding the reason for the diet and guidelines for avoiding hyperallergenic foods. Chinese therapy may also be a possible solution.

Since hypoallergenic diets take time before visible effects are apparent, parents need reassurance that results may not be seen immediately. If airborne allergens also worsen the eczema, the family is counselled regarding measures to 'allergy proof' the home (see Bronchial Asthma, Chapter 26).

Perhaps it is because the physical problems seem insurmountable during periods of acute exacerbation that the emotional stress becomes so intense for the family members. They need time to discuss negative feelings and to be reassured that these feelings are expected, normal, acceptable, and healthy, provided there is an emotional outlet to dissipate the invested energy. During acute phases, relieving as much anxiety as possible in both parents and child has a beneficial emotional and physical effect, since stress tends to aggravate the severity of the condition.

Evaluation

The effectiveness of nursing interventions is determined by continual reassessment and evaluation of care based on the following observational guidelines and expected outcomes:

1. Observe the child's behaviour, clothing, and activities.
2. Examine the skin surface for evidence of dryness.
3. Examine skin lesions for evidence of secondary infection.
4. Interview the family and encourage dialogue regarding the child and aspects of care.

DISORDERS OF UNKNOWN AETIOLOGY

Several disorders may occur during early childhood in which the aetiology is unknown or speculative. However, two of these disorders, sudden infant death syndrome and autism, occur almost exclusively during infancy and generate tremendous stress for the family. In one, the family must cope with the loss of an infant; in the other, the family must deal with the stresses of caring for a severely disturbed child. Competent and sensitive nursing care can relieve some of the emotional burden.

SUDDEN INFANT DEATH SYNDROME

Sudden infant death syndrome (SIDS), also known by outdated terms such as cot death, is defined as 'the sudden death of an infant under one year of age that remains unexplained after a complete postmortem examination, including an investigation of the death scene and a review of the case history' (cited by Zylke, 1989). It was the leading cause of death in children between the ages of one month and one year, and claims the lives of 7,000 infants annually. Table 15-1 summarizes the major epidemiological characteristics of SIDS.

Since the introduction of the 'Back to Sleep' campaign by the Department of Health and the Foundation for the Study of Infant Death Syndrome in 1990, the reduction of sudden infant deaths has more than halved, down to 460 deaths per annum.

The guidelines state that babies should:

• be placed on their backs to sleep
• not be too warm
• not be exposed to a smoky atmosphere

AETIOLOGY

Numerous theories have been proposed regarding the aetiology of SIDS; however, the cause is unknown. The most compelling hypothesis is that SIDS is related to a brainstem abnormality in the neurological regulation of cardiorespiratory control. Abnormalities include prolonged sleep apnoea, increased frequency of brief inspiratory pauses, excessive periodic breathing, and impaired arousal responsiveness to increased carbon dioxide or decreased oxygen. A prominent aspect of the respiratory control hypothesis was the apnoea hypothesis, which proposed that SIDS victims experienced periods of prolonged apnoea during sleep and eventually died during one of these episodes because of a failure in the autonomic regulation of breathing (Hunt and Brouillette, 1987). However, apnoea of infancy is not the cause of SIDS. The vast majority of infants with apnoea do not die, and only a minority of SIDS victims have documented apparent life-threatening events.

Although the aetiology is unknown, autopsies reveal consistent pathologic findings, such as pulmonary oedema and intrathoracic haemorrhages, that confirm the diagnosis of SIDS. Consequently, all infants with suspected SIDS death should be autopsied, and these findings shared with the parents as soon as possible after the death.

FACTORS	OCCURRENCE
Incidence	2:1000 live births
Peak age	2 to 4 months; 90% occur by 6 months
Sex	Higher percentage of males affected
Time of death	During sleep
Time of year	Increased incidence in winter; peak in January
Socioeconomic	Increased occurrence in lower socioeconomic class
Birth	Higher incidence in:
	Premature infants, especially infants of low birth weight
	Multiple births
	Neonates with low Apgar scores
	Infants with central nervous system disturbances and respiratory disorders such as bronchopulmonary dysplasia
	Increasing birth order (subsequent siblings as opposed to firstborn child)
Siblings	May have greater incidence
Maternal	Younger age
	Cigarette smoking
	Drug addiction

Table 15-1 Epidemiology of SIDS.

CHILDREN AT RISK OF SIDS

Certain groups of children are at increased risk for SIDS. These groups include:

1. Infants with one or more severe apparent life-threatening events disorder requiring cardiopulmonary resuscitation (CPR) or vigorous stimulation
2. Preterm infants who continue to have pathological apnoea at the time of hospital discharge
3. Siblings of two or more SIDS victims
4. Infants with certain types of diseases or conditions, such as central hypoventilation

Home monitoring is recommended for these children, providing parents are familiar with resusitation techniques. No diagnostic tests exist to predict which infants, including those in the above groups, will survive or die, and home monitoring is no guarantee of survival (Bentele and Albani, 1988; Ward *et al*, 1986). Presently, strategies to prevent SIDS are best directed at decreasing known risk factors, such as mothers seeking adequate prenatal care and avoiding cigarette smoking and drug abuse both before and after the child's birth. Ensuring that the infant is positioned correctly in the cot (ideally lying on its back), the room is at a suitable temperature, and that the infant is not over-dressed may also help in the prevention of SIDS.

Whether subsequent siblings of the SIDS infant are at increased risk for SIDS is unclear. Even if the increased risk is correct, families have a 99% chance that their subsequent child will *not* die of SIDS. Home monitoring is not recommended for this group of children (Foundation for the Study of Infant Death, 1992). Home monitoring is an option that the parents and health visitor should discuss.

IMPLICATIONS FOR NURSING

Loss of a child from SIDS presents several crises with which the parents must cope. In addition to grief and mourning for the death of their child, the parents must face a tragedy that was extremely sudden, unexpected, and unexplained.

Finding the infant

Usually it is the mother who finds the child dead in the cot. Typically, the child is in a dishevelled bed, with blankets over its head.

Frequently the mother is alone and must deal with her initial shock, panic, grief, questions of the other siblings, and the decision of where to find help. The first persons to arrive may be the police and ambulance attendants. Hopefully, they will handle the situation by asking few questions, giving *no* indication of wrongdoing, abuse, or neglect, making sensitive judgements concerning the resuscitation efforts for the child, and comforting the members of the family as much as possible. These individuals should be properly informed about SIDS in order to recognize its characteristic signs and tell parents that their child probably died from a disease called sudden infant death syndrome, which cannot be predicted or prevented. A compassionate, sensitive approach to the family

during the very first few minutes can help spare them some of the overwhelming guilt and anguish that frequently follow this type of death.

Arriving at the accident and emergency department

The first contact nurses typically have with these families is in the accident and emergency department, when the infant is seen by a doctor in order to be pronounced dead. Usually, there is no attempt at resuscitation. During the time in casualty, several aspects warrant special consideration. Parents are asked only factual questions, such as when they found the infant, how he or she looked, and who they called for help. Any remarks that may suggest responsibility, such as why didn't they go in earlier, didn't they hear the infant cry out, was the head buried in a blanket, or were the other siblings jealous of this child, should be avoided.

The events that took place when help arrived should be discussed. If resuscitation was attempted, the infant may have fractured ribs, internal bleeding, and traumatic bruising, which can simulate physical abuse. The discussion of an autopsy should be presented at this time, emphasizing that a diagnosis cannot be confirmed until the postmortem examination is completed. Instructions about the autopsy and funeral arrangements may need to be repeated or put in writing. If the mother was breast-feeding, she needs information about abrupt discontinuation of lactation (Lawrence, 1989).

Another very important aspect of compassionate care towards these parents is allowing them to say good-bye to their child. Before they go into the examining room the body is covered partially with a sheet or blanket, and the room is put in order, especially if instruments and equipment were used. These are the parents' last moments with their child, and they should be as quiet, meaningful, peaceful, and undisturbed as possible. The child's belongings are packaged for the parents to take home if they wish. Because the parents leave the hospital without their infant, it is helpful to accompany them to the car or arrange for someone else to take them home (Woolsey, 1988).

Returning home

Parents are able to take their baby home when the death has been registered. On returning home, they should be visited by a general practitioner and a health visitor as soon after the death as possible. A referral should also be made to the local Foundation for Sudden Infant Death (FSID) (see useful addresses). Printed material that contains information about SIDS (available from FSID) should be provided.

During the initial home visit, one of the nursing objectives is to assess what the parents have been told, what they think happened, and how they have explained this to the other siblings. If parents have been told about SIDS, they may answer the questions factually and seem to understand and accept the diagnosis. Although this might be so, it is unusual for parents not to have second thoughts, doubts, and feelings of guilt. Pursuing the factual answer by asking about feelings or emotions may uncover repressed thoughts that, when once said aloud, can be dealt with.

The general practitioner or health visitor cannot deal with all the issues related to the child's death in one visit. During the initial visit, the general practitioner or health visitor may be doing most of the talking, as the parents are helped to gain an understanding of the disease. If the visit is made within a day or two of the death, the parents are in the impact phase of crisis, in which their thinking abilities are disorganized and distracted. It is difficult for them to deal with the crisis in concrete terms, especially in exploring problem-solving approaches.

During the second visit, the goal is to help the parents bring their feelings out into the open. During this session the parents are helped to explore their usual coping mechanisms and, if these are ineffectual, to investigate new approaches. It may be a time when parents are making rash decisions such as moving away to avoid questions or deciding never to have another child. This is not the time to decide these issues rationally and logically, but rather to acknowledge that they are unable to deal with them.

Because questions like these do arise and must be answered eventually, the number of visits and plan for intervention must be flexible. For example, the needs of the siblings must be considered. Although they may initially appear accepting of the explanation and well-adjusted, subsequent problems are common and may include: (1) changes in the parent-child interaction, such as increased anger towards the parent or increased discipline problems; (2) altered sleep patterns, including resistance to going to bed and bedtime fears; and (3) changes in social patterns, from withdrawn to aggressive behaviour (Mandell, McAnulty and Carlson, 1983). Children need an opportunity to talk about their perception of the death. With young children, the use of stories about death, drawing, or play is recommended. Parents should be aware that sibling grief often lasts as long as adult grief — typically longer than one year (Burns, House and Ankenbauer, 1986).

One of the important decisions for many parents is the question of a subsequent pregnancy and their concern regarding recurrent SIDS. The optimum timing for a subsequent pregnancy is not known, and many families have a strong desire to rebuild the family, often within the first year (Swoiskin-Schwartz, Deatrick and Hanson, 1988). If another pregnancy occurs before both parents are ready, they may be forced to deal with an additional crisis before resolution of the first. One of the dangers of having another child soon after the other's death is that this infant may become a 'replacement' child. Even when parents are well prepared for the birth of a subsequent child, they may have difficulty conceiving, have doubts about the child's well-being, be overprotective and view the child as more vulnerable, especially near the age of the other infant's death, and need support that these responses are normal. Health visitors can help families assess their readiness for another child and support them in their decision. The Care of the Next Infant (CONI) scheme enables health visitors to give intensive home support and help prepare families for the birth of their next child.

APNOEA OF INFANCY

Apnoea, the cessation of respirations, can be of three types (Brazy, Kinney and Oakes, 1987):

- **Central** — absence of airflow and respiratory effort
- **Obstructive** — absence of airflow, but presence of respiratory effort
- **Mixed** — absence of airflow and respiratory effort (central apnoea), followed by resumption of respiratory effort without airflow (obstructive apnoea)

Short periods of central apnoea (15 seconds) can be normal at any age. *Pathological apnoea* is a respiratory pause that is prolonged (20 seconds) or associated with cyanosis, marked pallor or hypotonia, or bradycardia. Apnoea of infancy (AOI) generally refers to pathological apnoea in infants greater than 37 weeks of gestation (see also discussion of apnoea of prematurity in Chapter 13). The clinical presentation of AOI is an apparent life-threatening event (ALTE) (previously referred to by the inaccurate and misleading expression, near-miss SIDS) (Box 15-9). AOI can be a symptom of many disorders, including sepsis, seizures, upper airway abnormalities, gastro-oesophageal reflux, hypoglycaemia or other metabolic problems, and impaired regulation of breathing during sleep or feeding. In rare instances, the ALTE may be the result of intentional poisoning by a caregiver suffering from Münchausen syndrome by proxy (Hickson *et al*, 1989). However, in about half the cases, no cause is identified. Infants with a history of ALTE are at increased risk of SIDS (Brooks, 1982; Oren, Kelly, Shannon, 1986), but these children constitute less than 7% of all SIDS victims (National Institutes of Health, 1986).

PROCESS OF DIAGNOSIS

Diagnostic procedures generally include close observation of the individual, and several tests (blood chemistry, chest radiograph, electrocardiography, and electroencephalography) to rule out specific, sometimes treatable causes, such as seizures. The most widely used test, however, is continuous recording

---

◆ **BOX 15-9**

Definition of an apparent life-threatening event

Frightening to the observer, who fears child died or would have died without vigorous intervention

Some combination of:

Apnoea — usually central, but occasionally obstructive

Colour change — cyanosis or pallor, but sometimes plethora

Marked change in muscle tone — usually extreme limpness

Choking or gagging

of cardiorespiratory patterns (cardiopneumogram or pneumo-cardiogram). Four-channel pneumocardiograms are commonly used; the four monitor channels are heart rate, respirations (chest impedance), nasal air flow, and oxygen saturation. A more sophisticated test, polysomnography ('sleep test'), also records brain waves, eye and body movements, oesophageal manometry, and end-tidal carbon dioxide measurements. However, none of these tests can predict risk. Some children with normal results may still have subsequent apnoeic episodes.

IMPLICATIONS FOR NURSING

The diagnosis of AOI engenders great anxiety and concern in parents, and the institution of home monitoring presents additional physical and emotional burdens. If monitoring is required, the nurse can be a major source of support to the family in terms of education about the equipment, observation of the infant's status, and immediate intervention during apnoeic episodes, including CPR.

Before the actual teaching begins, parents need an opportunity to discuss their feelings about the diagnosis, especially if another child has died from SIDS. Excessive fears and concerns, especially since monitoring offers no guarantees of survival, can impede their readiness to learn (Duncan and Webb, 1983).

Several types of home monitors are available, and most hospitals select the model that the infant will use at home. Nurses, especially community paediatric nurses and health visitors, must become familiar with the equipment, including its advantages and disadvantages. Guidelines for using apnoea monitors are described in Box 15-10.

Caregivers need detailed information regarding proper attachment of the electrodes to the infant. For home use, electrodes attached to a belt that is placed around the child's trunk are preferred. The belt is positioned so that the electrodes contact the skin in the same area.

Monitors are effective only if they are used. They do not prevent death, but alert the caregiver to the apparent life-threatening events in time to intervene. The need to use the monitor and to respond appropriately to alarms must be stressed. Noncompliance can result in the infant's death (Meny, Blackman and Fleischmann, 1988).

Family support

Although AOI is not a chronic illness, many of the stresses observed during the monitoring period are characteristic of families with chronically ill children. Parents report increased stress, anxiety, and fatigue, especially mothers who typically have to respond 24 hours a day and feel responsible for the infant's survival (DiMaggio and Sheetz, 1983).

To lessen the continuous responsibility of monitoring, other family members such as grandparents, or babysitters if applicable, should be taught how to manipulate the equipment, read and interpret the signals, and administer CPR. They are encouraged to stay with the infant for regular periods to allow parents respite. Support groups of other families who have successfully completed monitoring can also be of benefit.

INFANTILE AUTISM

Autism is a complex developmental disorder accompanied by severe and usually permanent intellectual and behavioural deficits. It occurs in 1:2500 children, is about four times more common in males than in females, although females are more severely affected, and is not related to socioeconomic level, race, or religion.

AETIOLOGY

The aetiology of autism is an unsolved and controversial question. However, considerable evidence supports a biological cause. Individuals with autism may have abnormal electroencephalograms, seizures, delayed development of hand dominance, persistence of primitive reflexes, metabolic abnormalities (elevated blood serotonin), and cerebellar vermal hypoplasia (part of the brain involved in regulating motion and some aspects of memory).

There is also strong evidence for a genetic basis. Twin studies demonstrate a very high concordance (96%) for monozygotic (identical) twins and a 24% concordance for dizygotic (non-

---

◆ **BOX 15-10**

Guidelines for using apnoea monitors

Use the monitor despite its shortcomings, such as false alarms.

Do not adjust the monitor to eliminate false alarms. Adjustments could compromise the monitor's effectiveness.

Place monitor on firm surface away from cot and covers; plug directly into wall socket.

Do not sleep in the same bed as a monitored infant. Moving the infant monitor could cause malfunctions.

Keep pets and children away from the monitor and infant.

Keep the monitor away from possible electrical interferences such as appliances (e.g., electric blankets, televisions).

Check the monitor several times a day to be sure the alarm is working and that it can be heard from room to room. Be sure caregiver can reach the monitor quickly (in less than 10 seconds).

Periodically check the monitor's breath detection indicator and battery or charger connections.

Read the monitor's user manual carefully; report problems promptly.

Inform local utility and rescue squads of home monitoring.

Keep emergency numbers near all phones in home.

Practise safety precautions:
  Remove leads when infant is not attached to monitor.
  Unplug power cord from electrical outlet when cord is not plugged into monitor.

If in doubt, check with the health visitor or community paediatric nurse.

identical) twins. These concordances are consistent with an autosomal recessive pattern of inheritance. In addition, between 5% and 16% of males with autism are positive for the fragile X chromosome (Chudley and Hagerman, 1987).

CLINICAL MANIFESTATIONS/ PROCESS OF DIAGNOSIS

Children with autism demonstrate several peculiar and bizarre characteristics, primarily in social interactions, communication, and behaviour. The majority of children with autism are mentally retarded, with scores typically in the moderate to severe range. More females than males tend to have very low intelligence scores. Despite relatively severe mental retardation, some children with autism excel in particular areas, such as art, music, memory, mathematical calculation, or perceptual skills, such as puzzle building. Instances of exceptional ability despite a low overall mental capacity are know as the *savant syndrome*. However, even children with exceptional abilities are rarely able to productively use their talents, because of their other severe deficits.

PROGNOSIS

Autism is a severe disabling condition. Only about 1-2% of the autistic population ultimately achieve independence, with the majority requiring lifelong supervision. Aggravation of psychiatric symptoms occurs in about half the children during adolescence, with girls having a tendency for continued deterioration. Prognosis is most favourable for children with communicative speech development by age six years and an intelligence quotient above 50 at the time of diagnosis (Gillberg and Steffenburg, 1987).

IMPLICATIONS FOR NURSING

Autism, like many other chronic conditions, involves the entire family and often becomes 'a family disease'. Parents need expert counselling early in the course of the disorder and should be referred to the National Autistic Society (see useful addresses), social services, and child and adolescent psychiatrists, who will provide information, support and advice.

When these children are hospitalized, they usually present many management problems. Decreasing stimulation by using a private or semiprivate room, avoiding extraneous auditory and visual distraction, and encouraging parents to bring in possessions the child is attached to may lessen the disruptiveness of hospitalization. Since physical contact frequently upsets these children, minimum holding may be necessary to prevent temper tantrums.

Care must be taken when performing procedures on, administering medicine to, or feeding these children, since they are either fussy eaters who may wilfully starve themselves or gag to prevent eating, or they are indiscriminate hoarders, swallowing any available edible or inedible items, such as a thermometer. Their disturbing sleep patterns may also pose problems in a hospital setting. A thorough assessment of the child's usual routine and activities can help maintain an environment that is more manageable and conducive to physical recovery.

A key principle in working with these children is establishing trust. They need to be introduced slowly to new situations, with visits with caregivers kept short whenever possible. Because these children have difficulty organizing their behaviour and redirecting their energy, they need to be told directly what to do.

As much as possible, the family is encouraged to care for the child in the home. With the help of family support programmes, families are often able to provide the home care and assist with the educational services the child needs. Family centres and residential or weekly homes can offer alternative methods of care. As the child approaches adulthood, the family may require assistance in locating a long-term placement facility for the affected adult (see also Chapter 22).

KEY POINTS

◆ Common nutritional disturbances of infancy include vitamin and mineral disturbances, some types of vegetarian diets, protein and caloric malnutrition, obesity and food intolerance.

◆ Mineral disturbances may be caused by mineral-mineral interactions and mineral-diet interactions.

◆ Vegetarians may be classified into four groups: lacto-ovovegetarians, lactovegetarians, pure vegetarians, and macrobiotics.

◆ Protein and energy malnutrition may occur as a complication of underlying disease, or as a result of fad diets, lack of parental education about infant nutrition, inappropriate management of food allergy, and incorrect preparation of formula.

◆ Food intolerance encompasses food allergies and food sensitivities, the most serious of which are cow's milk allergy and lactose intolerance.

◆ Treatment of colic may involve change in feeding practices, correction of stressful environment, and support of parent.

◆ Failure to thrive may be classified as organic, resulting from some physical cause, and nonorganic, resulting from psychosocial factors involving the child and caregiver (e.g., maternal deprivation), environmental causes (e.g., inadequate parental knowledge of child feeding), or unexplained causes.

◆ Sudden infant death syndrome is the leading cause of death in children between the ages of one month and one year.

◆ Children with apnoea of infancy receive home monitoring to alert the family to an apparent life-threatening event.

REFERENCES

Anderson J: The establishment of common language concerning adverse reactions to foods and food additives, *J Allergy Clin Immunol* 78(1, pt. 2):140, 1986.

Ayoub C, Milner J: Failure to thrive: parental indicators, types, and outcomes, *Child Abuse Neglect* 9:491, 1985.

Barr R *et al*: Feeding and temperament as determinants of early infant crying/fussing behavior, *Pediatr* 84(3):514, 1989.

Bentele K, Albani M: Are there tests predictive of prolonged apnoea and SIDS? A review of epidemiological and functional studies, *Acta Paediatr Scand* 342(suppl):1, 1988.

Brazy J, Kinney H, Oakes W: Central nervous system structural lesions causing apnea at birth, *J Pediatr* 3(2):163, 1987.

Brooks JG: Apnea of infancy and sudden infant death syndrome, *Amer J Diseases Children*, 136:1012, 1982.

Burns E, House J, Ankenbauer M: Sibling grief in reaction to sudden infant death syndrome, *Pediatr* 78(3):485, 1986.

Carpenter T *et al*: Severe hypervitaminosis A in siblings: evidence of variable tolerance to retinol intake, *J Pediatr* 111(4):507, 1987.

Chatoor I *et al*: A developmental classification of feeding disorders associated with failure to thrive: diagnosis and treatment. In Drotar D, editor: *New directions in failure to thrive*, New York, 1985, Plenum Press.

Chudley A, Hagerman R: Fragile X syndrome, *J Pediatr* 110(6):821, 1987.

Council on Scientific Affairs: Vitamin preparations as dietary supplements and as therapeutic agents, *JAMA* 257(14):1929, 1987.

Dewey K *et al*: Infant growth and breast feeding, *Am J Clin Nutr* 50:1116, 1989.

DiMaggio GT, Sheetz AH: The concerns of mothers caring for an infant on an apnea monitor, *MCN* 8(4):294, 1983.

Duncan JA, Webb LZ: Teaching families home apnea monitoring, *Pediatr Nurs* 9(3):171, 1983.

Foundation for the Study of Infant Death: *Fact file 3: Apnoea/respiration monitors*, London, 1992, Foundation for the Study of Infant Death.

Gillberg C, Steffenburg G: Outcome and prognostic factors in infantile autism and similar conditions: a population-based study of 46 cases followed through puberty, *J Autism Dev Disord* 17:273, 1987.

Hickson G *et al*: Parental administration of chemical agents: a cause of apparent life-threatening events, *Pediatr* 83(5):772, 1989.

Hill D *et al*: Manifestations of milk allergy in infancy: clinical and immunologic findings, *J Pediatr* 109(2):270, 1986.

Hill D *et al*: Recovery from milk allergy in early childhood: antibody studies, *J Pediatr* 114(5):761, 1989.

Hunt C, Brouillette R: Sudden infant death syndrome: 1987 perspective, *J Pediatr* 110(5):669, 1987.

Jarvis WT: Vitamin use and abuse, *Contemp Nutr* 9(10):1, 1984.

Lawrence RA: *Breastfeeding: a guide for the medical profession*, ed 3, St Louis, 1989, Mosby–Year Book.

Mandell F, McAnulty EH, Carlson A: Unexpected death of an infant sibling, *Pediatr* 72(5):652, 1983.

Meny R, Blackmon L, Fleischmann D: Sudden infant death and home monitors, *Am J Dis Child* 142:1037, 1988.

Morelli J, Weston W: Soaps and shampoos in pediatric practice, *Pediatr* 80(5):634, 1987.

Moss A *et al*: *Use of vitamin and mineral supplements in the United States: current users, types of products, and nutrients.* Advance data from vital and health statistics, No 174, Hyattsville, MD, 1989, National Center for Health Statistics.

National Institutes for Health: National Institutes of Health consensus development conference on infantile apnea and home monitoring: consensus statement, *Pediatrics* 79(2):292, 1987.

Oates RK, Peacock A, Forrest D: Long-term effects of nonorganic failure to thrive, *Pediatr* 75(1):36, 1985.

Olness KN: Nutritional consequences of drugs used in pediatrics, *Clin Pediatr* 24(8):417, 1985.

Oren J, Kelly D, Shannon DC: Identification of a high risk group for sudden infant death syndrome among infants who were resuscitated for sleep apnea, *Pediatrics* 77:495-499, 1986.

Sampson H, Scanlon S: Natural history of food hypersensitivity in children with atopic dermatitis, *J Pediatr* 115(1):23, 1989.

Sherman J, Alexander M: Obesity in children: a research update, *J Pediatr Nurs* 5(3):161, 1990.

Stunkard A *et al*: An adoption study of human obesity, *N Engl J Med* 314(4):193, 1986.

Stunkard A *et al*: The body-mass index of twins who have been reared apart, *N Engl J Med* 322(21):1483, 1990.

Swoiskin-Schwartz S, Deatrick J, Hanson D: Parents' views about having a child after a SIDS death, *J Pediatr Nurs* 3(1):24, 1988.

Walravens P, Hambidge M, Koepfer D: Zinc supplementation in infants with a nutritional pattern of failure to thrive: a double-blind, controlled study, *Pediatr* 83(4):532, 1989.

Ward S *et al*: Sudden infant death syndrome in infants evaluated by apnea programs in California, *Pediatr* 77(4):451, 1986.

Wilson N, Self T, Hamburger R: Severe cow's milk-induced colitis in an exclusively breast-fed neonate, *Clin Pediatr* 29(2):77, 1990.

Wishon PM, Kinnick VG: Helping infants overcome the problem of obesity, *MCN* 11(2):118, 1986.

Woolsey S: Support after sudden infant death, *AJN* 88(10):1347, 1988.

Zylke J: Sudden infant death syndrome: resurgent research offers hope, *JAMA* 262(12):1565, 1989.

FURTHER READING

Vitamin and Mineral Disturbances

Crombie I *et al*: Effect of vitamin and mineral supplementation on verbal and non-verbal reasoning of schoolchildren, *Lancet* 355:744, 1990

Holland P *et al*: Prenatal deficiency of phosphate, phosphate supplementation, and rickets in very-low-birthweight infants, *Lancet* 335:697, 1990.

Williams SR: *Nutrition and diet therapy,* ed 6, St Louis, 1989, Mosby–Year Book.

Vegetarian Diets

Rudy CA: Teaching families about the well-balanced vegetarian diet, *Child Nurse* 3(5):1, 1985.

Trahms C: Vegetarian diets for children. In Pipes P: *Nutrition in infancy and childhood,* ed 4, St Louis, 1989, Mosby–Year Book.

Obesity

Castiglia P: Obesity in infants and toddlers, *J Pediatr Health Care* 1(4):218, 1987.

Griffiths M *et al*: Metabolic rate and physical development in children at risk of obesity, *Lancet* 336(8707):76, 1990.

Morgan J: Prevention of childhood obesity, *Issues Compr Pediatr Nurs* 9(1):33, 1986.

Satter E: The feeding relationship, *J Am Diet Assoc* 86(3):352, 1986.

Food Sensitivity

Brill B: Oral rehydration, food allergy, and specialized nutrition, *Curr Opin Pediatr* 1:384, 1989

Feeding Difficulties: General

Satter E: Childhood feeding problems, *Feelings Med Signif* 32(2):5, 1990.

Walker M, Driscoll J: Sore nipples: the new mother's nemesis, *MCN* 14:260, 1989.

Failure to Thrive

Castiglia P: Failure to thrive, *J Pediatr Health Care* 2(1):50, 1988.

Klein M: The home health nurse clinician's role in the prevention of nonorganic failure to thrive, *J Pediatr Nurs* 5(2):129, 1990.

Colic

Gillies C: Infant colic: is there anything new? *J Pediatr Health Care* 1(6):305, 1987.

Hartsell M: New product to quiet baby's crying spells, *J Pediatr Nurs* 2(6):438, 1987.

Sampson H: Infantile colic and food allergy: fact or fiction? *J Pediatr* 115(4):583, 1989.

Schmitt B: When your baby has colic, *Contemp Pediatr* 7(2):85, 1990.

Skin Disorders

Antherton D: Controversies in therapeutics: role of diet in treating atopic eczema: elimination diets can be beneficial, *BMJ* 297(6661):1458, 1988.

Berg R: Etiology and pathophysiology of diaper dermatitis, *Adv Dermatol* 3:75, 1988.

Broadbent J, Sampson H: Food hypersensitivity and atopic dermatitis, *Pediatr Clin North Am* 35(5):1115, 1988.

Chandra R, Puri S, Hamed A: Influence of maternal diet during lactation and use of formula feeds on development of atopic eczema in high risk infants, *BMJ* 299:228, 1989.

Kramer M: Does breast-feeding help protect against atopic disease? Biology, methodology, and a golden jubilee of controversy, *J Pediatr* 112(2):181, 1988.

Lucas A *et al*: Early diet of preterm infants and development of allergic or atopic disease: randomised prospective study, *BMJ* 300:837, 1990.

Sudden Infant Death Syndrome

Balarajan R, Raleigh V, Botting B: Sudden infant death syndrome and postneonatal mortality in immigrants in England and Wales, *BMJ* 298(6675):716, 1989.

de Jonge G *et al*: Cot death and prone sleeping position in the Netherlands, *BMJ* 298(6675):722, 1989.

Gilbert R *et al*: Signs of illness preceding sudden unexpected death in infants, *BMJ* 300(6734):1237, 1990.

Grether J, Schulman J: Sudden infant death syndrome and birth weight, *J Pediatr* 114(4, pt 1):561, 1989.

Haglund B, Cnattingius S: Cigarette smoking as a risk factor for sudden infant death syndrome: a population-based study, *Am J Public Health* 80:29, 1990.

Jezierski M: Infant death: guidelines for support of parents in the emergency department, *J Emerg Nurs* 15(6):475, 1989.

Nelson E, Taylor B, Weatherall I: Sleeping position and infant bedding may predispose to hyperthermia and the sudden infant death syndrome, *Lancet* 1(8631):199, 1989.

Useful Addresses

La Leche League, BM 3424, London WC1N 3XX.

Foundation for Sudden Infant Death, 14 Halkin Street, London SW1X 7DP.

The National Childbirth Trust, Alexandra House, Oldham Terrace, London W3 6NH.

National Autistic Society, 276 Willesden Lane, London NW2 5RB.

Chapter 16

Health Problems of Early Childhood

LEARNING OUTCOMES

After studying this chapter you should be able to:

◆ Define child protection.
◆ Describe the different categories of abuse and neglect.
◆ Outline the main principles of the Children Act 1989.
◆ Identify the key child protection agencies in the United Kingdom.
◆ Identify ten possible indicators of abuse and neglect.
◆ Outline six characteristics of vulnerable families.
◆ Discuss the importance of the *Working Together* guidelines.
◆ Understand the local procedures for nursing staff where cases of child abuse and/or neglect are suspected.
◆ Describe the features of infectious diseases in childhood.
◆ Detail the supportive advice that may be given to parents caring for a child with an infectious disorder.
◆ Describe the nurse's role in the prevention of poisoning.
◆ Define the glossary terms.

GLOSSARY

child abuse A broad, socially constructed term that includes neglect, physical injury, sexual abuse or emotional abuse of children, usually by an adult

communicable disease Illness caused by a specific infectious agent or its toxic products through a direct or indirect mode of transmission of that agent from a reservoir

contact Person or animal that has been in association with an infected person, animal or contaminated environment that might transfer the infective agent

control measures Methods used to prevent the spread of an organism

direct transmission Direct and immediate transfer of infectious agents, either by direct contact or by droplet spread

enanthema Eruption on mucous surface

exanthema Eruptive rash, fever

host Living person or animal that provides subsistence or lodging for an infectious agent under natural conditions

incest Any physical sexual activity between family members; blood relationship is not required (e.g., step parents)

incubation period Time between infection or exposure to disease and appearance of initial symptoms

isolation Separation of infected persons from non-infected persons for the period of communicability under conditions that prevent transmission of the aetiological agent

period of communicability Time or times during which an infectious agent may be transferred directly or indirectly from an infected person to another person

prodromal period Interval between early manifestations of disease and overt clinical syndrome

quarantine Restriction of activities of persons who have been exposed to a communicable disease until the incubation period has expired

his chapter describes some of the health problems of early childhood. Such problems include child abuse and neglect, infectious disorders and poisoning.

CHILD ABUSE

Child abuse is a broad, socially constructed term that includes neglect, physical injury, sexual abuse or emotional abuse of children, usually by an adult. It is one of the most significant social problems affecting children. The National Society for the Prevention of Cruelty to Children estimates that 150-200 children in England and Wales die each year from the effects or consequences of child abuse and neglect. Although statistics only partially reflect the true incidence of child abuse and neglect, figures for England taken from Area Child Protection Committee Child Protection Registers in the year ending 31 March, 1993, indicate a registration rate of 29.6 children per 10,000 population under the age of 18. Importantly, younger children are more likely to be on the registers than older children; 68% of the children on the registers at 31 March, 1992 were aged under 10 years (Department of Health, 1994).

Child protection is the promotion of decisive action to protect children from abuse and neglect (Home Office *et al*, 1991). The widespread introduction of a concept of child protection was introduced in the United Kingdom following the recommendations of the Beckford Report (London Borough of Brent, 1985). This report into the death of a child in care of a Local Authority was unequivocal in its view that the central task of Social Services in cases of child abuse was to protect children. The resultant *Working Together* guidelines emphasize the need for inter-agency cooperation in child protection work (Department of Health and Social Security, 1988; Home Office *et al*, 1991).

Official definitions of abuse and neglect are provided in the *Working Together* guidelines. Four categories of abuse are identified: neglect, physical injury, sexual abuse and emotional abuse. The definitions provide a useful starting point in outlining the different forms of abuse.

NEGLECT

Neglect has been defined as the persistent or severe neglect of a child or the failure to protect a child from exposure of any kind of danger, including cold or starvation, or extreme failure to carry out important aspects of care, resulting in the significant impairment of the child's health or development, including non-organic failure to thrive (Home Office *et al*, 1991).

Approximately one-quarter of children on Child Protection Registers are registered under this category (Department of Health, 1994). Neglect is generally considered an omission, rather than a commission, of a direct act or behaviour that has a detrimental effect on the child's physical and psychological development.

Many risk factors identified with physical abuse (see discussion on page **310**) apply to neglect, as well. For example, neglectful parents often demonstrate a lack of knowledge of parenting skills. They may be unaware that an infant needs to be fed every 3-4 hours, be unable to cook a meal, or not know what constitutes a balanced meal. The most serious lack of knowledge is failure to recognize emotional nurturing as an essential need of children.

IDENTIFICATION OF NEGLECT

Neglect from deprivation of necessities is easier to identify than emotional abuse or neglect, because physical signs of neglect are usually evident (Box 16-1).

IMPLICATIONS FOR NURSING

Nursing goals are similar to those discussed under physical abuse, with identification and prevention as priorities. Often, neglect is caused by ignorance. Early education of caregivers regarding children's basic physical and emotional needs can avert serious problems. Any persistent change in children's behaviour is a clue to unsatisfactory situations and must be taken seriously. Nurses can be alert to such problems by routinely incorporating questions about children's activities into their assessment and by referring any concerns or suspicious complaints to a Social Services department. Local child protection policies and procedures documents provide guidelines for referral. These should be readily available to health care staff.

PHYSICAL INJURY

Physical injury is defined as the actual or likely physical injury to a child, or failure to prevent physical injury (or suffering) to a child including deliberate poisoning, suffocation and Munchausen's syndrome by proxy (Home Office *et al*, 1991). Approximately one-third of children on Child Protection Registers are registered under this category. Physical injury has received more attention than other types of abuse, particularly following the coining of the term 'battered child syndrome' by Kempe *et al* in 1962. However, no single definition of the term is universally accepted.

The exact cause of child abuse is not known, but three major criteria seem to predispose children to physical injury by their parents or other caregivers: these include parental characteristics, characteristics of the child, and environmental characteristics. No single aetiological factor can be isolated as responsible for abuse: the greater the number of variables, the greater the risk. Different variables may be responsible for certain types of abuse. For example, poverty may be more strongly associated with neglect, whereas parental characteristics maybe more strongly related to physical abuse. One combination of risk factors predisposing to physical abuse is poor nurturing during the parent's own childhood, negative feelings towards the pregnancy, and birth of a temperamentally difficult child who is developmentally delayed and/or in poor health (Browne and Saqi, 1988).

280

PARENTAL CHARACTERISTICS

Extensive research has focused on parental characteristics which distinguish abusive parents from non-abusive parents. While physical punishment tends to occur often in abusive parents' childhoods, most of the parents were not physically abused as children. Abusive parents tend to have difficulty controlling aggressive impulses, and the free expression of violence is one of the most consistent qualities of these families (Altmeier *et al*, 1982).

Another finding is that abusive families are often more socially isolated and have fewer supportive relationships than non-abusive parents. With little or no available support system, and the presence of concurrent stresses imposed by the child or the environment, these parents are extremely vulnerable to crises of any nature. They literally strike out at the child as a method of releasing their increasing frustration and anxiety. Some studies suggest that the level of social support is an important factor in identifying potential abusers, and that enhancement of the person's support system may be a prevention or intervention strategy for abuse (Browne and Saqi, 1988).

Another characteristic of some abusing parents is inadequate knowledge of normal developmental expectations. Thus, they expect their children to nurture and parent them, in the same way their parents demanded similar behaviour.

Other factors identified in abusive parents include low self-esteem, less adequate maternal functioning, untruthfulness, poor rapport in the interviewing situation, and negative attitude towards the pregnancy.

CHARACTERISTICS OF THE CHILD

The child's temperament, position in the family, additional physical needs if ill or cognitively impaired, activity level or degree of sensitivity to parental needs, all contribute to the potential for physical abuse. For example, the firstborn may not be abused if he or she fits into the easy child pattern and demands little, other than routine feeding and nappy changing.

Not infrequently, the affected child is illegitimate, unwanted, brain damaged (especially in situations where the parents cannot accept the learning difficulties), hyperactive, physically disabled or from a broken home. Sometimes, children are abused because they remind the parent of someone the parent dislikes, such as a younger brother or sister who received all the attention from their own parents. Pre-term infants may be at risk from abuse due to a lack of parent-child bonding during early infancy. Often a difficult pregnancy, labour or delivery is a predisposing factor in abuse, especially when the infant is born prematurely or with congenital anomalies.

Although one child is usually the victim in an abusing family, removing that child from the home often places the other siblings at risk for abuse. Therefore, no child is safe if left in the abusing environment unless the parents can be helped to learn new parenting skills, and assisted to meet their needs and release their frustration through alternatives other than attacking their children.

ENVIRONMENTAL CHARACTERISTICS

The environment is an integral part of the potential abusing situation. Typically, the environment is one of chronic stress, including problems of divorce, extramarital relationships, financial difficulties, unemployment, poor housing, alcoholism and drug addiction. There is often lack of a social support system and the environment becomes a trap from which there is no emotional exit, except to direct the anger and frustration towards a helpless victim — the child.

Although most of the reporting has been from lower socio-economic groups, child abuse is not a problem of any one societal group. It spans all educational, social and economic levels. Certainly, stresses imposed by poverty predispose lower socioeconomic families to abusive situations, and abuse in these groups is more likely to be reported. However, concealed crises can also be present in upper-class families.

IDENTIFICATION OF PHYSICAL ABUSE

One of the most critical responsibilities of health professionals is identifying abusive situations as early as possible. The characteristics discussed above can serve as a framework to assess the vulnerability of families to abuse, but never to predict actual abuse. Rather, a thorough physical examination and a careful, detailed history are the diagnostic tools to identify the possibility of abuse. Recognition of abuse or neglect necessitates a familiarity with both physical signs and behavioural indicators (see Box 16-1). Not all forms of abuse demonstrate obvious signs. Violent shaking of children can cause fatal intracranial trauma without signs of external head injury (Alexander *et al*, 1990).

In the United Kingdom, the statutory agencies responsible for investigating abuse and neglect are the Social Services and, in some areas, the National Society for the Prevention of Cruelty to Children (NSPCC). The nurse may be the first person to identify a child who is in need, and should act to bring the child to the attention of social services (Department of Health, 1992). Nurses, midwives and health visitors may contribute to inter-agency working to protect children through their contribution to strategy discussions and child protection case conferences (Home Office *et al*, 1991).

Munchausen syndrome by proxy

One of the most unusual and perplexing types of abuse is Munchausen syndrome by proxy (MSbP), which refers to illness that one person fabricates or induces in another person. In children, it is usually the mother who fabricates signs and symptoms of illness in her child, the proxy, to gain attention from the medical staff. MSbP can take many forms, such as adding maternal blood to the child's urine to simulate haematuria, presenting a fictitious medical history, chronic poisoning of the child, or suffocating the child to cause apnoea and seizures. Another form of MSbP is alleging that the child has

---

◆ **BOX 16-1**

Clinical manifestations of child abuse

Neglect
Physical signs:
Failure to thrive
Signs of malnutrition, such as thin extremities, abdominal distension, lack of subcutaneous fat
Poor personal hygiene, especially of teeth
Unclean and/or inappropriate dress
Evidence of poor health care, such as poor immunization status, untreated infections, frequent colds
Frequent injuries from lack of supervision
Behavioural indicators:
Dull and inactive: excessively passive or sleepy
Self-stimulatory behaviour, such as finger sucking or rocking
In older children: begging or stealing food, absenteeism from school, drug or alcohol addiction, vandalism or shoplifting

Physical Injury
Physical signs:
Bruises and welts - on face, lips, mouth, back, buttocks, thighs or torso; regular patterns descriptive of objects used, such as belt buckle, hand, wire hanger, chain, wooden spoon, squeeze or pinch marks. May be present in various stages of healing.
Burns - on soles of feet, palms of hands, scalp, back or buttocks; patterns descriptive of object used, such as round cigar or cigarette burns; glove-like, sharply demarcated areas from immersion in scalding water; rope burns on wrists or ankles from being bound; burns in the shape of an iron, radiator, or electric stove ring; absence of 'splash' marks and presence of symmetrical burns.
Fractures and dislocations - skull, nose or facial structures. Injury may denote type of abuse, such as a spiral fracture or dislocation from twisting of an extremity, or whiplash from shaking the child. Multiple new or old fractures in various stages of healing.
Lacerations and abrasions - on backs of arms, legs, torso, face or external genitalia. Unusual symptoms, such as abdominal swelling, pain, and vomiting from punching. Descriptive marks such as from human bites or pulling out the hair.
Chemical - unexplained repeated poisoning, especially drug overdose. Unexplained sudden illness, such as hypoglycaemia from insulin administration.
Behavioural indicators:
Wary of physical contact with adults
Apparent fear of parents or going home
Frozen watchfulness
Inappropriate reaction to injury, such as failure to cry from pain
Lack of reaction to frightening events
Apprehensive when hearing other children cry
Indiscriminate friendliness and displays of affection
Superficial relationships
Acting out behaviour, such as aggression, to seek attention
Withdrawal behaviour

Sexual Abuse
Physical signs:
Bruises, bleeding, lacerations or irritation of external genitalia, anus, mouth or throat
Torn, stained or bloody underclothing
Pain on urination or pain, swelling, and itching of genital area
Penile discharge
Sexually transmitted disease, non-specific vaginitis, or venereal warts
Difficulty in walking or sitting
Unusual odour in the genital area
Recurrent urinary tract infections
Pregnancy in young adolescent
Foreign bodies in the urethra, bladder, vagina or anus
Behavioural indicators:
Sudden emergence of sexually related problems, including excessive or public masturbation, age-inappropriate sexual play, promiscuity or overtly seductive behaviour
Withdrawn, excessive daydreaming
Preoccupation with fantasies, especially in play
Poor relationship with peers
Sudden changes such as anxiety, weight changes; bulimia/anorexia nervosa
In incestuous relationships, excessive anger at mother for not protecting daughter
Regressive behaviour such as bed-wetting or thumb sucking
Sudden onset of phobias or fears, particularly fears of the dark, men, strangers, or particular settings or situations (e.g., undue fear of leaving the house, staying at the child-minders or play group)
Running away from home
Substance abuse, particularly of alcohol or mood elevating drugs
Profound and rapid personality changes, especially extreme depression, hostility, and aggression (often accompanied by social withdrawal)
Rapidly declining school performance
Suicide attempts

Emotional Abuse
Physical signs:
Failure to thrive
Feeding and eating disorders
Enuresis
Sleep disorders
Behavioural indicators:
Self-stimulatory behaviour such as biting, rocking, sucking
In infants, lack of social smile and stranger anxiety
Withdrawal
Unusual fearfulness
Antisocial behaviour such as stealing, destructiveness, cruelty
Extremes of behaviour, such as over compliant and passive or aggressive and demanding
Emotional and intellectual developmental delay, especially language
Suicide attempts

been sexually abused by someone else, in order to gain recognition as the child's protector.

Such cases are often difficult to confirm and require a high index of suspicion in order to protect the children (Box 16-2). Nurses play an important role in monitoring the parent's activities to identify instances of causing the children's symptoms. The parent's actions may induce a serious illness in children—one that may even be fatal. Children may develop chronic invalidism, accepting the illness story and believing themselves to be ill (Meadow, 1989).

History pertaining to the incident
Aside from observable evidence of physical abuse, the type of history revealed by parents or other caregiver, such as the babysitter or mother's boyfriend, is a significant diagnostic factor. Areas of the history that should arouse suspicion of abuse are summarized in Box 16-3. Incompatibility between the history and the injury is probably the most important criterion on which to base the decision to report suspected abuse.

An important point to remember when taking a history is that abused children rarely betray their parents by confessing to the abuse they received. If questioned, they will repeat the same story as the parents and try to defend the parent's actions. Children fear losing whatever security and love they have. Between abusive acts, children may receive some measure of attention and love from the parents. If they betray the parents, they may lose this and be uncertain or fearful of the consequences, such as foster care. Preserving the present situation may be less frightening than the unknown future.

Parental behaviours
Certain behavioural responses of the parents to their child and to the interviewer may alert the nurse to the possibility of abuse. The parent's perception of the incident is in terms of how it affects them, not the child, which indicates their pre-occupation with their own needs and their inability to support others.

In cases of family violence where the wife is also abused, the mother may appear to be more concerned about her mate's needs, in order to keep him happy, and may be less focused on the child. The couple may even appear to be very loving. In these instances, the abused child may also appear to be greatly attached to the mother, to protect the mother from being assaulted when she returns home.

In contrast to parents who seem overtly aloof, many abusive parents also show great concern for their children. Therefore, while certain behavioural characteristics of parents may arouse suspicion, their attitude towards the child is not diagnostic of abuse.

Child behaviours
Although no single pattern is typical, extremes of behaviour may be observed. Children may be very unresponsive to the parent or may be excessively clinging and intolerant of separation. There may be over attachment to the abusing parent, possibly in the hope of preventing any upset that may precipitate anger and another attack. Some children shy away from strangers as if frightened, whereas others are unusually affectionate and outgoing.

IMPLICATIONS FOR NURSING

Nursing care involves several important areas, ideally beginning with prevention of abuse and neglect and, following an abusive act, the identification, referral and protection of the child from further abuse.

Prevention
Home visiting in the pre- and postnatal period by midwives and primary health care nurses, such as health visitors, helps to identify families at high risk and provides the opportunity to offer programmes of support (see Boxes 16-4 and 16-5).

Nurses can also provide information about normal childhood growth and development, and routine health care needs. In addition, nurses can help teach parents appropriate methods of bathing, feeding, toileting, disciplining and accident prevention, while stressing children's normal needs and developmental characteristics. Where needs for assistance are identified, the nurse, midwife or health visitor may act as a source of referral to other agencies.

Identification and protection from further abuse
Initially, identification of instances of suspected abuse or neglect is essential. The nurse may come into contact with abused children in the accident and emergency department, general practitioner's surgery, home or school. Signs that indicate possible abuse (see Box 16-1) must be recognized.

The nurse should also be aware of the local policies and procedures for dealing with cases of suspected abuse or neglect, and the mechanisms of referral to the statutory agencies. In an emergency situation, the police have powers to ensure the child's safety. *The Children Act 1989* (Box 16-6) contains several provisions which enable local authorities to take action in an emergency situation in order to protect a child. However, the *Act* prohibits the court from making any order unless it is satisfied that it will be better for the child than making no order at all.

Although the *Act* is mainly addressed to the courts and Social Services departments, there are several important implications for health professionals. The need for health professionals to cooperate in child protection investigations and to collaborate in meeting health needs of children looked after by Social Services are central to meeting the guiding principles of the *Act*.

Nurses may be asked to contribute to strategy discussions and child protection conferences (see Box 16-7). When the courts are involved, they usually require first-hand testimony by the referring parties. This may mean that nurses in the school, hospital, or community health agency are subpoenaed or that their records are introduced as evidence. Nurses have a great responsibility in reporting facts. Therefore, accurate nurse's notes are critical in any suspected abusive situation. Colour of bruises can be important in evaluating time of injury (see Table 16-1). Behaviours are described, rather than interpreted, and conversations between the nurse, child and parent are recorded in quotation form as much as possible. The nurse must bear in mind that the record of the hospital or home visit may be the most supporting evidence available. Part of the long-term plan is help for the parents, but the priority must be the welfare and protection of the child.

Care of the child

Frequently, children suspected of abuse are hospitalized for medical management of their injuries. All abuse and neglect cases are managed by a multidisciplinary team including at least a doctor, nurse, social worker and police officer. These children's needs are the same as those of any hospitalized child, but are multiplied by their situation.

The goal of the consistent nurse-child relationship is to provide a role model for parents. The nurse helps them to relate positively and constructively to their child, and to foster a therapeutic environment during the child's reprieve from the abusive situation.

Placement on discharge may be a return to the parents, a temporary foster home, or permanent termination of parental rights. No matter how severe the abuse, children will usually mourn the loss of their parents. They need help to understand why they must not return home and that the new home is not a punishment. Whenever possible, foster parents should be encouraged to visit, and the nurse should take an active role in helping these parents understand the child.

Care of the family

The relationship of professionals with the parents or caregivers must be one of genuine concern and treatment, not of accusation and punishment. In some way, such as group discussion, nurses and other workers must come to an understanding of their feelings, in order to be effective with abusive parents. Unless the nurse's attitude is positive, abusing parents will not be motivated to change, since they will not be working with a trusting person who demonstrates the behaviour being asked of them.

Since some parents have unrealistic expectations of children's capabilities, the nurse also fosters knowledge and

---

◆ BOX 16-2

The Allitt case

Early in 1991, on a children's ward in a general hospital in the United Kingdom, three children died suddenly and one baby died shortly after discharge from the ward. All the deaths were unexpected. In addition, nine other children from the ward collapsed unexpectedly during this time. A state enrolled nurse, Beverly Allitt, was subsequently convicted of murdering four children, attempting to murder three more and of causing grievous bodily harm to six other children in her care. The inquiry that followed made 13 recommendations; these are of importance to all nurses working in the field of child health:

That, for all those seeking entry to the nursing profession, in addition to routine references, the most recent employer or place of study should be asked to provide at least a record of time taken off on the grounds of sickness.

That in every case, coroners should send copies of post-mortem reports to any consultant who has been involved in the patient's care prior to death.

That the provision of paediatric pathology services be reviewed with a view to ensuring that such services be engaged in every case in which the death of a child is unexpected or clinically unaccountable.

That no candidate for nursing in whom there is evidence of a major personality disorder should be employed in the profession.

That nurses should undergo formal health screening when they obtain their first posts after qualifying.

That the possibility be reviewed of making available to occupational health departments any records of absence through sickness from any institution which an applicant for a nursing post has attended or has been employed by.

That procedures for management referrals to occupational health departments should make clear the criteria which trigger such referrals.

That consideration be given to how GPs might, with the candidate's consent, be asked to certify that there is nothing in the medical history of a candidate for employment in the NHS which would make them unsuitable for their chosen occupation.

That the Department of Health should take steps to ensure that its guide *Welfare of Children and Young People in Hospital* is more closely observed.

That, in the event of failure of an alarm on monitoring equipment, an untoward incident report should be completed and the equipment serviced before it is used again.

That reports of serious untoward incidents to District and Regional Health Authorities should be made in writing and through a single channel.

That the Grantham disaster should serve to heighten awareness in all those caring for children of the possibility of malevolent intervention as a cause for unexplained clinical events.

(Clothier et al., 1994).

understanding of normal growth and development. As abusing parents are often very sensitive to criticism or domination, and may possess a low self-esteem, any competent parenting abilities they demonstrate should be praised in an attempt to promote their sense of parental adequacy. Abusing parents desperately need 'mothering' to be able to parent their own children. Home visits may be planned at a time when the children are at school, with a friend or asleep to allow maximum attention to the parent.

SEXUAL ABUSE

Sexual abuse has been defined as the 'actual or likely sexual exploitation of a child or adolescent. The child may be dependent and/or developmentally immature.' (Home Office *et al*, 1991). Approximately one-quarter of children on Child Protection Registers are registered under this category. Child sexual abuse has become a major concern in the United Kingdom in recent years, with increased reporting and registrations in this category (Wynne, 1992). Sexual abuse includes several types of sexual maltreatment, including incest, molestation, exhibitionism, child pornography, child prostitution and paedophilia.

IDENTIFICATION OF SEXUAL ABUSE

Unlike physical abuse or neglect, sexual abuse may occur with few, if any, obvious indications of the activity. Children may reveal the fear that their parents would not believe them, especially if the offender is a trusted member of the family. Some children fear they will be blamed for the situation. Many young children with limited vocabulary have difficulty describing the activity, when they do have the courage or opportunity to complain. Consequently, the abuse is perpetuated over a prolonged period.

No typical profile of the victim exists, and nurses must have a high index of suspicion to identify these children. Physical signs vary and may include any of those listed in Box 16-1 for sexual abuse. When it is suspected, other children in the family should also be checked. The victim may exhibit various behav-

---

◆ BOX 16-3

Warning signs of physical abuse

Physical evidence of abuse and/or neglect, including previous injuries

Conflicting stories about the 'accident' or injury from the parents or others

Cause of injury blamed on sibling or other party

An injury inconsistent with the history, such as a concussion and broken arm from falling off a bed

History inconsistent with child's developmental level; such as a 6-month-old turning on the hot water

A complaint other than the one associated with signs of abuse; for example, a chief complaint of a cold when there is evidence of first- and second-degree burns

Inappropriate parental concern for the degree of the injury, such as an exaggerated or absent emotional response

Refusal of the parents to sign for additional tests or agree to necessary treatment

Excessive delay in seeking treatment

Absence of the parents for questioning

Inappropriate response of child, such as little or no response to pain, fear of being touched, excessive or lack of separation anxiety, indiscriminate friendliness to strangers

Previous reports of abuse in the family

Repeated visits to emergency facilities with injuries

◆ BOX 16-4

Observations of parents-to-be during antenatal care

1. Are the parents overconcerned with the baby's sex?
2. Are the parents overconcerned with the baby's performance? Do they worry that the infant will not meet the standard?
3. Is there an attempt to deny that there is a pregnancy (mother not willing to gain weight, no plans whatsoever, refusal to talk about the situation)?
4. Is this child going to be one child too many? Could he or she be the 'last straw'?
5. Is there great depression over this pregnancy?
6. Is the mother alone and frightened, especially by the physical changes caused by the pregnancy? Do careful explanations fail to dissipate these fears?
7. Is support lacking from the husband and/or family?
8. Where are the parents living? Do they have a listed telephone number? Are their relatives and friends nearby?
9. Did the mother and/or father formerly want an abortion but not go through with it or wait until it was too late?
10. Have the parents considered relinquishment of their child? Why did they change their minds?

Modified from Kempe, 1976. Copyright 1976, American Medical Association.

◆ **BOX 16-5**

Observations to be made at postpartum and paediatric check-ups

1. Do the parents have fun with the baby?
2. Do the parents establish eye contact (direct-face position) with the baby?
3. How do the parents talk to the baby? Is everything they express a demand?
4. Are most of their verbalizations about the child negative?
5. Do they remain disappointed over the child's sex?
6. What is the child's name? Where did the name come from? When was the child named?
7. Are the parents' expectations for the child's development far beyond the child's capabilities?
8. Are the parents very bothered by the baby's crying? How do they feel about the crying?
9. Do the parents see the baby as too demanding during feedings? Are they repulsed by the messiness? Do they ignore the baby's demands to be fed?
10. What are the parents' reactions to the task of changing nappies?
11. When the baby cries, are the parents able to comfort him or her?
12. What are other family members' reactions to the baby?
13. What types of support is the mother receiving?
14. Are there sibling rivalry problems?
15. Is the husband jealous of the baby's drain on the mother's time and affection?
16. When the parents bring the child to the practitioner's office, do they get involved and take control over the baby's needs and what's going to happen (during the examination and while in the waiting room), or do they relinquish control to the doctor or nurse (e.g., undressing, holding, or allowing the child to express fears)?
17. Can attention be focused on the child in the parents' presence? Can the parents see something positive for them in that?
18. Do the parents make nonexistent complaints about the baby? Do they call with strange stories that the child has, for example, stopped breathing, turned colour, or is doing something 'on purpose' to aggravate the parent?
19. Do the parents make emergency calls for very small things, not major things?

Modified from Kempe, 1976. Copyright 1976, American Medical Association.

◆ **BOX 16-6**

The Children Act 1989

The Children Act 1989, took effect on October 14th, 1991. This *Act* is widely described as the most comprehensive piece of legislation Parliament has ever enacted about children. The main principles of the *Act* embody the notions of the welfare of the child as paramount in court proceedings, partnership with the child and parents and parental responsibility. The *Act* also seeks to ensure that the provision of services to the child and his or her family reflect individual, identified needs that are appropriate to the child's race, culture, religion and language (Department of Health, 1989). In intervening to protect children, the *Act* considers the concept of 'significant harm':

Where the question of whether harm suffered by the child is significant turns on the child's health and development, his health or development shall be compared with that which could be reasonably expected of a similar child.

[*The Children Act 1989* — Section 31 (10)]

ioural manifestations; however, none of these are diagnostic of sexual abuse (Legrand *et al*, 1989). Signs may be incorrectly attributed to the normal stresses of childhood, especially in older children or adolescents. Even those signs considered most predictive of sexual abuse, such as sexually inappropriate behaviour for age, enactment of adult sexual activity, and intense focus on sexual activity (e.g., masturbation), do not always indicate that sexual abuse has occurred.

The disclosure comes about in a variety of ways: the act is observed by others; the child tells someone, such as a parent of a friend; visible clues of the relationship are observed, such as the accumulation of money, gifts or sweets; obvious clues are seen, such as the child coming home dishevelled or becoming pregnant; and physical signs or behavioural indicators are observed.

IMPLICATIONS FOR NURSING

Nursing care of sexually abused children involves the same objectives as those discussed for physically abused children: prevention, identification and protection. Many of the interventions are identical, such as referring the child and family to Social Services. The child may be interviewed as part of a joint investigation procedure and the interview will be conducted by an experienced social worker and police officer. Medical examinations are carried out by a police surgeon or specially trained paediatrician, and forensic evidence may be obtained. Where possible, all care is provided in the community setting.

Prevention programmes are directed at teaching children to recognize situations that increase the risk of sexual abuse and

◆ BOX 16-7

Child protection meetings

Strategy Meeting/Discussion

The strategy meeting or discussion is held to plan the details of a joint investigation into allegations or suspicions of child abuse by social workers and police officers so that all action is coordinated. Professionals who are in possession of important information about the suspected abuse may be asked to attend. Parents and children are not asked to attend strategy meetings.

Child Protection Conference

Initial Child Protection Conferences are usually held within eight working days of a referral to the Statutory Agencies. Here, family information, the allegations of abuse and the subsequent medical, police and social work investigations will be available to all the professionals involved. The recent *Working Together* (1988) guidelines assert that parents, and where appropriate children, should also attend. A decision will be made as to whether the child's (and any siblings) name will be entered on the Child Protection Register. If a child's name is placed on the register, then a Child Protection Plan will be formulated in order to provide for the child's future protection and well-being. Review Child Protection Conferences will then take place at a minimum of every six months.

COLOUR	AGE OF BRUISE
Red to red-blue	Less than 24 hours
Purple to dark blue	1 to 4 days
Green to yellow-green	5 to 7 days
Yellow to brown	7 to 10 days
Disappearance	1 to 3 weeks

Table 16-1 Stages of healing noted in bruises.

to respond in ways that reduce the risk. The nurse may be in a position to discuss this topic with parents as part of health maintenance programmes (see Parent Guidelines).

EMOTIONAL ABUSE

Emotional abuse is defined as the 'actual or likely severe adverse effect on the emotional and behavioural development of a child caused by persistent or severe emotional ill-treatment or rejection. All abuse involves some emotional ill-treatment. This category should be used where it is the main or sole form of abuse.' (Home Office *et al*, 1991.)

Approximately one-tenth of children on child protection registers are registered under this category. Emotional abuse refers to an adult's concerted attack on a child's development of self and social competence; it is a pattern of psychically destructive behaviour. Emotional abuse may also be seen as isolating, terrorizing, ignoring and corrupting the child (Garbarino *et al*, 1986).

IDENTIFICATION OF EMOTIONAL ABUSE

Emotional abuse may be readily suspected, but it is very difficult to substantiate. Physical signs are often non-specific and nurses must rely on suggestive behaviours, which range from depression to acting out behaviour, to help to identify a possible abusive situation (see Box 16-1). Although primary caregivers are generally responsible for instances of emotional abuse, this is not always the case. School teachers also can inflict emotional abuse on pupils. Indications of teacher abuse include excessive worry about school performance; expressed fear of the teacher; negative perception of self and school; excessive crying, nightmares, headaches and stomach-aches; and decreased attendance.

IMPLICATIONS FOR NURSING

Nursing goals are similar to those discussed under physical injury and neglect, with identification and prevention as priorities.

INFECTIOUS DISEASES

Young children may be particularly susceptible to infectious disease. This is because they may have low resistance to infectious agents at a time when they are increasing social contacts outside the home. Such problems include the typical childhood communicable diseases: conjunctivitis, stomatitis and intestinal parasitic diseases.

COMMUNICABLE DISEASES

The incidence of common childhood communicable diseases has declined following the advent of immunizations. In cases where the diseases still present, complications have been reduced through the use of antibiotics. Although some of these diseases are now rare, nurses needs to be able to recognize the signs of such diseases (see Table 16-2).

IMPLICATIONS FOR NURSING

Primary health care nurses and nurses working in accident and emergency departments may be the first to see the signs of a communicable disease. Nursing assessment of a child presenting with symptoms such as a sore throat or rash should include taking a history of any recent contact with a communicable disease. The nurse should also note immunization status and history of having the disease, as the possibility of many infectious diseases can be eliminated by these two criteria.

In most cases, the child will be cared for at home. The principal goals of nursing care include:
1. Preventing the spread of infection to others.
2. Prevention of complications.
3. Maintaining comfort.
4. Supporting the child and family.

Prevention

Primary prevention occurs almost exclusively through immunization. Prevention of spread includes appropriate techniques to reduce cross-infection. If a child is hospitalized, then local infection control policies are implemented. Hand washing is particularly important.

Prevention of complications

Most children recover from these illnesses without difficulty, and treatment is generally supportive. However, antibiotic therapy may be indicated in some cases and the nurse can help to ensure compliance.

Children who are immunosuppressed through steroid or other immunosuppressive therapy, those with a generalized malignancy such as leukaemia, and those with an immunologic disorder are at greater risk from communicable diseases. This is especially true of chicken pox and erythema infectiosum (EI). In addition, children with haemolytic disease, such as sickle cell anaemia, are considered to be at particular risk from EI.

High-risk children who have signs of a communicable disease should be referred to their medical practitioner. Primary health care nurses need to be aware of high-risk children and should alert parents to any local outbreaks of communicable diseases. In most cases, these children are kept at home until the outbreak is over. Immunoglobulin may be prescribed.

Maintaining comfort

The main problem is associated with skin manifestations. The use of cool baths and calamine lotion may be helpful in relieving itching. The child should be nursed in a cool environment. Lightweight, loose clothing also helps to control itching. Antipuritic medication may be prescribed.

Pyrexia is common and measures for controlling temperature may be necessary. Lozenges, analgesics and rinses may be offered for relief of a sore throat. A light, bland diet and increased fluids should be provided. Bed rest may be indicated (see Table 16-2). Quiet activity helps distract children from discomfort.

Supporting the child and family

Although most cases of communicable disease are benign, parents may need support and help in coping with manifestations of the disease, such as itching. Primary health care nurses have a role in helping support the family in the community, where necessary.

Parent Guidelines

Preventing or Dealing with Sexual Abuse

Sexual assault of children occurs more frequently than most of us realize. It may be preventable if children have good preparation. *To provide protection and preparation,* as parents we can:

Pay careful attention to who is around our children. (Unwanted touch *may* come from someone we like and trust.)

Back up a child's right to say 'No'.

Encourage communication by taking seriously what our children *say*.

Take a second look at signals of potential danger.

Refuse to leave our children in the company of those we do not trust.

Include information about sexual assault when teaching about safety.

Provide specific definitions and examples of sexual assault.

Remind children that even 'nice' people sometimes do mean things.

Urge children to tell us about *anybody* who causes them to be uncomfortable.

Prepare children to deal with bribes, threats, and, as well as possible, physical force.

Eliminate secrets between us and our children.

Teach children how to say 'no', ask for help, and control who touches them and how.

Model self-protective and limit-setting behaviour for our children.

Should it ever become necessary *to help a child recover from a sexual assault,* as parents we can:

Listen carefully and understand how children tell us.

Support the child for telling by praise, belief, sympathy and lack of blame.

Know local resources, and choose help carefully.

Provide opportunities to talk about the assault.

Provide opportunities for the entire family to go through a recovery process.

Sexual assault affects all of us, whether or not our own children are assaulted. *To help deal with this social problem,* all of us can:

Provide sympathetic care and support to those who have been victimized.

Recognize that offenders do not change without intervention.

Organize neighbourhood programmes to support each other's efforts to protect children.

Encourage schools to provide information about sexual assault as a problem of health and safety.

Organize community groups to support educational, treatment, and law enforcement programmes.

From Adams and Fay, 1981.

CONJUNCTIVITIS

Acute conjunctivitis (inflammation of the conjunctiva) is a common condition in children. The usual causes are viral, bacterial, allergic or related to a foreign body. Recurrent conjunctivitis in infants may indicate nasolacrimal duct obstruction. Although diagnosis is usually made from the clinical picture, eye swabs may be taken for culture (Box 16-8).

IMPLICATIONS FOR NURSING

Nursing care includes administration of medication and keeping the eye clean. Treatment of conjunctivitis is usually with medicated eye drops by day and ointment at night. Supportive treatment includes removal of accumulated secretions by wiping from the inner canthus downward and outward away from the opposite eye. Warm moist compresses are helpful in removing crusts.

Prevention of cross infection is important. The child's flannel and towel should be kept separate, and tissues used to clean the eye should be properly disposed. The child should not rub the eyes and should be taught correct hand washing technique.

STOMATITIS

Stomatitis is the inflammation of the oral mucosa. Children with immunosuppression and those receiving chemotherapy or head and neck radiotherapy are considered high risk for developing mucosal ulceration and herpetic ulceration.

Herpes stomatitis, caused by the herpes simplex virus (HSV), may occur as a primary infection or may recur as a less severe form commonly known as 'cold sores'.

IMPLICATIONS FOR NURSING

Nursing care of children with herpetic stomatitis is concerned with pain relief and preventing the spread of infection. In severe cases, acyclovir may be prescribed. Analgesic and topical anaesthetics are used to provide relief, especially before meals. Drinking bland fluids through a straw may be particularly helpful in avoiding painful lesions. Mouth care may include mouthwashes and the use of a very soft toothbrush or foam stick.

Local hospital policies for prevention of spread should be followed. Careful hand washing is essential and since the infection is auto-inoculable, care should be taken to ensure that children do not infect other parts of the body. All articles placed in the mouth should be cleaned thoroughly.

INTESTINAL PARASITIC DISEASES

Intestinal parasitic diseases are the most common infections in the world. Although many are concentrated in the tropical regions, several are encountered relatively frequently in the United Kingdom. This section considers two common parasitic infections in children: giardiasis and enterobiasis (threadworms).

GIARDIASIS

Giardiasis is caused by the protozoan *Giardia lamblia* (Hill, 1993). Although individuals infected with giardiasis may be asymptomatic, young children, especially infants, may manifest symptoms such as diarrhoea, vomiting, anorexia and failure to thrive. Children older than five years of age may complain of abdominal pain, intermittent loose stools and constipation. The stools may be watery, malodorous and greasy. Most infections resolve spontaneously, but the infection may become chronic and may last for months or years.

IMPLICATIONS FOR NURSING

The key role of nurses is prevention. Parents and caregivers may require education in hygienic nappy changing practices. Metronidazole is the drug of choice.

ENTEROBIASIS

Enterobiasis (commonly known as threadworm in the United Kingdom) is caused by the nematode *Enterobiasis vermicularis*. Infection begins when the eggs are ingested or inhaled. The typical hand-to-mouth activity of children makes them especially prone to continual re-infection. The principal symptom is intense perianal itching. However, young children may display irritability, sleep problems and bed wetting. In females, the worms may migrate to the vagina and urethra to cause infection. Diagnosis is by 'tape test' where sticky tape, pressed against the perianal area, is used to show the presence of threadworms on microscopic examination.

IMPLICATIONS FOR NURSING

Nursing care is directed at identification, eradication and prevention of re-infection. The nurse may also help teach good hygiene in toilet use and nappy changing practices. The drug of choice is usually mebindazole, although this cannot be given to children under the age of two years. Treatment is usually indicated for the whole family.

POISONING

The developmental characteristics of young children means that they may be susceptible to accidental poisoning by ingestion. Despite the impact of childproof containers, poisoning remains a common problem in the United Kingdom. Occasionally, children are poisoned deliberately by their parents or caregivers (non-accidental poisoning). This section is concerned with the role of nurses in preventing accidental poisoning, and the principles of emergency treatment in cases of acute poisoning.

Substances taken in accidental child poisoning include medicines, household products and plants. Not all substances taken by children are toxic, for example crayons, plant foods and vitamin preparations (without iron). Many products are

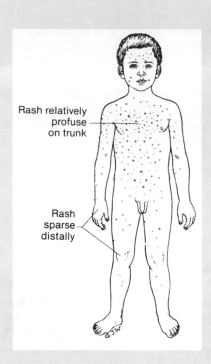

Fig 16-1 Chickenpox (varicella).

Rash relatively profuse on trunk

Rash sparse distally

DISEASE

CHICKENPOX (varicella) (Fig. 16.1)
Agent: varicella zoster
Source: primary secretions of respiratory tract of infected persons; to a lesser degree skin lesions (scabs not infectious)
Transmission: direct contact, droplet spread, and contaminated objects
Incubation period: 2 to 3 weeks, usually 13 to 17 days
Period of communicability: probably 1 day before eruption of lesions (prodromal period) to 6 days after first crop of vesicles when crusts have formed

DIPTHERIA
Agent: *Corynebacterium diptheriae*
Source: discharges from mucous membranes of nose and naspharynx, skin and other lesions of infected person
Transmission: direct contact with infected person, a carrier, or contaminated articles
Incubation period: usually 2 to 5 days, possibly longer
Period of communicability: variable; until virulent bacilli are no longer present (identified by three negative cultures); usually 2 weeks but as long as 4 weeks

Table 16-2 Communicable diseases of childhood.

CLINICAL MANIFESTATIONS	THERAPEUTIC MANAGEMENT/ COMPLICATIONS	NURSING CARE
Prodromal stage: slight fever, malaise, and anorexia for first 24 hours; rash highly pruritic; begins as macule, rapidly progresses to papule and then vesicle (surrounded by erythematous base, becomes umbilicated and cloudy, breaks easily and forms crusts); all three stages (papule, vesicle, crust) present in varying degrees at one time **Distribution:** centripetal, spreading to face and proximal extremities but sparse on distal limbs **Signs and symptoms:** pyrexia, irritability from pruritus	**Specific:** usually none; antiviral agent (acyclovir) for infected high-risk children; varicella-zoster immune globulin (VZIG) after exposure in high-risk children **Supportive:** diphenhydramine hydrochloride to relieve itching; skin care to prevent secondary bacterial infection **Complications:** Secondary bacterial infections (abscesses, cellulitis, pneumonia, sepsis) Encephalitis Varicella pneumonia Hemorrhagic varicella (tiny hemorrhages in the vesicles and numerous petechiae in the skin) Chronic or transient thrombocytopenia	Maintain *strict* isolation in hospital Isolate child in home until vesicles have dried (usually 1 week after onset of disease) and isolate high-risk children from infected children Administer skin care: give bath and change clothes and linens daily; administer topical application of calamine lotion; keep child's fingernails short and clean; apply mittens if child scratches. Lessen pruritus; keep child occupied Remove loose crusts that rub and irritate skin Teach child to apply pressure to pruritic area rather than scratch it If older child, reason with child regarding danger of scar formation from scratching Paracetamol
Vary according to anatomical location of pseudomembrane **Nasal:** resembles common cold, serosanguinous mucopurulent nasal discharge; may be frank epistaxis **Tonsillar/pharyngeal:** malaise; anorexia; sore throat; low-grade fever; pulse increased above expected for temperature within 24 hours; smooth, adherent, white or grey membrane; lymphadenitis possibly pronounced (bull's neck); in severe cases, toxaemia, septic shock, and death within 6 to 10 days **Laryngeal:** fever, hoarseness, cough with or without previous signs listed; potential airway obstruction, apprehensive, dyspnoeic retractions, cyanosis	Antitoxin Antibiotics (penicillin or erythromycin) Complete bed rest (prevention of myocarditis) Tracheostomy for airway obstruction Treatment of infected contacts and carriers **Complications:** Myocarditis (second week) Neuritis	Maintain *strict* isolation in hospital Participate in sensitivity testing; have adrenaline available Administer antibiotics; observe for signs of sensitivity to penicillin Administer *complete* care to maintain bed rest Use suctioning as needed Humidity for loosening of secretions Observe respirations for signs of obstruction

(cont.)

Table 16-2 Communicable diseases of childhood (continued).

DISEASE

ERYTHEMA INFECTIOSUM (slapped cheek disease)

Agent: human parvovirus B19 (HPV)

Source: infected persons

Transmission: unknown; possibly respiratory secretions and blood

Incubation period: 4 to 14 days, maybe as long as 20 days

Period of communicability: uncertain but before onset of symptoms in most children

EXANTHEMA SUBITUM (roseola)

Agent: human herpes virus type 6

Source: unknown

Transmission: unknown (virtually limited to children between 6 months and 2 years of age)

Incubation period: unknown

Period of communicability: unknown

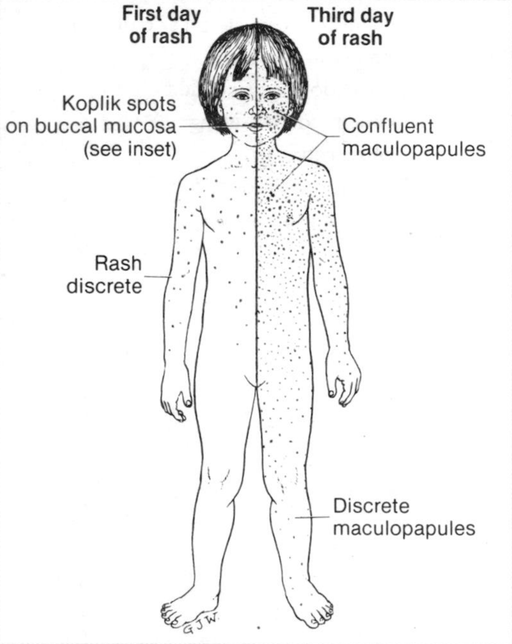

Fig 16-2 Measles (rubeola).

MEASLES (rubeola) (Fig. 16.2)

Agent: virus

Source: respiratory tract secretions, blood, and urine of infected person

Transmission: usually by direct contact with droplets of infected person

Incubation period: 10 to 20 days

Period of communicability: from 4 days before to 5 days after rash appears, but mainly during prodromal (catarrhal) stage

Table 16-2 Communicable diseases of childhood (continued).

CLINICAL MANIFESTATIONS	THERAPEUTIC MANAGEMENT/ COMPLICATIONS	NURSING CARE
Rash appears in three stages: *I* – erythema on face, chiefly on cheeks, 'slapped face' appearance; disappears by 1 to 4 days *II* – about 1 day after rash appears on face, maculopapular red spots appear, symmetrically distributed on upper and lower extremities; rash progresses from proximal to distal surfaces and may last a week or more. *III* – rash subsides but reappears if skin is irritated or traumatized (sun, heat, cold, friction). In children with aplastic crisis, rash is usually absent and prodromal illness includes fever, myalgia, lethargy, nausea, vomiting, and abdominal pain	None necessary **Complications:** Self-limited arthritis and arthralgia May result in fetal death if mother infected during pregnancy, but no evidence of congenital anomalies Aplastic crisis in children with haemolytic disease or immune deficiency	Reassure parents regarding benign nature of condition in affected child; isolation of child not necesssary. Place hospitalized child (immunosuppressed or with aplastic crises) suspected of HPV infection in isolation. Pregnant women: need not be excluded from workplace where HPV infection; should not care for patients with aplastic crises; explain low risk of fetal death to to those in contact with affected children
Persistent high fever for 3 to 4 days in child who appears well Precipitous drop in fever to normal with appearance of rash **Rash:** discrete rose-pink macules or maculopapules appearing first on trunk, then spreading to neck, face and extremities; nonpruritic, fades on pressure, lasts 1 to 2 days **Associated signs and symptoms:** cervical/postauricular lymphadenopathy, injected pharynx, cough, coryza	Nonspecific Antipyretics to control fever Anticonvulsives for child with history of febrile convulsions **Complications:** Febrile convulsions	Teach parents measures for lowering temperature (antipyretic drugs) If child is prone to convulsions, discuss appropriate precautions Reassure parents regarding benign nature of illness
Prodromal (cartarrhal) stage: fever and malaise, followed in 24 hours by coryza, cough, conjunctiviitis, Koplik spots (small, irregular red spots with a minute, bluish-white centre, first seen on the buccal mucosa opposite the molars 2 days before rash); symptoms gradually increase in severity until the second day after rash appears, when they begin to subside **Rash:** appears 3 to 4 days after onset of prodromal stage; begins as erythematous maculopapular eruption on face and gradually spreads downward; more severe in earlier sites (appears confluent) and less intense in later sites (appears discrete); after 3 to 4 days, assumes brownish appearance and fine desquamation occurs over areas of involvement **Symptoms:** anorexia, malaise, generalized lymphadenopathy	Vitamin A supplementation **Supportive:** bed rest during febrile period, antipyretics Antibiotics to prevent secondary bacterial infection in high-risk children **Complications:** Otitis media Pneumonia Bronchitis Obstructive laryngitis and laryngotracheitis Encephalitis	Isolation until fifth day of rash; if hospitalized, institute respiratory precautions Maintain bed rest during prodromal stage; provide quiet activity. **Fever:** instruct parents to administer antipyretics; avoid chilling; if child is prone to convulsions, institute appropriate precautions (fever spikes to 40°C between fourth and fifth days) **Eye care:** dim lights if photophobia present; clean eyelids with warm saline solution to to remove secretions or crusts; keep child from rubbing eyes; examine cornea for signs of ulceration **Coryza/cough:** humidified air; protect skin around nares; encourage fluids and soft, bland foods **Skin care:** keep skin clean; use tepid baths as necessary *(cont.)*

Table 16-2 Communicable diseases of childhood (continued).

DISEASE

MUMPS
Agent: paramyxovirus
Source: Saliva of infected persons
Transmission: direct contact with or droplet spread from an infected person
Incubation period: 14 to 21 days
Period of communicability: most communicable immediately before and after swelling begins

PERTUSSIS (whooping cough)
Agent: *Bordetella pertussis*
Source: discharge from respiratory tract of infected persons
Transmission: direct contact or droplet spread from infected person; indirect contact with freshly contaminated articles
Incubation period: 5 to 21 days, usually 10
Period of communicability: greatest during catarrhal stage before onset of paroxysms and may extend to fourth week after onset of paroxysms

POLIOMYELITIS
Agent: enteroviruses, three types; type 1 - most frequent cause of paralysis, both epidemic and endemic, type 2 - least frequently associated with paralysis, type 3 - second most frequently associated with paralysis
Source: faeces and oropharyngeal secretions of infected persons, especially young children
Transmission: direct contact with persons with apparent or unapparent active infection; spread is via faecal-oral and pharyngeal-oropharyngeal routes
Incubation period: usually 7 to 14 days, with range of 5 to 35 days
Period of communicability: not exactly known; virus is present in throat and faeces shortly after infection and persists for about 1 week in throat and 4 to 6 weeks in faeces

Table 16-2 Communicable diseases of childhood (continued).

CLINICAL MANIFESTATIONS	THERAPEUTIC MANAGEMENT/ COMPLICATIONS	NURSING CARE
Prodromal stage: fever, headache, malaise, and anorexia for 24 hours, followed by 'earache' that is aggravated by chewing **Parotitis:** by third day, parotid gland(s) (either unilateral or bilateral) enlarges and reaches maximum site in 1 to 3 days, accompanied by pain and tenderness **Other manifestations:** submaxillary and sublingual infection, orchitis, and meningo-encephalitis	**Symptomatic and supportive:** analgesics for pain and antipyretics for fever Intravenous fluid may be necessary **Complications:** Meningo-encephalitis, sensorineural deafness, postinfectious encephalitis, myocarditis, Arthritis, Hepatitis, lymphocytic meningitis, pancreatitis and orchitis (rare before puberty)	Isolation during period of communicability; institute respiratory precautions during hospitalization Maintain bed rest during prodromal phase until swelling subsides Give analgesics for pain Encourage fluids and soft, bland foods Apply hot or cold compresses to neck, (whichever is more comforting) To relieve orchitis, provide warmth and local support with tight-fitting underpants
Cartarrhal stage: begins with symptoms of upper respiratory infection, such as coryza, sneezing, lacrimation, cough and low-grade fever; symptoms continue for 1 or 2 weeks, when dry, hacking cough becomes more severe **Paroxysmal stage:** cough most often occurs at night and consists of short, rapid coughs followed by sudden inspiration associated with a high-pitched crowing sound or 'whoop'; during paroxysms, cheeks become flushed or cyanotic, eyes bulge and tongue protrudes; paroxysm may continue until thick mucous plug is dislodged; vomiting frequently follows attack; stage generally lasts 4 to 6 weeks, followed by convalescent stage	Antimicrobial therapy (e.g. erythromycin) Administration of pertussis-immune globulin **Supportive treatment:** hospitalization required for infants, children who are dehydrated or who have complications Bed rest Increased oxgen intake and humidity Adequate fluids Intubation possibly necessary **Complications:** Pneumonia (usual cause of death), atelectasia, bronchiolitis, otitis media, convulsions, haemorrhage (subarachnoid, subconjunctival, epistaxis) weight loss and dehydration, hernia, prolapsed rectum	Isolation during catarrhal stage; if hospitalized, institute respiratory precautions Maintain bed rest during fever Keep child occupied during day (interest in play associated with fewer paroxysms) Reassure parents during frightening episodes of whooping cough Provide restful environment and reduce factors that promote paroxysms (dust, smoke, sudden change in temperature, chilling, activity, excitement); keep room well ventilated Encourage fluids; offer small amount of fluids frequently; refeed child after vomiting Provide high humidity (humidifier or tent); suction gently but often to prevent choking on secretions Observe for signs of airway obstruction (increased restlessness, apprehension, retractions, cyanosis)
May be manifest in three different forms: **Abortive or unapparent**—fever, uneasiness, sore throat, headache, anorexia, vomiting, abdominal pain; lasts a few hours to a few days **Nonparalytic** - same manifestations as abortive but more severe, with pain and stiffness in neck, back, and legs **Paralytic** - initial course similar to non-paralytic type, followed by recovery and then signs of central nervous system paralysis	Complete bed rest during acute phase Assisted respiratory ventilation in case of respiratory paralysis Physiotherapy for muscles following acute stage **Complications:** Permanent paralysis Respiratory arrest Hypertension Kidney stones from demineralization of bone during prolonged immobility	Maintain complete bed rest Administer mild sedatives as necessary to relieve anxiety and promote rest Participate in physiotherapy procedures (use of moist hot packs and range of motion exercises) Position child to maintain body alignment and prevent contractures or pressure sores; use footboard Encourage child to move, administer analgesics for maximum comfort during physical activity Observe for respiratory paralysis; report such signs and symptoms to practitioner; have tracheostomy set at bedside *(cont.)*

Table 16-2 Communicable diseases of childhood (continued).

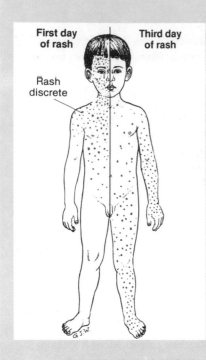

First day of rash

Third day of rash

Rash discrete

Fig 16-3 Rubella (German measles).

DISEASE

RUBELLA (German measles)
Agent: rubella virus

Source: primarily nasopharyngeal secretions of person with apparent or unapparent infection; virus also present in blood, stool, and urine

Transmission: direct contact and spread via infected person; indirectly via articles freshly contaminated with nasopharyngeal secretions, faeces, or urine

Incubation period: 14 to 21 days

Period of communicability: 7 days before to about 5 days after appearance of rash

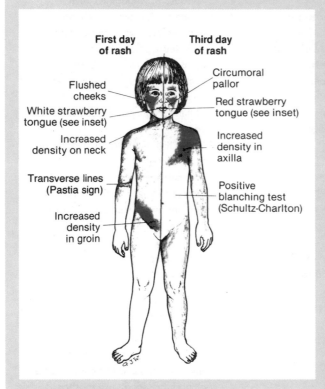

First day of rash

Third day of rash

Flushed cheeks

White strawberry tongue (see inset)

Increased density on neck

Transverse lines (Pastia sign)

Increased density in groin

Circumoral pallor

Red strawberry tongue (see inset)

Increased density in axilla

Positive blanching test (Schultz-Charlton)

Fig 16-4 Scarlet fever.

SCARLET FEVER
Agent: group A β-haemolytic streptococci

Source: usually from nasopharyngeal secretions of infected persons and carriers

Transmission: direct contact with infected person or droplet spread; indirectly by contact with contaminated articles, ingestion of contaminated milk or other food

Incubation period: 2 to 4 days, with range of 1 to 7 days

Period of communicability: during incubation period and clinical illness approximately 10 days; during first 2 weeks of carrier phase, although may persist for months

Table 16-2 Communicable diseases of childhood (continued).

CLINICAL MANIFESTATIONS	THERAPEUTIC MANAGEMENT/ COMPLICATIONS	NURSING CARE
Prodromal stage: absent in children, present in adults and adolescents; consists of low-grade fever, headache, malaise, anorexia, mild conjuncvtivitis, coryza, sore throat, cough, and lymphadenopathy; lasts for 1 to 5 days, subsides 1 day after appearance of rash **Rash:** first appears on face and rapidly spreads downward to neck, arms, trunk, and legs; by end of first day body is covered with a discrete, pinkish-red maculopapular exanthema, disappears in same order as it began and is usually gone by third day **Constitutional signs and symptoms:** occasionally low-grade fever, headache, malaise, and lymphadenopathy	No treatment necessary other than antipyretics for low-grade fever and analgesics for discomfort **Complications:** Rare (arthritis, encephalitis, or purpura); most benign of all childhood communicable diseases; greatest danger is teratogenic effect on fetus	Reassure parents of benign nature of illness in affected child Employ comfort measures as necessary Isolate child from pregnant women
Prodromal stage: abrupt high fever, pulse increased out of proportion to fever, vomiting, headache, chills, malaise, abdominal pain **Enanthema:** tonsils enlarged, oedematous, reddened, and covered with patches of exudate; in severe cases appearance resembles membrane seen in diphtheria; pharynx is oedematous and bright red; during first 1 to 2 days tongue is coated and papillae become red and swollen (white strawberry tongue); by the fourth or fifth day white coat sloughs off, leaving prominent papillae (red strawberry tongue); palate is covered with erythematous punctate lesions **Exanthema:** rash appears within 12 hours after prodromal signs; red pinhead-sized punctate lesions rapidly become generalized but are absent on the face, which becomes flushed with striking circumoral pallor; rash is more intense in folds of joints; by end of first week desquamation begins (fine, sandpaper-like on torso, sheet-like sloughing on palms and soles), which may be complete by 3 weeks or longer	Treatment of choice is a full course of penicillin (or erythromycin in penicillin sensitive children), fever should subside 24 hours after beginning therapy Antibiotic therapy for newly diagnosed carriers (nose or throat cultures positive for streptococci) **Supportive measures:** bed rest during febrile phase, analgesics for sore throat **Complications:** Otitis media Peritonsillar abscess Sinusitis Glomerulonephritis Carditis, polyarthritis (uncommon)	Institute respiratory precautions until 24 hours after initiation of treatment Ensure compliance with oral antibiotic therapy (intramuscular penicillin G may be given if parents' reliability in giving oral drugs is questionable) Maintain bed rest during febrile phase; provide quiet activity during convalescent period Relieve discomfort of sore throat with analgesics, gargles, lozenges, antiseptic throat sprays and humidity Encourage fluids during febrile phase; avoid irritating liquids (citrus juices) or rough foods; when child is able to eat, begin with soft diet Advise parents to consult practitioner if fever persists after beginning therapy Discuss procedures for preventing spread of infection

Table 16-2 Communicable diseases of childhood.

◆ **BOX 16-8**

Clinical manifestations of conjunctivitis

Bacterial Conjunctivitis (Pink Eye)
Purulent drainage
Crusting of eyelids, especially on awakening
Inflamed conjunctiva
Swollen lids
Usually both eyes infected
Viral Conjunctivitis
General
Usually occurs with upper respiratory infection
Serous (watery) drainage
Inflamed conjunctiva
Swollen lids
Haemorrhagic
Caused by specific virus, enterovirus 70

Severe inflammation
Subconjunctival haemorrhage
Conjunctivitis Caused by Foreign Body
Tear production
Pain
Inflamed conjunctiva
Usually only one eye affected
Photophobia
Allergic Conjunctivitis
Itching
Watery to viscous stringy discharge
Inflamed conjunctiva
Swollen lids

---

unlikely to be harmful in the small quantities taken by children and hospitalization is not always indicated. However, a few children die from accidental poisoning each year and a few would die without expert medical care. Sibert and Routledge (1991) have classified the most commonly taken substances according to level of toxicity (see Table 16-3).

IMPLICATIONS FOR NURSING

Nurses have a role in prevention and need to know the principles of emergency treatment.

Prevention

Health visitors and other primary health care nurses have a key role in educating parents and caregivers in aspects of home safety and accident prevention (Robertson, 1991). Programmes of health education include raising awareness of safe storage and labelling of cleaning products, medicines and gardening supplies. Medicines kept in handbags may pose particular problems, as do household products kept under the sink. Knowledge of both toxic and non-toxic plants, the use of high shelves and hanging baskets for house plants, and teaching children never to eat anything without parental permission may help reduce poisoning by plants.

As part of their routine care, nurses or health visitors may discuss the difficulties of constantly watching and safeguarding young children. This approach facilitates a discussion of family stresses that may be a contributing factor to accidents. The *Inequality in Health* reports (Townsend *et al*, 1992) have highlighted a higher level of accidents in children from the lower social classes. The health visitor may target preventive care to such communities through local initiatives and links with other agencies.

Principles of Emergency Treatment

The first and most important principle in dealing with a poisoning is to treat the child first, not the poison. Common signs of poisoning are shown in Table 16-4.

Vital signs are taken and respiratory and/or circulatory support instituted as necessary. Mouth-to-mouth resuscitation and/or mechanical ventilation may be required. The condition of the child is monitored carefully. Since shock is a complication of several types of household poisoning, particularly corrosives, measures to reduce the effects of shock, such as raising the legs and head to the level of the heart to promote venous drainage, and warmth and rest are important.

The accident and emergency nurse's responsibility is to be ready for such interventions. Since time and speed are critical factors in recovery from serious poisonings, anticipation of potential problems and complications may mean the difference between life and death.

If possible, the poison should be identified. The nurse can help in this by questioning the victim and any witnesses, seeking evidence from containers and saving specimens of vomit or urine. Knowledge of the signs of common poisoning may be helpful. The United Kingdom has several Poison Information Services available 24 hours per day that may be consulted in cases where there is doubt about the degree of risk, or to seek advice concerning management (see Table 16-5).

The immediate treatment of ingestion may be to remove the poison from the stomach by induced emesis or gastric lavage. This treatment is usually limited to the first four hours following ingestion and is not used if the poison is a corrosive or a petroleum distillate, as this increases the risk of aspiration and further damage to the mucosa of the pharynx and oesophagus.

Low toxicity

Substances that come into this category include:

Medicines

Antibiotics (except ciprofloxacin, sul phasalazine, and chloramphenicol)

Antacids

Calamine

Oral contraceptives

Vitamin preparations which do not contain iron

Zinc oxide creams

Household products

Chalks and crayons

Emulsion paints and water paints

Fabric softeners

Plant foods and fertilizers

Silica gel

Toothpaste

Wallpaper paste

Washing powder (except dishwasher powder)

Plants

Begonia

Cacti

Cotoneaster

Cyclamen

Honeysuckle

Mahonia

Rowan

Pyracantha

Spider plant

Sweet pea

Intermediate toxicity

Substances that come into this category include:

Medicines

Antihistamines (most)

Cough medicines (most)

Fluoride

Ibuprofen

Laxatives

Lignocaine gel

Paracetamol elixir

Thyroxine

Salbutamol

Household products

Alcohol containing colognes, after shaves, and perfumes

Bleach

Detergents

Disinfectants (most)

Mercury thermometers

Nail varnish remover

Paints (oil based)

Pyrethrins

Talc (if not inhaled)

Rat or mouse poison

Window cleaners

Plants

Berberis

Fuchsia

Holly

Philodendron

Mistletoe

Dieffenbachia (dumb cane)

Potentially very toxic substances

Substances that come into this category include:

Medicines

Barbiturates

Benzodiazepines

Carbamazepine

Clonidine

Digoxin

Diphenoxylate (Lomotil)

Iron

Lithium

Mefenamic acid (Ponstan)

Metoclopramide

Mianserin (Bolvidon)

Paracetamol tablets

Phenothiazines

Phenytoin

Quinine

Opiates, including codeine and cough medicines containing codeine

Salicylates

Hyoscine

Tricylic antidepressants (including doth iepin and amtitriptyline) and monoamine oxidase inhibitors

Theophyllines

Household products

Alcoholic beverages

Acids

Alkalis (including dishwasher powder and denture cleaner)

Camphor and camphorated oil

Cetrimide

Carbon monoxide

Disc batteries

Bottle sterilizing tablets

Ethylene glycol (antifreeze)

Essential oils (for example, real turpen tine, pine oil, citronella, and eucalyptus)

Methanol

Methylene chloride (paint stripper)

Organochloride insecticides

Organophosphate and carbonate insecticides

Paradichlorobenzene moth balls

Petroleum distillates (white spirit, kerosene, or turpentine substitute)

Paraquat and other weedkillers (phenoxyacetic acids)

Phenotic compounds (that is, some disinfectants)

Slug pellets metaldehyde

Plants

Arum lily

Deadly nightshade

Laburnum

Yew

The table is produced with permission from 'accidents, poisoning and sudden infant death syndrome', by JR Sibert and P Davies in *Forfar and Ameul's Textbook of Paediatrics*, 4th Ed. Edited by AGM Campbell and N McIntosh, Edinburgh 1992 Churchill Livingstone.

Table 16-3 Guide to toxicity of substances taken in accidental child poisoning.

GENERAL SIGNS	SPECIFIC SIGNS
Gastrointestinal system	**Corrosives**
Abdominal pain	Severe burning pain in
Vomiting	mouth, throat, stomach
Diarrhoea	White, swollen mucous
Anorexia	membranes: oedema of
	lips, tongue, pharynx (res-
Respiratory/circulatory	piratory obstruction)
system	Violent vomiting, haemoptysis
Depressed respirations	Drooling and inability to clear
Laboured respirations	secretions
Unexplained cyanosis	Signs of shock
Signs of shock: increased,	Anxiety and agitation
weak pulse; decreased	
blood pressure; increased,	**Hydrocarbons**
shallow respiration; pallor;	Gagging, choking, coughing
cool, clammy skin	Nausea
	Vomiting
Central nervous system	Alterations in sensorium,
Convulsions	e.g., lethargy
Overstimulation	Weakness
Sudden loss of	Respiratory symptoms of
consciousness	pulmonary involvement
Dizziness	Tachyapnoea
Stupor, lethargy	Cyanosis
Coma	Retractions
	Grunting
	Salicylates
	Nausea
	Disorientation
	Vomiting
	Dehydration
	Diaphoresis
	Hyperapnoea
	Hyperpyrexia
	Oliguria
	Tinnitus
	Coma
	Convulsions

Table 16-4 Common signs of poisoning.

London:	
Guy's Hospital	0171 955 5000 or 0171 635 9191
Edinburgh	0131 229 2477
Cardiff	01222 709901
Belfast	01232 240503
Dublin	0001 379964
Birmingham	0121 554 3801
Leeds	01532 430715
Newcastle	0191 232 5131

Table 16-5 Poison Information Services in the United Kingdom.

In a conscious patient, vomiting is induced by administering paediatric ipecacuanha syrup followed by a tumbler full of water. The dose can be repeated after 20 minutes, if necessary. Gastric lavage is indicated for infants in whom ipecacuanha is contraindicated. It is also the treatment of choice in cases where the patient is comatose, convulsing or requires a protected airway, or if the ingested poison is rapidly absorbed (e.g., strychnine or cyanide). The use of lavage in petroleum distillate poisoning remains controversial because of the danger of aspiration. When lavage is performed, the largest diameter tube that can be inserted is used to facilitate passage of gastric contents.

Activated charcoal, taken by mouth, is sometimes given to bind poisons in the stomach and reduce their absorption. Repeated doses of charcoal are given to enhance the elimination of some drugs (e.g., aspirin and barbiturates).

In a minority of poisonings, specific antidotes are available to counteract the poison. Examples include acetylcysteine and methionine for paracetamol poisoning, oxygen for carbon monoxide poisoning, and naloxone for opioid overdose. In cases of severe poisoning, active elimination techniques such as forced alkaline diuresis, haemodialysis and charcoal haemoperfusion may be used.

A poisoning is more than an emergency for the child. It usually represents an emotional crisis for the parents, particularly in terms of guilt and self blame at their failure to protect the child. The nurse has a role in supporting the family, while exploring the circumstances of the incident. The accident and emergency department or liaison health visitor should contact the family health visitor who will arrange a follow-up visit at home.

REFERENCES

Adams C, Fay J: *No more secrets: protecting your child from sexual assault* San Louis Obispo, CA, 1981, Impact.

Alexander R et al: Incidence of impact trauma with cranial injuries ascribed to shaking, *Am J Dis Child* 144:724, 1990.

Altemeier WA et al: Antecedents of child abuse, *J Pediatr* 100(5):823, 1982.

Browne K, Saqi S: Approaches to screening for child abuse and neglect. In Browne K, Davies C, Stratton P, editors: *Early prediction and prevention of child abuse,* Chilchester, 1988, Wiley.

Clothier C, MacDonald CA, Shaw DA: *The Allitt inquiry: independent inquiry relating to deaths and injuries on the children's wards at Grantham and Kesteven General Hospital during the period February to April 1991,* London, 1994, HMSO.

Department of Health: *An Introduction to the Children Act 1989,* London, 1989, HMSO.

Department of Health: *Child protection: guidance for senior nurses, health visitors and midwives,* ed 2, London, HMSO, 1992.

Department of Health: *Children and young people on child protection registers; year ending 31 March 1993: England,* London, 1994, HMSO.

Department of Health and Social Security: *Working together: a guide to inter-agency co-operation for the protection of children from abuse,* London, 1988, HMSO.

Garbarino J, Guttmann E, Seeley J: *The psychologically battered child,* San Francisco, 1986, Jossey-Bass.

Hill DR: Giardiasis: issues in diagnosis and management, *Infect Dis Clin North Am* 7(3):503, 1993.

Home Office, Department of Health, Welsh Office et al: *Working together under the Children Act 1989; a guide to arrangements for inter-agency co-operation in child protection,* London, 1991, HMSO.

Kempe CN: Approaches to preventing child abuse, *Am J Dis Child,* 130:941, 1976.

Kempe CN et al: The battered child syndrome, *JAMA* 181:17, 1962.

Legrand R, Wakefield H, Underwager R: Alleged behavioral indicators of sexual abuse, *Issues Child Abuse Accus* 1(2):1, 1989.

London Borough of Brent: *A child in trust - the report of the panel of inquiry into the circumstances surrounding the death of Jasmine Beckford,* London Borough of Brent in Corby, 1993.

Meadow R: Munchausen syndrome by proxy, *BMJ* 299:248, 1989.

Robertson C: *Health visiting in practice,* ed 2, Edinburgh, 1991, Churchill Livingstone.

Sibert JR, Routledge PA: Accidental poisoning in children: can we admit fewer children with safety? *Arch Dis Child* 66:263, 1991.

Townsend P, Davidson N, Whitehead W: *Inequalities in Health - revised edition,* Harmondsworth, 1992, Penguin.

Wynne J: The construction of child abuse in the accident and emergency department. In Cloke C, Naish J: *Key issues in child protection for health visitors and nurses,* Essex, 1992, Longman.

FURTHER READING

Corby B: *Child abuse: towards a knowledge base,* Buckingham, 1993, Open University Press.

Ferguson JA, Sellar C, Goldacre MJ: Some epidemiological observations on medical and non-medical poisoning in pre-school children, *J Epidemiology Community Health* 46:207, 1992.

Owen H, Pritchard J: *Good practice in child protection - a manual for professionals,* London, 1993, Jessica Kingsley.

Olds DL, Henderson CR, Kitzman H: Does prenatal and infancy nurse home visitation have enduring effects on qualities of parental caregiving and child health at 25 to 50 months of life? *Pediatrics* 93(1):89-98, 1994.

Pound R: Children's rights and the health of the nation, *Health Visitor* 67(6):192, 1994.

Seidl AH et al: Nurses attitudes toward the child victims and the perpetrators of emotional, physical and sexual abuse, *Issues Child Abuse Accus* 5(1):28, 1993.

Chapter 17

Health Problems of Middle Childhood

LEARNING OUTCOMES

After studying this chapter you should be able to:

- ◆ Discuss expectations of health status in middle childhood.
- ◆ Define potential deviations from health.
- ◆ Describe the factors to take into consideration when assessing children.
- ◆ Identify goals/outcomes of nursing care for each health care problem.
- ◆ Discuss information utilized to prepare families for discharge.
- ◆ Consider overall holistic nursing care plans to meet the needs of children and their families.
- ◆ Define the glossary terms.

GLOSSARY

AD-HD Attention deficit-hyperactivity disorder

ecchymoses (bruises) Localized red or purple, discolourations caused by extravasation of blood into dermis and subcutaneous tissues

erythema A reddened area caused by increased amounts of oxygenated blood in the dermal vasculature

petechiae Tiny (pinpoint size) and sharply circumscribed spots in the superficial layers of the epidermis

primary lesions Skin changes produced by some causative factor

PTSD Post-traumatic stress disorder

RAP Recurrent abdominal pain

secondary lesions Skin changes that result from alteration in primary lesions

SPF Sun protective factor

UVA Ultraviolet A

UVB Ultraviolet B

As a group, school-aged children are fairly healthy when compared with children in infancy and early childhood, and the ages of 9-12 are usually the healthiest years. Respiratory illnesses (the leading cause of morbidity) and gastrointestinal upsets are the most common conditions. A factor contributing to this overall healthy state is the quantity of lymphoid tissue. At this age, children can have up to twice the amount of the young adult, helping to fight infection and ward off disease.

Most children in this age group have either contracted the communicable diseases of childhood or been immunized against them. Their excellent appetites, adequate rest, and sufficient physical exercise further contribute to their general good health. The common health problems of school-aged children are usually amenable to therapy. Conditions that are not uncommon in middle childhood are dental problems and emotional or behavioural disorders. Allergic manifestations, especially asthma, may reach a peak during the middle childhood years, and a variety of other serious disorders make a significant contribution to childhood morbidity. These will be considered as appropriate in relation to ill children.

DISORDERS AFFECTING THE SKIN

Skin disorders are common at all ages, with many limited to a specific age group. Examples are birthmarks in the newborn, nappy rash and eczema in infancy, and acne during adolescence.

THE SKIN

The skin and its component and associated structures constitute the integumentary system. The largest organ in the body, the skin is a thin structure (only about 1 mm thick at birth, increasing to approximately twice that thickness at maturity) that serves primarily as an insulator, not as an organ of exchange.

Anatomically and physiologically, the skin differs markedly in various areas of the body, to enable it to meet special stresses. Regions such as the soles of the feet, the eyelids, and the back vary in skin thickness, looseness, and overall composition of sweat glands and hair follicles. These variations are the basis for the localization of many disorders to specific areas and for the distribution of certain eruptions in characteristic patterns.

PURPOSES OF THE SKIN

The skin provides several physical functions essential to life.

Protection
The skin serves as protection against trauma, including mechanical, thermal, chemical, and radiant. The intact tough outer layer is a mechanical barrier. Organisms and chemicals penetrate it with difficulty, and it is further protected by the oily and slightly acid secretions of its sebaceous glands, which limit the growth of bacteria.

Impermeability
The outer side of the upper layer, with its low water content, is in equilibrium with the viable cells underneath. It protects against loss of essential body constituents to the environment. The effectiveness of this impermeable membrane is demonstrated by the profuse fluid loss that follows damage to the epidermis by superficial burns and injury. Loss of water and some electrolytes takes place only through pores in this effective barrier.

Heat regulation
The skin adjusts heat loss to heat production, to maintain the thermal balance of the body. This is accomplished primarily through functioning of cutaneous blood vessels and sweat glands. The vascular supply to the skin, much more extensive than needed for tissue nourishment, is regulated by way of central and local neural and hormonal processes.

Sensation
As a sensory organ, perceptions (touch, pain, heat, and cold) are registered through the nerves that permeate the skin. To some extent, skin is also an organ of expression that betrays strong feelings: blushing (shame or embarrassment), redness (anger), blanching (fear), and sweating (anxiety).

SKIN LESIONS

Lesions of the skin can result from a wide variety of specific aetiological factors. In general, skin lesions originate from: (1) contact with injurious agents such as infectious organisms, toxic chemicals, and physical trauma, (2) hereditary factors, (3) some external factor that produces a reaction in the skin (for example, allergens), or (4) a systemic disease of which the lesions are a cutaneous manifestation (e.g., measles, lupus erythematosus). Such responses are highly individual. An agent that may be harmless to one individual may be damaging to another, and a single agent may produce various types of responses in different individuals.

The school-aged child is susceptible to ringworm of the scalp, and acne is a characteristic skin disorder of puberty. Although less common in children, tension and anxiety may produce, modify or prolong many skin conditions.

PATHOPHYSIOLOGY OF DERMATITIS

Over half of dermatological problems are various forms of dermatitis. This implies a sequence of inflammatory changes in the skin that are grossly and microscopically similar, but diverse in course and causation. Acute responses produce intercellular and intracellular oedema, the formation of intradermal vesicles, and an initial minimum infiltration of inflammatory cells into the epidermis. In the dermis there is oedema, vascular dilation, and early perivascular cellular infiltration. The location and manner of these reactions produce the lesions characteristic of

SECONDARY SKIN LESIONS

Mound of flaky, dead, cornified tissue shed from the skin; irregular shape; variabl thickness and diameter; dry or oily; silver, white, or tan colour
Example: Psoriasis, ringworm

Scale

Crust

Dried masses of serum, pus, dead skin, and debris that can be found surmounting any lesion; slightly elevated; brown, black, tan or straw-coloured
Example: Impetigo, scab, eczema

Irregularly shaped, concave, excavation with loss of epidermis and dermis; variable size; exudative; red or reddish blue
Example: Decubiti

Ulcer

Fissuere

Deep linear split through epidermis into dermis; small; deep; red
Example: Chapping, tinea pedis

Permanent thick to thin fibrous tissue that replaces damaged corium by production and deposition of collagen; irregular shape; red, pink, or white; atrophic or hypertrophic
Example: Vaccination, healed wound, abrasion, laceration

Scar

Excoriation

Rough, thickened, and hardened epidermis with accentuated skin markings
Example: Result of chronic dermatitis, such as eczema

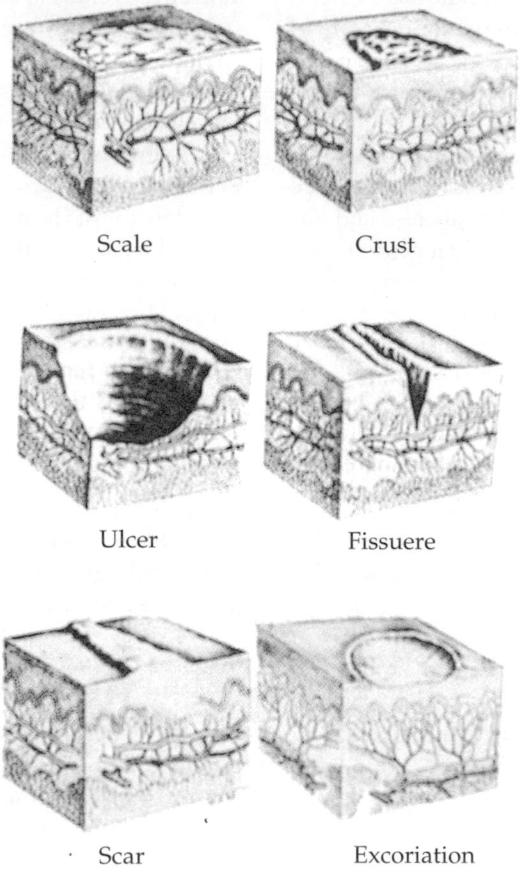

Fig. 17-1 Secondary skin lesions.

each disorder. The changes are reversible, and the skin ordinarily recovers without blemish and completely intact unless complicating factors such as ulceration from the primary irritant, scratching, and infection are introduced or underlying vascular disease develops. In chronic conditions, permanent effects are seen that vary according to the disorder, the general condition of the affected individual, and available therapy.

Subjective symptoms

Many cutaneous lesions are associated with local symptoms, the most common being itching, which varies in kind and intensity. Pain or tenderness often accompanies some skin lesions, and other sensations may be described as burning, prickling, stinging, or crawling. Alterations in local feeling or sensation include anaesthesia (absence of sensation), hyperaesthesia (excessive sensitivity), and hypaesthesia or hypoaesthesia (diminished or lessening of sensation). These symptoms may remain localized or may migrate, may be constant or intermittent, and may be aggravated by a specific activity or circumstance, such as exposure to sunlight.

Lesion

Skin lesions are classified as:
- Primary lesions — skin changes produced by some causative factor
- Secondary lesions — changes that result from alteration in the primary lesions, such as those caused by rubbing, scratching, medication, or involution and healing (Fig. 17-1)

Distribution pattern

How lesions are distributed over the body is a useful aid in diagnosis. Local processes are distinguished from generalized ones. Many lesions are primarily associated with specific areas, such as extensor areas in atopic dermatitis or uncovered areas that allow exposure to sun; others are related to location of specific cutaneous appendages, such as the unique sebaceous gland distribution of acne.

Configuration and arrangement

The size, shape, and arrangement of a lesion or groups of lesions assist in diagnosis. *Discrete* (individually distinct) lesions are distinguished from clustered (appear close together), *diffuse* (scattered), or *confluent* (running together) configurations. *Grouped* or *clustered* lesions are characteristic in herpes eruptions; *annular* (ringed) or *arciform* lesions are typical of ringworm and diseases resulting from vascular reactions, such as urticaria or drug reaction; linear arrangements usually represent an exogenous influence that has either caused the process or contributed to its spread, such as scratching.

PROCESS OF DIAGNOSIS

It is important to determine whether the child has had an allergic condition, such as asthma or hay fever, or has had previous skin disease. Eczema, often associated with allergies, frequently begins in infancy. It should be determined when the lesion or symptom first became apparent, as well as whether it is related to ingestion of a food or other substance, including any medication the child might be taking. It may be related to some activity, such as contact with plants, insects, or chemicals.

When it is suspected that a skin problem might be related to a systemic disease, such as one of the collagen diseases or immune deficiency disease, studies are carried out. Microscopic examination, cultures, skin biopsy, patch testing, allergic skin testing and various other laboratory tests (blood count, sedimentation rate) are employed when indicated.

THERAPEUTIC MANAGEMENT

The human body tends to heal; therefore treatment is directed towards eliminating or ameliorating influences that interfere with normal healing processes. Some disorders may demand aggressive therapy, but the major aim of any treatment is to prevent further damage, eliminate the cause, prevent complications and provide relief from discomfort while the tissues heal. Factors that contribute to the dermatitis and prolong the course of the disease must be eliminated when possible. The most common offenders in paediatrics are environmental factors (such as soaps, bubble baths, shampoos, rough or tight clothing, blankets, and toys) and the natural elements (such as dirt, sand, heat, cold, moisture, and wind). Dermatitis can also be aggravated by home remedies and medications.

Dressings are frequently applied to skin lesions and are universally used for wound management. Dressings serve several useful functions. They are used to:
- protect the wound from infection
- protect the wound from trauma
- provide compression in the event of anticipated bleeding or swelling
- apply medication
- absorb drainage and/or debride necrotic tissue (Sieggreen, 1987).

Most skin disorders respond to topical therapy; that is, application of an active ingredient directly to the affected areas, with physical properties that protect, soothe or cleanse.

However, there are occasions when therapeutic agents are systemically administered.

Topical applications
Several basic concepts should be followed during treatment. Overtreatment should be avoided. For example, when the dermatitis is acute, the applications should be mild and bland to avoid further irritation. Broken or inflamed skin, especially in children, is more absorbent than intact skin, and chemicals that are nonirritating to intact skin may be very irritating to inflamed skin. The dermatitic skin is also more likely to develop allergic contact-type sensitization to substances applied as medication or base.

Topical applications may be applied to treat the disorder, reduce the itching associated with many diseases, decrease external stimuli, or apply external heat or cold. The emollient action of soaks, baths, and lotions provides a soothing film over the skin surface that reduces external stimuli. Application of heat tends to aggravate most conditions, and its use is usually reserved for reducing specific inflammatory processes, such as folliculitis and cellulitis. Ordinarily applications offer greatest relief when they are lukewarm, tepid, or cool.

The most frequent means for topical treatment of skin disorders are wet dressings, soaks, lotions and shake solutions, baths, creams and ointments, sprays and aerosols, pastes, powders, occlusive dressings, soaps and shampoos, other topical treatments, and topical corticosteroid therapy.

Topical corticosteroid therapy
Glucocorticoids (a type of corticosteroid) are the therapeutic agents used most widely for skin disorders. Their local anti-inflammatory effects are merely palliative, so the medication must be applied until the disease state undergoes a remission or until the causative agent is eliminated. Corticosteroids are applied directly to the affected area and, because they are essentially nonsensitizing and have only minor side effects, they can be applied over prolonged periods with continuing effectiveness. As with the use of any steroids, in large amounts they may mask signs of infection, and there may be exacerbation of symptoms following termination of the drug.

Hydrocortisone preparations are available in sprays, lotions, creams, ointment, gels, suspension, and powders. They may cause worsening of inflammation caused by fungus or bacteria, and it is both effective and economical to apply only a thin film and massage it into the skin.

Other topical therapies
Other topical treatments include chemical cautery (especially useful for warts), ultraviolet therapy (primarily used in psoriasis and acne), laser therapy, and special acne therapies such as dermabrasion and acne 'surgery'.

Systemic therapy
Therapeutic agents are often used as an adjunct to topical therapy in dermatological disorders, and those most frequently used are

the corticosteroids and antibiotics. Corticosteroid hormones, with their capacity to inhibit inflammatory and allergic reactions, are valuable in the treatment of severe skin disorders. Dosage is carefully adjusted and gradually tapered to the minimum that is effective and tolerated. In infants and children, the dosage is larger than is usually calculated from body-weight ratios. Protracted use may temporarily suppress growth, however.

Antibiotics, which interfere with the growth of micro-organisms, are used in severe or widespread skin infections. The danger inherent in the use of antibiotics is their tendency to produce a hypersensitivity in the patient; therefore they are used with caution. Antifungal agents are the only means for treating systemic fungal infections.

Assessment To assist in establishing a diagnosis, it is important for nurses to accurately describe any deviation in the character of the skin, using both inspection and palpation. The colour, shape, and distribution of the lesions are noted, including absence of pigment (vitiligo). The individual lesions are described according to the accepted terminology and may involve more than one type, such as a maculopapular rash.

The skin should be checked for characteristics such as temperature, moisture, texture, elasticity, and presence of oedema. It should be indicated whether the findings are restricted to the area of the lesion(s) or are generalized.

The child's subjective symptoms provide additional information. Older children are able to describe the condition as painful, itching, tingling, or in other descriptive terms. However, much can be determined by observation of the younger child's behaviour and the parents' account of these reactions. Does the child scratch? Is the child restless or irritable? Does the child favour or avoid using a part? A careful history may provide clues. Has the child had access to chemicals or been taking medication? Has the child any known allergy? Do any playmates have a similar lesion? A doubtful diagnosis is frequently confirmed on the basis of history.

Planning The goals of care for the child with a skin condition are:
1. Prevent secondary damage to the lesions(s).
2. Relieve discomfort.
3. Educate and support the child and family.

Therapeutic programmes are usually designed to provide general measures such as rest, protection, relief from discomfort, and specific treatments such as a definitive medication or physical technique. Since only a few skin diseases are contagious, it is usually not necessary to isolate the affected child unless there is a danger of acquiring a secondary infection; for example, the child who is receiving large doses of corticosteroids or other immunosuppressant drugs, or the child with an immunological deficiency disorder. If the skin manifestation is caused by a virus, such as measles or chicken pox, the child should be prevented from exposing other susceptible children.

Self-infection is a constant hazard in some disorders such as impetigo or (to a lesser extent) warts. Measures are imple-mented to lessen the itching sensation and to reduce scratching. Such methods, along with general cleanliness and hygiene, also reduce the likelihood of secondary infection of a primary lesion.

Relief of symptoms
Most of the therapeutic treatments are directed towards relief of pruritus, the most common subjective complaint. Itching is believed to result from stimulation of C fibres at the dermoepidermal junction. These fibres are similar to, but distinct from, pain fibres. Substances released within the skin (histamine and endopeptidases) also elicit itching, although their release triggers are unknown (Barnett, 1987).

Cooling the affected area and increasing the skin pH make conditions for enzymatic action less favourable (Madden, 1986). Such measures include cool baths or compresses to reduce external stimuli to the area. Maintenance of cleanliness and good aeration improve comfort. Clothing and bed linen should be soft and lightweight to decrease the irritation from friction and stimulation.

Preventing scratching is of primary importance. The cooperation of older children can be obtained, although they may need reminding to stop scratching or rubbing. In smaller and uncooperative children, the use of techniques and devices such as mittens (especially during sleep), or special coverings is required. Keeping fingernails short, well-trimmed, and clean helps reduce the chance of secondary infection.

Antipruritic medications may be prescribed for severe itching, especially if it disturbs the child's rest. Pain and discomfort are usually managed with nonpharmacological measures and mild analgesia; severe pain may require more potent medication (see Pain Management, Chapter 3).

Topical therapy
Nurses and parents are responsible for the application of topical therapeutic agents and the administration of systemic medications. Therefore, an understanding of the various methods of application, the type and consistency of the preparation, and their purposes and uses is needed for effective application.

It is especially important to wash the hands before and after application of topical therapies. The skin should be assessed before the treatment or application of medication and reassessed after the treatment is completed. Any observed changes are noted and described.

Wet compresses Wet compresses or dressings are probably the mildest form of topical therapy. They cool the skin by evaporation, relieve itching and inflammation, and cleanse the area by loosening and removing crusts and debris.

Dressings immersed in the desired solution are wrung out slightly and applied to the affected area wet, but not dripping. They are applied flat and smooth and in such a way that motion is not totally restricted — fingers are wrapped separately, and arms and legs are wrapped so that elbows and knees can bend. When evaporation begins to dry them, the dressings are removed, rewet in the solution, and reapplied to the area using aseptic technique. The solution is not poured or syringed directly over the dressings. As fluid evaporates, the solution becomes increasingly concentrated and thus stronger, which may be damaging to sensitive lesions.

Water is the most important ingredient in wet dressings, and evaporation is primarily responsible for the symptomatic relief experienced by the patient. The most common solution used for wet dressings is normal saline, which is applied to cleanse and disinfect open, oozing, crusting, and/or secondarily infected lesions. Sometimes, fresh warm or tepid tap water is used alone or in conjunction with topical steroids.

Fresh solution at room temperature is applied at 2-, 3-, or 4-hour intervals and is allowed to remain on the lesion from 30 minutes to 1.5 hours. Wet dressings are seldom continued after about 48 hours. The child must be guarded against chilling during treatment, and no more than 20% of the body should be covered at one time to avoid the risk of hypothermia. After treatment, the skin is dried thoroughly by patting with a towel. Lotion or other medication may then be applied.

Moist dressings Dry dressings are commonly used only on wounds that produce considerable exudate. Dry dressings adhere to the wound surface, damaging newly forming tissue. Skin lesions heal in a moist environment. Transparent dressings also function as moist dressings. The adhesive sticks to intact epithelium, but not to new epithelium. Because they are transparent, they allow for wound assessment and require fewer changes than do traditional moist dressings.

Soaks Gaining young children's cooperation for hand or foot soaks is difficult, unless the procedure is made attractive to them through play. The older child is able to cooperate, but may need something to do during the procedure, such as listening to music, reading a story, or watching television.

Baths Baths are especially useful in the treatment of widespread dermatitis as they evenly distribute the soothing antipruritic and anti-inflammatory effects of the solution. The solution is added to a tub of lukewarm water. The temperature of the bath is tepid, and the duration of treatment is usually 15 to 30 minutes. Therapeutic baths are always more interesting when the child is accompanied by toys or other items for water play.

Discharge planning and family support

Childhood dermatological conditions always involve the family. Since few situations require hospitalization and children who are hospitalized will complete a therapy program at home, the family must carry out the treatment plan; therefore, their cooperation is essential. Child and parents are more likely to be motivated if they are told why something is being done in a certain way. Success of treatment depends on the correct interpretation of instructions, and it is often the nurse's responsibility to teach the parent how to carry out the instructions, and to offer encouragement, support and assistance in solving problems.

One of the most difficult areas to deal with is the child's irritability and tendency to disturb dressings and scratch or pick

at lesions. Nurses can help parents devise distracting activities for the child.

Since the skin is the most visible portion of the body, defects in its surface that alter its appearance are sometimes an additional source of distress to the affected child and the family. Unsightly lesions or medicinal preparations applied to the skin are often sources of revulsion and rejection by others. Other children will make derogatory comments and may even reject the affected child. Parents of other children may fear that their children will 'catch' the disorder. Chronic conditions can create problems in development of a positive self-concept.

Evaluation

The effectiveness of nursing interventions is determined by continual reassessment and evaluation of care. Monitor the child's lesions, reactions to therapies and relief from discomfort. Lesions should the be reassessed, and the child and family observed and interviewed for compliance with therapy.

WOUNDS

Wounds are produced in a variety of ways, and the manner and extent of the injury determines the manner of healing and the form of management. In general, wounds are classified as open if the skin has been divided or disrupted and closed if the skin surface remains intact (Box 17-1). Wounds can also be superficial, involving only the epidermis, or deep, involving the dermis, subcutanous tissue and deeper structures.

◆ **BOX 17-1**

Types of wounds

Closed Wounds

Blister — raised circumscribed area of epidermis containing serum

Contusion - injury to subcutaneous tissues without disrupting the skin

Sprain — disruption in continuity of a ligament

Fracture — discontinuity of bone tissue

Open Wounds

Abrasion — removal of the superficial layers of skin by rubbing or scraping

Evulsion — forcible pulling out or extraction of tissue

Laceration — torn or jagged wound; accidental cut wound

Incision — a division of the skin made with a sharp object; cut

Penetrating wound — disruption of the skin surface that extends into underlying tissue or into a body cavity

Puncture — a wound with relatively small opening compared to the depth

EPIDERMAL INJURIES

Abrasions are the most common epidermal wounds of childhood, usually in the form of a skinned knee or elbow. In most injuries, the margins of the abraded area are superficial, involving only the outer layers of epidermis, although the central portion may extend into the dermis. Initially, the defect is filled by a blood clot and necrotic debris, which subsequently dehydrate to form a scab. Epithelial tissue is composed of labile cells, which are constantly destroyed and replaced throughout life. Injury to these tissues is accomplished by regeneration; that is, rapid replacement by similar cells. When coverage of the wound surface is completed, the scab sloughs off, and keratinization begins.

An abrasion from which the dirt cannot be removed will require abrading under topical anaesthesia, and those covering a very large area (more than 15% of the body) will need medical attention.

INJURY TO DEEPER TISSUES

Tissues composed of *permanent* cells, such as muscle and nerve cells, are unable to regenerate. Therefore these tissues *repair* themselves by substituting fibrous connective tissue for the injured tissue. This fibrous tissue, or scar, serves as a patch to preserve or restore the continuity of the tissue. Wounds involving permanent cells include surgical incisions, lacerations,

ulcers, evulsions, and full-thickness burns. Injured cells of glandular organs and bones, composed of *stable* cells, multiply less vigorously and heal more slowly (see Bone Healing and Remodelling, Chapter 33).

Process of wound healing
The nonspecific repair mechanism of wound healing with scar formation involves the processes of *inflammation, fibroplasia, contraction,* and *scar maturation*. Table 17-1 summarizes the healing process.

Wounds that often become chronic skin injuries are burns and pressure ulcers, a localized area of cellular necrosis that develops when soft tissue is compressed between a bony prominence and a firm surface (Hagelgans, 1993).

FACTORS THAT INFLUENCE HEALING

In general, wounds in children heal more rapidly because of children's increased metabolism and good circulation. Factors that delay wound healing are outlined in Table 17-2.

IMPLICATIONS FOR NURSING

Small injuries to the skin are cleaned with soap and water and may be left exposed to the air, or covered with a sticking

PHASE	ACTIVITY	COMMENTS
1 Inflammation (3 to 5 days)	Clot formation as meshwork for capillary growth Inflammation with phagocytosis; wound debris removed Epithelial cell migration	Wound weakest during this phase
2. Fibroplasia (5 days to 4 weeks)	Granulation tissue formed Migration of fibroblasts Secretion of collagen Abundant capillary buds	Wound fragile Granulation tissue bleeds profusely if disturbed
3. Scar contracture (1 to 6 weeks)	Continued deposition of collagen Further organization and remodelling Blood vessels compressed Healing area contracts Blood flow across wound gradually ceases	Appears as broad, pinkish, raised scar Heavy use of any affected muscles is discouraged
4. Scar maturation (several months)	Formation of mature scar Shrinkage of wound Contracture deformity can occur if wound is near a joint	Scar is acellular and avascular tissue pale in colour Does not tan when exposed to sunlight Will not sweat or produce hair May cause itching

Table 17-1 Summary of wound healing process.

FACTOR	EFFECT ON HEALING
Nutritional deficiencies	
Vitamin C	Inhibits formation of collagen fibres and capillary development
Protein	Reduces supply of amino acids for tissue repair
Zinc	Impairs epithelialization
Impaired circulation	Reduces supply of nutrients to wound area
	Inhibits inflammatory response and removal of debris from wound area
Corticosteroids	Impair phagocytosis
	Inhibit fibroblast proliferation
	Depress formation of granulation tissue
	Inhibit wound contraction
Foreign bodies	Inhibit wound closure
	Increase inflammatory response
Infection	Increases inflammatory response
	Increases tissue destruction
Mechanical friction	Damages or destroys granulation tissue
Fluid accumulation	Accumulation in area inhibits tissues from approximating
Radiation	Inhibits fibroblastic activity and capillary formation
	May cause tissue necrosis
Diseases	
Diabetes mellitus	Inhibits collagen synthesis
	Impairs circulation and capillary growth
	Hyperglycaemia impairs phagocytosis
Anaemia	Reduces oxygen supply to tissues

Table 17-2 Factors influencing wound healing.

plaster to prevent dirt from entering the wound. Cuts on the face, a gaping cut longer than 0.5 cm, or one that bleeds persistently should be evaluated for possible suturing. Those covering a very large area (more than 15% of the body) will need medical attention.

Abrasions are cleaned in the same manner as wounds, except that any foreign matter must be removed with clean tweezers, and loose skin should be cut off with sterile scissors.

Lacerations present a special challenge. The injured child and family are usually very distressed by the bleeding, variable degrees of shock, and the guilt that usually accompany the injury. Because scalp lacerations bleed so profusely, they are especially frightening. Apply pressure to the area and attempt to calm the child before undertaking further examination. Unless there is bleeding from a severed artery, the wound can be cleansed with a forced jet of sterile tepid water or saline (via syringe) and examined for extent, depth, and presence of foreign material such as dirt, glass, or fabric fragments. The location of the wound also dictates assessment. For example, wounds over bony areas may contain bone chips, and clear fluid seeping from severe head wounds may indicate cerebrospinal fluid. (See also Trauma Management, Chapter 33, and Head Injury, Chapter 31.) A pressure dressing is applied in preparation for suturing.

For many children, the use of topical anaesthesia for repair of lacerations has reduced the discomfort and anxiety generated by injected anaesthesia (Bonadio and Wagner, 1988). Emla cream may be used in this instance.

Puncture wounds that do not require a tetanus booster (see Chapter 33) should be soaked in warm water and soap for 15 minutes. The wound is carefully observed for signs of infection from dirt and bacteria that might be trapped beneath the wound surface. Puncture wounds of the head, chest or abdomen, or those that could still contain a portion of the puncturing object, must be evaluated.

Open wounds
Open wounds are managed by application of moist dressings or synthetic plastic-film dressings. Because dehydration damages tissues in the wound bed, the injured tissues are not allowed to dry completely. Crusts impede epithelial migration and thus delay healing. (See Burns, Chapter 24.)

FOREIGN BODIES

Small wooden splinters can be removed by parents with a needle and tweezers that have been sterilized with alcohol or a flame. The area around the sliver should be washed with soap and water before attempting the removal. Some foreign bodies should have medical evaluation; these include a fishhook, a deeply imbedded object such as a needle in a foot or near a joint, glass splinters, or other objects that are difficult to see.

Much research is investigating new methods of promoting wound healing. Some research has indicated that a topical application of epidermal growth factor (EGF) significantly accelerated the rate of wound healing (Brown *et al*, 1989). Numerous factors have been identified that delay healing (Table 17-2). Many traditional practices, such as the application of antiseptic hydrogen peroxide and povidone iodine (Betadine solutions), would have only a minimal disinfectant effect, may have a cytotoxic effect on healthy cells, and in the case of povidone iodine, may be absorbed through the skin, especially in neonates and young children (LeVeen, LeVeen and LeVeen, 1993). It should be used cautiously in anyone with thyroid or renal disorders (Welch, 1992).

INFECTIONS OF THE SKIN

Dermatological infections and other disorders of the skin occur frequently in school children, as their social nature and proximity to other children render them highly susceptible to communicable diseases, including those caused by parasites. Most are troublesome ailments and are the source of considerable physical and emotional discomfort. For most of the disorders, the diagnosis and treatment are relatively simple; for others, the management is more complex and puzzling.

BACTERIAL INFECTIONS

Normally, the skin harbours a variety of bacterial flora, including the major pathogenic varieties of staphylococci and streptococci. The degree of their pathogenicity depends on the specific organism's invasiveness and toxigenicity, the integrity of the skin, the barrier of the host, and the immune and cellular defences of the host. Children with immune deficiency states are highly susceptible to bacterial invasion. This includes infants, children with congenital immune deficiency disorders, children in a debilitated condition, those on immunosuppressive therapy, and those with a generalized malignancy such as leukaemia or lymphoma.

Because of the characteristic 'walling-off' process of the inflammatory reaction (abscess formation), staphylococci are more difficult to treat and the local infected area is associated with an increase in numbers of bacteria all over the skin surface that serve as a source of continuing infection. Staphylococcal infections occur most often in younger children and the incidence decreases with advancing age. All of these factors emphasize the importance of careful handwashing when caring for infected children, and as an essential prophylactic measure when caring for infants and small children. Common bacterial skin disorders are listed in Table 17-3.

IMPLICATIONS FOR NURSING

The major nursing functions related to bacterial skin infections are to prevent the spread of infection and to prevent complications. Handwashing is mandatory before and after contact with an affected child, and is emphasized to both the child and the family. The child should be provided with towels separate from other family members. Impetigo contagiosa is easily spread by self-inoculation; therefore, the child must be cautioned against touching the involved area. This is difficult to accomplish. Distraction or reminders are useful, but are not helpful when the child is alone, such as at bedtime.

Children and parents are often tempted to squeeze follicular lesions. They must be warned that squeezing will not hasten the resolution of the infection and that there is a risk of making the lesion worse or spreading the infection. No attempt should be made to puncture the surface of the pustule with a needle or sharp instrument. Children with extensive cellulitis, especially around a joint with lymphadenitis or on the face, are usually admitted to the hospital for parenteral antibiotics.

VIRAL INFECTIONS

Viruses are intracellular parasites that produce their effect by using the intracellular substances of the host cells. Composed of only a DNA or RNA core enclosed in an antigenic protein shell, viruses are unable to provide for their own metabolic needs or to reproduce themselves. After a virus penetrates a cell of the host organism, it sheds the outer shell and disappears within the cell, where the nucleic acid core stimulates the host cell to form more virus material from its intracellular substance. In a viral infection, the epidermal cells react with inflammation and vesiculation (as in herpes simplex) or by proliferating to form growths (warts).

Most of the communicable diseases of childhood are associated with rashes, and each rash is characteristic. The type of lesion and the configuration of rubeola, rubella, scarlet fever, and chickenpox are described in Table 16-2. Other common viral disorders of the skin are outlined in Table 17-4.

DERMATOPHYTOSES (FUNGAL INFECTIONS)

The dermatophytoses (ringworm) are infections caused by a group of closely related filamentous fungi that invade primarily the stratum corneum, hair, and nails. These are superficial infections that live on, not in, the skin. Confined to the dead keratin layers, the fungus must multiply at a rate that equals the rate of keratin production to maintain itself; otherwise, the infection would be shed with the discarded skin cells.

Three principal types of fungi are responsible for dermatophyte infections: *Trichophyton, Microsporum,* and *Epidermophyton.* They are designated by the Latin word tinea, with further designation related to the area of the body where they are found; for example, tinea capitis (ringworm of the scalp). Most often transmitted from one person to another or from infected animals to humans, fungi exert their effect via an enzyme that digests and hydrolyses the keratin of hair, nails, and the stratum corneum. Dissolved hair breaks off to produce the bald spots characteristic of tinea capitis. Diagnosis is made from microscopic examination of scrapings taken from the advancing periphery of the lesion, which almost always produces scale.

IMPLICATIONS FOR NURSING

When teaching families regarding the care of children with ringworm, it is important to emphasize good health and hygiene. Because of the infectious nature of the disease, several basic hygienic measures are particularly pertinent. Affected children are not to exchange with other children any grooming items, headgear, scarves, or other articles of apparel that have been in proximity to the infected area. Affected children are

DISORDER/ ORGANISM	MANIFESTATIONS	MANAGEMENT	COMMENTS
Impetigo contagiosa *Staphylo coccus, Strep- tococcus-*	Begins as a reddish macule Becomes vesicular Ruptures easily, leaving superficial, moist erosion Tends to spread peripherally in sharply marginated irregular outlines Exudate dries to form heavy, honey-coloured crusts Pruritus common Systemic effects: minimal or asymptomatic See Chapter 9 for bullous impetigo	Careful removal of undermined skin, crusts and debris by softening with 1:20 Burow solution compresses Topical application of bactericidal ointment Systemic administration of oral or parenteral antibiotics (penicillin) in severe or extensive lesions	Tends to heal without scarring unless secondary infection Auto-inoculable and contagious Very common in toddler, preschooler
Pyoderma - *Staphylo- coccus, Strep- tococcus*	Deeper extension of infection dermis Tissue reaction more severe Systemic effects: fever, lymphangitis	Soap and water cleansing Wet compresses Bathing with antibacterial soap as prescribed	Auto-inoculable and contagious May heal with or without scarring
Folliculitis (pimple), furuncle (boil), carbuncle (multiple boils) - *Staphylo- coccus aureus*	Folliculitis: infection of hair Furuncle: larger lesion with more redness and swelling at a single follicle Carbuncle: more extensive lesion with widespread inflammation and 'pointing' at several follicular orifices Systemic effects: malaise, if severe	Skin cleanliness Local warm moist compresses Topical application of antibiotic agents Systemic antibiotics in severe cases Incision and drainage of severe lesions, followed by wound irrigations with antibiotics or suitable drain implantation	Auto-inoculable and contagious Furuncle and carbuncle tend to heal with scar formation A lesion should *never* be squeezed
Cellulitis - *Streptotoccus, Staphylo- coccus, Haemophi- lus influenzae*	Inflammation of skin and subcutaneous tissues with intense redness, swelling, and firm infiltration Lymphangitis 'streaking' frequently seen Involvement of regional lymph nodes common May progress to abscess formation Systemic effects: fever, malaise	Oral or parenteral antibiotics Rest and immobilization of both affected area and child Hot moist compresses to area	Hospitalization may be necessary for child with with systemic symptoms Otitis media may be associated with facial cellulitis
Staphylococcal scalded skin syndrome - *Staphylococcus aureus*	Macular erythema with 'sandpaper' texture of involved skin Epidermis becomes wrinkled (in 2 days or less) and large bullae appear	Systemic administration of antibiotics Gentle cleansing with saline, Burow solution, or 0.25% silver nitrate compresses	Infant subject to fluid loss, impaired body temperature regulation, and secondary infection such as pneumonia, cellulitis, and septicaemia Heals without scarring

Table 17-3 Bacterial infections.

provided with their own towel and directed to wear a protective cap at night to avoid transmitting the fungus to bedding, especially if they sleep with another person. Since the infection can be acquired by animal-to-human transmission, all household pets should be examined for the presence of the disorder. Other sources of infection are seats with headrests, such as seats in public transportation.

Treatment with the drug griseofulvin frequently lasts for weeks or months, and, because subjective symptoms subside, children or parents may be tempted to decrease or discontinue the drug. The nurse should impress on members of the family the importance of maintaining the prescribed dosage schedule. They are also instructed regarding the possibility of side effects from the drug such as headache, gastrointestinal upset, fatigue, insomnia, and photosensitivity. For children who take the drug over many months, periodic testing is required to monitor leukopenia and to assess liver and renal function.

DISEASE	MANIFESTATIONS	MANAGEMENT	COMMENTS
Verruca (warts)	Small, benign tumours Usually well-circumscribed, grey, or brown, elevated firm papules with a roughened, finely papillomatous texture Occur anywhere but usually appear on exposed areas such as fingers, hands, face, and soles May be single or multiple Asymptomatic	Not uniformly successful Local destructive therapy individualized according to location, type, and number - surgical removal, electro-cautery, curetage, cryotherapy (liquid nitrogen), caustic solutions (lactic acid and salicylic acid in flexible collodion, retinoic acid, salicylic acid plasters), x-ray treatment Hypnotherapy may be effective	Common in children Tend to disappear spontaneously Course unpredict-able Most destructive techniques tend to leave scars Auto-inoculable Repeated irritation will cause to enlarge
Variants: Verruca vulgaris (common wart)	A skin-coloured to brown, rough-surfaced epithelial growth May be single or multiple Asymptomatic Most frequent sites are dorsal and palmar surfaces of hands, fingers, and around nails		
Verruca plana juvenilis (juvenile wart)	Flat, skin-coloured to brown, slightly raised, smooth lesion Asymptomatic Lesions multiple Commonly located on face and dorsum of hands		
Verruca plantaris (plantar wart)	Located on plantar surface of feet and, because of pressure, are practically flat; may be surrounded by a collar of hyperkeratosis	Apply caustic solution to wart, wear foam insole with hole cut to relieve pressure on wart; soak 20 min after 2-3 days. Repeat until wart comes out	Destructive techniques tend to leave scars, which may cause problems with walking
Human papilloma-virus			*(cont.)*

Table 17-4 Viral infections.

DISEASE	MANIFESTATIONS	MANAGEMENT	COMMENTS
Herpes simplex virus Type I (cold sore, fever blister) Type II (genital)	Grouped, burning, and itching vesicles on inflammatory base, usually on or near mucocutaneous junctions (lips, nose, genitals, buttocks) Vesicles dry, forming a crust, followed by exfoliation and spontaneous healing in 8-10 days May be accompanied by regional lymphadenopathy	Avoidance of secondary infection Burow solution compresses during weeping stages Topical therapy has proved to have effect on recurrences Oral antiviral (acyclovir) for initial infection or to reduce severity in recurrence	Heal without scarring unless secondary infection Aggravated by corticosteroids Positive psychological effect from treatment May be fatal in children with depressed immunity
Varicella zoster virus (herpes zoster; shingles)	Caused by same virus that causes varicella (chickenpox) Virus has affinity for posterior root ganglia, posterior horn of spinal cord, and skin; crops of vesicles usually confined to dermatome following along course of affected nerve Usually preceded by neuralgic pain, hyperaesthesias, or itching May be accompanied by constitutional symptoms	Symptomatic Analgesics for pain Mild sedation sometimes helpful Local moist compresses Drying lotions may be helpful Ophthalmic variety: systemic corticotropin (ACTH) and/or corticosteroids Acyclovir	Pain in children usually minimal Postherpetic pain does not occur in children Chickenpox may follow exposure; isolate affected child from other children in a hospital or school May occur in children with depressed immunity; can be fatal
Molluscum contagiosum	Flesh-coloured papules with a central caseous plug (umbilicated) Usually asymptomatic	Cases in well children resolve spontaneously in about 18 months Treatment reserved for troublesome cases Curettage or cryotherapy	Common in school-age children Spread by skin-to-skin contact, including auto-inoculation and fomite-to-skin contact

Table 17-4 Viral infections (continued)

SCABIES

Scabies is an endemic infestation caused by the scabies mite, *Sarcoptes scabiei*, which becomes pandemic at 30-year cyclic intervals, with each incidence lasting approximately 15 years. The current pandemic is nearing completion. Lesions are created as the impregnated female scabies mite burrows into the stratum corneum of the epidermis (never into living tissue) where she deposits her eggs and faecal material. These burrows form minute, linear, greyish-brown thread-like lesions that are often difficult to see.

CLINICAL MANIFESTATIONS

The reaction causes intense pruritus that leads to punctate discrete excoriations secondary to the itching. Maculopapular lesions are characteristically distributed in intertriginous areas: skin folds, interdigital surfaces, the axillary-cubital area, popliteal folds, and inguinal region. However, there is large variability in type of lesions. Infants often develop an eczematous eruption; therefore, the observer must look for discrete papules, burrows, or vesicles. A mite is identified as a black dot at the end of a burrow. In children over two years of age, the largest percentage of eruptions are found in the hands and wrists and, in children less than two years, on feet and ankles. Children with Down syndrome do not complain of itching, and therefore they can get a severe infestation before it is recognized.

The inflammatory response and itching occur after the host becomes sensitized to the mite, approximately 30-60 days following initial contact. (In persons previously sensitized to the mite, the inflammatory response occurs within 48 hours after exposure.) After this time, anywhere the mite has travelled will begin to itch and develop the characteristic eruption. Consequently, mites will not necessarily be located at all sites of eruption. Also, a person needs prolonged contact with the mite to become infested. Since it takes about 45 minutes for the mite to burrow under the skin, transient body contact is less likely to cause transfer of the mite.

THERAPEUTIC MANAGEMENT

The diagnosis is made by microscopic identification from scrapings of the burrow. Treatment is application of 0.5% aqueous malathion in a vanishing cream base. Permethrin (Nix), a standard therapy for pediculosis, is approved for use for scabies. Because of the length of time between infestation and physical symptoms (30-60 days), all those who were in close contact with the affected child will need treatment. This may include people such as boyfriends or girlfriends, babysitters, and grandparents, as well as immediate family members. The objective is to treat as thoroughly as possible the first time.

IMPLICATIONS FOR NURSING

Nurses instructing families in use of the scabicide should emphasize the importance of following the directions accurately. It should be applied to cool, dry skin — not following a hot bath. It is applied over the entire cutaneous surface from the neck down and left on for the recommended time, usually four hours for infants and six hours for older children and adults. Since it is a superficial skin disorder, penetration need not be promoted. One liberal application is sufficient. The doctor usually prescribes enough medication for the entire family, allowing two ounces (56 g) for adults and one ounce (28 g) for each child.

Touching and holding the affected child should be minimized until treatment is completed, and hands should be washed carefully after contact is made. Nurses in hospitals are to wear gloves when caring for an affected child. Following treatment, freshly laundered bed linen and underclothing are used, and previously worn clothing is washed in very hot water and ironed. Families need to know that, although the mite will be killed, the rash and the itch will not be eliminated until the stratum corneum is replaced, which takes approximately 2-3 weeks. Soothing ointments or lotions can be used for pruritus.

PEDICULOSIS CAPITIS

Pediculosis capitis (head lice) is an infestation of the scalp by *Pediculus humanus capitis,* a very common parasite, especially in school-aged children. These lice infestations are not a major health threat, but they are highly communicable and create embarrassment and a panic reaction in the family and community. They can also cause a child to be ridiculed by other children.

The louse is a blood-sucking organism that requires approximately five meals a day. The adult louse lives only about 48 hours when away from a human host, and the life span of the average female is only one month. The female lays her eggs at night at the junction of a hair shaft and close to the skin, because the eggs need a warm environment.

Nurses or parents should carefully inspect the head of a child who scratches the head more than usual for bite marks, redness, and nits. Lice are visible to the naked eye. The nits, or eggs, hatch in approximately 7-10 days; therefore the egg is about 4 mm from the scalp at the time of hatching and appears as a tiny whitish oval speck adhering to the hair shaft. The adherent nature of the nits distinguish them from dandruff, which falls off readily. Empty nit cases, indicating hatched lice, are translucent rather than white and are usually located more than 0.5 cm from the scalp.

CLINICAL MANIFESTATIONS

Itching, caused by the crawling insect and insect saliva on the skin, is usually the only symptom. Common sites of involvement are the occipital area, behind the ears, at the nape of the neck, and (occasionally) the eyebrows and eyelashes. Scratch marks and/or inflammatory papules caused by secondary infection may also be found on the scalp in the vulnerable areas.

THERAPEUTIC MANAGEMENT

Malathion shampoo is applied as prescribed and repeated in 7-10 days to kill the hatching nymphs. A commercial preparation of 0.5% malathion lotion (Ovide lotion) is also available for treatment of pediculosis. Malathion was shown to be superior to other preparations because of its effectiveness and low toxicity. However, to be effective, any treatment should be accompanied by an educational and reinfestation-prevention programme.

Application

Treatment should not be administered after a warm bath or shower, because vasodilation from the heat increases skin absorption of chemicals. For the same reason, use of a hair dryer is avoided.

The pediculocide must remain on the scalp and hair for several minutes and the child is instructed to close the eyes tightly during application. The child can be provided with a towel or washcloth with which to cover the eyes. If eye irritation occurs, the eyes must be flushed well with tepid water. Because most of the application times are ten minutes, some diversional activity should be provided for the child.

Nit removal

Instructions on the labels indicate that dead lice and remaining nits are removed with an extra fine-tooth comb while the hair is still damp. All detectable nits and nit cases are removed because it is almost impossible to distinguish viable from non-viable nits with the naked eye. The child is examined daily for evidence of newly laid nits for at least two weeks following treatment.

Environmental management
Live lice will survive for up to 48 hours away from the host, but nits are shed into the environment and capable of hatching in 7-10 days. Therefore, measures must be taken to prevent further infestation (see Parent Guidelines).

Prevention
The increasing incidence of pediculosis in school children has become a serious concern for school nurses, parents, and community health agencies. Suggestions include encouraging parents to notify others if a child becomes infected and preventing children from re-entering school until they are completely free of nits.

Psychological aspects
It should be emphasized that *anyone* can get pediculosis. It has no respect for age, socioeconomic level, or cleanliness. The louse does not jump or fly, but it can be transmitted from one person to another on personal items. Lice are not carried or transmitted by household pets.

The psychological effects of lice infestations can be highly stressful to children. They are influenced by the reactions of others, including their parents, and may be made to feel ashamed or guilty. Parents are strongly cautioned against cutting a child's hair or, worse, shaving a child's head. Lice infest short hair as readily as long hair, and these actions only compound the child's distress and serve as a continual reminder to peers, who are always ready to taunt another with something out of the ordinary (McLaury, 1983).

SKIN DISORDERS RELATED TO CHEMICAL OR PHYSICAL CONTACTS

Children come into contact with an endless variety of substances and objects in day-to-day activities, including sunshine. Some children are troubled very little by these encounters; others are sensitive to many commonplace substances.

CONTACT DERMATITIS

The most common contact dermatitis in infants occurs on the convex surfaces of the nappy area as a result of chemical irritation from ammonia, putrefactive enzymes acting on urinary amino acids, or, less often, laundry products (see Nappy Rash, Chapter 15). Other agents that frequently produce dermatological responses from contact are animal irritants such as wool, feathers, and furs; oils, and turpentine; and chemicals of all kinds, including synthetic fabrics (e.g., shoe components), dyes, metals, cosmetics, perfumes, and soaps (including bubble baths). The list is endless.

IMPLICATIONS FOR NURSING

Nurses frequently detect evidence of contact dermatitis during routine physical assessments. Skin manifestations in specific areas suggest limited contact, such as around the eyes (mascara), areas of the body covered by clothing but not protected by undergarments (wool), or areas of the body not covered by clothing (ultraviolet injury). Generalized involvement is more likely to be bubble bath or soap. If the lesions persist, are extensive, or show evidence of infection, medical evaluation is indicated.

SUNBURN

Sunburn is a very common skin injury caused by overexposure to ultraviolet light waves — either sunlight or artificial light in the ultraviolet range. Ultraviolet A (UVA) waves cause only minimum burning, but play a significant role in photosensitive and photoallergic reactions. They are also responsible for premature ageing of the skin. Ultraviolet B (UVB) waves are responsible for tanning, burning, and most of the harmful effects attributed to sunlight, especially skin cancer.

Some individuals are more susceptible to sunburn than others. Protection from effects of the sun is provided by the fibrous keratin of the outer epidermis and the pigment melanin, produced by the melanocytes of the innermost, or basal, layer of the epidermis. Areas of the body with thick keratin layers (palms and soles) offer the greatest protection. The protective pigment layer decreases the intensity of all ultraviolet light by physically blocking and scattering the radiation. Ultraviolet rays stimulate the melanocytes to produce more melanin, turning the skin darker. After several days of exposure, the dark melanin is able to absorb most of the incoming ultraviolet radiation before the rays can cause further damage.

People with light skin and eyes produce melanin slowly and are more prone to burn, while very dark-skinned people are able to tolerate more rays without damage. Sunlight penetrates the atmosphere even on hazy days.

Other factors can play a role in sensitivity to ultraviolet rays. People with certain diseases (e.g., porphyria, lupus erythematosus) are more sensitive to the sun's rays. Some substances increase the skin's sensitivity, for example, numerous medications (e.g., barbiturates, oral contraceptives, sulphonamides, anticonvulsants), topical products (e.g., antiseptic soap, after-shave lotions, colognes), and certain foods containing photosensitizing chemicals (e.g., carrots, parsley, limes).

Ultraviolet rays penetrate the skin surface, where they precipitate a chemical change in the cell molecules, producing toxic by-products that irritate surrounding tissues. The result is redness, tissue swelling, increased capillary permeability, and the tenderness characteristic of superficial (first-degree) burns and the coagulation, necrosis, and blistering of partial thickness (second-degree) burns (see Burns, Chapter 24). Sunburned skin is exquisitely sensitive, and severe sunburn may be accompanied by nausea, chills, fever, abdominal cramping, and headache. Dehydration may also occur.

Excessive or long-term exposure to the sun causes permanent damage to the skin. Ninety percent of skin cancers occur in areas that are exposed to sunlight, and rates of skin cancers are higher in parts of the world where sunlight is more intense. Studies have also shown that childhood is a crucial time for sun exposure. Children who emmigrate to sunny climates after ten years of age develop cancer at lower rates than native-born children. In general, children receive three times as much sun exposure as adults, and teenagers are a high-risk group, with their emphasis on the desirability of a tanned skin.

IMPLICATIONS FOR NURSING

Treatment involves stopping the burning process, decreasing the inflammatory response and rehydrating the skin. Local application of cool tap water soaks or immersion in a tepid water bath for 20 minutes or until the skin is cool, limits tissue destruction and relieves the discomfort. After the cool applications, a bland oil-in-water moisturizing lotion can be applied, but petrolatum-based products that trap radiant heat in the tissues should be avoided (Anders and Leach, 1983).

Prevention

Protection from sunburn is the major goal of management. The harmful effects of the sun on the delicate skin of infants and children are receiving increased attention. Protection can be achieved by physical means, such as protective clothing and a hat, or by chemical means. Two types of products are available for sun protection: topical sunscreens, which partially absorb ultraviolet light, and sun blocks, which block out ultraviolet rays by reflecting sunlight.

Some chemicals have the capacity to absorb certain wavelengths of light and thus provide protection to the cutaneous surface when applied to the skin. Sunscreens are products containing a sun protective factor (SPF) based on evaluation of effectiveness against ultraviolet rays. The SPF is indicated by

number, such as 15, which indicates that, if a person normally burns in 10 minutes without a sunscreen, use of sunscreen with SPF 15 will allow them to remain in the sun for 15 times 10 or 150 minutes (2.5 hours) before acquiring the same degree of erythema or burn.

There is disagreement regarding the frequency of application. One opinion is that reapplication of sunscreen does not extend the period of protection; the protection will remain the same no matter how many times it is reapplied (Nicol, 1989). However, the predominant view is that sunscreen should be applied 15-20 minutes before exposure (so that the protective chemicals can penetrate the upper skin layers) and reapplied frequently and liberally (Coody, 1987; Hurwitz, 1989).

Most chemical sunscreens are available with SPF ranging from 2 to over 30; the higher the number, the greater the protection. A minimum SPF of 15 is recommended.

Individuals who care for or work with children, such as teachers, daycare workers, coaches, youth group leaders and relatives, should be made aware of sun safety for children. Sun damage is cumulative. Although most long-term effects (cancer, wrinkling) are not evident until adulthood, skin care must begin in childhood. Application of a sunscreen product is recommended for children after six months of age; infants less than six months of age should be kept out of the sun. It should be the goal of every nurse to teach skin care as a basic practice that becomes a routine part of a child's life, much the same as tooth care (see Parent Guidelines).

SKIN DISORDERS RELATED TO DRUG SENSITIVITY

Adverse reactions to drugs are seen more often in the skin than in any other organ, although any organ of the body can be affected. The reaction may be a result of toxicity related to drug concentration, individual intolerance to the average dosage of the drug, or an allergic or idiosyncratic response.

DRUG REACTIONS

Some drugs have a tendency to produce a particular reaction consistently, and some are more likely than others to produce an untoward effect. Many of these effects are allergenic responses following a prior administration of the drug, even a topical application. However, other factors also influence a drug response in a particular individual. For example, drug eruptions occur less frequently in children than in adults, the incidence increases with the number of drugs being given, climate may be a factor if light sensitivity produces a response on sun-exposed surfaces, and it is well known that genetic factors affect the way in which some individuals are able to metabolize specific drugs.

Manifestations of drug reactions may be delayed or immediate. Seven days are usually required for a child to develop sensitivity to a drug that has not been administered previously. With prior sensitivity, the manifestations appear almost

---

Parent Guidelines

Preventing the Spread and Recurrence of Pediculosis

Machine wash all washable clothing, towels, and bed linens in hot water and dry in a hot dryer for at least 20 minutes. Dry-clean nonwashable items.

Thoroughly vacuum carpets, car seats, pillows, stuffed animals, rugs, mattresses and upholstered furniture.

Seal nonwashable items in plastic bags for 14 days if parents are unable to afford dry cleaning and do not have a vacuum cleaner.

Soak combs, brushes, and hair accessories in lice-killing products for one hour or in boiling water for ten minutes.

From Clore 1989.

immediately. In children, rashes are the most common manifestation — exanthematous, urticarial, or eczematoid. However, individual drug reactions may vary from a single lesion to extensive, generalized epidermal necrosis. With few exceptions, the distribution of a drug eruption is widespread, since it results from a circulating agent, appears as an inflammatory response with itching, is sudden in onset, and may be associated with constitutional symptoms such as fever, malaise, gastrointestinal upsets, anaemia, or liver and kidney damage.

In most cases, treatment consists of discontinuation of the drug. Sometimes a decision is made to continue the drug (such as an antibiotic in an infant or small child) until the cause of the rash is clearly indicated. In urticarial-type eruptions antihistamines may be ordered, and for widespread and severe lesions corticosteroids are beneficial. Severe anaphylactic reactions are a medical emergency (see Anaphylaxis, Chapter 24).

IMPLICATIONS FOR NURSING

The most effective means of management is prevention. Parents always remember a severe response. A careful history will elicit evidence of a previous drug reaction. The history should include the name of the drug, nature of the reaction, drug dose, and how soon after administration the reaction occurred.

Nurses who suspect that a rash is caused by a medication should withhold any further dose and report the eruption to medical staff. The most frequent offenders in drug reactions are penicillin and sulphonamides, and nurses must be alert to this possibility. However, even commonplace drugs – including barbiturates, chemical agents in a number of foods, flavouring agents and preservatives – are capable of producing an undesired response. People who have severe reactions are reminded to obtain and wear an identification bracelet or chain in case of emergency or inadvertent administration of the offending drug.

MISCELLANEOUS SKIN PROBLEMS

INSECT STINGS AND BITES

Children at play may be particularly vulnerable to stings and bites, especially during the summer months, and due to their inquisitive nature and curiosity.

INSECT STINGS

When an insect stings, its stinger often remains imbedded in the skin. Since bees have barbed stingers that penetrate the skin, any pressure on the venom sac at the tip of the barb pushes more venom into the skin. The best approach is to flick the stinger off with the fingernail or knife blade — never squeeze the area. Another method is to cover the area with transparent tape and then peel off the tape. The stinger should come off with the tape (Gorrell, 1985).

ANIMAL BITES

Animal bites are common injuries, and young adults are the most frequent victims (Chun, Berkelhamer, and Herold, 1982). Contrary to accepted belief, stray dogs are seldom involved in the attacks; most of the dogs are owned by the family of the victim or a neighbour (Elliot *et al*, 1985).

Animal bites are potentially serious because of the likelihood of significant infection — 5% of dog bites and 20-50% of cat bites (Baker, 1989). Injuries vary in intensity from small puncture wounds to complete evulsion of tissue that can be associated with significant crush injury. Dog bites generally present as lacerations or evulsions; cats exert less biting force, but their sharp teeth penetrate more deeply, inoculating organisms deep into tissues.

The location of a bite influences the incidence of infection. Injuries to the arm and hand tend to become infected more often than those on legs, scalp, and face. Redness, swelling and tenderness develop around the site of injury, often accompanied by purulent or serosanguineous drainage. It may be difficult to assess hand infection, since most lymphatic drainage is contained in the dorsal subcutaneous space, and swelling occurs in this area when the injury may be elsewhere (Baker, 1989).

THERAPEUTIC MANAGEMENT

General wound care consists of rinsing the wound with copious amounts of a solution, such as salvodine, and washing the surrounding skin with mild soap. A clean pressure dressing is applied, and medical evaluation determines the use of antibiotic dressings.

Prophylactic antibiotics are indicated for puncture wounds and wounds in areas that may prove to be cosmetically or functionally impaired if infected. Extensive lacerations are debrided and loosely sutured to allow for drainage in the event of infection. Primary closure of jagged, irregular wounds with associated crush injury and devitalized tissue is contraindicated, except for facial wounds because of cosmetic reasons (Avery and First, 1989). Tetanus toxoid is administered according to standard guidelines. Injuries to poorly vascularized areas, such as the hands, are more likely to become infected than those in more vascularized areas such as the face; puncture wounds are more likely to become infected than are lacerations.

IMPLICATIONS FOR NURSING

The most important aspect related to animal bites is prevention. It is important that children understand animal behaviour and develop an honest respect for all animals.

Parents who are contemplating a pet, especially a dog, for themselves or their children should receive some advice about the dog that is least likely to be a danger to their children.

HUMAN BITES

Children often acquire lacerations from the teeth of other humans in rough play, during fights, or as victims of child

Parent Guidelines

Sun Exposure

Remember that tanning indicates sun injury and risks of skin cancer begin in childhood.

Keep infants and children out of the sun as much as possible.

Use prams with hoods when taking infants outdoors.

Use canopy on pushchairs for older infants.

Schedule child's activities to avoid sun exposure between 10 AM and 3 PM whenever possible.

Take increased precautions when living or taking a holiday in the mountains or the tropics.

Protect child with clothing when outdoors (sun hat, long-sleeved shirt, long trousers).

Apply sunscreen with SPF of at least 15.

Apply sunscreen to exposed areas:

Before every exposure

On cloudy as well as sunny days

Even when child plays in shade; sun reflects from sand, snow, cement, and water

Reapply liberally every 2-3 hours and whenever child goes in the water or sweats heavily.

Check with child's GP regarding any medications the child is taking and observe for any evidence of side effects (rash, redness, swelling).

Examine skin regularly for signs of any change in pigmented naevi (rapid growth, crusting, ulceration, bleeding, change in pigmentation, development of inflamed satellite lesions, loss of normal skin lines) or subjective symptoms (tenderness, pain, itching).

Prohibit child from using sunbeds.

Set a good example by following the above guidelines.

Modified from *For every child under the sun*, The Skin Cancer Foundation, 245 Fifth Avenue, Suite 2402, New York, NY 10016

abuse. Many preschool children bite others out of frustration or anger. Most childhood bites by humans are superficial and rarely become infected when the child receives early treatment (Baker and Moore, 1987; Esposito and Adams, 1989). Because human dental plaque and gingiva harbour pathogenic bacteria, all human bites should receive prompt attention - delayed treatment increases the risk of infection.

The wound should be washed vigorously with soap and water, and a pressure dressing applied to stop bleeding. Ice applications minimize discomfort and swelling. Increased pain or redness at the wound site is an indication that the child should receive medical attention for antibiotic therapy. Tetanus toxoid is needed if more than five years has elapsed since the last immunization.

DENTAL DISORDERS

Since all of the permanent teeth (except the wisdom teeth) erupt during middle childhood, dental health is particularly important. Ideally, children should receive regular preventive dental care and supervision in daily hygienic care from the time the teeth begin to erupt (see Chapter 11). The importance of dental care is undisputed; however, limited or inadequate dental care results in the most prevalent of all childhood health problems, chiefly dental caries, malocclusion, periodontal disease and trauma. Although these conditions are not considered illnesses, they have harmful long-range effects on children's health.

DENTAL CARIES

Dental caries is one of the most common chronic diseases that affects individuals at all ages. Although 100% preventable, dental caries is the principal oral problem in children and adolescents. Although the overall incidence of dental caries in children has decreased since the introduction of fluoridation, it is still an important health problem. Reducing the incidence and consequences of the disorder is of primary importance in childhood because dental caries, if untreated, results in total destruction of involved teeth. The ages of greatest vulnerability are 4-8 years for the primary dentition and 12-18 years for the secondary or permanent dentition.

Host

The areas most subject to attack by bacteria are (in order of difficulty of complete cleansing) grooves and fissures, interdermal areas, gum margins and other smooth surfaces. Newly erupted teeth that have not yet acquired sufficient surface minerals are more susceptible to decay than those that have been erupted for two or more years. Undoubtedly, hereditary factors influence resistance and susceptibility, since similar patterns and anatomical characteristics are seen in successive generations. Salivary flow can mechanically clean away bacteria and food debris. It also contains buffering systems, lysozymes, peroxidases, and immunoglobulins that influence the development of caries.

Substrates

Caries formation is strongly influenced by two concurrent processes that continually operate on enamel surfaces — acid production and acid neutralization by saliva. Sucrose has been consistently implicated as the most cariogenic substance. Sucrose-containing substances, especially in tenacious forms that cling (such as chewy candy) or that promote prolonged contact with the teeth (such as chewing gum, hard candy, and lollipops), when ingested between meals, contribute markedly to the development of dental caries. Saliva and other foods that are ingested at mealtime tend to help neutralize much of the acid formed from sucrose.

Time and other factors

Bacterial enzymes act on salivary glycoproteins to produce a tenacious protein matrix on the tooth surface. This substance, along with the micro-organisms, forms *dental plaque*. If plaque removal is inadequate or nonexistent for a significant length of time (a few days), the plaque is metabolized by the bacteria to form acid, which initiates the demineralization of enamel (Rule, 1982).

The susceptibility to dental decay may be influenced by the general health of the child. Children who suffer from chronic debilitating disease show increased caries activity, as do children with systemic conditions that alter the quality and quantity of saliva produced.

PROCESS OF DIAGNOSIS

Because the permanent teeth erupt during middle childhood, children are more susceptible to development of dental caries during this time than at any other age. Caries penetrate the vulnerable teeth rapidly at this age, as opposed to the slower, intermittent activity characteristic at later ages.

THERAPEUTIC MANAGEMENT

Prophylaxis is the major thrust of dental treatment, including hygiene and fluoride treatment. Treatment of dental caries involves removal of all carious portions of teeth as soon as detected, preparation of a retentive cavity, and replacement of the lost portion of the tooth with a material that is durable in the mouth environment. This restoration of involved teeth not only prevents progression of established caries, but also reduces the number of bacteria in the oral cavity to decrease the danger to uninvolved teeth.

IMPLICATIONS FOR NURSING

Oral inspection is an integral part of the nursing assessment of the child in any setting. If there is any evidence of dental caries or other unhealthy state, the child is referred for dental services. Nurses can be active members of preventive educational programmes and can counsel families regarding the importance of regular dental care, oral hygiene and dietary management.

Nurses can encourage good oral hygiene by teaching correct tooth cleaning to children and their parents. The random brushing allowed during the early childhood years should be replaced by more careful and methodic cleansing techniques.

School nurses have an excellent opportunity to engage in detection of dental needs, educating children in dental hygiene and preventing dental problems, making referrals, and motivating children to comply with prophylaxis and treatment.

Children should be prepared for dental services in such a way that visits to the dentist are a positive experience. Keeping appointments and following through on recommended treatments and practices are habits that extend beyond childhood.

PERIODONTAL DISEASE

Periodontal disease, inflammatory and degenerative conditions involving the gums and tissues supporting the teeth, often begins in childhood and accounts for a significant amount of

tooth loss in adulthood. The more common periodontal problems are *gingivitis* (simple inflammation of the gums) and *periodontitis* (inflammation of the gums and loss of connective tissue and bone in the supporting structures of the teeth).

Management is directed towards prevention, by conscientious brushing and flossing, and by depriving the bacteria of the substrates required to produce the disease. The implementation and maintenance of preventive dental practice, including use of fluoride, plus good dental hygiene are effective in preventing both caries and periodontal disease.

MALOCCLUSION

When teeth of the upper and lower dental arches approximate in the proper relationships, the physiological function of mastication is more effective, and the cosmetic effect is more pleasing. Teeth that are uneven, crowded, overlapping or that otherwise interfere with their ability to meet their opponents in the opposite jaw in the appropriate relationships, may be predisposed to dental disease.

The most common cause of malocclusion is hereditary factors, but abnormal growth and habits, such as thumbsucking and tongue thrusting, also contribute to the disordered alignment and occlusion of the teeth. The trend is towards early correction to prevent problems if the irregularity interferes with normal function and speech; therefore, referral should be made as soon as malocclusion is evident.

TRAUMA

Injury to the teeth is not an uncommon occurrence in childhood (Box 17-2). This includes fractures of varying degrees of severity, chipping, dislocation, or evulsion. All tooth injuries require prompt treatment by a competent dentist in order to prevent permanent displacement or loss.

Boys experience injury to permanent teeth much more frequently than girls, although this observation is not supported in all studies. A tooth that is evulsed ('knocked out') can be reimplanted and retained permanently if replaced without delay (Krasner, 1990).

IMPLICATIONS FOR NURSING: TOOTH EVULSION

A permanent tooth that is separated should be replanted by the child, parent, or nurse and stabilized as soon as possible so that the blood supply to the tooth can be re-established and the tooth kept alive. If the tooth is replaced within 30 minutes, there is a 70% chance that it will become reattached and roots will not resorb or the crown exfoliate. Separated primary teeth are usually not reimplanted.

Before reimplantation, it is important to carefully rinse a dirty tooth in milk, saline solution, or under running water to avoid disturbing the adhering periodontal membrane, which is essential to the success of the reimplantation. The tooth is

---

◆ **BOX 17-2**

Periods for increased frequency of dental trauma

Preschool (1-3 years) — injury usually secondary to falls or child abuse

School aged (7-10 years) — injury more often following bicycle and playground accidents

Adolescence (16-18 years) — injury generally sustained secondary to fights, athletic injury, and automobile accidents

Data from Berkowitz and Ludwig Johnson 1980.

---

held by the crown, not the root, while rinsing, and is then fitted back into its socket the best way possible, even if it means placing it backward or at an angle (Kochman, 1989). If the tooth is reimplanted almost immediately, excessive pressure is not needed; however, it becomes extremely difficult after clot formation (in approximately 10 minutes). The tooth is held in place by the child during transportation to a dentist. Care is taken to avoid sudden stops or turns that might cause the child to swallow or aspirate the loose tooth.

If the child or parents are reluctant to reimplant the tooth, the next best alternative is to place the tooth in cold milk, contact lens solution, or saline for transport to the dentist. Cold milk has precisely the osmolality to maintain fluid balance within the tissues surrounding the tooth. Tap water is not recommended (Kochman, 1989).

As with all mouth trauma, a separated tooth causes a large amount of bleeding, which may distress the child. Using a calm approach and providing gentle reassurance helps reduce anxiety.

DISORDERS OF CONTINENCE

Disorders involving elimination and continence are common in childhood, especially diarrhoea; constipation is observed less frequently (see also Chapter 27). More troublesome problems of elimination are enuresis and encopresis.

ENURESIS

Enuresis (bed-wetting) is a common and troublesome disorder that is difficult to define because of the variable ages at which children achieve bladder control. Bladder control depends on several factors, including the child's developmental stage, the manner in which training is carried out, the personality of the child, and the emotional climate of the home environment. In a broad sense, enuresis can be defined as repeated involuntary urination (usually nocturnal) in children who are beyond the age when voluntary bladder control should normally have been acquired. Some authorities place four years as an arbitrary age by

which diurnal and nocturnal bladder control is normally accomplished, although five years of age is probably more accurate.

Enuresis can be defined as *primary*, bed-wetting in children who have never been dry for extended periods, or *secondary*, the onset of wetting after a continuous dry period of more than one year (American Psychiatric Association, 1994). The incidence is approximately 5-17% in otherwise normal children from 3-15 years of age (Box 17-3).

The prevalence of enuresis at 5 years of age is 7% for males and 3% for females; at the age of 10 years the prevalence is 3% for males and 2% for females. At the age of 18 years, the prevalence is 1% for males and less among females (American Psychiatric Association, 1994).

No clear aetiology for enuresis, as a distinct entity, has been determined. A high frequency of bed-wetting has been observed in parents, siblings, and other near relatives of symptomatic children, and is supported by a high concordance rate in enuretic monozygotic twins. Family studies indicate that the closer the relationship, the higher the incidence of enuresis (Friman, 1986). Approximately 75% of all children with functional enuresis have a first-degree relative who has, or has had, the disorder (American Psychiatric Association, 1994). It appears that these persons have difficulty in inhibiting the mechanisms that regulate the emptying of the bladder.

Enuresis is more common in boys than in girls, but the reason for this is not clear. Other factors include a higher frequency in children in lower socioeconomic groups and in black children. An increased prevalence has also been observed among late-maturing adolescents, both male and female, than early or midmaturers, and the children describe themselves as tense, having difficulty sleeping, and having bad dreams. Children aged 6-11 have temperaments described as highly strung and lose their temper easily (Levine, 1983). Enuretic children are more likely to be afraid of the dark.

PATHOPHYSIOLOGY

Enuresis is primarily a problem of delayed or incomplete neuromuscular maturation of the bladder and as such is benign

---

◆ **BOX 17-3**

Cultural awareness: enuresis

The age at which children attain urinary continence varies widely. For example, white children in the United States tend to achieve continence earlier than do Afro-American children. Children in the United Kingdom and Sweden appear to attain continence slightly earlier than do children in the United States, and in the extreme, the East African Digos often achieve bladder control by the age of 12 months. Therefore, practitioners must be sensitive to the differences among groups before labelling a child enuretic (Rappaport, 1992).

---

and self-limiting. There are children who exhibit temporary regressive behaviour after the birth of a sibling or who have occasional 'accidents' when they become involved in play to such an extent that they are unaware of a full bladder, become excited, or 'forget' to empty the bladder. In other children, enuresis may be caused by problems associated with toilet training that are related to the age at which training is begun, the emotional atmosphere that surrounds the training situation, or an excessive amount of emotional dependence on the mother. In some children, enuresis is one behavioural manifestation of a personality disorder. However, behavioural problems associated with enuresis are probably a result rather than a cause of the enuresis.

A significant number of nocturnal enuretic episodes were thought to be related to deep sleep. These children seemed to sleep more soundly than others and not to waken from either external or internal stimuli. Many of these children demonstrated increased frequency and magnitude of spontaneous bladder contractions during the non-rapid-eye-movement (N-REM) stage of sleep preceding bed-wetting. Bed-wetting appeared to occur as the child moved from the deeper stages of non-REM sleep into the REM stage.

However, recent research suggests, however, that depth of sleep as measured by electroencephalogram is not the cause of noctural enuresis (Rappaport, 1993). However, this 'theory' continues to prevail in many treatment regimes.

Enuresis has a strong familial tendency and seems to be associated with a developmental delay that causes such intense urgency that the child is unable to inhibit bladder contraction after the bladder is distended beyond a certain volume. Such children acquire bladder control with difficulty and, even after control, are more prone to enuresis when subjected to stress than are other children. Although there is evidence that some children with enuresis have smaller bladder capacities than nonaffected children, evidence suggests that is not the cause. For example, children without enuresis but with smaller bladder capacity awaken during the night to void, as opposed to children with enuresis who do not awaken.

The *nocturnal polyuria theory* currently offers the most promising aetiology of nocturnal enuresis. It suggests that the kidneys of these children fail to concentrate urine during sleep because of insufficient *antidiuretic hormone* (ADH). One study showed that serum levels of ADH and urine osmolality were higher at night in children without enuresis than in children with enuresis (Rettig *et al*, 1989). This finding suggests that the ADH circadian rhythm may be a significant biological marker in enuresis, but additional research must be conducted to further clafify its role.

CLINICAL MANIFESTATIONS

The predominant symptom is urgency that is immediate and accompanied by acute discomfort, restlessness, and sometimes urinary frequency. Nocturnal enuresis is most common and is occasionally accompanied by diurnal wetting; diurnal bed-wetting without nocturnal bed-wetting is unusual. In most affected children, nocturnal bed-wetting is a primary matu-rational problem and usually ceases between ages six and eight, although it may continue into adolescence.

PROCESS OF DIAGNOSIS

Organic causes that may be related to enuresis should be ruled out before psychogenic factors are considered. These include structural disorders of the urinary tract, urinary tract infection, major neurological deficits, nocturnal epilepsy, disorders such as diabetes mellitus and diabetes insipidus that increase the normal output of urine, and disorders such as chronic renal failure or sickle cell disease that impair the concentrating ability of the kidneys. In other cases the enuresis is influenced by emotional factors, although it is doubtful that they are aetiological factors.

In older children, routine examinations are carried out to rule out infection, and bladder capacity is determined by having the children hold off voiding until they feel urgency, at which time they void into a measured container. A bladder volume of 300-350 ml is sufficient to hold one night's urine.

THERAPEUTIC MANAGEMENT

Enuresis not resulting from organic causes can be approached in several ways. No method is so successful as to achieve universal endorsement; however, some have proved helpful in keeping the child dry during the night. Frequently, more than one technique is employed

Bladder retention training

Most children with enuresis have smaller functional bladder capacities. Bladder training is aimed at stretching the bladder to accommodate increasingly larger volumes of urine. After taking fluids, the child is instructed to postpone voiding as long as can be tolerated before emptying the bladder. The heightened threshold for retention allows the child to remain dry throughout the night.

Motivational therapy

Motivational therapy involves a series of counselling interviews designed to encourage the child to assume responsibility for the disorder and the necessary learning. Approaches include reassurance, guilt removal, and emotional support by the family and health personnel. The emphasis is on promoting the development of a positive parent-child relationship and reinforcement for progress, ranging from verbal praise to material rewards. Punishment for bed-wetting is discouraged.

This responsibility-reinforcement therapy emphasizes 'sensation awareness' of bladder fullness and positive reinforcement for progressive steps towards the ultimate goal of being dry. Such response shaping requires considerable input by a supportive family and health professionals (Rushton, 1989).

Behaviour modification (conditioning) therapy

Several electrical devices are available that are based on the conditioned reflex response. These consist of a wire pad attached

Evulsed Tooth

Recover tooth.

Hold tooth by crown; avoid touching root area.

If tooth is dirty, rinse it gently under running water or saline; be sure to insert stopper in sink or basin (to avoid tooth loss).

Insert tooth into socket.

Have child maintain tooth in place.

Transport child to dentist immediately.

Avoid sudden stops or sharp turns to prevent dislodging tooth.

If reluctant to reimplant tooth:

Place evulsed tooth in suitable medium for transport:

a. Cold milk

b. Saliva — under the child's or parent's tongue

If child is holding tooth in the mouth, avoid sudden stops to prevent swallowing tooth.

DON'T FORGET TO TAKE TOOTH

to a bell or buzzer that wakens the child as soon as the first drops of urine create a closed circuit. The child is thus conditioned to waken at the initiation of micturition or to the stimulus of the bell or buzzer. Most have reported a substantial success rate with the device. There appear to be no undesirable emotional effects, although this is debatable.

There are disadvantages to the use of electrical devices. A practical problem is the disturbance it may create when other children sleep in the same room or in the same bed. The child may be too sleepy or forget to reset the alarm following its activation to render it effective for the remainder of the night. There may be a risk of ulceration and scarring caused by slow electrolysis of tissue cells when the child does not hear the alarm or turns the alarm off without waking while the current continues to flow or when the batteries have run down to a feeble point where the alarm is insufficiently loud.

The success rate of the urine alarm is higher than other methods, consistently producing approximately 75% success rate and a lower relapse rate of approximately 41% (Friman and Warzak, 1990). Relapse is addressed by reinstituting the alarm during sleep many times, producing longer lasting results. Some studies have shown that using an intermittent alarm schedule can reduce the relapse rate to as low as 17% (Friman and Warzak, 1990) or, by coupling alarm use with other behavioural procedures, can reduce the relapse rate to 15–25% (Houts, 1991). This method is inexpensive compared to drug therapy and has no side effects.

Drug therapy

Several pharmacological agents can be used in the treatment of enuresis, either alone or in combination with other techniques. The selection depends on the interpretation of the cause. The drug used most frequently is the tricyclic antidepressant drug imipramine, which exerts an anticholinergic action on the bladder to inhibit urination. The dosage and time of administration are individualized, and the drug is given in amounts sufficient to lighten sleep but not to cause wakefulness. The suggested length of treatment is 6-8 weeks, followed by gradual withdrawal over four weeks. Since this drug is dangerous in overdosage, parents must be cautioned about judicious use and keeping supplies of the drug far from the reach of younger siblings.

Anticholinergic drugs, especially oxybutynin, reduce uninhibited bladder contractions and may be helpful for children with daytime urinary frequency. Some success has also been achieved with desmopressin (DDAVP) nasal spray, an analogue of vasopressin, which reduces night-time urine output to a volume less than functional bladder capacity. Although DDAVP is very effective in reducing the number of wet nights, only about 25% of children may become completely dry. Information on the long-term effects of the drug are not known (Moffatt *et al*, 1993).

Miscellaneous therapies

Restricting or eliminating fluids after the evening meal is aimed at decreasing the output of urine during the night. This method has proved to be of questionable value.

Having the child void before retiring and then wakened and taken to the bathroom has met with limited success. Favourable responses are probably a result of the focused concern by both parents and child, and of the positive behavioural reinforcement it provides. For this to be effective, the parent should be sure that the child is fully awake when the bladder is emptied.

Other therapies include psychotherapy, hypnotherapy, and diet therapy. These therapies have been used in special cases and with varying success.

IMPLICATIONS FOR NURSING

No matter which of the various techniques are used, the nurse can help both children and parents to understand the problem of enuresis, the treatment plan, and the probable difficulties they may encounter in the process. Essential to the success of any method is the supportive management of parents and their children. Both need encouragement and patience. The problem is discussed with the parents, and, since any treatment involves and requires the child's active participation, children are included as well. The most important predictor for the outcome of treatment is family difficulties. Family disturbances influence the initial arrest of the enuresis, the relapse rate, and the long-term success rate (Dische *et al*, 1983).

Many parents believe that enuresis is caused by an emotional disturbance and fear that they have somehow produced the situation by imprudent childrearing practices. They need reassurance that the bed-wetting is not a manifestation of emotional disturbance nor does it represent wilful misbehaviour. They should be informed about the nature of enuresis and cautioned against scolding, shaming, threatening and punishing a child, which are useless and harmful.

Communication with children is directed towards eliminating the emotional impact of the problem by relieving them of feelings of shame, guilt, and the burden of parental disapproval and towards increasing their self-confidence and motivating them towards independent control. More important, the nurse can provide consistent support and encouragement to help sustain them through the inconsistent and unpredictable treatment process. Children need to believe that they are helping themselves and to sustain feelings of confidence and hope. Children who have mastered bed-wetting demonstrate an improvement in self-concept (Moffatt, Kato, and Pless, 1987).

ENCOPRESIS

Encopresis is repeated voluntary or involuntary passage of faeces of normal or near-normal consistency into places not appropriate for that purpose in the individual's own sociocultural setting (American Psychiatric Association, 1994). The disorder is less common than enuresis, but the two may coexist. It may not be an isolated symptom, but clustered with other somatic symptoms — social withdrawal, antisocial-aggressive behaviours, affective-dependent behaviours, and somatic manifestations. Although many children demonstrate significant behaviour problems, most children with encopresis do not (Friman *et al*, 1988).

A child who has not achieved faecal continence by four years of age is said to have primary, or continuous, encopresis. This type is more frequently observed as a result of neglect, lax training methods, and familial causes in children with learning disabilities. Secondary, or discontinuous, encopresis is faecal incontinence occurring in a child over four years of age preceded by at least one year of faecal continence (American Psychiatric Association, 1994). The disorder is more common in males than in females.

Because chronic soiling is now considered to be physiological as well as behavioural, the term *idiopathic faecal incontinence* (IFI) has been suggested as a more descriptive term and should be used except when psychiatric dysfunction contributes to the soiling (Stroh, Stern, and McCarthy, 1989).

AETIOLOGY

One of the most common causes of encopresis is constipation, which may be precipitated by environmental change, such as birth of a new sibling, moving to a new house, changing schools, or even having to use new or unfamiliar toilet facilities (Johns, 1985). Voluntary retention usually follows a painful incident with voluntary suppression of defecation (e.g., a child with anal fissures). Involuntary retention may be produced by emotional problems caused by the encopresis that sets up a fear-pain cycle and results in a learned process of abnormal defecation patterns. Psychogenic encopresis, in which the soiling is caused by emotional problems, is often related to a disturbed mother-child relationship.

During school years, children may experience exacerbations at the transition to school. Some of the reasons for developing retentive tendencies at this time are fear of using school bathrooms, a busy schedule, and the interruption of an established time schedule for bowel evacuation. Children at any age may react to stress with bowel dysfunction.

CLINICAL MANIFESTATIONS

The manifestation of simple constipation is painful expulsion of hard, pellet-like stools. Voluntary retention is usually temporary, and there is a history of a painful precipitating episode and blood-streaked stools. Involuntary retention is associated with a history of abdominal pain, distention, moodiness, poor appetite, and accumulation of stools with periodic passage of voluminous stools. Children display a characteristic posturing during suppression of colonic signals to defecate—stiffening, standing in a corner with straight legs and a bright-red face, 'doing a little dance', 'crawling', or hiding behind furniture or a tree when playing outdoors (Rappaport and Levine, 1986; Younger and Hughes, 1983). They typically hide soiled underwear. It is not unusual for soiling to take place after bathing, because of reflex stimulation.

School performance and attendance are affected, as the child's offensive odour becomes a target for scorn and derision from classmates. The child is not well-liked by peers because of it, and may be severely rejected by the parents as a result of the symptom. The rejection by peers and parents causes further withdrawal and other behavioural manifestations.

THERAPEUTIC MANAGEMENT

Treatment is directed towards the cause of the soiling. Diet, lubricants, and a toilet ritual that encourages the child to establish normal defecation are used (Younger and Hughes, 1983). Faecal impaction is relieved by suppositories, phosphate enemas, and or oral aperient. Customary dosages are usually insufficient. Dietary changes may be helpful, such as elimination of milk and dairy products and increased amounts of high-fibre foods, such as fruits, vegetables, and cereals, as well as increased fluids. Behaviour therapy may be indicated to eliminate any fear that has developed as a result of painful defecation. Frequently, psychotherapeutic intervention with the child and the family becomes necessary.

IMPLICATIONS FOR NURSING

The prevailing attitude of nurses towards the family of a child with encopresis is one of no-fault, thus relieving the guilt of both parents and child. A thorough history of the soiling is essential — when soiling began, how often it occurs, under what circumstances, and if the child uses the toilet successfully at all (Stroh, Stern, and McCarthy, 1989). Since parents and children are reluctant to volunteer information, direct questioning about the soiling is more successful. Following the history, a complete physical assessment is performed.

Education regarding the physiology of normal defecation, toilet training as a developmental process, and the treatment outlined for the particular family is prerequisite to a successful outcome. Parents are relieved to know that other parents share this problem and are surprised to know that functional changes that take place as the condition develops make control of seepage impossible. Many parents complain that their children soil because they do not take time from play for a bowel movement. Actually, the child may be unaware of a prior sensation and unable to control the urge once it begins. They may be so accustomed to bowel accidents that they are unable to smell or feel it and even deny soiling when it occurs (Stroh, Stern, and McCarthy, 1989).

The regimen prescribed for stimulating elimination is outlined and explained to parents. Sitting the child on the toilet at routine intervals is not recommended, because it may intensify parent-child conflict and result in a power play. Enemas may be needed for impactions, but long-term use prevents the child from assuming responsibility for defecation (Johns, 1985). Initially, lubricants are given liberally, but these stimulants often cause abdominal cramps that can be a frightening experience for a child.

Family counselling is directed towards reassurance that most problems resolve successfully, although the child may have relapses during periods of stress, such as vacation or illness. If encopresis persists beyond occasional relapses, the condition will need to be re-evaluated. Behaviour modification techniques are explained, and the family is assisted with a plan suited to their particular situation.

BEHAVIOURAL DISORDERS IN SCHOOL-AGED CHILDREN

Several classification systems have been employed to outline the various problems of middle childhood that interfere with development, learning and social relationships. Although there is no universal categorization, most authorities seem to broadly classify behavioural disorders in some manner that identifies mental subnormality, learning disabilities, neuroses, psychoses and antisocial behaviour. Many disorders have a major organic or developmental component, whereas others are seen almost exclusively in children of school age. Still others are primarily problems of adolescence, and many extend throughout the course of childhood. Very often, an organic disease (at other times, emotional problems) produce somatic symptoms of greater or lesser seriousness.

The variety and extent of emotional and behavioural disorders of childhood are too numerous to be considered here; some are discussed elsewhere (for example, mental retardation in Chapter 22 and sensory impairment in Chapter 23).

ATTENTION DEFICIT–HYPERACTIVITY DISORDER

Attention deficit–hyperactivity disorder (AD-HD) is the latest term applied to various behaviour problems that in some way impair the child's capacity to profit from new experiences.

The syndrome of manifestations affects a significant number of children and is ten times more frequent in boys than in girls. The difficulties are most often school related, behavioural or academic, and difficulties with social relationships in general are often manifested by aggressive behaviour and mood lability that interferes with peer relationships and makes disciplining difficult.

Considerable confusion and disagreement exist regarding AD-HD [previously known as attention deficit disorder (ADD)] with or without hyperactivity, hyperactivity, minimal brain damage (MBD), and hyperkinesis. Not all children display hyperactivity. In addition, there are individuals who evidenced AD-HD at an earlier age but who no longer demonstrate the hyperactivity. Many of the children have specific learning disabilities.

Early identification of affected children is needed, since the characteristics of the disorder significantly interfere with the normal course of emotional and psychological development. In an attempt to cope with attention deficit, many of these children develop maladaptive behaviour patterns that are a deterrent to psychosocial adjustment. Their behaviour evokes negative responses from others, and repeated exposure to negative feedback adversely affects the child's self-concept.

The term *specific learning disabilities* refers to the behavioural outcomes of impaired functioning in central processing such as dyslexia, dysphasia, and inability to calculate or draw. It is primarily an educational concern and mentioned briefly at the conclusion of this segment.

AETIOLOGY

The aetiology of AD-HD is uncertain, obscure, and often speculative. As the definition implies, it may be related to virtually any illness or trauma affecting the brain that occurs at any stage of development — before, during, or after birth. Multiple causes, including psychosocial factors, are probably involved.

Behavioural and learning disorders have been noted in children with some of the sex chromosomal abnormalities. For example, in girls with Turner syndrome there is a high incidence of impaired spatial abilities and right-left directional sense, and a large number of boys with Klinefelter syndrome have learning, behavioural, or peer problems. A sex-linked factor may be operating, because the hyperkinetic syndrome is much more common in boys than in girls.

A popular theory is the concept of a developmental lag. Distractibility, short attention span, and impulsiveness are all normal characteristics of children at a much younger developmental level. Since the symptoms tend to diminish with age, it is postulated that this may have an anatomical basis; that is, a maturational lag in myelination of the prefrontal cortex that takes place through adolescence. In addition, hyperactivity may be merely a normal variant of innate temperament in some children who represent the extreme end of the normal distribution curve for activity.

Support for a biochemical aetiology is suggested by the way in which a majority of hyperactive children respond to central nervous system stimulant drugs. In these children, there appears to be an absence or insufficiency of norepinephrine, a neurotransmitter that normally appears in high concentrations in areas of the brain that are associated with activity level, mood and awareness. Another theory suggests some alteration in the reticular activating system of the midbrain, a key area for controlling consciousness and attention, that interferes with its function of filtering out extraneous stimuli. Consequently, these children are unable to focus on one stimulus, but are compelled to respond to every stimulus in the environment. Central nervous system stimulants that increase the level of norepinephrine and/or activate the reticular activating system cause a reduction in the undesired behaviour. The fact that these children show few, if any, symptoms in a stress situation (such as the clinician's or principal's office) provides additional support to this hypothesis, because stress increases the level of norepinephrine.

Interest in diet as a factor in hyperactivity continues to generate controversies. There are those who believe that the observed behavioural patterns are related to an innate sensitivity to certain food items and/or food additives. Although this theory does not have wholehearted support, some children do show improvement when certain foods are eliminated from their diet, particularly those containing salicylates, those with specific additives such as artificial colouring, sweeteners and preservatives, and those that are more hyperallergic, such as chocolate, cow's milk, and eggs (Egger, Stolla, and McEwen, 1992). Others have no adverse effects from sucrose or aspartame (the artificial sweetener Nutrasweet or Equal) (Shaywitz *et al*, 1994; Wolraich *et al*, 1994).

CLINICAL MANIFESTATIONS

The behaviours exhibited by the child with AD-HD are not unusual aspects of child behaviour. The difference lies in the quality of motor activity and developmentally inappropriate inattention, impulsivity and hyperactivity the child displays. The manifestations may be numerous or few, mild or severe, and will vary with the developmental level of the child. Any given child will not have every manifestation that is characteristic of a syndrome, and the degree of severity is highly variable. Mild manifestations of the symptoms may not be apparent in a good educational and family environment, whereas severe symptomatology will be recognizable even in the most healthy and accommodating environment. Every dysfunctional child is, in some respects, different from all other children with AD-HD.

Most behavioural manifestations are apparent at an early age, but the learning disabilities may not become evident until the child enters school. The symptoms are more prominent before age ten, after which they become more subtle, tending to diminish with advancing age. The disorder is unpredictable; it may remit spontaneously at any age, and the number of years a child will require treatment is unknown. Although it appears that most characteristics of AD-HD do not extend into adolescence, increasing evidence indicates that hyperactive children

do not necessarily outgrow their symptoms (Brown, 1986). Concomitant emotional difficulties are frequent, and there are indications of continued difficulties in school, difficulties with peers and authority figures, and continued aggressive behaviour.

Children who are unable to function normally in their home and school environment will meet with constant failure and rejection and will react with hostility or other inappropriate behaviours. Their frequent recognition that they are 'bad' or not 'right inside' will produce a negative self-concept and reactive hostility.

The basic characteristics outlined in Box 17-4 reflect disturbances in central processing. These criteria are the basis for establishing a diagnosis of AD-HD. Research has found that children with AD-HD exhibit attention, behavioural and cognitive impairments, whereas children with AD-HD without hyperactivity show deficits in an attention/cognitive dimension (Berry, Shaywitz, and Shaywitz, 1985). Management problems and antisocial behaviour are associated with hyperactivity: increased impulsivity is not associated with attention deficits in the absence of hyperactivity.

The same researchers found that there are sex differences in children with AD-HD. Disruptive, uncontrolled behaviours are more frequent among boys; girls with AD-HD without hyperactivity display poor self-esteem and are significantly older than boys with the same type of AD-HD. Girls with AD-HD with or without hyperactivity are more likely to suffer peer rejection than boys. Girls may not be diagnosed as readily as boys, and cognitive deficits play a more prominent role with girls; behavioural disturbances increase the likelihood of identification for boys.

PROCESS OF DIAGNOSIS

Neurological and psychological examinations are useful in detecting specific defects, and observations made in a familiar environment may help confirm suspicions. However, it is the history that ultimately determines the diagnosis. The child seldom displays symptoms in the practitioner's office and acts reasonably normal in a one-to-one relationship.

A history (medical and developmental) and description of the child's behaviour should be obtained from as many observers of the child as possible, including parents, teachers, and health professionals. It should include descriptions of the child's behaviour in home and school situations. In obtaining descriptive material, the interviewer must question the observers carefully, because some people, especially parents, may be so concerned with gross behaviours that they overlook less distressing but equally important symptoms. For example, parents may report a 'colicky' infant, a child who began to run as soon as he walked, a toddler who is compelled to touch everything in sight, and a child who resists sleep until exhausted. A history of delayed or atypical language development is associated with specific learning disabilities. A pregnancy and birth history may provide clues to a situation that might have produced an episode of hypoxia.

◆ **BOX 17-4**

Diagnostic criteria for attention deficit – hyperactivity disorder

Note: Consider a criterion met only if the behaviour is considerably more frequent than that of most people of the same mental age.

A. A disturbance of a least six months during which at least eight of the following are present:

(1) Often fidgets with hands or feet or squirms in seat (in adolescents, may be limited to subjective feelings of restlessness)

(2) Has difficulty remaining seated when required to do so

(3) Is easily distracted by extraneous stimuli

(4) Has difficulty awaiting turn in games or group situations

(5) Often blurts out answers to questions before they have been completed

(6) Has difficulty following through on instructions from others (not due to oppositional behaviour or failure of comprehension), e.g., fails to finish chores

(7) Has difficulty sustaining attention in tasks or play activities

(8) Often shifts from one uncompleted activity to another

(9) Has difficulty playing quietly

(10) Often talks excessively

(11) Often interrupts or intrudes on others, e.g., butts into other children's games

(12) Often does not seem to listen to what is being said to him or her

(13) Often loses things necessary for tasks or activities at school or at home (e.g., toys, pencils, books, assignments)

(14) Often engages in physically dangerous activities without considering possible consequences (not for the purpose of thrill-seeking), e.g., runs into street without looking

Note: The above items are listed in descending order of discriminating power based on data from a national field trial of the DSM-III-R criteria for Disruptive Behaviour Disorders.

B. Onset before the age of seven

C. Does not meet the criteria for a Pervasive Developmental Disorder

Criteria for Severity of Attention Deficit—Hyperactivity Disorder:

Mild: Few, if any symptoms in excess of those required to make the diagnosis and only minimal or no impairment in school and social functioning

Moderate: Symptoms or functional impairment intermediate between 'mild' and 'severe'

Severe: Many symptoms in excess of those required to make the diagnosis and significant and pervasive impairment in functioning at home and school and with peers

From American Psychiatric Association, 1987.

A physical examination, including a detailed neurological evaluation, will help rule out any severe neurological disorders. Psychological testing, especially projective tests, is valuable in determining visual-perceptual difficulties, problems with spatial organization, and other phenomena that suggest cortical or diencephalic involvement, and it helps to identify the child's intelligence and achievement levels. Psychiatric and other disorders are ruled out, including lead poisoning, petit mal seizures, partial hearing loss and psychosis.

THERAPEUTIC MANAGEMENT

Management of the child with AD-HD usually involves a multiple approach that includes family education and counselling, medication, proper classroom placement, environmental manipulation and sometimes psychotherapy.

Behavioural therapy and psychotherapy

Behavioural therapy is often successful for the child whose behaviour, mood and reality-perception disturbances are not severe. This consists of a relatively controlled environment in conjunction with behaviour modification techniques, family counselling and/or psychotherapy (see Implications for Nursing). Diet modification has proved to be effective for some children, but is not a standard treatment.

IMPLICATIONS FOR NURSING

Nurses, especially school nurses, are active participants in all aspects of management of the child with AD-HD. Nurses in the community setting work with families in the home on a long-term basis to help plan and implement therapeutic regimens and to evaluate the effectiveness of therapy. They are in the best position to coordinate services and to liaise between other health and education professionals directly involved in the child's therapy programme. School nurses have an understanding of the child's special needs and work with teachers. The nurse in any setting (community, school, hospital) can provide support and guidance to children and families during the difficult tasks associated with growing up with a disabling condition.

The management of the child with AD-HD begins with an explanation to the parents and the child about the diagnosis, including the nature of the problem and the concept of the underlying central nervous system basis for the disorder. Most parents are confused and feel some measure of guilt. To some, it is confirmation of the fear that the child may be 'crazy' or has some irreversible, serious disease; to others, it is a relief. They need the opportunity to express their feelings and suspicions. A common complaint of parents is that health professionals have not listened to what they have to say about their child.

The parents need information about the prognosis and an understanding of the treatment plan. The greater their understanding of the disorder and its effects, the more likely they will be to carry out the recommended programme of therapy. It is important that they understand that the therapy is not necessarily a panacea and that it will extend over a long period.

This has particular significance for changes they need to make in environmental management. Reading material to help the child and family can be obtained from a variety of sources.

Medication

Parents are reminded that some medications require 2-3 weeks to achieve an effect. Other medications are begun at low dosage and increased until the desired effect is attained. When evaluating the child's response to the medication, it is helpful to obtain reports from the teacher as well as from the parents, since the parents may see the child when the effects of the drug are wearing off. Observing the child's behaviour through visits to home and school is useful for assessing attention span, interactional patterns with others at school, and behaviours with academic tasks. The nurse can consult with the teacher about the child's behaviour in general. This information provides data needed to regulate dosage based on recorded, systematic observations of the child's behaviours in at least two settings.

Parents need to be informed of the possible side effects of the medication — anorexia, blurred vision, and sleeplessness — which usually disappear after several weeks. A common complaint is that the child becomes quiet and very sensitive, crying at the slightest provocation. Sleeplessness is reduced by administering the medication early in the day. Another troublesome side effect is depressed growth, probably caused by interference with the release of growth hormone; therefore, the doctor may sometimes discontinue the drug on weekends or on vacations to allow for some catch-up growth, although some believe there is no theoretical or practical advantage to this practice (Brown, 1986).

Children on tricyclic antidepressants display a dramatic increase in the incidence of dental caries (Slome, 1984). The marked anticholinergic action of the drugs increases saliva viscosity and produces a dry mouth. Emphasis on rigorous dental hygiene, conscientious home fluoride treatment, regular visits to the dentist, limited intake of refined carbohydrates and use of artificial saliva is an important nursing function. The child should be kept well hydrated.

In children in whom a salicylate-free diet relieves the disordered behaviour, which is caused by an allergic reaction to food additives, the parents may need help with the child's diet; for example, it is the nurse's responsibility to find out what the child can eat and help the parents find sources for the proper foods, especially if the child is on a special metabolic diet.

Psychiatric, psychological and social therapies

Generally, psychotherapy is relatively unsuccessful in the treatment of the basic characteristics of AD-HD. However, psychotherapy is sometimes useful in children who have suffered negative experiences to the extent that their self-image is threatened. Often, children with this disorder describe themselves as stupid or 'mentally retarded'. They are different from other children and they know it. Although they have strengths, they seldom have an opportunity to demonstrate them. Consequently, they develop coping mechanisms to deal with their negative self-image. They are restless and disruptive, resort to clowning, and develop somatic symptoms. They may become apathetic, resort to daydreaming, appear 'not to care', or display perfectionistic perseverance in the attempt to do well. Shy children may withdraw. The child with behaviour problems is the one who will get help earlier than the quiet child. Therefore, the quiet child may not receive help until the problem is well advanced, which is a disadvantage because remediation takes longer when it is begun with older children. Both child and family may need help during certain periods of stress.

SPECIFIC LEARNING DISABILITY

Learning-disabled children are those who exhibit a disorder in one or more of the basic psychological processes involved in understanding or in using spoken or written language. The disability may be manifested in disorders of listening, thinking, talking, reading, writing, spelling or calculating. They include conditions that have been referred to as perceptual disabilities and developmental aphasia. They do not include learning problems, which result primarily from visual, hearing, or motor disabilities, mental retardation, emotional disturbances or environmental disadvantage.

Learning disabilities occur frequently in children diagnosed with AD-HD with or without hyperactivity. *Learning disability is an educational term, and schools, recognizing this disability, provide services for affected children.* The types of disabilities include *dyslexia* (difficulty with reading), *dysgraphia* (difficulty with writing), *dyscalculia* (difficulty with calculation), right-left confusion, and short attention span. Most affected children are hypoactive, and their needs are frequently overlooked or their behaviour is mistaken for retardation. Special education classes offer help and encouragement for these children and their parents, and early recognition facilitates the process of gaining the special assistance needed to function in the school situation.

TIC DISORDERS

A tic is an involuntary, recurrent, random, rapid, highly stereotyped movement or vocalization, occurring in 10-35% of all children. Tics can be simple or complex and involve motor movements, eye movements or vocalizations. Tics decrease during concentration, are markedly diminished during sleep, and become more exaggerated when the affected children are under stress or excitement. Obsessive-compulsive behaviours, in the form of ritualistic activities, also may be present and can occur in individuals free of tics. No major psychological components are evident (Golden, 1987). Many medications can precipitate tics.

Almost all mild *transient tic disorders* of childhood are self-limited and disappear within a few months, usually less than a year. The most common tics involve the eyes, head and face, and treatment does not affect recovery. Tic disorders can begin at any time during childhood. Boys are affected at least three times as often as girls and, in over 50% of cases, tics are observed in other family members (Avery and First, 1989).

Tic disorders that persist beyond one year are considered to be chronic and consist of one form of either motor or vocal manifestations but not both (Erenberg, 1988). The most severe of the chronic tics is Gilles de la Tourette's syndrome.

Diagnosis of a tic disorder is based on clinical observations. Most tic disorders resolve by late childhood or adolescence without treatment, and cause no physical harm to the child. Therapeutic management consists primarily of support to the child and family, reassurance about prognosis, and education regarding expectations (of the child) for control. Although the child is able to suppress the manifestations to some degree, persistent pressure for control constitutes an additional stress to an affected child.

EMOTIONAL DISORDERS OF CHILDHOOD

Some disorders affecting children produce distress to both children and their families. No organic basis can be detected in most situations. Some are amenable to interventions by health professionals.

POST-TRAUMATIC STRESS DISORDER

It is now believed that children do not outgrow the fear that follows a traumatic shock (Terr, 1989). Seemingly alright following a traumatic event, children tend to relive or visualize these experiences for years and retain some fear specific to the event. They continue to function in school as always, but have a feeling of foreboding regarding the future. It is important for children to talk about their experience and fears, and to be reassured regarding the randomness of such events.

The way in which children react depends on what resources the individual child brings to the situation — coping strategies used, defence mechanisms summoned, and the child's social environment. Post-traumatic stress disorder (PTSD) has also been observed in physically abused children (McCormack, Burgess, and Hartman, 1989). Each individual reacts differently. Although most children rapidly adapt, studies indicate that children do not outgrow the trauma, but can be helped to overcome their sense of hopelessness (Terr, 1989).

The initial response to the stressor is intense arousal, which usually lasts for a few minutes to one or two hours, depending on the stressor and the individual. The stress hormones are at the maximum as the individual prepares for 'fight' or 'flight'.

The second phase, which lasts approximately two weeks, is one in which defence mechanisms are mobilized. It is a period of quiescence in which the event appears to have produced no impression. The victims feel numb, and stress hormone secretion is absent. The reaction is outside their awareness, not well controlled, and involves some type of behavioural pattern. Defence mechanisms are less adaptive to specific situations and may not be what the situation demands.

Denial that anything is wrong is a frequently observed defence mechanism.

The third phase is one of coping, which normally extends over 2-3 months. It is one of consciously directed inquiry. The victims want to know what happened and appear to be getting worse, when actually they are getting better. Numerous psychological symptoms may be apparent, such as depression, repetitive phenomenon, or phobic and anxiety symptoms. Children frequently display repetitive actions. They play out the situation over and over again in an attempt to come to terms with their fear. Flashbacks are common. This phase can be self-perpetuating, and a prolonged reaction can develop into an obsession with the traumatic event. Some traumatic effects remain indefinitely (Terr, 1989). Researchers have also found that children with PTSD have impaired startle inhibition, indicating long-lasting alteration in the brainstem circuits that help startle modulation (Ornitz and Pynoos, 1989).

IMPLICATIONS FOR NURSING

Children need to deal with any traumatic event; much depends on the intensity of the event and their reaction to it. Their reactions depend heavily on their social environment and the way in which their caretaking adults react to the event. Children usually react in much the same manner as their caregivers (contagious pathology); therefore, it is important to be aware of these reactions also. In the second, or defence, phase of the PTSD the appropriateness of the defence mechanism must be assessed, and children must be assisted in application of their defence. If children do not engage in some catharsis or if their defence phase is prolonged, they may need referral for special psychological help.

Coping is a learned response, and children in the third phase can be helped to use their coping strategies to deal with their fear. Children usually are willing to accept reasoning. Those who are assisted in their catharsis and allowed expression will survive without serious lasting effects. They should be encouraged to play out the stress and/or discuss their feelings about the event. If they are unable to do this, they may become obsessed with the traumatic event and may need professional help.

Children need professional help if any of the phases of PTSD are prolonged. Boys tend to be more likely to have a prolonged defence phase than girls. Occasionally, the event will be unrecognized, and the affected child will engage in what is considered to be unusual behaviour. In the case of any sudden change in behaviour, the child needs to be assessed for a traumatic event — 'Did something happen?' When the change in behaviour is determined to be due to a traumatic event, treatment can be implemented.

SCHOOL PHOBIA

School phobia is a term used to describe children, other than beginning students, who resist going to school because of dread of the school situation, concerns with leaving home, or both. As a rule children below the age of 13 who fear school tend to be separation-anxious — children who are afraid of leaving the people they love. For these children, the term 'school refuser' is rapidly replacing 'school phobia', which is more accurate after the age of 13 years. By this time, children have worked through immature separation fears (Last *et al*, 1987). Children may also fear going to school because of a threatening relationship with a 'bully' or teacher.

Anxiety that frequently verges on panic is a constant manifestation, and children can develop symptoms as a protective mechanism to keep them from facing the situation that distresses them. Physical symptoms are prominent and may affect any part of the body — anorexia, nausea, vomiting, diarrhoea, dizziness, headache, leg pains, or abdominal pains, to name a few. They may even develop a low-grade fever. A striking feature of school phobia is the prompt subsiding of symptoms when it is evident that the child can remain at home. Another significant observation is absence of symptoms on weekends and holidays, unless they are related to other places such as Sunday school or parties. Occasional mild reluctance is not uncommon among school children, but if the fear continues for longer than a few days, it must be considered a serious problem — a warning of an important personality problem.

Unlike most other behaviour problems of children, school phobia is more common in girls than in boys. There is no relationship to socioeconomic status, ethnic origin or other subcultural affiliation, and no particular age predominates. The onset is usually sudden and precipitated by a school-related incident. A poor attendance record for trivial reasons can be elicited by a careful history.

AETIOLOGY

School phobia can be caused by several factors. Sometimes the complaints can be related to a transient, specific cause such as fear of a mismatched or overcritical teacher, fear of failing an examination or giving an oral recitation for a painfully shy child, or discrimination based on race, dress, or physical defect. Sometimes it may be related to a school bully or threatening gang. An insecure home situation in which the child fears that he may be deserted by a parent while he is gone may be the basis of anxiety, especially if the parent has previously threatened to leave for some reason.

A frequent source of fear is separation anxiety based on a strong dependent relationship between the mother and child, in which the child is reluctant to leave the mother and she is equally reluctant (even though this may be unconscious) to have the child leave her. The intense need for closeness between mother and child is normal in infancy, but the persistence of this type of relationship into childhood is inappropriate. Characteristically, these children are not afraid to go to school, but rather they are afraid to leave home. They fear something dreadful might happen while they are separated from their families. No event is required to trigger the associated behaviours. However, symptoms may be precipitated by a situation that intensifies the mutual dependency between the mother and the child, such as illness, arrival of a new baby, move to a strange neighbourhood or a new school, or parental discord.

In some instances, children have an unrealistic, exaggerated view of their abilities and achievements. When they feel threatened by incidents that challenge their estimation of themselves, such as a minor episode that leads to embarrassment, return to school after an absence, transfer to another class, or even imagined social or academic failure, they become anxious, withdraw and frequently seek proximity to the mother. Sometimes the step-up in expectations at school or change of important personnel at school (e.g., teacher or principal) is a contributing factor. Occasionally, the child may be suffering from an undiagnosed learning disability.

THERAPEUTIC MANAGEMENT

The treatment for school phobia depends on the cause. The children really *want* to go to school, but cannot force themselves to do so. They are not delinquent children; they are anxious, tense, and distressed because they are unable to muster enough courage to attend school. If the cause of the problem is an examination, relationships with a bully, or a mismatch between teacher and child, it can be dealt with accordingly. When the child is helped to understand and cope with the fear, the symptoms usually disappear. In severe cases, when returning to school is unsuccessful, professional psychiatric consultation is usually desirable to help identify possible distorted family relationships or a personality disturbance in the child, and to help both child and family understand the sources of the problem.

IMPLICATIONS FOR NURSING

The primary goal for the child with school phobia is to *return the child to school*. The longer the child is permitted to stay out of school, the more difficult it is to re-enter. Well-meaning parents or others who permit the child to stay away from school and support any efforts with written excuses only confirm the child's feelings of worthlessness and inability to cope. Parents must be convinced gently, but firmly, that *immediate* return is essential and that they are the ones who must insist upon the child's return for it to be effective.

Some modifications in school attendance might be necessary for the child with severe symptoms. The child who is unable to return to regular classes may be allowed to go to school on a part-time basis, and it may be necessary to transport the child to and from school or even have a parent attend class with the child. However, this practice is not allowed to continue for an unlimited time, and the time limit should be agreed beforehand. The essential factor is that the child must return to school right away, maintain the pattern of going, and remain there even while a solution is being worked out. The school nurse can provide both teacher and parents with support in carrying out this plan.

Prevention

Certain clues indicate that a child may be subject to first-time fear; thus children can be helped to adjust to it. Extra preparation may be needed for children who are very fearful, have trouble adjusting to new situations, or are very clinging (Last *et al*, 1987). Many individuals continue to manifest some form of fear throughout their school careers. When the problem is identified early, treated effectively, and negative emotions surrounding school minimized, a child is less likely to carry residual fears throughout life.

Parents who suspect that their child may be especially frightened may want to accompany the child to school and wait outside the classroom the first day. A gradual breakaway over succeeding days should relieve their child's and their own anxiety. If the distress extends beyond two weeks, professional help may be needed (Last *et al*, 1987).

CHILDHOOD DEPRESSION

Depression in childhood is often difficult to detect, because children may be unable to express their feelings and tend to act out their problems and concerns. Authorities agree that childhood depression exists, but they do not agree whether or not it is the same as adult depression. The characteristics of depression are largely determined by parallel developments in symbolism, language and cognitive development (Aylward, 1985). Younger children demonstrate a more cause-and-effect relationship between the stressors and the depressive manifestations, which are primarily the biological deprivation syndromes. As children develop, the relationships between stressful events and depression are less clear. Their reactions are less physiological and more cognitively complex, and the observed behaviours tend to be age specific (Herzog and Rathburn, 1982). Depressed children exhibit a distinctive style of thinking characterized by low self-esteem, hopelessness and a tendency to explain negative events in terms of personal shortcomings (McCauley *et al*, 1988).

Some states of depression are temporary; for example, acute depression precipitated by a traumatic event. This might include a period of hospitalization, loss of a parent through death or separation, or loss of a significant relationship with something (a pet), someone (a friend or family member), or a place (move from a familiar home, neighbourhood, or city). The easily identified manifestations include a sad, downcast face, tearfulness, irritability, and withdrawal from previously enjoyed activities and relationships. The child tends to spend more time in solitary activities, especially television viewing, and schoolwork is impaired. Some children become more dependent and clinging; others become more aggressive and disruptive. Sleeplessness and/or loss of appetite are not common reactions. Responses are not sustained and can be modified with social and family support.

More serious and less common are depressive responses to more chronic stress and loss; these are frequently observed in children with chronic illness or disability. There is no apparent precipitating event, but there is often a history of frequent disruptions in important relationships. Commonly, there is also a history of depressive illness in one or both parents during the child's lifetime. The manifestations are similar to responses to acute reactions. Some of the primary and associated symptoms that are observed in depressed children and the DSM-III criteria currently used for establishing a diagnosis of major depression are outlined in Box 17-5. There are several similarities among major depressive disorders in childhood and some other psychological disorders.

◆ BOX 17-5

Primary and associated symptoms of depression in children

Primary Symptoms
- Depressed affect (dysphoric mood)
- Anhedonia (loss of pleasure)
- Self-deprecatory ideation
- Tearfulness
- Low sense of self-worth/self-esteem
- Social withdrawal
- Impairment of schoolwork
- Psychomotor retardation
- Difficulty with biological functions (sleeping, eating)
- Morbid ideation/suicide attempts

Associated Symptoms
- Irritability
- Moodiness
- Social interactive difficulties
- Pathological guilt
- Fatigue
- Somatic complaints
- Anxiety, decreased concentration
- Obsessive rumination and thoughts
- Attention deficit
- Feelings of helplessness/hopelessness
- Enuresis/encopresis
- Aggressive and explosive behaviors

From Aylward, 1985.

THERAPEUTIC MANAGEMENT

Depressed children are managed by a health team specially prepared in the care of children with mental disorders. Treatment of depression should be undertaken in the least constrictive environment, usually outpatient management. Suicidal children are admitted to hospital for protection if the family is unable to provide constant monitoring. For children with associated disruptive behaviour, such as fighting with peers or family, hospitalization may be advised. Most therapeutic regimens focus on pharmacotherapy with tricyclic antidepressants as the most commonly prescribed medication. Other medications include monoamine oxidase inhibitors and lithium (Weller and Weller, 1989).

IMPLICATIONS FOR NURSING

Management of childhood depression is usually psychotherapeutic and highly individualized. Nurses should be aware that depression is a problem that can easily be overlooked in the school-aged child and can interrupt normal growth and development. Recognizing depression and making appropriate referrals is an important nursing function. Identification of the depressed child requires a careful history (health, growth and development, social and family health), interviews with the child, and observations by the nurse, parents and teachers. If the child is placed on antidepressants, the child and family must be instructed to monitor the child for side effects of the specific drug prescribed. (See Chapter 19 for a more definitive discussion of depression and suicide.)

KEY POINTS

- Middle childhood is a relatively healthy period and most problems encountered are not considered serious.
- The skin serves several important functions: protection, prevention of loss of body fluids, heat regulation and sensation.
- It is important for nurses to be able to describe skin lesions accurately.
- The stages of wound healing consist of inflammation, fibroplasia, scar contraction and scar maturation.
- Wound healing occurs by primary, secondary or tertiary intention.
- Bacterial, viral and fungal infections are common in childhood.
- Prevention of infection or reinfection is the primary goal in management of pediculosis.
- Contact dermatitis may involve a reaction to a primary irritant or sensitization.
- Teaching prevention of thermal injury, especially sunburn, is an important nursing function.
- Adverse reactions to drugs occur more often in the skin than in any other organ.
- Dental care continues to be important; most frequent problems that arise are dental caries and malocclusion.
- The behavioural disorders of childhood are primarily attention deficit-hyperactivity disorder and tic disorders.
- Some of the major emotional disorders involving school-aged children include school phobia and depression.

REFERENCES

American Psychiatric Association: *Diagnostic and statistical manual of mental disorders*, ed 4 (DSM-IV), Washington, DC, 1994, American Psychiatric Association.

Anders JE, Leach EE: Sun versus skin, *AJN* 83:1015,1983.

Avery ME, First LR (eds): *Pediatric medicine*, Baltimore, 1989, Williams & Wilkins.

Aylward GP: Understanding and treatment of childhood depression, *J Pediatr* 107:1, 1985. As modifiied *from Diagnostic and statistical manual of mental disorders*, ed 3—revised (DSM-III-R), Washington, DC, 1987, American Psychiatric Association.

Baker MD, Moore SE: Bites and scratches: when pets fight back, *Contemp Pediatr* 6(6):76, 1989.

Baker MD, Moore SE: Human bites in children, *Am J Dis Child* 141:1285, 1987.

Barnett NK: Pruritus. In Hoekelman RA, editor: *Primary pediatric care*, St Louis, 1987, Mosby-Year Book.

Berkowitz R, Ludwig S, Johnson R: Dental trauma in children and adolescents, *J Pediatr* 19:166, 1980.

Berry CA, Shaywitz SE, Shaywitz BA: Girls with attention deficit disorder: a silent minority? A report on behavioral and cognitive characteristics, *Pediatr* 76:801, 1985.

Bonadio WA, Wagner V: Efficacy of TAC anesthetic for repair of pediatric lacerations, *Am J Dis Child* 142:203, 1988.

Brown G et al: Enhancement of wound healing by topical treatment with epidermal growth factor, *N Engl J Med* 321:76, 1989.

Brown GL: Attention deficit disorder. In Gellis SS, Kagan BM: *Current pediatric therapy 12*, Philadelphia, 1986, WB Saunders.

Chun Y-T, Berkelhamer JE, Herold TE: Dog bites in children less than 4 years old, *Pediatr* 69:119, 1982.

Clore ER: Dispelling the common myths about pediculosis, *J Pediatr Health Care* 3:28, 1989.

Coody D: There is no such thing as a good tan, *J Pediatr Health Care* 1:125, 1987.

Dische S et al: Childhood nocturnal enuresis: factors associated with outcome of treatment with an enuresis alarm, *Dev Med Child Neurol* 25:67, 1983.

Egger J, Stolla A, McEwen LM: Controlled trial of hypersensitisation in children with food-induced hyperkinetic syndrome, *Lancet* 339(8802):1150, 1992.

Elliot DL *et al*: Pet-associated illness, *N Engl J Med* 313:985, 1985.

Erenberg G: Identification and management of patients with tics/Tourette syndrome, *Feelings* 30:21-24, 1988.

Esposito AL, Adams D: Infection of skin and subcutaneous tissue. In Eichenwald HF, Stroder J (eds): *Current therapy in pediatrics-2*, Toronto, 1989, BC Decker, Inc.

Friman PC: A preventive context for enuresis, *Pediatr Clin N Am* 33:871, 1986.

Friman PC *et al*: Do encopretic children have clinically significant behavior problems? *Pediatr* 82:407, 1988.

Friman P, Warzak W: Nocturnal enuresis: a prevalent, persistent, yet curable parasomnia, *Pediatrician* 17:38, 1990.

Golden GS: Movement disorders: sorting the benign from the serious, *Contemp Pediatr* 4(5):77, 1987.

Gorrell R: Practical pointers, *Consultant* 25:154, 1985.

Hagelgans NA: Pediatric skin care issues for the home care nurse, *Pediatr Nurs* 19(5):499, 1993.

Herzog GB, Rathburn JM: Childhood depression, *Am J Dis Child* 136:115, 1982.

Houts AC: Noctural enuresis as a biobehavioral problem, *Behav Ther* 22(2):133, 1991.

Hurwitz S: That summer rash could be Lyme disease, *Contemp Pediatr* 5(6):74-82, 1988.

Johns C: Encopresis, *AJN* 85:153, 1985.

Kochman, Doron: What to do about facial trauma, *Contemp Pediatr* 6(7):72, 1989.

Krasner PR: The treatment of avulsed teeth, *J Pediatr Health Care* 4:86, 1990.

Last CG *et al*: Separation anxiety and school phobia: a comparison using DSM-III criteria, *Am J Psychiatry* 144:653, 1987.

LeVeen HH, LeVeen RF, LeVeen EG: The mythodology of povidone-iodine and the development of self-sterilizing plastics, *Surg Gynecol Obstet* 176(2):183, 1993.

Levine MD: Disordered processes of elimination. In Levine MD *et al*: *Developmental-behavioral pediatrics*, Philadelphia, 1983, WB Saunders.

Madden EJA: Itch, *J Pain Sympt Manag* 1(2):97, 1986.

McCauley E *et al*: Cognitive attributes of depression in children and adolescents, *J Consult Clin Psychol* 56:903, 1988.

McCormack A, Burgess AW, Hartman C: Familial abuse and post-traumatic stress disorder, *J Traumatic Stress* 1:231, 1989.

McLaury P: Head lice - pediatric social disease, *AJN* 83:1300-1303, 1983.

Moffatt MEK, Kato C, Pless IB: Improvements in self-concept after treatment of nocturnal enuresis: randomized controlled trial, *J Pediatr* 110:647, 1987.

Moffatt MEK *et al*: Desmopressin acetate and noctural enuresis: how much do we know? *Pediatrics* 92(3):420, 1993.

Nicol NH: What's new with sunscreens? Choices - choices - choices, *Pediatr Nurs* 15:417-418, 1989.

Ornitz EM, Pynoos RS: Startle modulation in children with post-traumatic stress disorder, *Am J Psychiatry* 146:866, 1989.

Rappaport LA: Enuresis. In Levine M *et al*: *Developmental-behavioral pediatrics*, ed 2 , 1992, WB Saunders.

Rappaport LA: The treatment of nocturnal enuresis (where we are now), *Pediatrics* 92(3):465, 1993.

Rettig S *et al*: Abnormal diurnal rhythm of plasma vesopressin and urinary output in patients with enuresis, *Am J Physiol* 256(4, pt 2): F664, 1989.

Rule JTD: Recognition of dental caries, *Pediatr Clin North Am* 29:439, 1982.

Rushton HG: Nocturnal enuresis: epidemiology, evaluation, and currently available treatment options, *J Pediatr* 114 (Suppl):691, 1989.

Shaywitz DA *et al*: Aspartame, behavior, and cognitive function in children with attention-deficit disorder, *Pediatrics* 93(1):70, 1994.

Shaywitz SE, Shaywitz BA: Neurochemical correlates of attention deficit disorder, *Pediatr Clin North Am* 31:387, 1984.

Sieggreen MY: Healing of physical wounds, *Nurs Clin North Am* 22:439, 1987.

Slome B: Rampant caries: a side effect of tricyclic antidepressant therapy, *Genet Dent* 32:494, 1984.

Terr L: Traumatic events in childhood have lasting effects, *AAP News* 5(5):1, 1989.

Weller EB, Weller RA: Pediatric management of depression, *Pediatr Ann* 18:104, 1989.

Welch JS: Efficacy and safety of povidone-iodine underscored, *J Emerg Nurs* 18(3):191, 1992.

Wolraich ML *et al*: Effects of diets high in sucrose or aspartame on the behavior and cognitive performance of children, *N Engl J Med* 330(5):301, 1994.

Younger JB, Hughes LS: No-fault management of encopresis, *Pediatr Nurs* 9:185, 1983.

FURTHER READING

Skin Disorders: General

Gelfant BB: Healing skin wounds, *Point of View* 23(3):6, 1986.

Parker F: The skin and the elements: sun, plants, and stinging and biting organisms, *Emerg Care Q* 4(3):21, 1988.

Infections

Brady M: Common viral skin problems of childhood: warts and molluscum, *J Pediatr Health Care* 2:208, 1988.

Caputo RV: Fungal infections in children, *Dermatol Clin North Am* 4:137, 1986.

Scabies and Pediculosis

Brimhall CL, Esterly NB: Uninvited guests: skin infestations of childhood, *Contemp Pediatr* 7(1):18, 1990.

Lane AT: Scabies and head lice, *Pediatr Ann* 16:51, 1987.

Malathion for head lice, *Med Lett Drugs* Ther 31:110, 1989.

Park BR, Smith D: Treatment of head lice and scabies in children, *Pediatr Nurs* 15:522, 1989.

Systemic Disorders

Elliot DL *et al*: Pet-associated illness, *N Engl J Med* 313:985, 1985.

Chemical and Physical Injuries

Hurwitz S, Rhodes A, Wiley H: *For every child under the sun: a guide to sensible sun protection*, New York, 1986, The Skin Cancer Foundation.

Moss JR: Playing it safe in the sun, *Child Nurse* 4(3):1,1986.

Miscellaneous Skin Disorders

Datloff J, Esterly NB: A system for sorting out pediatric alopecia, *Contemp Pediatr* 3(10):53, 1986.

Pau AK *et al*: Drug allergy documentation by physicians, nurses, and medical students, *Am J Hosp Pharm* 46:558, 1989.

Rasmussen JE: Psoriasis in childhood, *Dermatol Clin North Am* 4:99, 1986.

Bites and Stings

Adamski DB: Assessment and treatment of allergic response to stinging insects, *J Emerg Nurs* 16:77, 1990.

Dental Problems

Featherstone JDB: The mechanism of dental decay, *Nutr Today* 22(3):10, 1987.

Feldman AL, Aretakis DA: Herpetic gingivostomatitis in children, *Pediatr Nurs* 12:111, 1986.

Herrmann HJ, Roberts MW: Preventive dental care: the role of the pediatrician, *Pediatr* 80:107, 1987.

Kronmiller JE: Oral soft tissue abnormalities in children, *Pediatr Nurs* 13:161, 1987.

McDonald RE, Avery DR: *Dentistry for the child and adolescent,* ed 8, St Louis, 1988, Mosby-Year Book.

McGuire S: Fluoride content of bottled water, *N Engl J Med* 321:836, 1989.

Robertson JS, Maddux JE: Compliance in pediatric orthodontic treatment: current research and issues, *Child Health Care* 15:40, 1986.

Weinstein LB, Abrams RA, Ayers CS: Increasing awareness of sugar ingestion among children, *Pediatr Nurs* 14:277, 1988.

Elimination Disorders

Ack M, Norman ME, Schmitt BD (in discussion): Enuresis: the role of alarms and drugs, *Patient Care* 19:75, 1985.

Castiglia PT: Encopresis, *J Pediatr Health Care* 1:335, 1987.

Castiglia PT: Nocturnal enuresis, *J Pediatr Health Care* 1:280, 1987.

Friman PC, Warzak WJ: Nocturnal enuresis: a prevalent, persistent, yet curable parasomnia, *Pediatrician* 17:38, 1990.

Gibson LY: Bedwetting: a family's recurrent nightmare, *MCN* 14:270, 1989.

Johns C: Encopresis, *AJN* 85:153, 1985.

Novello AC, Novello JR: Enuresis, *Pediatr Clin North Am* 34:719, 1987.

O'Regan S et al: Constipation: a commonly unrecognized cause of enuresis, *Am J Dis Child* 140:260, 1986.

Rushton H: Nocturnal enuresis: epidemiology, evaluation, and current available treatment options, *J Pediatr* 114:691, 1989.

Shapiro SR: Enuresis: treatment and overtreatment, *Pediatr Nurs* 11(3):203, 1985.

Stadtler AC: Preventing encopresis, *Pediatr Nurs* 15:282, 1989.

Attention Deficit–Hyperactivity Disorder

Anderson V, Oberklaid F: Developmental dysfunction: learning disabilities and attention deficits in children and adolescents, *Curr Opinion Pediatr* 1:156, 1989.

Golden GS: A hard look at fad therapies for developmental disorders, *Contemp Pediatr* 4(10):47, 1987.

Kelly PC *et al*: Self-esteem in children medically managed for attention deficit disorder, *Pediatr* 83:211, 1989.

Levine MD, Melmed RD: The unhappy wanderers: children with attention deficits, *Pediatr Clin North Am* 29:105, 1982.

Niebuhr VN, Smith KE: Simple tests to assess behavior problems, *Contemp Pediatr* 7(1):117, 1990.

Behaviour Disorders

Cowell JM: Dilemmas in assessing the health status of children with learning disabilities, *J Pediatr Health Care* 4:24, 1990.

Epstein M, Cullinan D: Depression in children, *J School Health* 56:10, 1986.

Finn PA: Self-destructive behavior in school-age children: a hidden problem? *Pediatr Nurs* 12:198, 1986.

Gilligan J: Understanding learning disabilities, *School Nurse* 3(4):22, 1987.

Kenealy P: Children's strategies for coping with depression, *Behav Ther* 27:27, 1989.

Emotional Disorders

Dolgan JI: Depression in children, *Pediatr Ann* 19:45, 1990.

Mitchell J, Varley C, McCauley E: Depression in children and adolescents, *Child Health Care* 16:290, 1988.

Nelms BC: Assessing childhood depression: do parents and children agree? *Pediatr Nurs* 12:23, 1986.

Page-Goertz S: Recurrent abdominal pain in children, *Issues Compr Pediatr Nurs* 11:179, 1988.

Porter E: The school nurse's role in school phobia, *School Nurse* 3(4):8, 1987.

Promoting emotional health—role of the nurse practitioner, *J Pediatr Health Care* 2:1-2, 1988.

Rhyne MC *et al*: Children at risk for depression, *AJN* 12:1379, 1986.

Schmitt BD: School refusal, *Pediatr Rev* 8:99, 1986.

Simmons JE: When to refer to a child psychiatrist, *Contemp Pediatr* 4(2):77, 1987.

Sledden EA, Maddux JE, Katnick RJ: Psychological assessment and consultation in pediatric neurology, *Child Health Care* 16:43, 1987.

Chapter 18

Physical Health Problems of Adolescence

LEARNING OUTCOMES

After studying this chapter you should be able to:

◆ Identify the common physical problems of adolescence.
◆ Outline generalized measures the adolescent suffering from acne can implement to reduce the inflammatory process and improve the appearance of acne.
◆ Define Turner syndrome.
◆ Define Klinefelter syndrome.
◆ Identify the two most common infections of the male reproductive system, noting the differences.
◆ Define delayed menarche/amenorrhoea.
◆ Discuss human immunodeficiency virus infection and the adolescent.
◆ Give an explanation of the term PID.
◆ Define the glossary terms.

GLOSSARY

comedone Blackhead associated with acne

diabetogenic state A health condition manifested by signs and symptoms of diabetes mellitus

IUD Intrauterine device

IVDU Intravenous drug user

miscarriage Spontaneous abortion

PID Pelvic inflammatory disease

PIH Pregnancy-induced hypertension

STD Sexually transmitted disease

A dolescence is a period of rapid biological growth and psychosocial transition. Atkinson *et al* (1993) defined it in this way:

Adolescence refers to the period of transition from childhood to adult-hood. Its age limits are not clearly specified, but it extends roughly from age 12 to the late teens, when physical growth is nearly complete. During this period, the young person develops to sexual maturity and establishes an identity as an individual apart from the family (Atkinson *et al*, 1993).

It is frequently perceived as a time of optimum wellness. Logically, promotion of optimum wellness, which emphasizes not only absence of disease but also a positive sense of well-being and personal achievement, should have its inception during this developmental stage. However, a noticeable increase in risk-taking behaviours occurs with adolescents. This can lead to death or disability during this otherwise generally healthy time of life. Examination of information about the health status of adolescents has lead to increasing concern among many health professionals (e.g., nurses, doctors, psychologists, social workers, nutritionists, educators) who are involved with research or delivery of health services to this group (Millstein, 1989).

Efforts to combat the magnitude of health problems that occur during adolescence have never been sufficient. Surveys reveal that most health care professionals believe they received inadequate educational preparation to deal with the complexity of health and behavioural issues experienced by teenagers. Nurses have not been exempt from this void in professional education (Bearinger and Gephart, 1987). The emphasis of this chapter is on the physical problems of adolescence and the nurse's role in health management.

COMMON HEALTH PROBLEMS OF ADOLESCENCE

There are several health problems that have their onset in adolescence or are more prominent at this stage of development than at earlier or subsequent ages.

ACNE

Adolescents are subject to the same skin conditions that affect school-aged children, such as bacterial, viral, and fungal infection; contact dermatitis; and drug reactions. However, there is one skin disorder, acne vulgaris (common acne), that is not limited to adolescents, but appears predominantly at this time (Fig. 18-1). Acne is an almost universal occurrence during these years and involves anatomical, physiological, biochemical, genetic, immunological and psychological factors of significant import.

It is estimated that about 70% of the population will have had acne by the end of the teenage years, and as many as 25-50% of children before the age of ten have evidence of the disorder. However, the peak incidence is in late adolescence,

at about age 16-17 in girls and 17-18 years in boys. The disorder is more common in males than in females (Rothman and Lucky, 1993). After this, the disease usually decreases in severity, but may persist into adulthood. The degree to which an individual is affected may range from a few isolated comedones to a severe inflammatory reaction. Although the disease is self-limited and is not life-threatening, its significance to the affected adolescent is immense, and it is a mistake to underestimate the impact that it can have on young persons.

AETIOLOGY

The aetiology of acne is still unclear, although several factors appear to be related to its development. Its distribution in families and a high degree of concordance in identical twins suggest that hereditary factors predispose to susceptibility to acne. Androgens are implicated, since observations indicate a diminished effect on acne during pregnancy, its virtual absence

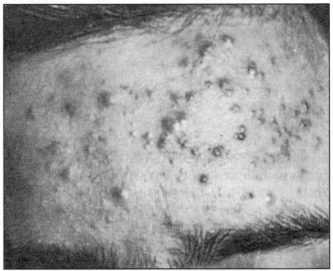

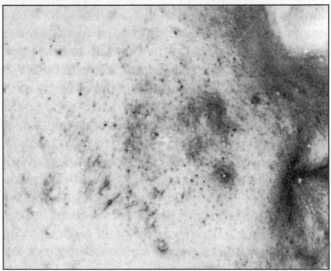

Fig. 18-1 *Acne vulgaris.* Papular pustules and comedones. From Stewart WD, Danto JL, Maddin S: *Dermatology: diagnosis and treatment of cutaneous disorders,* ed 4, St Louis, 1978, Mosby–Year Book Inc.

in castrated males and young children, and its higher incidence in adolescent males. The disease seems to be aggravated by emotional stress; hot, humid environments; some stimulant drugs; and the premenstrual period. There is no positive evidence that any specific foods are factors, except perhaps with individual youngsters.

THERAPEUTIC MANAGEMENT

There is little evidence that treatment shortens the duration of the entire course of the disease. However, much can be done to control acne, reduce the inflammatory process and scarring, and improve the appearance. All too often parents and health professionals have a tendency to dismiss acne as a normal part of 'growing up'.

The treatment of acne requires long-term management with patience and perseverance from the patient, family, and health professionals. Unlike many dermatological conditions the acne lesions resolve slowly, and improvement may not be apparent for many weeks. Also, in early stages of treatment the persistent postinflammatory erythematous macules may lead the patient to believe the therapy has been ineffective.

No single therapeutic agent is effective in the management of acne except in a few mild cases. It is usually more effective to employ a combination of therapies. The treatment most commonly consists of measures directed towards improving the general health of the youngster, removing comedones, preventing their formation, controlling excessive sebaceous gland activity, controlling infection and preventing scar formation. The treatment consists of general measures of care and specific treatments, largely determined by the type of lesions involved and the preference of the practitioner. Although the combination of therapies and brands selected vary, the objectives are similar.

General measures

A general explanation of the disease process and the plan of care is given to the youngster, with emphasis on compliance to carry out the programme faithfully for as long as the process persists.

Improvement of the adolescent's overall health status is part of the general management. Adequate rest, moderate exercise, a well-balanced diet, reduction of emotional stress and elimination of any foci of infection are all part of general health promotion. There is no convincing evidence to implicate any single dietary item or combination of foods in the exacerbation of acne, with the possible exception of iodides and bromide in therapeutic amounts. Occasionally, a youngster will demonstrate an aggravation of symptoms after each ingestion of a given food. In such instances, the food is eliminated for a time to assess its influence on the disease.

ALTERATIONS IN GROWTH AND MATURATION

The absence of sexual maturation at a time when other children are experiencing positive evidence of sexual development and its associated spurt in growth and physical strength is a matter of concern to both parents and affected child. In most instances, the slow growth is a simple physiological or constitutional delay that merely represents one end of the normal, genetically influenced variation of pubertal growth. These children will go through normal puberty in their late teens and catch up with their more rapidly developing peers. However, this becomes a psychosocial problem for some young people.

Less benign is delayed development caused by endocrine disorders or chromosomal aberrations. In other situations, delayed development may be a result of malnutrition or chronic diseases that are serious enough to retard the developmental process, such as malabsorption, chronic asthma, and poorly controlled diabetes mellitus.

ASSESSMENT

Serial measurements of growth are plotted periodically on standard growth charts to determine the pattern of growth and to compare the individual child with the norm for that particular age group. When assessing children in the extremes of height ranges, it is important to compare their height with the height of their parents and siblings. As a whole, children usually can be categorized into one of six groups according to their pattern of maturation (Box 18-1).

PROCESS OF DIAGNOSIS

Clinical diagnosis of delayed development can usually be determined with relative ease on the basis of the simple criteria outlined in Box 18-2.

◆ BOX 18-1

Categories of growth according to pattern of maturation

Average children—closely approximate the mean for height and weight at all ages

Early-maturing children—tall in childhood but not unusually tall adults

Early-maturing children who are also genetically tall—above the mean at all ages

Late-maturing children—shorter than average in childhood but not necessarily short adults

Late-maturing children who are also genetically short—below the mean at all ages

Children who deviate significantly from the normal growth curve—very rapid- and early-maturing children; much later- and slower-maturing children

---

SHORT STATURE

Short stature is a nonspecific finding that may be the first manifestation of a serious disorder, or it may be of no consequence medically. It is often the reason an adolescent is brought to the attention of health professionals.

The problem is more distressful to boys than to girls. Therefore, it is boys who more often seek assistance. Since the psychosocial factors are of importance, and there are rare situations in which delayed development is caused by a pathogenic condition, it is important to determine the reason for the short stature.

In most instances the cause of short stature is either *familial short stature* or a simple *constitutional growth* delay in which the child appears to be delayed because development is behind that of age-mates. Familial short stature refers to otherwise healthy children who have ancestors with adult height in the lower percentiles, and whose height during childhood is appropriate for genetic background.

Constitutional growth delay refers to individuals (usually boys) with delayed linear growth, in whom commensurate delays in skeletal and sexual maturation suggest that they will reach normal adult height.

Often, there is a history of a similar pattern of growth in one of the parents or other family members of children with constitutional growth delay. The untreated child will proceed through normal changes as expected on the basis of bone age. These changes, although occurring later than in the average child, will appear in normal sequence and manner, and treatment is not usually indicated.

THERAPEUTIC MANAGEMENT

Management consists of continued medical observation, attention to general health and nutrition, and psychological support. Further assurance can be provided by predicting the youngster's adult height from available tables and other criteria devised from comprehensive studies of child development.

◆ BOX 18-2

Diagnosis of delayed development

Family History
History of similar delayed growth and maturation in parents and/or other relatives
Height and weight of siblings at comparable ages and their present measurements are helpful
Child's History
Prenatal—factors that could influence normal growth
Birth—height and weight (usually appropriate for gestational age)
Concurrent chronic diseases
Past illnesses such as head injuries and gastrointestinal, renal, or neurological disorders
Dietary habits
Strength and stamina
Susceptibility to infection
Attainment of development milestones
School progress
Emotional problems or problems of social adjustment, especially those that may indicate past family instability (prolonged emotional upset has a significant influence on growth)
Previous Growth Pattern
Records available:
Decrease during any year or period (e.g. second year of life, just before puberty)
Remained relatively small throughout growth period with a growth curve parallel to or slightly below 3rd percentile
Records not available:

Determine when first noticed that the child was small compared with other children
Physical Examination
Accurate measurements of height and weight (child stripped to underclothing)
Measurement of body proportions
Crown to pubis
Pubis to heel
Signs of sexual development using standard criteria
Breast budding in girls
Testicular enlargement (testicular volume greater than 2 ml) in boys
If present, normal sexual development can be expected to follow in 1 to 2 years
Bone Age
Assessed from wrist x-ray films (always delayed)
Endocrine Studies
Hormonal investigations essentially normal
Growth hormone (GH) response
Gonadotropin levels
Gonadotropin-releasing factor (GnRF) responses
Usually low for the child's chronological age but consistent with bone age
Plasma testosterone and oestrogen levels consistent with bone age
Urinary excretion of 17-ketosteroids consistent with bone age
Corresponding change in endocrine response consistent with normal pubertal changes occurs with maturation

Very often, the longer a youngster takes to pass through puberty, the better are the prospects for achieving an acceptable adult height, since epiphyseal fusion is more advanced in youngsters who mature earlier.

Most youngsters can be managed with detailed explanation, reassurance and observation. Unlike growth hormone deficient children, who do not usually demonstrate maladjustment, children with constitutional delay often display characteristic behavioural difficulties.

Where the growth delay is accompanied by poor self-esteem and incompetence, the psychosocial situation is such that for the youngster (usually a boy) who is miserable as a result of peer ridicule and indignities, hormonal therapy in addition to psychological support has proved to be advantageous, and many authorities recommend treatment in these instances.

Often, a brief course of androgen therapy induces rapid development of secondary sexual characteristics. Lengthy treatments or large doses affect epiphyseal closure; therefore, criteria for selection of candidates must be precise. Treatment usually results in excellent growth, a significant improvement in self-image adjustment, and a dramatic increase in both school-related and extraschool social activity (Rosenfeld, Northcraft and Hintz, 1982; Wilson and Rosenfeld, 1987).

Thyroid hormone is of no value unless hypothyroidism is present; and human growth hormone, although capable of increasing height, is expensive and generally confined to the treatment of growth hormone deficiency.

The dangers of therapy are a possible diabetogenical effect and overuse in the treatment of short stature. There may be pressures from parents who want their children to be taller than they are genetically constituted.

IMPLICATIONS FOR NURSING

Deviation from the normal course of puberty is always of concern to affected adolescents, and to some it assumes monumental proportions.

Most of the problems of delayed development are caused by simple constitutional delay of puberty, and in this situation the child can be assured that the normal course of events will eventually occur. This is not always reassuring to such children. They are impatient to grow and are not easily convinced. Even after direct and thorough discussion of growth and the normal variations in rate and timing of maturation, they often doubt that they will grow. It is important to maintain contact with these children, convey to them a concern about their feelings, and let them know that they are accepted as they are.

One of the difficulties related to a size that is incongruent with chronological and mental age is the manner in which others, especially adults, relate to the child. People quite naturally respond to children with short stature as though they are younger than their age. Consequently, these children often react with babyish or juvenile behaviour, thus setting in motion a circular pattern of behaviour and response. Conversely, children who are tall or physically advanced for their age are treated as though they are more advanced than their years.

> ## ◆ BOX 18-3
>
> ### Characteristics of Turner syndrome
>
> Significant short stature, which is common to all (many adults are less than 150 cm, or 5 feet, tall) and begins to be apparent at about 4 years, becoming more severe by 8 years of age
>
> Redundant skinfolds on the neck (webbed neck) with low posterior hairline (present in 40% to 50% of cases)
>
> Multiple pigmented nevi
>
> Rather 'old' facial appearance with micrognathia and low-set and sometimes malformed ears
>
> Shield-shaped chest with widely spaced hypoplastic nipples
>
> Increased carrying angle at the elbow (cubitus valgus)
>
> Cardiac anomalies, principally coarctation of the aorta or aortic valvular stenosis
>
> Moderate degrees of learning difficulty (poor spatial perception)
>
> Abnormal growth patterns: absence of normal growth spurts and sexual development at puberty with primary amenorrhoea and sterility; sparse pubic and axillary hair; gonads replaced by fibrous streaks

They are often considered to be retarded or behaviourally immature when they actually perform according to the normal behavioural expectations for their age.

Listening to distressed adolescents and conveying to them genuine interest and concern are prerequisites to any successful intervention. Counselling and therapy are individualized to meet the needs of each youngster and his or her problems. Encouraging these children to accentuate the positive aspects of their bodies and personalities with sound health practices and good grooming helps foster a more positive self-image.

TALL STATURE

Tallness is rarely a problem to boys, but for girls it can be a source of acute distress. Although the average height for both boys and girls is steadily increasing, there is still a small group of children who are excessively tall when compared with their contemporaries. In almost all cases, the tall girl is expressing an expected genetically determined growth pattern. Many girls like the idea of being tall and manage to cope effectively with any height-related problems that may arise. For others, it can be a source of intense anxiety and a severe social handicap.

IMPLICATIONS FOR NURSING

Nursing intervention with a girl of tall stature has much in common with that for children with short stature. It is primarily directed towards support of the child and the family. Sometimes the concern is primarily that of the parent, especially a tall mother who does not wish to have her daughter experience the same distress as the mother did as a child. The child may not view it as a problem. Therefore, the initial goal of care is to determine the source and extent of the perceived problem. Some teenage girls are overwhelmed by a height of 170 cm, whereas most youngsters are well adjusted and happy with a height of 178 cm. Much depends on the social attitudes that affect what is considered to be a desirable or acceptable body image.

TURNER SYNDROME

Although Turner syndrome is often recognized at birth, it is diagnosed most frequently at puberty because of three outstanding features: short stature, sexual infantilism and amenorrhoea. The incidence of the condition in the population is considered to be from 1:2500 to 1:8000 live female births (Cohen, 1984).

AETIOLOGY

Turner syndrome is caused by absence of one of the X chromosomes. Consequently, the number of chromosomes in these girls is 45 [44 pairs of autosomes and one X chromosome (45,X)]. The reason for the growth retardation is unknown. The child's growth is usually normal until three years of age then slows, gradually drifting away from the normal growth curve. There is no prepubertal growth spurt.

CLINICAL MANIFESTATIONS

A tentative diagnosis can be made on the physical appearance in most instances. Only a few persons with this syndrome manifest all the possible clinical features listed in Box 18-3 (Fig. 18-2). Girls with Turner syndrome have been found to have difficulty with peer relationships and understanding social cues. They exhibit more behavioural problems, especially in relation to immature, socially isolated behaviour (McCauley, Ito, and Kay, 1986).

PROCESS OF DIAGNOSIS

Diagnosis can be suspected in the newborn period by the presence of lymphoedema and characteristic hairline, in childhood by short stature, and at puberty by delayed development. Absence of a Barr body, or negative chromatin, is consistent with the disorder. Definitive diagnosis is confirmed by chromosome analysis.

THERAPEUTIC MANAGEMENT

Therapy is always individualized for these girls and consists primarily of hormone treatment and psychological counselling for both child and parents. When the diagnosis is made early enough, growth is stimulated with administration of androgen therapy with or without growth hormone at about 10-11 years

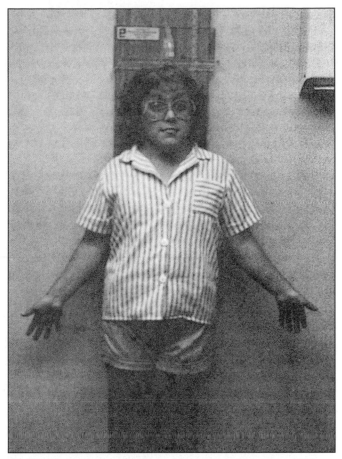

Fig. 18-2 Turner syndrome in 13-year-old girl. Note short stature (126 cm; weight, 37.2 kg), webbed neck, increased carrying angle, and broad chest.

of age. Androgen therapy is followed at about age 14 or 15 by oestrogen therapy, to promote the development of secondary sex characteristics. When linear growth begins to level off, the dosage is increased and combined with progesterone to effect a normal cyclic pattern. Responses to oestrogen therapy vary.

IMPLICATIONS FOR NURSING

Most of the nursing interventions described for the youngster with short stature apply to the girl with Turner syndrome. The diagnosis should be made as early as possible so that she and her parents can be counselled regarding what to expect. The girl is given some idea of the final height projected in her particular case and the expectations for developing secondary sex characteristics as a result of successful treatment. The girl and parents should understand that the short stature will probably remain despite hormone therapy. It is often reassuring for them to see others who have undergone successful treatment and who are able to adapt to the compromised stature.

It is important that families understand some of the health problems associated with the disorder. The tendency towards obesity may require special attention to diet. The increased tendency for otitis media presents the need for prompt treatment of respiratory infections and regular hearing tests. Other complications commonly associated with Turner syndrome that should be evaluated periodically include hypertension, cardiac anomalies, thyroid disorders, inflammatory bowel disease and urinary tract anomalies.

Because children with Turner syndrome may have more difficulty with peer relationships and in understanding social cues, and may have more behaviour problems, they often require more structure to socialize and complete tasks.

KLINEFELTER SYNDROME

Young boys with Klinefelter syndrome are seldom seen before puberty, at which time varying degrees of failure of adolescent virilization occur. Some males are not detected until they appear for evaluation for infertility. All have absence of sperm in the semen (azoospermia), small testes, and defective development of secondary sex characteristics.

AETIOLOGY

Klinefelter syndrome is the most common of all chromosomal abnormalities and is caused by the presence of one or more additional X chromosomes.

CLINICAL MANIFESTATIONS

There are no physical characteristics that are helpful in detecting Klinefelter syndrome before the advent of puberty, with the possible exception of mental retardation. Mental impairment of varying degrees is a frequent finding and appears to have a direct relationship to the number of X chromosomes in the cells. The severity of retardation increases with the number of X chromosomes. Characteristic features of the Klinefelter syndrome are listed in Box 18-4.

Boys with Klinefelter syndrome have essentially normal intelligence, but may have gross motor skill difficulties, developmental language delay, poor verbal skills, and reduced auditory memory. Shyness, passivity, behavioural problems, and school difficulties are often associated with the disorder, but this may be related to the difference in body build, delayed development, and tendency towards clumsiness (Bender *et al*, 1983; Walzer *et al*, 1982).

PROCESS OF DIAGNOSIS

Diagnosis is suspected on the basis of clinical manifestations, and the extra chromosome is apparent on chromosomal analysis.

THERAPEUTIC MANAGEMENT

The major effort in medical treatment is directed towards enhancing the masculine characteristics through administration of male hormones, principally testosterone. Cosmetic surgery will eliminate embarrassment for a boy with gynaecomastia. As with other pubertal development, psychological counselling and support are considered along with psychological problems associated with developmental difficulties.

◆ **BOX 18-4**

Characteristics of Klinefelter syndrome

Tall, eunuchoid figure with legs disproportionately long in relation to the trunk

Sparse facial and pubic hair, often with female distribution pattern

Gynaecomastia of some degree (seen in half the cases and often the reason for seeking medical advice)

Small, firm, and insensitive testes; small penis in childhood (usually normal at adolescence)

Aspermia or oligospermia

IMPLICATIONS FOR NURSING

Special nursing considerations in the care of the youngster with Klinefelter syndrome include counselling or referral for problems associated with peer relationships, techniques for handling difficult social situations, and increasing self-esteem (Cohen and Durham, 1986).

DELAYED DEVELOPMENT CAUSED BY PATHOLOGICAL CONDITIONS

A small number of children suffer delay of growth or onset of adolescence because of disorders that may or may not be amenable to treatment. From a worldwide point of view, the most common cause of short stature and/or delayed development is probably inadequate nutrition; however, the major disorders that produce delayed development are most often caused by chronic diseases, endocrine dysfunction, and primary gonadal dysgenesis, usually Turner or Klinefelter syndromes.

CHRONIC DISEASES

Chronic diseases can interfere with growth, but unless the illness is unduly prolonged, catch-up growth will occur. There are several chronic illnesses that fit in this category, and these are discussed where appropriate. Those encountered most frequently are respiratory disorders such as asthma, cystic fibrosis, and recurrent upper respiratory infection; illnesses caused by defective organ or disturbed immune mechanisms; gastrointestinal diseases such as parasitic infestations, cystic fibrosis, and other malabsorption syndromes; cardiac anomalies and blood dyscrasias such as sickle cell anaemia; and chronic renal disturbances, especially renal tubular acidosis. It appears that the duration of the illness is more significant than the intensity in its effect on growth, although the precise length of time necessary to affect growth permanently has not been determined.

SKELETAL DEFECTS

Skeletal disorders that affect growth in stature are principally those described as dwarfism. Most are caused by a variety of congenital defects and disorders, such as achondroplasia, and some of the inborn errors of metabolism, such as Hurler or Hunter syndrome. Whereas some are readily apparent at or shortly after birth, milder cases may not be recognized until later in life and are diagnosed by x-ray and biochemical examinations.

ENDOCRINE DYSFUNCTION

The major hormones that promote physical growth are thyroid hormone, growth hormone and sex hormones. Insulin can be said to promote growth by its effect on carbohydrate metabolism, whereas cortisol inhibits growth. Therefore deficiencies of growth-promoting hormones or an excess of cortisol can cause growth retardation in children. Endocrine deficiencies can be the result of abnormal secretory function in the glands responsible for their production, the pituitary hormones that stimulate their secretion, or the releasing factors from the hypothalamus. In some instances, growth retardation may be the result of increased production of factors that inhibit hormone secretion.

Sex hormone deficiency

Sex hormone deficiency that causes delayed puberty can occur as a result of either pituitary dysfunction or hypogonadism. A hypofunctioning pituitary gland can produce a deficiency in either the gonadotropic hormones, which retards maturation of the gonads, or growth hormone, which will diminish total growth during childhood. In addition, there is a large variety of disorders that cause absence or deficiency of sex hormone secretion by their effect on the gonads directly. These may be genital abnormalities that are related to defective gonadal differentiation or those that are associated with functional abnormalities of the already differentiated fetal gonad. The largest group of disorders in which deficient gonadal development is a prominent feature includes the sex chromosomal aberrations.

HEALTH PROBLEMS OF THE MALE REPRODUCTIVE SYSTEM

It is fortunate for the male that most of the parts of the reproductive system are external and therefore visible and palpable. In most instances, obvious anomalies have been identified and corrective measures instituted during childhood. A number of the conditions present in the newborn or young child can affect the development of appropriate sexuality during adolescence. Functional disorders such as enuresis may persist, and gynaecomastia, a cause of concern in the pubescent male, may become a problem. Conditions related to urinary function frequently involve the renal system as a whole. Some conditions are related to trauma; others are associated with sexually transmitted diseases.

INFECTIONS

The two most common infections in adolescent males are urethritis and epididymitis. Although both types of infection may be distressing for the adolescent male, a course of antibiotic therapy and reassurance by the health worker is generally all the treatment required.

URETHRITIS

Urethritis is the most common genital tract infection occurring among adolescent males. Symptoms of dysuria, penile discharge, and itching on urination are the result of urethral inflammation. Most urethral infections among adolescent males are related to sexual contact. Infections caused by coliform bacteria are usually the result of congenital anomalies in the urogenital tract, most of which are identified in childhood. Therefore among sexually active males, *Neisseria gonorrhoeae*, *Chlamydia trachomatis*, and *Ureaplasma urealyticum* are the most common aetiological agents. Other less frequently implicated organisms are *Trichomonas vaginalis*, yeast, herpes simplex virus (HSV), *Staphylococcus saprophyticus*, and *Escherichia coli* (Bowie, 1990; Larson and Shapiro, 1988).

Concerns about asymptomatic urethritis among adolescent males have received greater attention. Although men with new gonococcal infections are asymptomatic, some may complain of mild burning and discharge, which are difficult to ignore. Since asymptomatic males remain sexually active, they may continually transmit these bacteria to their female partners. Also, complications such as epididymitis can occur as a result of these sexually transmitted pathogens. Routine urinalysis of the first 10-15 ml of voided urine from the sexually active male has been advocated to screen for the presence of asymptomatic urethritis.

Diagnosis is usually made through laboratory techniques, such as urethral Gram stain or appropriate cultures. Treatment is administration of a suitable antibiotic.

EPIDIDYMITIS

Epididymitis is an inflammatory reaction of the epididymis of the testicle as a result of either infection or, occasionally, local trauma. The clinical presentation is a sudden onset of unilateral scrotal pain, redness, and swelling. Associated symptoms include urethral discharge, dysuria, fever, and pyuria. The diagnosis is made on the basis of urinalysis, Gram stain, and urethral culture. Mild presentation of symptoms may mimic testicular torsion, which requires immediate surgical intervention. Therefore immediate evaluation by a practitioner is indicated. Treatment consists of analgesics, scrotal support, bed rest, and initiation of appropriate antibiotic therapy. For males with a culture-verified sexually transmitted disease, treatment of their sexual partners is also indicated.

PENILE PROBLEMS

Common congenital anomalies of the penis are almost always detected and corrected in infancy or early childhood, although some boys who need several operative procedures to repair a hypospadias (the most common congenital deformity of the penis) reach adolescence with a penis that looks different from those of their friends. A few who have received no medical care have uncorrected deformities that can cause serious psychological problems during this sensitive period of development, when being different is intolerable. These young boys need to be identified for surgical repair of the defect.

Uncircumcized males may encounter some problems during adolescence. Some young men have tight foreskins that cannot be retracted over the enlarging glans; some may not cleanse the area properly even though they know that the foreskin should be retracted and the penis bathed regularly. These boys suffer more frequently from infection. *Penile carcinoma* occurs almost exclusively in uncircumcised people and is more common in those in whom circumcision was delayed until adolescence.

Trauma to the penis may occur in various ways, including burns and accidental injuries. The frenulum (the fold on the lower surface of the glans that connects it with the prepuce) can be torn after retraction of the foreskin, masturbation, or coitus. It can be terrifying to the young boy, but usually heals spontaneously with minimum care. However, any extensive bleeding may require suturing of the tissues.

Other problems include an *adherent penis*, a common condition in which the ventral surface of the penis adheres to the scrotum, producing a severe ventral curvature during erection, thus preventing satisfactory coitus; and *priapism*, a rarer disorder consisting of painful, sustained penile erection without sexual desire. The adherent penis can be surgically corrected; treatment of priapism is directed towards treating conditions with which it is often associated, such as sickle cell disease, leukaemia, the use of certain medications, and central nervous system lesions.

A frequent concern of adolescent males is *penile size*. Many boys erroneously assume that the size of the penis is directly related to virility and male prowess; the boy with a small penis is often the object of remarks from more amply endowed agemates. A concerned young man can also be reassured that the size of the flaccid penis is unrelated to the size of the erect penis and that the length is usually adequate for satisfactory coitus.

TESTICULAR TUMOURS

Tumours of the testes are not a common condition, but when manifested in adolescence they are generally malignant. The usual presenting symptom is a heavy, hard, painless mass, palpable on the anterior or lateral aspect of a testis. The tumour may be smooth or nodular and does not transilluminate unless accompanied by a hydrocele. The involved testicle hangs lower and is therefore more susceptible to trauma. Although not all scrotal masses are malignant, any firm swelling of the testis demands immediate evaluation. If a firm swelling is noted, the youth should be subjected to a minimum of preoperative palpation and referred immediately for surgical exploration. There is seldom delay in seeking medical advice if the mass is painful, but in the absence of pain the condition may go unattended for some time.

Treatment for testicular cancer consists of surgical removal of the affected testicle (orchiectomy) and the adjacent lymph nodes, if affected. If metastases are evident in more distant nodes or organs, chemotherapy and radiation therapy are implemented.

VARICOCELE

A varicocele most often appears as a scrotal mass and is characterized by elongation, dilation, and tortuosity of the veins of the spermatic cord superior to the testicle. It is ordinarily small and requires no treatment. Varicoceles are found most often on the left side because of the greater length of the left spermatic vein and its entry into the left renal artery; the right spermatic vein enters the vena cava directly and at a lesser angle, which may be a source of future difficulty (Sawczuk *et al*, 1993). A varicocele can be palpated as a worm-like mass situated above the testicle that decreases in size when the youth is recumbent and becomes distended and tense when he is upright. There may be discomfort during sexual stimulation in some males. The condition frequently improves spontaneously. Surgical ligation of the varicocele is recommended when there is volume loss of the ipsilateral testis; in other cases periodic re-examination is the usual suggested approach (Nagar and Levran, 1993).

TESTICULAR TORSION

Torsion of the testicle is a condition in which the tunica vaginalis, which normally encases the testicle, fails to do so and the testis hangs free from its vascular structures. This condition can result in partial or complete venous occlusion with rotation around this vascular axis. In severe torsion, the organ can become swollen and painful; the scrotum becomes red, warm, and oedematous and appears to be immobile or fixed as a result of spasm of the cremasteric fibres.

Typically, the onset is acute and frequently follows intense activity or trauma. Often, the patient has a history of a similar pain that was shorter in duration and less intense. An increased incidence of testicular torsion has also been observed in cold weather, presumably caused by contraction of the cremaster muscle (Williamson, 1983). The cold-related torsion is more common in younger than in older children because of the more reactive reflex in young children. Nausea, vomiting, abdominal pain and a slight fever may accompany the pain. Surgical intervention is mandatory to prevent haemorrhagic necrosis.

HEALTH PROBLEMS OF THE FEMALE REPRODUCTIVE SYSTEM

Unlike the male, the reproductive organs of the female are located internally; therefore, abnormalities are less apparent and more difficult to detect. Infections are a major source of morbidity, especially those described as sexually transmitted diseases. However, the problems most often brought to the attention of health professionals are those related to menstruation — menstrual delay, irregularities or discomfort. Any concern is worthy of consideration and understanding from health professionals.

THE GYNAECOLOGICAL EXAMINATION

One of the most difficult experiences the adolescent girl may face is the gynaecological examination (Box 18-5). Whether it is her first experience or not, she is most likely to be apprehensive. Almost all adolescent girls are extremely self-conscious about their bodies and the changes taking place. The girl will need continuing support in the form of anticipatory guidance regarding what she can expect, and suggestions of what she can do to help herself relax during the procedure.

The teenager is usually given the option of choosing a supportive person to be present during the pelvic examination. Suggested individuals might include a parent (usually the mother), best friend, boyfriend, or other health professional, such as the nurse or medical assistant.

Description of the examination includes information about the procedure, and words that describe anticipated feelings and

---

◆ **BOX 18-5**

Indications for pelvic examination of adolescent females

Menstrual disorders:

Amenorrhea

Irregular uterine/vaginal bleeding

Dysmenorrhea unresponsive to therapy

Undiagnosed abdominal pain

Any sexually active adolescent

Request for a prescription method of birth control

Suspected pelvic mass

Rape

Request by patient

---

sensations experienced during the examination have been demonstrated to reduce anxiety. Of major concern to the adolescent is fear of discovery of pelvic pathology. Reassurance regarding normal physical findings is extremely important (Millstein, Adler and Irwin, 1988).

Usually, the stressful experience of being placed in stirrups in the traditional lithotomy position can be avoided. Most girls favour a semi-sitting position, which has the additional advantage of allowing eye contact during the procedure. The youngster who is relaxed may be examined in the supine position. Girls experiencing their first pelvic examination have been found to be more relaxed when examined by a female.

DELAYED MENARCHE/AMENORRHOEA

It is not unusual for an adolescent to skip a menstrual period or two when establishing normal menstrual and ovulatory cycles. Two-thirds of adolescent females will establish regular menstrual cycles by two years after menarche. This is of little concern unless it creates undue anxiety on the part of the girl and her parents, which can ordinarily be allayed by explanation and reassurance. Careful examination will reveal any congenital defects of the genital tract (a rare cause).

Amenorrhoea is considered to be *primary* when menarche is delayed beyond age 17, although some prefer the term *delayed menarche*. Secondary or *postmenarchal* amenorrhoea is prolonged absence of menstruation for six months or more between periods in the first two years after menarche, or when more than three periods have been missed after menses have become established.

DELAYED MENARCHE

Delayed menarche may be the result of absence or malformation of the female genital structures or the inability of normal structures to respond to hormonal stimulation. This can be of hypothalamic, pituitary, ovarian or uterine origin, and can include hypopituitarism, Turner syndrome, tumours and infections. Primary amenorrhoea resulting from congenital anomalies, which obstruct the outflow of menses, can be caused by imperforate hymen or transverse vaginal septum. Imperforate hymen and transverse vaginal septum are unusual causes of absent menses in a girl who exhibits all the evidences of oestrogen production and sexual maturation, and who complains of periodic (usually monthly) lower abdominal pain. The treatment is simple surgical perforation and drainage.

A group of systemic disorders that may affect the functions of the reproductive tract are thyroid hypofunction or hyperfunction, prolonged or severe infections, adrenal hyperplasias, diabetes mellitus and other chronic diseases. Obesity, malnutrition (including protein, vitamin, or iron deficiencies), or any rapid change in weight (up or down) can produce amenorrhoea. A common cause of delayed menarche is strenuous physical activity sufficient to reduce body fat content (Theintz *et al*, 1993).

SECONDARY AMENORRHOEA

The most common cause of secondary amenorrhoea in adolescence is pregnancy. Other factors, which disturb the hypothalamic-pituitary-gonadal axis and cause secondary amenorrhoea, include immaturity, extreme physical stress, severe emotional stress, sudden environmental change, hyperthyroidism or hypothyroidism, chronic systemic illness, extreme weight loss or gain, anorexia nervosa (even before marked weight loss), ovarian disturbance and extrinsic pharmacological agents (Greydanus and Shearin, 1990).

DYSMENORRHOEA

A certain amount of discomfort during the first day or two of the menstrual flow is common. Most girls experience cramping, abdominal pain, backache, and leg ache, but in a few the pain is intolerable and incapacitating. The term *primary dysmenorrhoea* is applied to these symptoms when there is no pelvic disease to account for cramping discomfort that is severe enough to interfere with normal activity. Primary dysmenorrhoea occurs almost always in ovulatory cycles and commonly appears within 6-12 months of the onset of menarche, when ovulatory cycles are usually established. Primary dysmenorrhoea is the most common gynaecological complaint.

Dysmenorrhoea beginning more than two years after menarche is more suggestive of *secondary dysmenorrhoea* - painful menstruation secondary to pelvic pathology. Endometriosis and pelvic inflammatory disease (PID) are the most frequent causes of secondary dysmenorrhoea in adolescents.

CLINICAL MANIFESTATIONS

Typical complaints of the girl with dysmenorrhoea are lower abdominal cramping, pain or discomfort, and nausea (often with vomiting), diarrhoea and fatigue. Sometimes syncope and collapse occur. The pain usually begins some hours before the appearance of visible vaginal bleeding, is most severe on the first day of menstruation, and may last from a few hours to a day, but seldom exceeds 2-3 days. The symptoms and degree of discomfort vary considerably from one individual to another and from one period to another in the same person.

Mittelschmerz, a symptom observed in some girls, is a midcycle lower quadrant pain that sometimes occurs in association with ovulation and is believed to be caused by pelvic irritation from discharged ovarian follicular contents. The discomfort is unilateral and on alternate sides each month, often accompanied by mild bleeding or changes in vaginal secretions. The discomfort may last from several hours to 3-4 days.

THERAPEUTIC MANAGEMENT

A thorough gynaecological examination is carried out to exclude any pelvic abnormalities, and a careful history is taken regarding the type and duration of pain, its relationship to menstrual flow, and any associated symptoms. These questions not only provide information to the examiner, but also serve to provide the girl with evidence that her problem is being taken seriously. An explanation of the physiology of menstruation helps to give reassurance.

The treatment of choice for adolescents is the administration of nonsteroidal anti-inflammatory drugs, the drugs that block the formation of prostaglandins (called antiprostaglandins, prostaglandin inhibitors, or prostaglandin synthetase inhibitors). Antiprostaglandins are taken for only 2-3 days of the menstrual cycle. Prophylactic aspirin has proved effective when begun a few days before the onset of the menses — approximately 11 days after ovulation. The relief appears to be the result of prostaglandin-inhibitory (rather than analgesic) effect.

PREMENSTRUAL TENSION SYNDROME

Premenstrual tension syndrome (PMS) is a loosely defined congestive dysmenorrhoea (sometimes called pelvic congestion syndrome) that begins approximately 7-10 days before and ends at the onset of menses. The manifestations most frequently cited are headache, backache, increased fatigue, weight gain, irritability, crying spells, depression, bloating and breast congestion before menstrual flow (Allen, McBride, and Pirie, 1991).

The aetiology is unclear, but water and sodium retention as a result of progesterone production after ovulation appear to be factors. Characteristically, these symptoms are present several days before the menstrual period and are relieved at the onset of the menstrual flow.

ENDOMETRIOSIS

Endometriosis is much more common in adolescents than had previously been thought. This painful disorder is caused by the presence of endometrial tissue refluxed from the fallopian tubes during menstruation or developing from embryonic rests that are seeded anywhere in the pelvis. This ectopic tissue forms multiple small cysts on the ovaries, uterine surface, pelvic ligaments, or peritoneum that swell during the menstrual cycle, irritating nerve endings or creating adhesions between pelvic structures. The resulting pain is localized in the lower abdomen, back, groin, thigh, and/or deep pelvis and can be cyclic or acyclic. It is aggravated by coitus, but usually relieved by rest.

Laparoscopic examination confirms the diagnosis. Treatment consists of cyclic hormone administration for 3-6 months. However, the disorder tends to become a chronic, recurring condition. Continuing management is usually referred to a gynaecologist, and surgical intervention may be required.

DYSFUNCTIONAL UTERINE BLEEDING

Dysfunctional uterine bleeding (DUB) is abnormal vaginal bleeding that occurs in the absence of pregnancy, infection, neoplasms, or any other demonstrable pathological condition or disease (Anderson, Irwin, and Snyder, 1986). During adolescence, abnormalities in the timing (intervals of less than 20 days or greater than 40 days), length (greater than 8 days' duration), and amount (more than 80 ml) of menstrual flow can occur frequently. This irregularity is usually attributed to immaturity of the positive feedback mechanism between the hypothalamic-pituitary-gonadal axis and absence of the luteinizing hormone (LH) surge late in the menstrual cycle. This results in anovulatory cycles, which occur at unpredictable intervals ranging from continual spotting to heavy vaginal bleeding (Polaniczky and Slap, 1992).

VAGINITIS AND VULVITIS (VULVOVAGINITIS)

A small quantity of vaginal mucus is normal, and in adolescent girls usually increases at the time of ovulation and before the onset of menstruation. It is characteristically clear and, except in rare instances when it appears in large amounts, causes no discomfort. However, some teenagers mistakenly believe it to be a sign of vaginal infection. After an examination, the girl can generally be reassured. Since increased secretions may be associated with sexual excitement, this association with lovemaking should be discussed with the girl.

Leukorrhoea is the term used to describe a glutinous, greywhite discharge, which can be caused by physical, chemical or infectious agents (Sparks, 1991). Physical causes include foreign bodies (especially in prepubertal girls), a forgotten tampon, an intrauterine device, or even tight jeans. It can also be caused by irritation from pinworms, bubble bath, feminine hygiene products, or improper wiping after defecation. The resulting discharge is purulent, blood-tinged, or brown, with an offensive odour. Removal of the foreign material and the use of an acidifying vaginal treatment is all that is usually needed.

IMPLICATIONS FOR NURSING

Health teaching is important in the prevention and management of vaginitis. Girls should be taught at an early age the proper hygiene after toileting; that is, wiping from front to back. A careful history can often elicit other causes such as use of irritating substances, foreign bodies, or sexual activity that may be divulged to a sensitive and sympathetic examiner.

HEALTH PROBLEMS RELATED TO SEXUALITY

The biological maturation that forms the foundation of adolescent development and the transition to adulthood is accompanied by conflicting feelings, attitudes, and social practices related to the developing sexuality (Gillmore *et al*, 1992).

ADOLESCENT PREGNANCY

Today, in most cases teenage pregnancy is no longer considered to be biologically disadvantageous to the conceptus, but it is still regarded as socially, educationally, psychologically and economically disadvantageous to the mother.

MEDICAL ASPECTS

With better facilities available for care, the mortality for teenage pregnancies is decreasing, but the morbidity remains high. Teenage girls and their unborn infants are at greater risk for complications of both pregnancy and delivery. The most frequent complications are premature labour and infants of low birth weight, high neonatal mortality, pregnancy-induced hypertension (PIH), iron deficiency anaemia, fetopelvic disproportion, and prolonged labour. It now appears that the major obstetric difficulties are related to the smaller maternal size rather than the younger age or developmental immaturity.

Although teenagers have special needs, the obstetric risk should be no greater than for any pregnant woman. When quality antenatal care is available early in the pregnancy, the progress and outcome of teenage pregnancies compare favourably with the obstetric performance of older women (Pope *et al*, 1993).

IMPLICATIONS FOR NURSING

Basic to the implementation of any programme of care is communication and the establishment of a trusting relationship. Initially, the adolescent girl frequently appears apathetic and displays little interest in discussing her pregnancy. She may be abrupt, impatient, defensive, hostile or indifferent. It is important for the nurse to make every effort to put the youngster at ease and avoid undue pressure until a rapport can be developed, so that the girl is comfortable in sharing her feelings and concerns. Conveying a non-judgemental and genuine caring acceptance of the girl and her goals will assist the nurse in gaining her confidence and trust. The girl may have encountered rejection and open criticism from authority figures and peers, depending on the social and cultural attitudes of the school, the community, and her own family structure.

Communication takes time and patience. Asking open-ended questions and listening for cues will help identify physical, emotional, social and cultural influences that might affect the adolescent's progress through the maternity cycle. For example, various cultural groups have different attitudes towards unsanctioned pregnancies, and it is important to determine other sources of support, such as the family. Factors that might affect her physical status, such as smoking, drug use, and nutritional state and habits, need to be explored and confronted. Each teenager presents a unique situation in relation to background, life-style, support structure, and coping mechanisms.

Nutrition assessment should focus on the dietary adequacy of iron and calcium; multivitamins with folic acid are prescribed (Stevens-Simon and McAnarney, 1992).

The young girl needs to know what is happening to her, what is expected of her, and how she can help in developing a plan of care. Adolescents have their own ideas of the type of help they need and support that would be beneficial. They should be consulted, and encouraged to share their ideas and to feel they make an important contribution to planning their care.

ADOLESCENT ABORTION

Although abortion is a controversial and emotional issue, health care professionals involved in delivery of services to pregnant adolescents are confronted with this reality frequently. Counselling the adolescent about pregnancy options in a non-judgemental way is essential.

Concerns regarding the psychological impact of the abortion decision have been raised. Studies have revealed that although teenagers may delay a decision and may find it more difficult, they suffer no long-term negative psychological sequelae (Adler and Dolcini, 1986). Active involvement in the decision-making process and perception of having made the choice personally can contribute to the adolescent's psychological growth.

IMPLICATIONS FOR NURSING

For the adolescent who chooses to continue the pregnancy, prenatal care referral should be initiated as soon as possible. For the adolescent who elects abortion as an option, referral should be initiated quickly to ensure that the procedure is performed during the first trimester, when complications are reduced. Pelvic ultrasound may be indicated to assess gestational age correctly for girls who cannot recall the date of their last menstrual period and when a bimanual pelvic examination is inconclusive. Appropriate pre-operative counselling is also indicated (Russo and Zierk, 1992).

Prior to the procedure, patient education regarding the medical aspects of the abortion should be conducted verbally and the patient should be given written instructions.

SEXUALLY TRANSMITTED DISEASES

The area of sexually transmitted disease (STD) diagnosis and treatment has become exceedingly complex with the expansion from the five traditional venereal diseases (VDs) to the expanded nomenclature of STD in the mid-1970s, which includes more than 20 different infections and associated syndromes.

Several unique characteristics — biological, developmental, and environmental — place adolescents at risk for acquisition of STDs. Biologically, the immature adolescent female undergoes major physiological transformation in the area of the endocervix. The thin layer of columnar cells appears to favour attachment of infectious agents (e.g., *Chlamydia trachomatis*, wart viruses, papillomavirus), which accounts in part for the increased prevalence of these infections in adolescents. The unchallenged immune system does not provide localized antibody response at the cervical level when exposed repeatedly to infectious agents. During anovulatory cycles, oestrogen

predominates, as demonstrated by the clear and watery cervical discharge. This may facilitate the transport of pathogens to the upper genital tract (Biro, 1992).

Developmentally, teenagers experience biological discontinuities wherein pubertal maturing precedes psychological and cognitive maturity.

The absence of future planning is often evident in their failure to see the implications of current behaviour on future outcome, such as condom use to prevent STD or pregnancy, or the need to return for follow-up visits for contraceptive refill or STD treatment. During this time of evolving identity and emerging sexuality, the outcome is teenagers who have reproductive capabilities, but insufficient maturity and absent social sanctions to be open and responsible about their sexual behaviour (Box 18-6).

HUMAN IMMUNODEFICIENCY VIRUS INFECTION AND ACQUIRED IMMUNE DEFICIENCY SYNDROME

Health professionals caring for teenagers have expressed growing concern regarding the transmission of human immunodeficiency virus (HIV), which eventually causes acquired

---

◆ **BOX 18-6**

Reasons for not seeking or using birth control

Responses of teenagers at initial interview for contraception in order of frequency:

Didn't get around to it

Afraid family would find out

Waiting for closer relationship with partner

Thought birth control dangerous

Afraid of examination

Thought it cost too much

Didn't think had sex often enough to get pregnant

Never thought of it

Didn't know where to get birth control

Thought had to be older to get birth control

Didn't expect to have sex

Thought too young to get pregnant

Thought birth control wrong

Partner objected

Thought wanted pregnancy

Thought method used good enough

Modified from Tyrer, Rothbart and Anderson, 1989; with data from Alan Guttmacher Institute, 1981.

immune deficiency syndrome (AIDS) among specific sub-groups of adolescents. Presently, this virus is considered to be universally fatal. Its ability to overwhelm the individual's immune system causes death through a variety of diseases. Transmission of the virus takes place through sharing body fluids infected with the HIV. Major mechanisms of transmission are through exchange of sexual fluids (semen, vaginal fluid, menstrual fluid, and blood); receiving blood or blood products infected with HIV (intravenous drug users [IVDUs] sharing unclean needles); and passage of the virus from an infected mother to her unborn child. Consequently, HIV has been called the primary public health problem facing the United States, although the total number of AIDS cases among teenagers is very small (less than 2%) when compared with all other age-groups with the disease.

Reason for concern about AIDS in teenagers is related to several factors. Sexual partners of female adolescents are often several years older and may have been already infected. The known high prevalence rates of other STDs and pregnancy among adolescents document that adolescents are sexually active, but do not take precautions to protect themselves against HIV infection.

A long latency period between infection and the development of clinical AIDS has been demonstrated (average duration, 7 years). Since the greatest number of reported AIDS cases occur among young adults in their twenties, it can be inferred that many of these infections were acquired in adolescence. Transmission of HIV occurs while affected individuals are asymptomatic for AIDS, and adolescents infected with the virus can continue to spread the infection without ever knowing they have the disease (Hein, 1989; Hein and Hurst, 1988).

Degrees of risk have been identified for adolescents related to AIDS, with specific recommendations for education and intervention (Box 18-7).

HEPATITIS B

Hepatitis B virus (HBV) is an infection of the liver. Major concerns have been voiced because of the increased rate of infection, particularly among high-risk populations.

Another area of concern is transmission of HBV from pregnant women to their infants. It is estimated that infants whose mothers are positive for HBV will have a 70-90% chance of becoming infected, and nearly all these infants will develop chronic HBV carrier status.

Many potential negative outcomes can be avoided with primary prevention, which is adequately achieved through immunization.

PELVIC INFLAMMATORY DISEASE

Pelvic inflammatory disease (PID) is an infection of the upper genital tract (endometrium and fallopian tubes), most commonly caused by sexually transmitted bacteria, such as *N. gonorrhoeae*, *C. trachomatis*, and a variety of other anaerobic bacteria. PID represents one of the most serious complications of STDs among adolescent females because of the damage that can occur from tubal scarring. Contraceptives, such as barrier methods (condoms) or spermicides, which protect against STDs, are used inconsistently by teenagers. Biologically, the immature adolescent cervix is in the process of undergoing considerable change, and the area of transformation (ectopy) at the endocervical os seems less resistant to attack by infectious agents (Shafer and Sweet, 1989).

◆ **BOX 18-7**

Degrees of HIV risk and interventions among adolescents

Category 1

Teenagers who are currently not at risk for AIDS because of current life-style or absence of virus within their sphere of activities; very young, virginal; have received no transfusions; are not IV substance abusers

Issues:

Worried but healthy; need to learn how to live in atmosphere of concern and maintain appropriate level of concern without undue anxiety; need help to differentiate between myths and facts

Need for information on casual contacts; encourage to engage in activities that do not place them at risk

Support decision making about sexual activities

Category 2

Sexually active teenagers who have not yet been exposed to HIV

Issues:

Knowing (or not being able to 'know') their partners

Reconsider patterns of sexual behaviour

Use of contraceptives in general and condoms in particular

Category 3

Teenagers at risk for HIV acquisition because of exposure to infected individuals (IV drug users, sexual partners of IV drug users, homosexuals or bisexuals, sex partners of homosexuals or bisexuals)

Issues:

Decisions about HIV testing

Knowledge of serostatus of partner(s)

Need for barrier methods of contraception

Reconsideration of patterns of sexual behaviour

Decision about continuing pregnancy

Need for services geared to adolescent age-group for crisis intervention and follow-up of HIV-infected teenagers and partners

Modified from Hein, 1989.

Presenting symptoms in the adolescent may be generalized, with fever, abdominal pain, urinary tract symptoms, and vague influenza-like manifestations, such as malaise, nausea, diarrhoea, or constipation. A pelvic examination is indicated for every sexually active female who complains of lower abdominal pain, to evaluate the possibility of PID.

Approximately 25% of women experiencing PID may have short-term complications, such as acute abscess formation in the fallopian tubes (tubo-ovarian abscess), or long-term complications, such as chronic pelvic pain, dyspareunia (painful coitus), or formation of adhesions. Most significant, however, is the increased risk for ectopic pregnancy and/or infertility, which results from tubal scarring.

Prevention is the primary concern of health care professionals. Use of barrier contraceptive methods, such as condoms with addition of spermicide, seem to offer the best protection for preventing STDs and this serious complication. Sexually active teenage females should be screened routinely to detect those with asymptomatic STDs, and treatment is needed to prevent PID and all associated complications.

IMPLICATIONS FOR NURSING

Delivery of care to adolescents requires a developmental perspective. Understanding the biological, psychosocial, and legal issues affects the delivery of health care to adolescents and their families.

KEY POINTS

- Typical adolescent health-seeking behaviours centre on skin problems, obesity, headaches, abdominal discomfort, menstrual symptoms, and anxieties about physical development and sexual change.
- Acne is prevalent in the teen years; medication and hygiene are the treatments of choice.
- Alterations in growth and maturation may be manifest in short stature; tall stature; precocious puberty; Turner syndrome; Klinefelter syndrome; pathological conditions such as chronic disease, skeletal defects, endocrine dysfunction, and cortisol excess; and psychosocial dwarfism.
- Assessment of growth consists of taking a family history, determining previous growth patterns, conducting a physical examination, determining bone age and conducting endocrine studies.
- The most frequent problems related to the male reproductive system are infections, scrotal conditions and gynaecomastia.
- The most frequent problems of the female reproductive system involve menstruation — delays, irregularities, discomfort — and infections.
- Adolescent pregnancy has profound social, educational, psychological, and economic ramifications; physiologically, the pregnancy necessitates special attention to nutrition and psychological and emotional support for the mother and father.
- Abortion, as an alternative to birth, has been determined to have no long-term psychological sequelae.
- Contraception is often not used because of lack of information, anxiety regarding use, conflict over sexual activity, and desire for pregnancy.
- Sexually transmitted diseases are the most frequently occurring infectious diseases and a major cause of adolescent morbidity.

REFERENCES

Adler NE, Dolcini P: Psychological issues in abortion for adolescents. In Melton GB (ed): *Adolescent abortion: psychological and legal issues*, Lincoln, NE, 1986, University of Nebraska Press.

Alan Guttmacher Institute: *Teenage pregnancy: the problem that hasn't gone away*, New York, 1981, Alan Guttmacher Institute.

Allen SS, McBride CM, Pirie PL: The shortened premenstrual assessment form, *J Reprod Med* 36:769, 1991.

Anderson MM, Irwin CE, Snyder DL: Abnormal vaginal bleeding in adolescents, *Pediatr Ann* 15:697, 1986.

Atkinson *et al*: *Introduction to psychology*, ed 11, London, 1993, Harcourt Brace.

Bearinger L, Gephart J: Priorities for adolescent health: recommendations of a national conference, *MCN* 12:161, 1987.

Biro FM: Adolescents and sexually transmitted diseases, *Matern Child Health* (technical bulletin), August, 1992.

Bender B *et al*: Speech and language development in 41 children with sex chromosome anomalies, *Pediatrics* 71:262, 1983.

Bowie WE: Urethritis in males. In Holmes KK *et al*: *Sexually transmitted diseases*, ed 2, New York, 1990, McGraw-Hill.

Cohen FL: *Clinical genetics in nursing practice*, Philadelphia, 1984, JB Lippincott.

Cohen FL, Durham JD: Children with sex chromosome variations: implications for pediatric nursing practice, *J Pediatr Nurs* 1:12, 1986.

Gillmore MR *et al*: Substances use and other factors associated with risky sexual behaviour among pregnant adolescents, *Fam Plann Persp* 24:255, 1992.

Greydanus DE, Shearin RB: *Adolescent sexuality and gynecology*, Philadelphia, 1990, Lea & Febiger.

Hein K: Commentary on adolescent acquired immunodeficiency syndrome; the next wave of the human immunodeficiency virus epidemic? *J Pediatr* 114:144, 1989.

Hein K, Hurst M: Human immunodeficiency virus infection in adolescence: a rationale for action, *Adolesc Pediatr Gynecol* 1:73, 1988.

Larson RE, Shapiro MA: Sexually transmitted urogenital diseases, *Emerg Med Clin North Am*, 6:487, 1988.

McCauley E, Ito J, Kay T: Psychosocial functioning in girls with Turner syndrome and short stature: social skills, behavior problems, and self-concept, *J Am Acad Child Psychiatry* 25:105, 1986.

Millstein SG: Adolescent health: challenges for behavioral scientists, *Am Psychol* 4:837, 1989.

Millstein SG, Adler NE, Irwin CE: Sources of anxiety about pelvic examinations among adolescent females, *Sex Active Teenagers* 2(2):66, 1988.

Nagar H, Levran R: Impact of active case finding on the diagnosis and therapy of paediatric variocele, *Gyn Obst* 177:3, 1993.

Polaniczky MM, Slap GB: Menstrual disorders in the adolescent: dysmenorrhoea and dysfunctional uterine bleeding, *Ped Review* 13:83, 1992.

Pope SK *et al*: Low birth-weight infants born to adolescent mothers, *JAMA* 269:1396, 1993.

Rosenfeld RG, Northcraft GB, Hintz RL: A prospective, randomized study of testosterone treatment of constitutional delay of growth and development in male adolescents, *Pediatr* 69:681, 1982.

Rothman KF, Lucky AW: Acne vulgaris, *Adv Derm* 8:347, 1993.

Russo NF, Zierk KL: Abortion, childbearing, and womens' well-being, *Prof Psychol Res Pract* 23:256, 1992.

Sawczuk IS *et al*: Varicoceles effect of testicular volume in prepubertal and pubertal males, *Urology* 41:466, 1993.

Shafer MA, Sweet RL: Pelvic inflammatory disease in adolescent females, *Pediatr Clin North Am* 36:513, 1989.

Sparks JM: Vaginitis, *J Reprod Med* 36:745, 1991.

Stevens-Simon C, McAnarney ER: Adolescent pregancy, gestestional weight gain and maternal and infant outcomes, *AJDC* 146:1359, 1992.

Theintz *et al*: title, *J Pediatr* 122:306, 1993.

Tyrer LB, Rothbart B, Anderson K: What every teen should know about contraceptives, *Contemp Pediatr* (10):68, 1989.

Walzer *et al*: Preliminary observations on language and learning in XXY boys, *Birth Defects Original Series* 18(18):185, 1982.

Williamson R: Cold weather and testicular torsion, *BMJ* 286:1436, 1983.

Wilson DM, Rosenfeld RG: Treatment of short stature and delayed adolescence, *Pediatr Clin North Am* 34:865, 1987.

FURTHER READING

Acne

Lucky AW: Update on acne vulgaris, *Pediatr Ann* 16:29, 1978.

Stone AC: Facing up to acne, *Pediatr Nurs* 8:229, 1982.

Altered Growth and Maturation

Bercu B: Growth hormone treatment and the short child: to treat or not to treat, *J Pediatr Health Care* 110:991, 1987.

Hall JG *et al*: Turner syndrome and its variants, *Pediatr Clin N Am* 37(6), 1990.

Lee PD, Rosenfeld RG: Psychosocial correlates of short stature and delayed puberty, *Pediatr Clin North Am* 34:851, 1987.

Mandoki M, Sumner G: Klinefelter syndrome: the need for early identification and treatment, *Clin Pediatr* 30(3):161, 1991.

Solomon SB: Children with short stature, *J Pediatr Nurs* 1:80, 1986.

Disorders of the Male Reproductive System

Casey MP: Testicular cancer: the worst disease at the worst time, *RN* 50(2):36, 1987.

Goldbloom RB: Self-examination by adolescents, *Pediatr* 76:126, 1985.

Schaufele B: Teaching testicular self-examination. In Glasper A: *Child care: some nursing perspectives*, London, 1991, Wolfe.

Disorders of the Female Reproductive System

Coupey SM, Ahlstrom P: Common menstrual disorders, *Pediatr Clin North Am* 36:551, 1989.

Gemberling CL: The adolescent gynecologic examination: an overview, *J Pediatr Health Care* 1:141, 1987.

Khoiny FW: Adolescent dysmenorrhea, *J Pediatr Health Care* 2:29, 1988.

Soules MR: Adolescent amenorrhea, *Pediatr Clin North Am* 34:1083, 1987.

Szydlo VL: Approaching an adolescent about a pelvic exam, *AJN* 88:1502, 1988.

Adolescent Pregnancy

DeAngelis C: Confronting the crisis of teenage pregnancy, *Contemp Pediatr* 4(9):68, 1987.

Heller RG: School-based clinics: impact on teenage pregnancy prevention, *Pediatr Nurs* 14:103, 1988.

Porter LS, Sobong LC: Differences in maternal perception of the newborn among adolescents, *Pediatr Nurs* 16:101, 1990.

Stephenson JN.: Pregnancy testing and counseling, *Pediatr Clin North Am* 36:681, 1989.

Contraception

Reis J, Herz L: Young adolescents' contraceptive knowledge and attitudes: implications for anticipatory guidance, *J Pediatr Health Care* 1:247, 1987.

Sexually Transmitted Diseases

Brown HP: Recognizing STDs in adolescents, *Contemp Pediatr* 6(1):17, 1989.

Hein K: Adolescent acquired immunodeficiency syndrome, *Am J Dis Child* 144:46, 1990.

Kegeles SM, Adler NE, Irwin CE: Adolescents and condoms, *Am J Dis Child* 143:911, 1989.

Rosenfeld WD, Clark J: Vulvovaginitis and cervicitis, *Pediatr Clin North Am* 36:489, 1989.

Steiner JD *et al*: Are adolescents getting smarter about acquired immunodeficiency syndrome? *Am J Dis Child* 144:302, 1990.

Unit Three

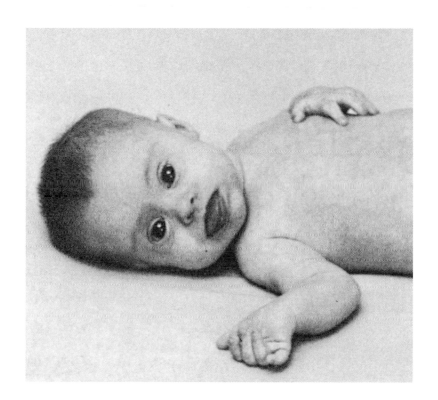

The Child with Special Needs

Chapter 19

Behavioural Health Problems of Adolescence

LEARNING OUTCOMES

After studying this chapter you should be able to:

◆ Understand adolescence as an individual developmental stage.
◆ Discuss behavioural problems which may arise in adolescence as a result of achieving the developmental tasks and adjustment required to maintain a state of social, physical and emotional health.
◆ Describe the onset and progress of obesity, anorexia and bulimia, giving relevant individual and familial/social factors.
◆ Describe the nursing practice issues in producing a therapeutic programme for anorexia, bulimia and obesity, including work with individuals and families.
◆ Discuss the incidence and problems of smoking in adolescence and outline issues for prevention.
◆ Describe the incidence and development of the abuse of drugs, including alcohol and other substances.
◆ Discuss preventive aspects and the therapeutic management of drug and alcohol abuse.
◆ Explain the difference between suicide, suicidal ideation, gesture and attempt.
◆ Be aware of the critical developmental and familial factors in any suicide attempt.
◆ Discuss the therapeutic management of depression and suicidal ideation or attempted suicide.
◆ Define the glossary terms.

GLOSSARY

AN Anorexia nervosa

drug abuse The regular use of drugs for other than accepted medical purposes, to the extent that it results in physical or psychological harm to the user and/or is used in a way that is detrimental to society

drug misuse The overzealous use of drugs or the exercise of bad judgement in their use

drug tolerance The clinical need to increase the dosage of a drug in order to attain the same desired effect; caused by an increased capacity to metabolize and eliminate the drug or the ability of the individual's tissues to adapt to the drug

narcotic addiction Behavioural pattern of overwhelming involvement with obtaining and using a narcotic for its psychic effects rather than for medical reasons, thereby eliciting social disapproval

physical dependence An adaptive physiological state that occurs when a drug is taken in increasing amounts and that is manifest by the development of physiological symptoms when the drug is withdrawn

suicidal attempt An act intended to cause injury or death

suicidal gesture An act made without any real attempt to cause serious injury or death

suicidal ideation Thoughts about or plans for suicide

dolescence is a time of transition, maturational crisis, and adjustment. The transition to adulthood is characterized by change, growth and stress. Ineffective and unsuccessful accomplishment of the developmental tasks of adolescence produces a sense of inadequacy within some adolescents, who may use faulty problem solving in their search for relief from the discomfort and stress of this transitional period of life.

EATING DISORDERS

Eating disorders are among the most frequently encountered health problems of adolescence. Overeating often begins in infancy and continues throughout childhood; deliberate undereating usually does not become apparent until later childhood or adolescence. Either overeating or undereating can have a detrimental effect on health and well-being and, if extreme, can be a threat to life.

The term *eating disorder* is often applied to the two major eating disorders, anorexia nervosa and bulimia. However, for the purpose of this discussion, the two are considered separately because of their age distribution and their characteristics.

OBESITY

Probably no problem related to adolescence is so obvious to others, is so difficult to treat, and has such long-term effects on psychological and physical health status as obesity. It is the most common nutritional disturbance of children, and one of the most challenging contemporary health problems at all ages. The prevalence of obesity has been determined to be 25-30% of prepubertal children and 18-25% of adolescents.

Obesity is an increase in body weight resulting from an excessive accumulation of fat or simply the state of being too fat. *Overweight* refers to the state of weighing more than average for height and body build, which may or may not include an increased amount of fat.

AETIOLOGY/PATHOPHYSIOLOGY

General body build seems to have some effect on obesity. However, it is almost impossible to distinguish between hereditary and environmental factors, since both may be operative in any situation, especially when other family members are also obese. Family eating patterns, ethnic diet, and psychological factors play an important role; to many persons, fat is still considered to be an indication of good health.

Sociocultural factors
Patterns of eating are culturally and socially based in most instances, and in some the food preferences of the culture contribute to the development of obesity.

Psychological factors
Psychological factors may provide a basis for eating patterns in childhood. In infancy, the child first experiences relief from discomfort through feeding and learns to associate eating with

feelings of well-being, security and the comforting presence of the mothering person.

OBESITY IN ADOLESCENCE

Adolescent-onset obesity appears to be closely related to an inability to master the developmental tasks of adolescence; as a result, children regress to the self-satisfying tactic of overeating to compensate.

Vulnerable personality
Obesity is most often a symptom in passive-dependent, compliant youngsters who are readily controlled by guilt and shame. They are easily influenced by outside forces (such as parents, peers and school) that they consider to be more powerful than themselves.

Self-concept and obesity
Obese adolescents score higher on depression-measurement tests than thinner teenagers and significantly lower on body-image tests, indicating a less positive or a more impaired body concept. (See Fig. 19-1 for complex relationships in adolescent obesity.)

PROCESS OF DIAGNOSIS

The presence of obesity is obvious from appearance alone, and a gross determination can be made by a rough comparison of height and weight with standard growth charts. Children who are 20% over normal for their height and weight should undergo further evaluation, including a height and weight history of the child, parents and siblings, as well as eating habits, appetite and hunger patterns, and physical activities. A careful history is taken regarding the development of the obesity, and a physical examination is carried out to help differentiate simple obesity from increased fat resulting from organic causes.

THERAPEUTIC MANAGEMENT

Because of the self-perpetuating nature of obesity, efforts to treat the condition have been universally disappointing. A high proportion of obese children become obese adults. Varying degrees of success have been achieved in some highly motivated individuals through weight-reduction techniques, including diet, exercise, behaviour modification and psychological support.

Diet
Diet modification is essential to any weight-reduction program. The ideal diet regimen for children and adolescents should meet the criteria listed in Box 19-1.

Exercise
Some type of regular exercise is incorporated in a weight-reduction programme. In the absence of exercise, both fat and lean body mass are generally lost and weight regained is primarily fat (Fox and Mathews, 1981).

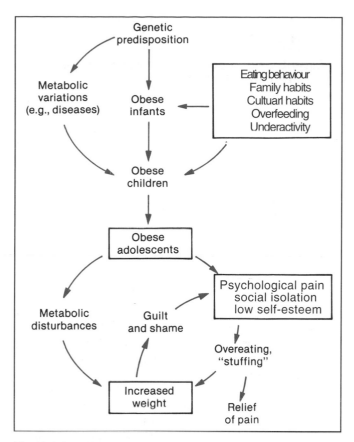

Fig. 19-1 Complex relationships in adolescent obesity.

Behaviour modification

Behaviour modification approaches to weight loss are based on the observation that obese individuals have abnormal eating practices that can be altered. The attention is focused not on food, but on the social and behavioural aspects surrounding food consumption. The technique has been used primarily with older children and adolescents.

Behaviour weight modification programmes appear to be more successful when the management includes a problem-solving component. Youngsters who are able to identify problems and determine possible solutions have significantly greater success with weight loss, both immediately following the programme and at follow-up evaluations (Graves, Meyers, and Clark, 1988).

Drugs

Prescribing appetite-suppressant drugs to children and adolescents is not favoured by most practitioners. There is little, if any, convincing evidence that they are more effective than diet and exercise in maintaining long-term weight loss.

IMPLICATIONS FOR NURSING

Although therapy involves a team approach that includes the doctor, dietitian, family and the children themselves, nurses play a dominant role in any regulated and promising programme of weight reduction. Interested nurse practitioners are able to evaluate, treat and follow overweight adolescents. They also assume an important position in recognizing potential

weight problems and in assisting parents and children in prevention programmes.

Nursing Interventions

Nursing objectives for the obese child include:
1. Modify diet to provide loss of fat content without interfering with growth, normal activity and psychological well-being.
2. Implement a regular exercise programme.
3. Modify eating behaviour.
4. Provide psychological support.

Implementation

The reasons behind the desire to lose weight need to be explored with youngsters, but success is rarely achieved unless they are motivated to lose weight and to take personal responsibility for dietary habits and exercise programmes. Teenagers who are forced by parents to seek help are seldom sufficiently motivated, become rebellious of parental nagging, and are unwilling to control dietary intake. A rigid approach or one based on parental enforcement of the regimen is usually doomed from the start.

Nutrition counselling

The most successful diets are those that use ordinary foods in controlled portions rather than diets that require the avoidance of any specific food. The youngster and parents are taught how to incorporate favourite foods into the diet and how to select substitutes that are also satisfying. The dieting youngster should eat what the rest of the family eats, but less of it. When parents buy and prepare smaller amounts, tempting second helpings and leftovers are eliminated. For older children, exchange diets are useful. There are a multitude of restricted calorie diets available from a number of sources, such as the British Dietetic Association, and the caloric values for a wide variety of commercial foods are available to facilitate meal planning.

No adolescent should be encouraged to initiate a reduction diet without health assessment, evaluation, and counselling. It is also important to emphasize the undesirable nature of the fad diets and crash programmes that continually appear in various publications.

Behaviour modification

Altering eating behaviour has been found essential to weight reduction, especially in maintaining long-term weight control. This approach emphasizes identification and elimination of inappropriate eating habits. Although the long-term effects of this method are still in need of evaluation, it appears promising for the treatment of obesity in adolescents. Behaviour modification programmes are based on various concepts; primarily those that incorporate (Taitz, 1983):
- A description of the behaviour to be controlled, such as eating habits
- Attempts to modify and control stimuli governing eating
- Development of eating techniques designed to control speed of eating
- Positive reinforcement for these modifications by a suitable reward system

Family-centred care

There is a definite connection between family environment and interaction, and obesity (Huse *et al*, 1982a, 1982b). Involving the family facilitates weight loss, but the nature and extent of the involvement are related to the age of the child. With adolescents, parents need education in the purposes of the therapeutic measures and their role in management. The family is given nutrition education and counselled regarding the reinforcement plan, altering the food environment, and maintaining proper attitudes. They assist in monitoring the child's eating behaviour, food intake, physical activity and weight changes. More success has been achieved when counsellors meet with adolescents and their parents separately (Brownell, Kelman, and Strunkard, 1983). Younger children and parents meet together, and parents are counselled alone when the children are very young.

Evaluation

The effectiveness of nursing interventions is determined by continual re-assessment and evaluation of care based on the following observational guidelines and expected outcomes:

1. Assess weight at regular intervals (usually weekly); discuss with the youngster his or her feelings, reactions, and concerns; analyse daily recordings of activities (eating, behaviour, exercise) and feelings.
2. Review exercise programme with the youngster.
3. Review log of eating behaviours; discuss the observations with the youngster.
4. Interview the youngster about the plan of care and progress towards short-term goals.

ANOREXIA NERVOSA

Anorexia nervosa (AN) is the term applied to a long-recognized disorder characterized by severe weight loss in the absence of obvious physical cause. The term *anorexia nervosa* inaccurately describes the disorder in which individuals do not lack hunger, but deny its existence. Emaciation occurs as a result of self-inflicted starvation. In Britain, the annual incidence of anorexia nervosa is estimated at 0.6-1.6 per 100,000 of the total population (Kendall *et al*, 1973). The incidence rate has been reported to be 1:250 in UK school girls aged 16 years and older, rising to 1% of girls in independent or boarding schools. Between 90-95% of anorexia nervosa suffers are female (Garfinkel *et al*, 1982).

AETIOLOGY/PATHOPHYSIOLOGY

The onset of AN has two peaks: between 12 and 14 and between 16 and 17 years of age (Herzog and Copeland, 1985). Young women who have this disorder are described as 'good children', perfectionists, academically high achievers, conforming and conscientious. Typical patients are female with high energy levels, despite marked emaciation. A strong extrinsic motive has, for some reason, suppressed the vital function of eating. Because the disorder predominately involves females, the feminine pronoun is used in the ensuing discussions.

◆ **BOX 19-1**

Essentials of a good dietary regime for children and adolescents

The diet should provide for:
- Rapid weight loss
- Lack of metabolic complications
- Lack of hunger
- Preservation of lean body mass
- Absence of psychiatric reactions

Psychological aspects

Dominating the psychological aspects of AN are a relentless pursuit of thinness and a fear of fatness. These are usually preceded by a period (1-2 years) of mood disturbances and behaviour changes. The weight loss is usually triggered by a typical adolescent crisis, such as the onset of menstruation or a traumatic interpersonal incident, that precipitates serious dieting, and this dieting continues out of control. Frequently, there is an exaggerated misinterpretation of the normal fat deposition characteristic of the early adolescent period, or someone may comment that the adolescent girl is putting on weight. The weight loss may be a response to teasing, some change in her life (such as changing schools or going to college), or an incident that requires an independent decision that she is unprepared to make (such as a career choice).

The current emphasis on slimness is a significant factor contributing to the increasing incidence of this disorder among young women. The standard for beauty is one exemplified by the models chosen for advertising clothing. The pressure to diet and be slim continues relentlessly. Youngsters entering the growth phase of puberty, when biological fat accumulation is the normal course of development, are particularly vulnerable.

The syndrome of AN consists of three major areas of disordered psychological functioning (Box 19-2). Some current evidence suggests that AN is a symptom of family psychopathology that is not usually apparent until the child has improved. These girls are usually strongly dependent on their parents, and frequently an ambivalent mother-daughter relationship is present. There is often a history of family strife, with the AN being a symptom of the family's problems. Families are usually rigid, incapable of resolving conflict, overly enmeshed, excessively controlling, and unable to display their feelings (Joffe, 1990).

Affected youngsters are model daughters who are afraid to assume adult responsibilities. They usually find it difficult to formulate an identity and feel ineffective in their personal lives, even if they appear successful and capable (Joffe, 1990). They usually feel out of control in all aspects of their lives and choose control of food intake to express their autonomy. Any interventions are viewed as an attempt to remove this control.

PROCESS OF DIAGNOSIS

The most obvious manifestation of this disorder is the severe and profound weight loss induced by self-imposed starvation. The youngsters identify with this skeleton-like appearance and do not regard it as abnormal or ugly. They attempt to hide their extreme thinness by wearing bulky sweaters and baggy pants. Girls with AN also tend to overestimate the size of others. Patients absolutely refuse to eat and have a repertoire of excuses for not eating. They display a marked preoccupation with food: preparing meals for others, talking about food and hoarding food. The youngsters become obsessed with fasting and engage in frequent strenuous exercise, self-induced vomiting, and/or taking laxatives in an attempt to speed up the weight-loss process.

These youngsters tend to withdraw from peer relationships and engage in self-imposed social isolation. They are continually striving for perfection, which may be demonstrated in other compulsive behaviours such as stinginess. They are usually overachievers, and their schoolwork is very important to them.

In the wake of the severe weight loss, these young girls exhibit physical signs of altered metabolic activity. They develop secondary amenorrhoea, bradycardia, lowered body temperature, decreased blood pressure and cold intolerance. They have dry skin and brittle nails, and develop lanugo hair. The changes are usually reversible with adequate weight gain and improved nutritional status. Table 19-1 lists the differences between AN and bulimia.

THERAPEUTIC MANAGEMENT

The treatment and management of AN involve three major areas: (1) reinstitution of normal nutrition or reversal of the severe state of malnutrition, (2) resolution of the disturbed patterns of family interaction and (3) individual psychotherapy to correct deficits and distortions in psychological functioning. Because of the psychogenic nature of the disorder, treatment is difficult and lengthy. Because most therapeutic interventions require a team approach, the bulk of management is discussed in relation to nursing considerations.

Nutrition

The initial goal is to treat the life-threatening malnutrition with strict adherence to dietary requirements, which sometimes necessitates intravenous and/or tube feedings, although such methods are usually reserved for severe situations. This is combined with resolution of the family interaction and psychotherapy to improve the underlying psychological misconceptions about the weight loss. Weight gain alone cannot be considered a cure for the disease, and is an unreliable sign of progress. Relapses are frequent as the young girl reverts to previous eating patterns when removed from the therapeutic environment.

There is a decided relationship between AN and depression. Decreasing the patient's consciousness of and vigilance about eating can make her less anxious and more amenable to other suggestions, and may include the administration of antidepressant or antianxiety agents. However, these drugs must be carefully monitored because of their cardiovascular side effects.

Some observations indicate that there may be a link between zinc and some aspects of AN. It is unclear whether the reduced serum zinc levels in these patients are secondary to the inadequate dietary intake or whether a premorbid zinc deficiency precipitates the eating behaviour (Bryce-Smith and Simpson, 1984).

Psychotherapy

Psychotherapy for the affected youngster is essential. The patient needs to be an active participant in the treatment process and to become aware of the impulses, feelings and needs originating within herself.

Children whose illness can be clearly related to a dysfunctional family situation respond to therapy best when separated from the family. Many of those whose therapy plan is implemented in the hospital need a continued behaviour modification programme after discharge in order to maintain the desired weight. Psychotherapy is aimed at helping the child

---

◆ **BOX 19-2**

Areas of disordered functioning in anorexia nervosa

1. Disturbed body image and deluded concept of body proportions. The young girl identifies with her emaciation, defending the skeleton-like appearance as normal, actively maintains it and denies that it is abnormal. She indicates that it is rewarding to achieve and maintain this emaciated state. She is increasingly fearful of weight gain and interprets the concern of others as attempts to make her fat.

2. Inaccurate and confused perception and interpretation of inner stimuli. Inaccurate hunger awareness is pronounced. The adolescent does not recognize signs of nutritional need in herself and is unable to assess the amounts of food taken. She may feel 'full' after only a few bites and derives pleasure from the refusal of food. A preoccupation and tremendous involvement with food and related activities are associated with this eating behaviour; the girl frequently assumes all meal planning and preparation for others. Girls with anorexia nervosa often increase their activity to help counteract the possibility of weight gain. This hyperactivity may continue until emaciation is far advanced.

3. Paralysing sense of ineffectiveness that pervades all aspects of daily life. Youngsters with anorexia nervosa are overwhelmed by a deep sense of ineffectiveness. They are convinced that they function only in response to demands and wishes of others, rather than doing as they want or choose. They have always been compliant children, but careful analysis reveals this to be mechanical obedience and overconformity that is not recognized as a reflection of a serious problem — a self-doubt regarding their ability to stand up for themselves or even the right for self-assertion.

Modified from Bruch, 1978.

FACTORS	ANOREXIA NERVOXA	BULIMIA
Food	Turns away from food to cope	Turns to food to cope
Personality	Introverted Avoids intimacy Negates feminine role	Extroverted Seeks intimacy Aspires to feminine role
Behaviour	'Model' child Compulsive/ obsessive	Often 'acts out' Impulsive
School	High achiever	Variable school performance
Control	Maintains rigid control	Loses control
Body image	Body distortion	Less frequent body distortion
Health	Denies illness	Recognizes illness
Weight	Less than 85% of expected norm	Within 5 to 15 lb of normal body weight
Sexuality	Not sexually active	Often sexually active

Table 19.1 Some characteristics of eating disorders.

resolve the adolescent identity crisis, particularly as it relates to a distorted body image.

PROGNOSIS

The complete recovery rate for AN is less than ideal. Only 15% of affected individuals attain full recovery; 50% improve substantially, although they may relapse during times of stress. A few report a more favourable outcome with a small number of patients (Kreipe, Churchill, and Strauss, 1989). The fatality rate for this disorder is approximately 5% and is almost always associated with long-standing symptoms (Comerci, 1988) and such factors as depression, bulimia, and vomiting. Although the changes are often reversible, long-term effects of severe malnutrition may be evident. For many, AN will be a lifelong problem. The prognosis is best for teenagers in whom the disorder is diagnosed at a relatively early age, before abnormal eating patterns and other weight-loss techniques are established and emaciation has set in (Joffe, 1990).

Evidence indicates that patients restored to normal weight still demonstrate a very low self-esteem, are highly sensitive to social interactions, and remain 'obsessive' (Toner, 1986). There is a strong underlying suicidal tendency, and although patients may not be aware of it, the efforts to starve themselves may be

a manifestation. This should be explored in psychotherapy.

Nurses need to adopt and maintain a kind, supportive, yet firm manner in managing the care of a child with AN, without creating a passive-dependent attitude in the child. The child requires sustained support and reassurance as she copes with ambivalent feelings related to her own body concept and the desire to see herself as cooperative, reliable and worthy of the kindness she receives. Encouraging the child with education and activities that strengthen her self-esteem facilitates her resocialization process and social acceptance among her peers.

Diet
Rapid weight gain should be avoided. It can be medically unsafe, and it overwhelms the patient, who feels out of control immediately. A safe and reasonable target weight is calculated by the doctor and dietitian. Initially, the child resists the target weight as 'too heavy', but without a target weight she feels out of control and believes people want her to gain weight indefinitely. Establishing a 'maintenance weight range' of 1kg over or under the target weight also helps the youngster feel in control and teaches how weight is maintained through good dietary habits (e.g., uncontrollable weight gain is not inevitable when an individual consumes a normal diet).

It is also important for nurses to be aware of some of the physical side effects of AN. Patients with AN often limit their fluid intake, which can lead to urinary tract problems. Ketones and proteins are frequently detected in the urine as a result of fat and protein breakdown. Vital sign instability can be severe, including orthostatic hypotension; the heartbeat becomes irregular and the pulse rate decreases markedly. The bradycardia and hypothermia can result in cardiac arrest.

Behaviour therapy
The behaviour modification approach to therapy has both supporters and detractors. Providing privileges or activities for weight gain or positive eating behaviours has had some success, although this approach alone ignores the youngster's individuality and does not address the conflict precipitating the disorder (Pipes, 1989). A clearly defined behaviour modification plan is communicated to the child and maintained through a unified team approach by all persons involved in care. Several aspects are essential: (1) constancy, with team members providing a united front to avoid manipulation, (2) involvement of all team members, (3) continuity of team members and (4) clear communication.

A *behavioural contract*, an agreement that the patient makes with the others involved to change a maladaptive behaviour, has been effective in some cases. The written contract, constructed by the therapeutic team, is approved and signed by the patient. Unless the patient agrees to its terms, the contract can become the source of a power struggle. However, it can be an effective tool by placing the responsibility on the patient for weight gain or other behaviour change (Carino and Chmelko, 1983).

Family-centred care
Family therapy seems to be effective when begun soon after

the onset of illness, but it is less successful when the condition has existed for some time. Therapy is directed towards disengagement and redirection of malfunctioning processes in the family, but this usually requires individual psychotherapy for family members (Russel *et al*, 1987).

Cognitive Behavioural Approach

There is a persistence of distorted thoughts and beliefs even after weight gain. Thus, there appears to be a role in the cognitive process in developing and maintaining anorexia nervosa. This includes:

- fostering a sound therapeutic relationship
- accepting the patient's beliefs as genuine
- introducing doubt about the basic premise of the belief (e.g., does it seem advantageous to maintain the values of thinness, considering the impact on the life of the young person in missing out on school, friends, etc.)
- leaving patient with some feeling of control; for example, using a step-by-step approach and trial periods
- educating the patient about AN
- raising patient awareness of cognitive behavioural techniques (e.g., rehearsing seeing number increase on bathroom scale in process of desensitization), thus enabling patient to develop a clear understanding of behaviours which constitute anorexic/dieting strategies (e.g., cutting food up into tiny amounts) and encouraging a nonanorexic approach to eating

Prevention

There are no easy ways to prevent AN. However, public and professional awareness of signs and symptoms can help identify patients early, so that treatment can be implemented in order to prevent or reduce the long-term adverse consequences. Some of the early signs of AN are outlined in Box 19 3. Education about the disorder may help prevent some cases.

Evaluation

The effectiveness of nursing interventions is determined by continual reassessment and evaluation of care based on the following observational guidelines and expected outcomes:

1. Perform nutritional assessment, measure weight; review diet and nutritional intake; interview child regarding food and eating behaviours; observe eating behaviours.
2. Interview the youngster regarding self-perceptions; observe behaviour; confer with psychologist and other members of the health team regarding evidence of progress.
3. Observe child's behaviour and interview the youngster regarding attitudes and concerns.
4. Interview family and confer with team members regarding progress; observe interpersonal interactions between child and others, especially family members.

BULIMIA

Bulimia (from the Greek meaning 'ox hunger') is the term applied to an eating disorder, similar to AN, that is characterized by binge eating. The binge behaviour consists of secretive, frenzied consumption of large amounts of high-calorie (or 'forbidden') foods during a brief period of time (usually less than two hours). The binge is counteracted by a variety of weight control methods (purging), including self-induced vomiting, diuretic and laxative abuse, and rigorous exercise. These binge/purge cycles are followed by self-deprecating thoughts, a depressed mood and an awareness that the eating pattern is abnormal.

CLINICAL MANIFESTATIONS

Bulimia is observed more frequently in older adolescent girls and young women. Male bulimics are uncommon. Dynamically, persons with bulimia have many issues in common with other eating disorders (control being a major issue). Many begin with only occasional binges and purges 'just for fun', enjoying the control over their weight while eating amounts of food that would normally produce obesity. As the disease progresses, the frequency of binges increases, the amount of food consumed increases, and the person gradually loses control over the binge/purge cycle. The binge/purge cycle provides relief from feelings of guilt resulting from the enormous amounts of

---

◆ BOX 19-3

Early signs of anorexia nervosa

The youngster:

Consumes an inappropriate diet (excessively strict) or may refuse to eat altogether

Develops peculiar eating habits such as toying with food, food 'rituals', preparing and forcing food on family members without eating any herself

Engages in excessive exercise, such as compulsive jogging, running up and down stairs, or other rigorous activities to burn off calories—often to the point of exhaustion

Withdraws from social interaction — starts to spend all her time in her room studying, exercising, or otherwise occupied

Ceases to have menstrual periods after sudden or excessive weight loss — sometimes almost as soon as dieting begins

Takes laxatives, diuretics or enemas to speed intestinal transit time to lose added weight and empty intestines to flatten abdomen

Vomits deliberately — may go to bathroom after a meal and turn on taps to avoid being heard

Denies hunger, even after eating practically nothing for days or weeks

Develops a distorted body image — states she 'feels fat' as she becomes increasingly thinner

Loses weight — growing girls fail to achieve the 25th percentile on normal growth curves

costly food consumed. The family becomes angry, and the individual with bulimia becomes frightened, frustrated and increasingly guilt-ridden, which only increases the symptoms in the self-destructive cycle.

The frequency of bingeing can be anywhere from once per week to seven or eight times per day. Because persons with bulimia usually binge on high-calorie foods, especially sweets, ice cream and pastries, insulin production is stimulated to cope with the added carbohydrates. When the food is vomited, the unused insulin stimulates hunger and the desire to eat. An intake of 20,000 to 30,000 calories per day is not unusual.

Characteristically, persons with bulimia are those who have been unsuccessful dieters, have low impulse control, and may have been self-conscious about overweight in childhood. They may consciously or unconsciously suppress their feelings, and have a strong desire to fit into the group.

Individuals with bulimia appear to fall into two categories: (1) those who consume vast quantities of food followed by purging but who, if unable to purge, still consume large amounts and (2) those who restrict their caloric intake, especially when unable to purge. Some bulimic women are of normal or (more often) slightly above normal weight; others become as underweight as individuals with AN. This latter type with a tendency to restrict intake is also called *bulimarexia*. (See Table 19-1 for a comparison of AN and bulimia.)

Complications

Women with bulimia suffer from several medical complications as a result of the frequent vomiting. Loss of fluids and electrolytes can occur very rapidly, as in any other disorder characterized by gastrointestinal losses. Potassium depletion causes diminished reflexes, fatigue, and, if severe, possible cardiac arrhythmias. Potassium losses are more likely to occur with diuretic abuse. Laxative abuse can interfere with absorption of fat, protein and calcium, as well as produce abdominal complaints, such as cramping and sluggish bowel function.

Vomiting produces several serious complications. Irritation from stomach acid causes erosion of tooth enamel and an increase in dental caries. Chronic oesophagitis, chronic sore throat, difficulty swallowing, inflammation and parotitis are frequent findings. Vomiting may be so severe that the patient suffers oesophageal tears, hiatal hernia and spontaneous bleeding in the eye. Anaemia is common.

PROCESS OF DIAGNOSIS

The diagnosis may be first suspected from the presence of complications. Final diagnosis is made on the basis of criteria established by the American Psychiatric Association (1987) (Box 19-4). Distinctive hand lesions have also been observed in bulimic persons. The backs of the hands are often scarred and cut from repeated abrasion of the skin against the maxillary incisors during self-induced vomiting (Williams, Friedman and Steiner, 1986).

THERAPEUTIC MANAGEMENT

Therapy is similar to the management of AN. Hospitalization may be required, especially for complications, which are treated symptomatically. Intravenous fluids and potassium replacement are the essential elements of care, and cardiac monitoring is indicated.

DESTRUCTIVE BEHAVIOURS

The turmoil and stress associated with the pubertal changes of adolescence, limited problem-solving capacity, and the struggle for independence experienced by many adolescents, make them vulnerable to superimposed stresses. Some youngsters who are unable to cope with these complex problems and feelings indulge in behaviours that are life-threatening or physically harmful.

SMOKING

The problem of smoking among teenagers is becoming increasingly serious. The habit appears to be spreading among teenagers even as the evidence of the relationship between smoking and health problems increases.

Findings in one area of the United States disclosed that 22% of the girls and 11% of the boys were smoking.

A preventive approach to teenage smoking is especially important. The World Health Organization has found there is a high probability that regular smoking in childhood leads to a lifetime habit with concomitant increases in morbidity and mortality.

Social factors

Social pressures to smoke include imitation of the smoking behaviour and attitudes of parents and other adults, and social pressure from advertisers who aim directly at members of this vulnerable age group.

◆ **BOX 19-4**

Diagnostic criteria for bulimia nervosa

1. Recurrent episodes of binge eating (rapid consumption of a large amount of food in a discrete period of time)
2. A feeling of lack of control over eating behaviour during the eating binges
3. Regularly engages in either self-induced vomiting, use of laxatives or diuretics, strict dieting or fasting, or vigorous exercise in order to prevent weight gain
4. A minimum of two binge eating episodes a week for at least three months
5. Persistent overconcern with body shape and weight

Modified from American Psychiatric Association, 1987.

Sociodemographic factors

Sociodemographic factors include socioeconomic status, sex, and performance in school. A consistent, negative association has been observed between socioeconomic status and smoking (especially among boys), and there is a consistent correlation between low academic goals and performance and smoking (cited in Flay *et al*, 1983).

Psychosocial factors

A primary feature of early adolescence is development of a positive identity and an autonomous self-concept. Cigarette smoking may be an attempt on the part of young people who are low achievers in school to emulate the personality traits of toughness, friendliness, confidence, attractiveness and enthusiasm — traits that are popularly attributed to smokers.

IMPLICATIONS FOR NURSING

Nurses in schools and other agencies of the community are in a position to implement and reinforce teaching, to serve as consultants and counsellors to student, teacher, and parent groups, and to be advocates in all areas in which antismoking campaigns might be effective. Several strategies are recommended (Box 19-6). A survey of adolescent smokers seen in general practice indicated that of those given counselling, 60% gave up smoking. General practice, therefore, seems to be an appropriate place to receive advice (Townsend *et al*, 1991).

SUBSTANCE ABUSE

The use of substances, primarily drugs, by children and adolescents to produce an altered state of consciousness is widespread. It is believed to reflect the variety of changes taking place in their lives and the stresses engendered by these changes. The difficulties associated with the growth and changes of this prolonged and intense transitional process, encourage the adolescent to search for relief, escape or self-exploration. To achieve relief, young people often turn to the exhilarating, mind-easing, euphoriant qualities of drugs.

PATTERNS OF DRUG USE

Many factors influence the extent to which drugs are used by teenagers. The type of drug used, mode of administration, duration of use, frequency of use and single or multiple drug use must be considered in determining the severity of the individual drug problem. Most drug use begins with experimentation. The individual may try a drug only once, it may be used occasionally, or it may become an integral part of a drug-centred lifestyle. Identification of the pattern of drug use in an individual facilitates the formulation of an approach to the problem. Patterns have been observed based on dose and frequency of use.

There are two broad categories of adolescents who use drugs: (1) the *experimenters* and (2) the *compulsive users*. With the exception of a 'bad trip' or accidental overdose, the experimenters present few medical problems, although they probably represent the bulk of adolescent drug users. Some of these youngsters, who have a predisposition to heavy drug use, proceed to compulsive use, but generally, they are the minority.

Between the experimenters and compulsive users is a broad range of *recreational* users of drugs. The groups of greatest concern to health workers are those whose patterns of use involve high doses with the danger of overdose, and compulsive users with the threat of dependence, withdrawal syndromes and altered life-style.

MOTIVATION

There are several common motives for drug use. Adolescents try drugs out of curiosity. Drugs produce, for some persons, a dreamy state of altered consciousness and a feeling of power, excitement, heightened acuity or confidence. Others seek visual hallucinatory experiences and sexual sensation. Many youngsters use drugs not only for the perceptual and sensory experiences, but also for the social aspects. An investigation into the significance of various factors as possible indicators of drug abuse (including previous drug use, suspension at school, law infringements, truancy, conflict with parents, and alcohol and cigarette use) found the most predictive factor was peer drug use. The more of the other factors present in the adolescent, the higher the risk of drug abuse.

TYPES OF DRUGS ABUSED

Any drug can be abused, and most are potentially harmful to adolescents still going through formative life experiences. Although rarely considered drugs by society, the chemically active substances most frequently abused are the xanthines and theobromines contained in chocolate and in common beverages such as tea, coffee and colas. Common analgesics, ethyl alcohol, and nicotine are others that, although recognized as drugs, are sanctioned by society. Any of these can produce mild to moderate euphoric and/or stimulant effects and can lead

---

◆ BOX 19-5

Stages of becoming a smoker

Preparation — early learning experiences provided in the environment (e.g., parent or sibling smokers in the family)

Initiation — trying the first cigarette; peer influences are more important than family influences in determining when cigarettes are first tried

Experimentation — learning to smoke by repeated experimentation: decision to quit or continue

Regular smoking — smoke sufficiently often to be considered a regular smoker

Data from Leventhal, Cleary, 1981.

◆ **B O X 1 9 - 6**

Recommended non-smoking strategies

- Provide only a cursory mention of long-term health consequences (e.g., cardiovascular and cancer risks)
- Discuss immediate physiological consequences in some detail (e.g., changes in heart rate and blood pressure, minor respiratory symptoms, and blood carbon monoxide concentrations)
- Mention alternatives to smoking for establishing a self-image that appears tough, independent, mature, or sophisticated (e.g., establishing a weight-lifting regime, jogging and dancing, joining a youth club, engaging in volunteer work for a hospital or political or religious group)
- Mention the negative effects of smoking (e.g., earlier wrinkling of skin, yellow stains on teeth and fingers, tobacco odour on breath and clothing)
- Mention the increasing ostracism of smokers by nonsmokers, both legal and informal, in places of work and public places
- Mention the increasing evidence that second-hand smoke is injurious to the health of nonsmokers who are regularly exposed, especially small children
- Acknowledge that many adults once believed that important social benefits were associated with smoking; but point out that the majority of adult smokers would now quit smoking if they could
- Arm the cooperative adolescent with arguments for dealing with peer pressure (e.g., by not smoking, a teenager demonstrates independence and nonconformity, traits normally prized by youth)
- Request posters and pamphlets from local voluntary agencies

Modified from Wong-McCarthy, Gritz, 1982.

◆ **B O X 1 9 - 7**

Problems related to drug use

Legal — the drug being taken is strictly controlled by law and Is accompanied by severe penalties for its use or possession.

Social — use of a substance leads to disruptive or bizarre behaviour that alienates the user from the rest of society; this results in a social problem.

Medical — current or continued use of a substance may adversely affect the physical or mental health of the youngster.

Individual — focuses on the role that drug use plays in the individual's life and factors that contribute to the individual's need for the drug.

---

and the nature of additives are highly variable. Many of the hazards associated with drug use are related to driving a car or operating equipment that may be harmful when carelessly used while under the influence of the drug.

Alcohol

Acute or chronic abuse of ethanol, a socially accepted depressant, is responsible for many acts of violence, suicide, and accidental injury and death. Ethanol reduces inhibitions against aggressive and sexual acting out. Abrupt withdrawal is accompanied by severe physical and psychological symptoms, and long-term use leads to slow tissue destruction, especially of the brain and liver cells.

Teenage drinking is not a new phenomenon, but because of its social acceptance, peer pressure, and easy accessibility, alcohol appears to have become the drug of choice. It is the most widely accepted drug, can be purchased legally by adults, is relatively inexpensive, is often used as part of a meal (wine, beer), and is approved by adults throughout the world when used in moderation. Youngsters may be afraid of hard drugs, but they feel comfortable with alcohol. Most have been exposed to alcohol all their lives.

Teenage alcoholics rely on alcohol as a defence against depression, anxiety, fear and anger. They become increasingly tolerant to the drug, and there is an increased use of sedatives with the alcohol. Not all of these characteristics are observed in the alcoholic, but if several of the signs are evident, the youngster should be considered at risk and detoxification therapy should be initiated to ensure safe and complete withdrawal from the drug.

Cocaine

Cocaine is the most potent antifatigue agent known, and although it is not a narcotic, it is legally categorized as such. 'Crack' or 'rock' is a newer, purer and more menacing form of

---

to physical and psychic dependence. The type of drugs used also varies according to geographic location, socioeconomic status, urban as opposed to suburban areas, and various times.

A drug that is popular with one 'generation' of adolescents may not be attractive to another, and changing trends are influenced by the adolescent's constant search for new and different experiences. The present concern is the use of alcohol, tobacco and cocaine.

Drugs with mind-altering capacity that are available on the black market and that are of medical and legal concern are the hallucinogenic, narcotic, hypnotic, and stimulant drugs. In addition, health professionals are concerned about use of various volatile substances, such as antifreeze, plastic model aeroplane cement, organic solvents, and typewriter correction fluid, that are inhaled to achieve altered sensation in the user. Drugs available on the street are often mixed with other compounds and fillers so that the purity of the drug, its strength,

the drug; it can be produced cheaply and smoked in either water pipes or mentholated cigarettes. The increased use of cocaine is related to its availability and affordability, the false perception of safety in its use, its association with persons in glamorous occupations, its snob appeal, its reputation as a sexually enhancing drug, and peer pressure.

Narcotics

Narcotic drugs include opiates such as heroin, morphine, meperidine hydrochloride and codeine. They produce a state of euphoria by removing painful feelings and creating a pleasurable experience of a specific quality, and a sense of success accompanied by clouding of consciousness and a dreamlike state. Physical signs of narcotic abuse include constricted pupils, respiratory depression, and, often, cyanosis. Needle marks may be visible on arms or legs in chronic users. Withdrawal from opiates is extremely unpleasant unless controlled with supervised substitution of methadone.

Health problems result from self-neglect of physical needs (nutrition, cleanliness, dental care), overdose, contamination and infection, including acquired immune deficiency syndrome (AIDS) and hepatitis.

Central nervous system depressants

A variety of hypnotic drugs that produce physical dependence and withdrawal symptoms on abrupt discontinuation may be used by adolescents. They create a feeling of relaxation and sleepiness, but impair general functioning. Drugs in this category include barbiturates and nonbarbiturates (e.g., methaqualone), as well as alcohol. Barbiturates combined with alcohol produce a profound depressant effect.

Central nervous system stimulants

Amphetamines and cocaine do not produce strong physical dependence and can be withdrawn without much danger. However, psychological dependence is strong, and acute intoxication can lead to violent, aggressive behaviour or psychotic episodes manifest by paranoia, uncontrollable agitation, and restlessness. When combined with barbiturates, the euphoric effects are particularly addictive.

Hydrocarbons and fluorocarbons

Glue 'sniffing' and the inhalation of plastic cement, typewriter correction fluid, and other volatile substances (e.g., petrol, gold and silver spray paint) that youngsters breathe directly, or place in paper or plastic bags from which they rebreathe the fumes, produce an immediate euphoria and altered consciousness. The substances are extremely hazardous to the individual, causing rapid loss of consciousness and respiratory arrest. Many persons taking these drugs do not have time to remove the bag from their heads and quickly become asphyxiated.

Mind-altering drugs

Hallucinogens (psychedelic, psychotomimetic, psychotropic or illusionogenic) are drugs that produce vivid hallucinations and euphoria. These drugs do not produce physical depen-

dence, since they can be abruptly withdrawn without ill effect. However, acute and long-term effects are variable, and in some individuals the dissociative behaviour may be unduly protracted. This category includes cannabis (marijuana, hashish) and lysergic acid diethylamide (LSD).

Terminology

Drug users have developed a specialized vocabulary for the abused substances.

THERAPEUTIC MANAGEMENT AND IMPLICATIONS FOR NURSING

Nurses in almost every setting are increasingly likely to have contact with youthful drug abusers or to be in a position to serve as educator and patient advocate. They are often in a position to serve as listener, confidant and counsellor to troubled youngsters. Nurses are essential members of health teams whose efforts are directed towards short-term and long-term therapy for drug abusers.

Often, observation or a description of the behaviour is more valuable than a report by patients or their friends as to the chemical agent taken (see Box 19-8 for diagnostic criteria).

Stimulation should be kept to a minimum for agitated, frightened youngsters. Treatment or tests that are not required immediately are best postponed. These youngsters primarily need psychological support in a nonthreatening environment and close contact with a sympathetic person who can stay with them and help them maintain contact with reality.

Obstetric and nursery personnel sometimes encounter the problem of drug dependence and withdrawal in newborn infants or in a compulsive drug-using mother.

Long-term management

A major factor in the treatment and rehabilitation of young drug users is careful assessment, in the nonacute stage, to determine the function the drug plays in these youngsters' lives. Adolescents need help to identify the problem that motivated them to resort to drugs and to recognize their own role in self-destructive, inappropriate drug-abuse behaviour before they can embark on a rehabilitation programme.

This requires a trusting relationship between the youngster and the health team, and involves a thorough physical examination and assessment of physical, psychological, educational and vocational status. A realistic appraisal of the adolescent's potential and efforts, aimed at short-term goal satisfaction along with building self-esteem, lays the groundwork for a successful rehabilitation programme.

Rehabilitation begins when youngsters decide that with the help of concerned and supportive adults, they can and are willing to change. Rehabilitation implies not only environmental manipulation and involvement therapy, but also commitment on the part of the patient to substitute dependency on people for dependency on drugs and to explore alternative mechanisms for problem solving and coping with stress. Professionals working with troubled youths must be prepared for recidivism, or the tendency to relapse, and maintain a plan for re-entry into the treatment process.

Local drug and alcohol dependancy centres should be able to advise nurses on the available groups (e.g., Parent's Anonymous) which can help parents and youngsters cope with the problem of drug abuse.

Prevention

Drug abuse in adolescence is both an individual and a community problem, and nurses play an important role in education and legislation, as well as in individual observation, assessment, and therapy.

Researchers have observed that high levels of parental support and nurturance are associated with the lowest average number of alcohol problems, illicit drug use and deviant acts. Therefore, 'working with families to develop better parenting skills relevant to nurturance and control can have long-term benefits for adolescents, their families and society at large' (Barnes and Windle, 1987).

SUICIDE

The problem of suicide is worldwide and is increasing in many countries. A striking feature is the increase among younger people. It is the third leading cause of death among persons aged 15-24 years in the United States (Brent *et al*, 1988), claiming more than 6,000 youths annually. There are 50-220 suicide attempts for every completion (Shaw, Sheehan, and Fernandez, 1987).

Suicide is defined as the deliberate act of self-injury with the intent that the injury should kill. Most authorities distinguish between a suicidal ideation, gesture and attempt, and all three must be acknowledged. Suicidal *ideation* is thoughts about or plans for suicide. A *gesture* is made without any real attempt to cause either serious injury or death, but rather to send out a signal that something is wrong. An *attempt,* unlike a gesture, is intended to cause injury or death. Teenagers sometimes make several gestures to draw attention to the fact that they are unable to cope. If the signals are not detected and responded to promptly, they may escalate in seriousness until they become serious attempts or completed acts.

INCIDENCE

The true incidence of suicide in children and adolescents is not known because of general under-reporting. Frequently, deaths by suicide are reported as accidental because of pressures exerted by family and society to avoid the cultural and religious stigma associated with self-destruction. There also appears to be some degree of certainty that the high accident rate in persons in this age group may reflect suicides masked by accidental death or homicide.

There are some differences in suicides in relation to ethnic and racial factors. Girls make suicidal gestures or attempts four to eight times more often than boys and account for 90% of suicide attempts, whereas boys account for 70% of successful

---

◆ BOX 19-8

Diagnostic criteria for psychoactive substance dependence

Any person with a psychoactive substance abuse disorder will be diagnosed as 'dependent' if any three of the following criteria are met:

1. Frequent preoccupation with, seeking or taking the substance
2. Frequent use in larger amounts or over a longer period than intended
3. Need for increased amounts of the substance to achieve intoxication or desired effect, or diminished effect with continued use of the same amount
4. Display of characteristic withdrawal symptoms
5. Frequent use of the substance to relieve or avoid withdrawal symptoms
6. Persistent desire or repeated efforts to cut down or control substance use
7. Frequent intoxication or impairment from substance use when expected to fulfil social or occupational obligations, or when substance use is hazardous (e.g., driving when drunk)
8. Relinquishment of some important social, occupational, or recreational activity to seek or take the substance
9. Continuation of substance use despite a significant social, occupational or legal problem, or a physical disorder that the person knows is exacerbated by the use of the substance

Modified from American Psychiatric Association, 1987.

---

suicides (Raley, 1985). Gestures are made at home when someone else is nearby, usually in the evening or afternoon.

Individual factors

Adolescence has always been characterized by turmoil, heightened emotionality, and wide variations in mood. Youngsters display moods that range from the depths of depression to the heights of elation. It is sometimes difficult to determine whether a youngster is exhibiting a normal mood swing or is at risk for true depression and suicide. With limited capacities for problem solving and with fewer and less sophisticated resources for resolving difficulties, they may resort to methods of handling problems that were acquired at an earlier age. It often appears to adults that adolescents 'overreact' to situations. Actually, they experience emotions and react to events more intensely than adults.

Some teenagers have difficulty coping well with critical events, especially a situation that is forced on them, such as the death of a friend, parent or sibling.

A surprising number of children 5-9 years of age commit or attempt to commit suicide. This behaviour is often wrongly assumed to be accidental. Children in this age group are unable to think in abstract terms and therefore do not comprehend the permanence and irreversibility of death. Immature adolescents with poor ego development tend to react impulsively to situations much as they did at a younger age.

Gay and lesbian adolescents are at particularly high risk for suicide completion, especially those raised in an environment where they are denied support systems (Bidwell and Deyher, 1991). When a gay or lesbian young person grows up in a community and family that does not accept homosexuality, they are likely to internalize the the homophobia and feel self-hate, which often turns to suicidal feelings. In this alienating social context, self-esteem is challenged. Youths who recognise their homosexuality at an earlier age have been found to be more likely to attempt suicide than those who confront sexual orientation issues at a later age. Although similar data are not known for lesbian or bisexual young people studies indicate that as many as 3 in 10 gay youths attempt suicide during adolescence (Remafedi *et al*, 1991).

Family factors

Suicidal youngsters almost invariably come from a disturbed family situation, such as one experiencing economic stress, family disintegration, medical problems or psychiatric illness.

SUICIDAL METHODS

The most common method of suicide attempt is overdose or ingestion of a potentially lethal substance such as drugs. A study of adolescent suicide attempts found that 83% overdosed as a means of attempting suicide (Spirito *et al*, 1992). The second most common method of suicide attempt is self-inflicted laceration.

Sometimes, an adolescent will threaten suicide in order to manipulate the environment. Unfortunately, with no self-destructive intent, a youngster may make a half-hearted attempt that leads to death or permanent injury. A 'partial' or chronic suicide is illustrated by the adolescent with a chronic illness, such as diabetes, who refuses to comply with the prescribed medical regimen, the accident-prone adolescent, and the drug-abusing youngster.

MOTIVATION

Suicidal ideation is not uncommon in adolescents. It represents numerous fantasies, such as relief from suffering, a means to gain comfort and sympathy, or a means of revenge against those who have hurt them. The youngsters have the erroneous perception that the act of suicide will evoke remorse and pity and that they will be able to return and witness the grief. They expect people to care and be concerned. A frequent motive for suicide in children and younger adolescents is the desire to punish others who will be grieved by their death. Angry children who are unable to punish directly those who have injured or insulted them will take revenge on those who love them through self-destruction ("They'll be sorry when they find me dead"; "They'll be sorry they were unkind to me").

Occasionally, there are adolescents who are so severely depressed that suicide appears to them to be the only means of release from their despair. These youngsters rarely give evidence of their intent, concealing their suicidal thoughts for fear of outside intervention.

Adolescents often respond to feelings of anger, failure, or loss with overt flight reactions. Some of these adaptive techniques are rebellion, withdrawal into the self with silence, physical withdrawal, such as running away from home, or, the most drastic of all, suicide. Social isolation is seen in many suicidal adolescents, but it appears to be the most significant factor in distinguishing those who will kill themselves from those who will not. It is more characteristic of those who complete suicides than of those who make attempts or threats.

Although suicide is often linked to a specific event, such as a family fight, an important school examination, the death of a teen idol, or the breakup of a youthful romance, that produced an impulsive response in the child, careful analysis will usually reveal an ongoing depressive process that has been expressed periodically and behaviourally. Teachers often report changes in the behaviour of children who previously had not had behaviour problems. They may become easily irritated, demonstrate a low frustration point, or exhibit clowning and active, restless behaviour. Older children may begin using drugs and alcohol.

It has often been a general tendency to dismiss a suicide attempt as an impulsive act resulting from a temporary crisis or depression. If this drastic move fails to draw attention to their problems or makes them worse, adolescents may conclude that taking their lives is their only means to solve these escalating, unsolvable and unbearable problems.

DEPRESSION

Depression is a symptom common to all human beings. It is a normal part of life, and even adolescents who are healthy and happy experience alternating periods of depression and elation as a part of the growth process. When depression appears as a predominant mood, persists for a long time, or is so disabling that the adolescent is unable to fulfil the normal tasks of this period of life, the condition is serious and warrants special attention and intervention.

Depressed persons describe feelings of sadness, despair, helplessness, hopelessness, boredom, loss of interest, and isolation. They may also feel self-reproach, self-deprecation and guilt. These subjective symptoms are evidenced by changes in behaviour and attitude.

THERAPEUTIC MANAGEMENT

Suicidal threats should be taken very seriously. Most youngsters respond quickly to intervention. It offers them the opportunity to talk things out. Often the problems are very specific ones that environmental manipulation, such as a change of school or classroom or conferences with parents, can solve. Sometimes, simply forming an attachment to a sympathetic, caring adult figure (therapist, nurse or counsellor) is sufficient.

IMPLICATIONS FOR NURSING

Care of the suicidal adolescent includes early recognition, management and prevention. Probably the most important aspect of management is the recognition of prodromal signs that indicate that a youngster is troubled and might attempt suicide. Health professionals need to be alert to the signs of adolescent depression, and any youngster who exhibits such behaviour, subtle or overt, should be referred for thorough psychological assessment. Depression can be manifested in two different ways: youngsters who feel depressed may talk about suicide and feelings of worthlessness, or they may build themselves a solid defence against such intolerable feelings of depression with behavioural or psychosomatic disturbances.

NURSING ALERT

No threat of suicide should be ignored or challenged in any way. It is a symptom that must be taken seriously. Too often, suicidal threats or minor attempts are confused with bids for attention. It is also a mistake to be lulled into a false sense of security when the adolescent's depression is apparently relieved. The improvement in attitude may very well mean that the youngster has made the decision to carry out the threat.

As soon as the youngster who attempts suicide is out of danger from medical problems resulting from the attempt, the data-gathering process should begin. It should include information from several sources to help evaluate the extent to which the child is suffering, the direction for therapy, and the probability of a repeated attempt. At least 10-15% of adolescents who attempt suicide ultimately *do* commit suicide, and at least 25% who commit suicide have made previous attempts (Adolescent in despair, 1985).

The youngster should be questioned directly about the depression or suicidal behaviour — it should never be dismissed. Clues to a youngster's feelings may be elicited by questions such as, "You look so sad. What is troubling you?", or "Sometimes people feel life is no longer worth living. Have you had such thoughts?". Sometimes the youngster is relieved to know others have had similar thoughts. The important objective is to get the teenager to talk about thoughts and feelings. "Where do you see yourself 5 years from now?" may offer clues

---

◆ BOX 19-9

Guidelines for evaluating a suicide gesture or attempt

Social setting — determine what steps were taken to prevent rescue, if another person was present in the room or the house during the attempt, and if others were aware of the attempt either before or immediately after.

Intent — determine how detailed the suicidal plans were (if a suicide note or letter was written). Such communication often expresses the true depth of a youth's despair.

Method — examine the means selected and the youngster's understanding of the method (e.g., kind, number, and action of pills taken).

History — determine if the attempt was an isolated event and, if not, the number and nature of previous attempts or gestures. A family history of suicide is significant.

Stress — determine the nature of the precipitating event, the alternative courses of action available to the child, and previous methods of coping with stress.

Mental status — assess the present mental status of the youngster and compare it with pre-attempt status as described by others.

Support — evaluate the type of support that could be expected from the youngster's family, friends, peers, teachers

---

to future plans. "It's very sad you have thought about dying. Have you made any plans?", "What did [do] you think would [will] happen to you as a result of taking the medications [or other means]?", and "When something is not going well, is there someone you can go to?" are questions that provide clues regarding the seriousness of the intent (Box 19-9).

Follow-up care is of utmost importance. Although confidentiality is the usual approach with adolescent counselling, in the case of self-destructive behaviours this cannot be honoured. The suicidal behaviour is reported to the family and other professionals, and youngsters are informed that this will be done. They are told that the health professional cannot let the youngster do this! Such action conveys an important message to an attempter — that the professionals understand and that they care.

KEY POINTS

◆ The change, growth and stress accompanying the transition to adulthood may predispose adolescents to faulty problem solving.

◆ The major eating disorders of adolescence are obesity, anorexia nervosa and bulimia.

◆ Age of onset of obesity, presence of emotional disturbances or neuroses, and negative evaluation of obesity by others may all contribute to the development of a disturbed body image in the adolescent.

◆ Diet, exercise, and behaviour modification are the hallmarks of treatment for obesity.

◆ The nurse's involvement in obesity control includes nutritional counselling, behaviour modification, group programmes and family counselling.

◆ Anorexia nervosa, a disorder characterized by severe weight loss in the absence of obvious physical cause, consists of three areas of disordered psychological functioning: (1) disturbed body image and deluded concept of body proportions, (2) inaccurate and confused perception and interpretation of inner stimuli, and (3) paralysing sense of ineffectiveness that pervades all aspects of daily life.

◆ Bulimics fall into two categories: (1) those who consume vast quantities of food followed by purging but who, if unable to purge, still consume large amounts and (2) those who restrict their caloric intake, especially when unable to purge.

◆ Smoking is a widespread problem among teenagers; reasons for smoking include social pressure, mass media influence and a need to develop a self-concept.

◆ Substance abuse is a severe problem in adolescence, and abusers include experimenters and compulsive users.

◆ Suicide, the deliberate act of self-injury with the intent to kill, may occur in adolescents because of difficulties in coping with stress, disturbed family environment, and psychoses.

REFERENCES

Adolescent in despair, *Emerg Med* 17(9):51, 1985.

American Psychiatric Association: *Diagnostic and statistical manual of mental disorders*, ed 3 (DSM-III-R), Washington, DC, 1987, The Association.

Barnes GM, Windle M: Family factors in adolescent alcohol and drug abuse, *Pediatr* 14:13, 1987.

Brent DA *et al*: Risk factors for adolescent suicide, *Arch Gen Psychiatry* 45:581, 1988.

Brownell KD, Kelman JH, Strunkard AJ: Treatment of obese children with and without their mothers: changes in weight and blood pressure, *Am J Clin Nutr* 71:515, 1983.

Bragg C, Hughes SH: Understanding and managing patients who smoke, *Fam Comm Health* 7:12, 1984.

Bruch H: Anorexia nervosa, *Nutr Today* 13(5):14, 1978.

Bryce-Smith D, Simpson RID: Case of anorexia nervosa responding to zinc sulfate (letter), *Lancet* 2:350, 1984.

Carino CM, Chmelko P: Disorders of eating in adolescence: anorexia nervosa and bulimia, *Nurs Clin North Am* 18:343, 1983.

Comerci GD: Eating disorders in adolescents, *Pediatr Rev* 10:1, 1988.

Flay BR *et al*: Cigarette smoking: why young people do it and ways of preventing it. In McGrath PJ, Firestone P: *Pediatric and adolescent behavioral medicine: issues in treatment*, New York, 1983, Springer.

Fox EL, Mathews DK: *The physiological basis of physical education and athletics*, Philadelphia, 1981, WB Saunders.

Graves T, Meyers AW, Clark L: An evaluation of parental problem-solving training in the behavioral treatment of childhood obesity, *J Consult Clin Psychol* 56:245, 1988.

Guggenheim J *et al*: Changing trends of tobacco use in a teenage population in Western Pennsylvania, *Am J Publ Health* 76:196, 1986.

Herzog DB, Copeland PM: Eating disorders, *N Engl J Med* 313:295, 1985.

Hofmann AD, editor: *Adolescent medicine*, Menlo Park, CA, 1983, Addison-Wesley.

Huse DM *et al*: The challenge of obesity in childhood. I. Incidence, prevalence, and staging, *Mayo Clin Proc* 57:279, 1982a.

Huse DM *et al*: The challenge of obesity in childhood. II. Treatment guidance by stage, *Mayo Clin Proc* 57:285, 1982b.

Joffe A: Too little, too much: eating disorders in adolescents, *Contemp Pediatr* 7(3):114, 1990.

Kendell RE *et al*: The epidemiology of anorexia nervosa, *Psychol Med* 3:200, 1973.

Kreipe RE, Churchill BH, Strauss J: Long-term outcome of adolescents with anorexia nervosa, *Am J Dis Child* 143:1322, 1989.

Leventhal H, Cleary PD,: The smoking problem: a review of the research and theory in behavioural risk modification, *J Personality Soc Psychol* 88:370,1981.

Marty PJ *et al*: Patterns of smokeless tobacco use in a population of high school students, *Am J Public Health* 76:190, 1986.

National Center for Health Statistics, 1988

Pipes PL: Nutrition in infancy and childhood, ed 4, St Louis, 1989, Mosby-Year Book.

Raley G: Youth suicide: the federal response, *Soc Legis Bull* 29:65, 1985.

Ramafedi G, Farrow JA, Deisher RW: Risk factors for attempted suicide in gay and bisexual youth, *Pediatrics* 87:869, 1991.

Russel G *et al*: An evaluation of family therapy in anorexia nervosa and bulimia nervosa, *Arch Gen Psychiatry* 44:1047, 1987.

Shaw KR, Sheehan KH, Fernandez RC: Suicide in children and adolescents, *Adv Pediatr* 34:313, 1987.

Spirito *et al*: Adolescent suicide attempts: outcomes at followup, *Am J Orthopsychiatry* 62:464, 1992.

Taitz LS: *The obese child*, Boston, 1983, Blackwell Scientific.

Toner BB: Long-term follow-up of anorexia nervosa, *Psychosom Med* 48:520, 1986.

Townsend J *et al*: Adolescent smokers seen in general practice: health, lifestyle and response to antismoking advice, *BMJ* 303:947, 1991.

Williams JF, Friedman IM, Steiner H: Hand lesions characteristic of bulimia, *Am J Dis Child* 140:28, 1986

Wong-McCarthy WJ, Gritz ER: Preventing regular teenage cigarette smoking, *Pediatr Ann* 11:683, 1982.

FURTHER READING

General

Barker P: Basic child psychiatry, 1979, Granada Press.

Crisp AH *et al*: How common is anorexia nervosa?—a prevalence study, *Br J Psychiatry* 128(5):49, 1976.

Plant M *et al*: Young people and drinking: results of an English national survey, *Alcohol Alcohol* 25(6):685, 1990.

Russel GM: Anorexia and bulimia nervosa. In Rutter M, Hirson L, editors: *Child and adolescent psychiatry—modern approaches,* Oxford, 1985, Blackwell Scientific.

Smelden GI: Weight and food preoccupation in a population of English schoolgirls. In Bargman GJ: Understanding bulimia and anorexia nervosa, *Report of fourth Ross Conference on Medical Research,* Colombo, Ohio, 1983.

Obesity

Castiglia PT: Obesity in adolescence, *J Pediatr Health Care* 3:221, 1989.

Dietz WH, Gortmaker SL: Do we fatten our children at the television set? Obesity and television viewing in children and adolescents, *Pediatr* 75:807, 1985.

Rosenbaum M, Leibel RL: Pathophysiology of childhood obesity, *Adv Pediatr* 35:73, 1988.

Wadden TA *et al*: Obesity in black adolescent girls: a controlled clinical trial of treatment by diet, behavior modification, and parental support, *Pediatr* 85:345, 1990.

Anorexia Nervosa/Bulimia

Danziger Y *et al*: Parental involvement in treatment of patients with anorexia nervosa in a pediatric day-care unit, *Pediatr* 81:159, 1988.

Garner DM, Garfinkel PE: *Handbook of psychotherapy for anorexia nervosa,* New York, 1985, Guilford Press.

Lakin JA, McClelland E: Binge eating and bulimic behaviors in a school-age population, *J Community Health Nurs* 4:143, 1987.

Lucas AR: Update and review of anorexia nervosa, *Contemp Nutr* 14(9), 1989.

Smoking

Coe RM *et al*: Patterns of change in adolescent smoking behavior and results of a one year follow-up of a smoking prevention program, *J School Health* 52:348, 1982.

Goldstein AO *et al*: Relationship between high school student smoking and recognition of cigarette advertisements, *J Pediatr* 110:488, 1987.

McCaul KD *et al*: Predicting adolescent smoking, *J School Health* 52:342, 1982.

Perry CL, Silvis GL: Smoking prevention: behavioral prescriptions for the pediatrician, *Pediatr* 79:790, 1987.

Substance Abuse

Burpo RH: A step beyond 'just say no', *MCN* 13:428, 1988.

Hahn E, Papazian K: Substance abuse prevention with preschool children, *J Community Health Nurs* 4:165, 1987.

Isralowitz R, Singer M, editors: *Adolescent substance abuse: a guide to prevention and treatment,* New York, 1983, Haworth Press.

Richardson JL *et al*: Substance use among eighth-grade students who take care of themselves after school, *Pediatr* 84:556, 1989.

Swaim RC *et al*: Links from emotional distress to adolescent drug use: a path model, *J Consult Clin Psychol* 57:227, 1989.

Alcohol

Barnes GM, Farrell MP, Cairns A: Parental socialization factors and adolescent drinking behaviors, *J Marriage Fam* 8:27, 1986.

Casswell S *et al*: What children know about alcohol and how they know it, *Br J Addict* 3:223, 1988.

Cocaine

Acee AM, Smith D: Crack, *AJN* 87:614, 1987.

Brown BS *et al*: Kids and cocaine—a treatment dilemma, *J Subst Abuse Treat* 6:3, 1989.

Estroff TW, Schwartz RH, Hoffmann NG: Adolescent cocaine abuse, *Clin Pediatr* 28:550, 1989.

Heagarty MC: Crack cocaine: a new danger for children, *Am J Dis Child* 14:756, 1990.

Mofenson HC, Copeland P, Caraccio TR: Cocaine and crack: the latest menace, *Contemp Pediatr* 3(10):44, 1986.

Smith DE, Schwartz RH, Martin DM: Heavy cocaine use by adolescents, *Pediatr* 83:539, 1989.

Suicide

Bakkala CF: The role of the school nurse in suicide prevention, *School Nurse* 6(1):13, 1990.

Hoffman Y: Surviving a child's suicide, *AJN* 87:955, 1987.

Lamb JM: The suicidal adolescent: how you can help, *Nurs '90* 20(5):72, 1990.

Pfeffer CR: *The suicidal child,* New York, 1987, Atcom.

Valente S: Suicide in school aged children: theory and assessment, *Pediatr Nurs* 9:25, 1983.

USEFUL ADDRESSES

British Dietetic Association , 7th Floor, Elizabeth House, 22 Suffolk Street, Queensway, Birmingham B1 1LS.

Chapter 20

Impact of Chronic Illness or Disability on the Child and Family

LEARNING OUTCOMES

After studying this chapter you should be able to:

◆ Discuss the scope of the problem of families with a disabled or chronically sick child.
◆ Explain the concept of family-centred care as it relates to the family of a chronically sick or disabled child.
◆ Understand the principle of 'statementing' for Special Education Need.
◆ Discuss the concept of loss with regard to families of children with chronic illness or disability.
◆ State factors which contribute to stress in such families.
◆ Discuss likely effects on parental relationships and siblings of having a chronically ill or disabled child within the family.
◆ Explain the importance of continuous assessment of the child and family.
◆ Discuss ways of helping the family to cope.
◆ Explain why it is important for nurses to foster reality adjustment in these families.
◆ Discuss problems associated with the transition to adulthood.
◆ Define the glossary terms.

GLOSSARY

benevolent overreaction A cycle of overprotective, permissive parent and dependent, demanding child

chronic illness A condition that interferes with daily functioning for more than three months in a year, causes hospitalization of more than one month in a year, or (at time of diagnosis) is likely to do either of these (Hobbs and Perrin, 1985)

Congenital disability A disability that has existed since birth but is not necessarily hereditary

developmental delay A maturational lag – an abnormal, slower rate of development in which a child demonstrates a functioning level below that observed in most children of the same age

developmental disability Any mental and/or physical disability that is manifested before the age of 22 years and is likely to continue indefinitely

developmental model Focuses on the child's developmental needs rather than on the medical diagnosis

disability The restriction or lack of ability to perform normally as a result of impairment

handicap A disadvantage resulting from impairment or disability, which limits or prevents the fulfilment of a role that is normal for that individual, depending on age, sex, and social and cultural factors (WHO, 1992); individuals with chronic illnesses or disabilities are not necessarily handicapped

impairment Any loss of abnormality of psychological, physiological, or anatomical structure or function (WHO, 1992)

normalization Establishing a normal pattern of living; the principle that children and families should have access to services provided in as usual a fashion and environment as possible (Johnson, McGonigel, and Kaufmann, 1989)

technology-dependent child A child with a chronic disability that requires the routine use of a medical device to compensate for the loss of a life-sustaining body function; daily, ongoing care, and/or monitoring is required by trained personnel

I n a complex society, there are innumerable abilities necessary for functioning. Loss of any physical or cognitive power immediately poses an obstacle to a person's ability to meet societal expectations. With advances in early diagnosis and treatment of many chronic illnesses, and with improved technology for people with physical impairments, there is an increasing number of children who need care. Because nurses are intimately involved in care for every type of health deviation, it is inevitable that they will be responsible for some phase of care with families who have children with special needs imposed by a physical or mental limitation. This chapter is primarily concerned with families' responses to the disorder, the effects of chronic illness or disability on the child and family unit, and nursing interventions that promote the optimum adjustment of each family member and acceptance of the child as a unique individual with special attributes, as well as needs.

PERSPECTIVES IN THE CARE OF CHILDREN WITH SPECIAL NEEDS

Children with special needs comprise an increasingly important group of children who require both routine and specialized health care.

SCOPE OF THE PROBLEM

Exact definitions and incidence rates of chronic illness and disability do not exist. Statistics regarding chronic illness and disability are, at best, only estimates of the true incidence of the problem. These figures vary, according to the definitions used, the methods of study, and the population investigated. The prevalence rate for all children defined in the OPCS survey published in 1989 was 32:1000, or approximately 3%; however, figures of up to 16% have been quoted in earlier estimates, where a wider range of problems, such as impairments, have been included (OPCS, 1989).

The past 20 years have seen a dramatic change in the survival rates for some children with chronic and/or life-threatening diseases such as leukaemia, Hodgkin's disease, cystic fibrosis or spina bifida. For conditions such as asthma and muscular dystrophy, however, survival rates have changed little during the same period. The prognosis for the extremely low birth weight infant continues to improve annually (Cooke, 1994). However, the progress of these children at risk contributes to the growing number of children with chronic and/or disabling conditions, many of whom remain dependent on technology.

Most of these children live at home with their families. Considering that the average family in the United Kingdom has between three and four members, the number of individuals intimately affected by these children is staggering.

The numbers alone suggest that comprehensive nursing approaches are required to meet the immense needs of children, young people, and families. Nurses have a more crucial role than ever before, in early screening, identification of children in need, and assessment and diagnostic studies, as well as supportive interventions that minimize the disruptive effects of the condition on the family. Another major responsibility is preventing disabling disorders by eliminating their known causes. Nurses and health visitors have opportunities to influence uptake levels of immunization programmes, identify infants and mothers who may be at risk antenatally or postnatally, identify disability early, promote injury prevention policies and programmes, and implement innovative health education programmes.

CHANGING TRENDS IN CARE

In recent years, changes have occurred in providing services to children with special needs. Current practice avoids classifying needs and services by medical diagnoses, since most psychosocial and developmental needs of children with chronic conditions are not disease specific (Yoos, 1987).

DEVELOPMENTAL FOCUS

Using the developmental approach, rather than chronological age, emphasizes the child's abilities and strengths, rather than disabilities. In the past, health professionals have tended to view persons with a disability within a pathological framework, probing for weaknesses and negative features; consequently, insufficient attention has been paid to the child's individuality, personality, or strengths, or to the family's needs. Using a developmental model, attention is directed to the child's functional development and adaptation to the environment.

FAMILY DEVELOPMENT

A developmental focus also considers family development. A family member's serious illness or disability can cause significant stress or crisis at any stage of family development. Just as with individual development, family development may be interrupted or may regress to an earlier, inappropriate level of functioning. Nurses can use the concept of family development to plan meaningful interventions and to evaluate care.

FAMILY-CENTRED CARE

Family-centred care (see Chapter 3) is a philosophy of care that recognizes that the family is the constant in a child's life and that service systems and personnel must support, respect, encourage, and enhance the strength and competence of the family (Johnson, McGonigel, and Kaufmann, 1989). Families are supported in their natural caregiving and decision-making roles by building on their unique strengths as individuals and families. The needs of all family members, not just the child's, are considered.

Two basic concepts in this process are *enabling* and *empowerment*. Professionals *enable* families by creating opportunities for all family members to display their present abilities and to acquire new competencies necessary to meet the needs of the child and family. *Empowerment* describes the interaction of professionals with families in such a way that families maintain or acquire a sense of control over their family lives and that help families foster their own strengths, abilities, and actions.

The *parent–professional partnership* is a powerful mechanism for enabling and empowering families. Parents move from being the passive recipients of care for their child to serving as respected equals with professionals. Partnerships imply the belief that partners are capable individuals who become more capable by sharing knowledge, skills, and resources in a manner that benefits all participants. Collaboration is viewed as a continuum. Families have the option to be anywhere along that continuum, depending on the strengths and needs of the child, the family, and the professionals who are involved.

A significant number of families of children with special needs will bring a previous history of serious personal and/or family problems, and will need special help. However, *every* family has strengths as well as needs. The nurse can help identify their strengths and build on them. While family-centred care is an important concept in the care of all children, it is crucial to optimum care for children with chronic illnesses or disabilities. Elements of family-centred care include:

- Recognizing that the family is constant in a child's life, while the service systems (health, social services, education), and personnel within them, fluctuate.
- Recognizing family strengths and individuality, and respecting different methods of coping; involving the family to its level of coping and educating them towards total involvement in care.
- Facilitating parent and/or professional collaboration.
- Honouring racial, ethnic, cultural, and socioeconomic diversity.
- Sharing information with parents on a continuing basis.
- Encouraging and facilitating family-to-family support and networking.
- Designing accessible health care systems that are flexible and responsive to family-identified needs.

NORMALIZATION

Normalization refers to establishing a normal pattern of living. It implies child and family access to services in as usual a fashion and environment as possible (Johnson, McGonigel, and Kaufmann, 1989), and permits the child and family to become or remain part of the community. It means preparing the child and family in advance for changes that may occur, including the child, in as many decisions as possible, identifying areas where the child can be in control, and applying the same family rules to the child with a chronic illness or disability as to siblings.

CARE IN THE COMMUNITY

Concurrent with the trend towards normalization has been the earlier discharge of children from acute or chronic care facilities to the family and community, recognizing that family values are as important to the care of a child with a chronic health problem as they are to the care of other children (see

Chapter 4). The objectives are to:

- Normalize the life of a child with special needs, including those with technologically complex care, in a family and community context and setting.
- Minimize the disruptive impact of the child's condition on the family.
- Foster the child's maximum growth and development.

With appropriate training and support, families provide complex procedures and treatments in the home. Parents are challenged to retain a home-like setting among monitors, ventilators, and other sophisticated equipment.

INTEGRATION INTO MAINSTREAM EDUCATION

Just as the home is the natural environment for children, so school must also be included as an essential component of the children's overall physical, intellectual, and social development. Children who attend school have the advantages of learning and socializing with a wide group of peers.

'STATEMENTING'

As soon as it becomes evident that a child has special educational needs, a parent or professional may request an assessment of Special Educational Need (a 'Statement'). A nurse who knows the family may be well placed to support the parents in making this request. The *1993 Education Act* requires the Local Education Authority (LEA) to complete the process within six months of the request being made, no matter what the age of the child. The statement identifies areas in which additional support is needed, and how that support will be given. It is intended that most children will have their needs met within mainstream education, although they may need extra help in terms of environmental aids or specialist support staff.

Children in state schools must follow the National Curriculum; a Statement will specify if it is appropriate for a child to be following it in all areas. In some cases, it may be 'modified'; for example, a child who is physically unable to write may be allowed to dictate test or examination answers to a scribe; or 'differentiated'; that is, specific parts of the curriculum may be omitted.

SPECIAL SCHOOLS

A minority of children are recommended for special schools which address specific areas:

- Physical disability.
- Sensory disability.
- Cognitive disability.
- Medical needs.
- Behavioural and emotional difficulties.

The LEA must provide parents with a list of all appropriate schools — including independent schools — and must agree with the parents' preference, providing it is suitable for the child's age, ability, and special educational needs, and is an efficient use of the LEA's resources (Department for Education, 1994).

All children are entitled to a broad, balanced, and relevant curriculum within a school, no matter how complex their needs. In some cases of exceptional need, this may mean residential education. Both child and parents may need help accepting this as appropriate, recognizing that it may be the only way in which the family can continue to function as such, and may be the only way the child can receive education that meets his or her needs.

Nurses in residential schools have an important role to play, in conjunction with teaching staff, in encouraging families to remain closely involved with their child, to actively participate in the life of the school, and to continue the learning programmes while at home with their child. As it is often the nurse who is available by telephone or in person during out of school hours, he or she is frequently the most important link between the family and the school.

In non-residential schools, nurses have much to contribute to providing care for statemented children. Clinical skills and a traditional philosophy of family-focused care make them valuable contributors to interdisciplinary assessment and planning teams. Nurses and health visitors can assess children in preschool settings, provide ongoing family and staff education, coordinate care with other health care providers, and develop health promotion programmes for family and school staff.

PORTAGE

For some children whose needs are recognized early, education may begin prior to school age; for example, within Portage. This scheme is designed to help parents at home to teach their disabled child the early developmental skills which other children learn naturally. A Portage worker usually visits the family weekly with a checklist of developmental stages. Short-term goals are set at each stage, and ways to achieve the goals are discussed, together with access to appropriate materials (Glossop, 1989).

THE CHILD AND FAMILY WITH SPECIAL NEEDS

The family of the child with special needs faces the loss of a perfect child and must adjust to, and accept, the child and his or her condition. Nurses who understand the responses to the diagnosis and the effects the diagnosis commonly has on the family are able to emotionally support the family, anticipate and prevent potential problems, and foster development despite the disorder.

REACTIONS OF FAMILIES TO A CHRONIC ILLNESS OR DISABILITY

When the diagnosis of a disability or chronic illness is made,

the family progresses through a fairly predictable sequence of stages, regardless of the actual nature of the condition. The following discussion focuses on stages that are common to most families. Not all families experience this process, and each family member may vary widely in the time needed to progress through any of the stages.

The nurse must explore family reactions for all possible interpretations, not just negative ones, using a positive, supportive stance during interactions.

SHOCK AND DENIAL

The initial stage is a period of intense emotion and is characterized by shock, disbelief, and sometimes denial, especially if the disorder is not obvious, such as in chronic illness. Denial is a normal response to grieving any type of loss. Probably all family members experience various degrees of adaptive denial as they learn of the impact that the diagnosis has on their lives. Denial becomes maladaptive when it prevents recognition of treatment or rehabilitative goals necessary for the child's optimum survival or development. For example, protracted denial may be seen in the response of a family to learning disability. As long as the family can maintain normality, they may not recognize the diagnosis. Instead, the problem is explained as 'slow maturation'. The denial may be reinforced by the child's social development, which belies the degree of motor and speech retardation. This ability to rationalize delayed development is successful until the child enters school and the difference to the other children becomes evident. At this point, the family may begin to recognize the diagnosis as a crisis and react with shock and disbelief.

Shock and denial can last from days to months, sometimes even longer. Examples of denial that may be exhibited at the time of diagnosis include: 'doctor shopping'; attributing the symptoms of the actual illness to a minor condition; refusal to believe the diagnostic tests; refusing to tell or talk to anyone about the condition; insisting that no one is telling the truth; and asking no questions about the diagnosis, treatment, or prognosis. These mechanisms allow individuals to distance themselves from the emotional impact.

Partial denial, such as seeking additional professional consultations or occasionally acting as if nothing is wrong, is common for families with children who have life-threatening conditions. Without such a temporary protective mechanism, few people could survive the constant emotional drain of anticipating the death of their child.

In children, the importance of denial has repeatedly been demonstrated as a factor in their positive coping with the diagnosis. Children who use denial to cope with illness deal more positively with anxiety and have a productive attitude about life. Seriously ill adolescents may use denial to enable them to function adaptively and with hope. It allows them to maintain hope in the face of overwhelming odds. Like hope, denial may be an adaptive mechanism for dealing with loss that persists until a family or patient is ready or needs other responses.

ADJUSTMENT

Adjustment gradually follows shock and is usually characterized by an open admission that the condition exists. This stage is one of 'chronic sorrow' and only partial acceptance (Fraley, 1990) and is characterized by several responses, probably the most universal of which are *guilt* and *self-accusation*. Guilt is often greatest when the cause of the disorder is directly traceable to the parent, such as in genetic diseases or from accidental injury, but may occur without any realistic basis for parental responsibility. Frequently, the guilt stems from a fallacious assumption that the disability is a result of personal failing or wrongdoing. It may be related to thoughts of wishing the child dead, especially when the demands of care seem overwhelming and unrelenting. Guilt may also be associated with religious beliefs. Some parents are convinced that they are being punished for some previous misdeed, others that their religious strength and faith are being tested.

Children, too, may interpret their serious illness as retribution for past misbehaviour. The nurse should be particularly sensitive to the child who passively accepts all painful procedures. This child may believe that such acts are inflicted as deserved punishment. It is always vital to assure children that what happens to them during diagnosis or treatment is done to make them better.

Other common reactions are bitterness or anger. Anger directed inwards may be evident as self-reproaching or punitive behaviour, such as neglecting one's health and verbally degrading oneself. Anger directed outwards may be manifest in open arguments or withdrawal from communication, and may be evident in the person's relationship with individuals, such as the spouse, the child, and siblings. Passive anger towards the ill child may be evident in decreased visiting, refusal to believe how sick the child is, or inability to provide comfort. One of the most common targets for parental anger is members of staff; parents may complain about the nursing care or the insufficient time doctors spend with them.

It is important to recognize that the family's reactions may be strongly influenced by cultural beliefs and perceptions of the issues surrounding disability. A broad knowledge of the principal issues is essential for nurses working in an increasingly diverse society (Russel, 1992).

Children may react angrily to the restrictions imposed by their illness or disability, or to the feelings of being 'different'. Siblings may also feel anger and resentment towards the ill child and parents for the loss of routine and parental attention. It is difficult for older children and almost impossible for younger children to comprehend the plight of the affected child. Their perception is of a brother or sister who has the undivided attention of their parents, is showered with cards and gifts, and is the focus of everyone's concern.

Children of various ages manifest anger differently. Young children may yell, scream, and physically fight. Older children may use abusive language. Passive anger, expressed as, 'I don't know' or 'I don't care' often evokes aggressive anger in others. These reactions may be misinterpreted as sullen, obnoxious, or hostile reactions, and are effective in keeping people at a distance, when the hidden message is, 'I need to talk. Please help me understand what is happening'.

Several other reactions among parents may include:
- **Lowered self-esteem,** in which parents perceive a defect in their child as a defect in themselves.
- **Shame,** in which parents anticipate social rejection, pity, or ridicule.
- **Ambivalence,** in which the simultaneous experience of love and hatred normally experienced by parents towards their children is greatly intensified.
- **Depression,** in which parents experience chronic feelings of sorrow.

During the period of adjustment, four types of parental reactions to the child influence the child's eventual response to the disorder:
- **Overprotection,** in which the parents fear letting the child achieve any new skill, avoid all discipline, and cater to every desire to prevent frustration.
- **Rejection,** in which the parents detach themselves emotionally from the child, but usually provide adequate physical care or constantly nag and scold the child.
- **Denial,** in which parents act is if the disorder does not exist or attempt to have the child overcompensate for it.
- **Gradual acceptance,** in which parents place necessary and realistic restrictions on the child, encourage self-care activities, and promote reasonable physical and social abilities

A common initial response, especially among mothers, is *benevolent overreaction*. It is usually a consequence of unresolved guilt or fear, such as ambivalent feelings or not wanting the child during pregnancy, believing that the child would die at the time of birth or diagnosis, or reactivated feelings about a previous death. It results in a cycle of overprotective, permissive parent, and dependent, demanding child. It prevents the child from developing self-control, independence, initiative, and self-esteem. It is a reaction that responds to early intervention and prevention, but is resistant to change once firmly established. Overprotection is so common a parental reaction that it behoves the nurse to assess for its presence and to begin counselling as soon as possible (Box 20-1).

REINTEGRATION AND ACKNOWLEDGEMENT

For many families, the last stage is characterized by realistic expectations for the child and reintegration of family life with the illness or disability in proper perspective. Since a large portion of this phase is one of grief for a loss, total resolution is not possible until the child dies or leaves home as an independent adult.

This adjustment phase also involves social reintegration in which the family broadens its activities to include relationships outside the home, with the child as an acceptable and participating member of the group.

One of the most important aspects of acceptance for health professionals to understand is that it is not an 'all-or-nothing'

◆ BOX 20-1

Characteristics of parental overprotection

Sacrifices self and rest of family for the child

Continually helps the child, even when the child is capable

Is inconsistent with regard to discipline or employs no discipline; frequently different rules apply to the other siblings

Is dictatorial and arbitrary, making decisions without considering the child's wishes, such as keeping the child from attending school

Hovers and offers suggestions; calls attention to every activity, overdoing praise

Protects the child from every possible discomfort

Restricts play, often because of fear that the child will be injured

Denies the child opportunities for growing up and assuming responsibility, such as learning to give own medications or perform treatments

Does not understand the child's capabilities and sets goals too high or too low

Monopolizes the child's time, such as sleeping with the child, permitting few friends, or refusing participation in social or educational activities

◆ BOX 20-2

Stresses of families with a child with special needs

Day-to-Day Stresses

Reactions of other children and the larger community

Effect on siblings

Financial worries

Housing

Transport

Clothing and appliances

Need for support

Anticipated Parental Stress Points

Diagnosis of the condition — requires considerable learning, as well as dealing with emotional response

Developmental milestones — times children normally achieve walking, talking, self-care are delayed or impossible for the child

Subsequent pregnancies — whether coming child will also be affected, or whether they will be able to cope

Start of schooling — particularly stressful are situations in which appropriate education will not be in a mainstream school

Reaching the ultimate attainment — situations, such as realizing that ambulation will be impossible or that the child will not learn to read, must be handled

Adolescence — issues such as sexuality and independence become prominent

Future placement — decisions about placement must be made when the child becomes an adult or when the parents can no longer care for the child

Death of the child

Anticipated Sibling Stress Points

Birth of another child — may be the affected sibling or the subsequent birth of an unaffected child

Diagnosis of condition — in certain illnesses, times of remission and exacerbations are difficult

Start of schooling — particularly stressful if friends reject the child with special needs

Adolescence — may be embarrassed to bring friends home

Future placement — may worry about responsibility for the affected sibling, especially if the parents are ill or die

Death of the child

---

phenomenon. Rather, it is interspersed with periods of intensified sorrow for the loss. Consequently, even families who have achieved a high level of adjustment and acceptance are, at predictable times, in need of support from professionals or other families who have coped successfully with similar experiences (Box 20-2).

PLACEMENT AWAY FROM HOME

If strategies of coping cannot be employed to minimize the stress and disorganization of maintaining the child within the home to tolerable levels, the affected child may be permanently placed in an alternative residential setting. This may be the only option that will preserve the integrity of the family. Ageing parents may be forced to accept this alternative from progressive inability to meet the demands imposed by a severe disability. Relinquishing the role of primary caregiver is followed by an initial sense of loss, relief, guilt, and ambivalence.

IMPACT OF THE CHILD'S CHRONIC ILLNESS OR DISABILITY ON FAMILY MEMBERS

Each family who has a child with special needs is affected by the experience. The parents' responses directly influence other members' reactions, including the extended family. Their response, as well as the community's acceptance of the child, can further assist or hinder the family's coping with the stresses imposed upon them.

PARENTS

Besides grieving for the loss of a perfect child, parents may or may not receive positive feedback from interactions with their child. Many feel satisfaction and fulfilment from the parenting role. For others, parenting may be a series of unrewarding experiences, which continually reinforce feelings of inadequacy and failure. For example, they may become preoccupied with their ability to carry out certain procedures, overlooking the child's regular needs, or fail to offer praise for anything less than perfect cooperation or performance. As a result, the parent can become caught in a pattern of interaction that is mutually unrewarding and minimally productive. For these parents, it may be beneficial to reduce the quantity of time spent with the child and thus increase the quality of the relationship.

Parental roles

Excessive demands may be placed on parental time, energy, and financial resources. Depending on the roles assumed by each partner, the mother often receives the majority of the time and energy demands, and the father the financial responsibilities. However, these responsibilities may be shared or shifted more heavily to one member. It is important for nurses to realize that the absence of one parent from the hospital or clinic does not necessarily indicate that the shared parent pattern is not in effect (Clements, Copeland, and Loftus, 1990).

Relationship conflicts may arise if one partner views his or her share as unequal. The partner who is not included in the caregiving activities may feel neglected, since all the attention is directed towards the child, and resentful that he or she has not had the opportunity to become competent in the care of the child. Without active participation in the caring activities, the parent has little appreciation of the time and energy involved in performing them. When the less competent partner does attempt to participate, the other parent frequently criticizes the less skilful efforts. As a result, communication breaks down and neither is able to support the other. Unfortunately, these problems are seldom recognized until they are well established, rather than earlier, when intervention can be most effective.

The mother and father may experience distinct differences in adjusting and coping as parents of a child with special needs; the father struggling with issues that may be quite distinct from those of the mother. Herbert and Carpenter (1994) found that the father's needs were often not addressed, or even noticed, so that he may feel 'disabled' in the supportive role that he is expected to fill, not knowing how to help and unable to protect the family from the seemingly overwhelming recurring problems. Dreams of lineage, ego fulfilment, and athletic and vocational achievement are threatened and, in turn, may threaten the father's self-esteem.

Fathers worry about what the future holds for their children (Field, 1990), as well as their ability to manage the increasing financial burden. Some escape in their work as a means of dulling the pain. Others view all of the difficulties of having a child with special needs as challenges to overcome, and are not afraid to push limits and be assertive to acquire the needed services for their children (Davies and May, 1991).

Single-parent families

Single-parent families are of special concern (McCubbin, 1989). The absence of a parent may be due to divorce or death, or the parents may never have married. As the only parent of a child who may require extensive, sophisticated, and lifelong care, the single parent may feel an enormous burden. Nurses must recognize that external sources of support and personal inner strength are particularly crucial for single parents to enable them to care for their child (Clements, Copeland, and Loftus, 1990).

SIBLINGS

Siblings can be deeply affected yet their needs are often overlooked (Atkinson and Crawforth, 1995). Younger siblings may feel uprooted and displaced more than older children. For example, firstborn children with cognitive impairment become the 'youngest' by virtue of their developmental age. Conversely, second-born children become the oldest, often shouldering adult-like responsibilities and participating in the care of the disabled child.

Siblings often may show symptoms of irritability, social withdrawal, or fear for their own health. Healthy siblings may display a wide variety of physical complaints, such as headache, abdominal pain, or symptoms mimicking those of the sick or disabled child, as a reflection of their anxiety and fear. The level of their reactions to the child often do not mirror the severity of the condition.

Some specific behaviours may have a negative effect on the family, such as jealousy, increased competition and fighting, anger, hostility, social withdrawal, attention-seeking behaviour, and a decline in school performance. However, positive behaviours are also cited, such as increased nurturing, cooperation, sensitivity, compassion, and mastery of new skills (Gath, 1989).

Siblings reveal feelings of isolation, deprivation, inferiority, and inadequate knowledge about the child's condition. Their lives are most often affected in terms of the parent–child relationship and social restrictions, because of additional responsibilities in the home. Many siblings report receiving rewards in terms of 'bribes' to overlook shortcomings in their parent–child relationship, but few receive any reward in the form of praise, personal attention, or tangible items. They often feel left out and uninvolved in the child's care, especially when the child is treated or educated away from home.

The way family members feel about one another and cope with stress plays a major role in sibling adjustment (Lobato, 1990). Although positive, maturing attitudes can form in these siblings, the responsibility of health professionals is to involve the entire family unit in the adjustment process.

FACTORS AFFECTING THE FAMILY'S ADJUSTMENT

The diagnosis of a child with a serious health problem or disability is a major situational crisis that tremendously affects the entire family system. However, families can experience positive outcomes as they successfully deal with the many challenges that accompany a child with chronic illness or disability (Futcher, 1988). If they receive emotional support and guidance early, there is an increased likelihood that they will also cope successfully.

It is not necessarily the families of children with the most severe illnesses or disabilities that have the poorest adjustment. The family of a child with multiple disabilities demanding complex care — yet having many resources and coping skills — may adjust more successfully than the family of a child with a less serious condition but with fewer innate resources.

AVAILABLE SUPPORT SYSTEMS

Support systems may be available through a variety of relationships and may consist of one significant other, such as a marital partner, or a group, such as extended family or members of the health team. Support provided by professionals is different from that provided by family and friends. The most appropriate sources of informational support might include both professionals who have theoretical and practical knowledge and nonprofessionals — parents — whose experience equips them as experts. When professionals develop a strong therapeutic relationship with the family, they, too, can be appropriate sources of emotional support.

Status of the parental relationship

The parental relationship is a prime source of potential support and may be considered the best predictor of coping behaviour and adjustment. When the partners can openly discuss their feelings, there tends to be much less guilt, anger, blame, and indecision.

Alternative support systems

The single-parent family may have the support of extended family, such as that of the parent's own parents. Occasionally, parents may be able to communicate with each other, but are unable to talk with the child. This is particularly evident with very young children, who communicate least through verbalization, and with adolescents, who may be unwilling to discuss with or listen to adults. In this case, the child is left without an available support system.

Ability to communicate

Almost all methods of psychological intervention, such as support through active listening, counselling, or crisis intervention, require verbal communication between two individuals. The ability to verbalize about feelings such as anger, fear, guilt, or anxiety helps individuals cope with the particular emotion.

Not all individuals are able to communicate verbally. Some rely on religious faith and silent prayers for support. Others, such as children, communicate best through nonverbal methods, such as play, drawing, or writing. Some individuals may not be able to communicate with anyone because of their interpersonal withdrawal and social isolation. These individuals are most at risk because, even if a support system is available, they may be unable to share their problems with others.

Previous knowledge

Although family members may be shocked to learn that their child has a serious illness or disability, most will have some knowledge about the disorder from previous associations. It is important to explore the extent of that information, in order to understand what parents believe about their child's medical condition, and if these beliefs are based on accurate information (Austin, 1990).

Influence of religion

Religious beliefs and spirituality have various meanings for different people. For some, religion comprises the foundation of their support system. Healing and faith are synonymous, and any criticism of the family's spirituality can weaken their trust in the medical care. For others, it may intensify feelings of guilt, shame, bitterness, or punishment.

Imagined cause

Although the cause of many disorders is unknown, parents and children often supply their own answers. Children may interpret the reason for the illness as a punishment for not obeying others. Parents may be convinced that the disease was inherited, or brought on by curses, occult witchcraft, or devils. Once the fantasized cause is revealed, the person can be helped to deal with the irrationalities of that thinking.

COPING MECHANISMS

Coping mechanisms are behaviours aimed at reducing the tension caused by a crisis. *Approach behaviours* are coping mechanisms that result in movement towards adjustment and resolution of the crisis. *Avoidance behaviours* result in movement away from adjustment or maladaptation to the crisis. Several approach and avoidance behaviours used in coping with a chronic illness or disability are listed in Box 20-3.

Two long-term coping strategies of familial adaptation to chronic and severe childhood illness have been significantly associated with a high level of family functioning. The first is the parents' ability to endow the illness with meaning within an existing spiritual or medical and/or scientific philosophy of life. There is an optimistic belief that all things work out for the good and a focus on the positive qualities of the situation. Statements such as 'God has chosen our family to care for this special child' are reflective of the religious philosophy.

The second is an ability to share the burdens of the illness with individuals both inside and outside the family constellation. Intrafamilial relationships encourage togetherness of the family members and maintain a mutual acknowledgement that all members are important contributors to the family unit. Extrafamilial supports help preserve meaningful external contacts and provide needed help to the family.

REACTIONS TO THE CHILD

An awareness of the family members' reactions to the child is important and can uncover the type of childrearing practices or attitudes that may not only hamper the child's optimum development, but also influence the family's adjustment. Parental reactions are driven by feelings such as guilt, love, fear, power, shame, pride, pity, concern, and confusion. These reactions, in turn, affect attitudes and choice of childrearing practices, which can cause resounding effects throughout the family system.

AVAILABLE RESOURCES

Resources are the available means that exist or can be developed either within the family or in the community. Resources

---

◆ **BOX 20-3**

Guidelines for assessing coping behaviours

Examples of Approach Behaviours

Asks for information regarding diagnosis and child's present condition

Seeks help and support from others

Anticipates future problems; actively seeks guidance and answers

Endows the illness or disability with meaning

Shares burden of disorder with others

Plans realistically for the future

Acknowledges and accepts child's awareness of diagnosis and prognosis

Expresses feelings, such as sorrow, depression, and anger, and realizes reason for the emotional reaction

Realistically perceives child's condition; adjusts to changes

Recognizes own growth through passage of time, such as earlier denial and nonacceptance of diagnosis

Verbalizes possible loss of child

Examples of Avoidance Behaviours

Fails to recognize seriousness of child's condition despite physical evidence

Refuses to agree to treatment

Is angry and hostile to members of the staff, regardless of their attitude or behaviour

Avoids staff, family members, or child

Entertains unrealistic future plans for child, with little emphasis on the present

Is unable to adjust to or accept a change in progression of disease

Continually looks for new cures with no perspective towards possible benefit

Refuses to acknowledge child's understanding of disease and prognosis

Uses magical thinking and fantasy, may seek 'occult' help

Places complete faith in religion to point of relinquishing own responsibility

Withdraws from outside world; refuses help

Punishes self because of guilt and blame

Makes no change in life-style to meet needs of other family members

Resorts to excessive use of alcohol or drugs to avoid problems

Verbalizes suicidal intents

Is unable to discuss possible loss of child or previous experiences with death

---

within the family may include cohesion, adaptability, and hardiness — these are aspects of the family system that can help considerably in the family's adjustment.

Community resources, such as health care resources, parent support groups, availability of respite care, educational facilities, and recreational programmes, are key elements in family adjustment. These kinds of resources are better developed in some areas than others, meaning that what is available to a family depends largely on where they live. In an urban area, families of children with special needs may find a greater number of programmes and services for their children. The rural setting, however, may offer more social support because of a greater sense of community and less anonymity. Communities, like families, have different strengths which may vary also dependent upon the cultural background.

CONCURRENT STRESSES WITHIN THE FAMILY

The ability to deal with the already overwhelming stresses of a lifelong disability or illness is challenged when additional stresses are present. Ongoing stresses and strains in the family can accumulate, increasing the family's vulnerability and reducing its ability to adapt and adjust to a child with special needs.

Stressors may be situational or developmental. They may be related to relationship difficulties, financial pressures, housing problems or social isolation. With the alarming increase in substance abuse, it is reasonable to assume that some of the families may be struggling with a family member's alcohol or other drug problem. Even the more minor stresses ,such as arranging care for siblings, managing the home, and travelling to distant treatment centres, can jeopardize the family's ability to cope successfully (see also Box 20-2).

IMPACT OF CHRONIC ILLNESS OR DISABILITY ON THE CHILD

The child's reaction to chronic illness or disability depends to a great extent on his or her developmental level, temperament, and available coping mechanisms; on the reactions of significant others; and to a lesser extent on the condition itself. Knowledge of these variables is essential in providing the kind of support needed by these children to cope with a sometimes overwhelming situation.

DEVELOPMENTAL ASPECTS

The impact of a chronic illness or disability is influenced by the age of onset. Chronic illness affects children of all ages, but the developmental aspects of each age group dictate particular stresses and risks for the child. The nurse must also recognize that children need to redefine their condition and its implications as they develop and grow. An understanding of these factors facilitates planning care to support the child and minimize the risks (see Table 20-1).

Adolescence

The impact of illness or disability can be most detrimental during adolescence and it is therefore appropriate to look at this age in greater detail. Before this age, the child's self-image, self-esteem, and basic adjustment to life were primarily dependent on his or her relationship with the parents. A young child with impaired health reared in a home with loving parents who are sensitive to the child's needs generally copes well with the disorder. However, adolescence is different — even with all the benefits of parental love, the adolescent is striving for an independence away from parents and in many ways must deal with the impact of impairment alone.

For every adolescent, the major task is to establish an identity of their own. Pubertal changes must be integrated into the self-image while the teenager is gaining control and mastery over increased physical capabilities and sexuality. During early adolescence, this takes place primarily within the peer group. Illness or injury at this time interferes with teenagers' sense of mastery and control over a changing body. They are different at a stage of development when being different is unacceptable to the peer group. At no time of life is an individual so vulnerable to the emotional stress of impairment. Appearance, skills, and abilities are highly valued by peers; a teenager who is limited in any of these qualities is subject to rejection. This is especially marked when a physical disability interferes with sexual attractiveness.

These teenagers are faced with the task of incorporating their disability into the changing self-concept. The youngster who develops the illness or acquires the disability during the crucial adolescent years has greater difficulty than does the teenager who has been affected since childhood. The youngster with a newly acquired disorder will have the additional task of grieving for a lost 'perfection' while adjusting to the changes taking place as a natural course of events.

Adolescence is a time for achieving independence from the family, and planning for future goals and responsibilities. Adolescents with long-term chronic illness tend to be less future-directed and less independent than healthy peers (Blum *et al*, 1991). Enforced dependency from physical impairment can exacerbate the parent–child conflicts surrounding independence. The tendency towards rebellion may be directed at the disorder and reflected in decreased compliance with treatment, denying the disorder to preserve a sense of normalcy with peers, and risk-taking behaviour that can place the teenager in jeopardy. Such behaviours can further strain an already tense parent–child relationship.

COPING MECHANISMS

Children's innate and learned coping mechanisms are very important in their ability to deal with their disorder. Characteristics such as age, gender, temperament, sense of self-esteem, social skills, and intelligence may influence a child's ability to cope with stress. In addition, the social support afforded these children is critically important. Therefore, the better the family copes, the better the child is able to deal with the stressors imposed by the illness or disability.

Because it is often easier to recognize children who cope poorly with illness or disability, it is helpful to describe those behaviours typical of well-adjusted children. Well-adapted children gradually learn to accept their physical limitations, but find achievement in a variety of compensatory motor and intellectual pursuits. They function well at home, at school, and with peers. They have an understanding of their disorder that allows them to accept their limitations, assume responsibility for care, and assist in treatment and rehabilitation regimens.

They express appropriate emotions, such as sadness, anxiety, and anger at times of exacerbations, but confidence and guarded optimism during periods of clinical stability. They are able to identify with other similarly affected individuals, promoting positive self-images and displaying pride and self-confidence in their ability to master a productive, successful life despite the disability.

RESPONSES TO PARENTAL BEHAVIOUR

The parents' behaviour towards the child, especially in terms of childrearing, is one of the most important influencing factors in the child's adjustment. Children whose parents are overprotective tend to have marked dependency, especially on the mother, fearfulness, inactivity, and lack of outside interests. Children raised by oversolicitous and guilt-ridden parents are often overly independent, defiant, and high-risk takers. Children reared by parents who emphasize their deficits and tend to 'hide' or isolate them appear as shy and lonely individuals who harbour resentful and hostile attitudes. In contrast, children who are reared by parents who establish reasonable limits tend to develop independence that is appropriate for their age and achievement commensurate with their limitations. They often display pride and confidence in their ability to cope successfully with the challenges imposed by their disorder.

NURSING CARE OF THE FAMILY AND CHILD WITH SPECIAL NEEDS

The major nursing goal is to help the family remain intact and functioning at optimum levels throughout the child's life. This involves not merely supporting the child and family during the critical period when the child is being diagnosed. It involves forming parent–professional partnerships that invite the parents' early input, encourage them to be accountable and responsible for the child's care, and do not reinforce the dangerous attitude that the professional will 'fix' the child and give him or her back to the parents. It also reinforces the fact that it is not so much the condition itself that affects the child's progress and developmental outcomes, but the family's ability to cope successfully with the child's problems. Thus long-term, comprehensive, systematic, family-centred approaches must be applied.

AGE/ DEVELOPMENTAL TASKS	POTENTIAL EFFECTS OF CHRONIC ILLNESS OR DISABILITY	SUPPORTIVE INTERVENTIONS
■ Infancy		
Develop a sense of trust	Multiple caregivers and frequent separations, especially if hospitalized	Encourage consistent caregivers in hospital or other care settings
	Deprived of consistent nurturing	Encourage parents to visit frequently or stay and participate in care
Bond/attach to parent	Delayed because of separation, parental grief for loss of 'dream' child, parental inability to accept the condition, especially a visible defect	Emphasize healthy, perfect qualities of infant
		Help parents learn special care needs of infant for them to feel competent
Learn through sensori-motor experiences	Increased exposure to painful experiences over pleasurable ones	Expose infant to pleasurable experiences through all senses (touch, hearing, sight, taste, movement)
	Limited contact with environment from restricted movement or confinement	Encourage age-appropriate developmental skills, e.g., holding bottle, finger feeding, crawling
Begin to develop a sense of separateness from parent	Increased dependency on parent for care	Encourage all family members to participate in care to prevent overinvolvement of one member
	Overinvolvement of parent in care	Encourage periodic respite from demands of care responsibilities
■ Toddlerhood		
Develop autonomy	Increased dependency on parent	Encourage independence in as many areas as possible, e.g., toilet use, dressing, feeding
Master locomotor and language skills	Limited opportunity to test own abilities and limits	Provide gross motor skill activity and modification of toys or equipment, such as modified swing or rocking horse
		Give choices to allow simple feeling of control, e.g., choice of what book to look at or what kind of sandwich to eat
Learn through sensori-motor experience, beginning preopera-tional thought	Increased exposure to painful experiences	Institute age-appropriate discipline and limit-setting
		Recognize that negative and ritualistic behaviour are normal
		Provide sensory experiences, e.g., water play, sand-box, finger paint
■ Preschool		
Develop initiative and purpose	Limited opportunities for success in accomplishing simple tasks or mastering self-care skills	Encourage mastery of self-help skills
Master self-care skills		Provide devices that make task easier, e.g., self-dressing
Begin to develop 'peer' relationships	Limited opportunities for socialization with peers; may appear 'like a baby' to them	Encourage socialization, such as inviting friends to play, daycare experience, trips to park
	Protection within tolerant and secure family may cause child to fear criticism and withdraw	Provide age-appropriate play, especially associative play opportunities
Develop sense of body image and sexual identification	Awareness of body may centre on pain, anxiety, and failure	Emphasize child's abililties; dress appropriately to enhance desirable appearance
	Sex role identification focused primarily on mothering skills	Encourage relationships with same-sex and opposite-sex peers and adults
		Help child deal with criticisms; realize that too much protection prevents child from learning the realities of world
Learn through preop-erational thought (magical thinking)	Guilt (thinking he or she caused the illness/disability or is being punished for wrongdoing)	Clarify that cause of child's illness or disability is not his or her fault or a punishment

Table 20-1 Developmental aspects of chronic illness or disability on children.

AGE/ DEVELOPMENTAL TASKS	POTENTIAL EFFECTS OF CHRONIC ILLNESS OR DISABILITY	SUPPORTIVE INTERVENTIONS
■ School age		
Develop a sense of accomplishment	Limited opportunities to achieve and compete, e.g., many school absences or inability to join regular athletic activities	Encourage school attendance; schedule medical visits at times other than school; encourage to make up missed work Educate teachers and classmates about child's condition, abilities, and special needs
Form peer relationships Scouts,	Limited opportunities for socialization	Encourage sports activities, e.g., Special Olympics Encourage socialization, e.g., Cubs, Brownies, Guides, Youth groups, PHAB clubs
Learn through concrete operations	Incomplete comprehension of the imposed physical limitations or treatment of the disorder	Provide child with knowledge about his or her condition Encourage creative activities
■ Adolescence		
Develop personal and sexual identity	Increased sense of feeling different from peers and less able to compete with peers in appearance, abilities, special skills	Realize that many of the difficulties the teenager is experiencing are part of normal adolescence (rebelliousness, risk taking, lack of cooperation, hostility towards authority) Provide instruction on interpersonal and coping skills Encourage socialization with peers
Achieve independence from family	Increased dependency on family; limited job/ career opportunities	Provide information on decision making, assertiveness, and other skills necessary to manage personal plans Encourage increased responsibility for care and management of the disease or condition, such as assuming responsibility for making and keeping appointments (ideally alone), sharing assessment and planning stages of health care delivery, contacting resources
Form heterosexual relationships	Limited opportunities for heterosexual friendships; less opportunity to discuss sexual concerns with peers	
Learn through abstract thinking	Increased concern with issues such as why did he or she get the disorder, can he or she marry and have a family Decreased opportunity for earlier stages of cognition may impede achieving level of abstract thinking	Encourage activities appropriate for age, such as attending mixed-sex parties, sports activities, driving a car Be alert to cues that signal readiness for information regarding implications of condition on sexuality and reproduction Emphasize good appearance and wearing stylish clothes, use of make up Understand that the adolescent has same sexual needs and concerns as any other teenager Discuss planning for the future and how condition can affect choices

Table 20-1 Developmental aspects of chronic illness or disability on children (cont.).

ASSESS THE FAMILY'S STRENGTHS AND LEVEL OF ADJUSTMENT

Since the nurse may meet a family during any phase of the adjustment process, it is essential to assess the family members' individual strengths, coping mechanisms, and reactions to the disorder. Ideally, assessment should begin as soon as the family learns the diagnosis.

Assessment must be a continuous process, because approach behaviours during one phase of the illness do not ensure reciprocal coping mechanisms in subsequent phases. Since support systems may change and perception of events may be altered at any point during the illness, nurses must continually evaluate the effectiveness of their interventions.

The nurse also assesses the parents' reaction to the child: observing how parents interact with the child can provide valuable information, for example:

- Do the parents cuddle the infant during feeding or maintain distance by positioning the baby on a bed or infant seat?
- Do they touch or stroke an older child who is fed in a high chair, other than during actual feeding activities?
- During feeding, dressing, and play, do the parents periodically make direct eye contact with the child?
- Do the parents talk with the child and respond positively to vocalization?

The parents' and child's understanding of the condition is another significant assessment area. Parental knowledge fosters coping and is particularly important since most children seek information from the parents. One method of eliciting information is to ask how the person would explain the child's condition to a stranger.

While inquiring about the parents' level of understanding, the nurse also focuses on the child's and siblings' knowledge of the condition. It is not unusual for parents who appear well adjusted and knowledgeable to state that they have never told the children the truth. Although this is less of a problem when the condition is visible, conflict may arise when the child or siblings learn of the diagnosis from nonparental sources. (See also Informing Children of Life-Threatening Diagnosis, Chapter 21.)

There are special challenges in assessing children's feelings about having a disability. An approach to encourage children to discuss feelings about their diagnosis and future might include using drawing and play as a method of communication. This would be appropriate in the child who may lack verbal skills or for any child dealing with difficult feelings.

Traditionally, the mother and child have been active participants and receivers of professional care, whereas fathers and siblings have been excluded. However, to achieve the goal of optimum development for the family unit, each member must be included. This may involve arranging appointments and/or home visits at times when other family members can be present.

Ideally, a thorough assessment includes observing the child and family in a variety of settings, including the home and school, which is the second most important environment for a child. Teachers exert a tremendous influence on the child's developmental progress, feelings of self-esteem, learning capacity, and formation of social relationships. Whenever feasible, the nurse should visit the school to observe directly the child's behaviour and interaction among teachers and classmates.

PROVIDE SUPPORT AT THE TIME OF DIAGNOSIS

The impact of the crisis usually occurs at the time of diagnosis, which may be at the time of birth, following a long period

of physical and/or psychological testing, or immediately after a traumatic injury. It may begin before the diagnosis is made, when parents are aware that something is wrong with their child, but before medical confirmation.

The time of diagnosis is a critical time for parents (Leonard, 1994). Although they may not hear or remember all that is said to them, they frequently sense a certain attitude of acceptance, rejection, hope, or despair that may influence their ability to absorb the shock and to begin adapting to the family's altered future.

Although it is usually the doctor's responsibility to inform the family of the diagnosis, nurses are frequently responsible for giving follow-up information, and coordinating services with other agencies.

Parents are encouraged to be together when they are informed of their child's condition, thus avoiding the problem of one parent having to interpret complex findings and deal with the initial emotional reaction of the other. It also provides an opportunity to observe the interaction between the parents.

The informing session should take place in privacy, in a comfortable setting free of distractions and interruptions. The atmosphere should be one in which feelings can be expressed and acknowledged, so that the parents can be helped to deal openly with them. Their emotional needs are acknowledged by showing acceptance of such expressions as crying, sadness, anger, and disappointment. Emotional support is offered by demonstrating through facial and bodily language that this is a difficult and painful period. Although touching is a powerful expression of empathy, it must be used wisely. Nurses should also be aware of cultural issues regarding touching.

Most parents report wanting a clear, simple explanation of the diagnosis, a prediction of possible futures for the child, advice on what to do next, an opportunity to ask questions, a warm and sympathetic listener, and, most important, time (Leonard, 1994).

Finally, the session should not end with the presentation of devastating news. Instead, the child's strengths and potential for development are stressed, as well as available rehabilitation efforts or treatment. Parents are encouraged to view life with their child as very similar to life with other children. Their experiences should be thought of as a series of challenges that they are capable of handling, particularly with the available professional support. The parents are assured that the nurse will be available to answer questions and to provide further assistance as it is needed in the future.

ACCEPT THE FAMILY'S EMOTIONAL REACTIONS

One of the most supportive interventions is to accept the family's emotional reactions to the diagnosis in as nonjudgemental a manner as possible. Although all families respond differently and in varying degrees of intensity, three responses are so common and often so poorly handled that they deserve special consideration.

DENIAL

The most effective method of support is active listening. Silence neither reinforces nor rejects denial (or any other emotional reaction), but implies a willingness and acceptance of the person's need for this behaviour. However, silence alone can be misinterpreted.

To be effective, silence and listening must be accompanied by physical and mental concentration, and use of body language to communicate interest and concern. Direct eye contact, touch, physical closeness, and body posture, such as sitting and leaning slightly forwards, demonstrate silent but effective communication. Sometimes, accepting people where they are, from their own perspective, is likely to give them the acknowledgement necessary to become more aware of their motives and to consider change.

GUILT

Since guilt is such a common response and can cause family members tremendous anxiety, they should be told directly when there is no known cause of the disorder and that they are not to be blamed.

If family members are expressing feelings of guilt, it is important to allow them to talk about their feelings rather than quickly trying to dispel them with long 'scientific' explanations.

ANGER

Anger is one of the more difficult reactions to accept and to deal with therapeutically. The responses to anger may be reciprocal anger, fear, acceptance, and/or encouragement. The first two reactions close off communication and express disapproval and rejection of the person. They most commonly occur when the listener views the anger as a personal assault. The last two responses allow the individual to ventilate his or her feelings in an atmosphere of nonjudgemental acceptance. Two basic rules for dealing with the angry person are to avoid losing one's temper and to encourage the person to talk. See Box 20-4 for guidelines to encourage expression of emotions.

HELP THE FAMILY COPE

In order for the family to meet the stresses of optimally adjusting to the child's condition, each member must be individually supported so that the family system is strong. The nurse should bear in mind that the 'member in need' is not necessarily the affected child, but may be a parent or sibling who is dealing with stresses that require intervention.

PARENTS

The nurse can provide support by being attentive to families' responses to their children. Mothers and fathers need to experience success, joy, and pride in their children to give the support they need. Nurses must demonstrate belief that parents are equal to professionals and that parents are experts regarding their child. The partnership is based on trust. See Box 20-5 for guidelines for developing successful partnerships with parents.

Since the majority of parents of children with special needs have little or no experience with children who have chronic or disabling conditions, the nurse can role model appropriate interactions with the child. Above all, the nurse should ensure that the parents and siblings learn to perceive the child as a child first, with unique and individual needs. The nurse needs to convey a humanistic, accepting approach of the child so that the parents can observe this acceptance. This attitude of liking, concern for, and acceptance of the child should begin at the time of diagnosis and continue throughout the child's life.

Communication among all family members needs to be encouraged. Parent group sessions are helpful in assisting parents to verbalize thoughts and feelings to each other, but often do not take into account the siblings' or child's viewpoint.

Parents should be encouraged to discuss their feelings towards the child, the impact of this event on their relationship, and associated stresses, such as financial burdens. For most families, regardless of their income, financial concerns exist. The costs of caring for a child with special needs can be overwhelming: out of pocket expenses for non-prescription medication, special dietary needs, additional heating, washing and transport can consume a significant percentage of a family's income.

In addition, the family wage earner may have to sacrifice job opportunities to remain close to a specialized medical facility. They should be encouraged to consider financial and career planning at an early stage, and may find it helpful to take financial advice. Both parents should be encouraged to participate in meetings from the beginning, scheduling appointments to allow working parents time to make arrangements.

Policies for the inclusion of families in assessment and goal setting should be examined to ensure that they are flexible and offer genuine opportunities for both parents to participate actively. It is not unusual to find two parents who have opposing views of the child's abilities, especially in the area of developmental disabilities, and it is important to facilitate an open exploration of these differences.

Families may need help to find their way through the often confusing maze of benefits to which they may be entitled, of which some will be tax free and not means tested. The nurse needs to identify a reliable source of up-to-date information on benefits and services, including both statutory and independent service provision, and voluntary or charitable services, whether local or national (e.g., *Disability Rights Handbook*, *Voluntary Agencies Directory* — both annual publications). A useful source of grants for families of children with severe handicaps is the Family Fund, which will provide money for 'one-off' expenses, such as a holiday, bedding, or a washing machine.

Although community resources may exist, it is often very difficult for parents to locate suitable services, and coordination among agencies may be lacking (Social Services Inspectorate, 1994). Fragmented care is one of the chief complaints from families (Betts, Meyer, 1993), with specific problems of delayed referral and negative experiences with personnel from the various statutory authorities cited as other concerns. What is more services may not be available in the relevant language, or may inappropriate for the family's cultural or religious needs (Shah, 1992) consequently, community networking and the formation of pressure groups to bring about improved services may provide a positive outlet for families who, alone, feel powerless to influence local or national conditions.

Parent-to-parent support

The support a parent receives from another parent is unique and unobtainable from any other source. Just being with another parent who has shared similar experiences is helpful. A parent of a child with the same diagnosis is not always necessary, for parents in the process of adjusting to a child with special needs — or finding respite services, education or rehabilition services, special equipment, financial counselling — tread a common path. The nurse can offer information about self-help groups, who will often send information about their organization and local branch group meetings. Contact a Family, with its national help line Contact Line, is a useful umbrella organization which publishes a directory of specific conditions (Marsh, Partridge, and Youngs, 1994).

Group members feel less alone and have the opportunity to observe coping strategies in other members. Parents' groups are rich resources for information. Even if parents are unable to attend meetings, they can still benefit from group newsletters and other literature that often accompany membership. The nurse can foster parent participation in self-help groups by serving as a referral agent, a group advisory board member, a resource person, a group member, or an assistant in founding a group (Rollins, 1987). Sometimes all that is required in starting a group is identifying one or two parents as leaders, providing a venue for a first meeting, and, with the consent of other families, exchanging names, telephone numbers, and addresses.

THE CHILD

Through ongoing contacts with the child, the nurse (1) observes the child's responses to the disorder, ability to function, and adaptive behaviours within the environment and with significant others; (2) explores the child's own understanding of the nature of his or her illness or condition, and (3) provides support while the child learns to cope with his or her feelings. Children are encouraged to express their concerns rather than allowing others to express these for them, since open discussions may reduce anxiety. Howeverr, it should be remembered that in some cultures, families do not openly discuss certain topics and that common health care terms may be misinterpreted. The nurse needs to remain alert to these issues.

If the child cannot or will not talk, the child may have to play out his or her feelings. He or she can be provided with toys to express threatening or stressful emotions. The nurse may find that the child responds best to drawing pictures or telling stories (see Chapter 9). Puppets can also be used. By demonstrating to parents how useful these techniques are, the

---

♦ **BOX 20-4**

Guidelines for encouraging expression of emotion

Describe the behaviour: 'You seem angry with everyone'.
Give evidence of understanding: 'Being angry is only natural'.
Give evidence of caring: 'It must be difficult to endure so many painful procedures'.
Help focus on feelings: 'Maybe you wonder why this happened to your child'.

---

nurse also helps them learn new ways of communicating with the child. For youngsters with persistent maladjustment, psychiatric evaluation and management may be needed.

One of the most important interventions is alleviating the child's feeling of being different and normalizing his or her life as much as possible. The principles of 'normalization' are fundamental.

Children who are concerned that their condition detracts from their physical attractiveness need attention focused on the normal aspects of appearance and capabilities. Health professionals can help strengthen and consolidate the self-image by emphasizing the normal, while at the same time allowing children to express anger, isolation, fear of rejection, feelings of sadness, and loneliness. Anything that might improve attractiveness and contribute to a positive self-image is employed, such as make up for a teenager with a scar, clothing that disguises a prosthesis, or a hairstyle or wig to cover a deformity or lost hair.

Children, particularly adolescents, are sensitive to the presence or absence of hope. Nurses can influence hopefulness through interpersonal and environmental means such as:

- Giving honest reports of conditions or events.
- Encouraging and participating with the child in physical activities (e.g., arrange activities, play games, or go for walks together).
- Conveying a fond, personal interest in the child (give hugs, ask follow-up questions from previous discussions).
- Directing conversations to neutral, non-disease-related or less sensitive topics (discuss child's favourite sports, tell stories).
- Providing information about other children in similar situations who are doing well.
- Being lighthearted; initiating or responding to teasing or other playful interactions with the child, although it is important for the nurse to be sensitive to the child's mood and respond appropriately. Periods of sadness and anger are usual in the child's adjustment to chronic illness or disability, especially during exacerbations of the disorder.

SIBLINGS

Siblings may experience embarrassment associated with the stigma of a disorder such as a learning disability. Parents are

◆ BOX 20-5

Guidelines for developing successful parent-professional partnerships

Promote primary nursing. In nonhospital settings designate a case manager or key worker.

Acknowledge the parents' overall competence and their unique expertise with their child.

Respect the parents' time as having equal value to that of other members of the child's health care team.

Explain or define any medical, technical or discipline-specific terms.

Develop a glossary of commonly used terms, acronyms and abbreviations to distribute to parents. The list can stand alon or become part of patient or parent handbooks.

Tell families, "I am not sure" or "I don't know" when appropriate.

Facilitate the family's effectiveness in team meetings:

- Provide families the opportunity to decide on the appropriate family members and professionals to include in assessment conferences and other meetings.

- Provide information to parents in a face-to-face meeting before convening any formal decision-making meeting about their child.

- Distribute meeting agendas to all participants, including the family, before the date of the meeting. Families, like all other team members, should always be made aware of why a meeting is being held, who will be there and what to expect.

- Introduce other professionals who may be involved with the child to the parents before any group meeting.

- Provide parents with the same information as other participants so that they can contribute to any decision about their child (e.g., child development checklist, copies of assessment reports).

- Invite parents to speak first and often throughout any information-giving or decision-making meetings, to give their perspectives and describe their observations before professionals give theirs.

- Be open with families and with other professionals when there is disagreement about any aspect of assessment or programming.

then faced with the difficulty of responding to this embarrassment in an understanding and appropriate manner without punishing the siblings for feeling the way they do. Parents should talk with the siblings about how they view their affected sibling. For example, siblings of a child who is disabled may express fears about their ability to bear normal children. Adolescents, in particular, may not be able to discuss these vital issues with their parents and may prefer to consult with the nurse. Many siblings benefit from sharing their concerns with

other young people who are experiencing a similar situation. Support groups for siblings help decrease isolation, promote expression of negative feelings, and provide an opportunity to learn from each other.

Many parents express concern about when and how to inform other children in the family about a child who is disabled. It is usually best to inform siblings before a neighbour or other person does so: uninformed siblings may fantasize or develop apprehensions that are out of proportion to the child's actual condition. If parents choose to be silent or deceptive about the issue, they are setting a negative precedent for the siblings to follow, rather than encouraging them to cope with the experience in a healthy and nurturing way.

The nurse must be sensitive to the reactions of siblings who may, for example, mention that they are expected to take on additional responsibilities to help the parents care for the child. There may be a positive reaction to assuming the extra duties, but a negative response to feeling unappreciated for doing so. Such feelings can often be minimized by encouraging the siblings to discuss this with the parents and by suggesting to parents ways of showing gratitude; most significantly verbal praise (see Parent Guidelines).

FOSTER REALITY ADJUSTMENT

Fostering reality adjustment primarily involves family education regarding the disorder, as well as general health care, developmental needs of the child, and realistic goal setting. Education should be aimed at preventing problems (Pless *et al*, 1994).

EDUCATE ABOUT THE DISORDER AND GENERAL HEALTH CARE

Educating the family about the disorder involves not only supplying technical information, but also discussing how the condition will affect the child. Parents need to understand what the child can do in terms of self-help, academic learning, and independence. Similarly, the child must know the limitations his or her disability places on activity, as well as the available opportunities.

Parents also need guidance in how the condition may interfere with or alter activities of daily living, such as eating, dressing, sleeping, and toilet use. One area frequently affected is nutrition. Common problems are undernutrition as a result of food being inappropriately restricted, loss of appetite, vomiting, or motor deficits that interfere with feeding; and overnutrition, usually caused by a calorie intake in excess of energy expenditure — or consumed through boredom and lack of stimulation in other areas. Although the child requires the same basic nutrients as other children, the daily requirements may differ.

Another very important area in which modifications may be needed is car safety. Children with orthopaedic, neuromuscular, or respiratory problems often cannot safely use conventional car restraints. Modifications can be made to some commercial models, but should be undertaken only with informed professional advice. Children in travelling wheelchairs present special challenges. The posture harness supplied with the wheelchair must always be worn, *and* an approved harness anchoring the wheelchair and the child to the floor of the vehicle must be used (Medical Devices Directorate Report, 1992). The family should consult the wheelchair manufacturer for specific instructions regarding safe transport.

Children with special needs require all the usual health care recommended for any child. Attention to injury prevention, immunizations, and dental health is essential. Nurses and health visitors can play an important role in reminding parents of these aspects of care that are often neglected when the concern is focused on the child's illness or disability.

Parents also need to be aware of the importance of communicating the child's condition in the event of a medical emergency. Young children are unable to give information about their disorder and, although older children may be reliable sources, after an accident they may be physically unable to speak. Therefore, all children with any type of chronic condition that may affect medical care should wear some type of identification, such as a Medic-Alert bracelet, which lists the medical condition and a phone number for emergencies.

Children need information about their condition, its management, and how the disease or the therapy might affect their particular situation. Children nearing puberty also need to understand the maturation process and how their disability may alter this event. For example, the youngster with diabetes needs to know that hormonal changes and increased growth needs will alter food and insulin requirements at this time; and the sexually active girl who has sickle cell anaemia needs to be aware of the hazards of pregnancy. The information should not be given all at once, but timed appropriately to meet the changing needs of the youngsters.

The subject of sexuality related to the effects of the disorder is a prominent concern of adolescents, but they rarely initiate a discussion of this sensitive topic. Any probable interference in sexual function because of the disability should be discussed openly and candidly with the teenager. Unfortunately, many nurses are reticent to discuss sexual issues with adolescents. Adults often underestimate the degree to which adolescents engage in unrealistic fantasies regarding sexual activities and related matters, or sexual activity itself: parents are often unaware of their teenagers' sexual activity (Dragone, 1990).

Throughout the long process of caring for a child with special needs family members become expert in management of their child's care (Meyer, 1990). Unfortunately, this expertise is often not recognized by health professionals, who tend to be directive, rather than collaborative, in their approach to the family, particularly during periods of hospitalization, when they may be ignored as participants in care, especially during treatment procedures (Robinson, 1985). A supportive atmosphere must include coordination of care with family members, respect for their knowledge, and willingness to include their suggestions in the care plan.

PROMOTE NORMAL DEVELOPMENT

The family must be guided towards fostering appropriate development in their child; although each stage may take longer to achieve, parents are guided to helping the child fully realize potential in preparation for the next phase of development. See Table 20-2 for developmental aspects of chronic illness or disability and for supportive interventions.

Early childhood.

The affected child's early existence may be stressful, chaotic, and unsatisfying. Consequently, he or she may need more parental support and expressions of affection to achieve trust. Likewise, the parents require assistance in ways to meet the infant's needs, such as how to hold a rigid or flaccid infant, how to feed a child with tongue thrust or episodes of dyspnoea, and how to stimulate a child who seems incapable of achieving any skills. If hospitalizations are frequent or prolonged, a great deal of effort may be required to preserve the parent–child relationship (see also Chapter 5).

The natural parental response to having a sick child is overprotection. Parents need help in realizing the importance of brief separations from the child, of including others in the child's care, and of providing social experiences outside the home whenever possible. Respite care, which provides temporary relief for family members, is essential in allowing caregivers time away from the daily demands of caring for a child with special needs (Royal College of Nursing and The Spastics Society, 1993).

In spite of need, parents report extreme difficulty finding competent respite care. The responsibilities placed on local authorities by the *Children Act* (1989) and the NHS and *Community Care Act* (1990) have speeded up the process of development of small local respite care units and the provision of family based respite care. This remains the ideal of most local authority purchasers and the majority of families, although too many children with disabilities still receive respite care inappropriately within hospital wards. Children with profound and multiple disabilities, and those who also have challenging behaviour, are still poorly provided for in most areas (Robertson, Stalker, 1991; Robertson and Beckford, 1993).

Periodically, the child's developmental progress must be evaluated. Since each child develops at his or her own rate, there are no rigid guidelines for expecting when particular skills will be achieved, but lack of progress in any one area should be investigated. For example, sometimes a delay in self-feeding is not caused by lack of motor skill, but by the parents' impatience in waiting for the skill to develop. Cleaning up the spilled food may seem like one more unnecessary task unless the importance of using a cup or spoon is stressed. All that may be necessary to encourage parent participation are suggestions to avoid large accidents, such as pouring only a small amount of juice in a cup or having the child feed himself or herself mashed potatoes (a sticky food) rather than jelly (a slippery food).

Not all children with disabilities are capable of achieving normal developmental milestones. For example, the child

Parent Guidelines

Supporting Siblings

Promote healthy sibling relationships

Value each child individually, and avoid comparisons.

Create a climate in which children can achieve successes without feeling guilty.

Teach siblings ways to interact with the child.

Seek to be fair in terms of discipline, attention, and resources; require the affected child to do as much for himself or herself as possible.

Let siblings settle their own differences; intervene only to prevent siblings from hurting one another.

Respect a sibling's reluctance to be with or to include the child with special needs in activities.

Help siblings cope

Listen to siblings to let them know that their thoughts and suggestions are valued.

Praise siblings when they have been patient, have sacrificed, or have been particularly helpful. Do not expect siblings to always act in this manner.

Provide age-appropriate information about the child's condition, and update when appropriate.

Let teachers know what is happening so they can be understanding and helpful.

Schedule special time with siblings.

Encourage siblings to join or help establish a sibling support group.

Use the services of professionals when needed. If the parent feels that such a service is necessary, it should be provided in as vigorous a manner as a service for the child with special needs.

Involve siblings

Seek ways to realistically include siblings in the care and treatment of the child with special needs.

Limit caregiving responsibilities and give recognition when siblings perform them.

Develop a library of children's books on special needs.

Invite siblings to attend meetings to develop plans for the child with special needs.

Discuss future plans with them.

Solicit their ideas on treatment and service needs.

Help them develop competencies to teach the child new skills.

Provide opportunities for siblings to advocate for the child.

Modified from Powell T, Gallagher PA: Brothers and sisters — a special part of exceptional families, Baltimore, 1985, Paul H Brooks.

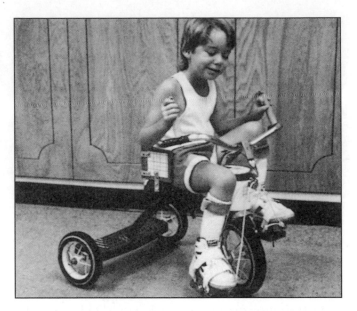

Fig. 20-1 A modified tricycle with block pedals, self-adhering straps for support, and modified seat and handlebars can help a child with disabilities gain mobility.

severely delayed achievement in one area, based on an understanding of normal development.

During early childhood, the basic innate drive for movement is dominant. Therefore, intervention must be based on providing activities that allow maximum motor development. For example, if a child has paraplegia, it is not sufficient to strengthen the upper extremities to compensate for the lower ones. Rather, the activity must take into account the child's need for social interaction, sense of control over the body, feeling of competence and achievement, and an outlet for aggression. Suitable activities may include ball throwing, swimming and water activities, such as races, bubble blowing, and splashing, building blocks, or pounding with a hammer.

With slight modifications, children with disabilities may be able to ride a tricycle by using self-adhering straps to secure the feet or hands (Fig. 20-1). With innovation, many such adaptations can be implemented in a child's environment to increase his or her mobility and independence. Technological advances are mushrooming, especially in the application of computers, and parents should be directed to the latest developments that may help their child.

Children with special needs derive enormous benefits from expressive activities, such as art, music, poetry, dance, and drama. With adaptive equipment and imagination, children can participate in a variety of activities.

Another critical component for normal child development is discipline. Unfortunately, this is one of the earliest child-rearing practices eliminated, as parents often become over-benevolent. Not only does lack of discipline destroy the child's security, because no boundaries exist on which to test behaviour, it also fails to teach the child socially acceptable behaviour and creates resentment and hostility among siblings and peers if different standards are applied. Parents may need help

with severe learning disability may never achieve cognitive skills above a preschool level. The child who is deaf may achieve only rudimentary verbal language. In these situations, adjustments must be made to compensate for the lack of or to learn successful methods of controlling behaviours before these become problems (Carr, 1987). Information on a toy library system for children with sensory deficits, motor disabilities and development delay is available from the National Association of Toy and Leisure Libraries.

School age

While the importance of school in the life of all children is generally acknowledged, studies indicate that school absences are significantly higher among children with chronic illness. The more school absences the child experiences, the more difficult it is to return, and 'school phobia' may result. Psychosocial factors that contribute to the risk of school phobia include depression, change in appearance, fear of separation (child and parents), and resistance on the part of school personnel. To prevent school phobia, the child should resume school as quickly as possible following diagnosis (Larcombe, 1991). (See also Chapter 17.)

Preparation for entry or resumption of school should entail a structured plan, with attention to those aspects of care that must be continued during school hours, such as administration of medication or other treatments. Teachers need to be aware of the child's abilities in order to set realistic academic and athletic expectations (Larcombe *et al*, 1991), and it is preferable to plan the school programme with as much participation and leadership from the child as possible.

Children need preparation before entering or resuming school. They need to think about the many questions others will ask. The nurse may be able to help the child to explore possible answers. If the child returns to school with some obvious physical change, such as hair loss, amputation, or visible scar, the nurse might ask questions about these alterations to prompt preparatory responses from the child.

Classroom peers need preparation too, and a joint plan between the school teacher, nurse, and child is best. At a minimum, the classmates should be given a description of the child's condition, prepared for any visible changes in the child, and allowed an opportunity to ask questions. The child should have the option of attending this session. As the child's condition changes, particularly if the condition is potentially fatal, school personnel, including the pupils, need periodic appraisal of the child's status and preparation for what to expect (see also Chapter 21).

Alternative activities may be substituted for those that are impossible or that place a strain on their condition. It is important for these children to have the opportunity to interact with healthy peers, as well as to engage in activities with groups or clubs composed of similarly affected children.

Adolescence

Adolescence can be a particularly difficult period. All the needs discussed before apply to this age group as well. Developing independence or autonomy, however, is a major task for the adolescent as planning for the future becomes a prominent concern. Even individuals with severe impairment can be viewed as autonomous if they perceive their own needs and

take responsibility for meeting them — either directly or by engaging the assistance of others. As adolescents become more autonomous, the nurse can help them discover and articulate how others can be of greatest assistance.

A sense of feeling different from peers can lead to loneliness, isolation, and depression. Participation in groups of teenagers with chronic conditions or disabilities can alleviate feelings of isolation and smooth the transition to meaningful relationships in adulthood.

Such questions have no clear-cut answers. Rather, adolescents should be encouraged to weigh decisions, investigate alternatives, and choose their own solution.

Consent and confidentiality are frequent dilemmas in providing care to any minor adolescent and are often made more complex by the teenager's health problem. For example, do these adolescents have the right to request health care without their parents' knowledge or permission? If they are engaging in potentially hazardous activities, such as the teenager with cystic fibrosis who begins to smoke or the young man with haemophilia who engages in contact sports or tests HIV positive and becomes sexually active, should parents be informed? Two principles may be used in resolving such ethical questions: the principle of *autonomy*, which states that a person should have a say in any action that will affect him or her, and the principle of *benevolence*, which states that whenever something beneficial can be done, it should be done. The *Children Act* (1989) supports the child's right to consult and to have their views taken into account in any procedures covered by the *Act* (White, Carr, and Lowe, 1990).

ESTABLISH REALISTIC FUTURE GOALS

One of the most difficult adjustments is setting realistic future goals for the child and for those involved in the child's continued care. Sometimes, the impact of this decision does not surface until the child finishes school or the parents near retirement, when a crisis can arise because all the family roles and relationships that maintained stability become disrupted.

Planning for the future should be a gradual process. All along, the parents should cultivate realistic vocations for the child. With prolonged survival for many chronic illnesses, surviving young people must deal with new decisions and problems, such as marriage, procreation, and employment. With appropriate guidance, many are capable of gainful employment and may marry and raise a family. For those whose conditions are genetic, there is the need for counselling regarding future offspring. Prospective partners often benefit from an opportunity to discuss their feelings regarding marriage to an individual with continued health needs and possibly a limited lifespan.

One approach that is gaining acceptance is transferring the older adolescent to adult care. The medical and psychosocial needs of adolescents approaching adulthood may be more easily managed by caregivers who are more familiar with adult issues, although arbitrary transfer to adult services based on age criterion alone can compromise both physical and psychosocial care for some young adults. Furthermore, age does not provide any information on how prepared the adolescent may be for transfer.

Many adolescents have received care in the same medical setting since birth and have established trusting and meaningful relationships with practitioners and staff members. Children's nurses can play a significant role in preparing adolescents and adult care providers for this important transition.

Unfortunately, vocational pursuits and independence are not realistic goals for all young people. Those with multiple or severe disabilities may require lifelong care and assistance.

In these situations, parents must look to the time when they will no longer be able to care for their child. Finding an appropriate residential placement may be very difficult. Admission to residential care should not be viewed as abandonment; not infrequently it is the only way to preserve the family unit. The nurse should help the family investigate suitable placements, discuss their feelings regarding this decision, and explore ways to maintain their relationships. The nurse can also help to prepare and educate the public to smooth the transition and help normalize the experience for the child, the family, and the community.

KEY POINTS

◆ Trends in the treatment of children with chronic illness have focused on developmental stages, the child's strengths and uniqueness, family relationships, establishment of normalization, early discharge, care in the community, and mainstream education.

◆ Families' reactions to disability or chronic illness are manifested in the following stages: shock and denial, adjustment, reintegration, and acknowledgement.

◆ In response to the child with chronic illness or disability, parents may be affected by feelings of inadequacy and failure; excessive demands on time, energy, and financial resources; and strain on relationships.

◆ Effects of chronic illness on siblings may include changes in role status, irritability and physical complaints, jealousy, competition, anger, hostility, attention-seeking behaviour, social withdrawal, and decline in school performance.

◆ Major factors affecting the family's adjustment to a child's chronic illness are the availability of a support system, their perception of the event, their coping mechanisms, reactions to the child, available resources, and concurrent stresses.

◆ The child's reaction to illness or disability depends on developmental level, coping mechanisms, others' reactions, and the illness itself.

◆ A family-centred approach to care that enables and empowers parents offers the greatest opportunity for appropriate interventions that meet the unique needs of all family members.

◆ To help parents cope with their child's chronic illness, nurses must offer attentiveness, humanistic support, solicitation of suggestions for care, facilitation of mutual participation in care by child and parent, and communication, verbalization of feelings, and referral to voluntary and community agencies.

◆ Supporting the child involves encouraging self-expression, alleviating feelings of being different, and strengthening self-image.

◆ Fostering reality adjustment entails supplying information about the disorder, promoting normal development, and establishing realistic future goals.

REFERENCES

Atkinson N, Crawforth M: All in the family: siblings and disability, London, NCH Action for Children, 1995.

Austin, J: Assessment of coping mechanisms used by parents and children with chronic illness, *MCN* 15(2):98, 1990.

Betts C C, Meyer G: Children with disabilities. In Glasper E A, Tucker A: *Advances in child health nursing*, London, 1993, Scutari.

Blum R W *et al*: Family and peer issues among adolescents with spina bifida and cereral palsy, *Pediatr* 88(2),1991.

Carr J: *Helping your handicapped child*, London, 1987, Penguin.

Clements D, Copeland L, Loftus M: Critical times for families with a chronically ill child, *Pediatr Nurs* 16(2):157, 224, 1990.

Cooke RWI: Factors affecting survival and outcome at three years in extremely premature infants, *Arch Dis Child* 71:F28, 1994.

Davies PB, May JE: Involving fathers in early intervention and family support programmes: issues and strategies, *Children's Health Care* 20(2):87, 1991.

Department for Education: *Special educational needs: a guide for parents*, London, 1994, HMSO.

Disability rights handbook, London, Annual publication.

Dragone M: Perspectives of chronically ill adolescents and parents on health care needs, *Pediatr Nurs* 16(1):45, 108, 1990.

Field SB: *Personal communication*, Aug 16, 1990.

Fraley A: Chronic sorrow: a parental response, *J Pediatr Nurs* 5(4):268, 1990.

Futcher J: Chronic illness and family dynamics, *Pediatr Nurs* 14(5):381, 1988.

Gath A: Living with a mentally handicapped brother or sister, *Arch Dis Child* 64:513, 1989.

Glossop C: Practical application of portage, *Health Visitor* 62(3):85, 1989.

Herbert E, Carpenter B: Fathers - the secondary partners: profcs sional perceptions and fathers' reflections, *Child society*, 8(1)31-44,1994.

Hobbs N, Perrin JM, editors: *Issues in the care of children with chronic illness*, San Francisco, 1985, Jossey-Bass.

Johnson B, McGonigel M, Kaufmann R, editors: *Guidelines and recommended practices for the Individualized Family Service Plan*, Washington, DC, 1989, Association for the Care of Children's Health.

Larcombe IJ *et al*: Child health: back to normality, *Nurs Times* 87:68, 1991.

Leonard A: *Right from the start*, London, 1994, The Spastics Society.

Lobato D: *Brothers, sisters, and special needs*, Baltimore, 1990, Paul H Brookes.

Marsh H, Partridge L, Youngs C, editors: *The CaF directory of specific conditions and rare syndromes in children with their family support networks*, London, 1994, Contact a Family.

McCubbin MA: Family stress and family strengths: a comparison of single- and two-parent families with handicapped children, *Res Nurs Health* 12:101, 1989.

Medical Devices Directorate Report 1992: *Safety guidelines for transporting children in special seats*, London, 1992, HMSO.

Meyer G: Who knows best? *Paediatric Nurs* 2(4): 1990.

OPCS (Office of Population Census and Surveys): Surveys of Disability in Great Britain. Report 3: *Prevalence of disability among children*, London, 1993a, HMSO.

OPCS (Office of Population Census and Surveys): Surveys of Disability in Great Britain 1989. Report 6: *Disabled children: services, transport and education*, London, 1993b, HMSO.

Pless I B *et al*: A randomized trial of a nursing intervention to promote the adjustment of children with chronic physical disorders, *Pediatrics* 94(1),1994.

Robinson C, Stalker K: *Respite care -summaries and suggestions. Final report to the Department of Health*, Bristol, 1991, Nora Fry Research Centre.

Robinson C, Beckford V: *Consolidation or change? A second survey of family based respite care services in the United Kingdom*, Bristol, 1993, Nora Fry Research Centre.

Robinson C: Double bind: a dilemma for parents of chronically ill children, *Pediatr Nurs* 11(2):112, 1985.

Rollins J: Self-help groups for parents, *Pediatr Nurs* 13(6):403, 1987.

Royal College of Nursing and the Spastics Society: *Day in, day out: a survey of views of respite care*, London, 1993, RCN/The Spastics Society.

Shah R: The silent minority: children with disabilities in Asian families, London, 1992, National Children's Bureau.

Social Services Inspectorate: *Services to disabled children and their families*, London, 1994, HMSO.

The voluntary agencies directory, London, Annual publication, NCVO.

White R, Carr P, Lowc N: *A guide to the Children Act 1989*, London, 1990, Butterworths.

WHO (World Health Organization): *Better opportunties for disabled people*, Geneva, 1992, WHO.

Yoos L: Chronic childhood illnesses: developmental issues, *Pediatr Nurs* 13(1)25, 1987.

FURTHER READING

Perspectives in the Care of Children with Special Needs

Barnes C. 1991 *Disabled People in Britain and Discrimination* London Hurst & Co.

Duffey T: *Focus on children with special needs: a guide to good practice for professionals*, Sevenoaks, 1994, Management Focus.

Gilbert P. 1993 *The A–Z Reference Book of Syndromes & Inherited Disorders* London Chapman & Hall.

Hammond HF: The handicapped child in an ordinary school, *Health at School* 4(7):211, 1989.

Hammond HF: The handicapped child in an ordinary school, *Health at School* 4(8):245, 1989.

Hammond HF: The handicapped child in an ordinary school, *Health at School* 4(9):274, 1989.

NCH Action for Children 1994 *Unequal Opportunities – Children with disabilities and their families speak out* London NCH Action for Children.

Office of Population, Census and Surveys: Surveys of disability in Great Britain. Report 6: *Disabled children: services, transport and education*, London, 1989, HMSO.

Pless IB: *The epidemiology of childhood disorders*, Oxford, 1994, Oxford University Press.

Westcott HL. 1993 *Abuse of Children and Adults with Disabilities* London NSPCC

Woodroffe C, Glickman M, Barker M and Power C. 1993 *Children, Teenagers & Health: The key data* Buckingham Philadelphia Open University Press.

The Child and Family with Special Needs

Austin JK: Family adaptation to a child's chronic illness, *Ann Review Nurs Research* 9:103, 1991.

Baldwin S, Carlisle J: *Social support for disabled children and their families: a review of the literature,* Edinburgh, 1994, HMSO.

Cohen MH: Diagnostic closure and the spread of uncertainty, *Issues Comp Pediatr Nurs* 16(3):135, 1993.

Council of Europe Steering Committee on Social Policy: *Report on the integration of disabled children into their family and society,* Strasbourg, 1989, Council of Europe.

Crowley A: Integrating handicapped and chronically ill children into day care centers, *Pediatr Nurs* 16(1):39, 1990.

Eiser C: *Growing up with chronic disease:the impact on children and their families,* London, 1993, Jessica Kingsley.

Eiser C, Havermaus T: Mothers and fathers coping with chronic childhood disease, *Psychol Health* 7(4):249, 1992.

Florian V, Kulik T: Loneliness and social support of mothers of chronically ill children, *Soc Sci Med* 32(11):1291, 1991.

Goodall J, Jones PW: Do disabled school children disable a marriage? *Matern Child Health* 18(5):151, 1993.

Klein SD & Maxwell JS (Eds). 1993 *It Isn't Fair! Siblings of Children with Disabilities* Westport, Conneticut Bergin & Garvey.

Leonard CJ: Parent/family reaction to childhood disability in families: three ethnic minority groups, *Int J Adv Counselling* 8(3):197, 1985.

Nursing Care of the Family and Child with Special Needs

Crittenden P: Toward a concept of autonomy in adolescents with a disability, *Children's Health Care* 19(3):162, 1990.

Deatrick JA, Knafle KA: Management behaviors: day-to-day adjustments to childhood chronic conditions, *J Pediatr Nurs* 5(1):15, 1990.

Duffy T. 1994 *Focus on children with special needs: a guide to good practice for professionals.* Sevenoakss, Management Focus.

Fitton P. 1994 *Listen to Me: Communicating the needs of people with profound intellectual & multiple disabilities* London Jessica Kingsley.

Hartman AF: Parent to parent support (for families of children with special needs), *Issues Comp Pediatr Nurs* 15(1):55, 1992.

Herbert E, Carpenter B: Fathers: the secondary partners: professional perceptions and fathers' reflections, Children & Society 8(1):31, 1994.

Hornby G. 1994 *Counselling in Child Disability – Skills for working with parents* London, Chapman & Hall.

Jackson PL and Vessey JA 1992 *Primary Care of the Child with a Chronic Condition* St Louis Mosby–Year Book.

LaMontague LL: Adopting a process approach to assess children's coping, *J Pediatr Nurs* 3(3):159, 1987.

McCarthy GT (Ed) 1992 *Physical Disability in Childhood – An interdisciplinary approach to management* Edinburgh Churchill–Livingstone.

Middleton L: *Children first: working with children and disability,* Birmingham, 1992, Venture Press.

Middleton L 1992 *Children First – Working with Children and Disability* British Association of Social Workers Birmingham Venture Press.

Perrin JM, Shayne MW and Bloom SR. 1993 *Home and Community Care for Chronically Ill Children* New York Oxford University Press.

Chapter 21

Impact of Life–Threatening Illness on the Child and Family

LEARNING OUTCOMES

After studying this chapter you should be able to:

◆ Discuss the understanding and reaction to death and dying of infants and toddlers, preschool children, school-aged children, and adolescents.

◆ Discuss the awareness of dying in children with a life-threatening illness.

◆ Discuss the implications of informing children of their life-threatening illness.

◆ Describe three theories of grief processes in expected and unexpected death.

◆ Discuss the concept of hospice care.

◆ Identify the important factors in supporting the parents of a child who is dying.

◆ Discuss the support of siblings of a child with a life-threatening disease during the stages of diagnosis, treatment, terminal stages, and after the death.

◆ State the potential reactions of the family during the treatment of a child with a life-threatening disease and following the death of a child.

◆ Discuss the reactions of nurses caring for a child with a life-threatening illness and the appropriate support methods.

◆ Define the glossary terms.

GLOSSARY

acute grief Somatic symptoms and intense subjective distress that occur within hours or days after a significant loss

anticipatory grief Grieving before an actual loss

bereavement Period of mourning

DNR Do not resuscitate

life-threatening illness Serious disorder with a potentially fatal outcome

mourning Prolonged process of resolving grief

terminal illness A condition wherein a life is near or approaching its end

Despite advances in the treatment of previously fatal childhood diseases, some children will still die. Health care professionals are faced with the challenge of providing the best care to meet the child's physical and psychological needs, as well as the psychological needs of the whole family.

There is probably no more difficult death to face than that of a child. Society is angry, shocked, and outraged (Judd, 1989) because the end of life is premature and parents are robbed of the fulfilment and joy of seeing their child grow. This chapter establishes some theoretical and practical guidelines for helping families cope with the loss of a child. An overview of children's concepts of death, the grieving process before and after death, each family member's reaction to a life-threatening illness, and nursing interventions to assist the family through each phase of the illness are presented. The chapter concludes with a discussion of the impact of caring for dying children on nurses.

CHILDREN AND DEATH

Children are naturally inquisitive concerning all aspects of life, including death. Despite adult attempts to protect them from learning about death, children encounter it in everyday experiences and therefore need help to make sense of it.

CHILDREN'S UNDERSTANDING OF AND REACTIONS TO DYING AND DEATH

The concept of death is acquired through the sequential development of cognitive abilities and follows closely Piaget's stages. Nurses require knowledge of the different stages of children's death-concept development and the fears associated with death at each stage.

Knowledge about preschool and older children's concept of death is primarily based on the work of Maria Nagy (1948) (Table 21-1).

INFANTS AND TODDLERS

Unless infants and toddlers have had previous experience, it is generally believed that preschool children have no concept of death. Toddlers' egocentricity and vague separation of fact and fantasy make it impossible for them to comprehend absence of life.

Reactions to dying
Children are astute observers and may perceive the seriousness of a situation from their parents' behaviour. Parents require appropriate support and education to stay with their child and must give age-appropriate explanations as to the reason for their distress.

Reactions to death
Toddlers may wish to talk about the dead person, keep all their belongings unchanged, and visit their grave regularly. They

COGNITIVE STAGE	CONCEPT
Sensorimotor (infancy, toddler)	No concept of death but reacts to loss
Preoperational thought (early childhood)	Death is temporary and reversible
	Death is seen as a departure or separation
Concrete operations (school age)	Death is irreversible but not necessarily inevitable
	Death may be personified and viewed as destructive
	Explanations for death are naturalistic and physiological
Formal operations (later school age, adolescence)	Death is irreversible, universal, and inevitable
	Death is still seen as a personal but distant event
	Explanations for death are physiological and theological

Table 21-1 Children's concept of death.

should receive honest, open explanations and reassurance at a level appropriate for their age and development.

PRESCHOOL CHILDREN

Preschool children are unable to differentiate physical cause from logical or psychological motivation. Their egocentricity may lead them to feel responsible for the death and to experience feelings of shame and guilt.

Concept of death
Children between ages three and five usually have heard the word 'death' and have some connotation of its meaning. They may recognize the fact of physical death, but do not separate it from living abilities. The dead person in the coffin still breathes, eats, and sleeps. Death is temporary; there is no real understanding of the universality and inevitability of death.

Reactions to dying
Children of all ages' greatest fear concerning death is separation from their parents.

Reactions to death
In relation to death, preschool children may engage in activities that seem strange or abnormal to adults. For example, if a pet dies, preschool children usually request a 'funeral' or some ceremony to symbolize their loss. After the 'funeral' and 'burial', the child may dig up the remains. This is to reassure themselves that the pet has not gone elsewhere. They still have no concept of irreversibility.

A common euphemism for death is 'gone to sleep'. Preschool children may attach the literal meaning of sleep to death and may fear going to sleep for fear of dying or never waking up.

Because of their fewer defence mechanisms for dealing with loss, young children may react to a less significant loss with more outward grief than to the loss of a very significant person. If the loss is so deep, painful, and threatening, the child may need to deny it, for the present, to survive its overwhelming impact. Behavioural reactions such as giggling, joking, attracting attention, or regressing to earlier developmental skills indicate children's need to distance themselves from the tremendous loss.

SCHOOL-AGED CHILDREN

Although school-aged children have a better understanding of causality, less egocentricity, and advanced perception of time, they still associate misdeeds or bad thoughts with causing death, and feel intense guilt and responsibility for the event.

Concept of death
Much of what pertains to the preschool period regarding the understanding of death also relates to school-aged children, particularly those near six or seven years of age. However, these children have a deeper understanding of death in the concrete sense.

By the age of nine or ten, most children have an adult concept of death. They realize it is inevitable, universal, and irreversible. Their attitudes towards death are greatly influenced by the reactions and attitudes of others, particularly their parents.

Reactions to dying
School-aged children's increased ability to comprehend and reason poses additional risks for them. They tend to fear the expectation of the event more than its realization. For this reason, anticipatory preparation is very necessary and effective. Inasmuch as the developmental task of this age is industry, helping children maintain control over their bodies by understanding what is happening to them and participating in what is done to them allows these youngsters to achieve independence, self-worth, and self-esteem, and to avoid a sense of inferiority.

Because dying is loss of control over every aspect of living, the realization of impending death or failing to recover is a tremendous threat to their sense of security and ego strength. These children are likely to exhibit their fear more through verbal uncooperativeness than actual physical aggression. Encouraging children to talk about their feelings and providing outlets for aggression through play are means of dealing with this type of uncooperativeness.

Reactions to death
School-aged children are very interested in postdeath services, such as wakes, funerals, and burials. They may be inquisitive about what happens to the body — who dresses it, how the body feels, or what happens in an autopsy. Such inquiries are children's way of assimilating all the facts about death into a concrete, logical framework.

ADOLESCENTS

By the time most children reach adolescence, they have a mature understanding of death and, as abstract thinking develops, there is more questioning of death and related topics, such as the religious meaning of afterlife. However, their other developmental needs, especially identity, make this an exceptionally difficult time for these young people to face their own impending death (Morgan, 1990). Adolescents may also have difficulty coping with the death of a loved one, and may experience feelings of guilt if they perceive the relationship as having been a difficult one.

Concept of death
Although adolescents have a mature understanding of death, they are still very much influenced by 'remnants' of magical thinking and are subject to the feelings of guilt and shame.

Reactions to dying
Adolescents have the most difficulty in coping with death. Although they have reached the level of adult comprehension of the concept of death, they are least likely to accept cessation of life, particularly if it is their own. Developmentally, the rejection of death is understandable because the adolescents' tasks are to establish an identity by finding out who they are, what their purpose is, and where they belong. Any suggestion of being different or nonbeing is a tremendous threat to the answers to such questions. Adolescents' concern is for the present much more than for the past or future.

Nurses are in an advantageous position in working with terminally ill adolescents; they can structure the hospital admission to allow for maximum self-control and independence, while allowing the adolescent the opportunity to learn to know the nurse. Answering adolescents' questions honestly, treating them as mature individuals, and respecting their needs for privacy, solitude, and personal expressions of emotions, such as anger, sadness, or fear, convey to adolescents the adult's true concern for their physical and emotional welfare. Nurses can help parents to communicate with their adolescent children by acting as role models, avoiding alliances with either parent or child, and allowing parents the opportunity to ventilate their feelings of frustration, incompetence, or failure in an atmosphere of acceptance and nonjudgement.

Reactions to death
The adolescent's reactions to death straddle the transition from childhood to adulthood. Although some teenagers are able to cope with death by expressing appropriate emotions, talking about the loss, and resolving the grief, others may appear undisturbed by the event, extremely angry, or unusually silent and withdrawn. Kuntz (1991) found that involving adolescents with the ritual surrounding death facilitates adaptive grieving.

IMPLICATIONS FOR NURSING

Nurses in almost any area of paediatrics have an opportunity to help children develop positive attitudes towards death. They can counsel parents regarding children's age-specific understanding of death, and appropriate ways to handle behaviours. Informed consent, especially concerning a child's choice for no further active treatment, is a sensitive issue and requires carefully planning communication strategies that maintain supportive relationships for all family members.

Nurses can also encourage parents to take advantage of 'small deaths' to help children become familiar and more comfortable with loss. The death of a pet, flowers, or a television character may present such an opportunity. Many children's books present death in a sensitive and non-threatening manner and, when read to children, offer opportunities for dialogue (Mattias and Spiers, 1990).

AWARENESS OF DYING IN CHILDREN WITH LIFE-THREATENING ILLNESS

One of the initial reactions of parents (and some health professionals) to the discovery of a life-threatening illness is to protect the child from the impact of the diagnosis. However, terminally ill children develop awareness of the seriousness of their diagnosis, even when protected from the truth (Waechter, 1985). Anxiety may not be attributable to fear of death, but may be demonstrated in relationship to separation, pain, intrusive procedures, bodily change or mutilation, loneliness, immobilization, and punishment. Children as young as two or three years of age perceive their parents' emotions and react accordingly.

Studies of children' experiences with life-threatening illness demonstrate that children learn about their situation through the acquisition of information, at which time they develop different conceptions of themselves. Five stages have been defined (Bluebond-Langner, 1978):
• **Stage I:** Disease is a serious illness. New identity of 'sick' child.
• **Stage II:** Discovery of the relationship of medication and recovery. Learns the taboos of disease and death.
• **Stage III:** Marked understanding of the purposes and implications of special procedures. Sense of well-being begins to fade and perceives self as different from other children.
• **Stage IV:** Illness is viewed as a permanent condition. Sense of always being sick and never getting better.
• **Stage V:** Realization that there is only a finite number of medications. Awareness (directly or indirectly) of their fatal prognosis.

Experience is considered the critical factor in the passage through these various stages. The experience of having a disease allows children to assimilate information by relating what they see and hear to what they feel and think. Experience also explains why age and intellectual ability are not related

to the speed or completeness with which children pass through the various stages of awareness. Some three- and four-year-olds of average intelligence know more about their prognosis than very intelligent nine-year-olds who are still in their first remission, have had fewer clinical experiences, and are aware only that they have a serious illness.

Time lapse between stages tends to be the same for all children regardless of age. Passage from the first stage to the second stage occurs rapidly on relapse. Passage through the second, third, and fourth stages takes somewhat longer, but passage to the fifth stage may take place as soon as the child learns of the death of another, and all knowledge from previous stages is quickly synthesized into a new self-awareness.

INFORMING CHILDREN OF LIFE-THREATENING DIAGNOSIS

All children should be told about the diagnosis by their parents alone or with the assistance of appropriate practitioners. Children need honest and accurate information about their illness, treatments, and prognosis. Appropriate literature about the disease is helpful. Providing an atmosphere of open communication early in the course of the illness facilitates answering difficult questions as the child's condition worsens (Lansky, List, and Ritter-Sterr, 1988).

Two important factors to consider when talking to children about a life-threatening illness are their age and level of development, and their previous knowledge (Chesterfield, 1992). Finding out what the child already understands, not just what he or she can repeat, is necessary before embarking on appropriate explanations.

Honesty is also very important. It not only deals with the present, but may act as a base for the future. Parents may be reluctant for their child to know the truth, for fear of them asking painful questions. As previously mentioned, children are astute observers and denying them the opportunity to ask questions may create a situation of mutual pretence, where everyone acts as if they are coping. Children require time to go through the grieving process, and they may also have final goals and objectives they wish to achieve (Lansky, List, and Ritter Sterr, 1988).

Informed consent, especially concerning the child's choice for no further action, is another sensitive issue that requires carefully planned communication stategies that maintain supportive relationships for all family members.

SIBLINGS' RESPONSES TO LIFE-THREATENING ILLNESS AND DEATH

The experience of a child with life-threatening illness and/or the child's death has profound effects on the family, including the siblings. Predominant feelings of children when the sibling's diagnosis is potentially fatal, such as cancer, include isolation, displacement, concern for their own health, guilt, and shame.

When a brother or sister dies, siblings grieve for the loss of the child, must deal with the stress of having grieving parents, and at times may feel like 'the replaced child' or the 'less special' child (Davies, 1987).

Some studies have reported a negative impact on children experiencing sibling death; however, positive benefits are also possible. Bereaved siblings can have higher self-concepts than their nonbereaved peers; they perceive that they have matured and grown psychologically as a result of the experience. Parents also report that the surviving siblings are more compassionate (Martinson, Davies, and McClowry, 1987). Factors influencing positive or negative adjustment are not fully understood, although open communication between the family and siblings, and increased involvement with the ill child's care and death are likely to aid in positive adjustment (Birenbaum, 1989; Lauer *et al*, 1985).

Children need information about the sibling's illness and death, especially if the death was unexpected. They need reassurance that they were not responsible for their sibling's death. Their fears of becoming ill or dying should be addressed and, whenever possible, the siblings should be involved in the child's care, praised for their cooperation, and made to feel involved. Parents are encouraged to spend quality time with the well children.

GRIEF PROCESS IN EXPECTED AND UNEXPECTED DEATH

In response to any loss, there is a grief reaction (Warden, 1991). *Acute grief* develops within hours to days and is characterized by somatic symptoms and intense subjective distress. *Grief work* or *mourning* refers to the lengthy process that begins with acute grief and extends into a period of reorganization of psychological life, with attachment to new people and interests. *Bereavement* often refers to the period of mourning, although grief, mourning, and bereavement are used interchangeably.

Numerous investigators have contributed greatly to the present understanding of grief and bereavement, and those whose work is considered classic are presented in the following paragraphs.

LINDEMANN: SYMPTOMATOLOGY OF GRIEF

Lindemann (1944) analysed and described the reactions of adult survivors following the loss of significant others and found that acute grief has the following characteristics:
1. It is a definite syndrome with psychological and somatic symptoms (Box 21-2).
2. The syndrome may appear immediately after a crisis, may be delayed, may be exaggerated, or may be apparently absent.
3. In place of the normal syndrome, there may appear distorted reactions that represent one special aspect of the syndrome.
4. Through intervention, distorted reactions can be transformed into normal grief work with successful resolution.

Health professionals should emphasize that grief reactions, such as hearing the dead person's voice, feeling distant from others, or seeking reassurance that they did everything possible for the lost person are normal, necessary, and expected.

PARKES: MOURNING

According to Parkes' findings, the grief process consists of at least four phases, which do not necessarily proceed in sequence and may recur at any time.

Resolution of grief may not always result in 'letting go' of the loved one. Many survivors describe the pressure of an 'empty space' in their lives nine years after the death of a child. Feelings of emptiness intensify around holidays and anniversaries, and with questions such as 'How many children are in the family?'.

SHOCK AND DISBELIEF

Shock, numbness, and disbelief are seen during the immediate phase of grief. This temporary numbness protects the survivors from the overwhelming pain associated with grief. Often, decisions are made automatically and only certain details are remembered.

EXPRESSION OF GRIEF

When the numbness fades, there begins a period of intense grief characterized by a yearning and loneliness for the deceased. During this stage, many of the signs of acute grief are evident, and physical complaints, such as inability to sleep, and appetite changes are common.

DISORGANIZATION AND DESPAIR

During this stage, the pain of the loss is replaced primarily by emptiness, apathy, and deep depression. There is a feeling that life has no meaning and that the pain will never end. Mothers often comment that they feel a great emptiness from suffering a double loss — loss of their child and loss of the mothering role (Wong, 1980).

REORGANIZATION

Reorganization refers to recovery from the loss. It is a very gradual process in which the survivors again find meaning in living, readjust to life without the deceased, develop new or renewed relationships, and learn to live with the memory of the deceased with much less pain.

EXPECTED VERSUS UNEXPECTED CHILDHOOD DEATH

Remarkably little research has been conducted comparing grief responses in survivors when the child's death was expected or unexpected. When death is expected, there is time for anticipatory grieving, and it has been suggested that this may

---

◆ **BOX 21-2**

Symptomatology of normal grief

Sensations of Somatic Distress
Feeling of tightness in the throat
Choking, with shortness of breath
Marked tendency to sighing
Empty feeling in abdomen
Lack of muscular power
Intense subjective distress described as tension or mental pain

Preoccupation with Image of the Deceased
Hears, sees, or imagines that the dead person is present
Slight sense of unreality
Feeling of emotional distance from others
May believe that he or she is approaching insanity

Feelings of Guilt
Searches for evidence of failure in preventing the death
Accuses self of negligence or exaggerates minor omissions

Feelings of Hostility
Loss of warmth towards others
Tendency to irritability and anger
Wish not be bothered by friends or relatives

Loss of Usual Patterns of Conduct
Restlessness, inability to sit still, aimless moving about
Continual searching for something to do or what he or she thinks should be done
Lack of capacity to initiate and maintain organized patterns of activity

Modified from Lindemann, 1944. Copyright 1944 American Psychiatric Association.

---

favourably affect the grief process. However, parents of children who died suddenly did experience more guilt, a prolonged period of numbness and shock, intense loneliness and emptiness, anxious fear that someone else would die, and intense anger at those responsible for the injury (Miles and Perry, 1985). Preliminary findings from a study done with Filipino children suggest that siblings of children who died suddenly may remain in the early stages of grief longer and may experience greater loneliness than siblings of children who died after an extended illness (Atuel, Williams, and Camar, 1988).

Although the grief process may be relatively unaltered by the timing of the child's death, there are differences for the families. In long-term, potentially fatal illnesses, the grief for anticipated loss becomes chronic. The parents mourn the loss of their child long before the death. Unlike parents who experience a sudden loss, these family members are unable to resolve their grief until the child is considered cured or is dead. Each time they see the pain the child must endure or anticipate the sudden loss of hope during a relapse, they are reminded of their child's uncertain future.

However, the prolonged period of chronic grief provides families with the precious opportunity to complete all 'unfinished business', such as helping the child and siblings understand and cope with a fatal prognosis.

In sudden, unexpected death, the family is deprived of any of the advantages of anticipatory grief. There is no opportunity to prepare oneself or others for the death; only the cruel reality that nothing remains of their child except memories (Black, 1991). Because of this lack of time to prepare, many families feel great guilt and remorse for not having done something additional or different with the child and may long grieve over missed opportunities (Kachoyeanos and Selder, 1993).

SPECIAL DECISIONS AT THE TIME OF DYING AND DEATH

Rarely are people prepared to cope with the numerous decisions that must be made when a loved one is dying or dies. When the death is expected, there is the opportunity to make plans in advance, such as where the child should spend the last days or what type of funeral arrangements are desired. When death is unexpected the shock is sufficient to render the survivors incapable of making even simple decisions. The following is a brief review of selected instances when nurses can help parents make decisions related to the expected or unexpected death.

HOSPICE OR HOSPITAL CARE

When the child is dying, parents should be given the choice of hospice or hospital care for the terminal stage of illness. Hospital care refers to the traditional practices of caring for dying patients; hospice is a concept, not necessarily a facility. Hospice is holistic care for the patient and family that is intended to maximize the present quality of life whenever there is no reasonable expectation of cure. Hospice intends for the child to live life to the fullest without pain, with choices and dignity, and with family support (Armstrong-Dailey, 1990; Corr and Corr, 1992). The three basic ways of providing hospice care are in a hospice, in a facility that employs the hospice concept, or in the child's home. If the home is chosen, the child may or may not die in the home. Reasons for final admission to a hospital vary, but may be related to the parent's or sibling's wish to have the child die outside the home, exhaustion on the part of the caregivers, physical problems, such as sudden, acute pain or respiratory distress, and insufficient nursing services in the home (Martinson, 1993).

Hospice care is based on a number of important concepts that significantly set it apart from hospital care (Copsey, 1981). First, the family are the principal caregivers, supported by a team of professional and volunteer staff. Second, the priority of care is comfort that considers the child's physical, psychological, social, and spiritual needs. Pain and symptom control are primary concerns, and no extraordinary efforts are used to attempt a cure or to prolong life. Third, the needs of the family are considered as important as those of the patient. Fourth, hospice is concerned with the family's postdeath adjustment, and care may continue for one year or more.

With children, home care has been the more common environment for implementing the hospice concept. This benefits the family in many ways. Children who are dying are allowed the opportunity to remain with those they love and with whom they feel secure. Many children who were thought to be in imminent danger of death have gone home and lived longer than expected. Siblings feel more involved in the care and have more positive perceptions of the death. Parental adaptation has been more favourable, as shown by their perceptions of how the experience at home affected their marriage, social reorientation, religious beliefs, and views on the meaning of life and death. They also feel significantly less guilt after the child's death than families whose child died in the hospital (Lauer *et al*, 1983).

Home care may engender stress for the family, particularly anxiety about what to expect at the time of death and how to provide the care. Parents providing home care may experience more physical fatigue than if the child receives hospital care (Birenbaum and Clarke-Steffan, 1992).

RIGHT TO DIE

One of the benefits of hospice has been the recognition of patients' right to die as they wish, with emphasis on the *quality* of life. Unfortunately, this is not always the focus of care, especially in the traditional hospital setting. Many families are not given the option to terminate treatment when cure is unlikely, and staff may be reluctant to make decisions about do not resuscitate orders (withholding cardiopulmonary resuscitation in response to cardiac arrest). Some of these situations, such as the dying child's right to refuse additional treatment, often pose difficult ethical questions (see Questions and Controversies).

As the health professionals who are most involved with families, nurses are in an excellent position to ensure that families are given the options available to them at the time of death. The nurse's first responsibility is to explore the family's wishes. Parents will require sensitive explanations concerning the meaning of no further active treatment and appropriate symptom management. An ethics consultant or committee may be called upon in the unusual situation where differing points of view cannot be resolved easily (Rushton and Hogue, 1993).

VISUALIZATION OF THE BODY

Although most institutions recognize the need for parents to hold and spend time with the dead child, a dilemma may arise when the body is mutilated. Although the memory of the child's disfigurement can be extremely upsetting and will generate concern for how much the child suffered, not seeing the body leaves the parents with imagined ideas of how their child looked, which can be worse than the reality and can delay the acceptance of the death (Miles and Perry, 1985). Families should be told what to expect and why certain parts of the body are covered or bandaged. Some people appreciate the presence of a nurse in the room with them; others desire privacy. Regardless of how badly the body is harmed, parents may want to hold the child. Such options are offered and respected.

Family members should be given as much time as they need to say good-bye; for many, viewing the body is a sign of closure to finish their good-byes and to leave the hospital (Jost and Haase, 1989).

TISSUE DONATION/AUTOPSY

A topic that is rarely considered when a child dies is tissue donation. However, for some families this may be a meaningful act — one that benefits another human being, despite the loss of their child. Unfortunately, initiating a discussion about tissue donation is often very stressful for staff, and there may be confusion regarding who is responsible for it.

Nurses need to be aware of common questions about organ donation to help families make an informed decision. Healthy children who die unexpectedly are excellent candidates for organ donation, although their age is a determinant of organ suitability. For example, very young donors present technical difficulties in organ removal (Williams, 1985). Children with cancer, chronic disease, or infection, or who have suffered prolonged cardiac arrest, may not be suitable candidates, although this is determined individually. The nurse should inquire if organ donation was discussed with the child or if the child ever expressed such a wish*. Several body tissues or organs can be donated (skin, eyes, bone, kidney, heart, liver, pancreas), and their removal does not mutilate or desecrate the body, or cause any suffering. The family may have an open casket, and there is no delay in the funeral. Most religions permit organ donation, although Orthodox Judaism forbids it (Gershan, 1985).

In cases of unexplained death, violent death, or suspected suicide, autopsy is required by law. In other instances it may

---

Questions & Controversies

Does the dying child have the right to refuse further treatment?

Traditionally, children (under the age of 16) have not had the legal right to give informed consent for treatment or to refuse treatment. However, there is a growing concern for children in the end stage of fatal disease to have a voice in their care during the terminal phase. One of the major issues is the age at which children have the cognitive ability to understand the medical information, consider and comprehend the consequences of the decision (death), and choose freely among the options. Bluebond-Langner (1978) found that fatally ill children progress through a series of stages that shape their understanding of their disease and death.

Staff need to assess each child's capacity to understand the implications of refusing treatment, with documentation of the child's words and actions that support their conclusions (Foley, 1985; *The Children's Act*, 1989).

Unit 3 The Child with Special Needs

be optional, and parents should be informed of this choice. The procedure, as well as forms that require signing, should be explained. The family should know that the child can be in an open casket following a post-mortem (Jost and Haase, 1989).

SIBLINGS' ATTENDANCE AT BURIAL SERVICES

One of the most frequent concerns of parents is whether young or school-aged children should attend funeral or burial services (see Questions and Controversies). Sharing moments of deep significance with parents helps children understand the experience and deal with their own feelings of shock, sorrow, and grief; depriving them of this opportunity may leave children with lifelong regrets (Fig. 21-1).

THE FAMILY OF THE CHILD WITH LIFE-THREATENING ILLNESS

In many respects, families who are experiencing life-threatening illness in their child respond to the diagnosis in much the same manner as families whose child has a chronic illness or disability.

REACTIONS OF THE FAMILY TO A LIFE-THREATENING ILLNESS

All families whose child has some type of physical or cognitive disability experience reactions to the loss of the 'perfect' child that are similar, despite the diagnosis. The following section focuses on five phases in which there are significant differences in reactions to chronic disease versus life-threatening illness, with cancer used as an example of life-threatening illness.

PHASE I — REVELATION AND DAWNING REALITY: DIAGNOSIS AND TREATMENT

When parents first learn of the diagnosis of cancer, their immediate reactions are similar to those of other families whose child has a chronic illness, except that the initial impact can be much more pessimistic and overwhelming because of the generally negative connotation regarding the disease. For children, principal concerns centre around the diagnostic tests and treatments and their effects.

With the commencement of treatment, families commonly react with quiet anger, depression, ambivalence, and bargaining (Stuart and Totterdell, 1990).

Shock and disbelief
Many parents relate that the shock of hearing the diagnosis prevents them from hearing everything else they are told. Some will disbelieve it, while others experience anticipatory grieving.

Anger
Children often may feel angry, particularly because of all the traumatic procedures done to them. Once they begin to feel better, they frequently express their anger through uncooperativeness. Overprotectiveness and permissiveness are typical reactions during remission, and helping parents deal with the child's anger constructively during the hospitalization also prevents some of the potential future problems.

Questions & Controversies

*S*hould children attend the funeral or burial services of a loved one?

This question generates much controversy among the general public and professionals. Many lay people feel it is too frightening for children to be exposed to the dead and that it is better for them to remember the loved person as he or she was when alive. There is a general attitude of protecting children from unhappy or distressing events. However, among health professionals involved with children there is a fairly general consensus that children should attend such services, and some authors suggest that no child is too young merely by virtue of age (Foley, 1986). Others recommend that the parents make the decision regarding attendance until children are six or seven years of age, at which time children should choose (Zelauskas, 1981). Children, like adults, have 'unfinished business', and visiting the dead person may represent an opportunity to complete those affairs. For example, the child may wish to say good-bye (verbally or written) or to leave a memento. Kübler-Ross (1983) tells of a seven-year-old child who chose a puzzle that her brother received shortly before he lost sight from a brain tumour. She matter of factly explained that he could finish it 'when he arrives in heaven'.

Unfortunately, little research has focused on the difference in adjustment between children who do or do not attend bereavement services. However, one study provides substantial evidence of the benefit of involving children in the experience of their dying sibling. Lauer et al (1985) compared children's perceptions of their sibling's death at home vs in the hospital. The home care group (ages five to 23 years) reported they were prepared for the impending death, received consistent information and support from their parents, were involved in most activities, found the funeral experience comforting, and viewed their own involvement as the most important aspect of the experience. The non-home care group (ages two to 26 years) had opposite perceptions. Another study found that greater participation in the child's care and death, including funeral attendance, was associated with higher self-esteem in the siblings (Michael and Lansdown, 1986). Thus it appears that *increased involvement* with the death rather than isolation and 'protection' benefits children.

398

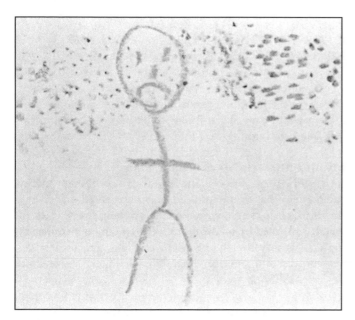

Fig. 21-1 Drawing, made by seven-year-old child whose sister died in a car crash, shows the boy sad and crying (dots are tears) because he was not allowed to see his dead sibling.

Reactions to altered body image

Alopecia has psychological implications for both the patient and his or her family.

Young children For young children, baldness has little significance. Preschool children may attach superficial concern to the hair loss, particularly if it affects their sex role image. This aspect can be difficult for the parents also.

School-aged children The reactions of school-aged children depend on their preparation for the loss and the type of parental adjustment. Telling children about this possibility before it occurs, stressing that it is temporary, and suggesting ways of camouflaging it, such as with a wig or other appropriate fashion accessories, fosters better adjustment to the altered body image.

Adolescents Adolescents have the most difficulty in accepting and adjusting to hair loss, because it occurs at a time when peer acceptance and group conformity are essential. They need the opportunity to express their anger and fears of rejection without being judged or reproached. Ritchie (1992) identified denial and rationalization as being the most frequently used coping mechanism.

Involving adolescents in selecting a wig or other means of camouflage *before* the hair falls out provides them with a feeling of participation and allows them to secure a wig that is most similar to their own hair. Altered body issues relating to weight loss or gain may require consultation with a dietitian experienced in working with adolescents. Most recent research

suggests that while adolescents with cancer are at most risk for psychological problems, most are generally well adjusted and meet developmental tasks (Ritchie, 1992).

Implications for Nursing

The time of diagnosis is a critical period for the development of therapeutic relationships. Ideally, the named nurse should be present with family members when the diagnosis is given. Parents want information that they consider critical information related to the diagnosis and prognosis, disease process, need for additional diagnostic tests, immediate therapeutic plan, and availability of the doctor. They value an open, sympathetic, direct and uninterrupted discussion, with sufficient time to hear the information and to ask questions. Information should be repeated and clarified (Woolley *et al*, 1989).

Encouraging parents and providing facilities to enable them to stay with the child and participate in their care, is important in restoring the parental role and in preparation for their discharge. Planning the child's care *with* family members is a most effective way of communicating genuine concern and providing ongoing education (Muller *et al.*, 1992).

Parents and children need thorough, detailed, and repeated explanations of the diagnostic tests and plan of therapy. They need reassurance that a change in the child's condition is most likely a result of therapy, not the disease. Decreasing the chance for the unexpected lessens the opportunities for increased anxiety.

PHASE II — REPRIEVE: REMISSION AND MAINTENANCE THERAPY

Once the child is in remission, there is a long period of hope for an eventual recovery and fear of a possible relapse. Parents commonly react with heightened vigilance by overprotecting the child, encouraging dependency, and liberalizing discipline. These reactions support the child's sick role and hinder optimum physical and emotional development. They may also give rise to feelings of sibling rivalry and resentment. Parents require support and education to help prevent this or to cope with such reactions.

Overprotectiveness

Although many children return home in relatively stable and much improved physical health, parents frequently treat them as invalids. One of the most common manifestations of overprotectiveness is parents' inability to set appropriate limits. For ill children, overprotection and 'special' treatment increase their fears of serious illness and failure to recover.

Dependency

Closely associated with the overprotectiveness is an increased dependency between parents and child. This is often evident in parents' unwillingness to send their child to school. Prior to the child's return to school, several issues should be addressed, including the course of the illness, susceptibility to common childhood diseases, other parents' questions about the disease (such as the chance of communicability), preparation of the class for expected physical changes, and possible future absences. During the terminal phase, the parents should also discuss the likelihood of the child's death and the need to discuss this with the other students. Teachers of siblings who attend the same school should also be included in the discussions.

Anxiety

In addition to the concerns discussed in the preceding paragraphs are many other anxiety-provoking stresses. The financial strain of a chronic illness is a constant worry. Job security is always a necessary consideration. There are also costs such as transportation to the hospital, meals away from home, baby-sitting for other siblings, or temporary housing for distant medical care. The nurse can provide assistance by referring the family to Social Services and other available organizations, such as the Leukaemia Research Fund or the Malcolm Sargent Cancer Fund for Children who may be able to provide financial support, information, and psychological support.

Nutrition is also a continuing concern. Many drugs cause severe nausea, vomiting, and alterations in taste, thereby decreasing the child's appetite. Growth may also be slowed during the treatment phase due to the various drugs and use of radiation. If parents are aware of some of these expected changes, they may be more accepting of the child's fluctuating appetite.

Implications for Nursing

Often, remission and 'going home' from the oncology centre or unit coincide, and several problems can be anticipated and often prevented by a thorough discussion at this time: maintenance of normal family patterns, school attendance, and relationships among family and friends (Lansky, 1985). Outpatient and/or day care visits should, where possible, be negotiated with the parent and the patient to minimize the disruption to the family routine.

Ongoing compliance with medical treatment is an important aspect of care, with prognosis closely related to treatments. Evening and Saturday clinics specifically for adolescents may help overcome this aspect. Strategies for enhancing compliance, especially in teenagers, are to include the patient in treatment discussions, assisting the family to set clear expectations and clarify roles, and provide written instructions (Lansky, List, and Ritter-Sterr, 1988).

To avoid unnecessary social isolation, the parents need to be prepared for common responses of friends and relatives. Families should take the initiative in informing others about the child's condition and asking directly that they remain in contact with each other. Many benefit from associating with other similarly affected families.

Where available, community liaison nurses act as the link between hospital, home, tertiary centres, and the community. Effective communication should be established before discharge to ensure continuity of care (Patel, 1990). If community liason nurses are not available, key workers for networks should be developed to establish links with the available resources in the community.

PHASE III — RECOVERY: CESSATION OF THERAPY AND POSSIBLE CURE

The maintenance period may be followed by cessation of therapy in the hope of a permanent recovery. Although this is a very happy time, it is mixed with feelings of grief, ambivalence, and concern for the future.

Denial and ambivalence

At the time the decision is made to terminate therapy, many parents deny that treatment is no longer warranted. In general, this reaction is characteristic of the grieving for the loss of security afforded by medical intervention and adjustment to the hazards of 'waiting it out' again. This long term anxiety can become disabling to some families (Faulker, Peace, and O'Keefe, 1993).

Overprotectiveness and concern for the future

Parents also relate a resurgence of the need to overprotect and isolate their child from any potential physical harm.

When cure is a realistic possibility, the family's concern for the *quantity* of life shifts to the *quality* of life. Children worry most about their psychological normalcy, schooling, and relationships with family and friends. They have concerns for the future about having children, transmitting cancer to their offspring, and recurrence of their disease or another cancer. Information concerning the effects of smoking and alcohol consumption on organs already compromised by radiation and chemotherapy should be provided (Hollen and Hobbie, 1993). Some worry about employment discrimination, and obtaining insurance and mortgages (Koocher, 1985).

Implications for Nursing

Probably the most important component of care is acceptance of the family's mixed reactions to cessation of treatment. Parents need to feel comfortable in phoning about any concern or problem. They also should be encouraged to talk about their feelings and thoughts of cessation of treatment. Follow-up clinics have now been established to address the long-term psychological and physical problems (Pinkerton, Cushing, and Sepion, 1994).

PHASE IV — RECURRENCE: RELAPSE AND DEATH

The most dreaded news, other than the initial diagnosis, is confirmation of a relapse. The family's reactions during the terminal stage are influenced by their previous acceptance or denial of the child's illness. It is a period of intense anticipatory grieving, characterized by the relapse reactions of depression, loss of hope, and possibly acceptance.

Loss of hope and depression

One of the most difficult realizations for the family is the knowledge that with each relapse the chances for eventual recovery diminish. Once another remission is attained, reason for hope is again present.

The usual reaction to loss of hope is depression. Nurses need to assess carefully the reason for the depression and plan intervention realistically.

Fear of death
The most prevalent fear is of death itself. Parents frequently ask about death through questions such as, 'What will he die from?', 'How will we know she is dying?', and 'What will happen when he dies?' (Kohler and Radford, 1985). It is important to listen sensitively to such questions, because the real concern may be hidden behind the question.

Fear of pain
The fear of uncontrollable pain is almost universal. Whatever bargaining occurs during the dying stage is for a peaceful, quiet, and quick death. It is important for nurses to understand that pain is much more than physical.

Fear of loss of control
A fear that is shared by the dying and the survivors is losing emotional and physical control as death approaches. Some parents attempt to cope with this fear by requesting that their child be heavily sedated during the terminal stage. However, the loss of control imposed by medication may make the child very distraught. Inasmuch as nurses usually regulate the administration of drugs, it is important for them to carefully assess the needs of both the child and the parents. Supporting parents at the time of impending death by being physically present, making the child as comfortable as possible, and talking to the awake child helps parents feel in control, without the need for sedating the child (Goldman, Beardsmore, and Hunt, 1990).

Fear of isolation and loneliness
Parents fear that their child will die when they are not present. Dying children often request that their parents stay with them, and this request should always be respected. Although everyone dies alone, no one need die in lonely isolation.

Implications for Nursing
Nurses can help parents and children formulate realistic, short-term goals and to establish reasonable priorities of care.

During the terminal stage, the fears of parents and children form the foundation for nursing care. These fears may be particularly worrisome for parents who have chosen home care, because they must assume primary responsibility for the child. The community liaison nurse's role includes preparing them to deal with each fear and providing assistance through home visits, telephone counselling, and the alternative of hospital admission at any time.

Both the family and the child may have heightened spiritual needs at the time of death. Spiritual support includes respect for the diverse beliefs of families, willingness to discuss matters of spirituality with them, and provision for the rituals and sacraments of organized religion (Conrad, 1985).

PHASE V — THE BEGINNING: POSTDEATH

The crisis of loss does not end with the child's death. In many ways, it only begins (Sarnoff Schiff, 1977).

Implications for Nursing
The optimum time and number of meetings and/or visits is not known. Follow-up can help the family understand the process of mourning, particularly its duration and pain, and can provide assistance in making decisions that involve the loss.

At times, family members may need assistance in their grieving. Mothers, in particular, often feel a great sense of loneliness and emptiness, and part of their resolving the grief is finding a substitute role that is fulfilling and rewarding. Nurses can be instrumental in this process by: (1) preparing the mother for anticipating the *normal* feelings of emptiness, loneliness, and sometimes even failure, (2) helping her re-evaluate her role as parent and spouse, (3) encouraging her to explore fulfilling activities that use her special interests, talents, and qualifications, and (4) supporting her as her role changes, particularly assisting with communication between affected family members (Wong, 1980).

Self-help groups, such as The Compassionate Friends, an international organization for bereaved parents and siblings, offer support to newly bereaved families. The siblings' reaction will depend upon many factors, including the circumstances of the death, the quality of the prior sibling relationship, parental reactions, and family communication patterns (Gibbons, 1992). Faulkner, Peace, and O'Keefe (1993) reported that siblings protect their grieving parents by suppressing their own feelings.

Nurses should also be aware of behaviours that indicate siblings' difficulty with resolving their grief, such as persistent blame and guilt, patterns of overactivity with aggressive and destructive outbursts, compulsive caregiving, persistent anxieties (such as fear of another family death or of their own), excessive clinging to the parent, difficulty with forming new relationships, problems at school (poor concentration, restlessness, preferring to be alone, not being liked by classmates), or delinquency (such as stealing) (Michael and Lansdown, 1986).

Communication with the bereaved family is essential. Regrettably, reports from bereaved families indicate that the majority (80%) consider the information or counselling from professionals to be inadequate and even harmful. Nurses require appropriate training if they are to provide this service, or should be aware of a trained specialist they can contact as required.

THE NURSE AND THE FATALLY ILL CHILD

It would not be complete to discuss the nurse's role in caring for the family and dying child without exploring the effects of this stressful, yet extremely rewarding, area of nursing practice on the caregiver. Recognition of the potential stresses is essential in coping with the emotional demands imposed by sharing the family's loss and grief (Brewis, 1990). Emery (1993) identified that death was the most stressful factor within the paediatric oncology critical care setting.

NURSES' REACTIONS TO CARING FOR FATALLY ILL CHILDREN

Nurses experience reactions to a fatal illness that are very similar to the responses of family members. Some of these help nurses provide care by protecting them from the emotional impact of the event. Others interfere with the establishment of a therapeutic relationship with family members. Analysis and understanding of these reactions are as important in providing effective care to the dying child as is the recognition of specific responses in the family.

DENIAL

When children are admitted to a paediatric unit with a suspected diagnosis of a serious illness, the initial response from some nurses is shock and denial. Their behavioural reaction may be withdrawal from the child and family. Because of their own dependency on denial, nurses may support denial in parents. There are several methods of conveying this message, such as emphasizing only optimistic 'survival statistics', negating the seriousness of the illness, focusing on 'cheering up' the family, and engaging in casual conversation to avoid meaningful dialogue.

Some denial is as important for nurses as it is for the child or parents; it protects nurses from the overwhelming reality of death. It would be extremely difficult to participate in the medical treatment plan without some expectation of a cure. Denial is also necessary to prevent feelings of failure (Hammer, Nichols, and Armstrong, 1992).

ANGER AND DEPRESSION

Some nurses may be angry for having been assigned to the child with leukaemia, because the very exposure to potential failure in a fatal illness is extremely threatening. Others may feel angry for having to subject the child to painful procedures or for being unable to relieve the child's physical and emotional suffering. Instead of anger, some nurses may feel depression for any of these reasons.

Depression also has adverse effects on a therapeutic relationship, because nurses may withdraw from the child and parents as a method of controlling their sadness. Unaware of the reason for the avoidance, family members interpret it as evidence of inadequate care. This reaction also fosters a nonsupportive cycle of avoidance, withdrawal, resentment, and frustration.

GUILT

Nurses who feel unable to deal with fatal illness in a child often experience guilt. They express guilt for having been intolerant of the child's or parents' behaviour and, even more important, realize the missed opportunity to provide these individuals with professional support and guidance.

Nursing staff may experience guilt even when they can deal effectively with the family. They may set expectations that are beyond anyone's ability to meet, such as the expectation that they are supposed to save lives, not let people die.

AMBIVALENCE

One of the most universal reactions of nurses is ambivalence in their feelings towards a dying child. There is the fluctuating adherence to hope for a cure and fear of a relapse.

Ambivalence may be demonstrated in a particular type of bargaining. Rather than bargaining for extra time, nurses may hope that their colleagues are assigned the patient, or that a death may occur on a shift other than their own. Bargaining for a temporary absence from the dying child is a healthy response, because it denotes nurses' awareness of their own emotional limits. Nurses who are unable to recognize their personal emotional limits are in danger of seeking from the professional relationship their own needs for gratification, achievements, and fulfilment. This results in the loss of an objective evaluation of therapeutic interventions and the increased potential for subjective overinvolvement with the family.

COPING WITH STRESS

One of the hazards of caring for dying children is the risk of *burnout*, a state of physical, emotional, and mental exhaustion. It occurs as a result of prolonged involvement with individuals in situations that are emotionally demanding.

Self-awareness and consciousness raising

The initial step in effectively caring for a dying child is making a deliberate choice to become involved. Many nurses react negatively to the word 'involvement' because they believe that professionals must remain uninvolved in order to maintain objectivity. Involvement does not displace objectivity. Maslach (1979) suggests that the achievement of *detached concern*, in which the health care practitioner provides sensitive, understanding care by being sufficiently detached to make objective, rational decisions, is the ideal.

Developing awareness requires the willingness to investigate one's motivations for choosing to work in such an area and an understanding of the stresses inherent in the role, to review one's resolution of past losses, and to contemplate one's own fears of death.

Knowledge and practice

Intervening therapeutically with terminally ill children and their families requires more than self-awareness. It also necessitates basing nursing practice on sound theoretic formulations and empirical observations that serve as a general, concise analysis of the typical reactions of families. Although every individual is different and responds to events or crises in a way that is influenced by all of his or her previous life's experiences, there must be some beginning point for understanding the more typical responses of individuals and for making some decision as to their importance in the eventual resolution of the crisis. In this way, nurses can plan care with the involvement of each family member in terms of prevention, as well as intervention, of problems.

Nurses must also explore ethical issues surrounding the definition of death, the use of extraordinary, lifesaving measures versus passive or active euthanasia, and patients' rights to know and choose their own destiny.

Support systems

Support systems, whether as part of the multidisciplinary team or from outside agencies, are essential for continued functioning in a high-stress environment. They allow for regeneration of energies by sharing feelings and concerns with others.

KEY POINTS

◆ To counsel families and children regarding death, nurses need to understand children's perceptions of death, the fears in each age group, and personal meanings of death and bereavement during developmental stages.

◆ Toddlers' egocentricity and separation of fact from fantasy make death incomprehensible; they may still refer to a dead person as if the person exists.

◆ Because of their sense of precausality and self-power, preschool children may believe that their thoughts actually cause another person's death.

◆ With their reasoning power and fear of the unknown, school-aged children may feel intense guilt and responsibility about someone's death.

◆ Adolescents have difficulty accepting death, because of their preoccupation with developing a sense of identity.

◆ Nurses may offer the following assistance in assessment and education about death: counselling parents about children's age-specific understanding of death, encouraging parents to help children become familiar and comfortable with loss, taking part in organized death education in schools, and serving as a resource to answer children's questions.

◆ What children are told about their serious illness is based on several general principles regarding developmental age, previous knowledge, and honesty.

◆ Kübler-Ross' stages of dying are denial, anger, bargaining, depression, and acceptance.

◆ Distorted reactions may represent one aspect of the syndrome and can be transformed into normal grief work.

◆ Parke's grief process consists of four phases that do not necessarily proceed in sequence and may recur at any time: shock and disbelief, expression of grief, disorganization and despair, and reorganization.

◆ Special decisions at the time of dying and death may involve hospital or hospice care, the child's right to die, visualization of the body, tissue donation and/or autopsy, and siblings' attendance at the funeral.

◆ In dealing with stress related to the dying patient, the nurse can cope successfully through self awareness, consciousness raising, knowledge and practice, available support system, maintaining general good health, and focusing on the positive rewards of involvement with dying children and their families.

REFERENCES

Armstrong-Dailey A: Children's hospice care, *Pediatr Nurs* 16(4):337, 1990.

Atuel TM, Williams PD, Camar MT: Determinants of Filipino children's responses to the death of a sibling, *Matern Child Nurs J* 17(2):115, 1988.

Birenbaum LK: The relationship between parent–sibling communication and coping of siblings with death experience, *J Pediatr Oncol Nurs* 6(3):86, 1989.

Birenbaum LK, Clarke-Steffan L: Terminal care cost in childhood cancer, *Paediatr Nurs* 18(3):285, 1992.

Black KJ: Sudden unexpected death: caring for the parents, *Paediatr Nurs* 17(6):571, 1991.

Bluebond-Langner M: *The private worlds of dying children,* Princeton, NJ, 1978, Princeton University Press.

Brewis EL: Care of the terminally ill child. In Thompson J, editor: *The child with cancer,* London, 1990, Scutari Press.

Chesterfield P: Communicating with dying children, *Nurs Stand* 6(20):30, 1992.

Conrad NL: Spiritual support for the dying, *Nurs Clin North Am* 20(2):415, 1985.

Copsey MK: Time to care, *Nurs Mirror* 153(22):38, 1981.

Corr CA, Corr DM: Children's hospice care, *Death Studies* 16(5):431, 1992.

Davies B: Family responses to the death of a child: the meaning of memories, *J Palliative Care* 3(1):9, 1987.

Emery JE: Perceived sources of stress amongst pediatric oncology nurses, *J Pediatr Oncol Nurs* 10(3):87, 1993.

Faulkner A, Peace G, O'Keefe C: Future imperfect, *Nurs Times* 89(51):40, 1993.

Foley G: Conflicts in practice: the argument for, *J Assoc Pediatr Oncol Nurs* 2(3):22, 1985.

Foley GV: Facilitating death discussions with children, *Pediatrics: nursing update,* lesson 19, Princeton, NJ, 1986, continuing Professional Education Corp.

Gershan JA: Judaic ethical beliefs and customs regarding death and dying, *Crit Care Nurs* 5(1):32, 1985.

Gibbons MB: A child dies, a child survives — the impact of sibling loss, *J Pediatr Health Care* 6(2):65, 1992.

Goldman A, Beardsmore S, Hunt J: Paliative care for children with cancer — home, hospital or hospice, *Arch Dis Child* 65:641, 1990.

Hollen PJ, Hobbie WL: Risk taking and decision making of adolescent long term survivors of cancer, *Oncol Nurs Forum* 20(5):769, 1993.

Jost KE, Haase JE: At the time of death: help for the child's parents, *Child Health Care* 18(3):146, 1989.

Judd D: *Give sorrow words*, London, 1989, Free Association Books.

Kachoyeanos MK, Selder FE: Life transitions of parents at the unexpected death of a school age and older child, *J Pediatr Nurs* 8(1):41, 1993.

Kohler JA, Radford M: Terminal care for children dying of cancer: quantity and quality of life, *Br Med J* 291:115, 1985.

Koocher G: Psychosocial care of the child cured with cancer, *Pediatr Nurs* 11(2):91, 1985.

Kübler-Ross E: *On children and death*, New York, 1983, Macmillan.

Kuntz B: Exploring the grief of adolescents after the death of a parent, *J Child, Adolescent Psychiatr Ment Health Nurs* 4(3):105, 1991.

Lansky SB, List MA, Ritter-Sterr C: Psychiatric and psychological support of the child and adolescent with cancer. In Pizzo P, Poplack D, editors: *Principles and practice of pediatric oncology*, Philadelphia, 1988, JB Lippincott.

Lansky SB: Management of stressful periods in childhood cancer, *Pediatr Clin North Am* 32(3):625, 1985.

Lauer ME *et al:* A comparison study of parental adaptation following a child's death at home or in the hospital, *Pediatr* 71(1):107, 1983.

Lauer ME *et al:* Children's perceptions of their sibling's death at home or hospital: the precursors of differential adjustment, *Cancer Nurs* 8(1):21, 1985.

Lindemann E: Symptomatology and management of acute grief, *Am J Psychiatry* 101:141, 1944.

Martinson IM: Hospice care for children past, present and future, *J Pediatr Oncol Nurs* 10(3):93, 1993.

Martinson IM, Davies EB, McClowry SG: The long-term effects of sibling death on self-concept, *J Pediatr Nurs* 2(4):227, 1987.

Maslach C: The burn-out syndrome and patient care. In Garfield C, editor: *Stress and survival: the emotional realities of life-threatening illness*, St Louis, 1979, Mosby–Year Book.

Mattias S, Spiers D: *A handbook on death and bereavement — helping children understand*, UK, 1990, National Library for the Handicapped Child.

Michael S, Lansdown R: Adjustment to the death of a sibling, *Arch Dis Child* 61:278, 1986.

Miles MS, Perry K: Parental responses to sudden accidental death of a child, *Crit Care Q* 8(1):73, 1985.

Morgan J: *The dying and the bereaved teenager*, Philadelphia, 1990, Charles Press.

Muller DJ, Harris PJ, Wattley L: *Nursing children: psychology and practice*, London, 1992, Harper & Row.

Nagy M: The child's view of death, *J Genet Psychol* 73:3, 1948.

Patel N: The child with cancer in the community. In Thompson J, editor: *The child with cancer*, London, 1990, Scutari Press.

Pinkerton CR, Cushing P, Sepion B: *Childhood cancer management — a practical handbook*, London, 1994, Chapman & Hall.

Ritchie MA: Psychosocial functioning of adolescents with cancer — a developmental perspective, *Oncol Nurs Forum* 19(10):1497, 1992.

Rushton CE, Hogue EE: When parents demand 'everything', *Pediatr Nurs* 19(2):180, 1993.

Sarnoff Schiff H: *The bereaved parent*, Great Britain, 1977, Souvenir Press.

Stuart A, Totterdell A: *Five and a half times three*, London, 1990, Hamish Hamilton.

Waechter E: Dying children: patterns of coping, *Issues Compr Pediatr Nurs* 8(1–6):51, 1985.

Warden JW: *Grief councelling and grief therapy*, New York, 1991, Springer Publishing.

Williams L: Organ procurement: what nurses need to know, *Crit Care Q* 8(1):27, 1985.

Wong D: Bereavement: the empty-mother syndrome, *MCN* 5(6):385, 1980.

Woolley H *et al:* Imparting the diagnosis of life threatening illness in children, *BMJ* 298(6688):1623, 1989.

Zalanskas B: Siblings: the forgotten grievers, *Issues Compr Pediatr Nurs* 5:45, 1981.

FURTHER READING

Bennet P: A care team for terminally ill children, *Nurs Times* 80(10):26, 1984.

Bond M: *Stress and self-awareness — a guide for nurses*, Oxford, 1986, Heinemann.

Brewis EL: Care of the terminally ill child. In Thompson J, editor: *The child with cancer — nursing care*, London, 1990, Scutari Press.

Brykczynska GM: *Ethics in paediatric nursing*, London, 1994, Chapman & Hall.

Buckman R: Breaking bad news: why is it still so difficult? *BMJ* 288:1597, 1984.

Burne SR, Dominica F, Baum JD: Helen House; a hospice for children — analysis of the first year, *BMJ* 289:1665, 1984.

Burton L: *Care of the child facing death*, Boston, 1974, Routledge & Kegan Paul.

Chambers EJ *et al:* Terminal care at home for children with cancer, *BMJ* 298:937, 1989.

Charles-Edward I: Who decides ethics? *Paediatr Nurs* 3(10):6, 1991.

Charles-Edward I, Casey A: Parental involvement and voluntary consent, *Pediatr Nurs* 4(1):16, 1992.

Dominica, Sister Francis: Reflections on death in childhood, *BMJ* 294:108, 1987.

Doyle B: I wish you were dead, *Nurs Times* 83(45):44.

Foster S: Explaining death to children, *BMJ* 282:540, 1981.

Goldman A: Care of the dying child. In Plowman PN, Pinkerton CR, editors: *Paediatric oncology — clinical practice and controversies*, London, 1992, Chapman & Hall.

Grogan LB: Grief of an adolescent when a sibling dies, *MCN* 15(1):21, 1990.

Hinds C: The needs of families who care for patients with cancer at home: are we meeting them? *J Adv Nurs* 10(6):575, 1985.

Johnson-Soderberg S: The development of a child's concept of death, *Oncol Nurs Forum* 8(1):23, 1981.

Kholer JA, Radford M: The dying child. In Lacey JH, Burns T, editors: *Psychological management of the physically ill*, Edinburgh, 1989, Churchill Livingstone.

Landsdown R, Goldman A: The psychological care of children with malignant disease, *J Child Psychol Psychiatr* 29:555, 1988.

Larcombe IJ, Walker J, Charlton A *et al:* Impact of childhood cancer on return to normal schooling, *BMJ* 301:169, 1990.

Oakhill A: *The supportive care of the child with cancer*, London, 1988, J Wright.

Papdatou D, Papadatos C: *Children and death*, New York, 1991, Hemisphere.

Patel N: The child with cancer in the community. In Thompson J, editor: *The child with cancer — nursing care,* London, 1990, Scutari Press.

Pettle Michael SA, Landsdown RG: Adjustment to the death of a sibling, *Arch Dis Child* 61:278, 1986.

Smith H: Physical, psychological and social aspects of childhood cancer, *Health Visitor* 61:221, 1988.

Thornes R: *Care of the dying child and their families,* London, 1988, King Edward Fund and National Association of Health Authorities.

Whiting M: Home care for children, *Nurs Standard* 4(22):52, 1990.

USEFUL ADDRESSES

British Organ Donor Society (Body), Balsham, Cambridge CB1 6DL and 6 Denmark Street, Bristol BS1 5DQ.

The Compassionate Friends, 53 North Street, Bristol, B53 1EN.

Hospice Information Service, 51–59, Lawrie Park Road, Sydenham, London SE26 6DZ.

Leukaemia Research Fund, 43 Great Ormond Street, London WC1N 3JJ.

Malcolm Sargent Cancer Fund for Children, 14 Abingdon Road, London W8 6AF.

Chapter 22

The Child with Learning Disabilities

LEARNING OUTCOMES

After studying this chapter you should be able to:

◆ Appreciate the wide range of needs of children with a learning disability.
◆ Identify criteria by which diagnosis of learning disabilities may be made.
◆ Discuss the major causes of learning disabilities and strategies of prevention.
◆ Identify areas of health need being met by nursing practice.
◆ Describe nursing approaches to meeting the needs of children with a learning disability.
◆ Understand the importance of the family context to successful nursing practice.
◆ Discuss particular needs of children with Down's syndrome and fragile X syndrome.
◆ Define the glossary terms.

GLOSSARY

adaptive behaviour Level of competence in everyday living skills

assessment tools Standardized frameworks to enable the assessment of individual needs

behaviour modification An approach and techniques for teaching skills; uses principles from learning theory, particularly reinforcement

Down's syndrome Autosomal abnormality, with a karyotype of 47

early intervention Strategies aimed to maximize learning in early years

fragile X syndrome Sex-linked chromosomal abnormality with unusual patterns of expression

IQ Intelligence quotient; score achieved on an intelligence scale

learning disability Term replacing 'mental handicap'; preferred term by the Department of Health

syndrome A set of signs and symptoms which indicate the presence of a disease or abnormal condition

WHO World Health Organization

terminal illness A condition wherein a life is near or approaching its end

t is estimated that one in every 50 people in the United Kingdom has some kind of learning disability. Within this group, approximately 15% are considered to have a severe learning disability (DoH, 1994).

Most people with learning disabilities have always lived within the community. However, recent social policy has consolidated the changing emphasis to provision of 'care in the community' which began in the 1950s. Particularly, this has begun to consider the needs of families for support and guidance, in enabling parents and their children with a learning disability to enjoy a reasonable quality of life. Nurses are in a strategic position to assume a vital role in meeting these needs, as traditional sites of practice expand to include the variety of settings of primary health care delivery. Increasingly, nurses are working in a much more flexible way. Inter- and intra-disciplinary boundaries are beginning to break down in response to local arrangements of services for people with learning disabilities, offered by local authorities, the National Health Service, and the private and voluntary sectors.

This chapter is an introduction to the complex problems encountered by families and children with learning disabilities — through considering its 'definition' and causes — and how nurses and families can work together. In addition, Down's syndrome, which is the single largest cause of severe learning disabilities, and fragile X syndrome will be briefly discussed in relation to nursing care. A review of Chapter 22 will provide details of the family's adjustment to disabilities in general.

PERSPECTIVES ON THE CARE OF CHILDREN WITH LEARNING DISABILITIES

'Learning disabilities' and 'learning difficulties' have recently become the favoured terms to replace 'mental handicap'. They are used to describe a group of people with lifelong intellectual impairment, originating within the developmental period, from conception to adulthood. Subdividing this group is the diversity of needs arising from associated physical, behavioural, and social problems. Professionals, service planners, and primarily service users themselves have advocated that the term 'mental handicap' has become prejudicial. Recent research supports this view (Eayrs *et al*, 1993). This term is also considered to attribute the problems people experience and their solutions solely to those individuals, without addressing the way society contributes to them.

The consequences of applying negative labels to children with learning disabilities were highlighted almost 20 years ago in a review of children's services, which stressed that children with learning disabilities should be seen as *children* first (Committee on Child Health Services, 1976). Since then, this philosophy has influenced the development of provision within this field. Fundamentally, children with learning disabilities have become incorporated into mainstream welfare provision; for example, as part of the group of 'children in need' within the *Children Act* (1989), which underwrites the practice of local

authority services for all children and their families, and within the *Education Act* (1981) (Middleton, 1992).

Families of children who have learning disabilities face more than the challenge of childrearing. There are educational dilemmas, the need for other special services, decisions regarding future care, and coping with a society which often denigrates anyone who is 'different'.

GENERAL CONCEPTS

As within other areas of health service provision, the medical model has been crucial to the development of approaches to meeting the needs of people with learning disabilities at all levels of service delivery. However, for the last three decades within the field of learning disabilities, behavioural psychology has also had a major influence within services. These two disciplines have, until recently, provided most of the research which has informed nursing practice.

As ideas about people with learning disabilities have changed, the value of these particular interventions has increasingly come into question. In response, professionals have used other frameworks to enrich their practice. Those which advocate for individual rights and integration into ordinary society have come to dominate; particularly the philosophy of 'normalization' (Wolfensberger, 1972). The set of ideas known as normalization have ensured that the concepts of integration and ordinary living are fundamental to service planning. It has created a common language within interdisciplinary and agency care provision for people with a learning disability. Nurses caring for children with a learning disability can utilize the following framework developed from these ideas to underpin the nursing process (O'Brien, 1987) (Box 22-1). It prompts the development of practical strategies which promote normalization by identifying aspects of life which are important to all individuals but which are often compromised as a consequence of disability.

Diagnosis and classification are fundamental to determining need. Within contemporary services, these processes inform decisions about the extent and nature of provisions available to people with learning disabilities. In the past, they have been central to a model of care which has involved the imposition of sanctions and segregated life-styles. It is perhaps this legacy which has attributed negative connotations to these two terms and some resistance to their use.

Historically, IQ tests have provided a basis for establishing the criteria for diagnosis and classification of people with intellectual impairment. Recent studies of populations with learning disabilities have shown that only a minority have had formal intelligence tests, indicating a move away from this method (Farmer *et al*, 1993).

It is generally considered, however, that the group of people with learning disabilities within the United Kingdom falls into two categories: people with severe learning disabilities with IQs under 50 (subgrouped moderate, severe, and profound), and people with mild learning disabilities with IQs of 50–70. The groupings correlate with classifications by the WHO

◆ BOX 22-1

Examples of strategies of normalization

Community presence
- advocate for children and parents wishing to use ordinary services, e.g. schools
- facilitate the use of local leisure opportunities
- encourage positive attitudes towards learning disabilities

Choices
- be responsive to the different methods by which children with a learning disability may communicate their choices
- maximize the range of experiences available to the child
- foster independence, e.g. by teaching self-help groups

Being competent
- recognize and build on a child's skills however limited they may seem
- adopt a systematic approach to the use of play in the child's normal development
- enable children and parents to take risks where appropriate

Respect and dignity
- plan interventions which take the child's age into account and avoid a child appearing different
- encourage the involvement of children and parents in decision making

Community participation
- recognize the importance of friendships with disabled and non-disabled people
- support family relationships and separations, e.g. when using short-term care

From O'Brien, 1987.

Expert Committee (1968) and within the International Classification of Diseases (ICD).

Physical and sensory handicaps are associated with severe learning disabilities and often necessitate a high level of long-term support. It is this association which makes the measurement of IQ relevant to determining the need of a local population.

The concept of 'adaptive behaviour' has also been influential in establishing a diagnosis of an individual's learning disability, but also in placing skill acquisition, use, and maintenance as a major focus to service development and evaluation. Several assessment tools have become available to determine an individual's level of ability to perform the skills necessary to function in a given environment. A summary of this approach and other assessments used with people with learning disabilities can be found in Hogg and Raynes (1988).

The aims of services for children with learning disabilities and their families have developed to include family support, promotion of quality life-styles, empowerment of individuals

and carers, and partnership between carers and professionals. Within educational, health, and social services, the planning, delivery, and evaluation of services at all levels has become informed by much broader diagnoses or assessments of *needs* — moving beyond a statement of what a person can or cannot do, or a measure of IQ.

Nurses working with children and their families do so in cooperation with other agencies and disciplines, and have a range of assessment data available to inform their own understanding of their client's situation and nursing diagnosis.

CAUSATION

The causes of learning disabilities can be broadly grouped as being either genetic, chromosomal or environmental in nature.

Genetic and/or chromosomal causes include chromosomal aberrations resulting from radiation, viruses, chemicals, parental age and genetic mutations, such as Down and fragile X syndromes. In addition, recessive gene abnormalities, such as inborn errors of metabolism, and (rarely) dominant gene abnormalities may cause learning disabilities.

Environmental causes affect the pattern of development after conception, during the antenatal, perinatal, and postnatal periods. During the antenatal period, causes include maternal nutrition, anoxia, infection, and intoxication. Perinatally, causes include birth injury (a major cause), prematurity, and low birth weight. Postnatal causes include childhood infection, such as encephalitis, cerebral trauma, and sensory and social deprivation.

Learning disabilities can be caused by either single or multiple factors. In most incidences, it is not possible to define an exact cause. However, a known cause is more often attributed in incidences of severe learning disability. Among individuals with severe learning disabilities, chromosomal abnormalities account for 20–25% of cases and the majority are Down's syndrome. Ten to twenty percent are associated with severe cerebral palsy, microcephaly, or epileptic seizures known as infantile spasms (Hall, 1984). The dominance of causes resulting in nervous system damage lead to high incidences of associated physical and sensory disability in people with severe learning disabilities.

Socially related factors, such as maternal life-styles and poor nutrition, predominate in incidences of mild learning disability, and link this to broader social and economic issues. Of the 1,000,000 or more people who fall within the mild learning disabilities group, fewer than one-half will have been specifically diagnosed as having an intellectual impairment (OHE/Mencap, 1986). Some will attend 'special schools', but most will not use any special services during adulthood.

PREVENTION

In 1971, a government report into the needs of people with learning disabilities recommended that research should be promoted into the causes of mental handicap and its prevention (DHSS, 1971). Despite the often controversial issues surrounding preventive measures within the field of learning disability, a wide range of services and interventions have developed. Preconceptual services include immunization against rubella, genetic counselling (especially in terms of Down's or fragile X syndrome), and general services to improve the health of potential mothers. These include education in the prevention of low birth weight, targeting alcohol consumption and smoking.

Family planning services can offer parents the opportunity for planned pregnancies and readiness for the demands of parenthood. During the antenatal period, some interventions are aimed at offering parents the choice of abortion on identification of conditions associated with learning disabilities. These include antenatal diagnosis or carrier detection of disorders, such as Down's syndrome. Procedures such as the examination of fetal cells will reveal genetic and/or chromosomal abnormalities and diagnostic ultrasound will reveal conditions such as hydrocephalus and placental abnormalities. Antenatal services may also target mothers most at risk.

Preventive interventions during the perinatal period include neonatal screening for phenylketonuria, and other inborn errors of metabolism. These strategies are designed to identify the condition early and to avert cerebral damage. Postnatally, strategies are aimed at preventing long-term consequences of conditions such as Down's syndrome, by treating coexisting problems. General strategies of support for families help overcome the consequences of environmental deprivation and incidences of mild intellectual disability.

IMPLICATIONS FOR NURSING

- To be aware of normal childhood development and the importance of recognition and referral of children who are not meeting developmental milestones.
- To utilise strategies to promote normalisation.
- To be aware of the roles of the multidisciplinary team in meeting the special needs of children with learning disabilities and their parents.
- To be knowledgeable about community support networks for the care of children with learning disabilities and their families.
- To provide family support and understand the need for respite care for some children with learning disabilities.
- To support parents and children in genetic counselling.

The child and their family — the early years

Most children with learning disabilities live either with their families or within families. As with other groups who may require long-term and continuing support, the needs of people with learning disabilities have gradually been redefined by policy initiatives as being social and educational issues. Nevertheless, there are a large number of adults and children in the United Kingdom with learning disabilities who have particular as well as general health care needs, often arising from the complexities of multiple disabilities.

Nurses working with children who have learning disabilities, and with their families, can contribute to maintaining and promoting health gain, and prevention of health loss by focussing on these particular needs. The diversity of children's individual physical, psychological, and social circumstances, and the complexities of service structures can be appreciated only through experience within the field. The following discussion explores general areas of need and approaches to meeting them, which have come to the forefront of nursing practice as a consequence of social policy, service provision, and a range of concepts and philosophies influencing the field.

Besides the responsibilities nurses have in meeting the long-term needs of families and their children with learning disabilities, they also play an important role both in preventive measures and in the initial identification and diagnosis of children's disabilities. Many of the strategies aimed at prevention have been discussed previously and, within these, nurses are involved in both education and counselling.

In some cases, a child's learning disability is identified at birth; for example, through recognition of distinct syndromes, such as Down's syndrome. However, in other instances the diagnosis is made after a period of suspicion by professionals and/or family that the child is failing to reach developmental milestones. Sometimes, a child's learning disability is first noticed through comparison to peers, when the child enters the educational system.

A complicating factor is that children with learning disabilities (as well as many without) have 'patchy' development; for example, a child may walk at the usual age, yet fail to develop recognizable speech and understanding.

The *Education Act* (1981) and the *Children Act* (1989) stress the importance of cooperation between professionals to establish systems for early identification and delivery of comprehensive services to minimize the effects of disability. Nurses working closely with children and families in many different settings are fundamental to these processes. An assessment of a child's health needs is a vital contribution, as are the nurse's skills in promoting the wishes of the family.

The major task of parenthood is participating in the development of the independence of the child. One of the first self-help skills that children learn is to feed themselves. It involves the integration of fine and gross motor skills, and visual perception. Children soon become independent in areas of personal hygiene, dressing, and continence.

Children with a learning disability experience difficulties in mastering the necessary skills which are almost automatically learned by other children. Research has indicated that the continuing dependence of children upon their parents to meet their basic self-help needs (beyond that normally expected), can significantly affect the family's ability to cope. The health of parents and other family members can become compromised, and the 'daily grind' of care may dominate family life (Ayer and Alaszewski, 1986). Ultimately, this will restrict the opportunities a child has to grow and develop as a whole, both within and outside the home. While it is possible to offer short-term relief to the family through, for example, respite care schemes, long-term benefits are gained by promoting independent self-help skills. Consequently, there has been considerable development in home teaching and support services by statutory and voluntary agencies. There are also many books that offer advice to parents on structured teaching of self-care and other skills.

One particular strategy which continues to be employed with children who have learning disabilities is 'early intervention'. Underpinning this is the belief that the early years of learning are of critical importance, and can be targeted to maximize the learning potential of these children (Wishart, 1991). This has proved successful in preventing learning disabilities, where a child is 'at risk' from an impoverished environment. However, if a child already has a learning disability, the criteria of success and failure are difficult to define and measure (Spitz, 1986). The input of a professional or adviser may not lead to a child learning new skills, but may alleviate the burden of care, physically and psychologically.

Parental involvement is considered to be integral to the process through which a child develops skills at any time (McConkey, 1985). Although education in self-help skills often takes place at school, children may have difficulty 'transferring' this learning to their home. The principles of behaviour modification have had a tremendous impact as an approach to teaching children with learning disabilities. These can be utilized within the home to teach self-help skills.

Using behaviour modification techniques, parents may work directly to teach skills. They may also have to overcome their child's difficult and obstructive behaviours which hinder learning (Yule and Carr, 1988). Using the technique of 'extinction' (systematically ignoring a behaviour), although effective, can be particularly difficult for many parents. Nurses can work together with parents to set realistic developmental targets for their child. A child with additional handicaps may have been assessed by other members of the multidisciplinary team, such as the speech therapist and physiotherapist. Parents may need help consolidating the information to inform their understanding of their child's needs. Nurses can also help parents overcome the sense of failure parents may feel, as most parents assume that they will be successful in teaching their children. Nurses can emphasize to parents elements of skills that their child may already have and thus help establish a 'positive' teaching environment.

Underpinning any successful teaching are the practicalities that a family faces in making these techniques work within the constraints of family life. The nurse, as a member of a multidisciplinary team, may play the role of key worker to the family. Within this role, it is possible to gain an understanding of the family as a whole. For example, who regularly cares for the child? Does the family have rigid routines and busy schedules to maintain? What other stresses affect the family? How motivated and able are the family to participate in teaching their child? Once any structured teaching begins, the nurse may be in an important position to give parents supportive feedback.

There are many other ways a nurse may be involved in the optimum development of the child with learning disabilities.

Acceptable social behaviour, feelings of self-esteem, worth, and security arise from a genuine caring and loving family environment and not simply from 'teaching programmes'. Often, it is the nurse who can provide continuing assistance in fostering these elements.

Enabling children to communicate their needs and wishes is fundamental to their welfare. Verbal skills are often delayed more than other physical skills; indeed, this is frequently the first clue to cognitive deficits. Speech requires the receptive skills of hearing and interpretation, and expressive skills such as facial muscle coordination.

For some children, especially those with severe cognitive and physical impairments, speech acquisition is not possible and communication is nonverbal. A nurse may interact with parents by giving support as they work to develop their child's speech. As learning is slower, their teaching must continue longer. They may feel like giving up and find it difficult to sustain the additional input their child needs. This may involve, for example, encouraging regular tongue exercises, or giving consistent reinforcement of attempts to vocalize a letter or intelligible syllable. They may also help to develop and maintain the use of nonverbal systems of communication, such as the sign language, makaton. Particularly, they may identify ways in which a child is attempting to communicate which have previously been unrecognized. In order for children with learning disabilities to communicate, others in their environment need to learn *how* they are communicating. The increasing emphasis upon child protection and the 'child's voice', driven by the *Children Act* (1989), gives the area of communication a particularly important focus to nursing practice.

The older child — looking beyond the family

In order for children to develop their potential for an independent and integrated life, they need opportunities to acquire social skills. These occur both within the home and, as they take part in social experiences, outside of it. The ability to behave in a socially acceptable way will make a major contribution to a child's future quality of life. Nurses may be involved directly in teaching these skills, using techniques such as role play or in supporting the parents in contributing to their child's socialization. Parents can be educated to see the importance of social skills; to say 'hello' and 'thank you', to respond when spoken to, to greet strangers without being overly affectionate.

When confronted with numerous other difficulties that face them, parents may fail to see the long-term implications of neglecting social skills. This is, in a sense, an aspect of teaching right and wrong, which is often one of the first childrearing practices neglected by parents who have a child with a disability. This can not only result in serious behaviour problems, but may also affect a child's developing sense of security and self-control.

For children with cognitive impairment, limit-setting measures must be consistent and simple. They may be unable to understand reasons behind requests and have limited self-awareness of the impact of their behaviour. Behaviour modification, reinforcing the child when he or she is obedient, and 'timeout' when he or she isn't, are still appropriate intervention strategies, despite concerns over misuse (Brigden and Todd, 1995).

Nurses can also help enable children to have peer experiences similar to those of other children, through which they can acquire social skills. In accessing associations, such as the Scouts and the Guides, careful planning may be needed to minimize risks, but still allowing them to be taken.

Adolescence may be a particularly difficult time. The young person will need social outlets for heterosexual experiences. The nurse can be instrumental in facilitating these by discussing with parents the sensitive issues surrounding their child's developing sexuality. The teaching of socially acceptable sexual behaviour is especially important in the promotion of sexual health, which is a target for nursing practice (DoH, 1993). Studies have highlighted the failure to use contraception as an issue for young people with learning disabilities who are having sexual intercourse. In addition, there are increased rates of sexual abuse or rape among adolescents with learning disabilities (Chamberlain *et al,* 1984). One factor that contributes to the vulnerability of children and adults with learning disabilities is their inability to understand the difficult concepts surrounding healthy sexual behaviour.

Nurses can assist parents in teaching sex education and preparing their child for physical and sexual maturity and expression. They can provide them with information that is geared to the child's developmental level. The young person with learning disabilities needs to be familiar with the names and functions of body parts and must have well-defined and concrete guidelines on the way to respond in certain situations. For example, while ideas of safety and familiarity may be difficult to grasp, a girl may be told that she should never go anywhere alone with any person she does not know.

The worry of pregnancy is often a parental concern, and may involve nurses in difficult moral and ethical decisions surrounding contraception and sterilization.

Another concern that nurses may help to address as a child reaches adolescence are future possibilities of marriage or long-term relationships. In many instances, marriage enables couples with learning disabilities to achieve mutually satisfying and supportive relationships. People with learning disabilities may also choose to become parents themselves, although this continues to be a controversial issue. There has been unjustified concern for the intellectual development of children attributed solely to the fact that their parents have a learning disability. The issue is complex; however, there is an increasing amount of research to inform nursing practice (Tymchuk and Andron, 1994).

The sharing of information, feelings, and attitudes within sex education creates an environment in which a teenager has the confidence to communicate any concerns with their parents (Craft and Hitching, 1989). Similarly, it allows the parents to explore and help prepare for this important aspect of their child's future well-being.

Working with families and their children, nurses help them to adjust to the many transitions in their lives. Not all families are able to cope with the demands of caring for their child, especially when their child has a severe intellectual and multiple disability.

Retirement or old age brings other difficulties to the emotional, social, and financial pressures parents often face. Questions of alternative and meaningful daytime activities, which provide, among other things, valuable time-out for families, also begin to arise as a child approaches school-leaving age (Bryne and Cunningham, 1985).

Families often have to make difficult decisions surrounding the need for residential services. A nurse may help parents and their child minimize the negative consequences of this major transition. This can be achieved through exploring the reasons which have lead to the need, and to affirm the importance of maintaining relationships. The nurse will need to work closely with other agencies and professionals at this time, particularly within the framework of the *NHS and Community Care Act* (1990). Through a knowledge of the family as a whole, the nurse can assist them in choosing available provisions through a multidisciplinary assessment of the child's needs. Provision may include several alternatives, ranging from foster care to group homes or semi-independent living schemes. Daytime occupation should then be considered as part of the total package of care.

Throughout childhood, a child with learning disabilities will access and use ordinary services, including generic health services. Sometimes the special needs of children with learning disabilities may be particularly challenging to health professionals. This includes nurses who work in hospital settings and have had little experience of learning disabilities. Rather than benefiting from the use of integrated services, there is a danger that children will become isolated as a result of staff insecurity and fear. This can affect a child's sense of self-esteem and overall development, and contribute to parents' inability to cope with a stressful experience. Structured approaches by nurses can be used to overcome these difficulties.

If a child needs to go into hospital, for example, a nurse may be able to make a prehospital visit to their home. This will enable the nurse to gather information about the child's usual environment, his or her abilities, special needs, and the way the family or other caregivers meet these needs. The assessment should include identifying special devices and aids the child uses, any unusual routines, and any particular ways the child is likely to communicate feelings. Continuity of care can be developed, and the family and child are provided with an opportunity to identify with someone when they go into hospital.

Both the unfamiliar surroundings and the nature of clinical interventions and procedures demand that nurses establish effective communication with any child. Nurses will need to use communication methods at the appropriate cognitive level of a child with learning disabilities.

Any experience is potentially able to lead to the healthy development of the child — even the experience of hospitalization. It can reinforce to parents the child's abilities, and can be an opportunity for social experiences with peers. It provides chances for children and their families to access other services and information that will help with long-term needs. It also may provide valuable respite to parents and their children from the everyday care responsibilities, and may provide opportunities to discuss their feelings with professionals.

Nurses contribute in many different ways to enhancing the quality of life of children with learning disabilities. Nursing practice is influenced by the many different approaches to defining the needs of people with learning disabilities which have developed over time. There is, however, a range of experiences that are essential to the healthy development of children with learning disabilities that are often overlooked.

Children with learning disabilities have the same need for play as any other children (Lear, 1993). It is essential to development and should, whenever possible, be an integral part of any nursing intervention. Because of the child's slower development, parents may be less aware of the need to continue appropriate stimulation. They may also feel inadequate in playing with the child, since the usual reciprocal satisfaction between child and parent may be slower in developing. Parents may be reluctant to take risks and may be overprotective.

The nurse should be involved in guidance towards the selection of suitable toys and activities. It is important that play is appropriate to the child's developmental age. For example, a child with a profound intellectual disability may need sensorimotor play for several years. Every opportunity should be used to expose the child to as many sounds, sights, and sensations as possible.

All children with learning disabilities should be treated as individuals. Before working with a child and family, the nurse will need to understand how each child's learning disability affects them as a whole. The following are examples of how some of the likely needs of children and their parents can be identified through the diagnosis and classification of a chromosomal syndrome.

SYNDROMES ASSOCIATED WITH LEARNING DISABILITIES

One of the major contributions of the medical and clinical approach within the field of learning disabilities has been the identification of signs and symptoms, including intellectual impairment, associated with a specific pathology. Thus, diagnosis of a syndrome gives parents and professionals a starting point for assessment, and can confirm and support long-term interventions. Each syndrome is described by its list of classic clinical features, although there are variations in the way these manifest.

DOWN'S SYNDROME

Down's syndrome (DS) is the most common chromosomal abnormality of a generalized syndrome. Its overall incidence is 1:700 (Smith and Berg, 1976) and research indicates an increase rather than a decrease in prevalence by the year 2000 (Nicholson and Alberman, 1992).

The cause of DS is not known, although several theories dominate. These include genetic predisposition to nondisjunction, radiation prior to conception, and infection. Studies support the concept of multiple causality.

The cytogenetics of DS are well established. Approximately 92–95% of all cases of DS are attributable to an extra chromosome 21, hence the name 'trisomy 21'. Children with trisomy 21 are born to parents of all ages, but there is a statistically greater risk to older women, particularly those over 35 years (Cuckle *et al*, 1987). However, most births overall occur at a younger maternal age; therefore, about 80% of all babies with DS are born to women under 35 years. Paternal age may account for 20–30% of trisomy 21 babies with DS. Four to six percent of the cases may be caused by translocation of chromosomes 15 and 21 or 22. This type of genetic abnormality is usually hereditary and is not associated with the age of parents. One to three percent of affected people demonstrate mosaicism, where cells have normal and abnormal chromosomes. The degree of physical and intellectual impairment is related to the ratio of normal to abnormal cells.

The mechanism by which the syndrome has occurred is significant to genetic counselling; whereas there is a low risk of recurrence of nondisjunction, translocation is more often hereditary. The following discussion will consider some general interventions a nurse may make, and provide an appreciation of the varied consequences of the genetic abnormalities of Down's syndrome. These affect both the physical and mental development of the child (Pueschel *et al*, 1987).

It is useful to consider the needs that Down's syndrome children have in two ways. The first is to ensure that health problems linked to Down's syndrome do not contribute to further developmental delay; the second is to consider appropriate education and opportunities for development (Wishart, 1993).

One of the ways a nurse can indirectly contribute to the latter is through the support that is given to the family at the time of diagnosis. Because of the characteristic facial and other physical characteristics, the infant with DS is usually diagnosed at birth. These characteristics include eyes which are usually upward and outward slanting, speckling of the iris (Brushfield spots), protruding tongue, a small round head, flat nasal bridge, mottled skin, and hypotonia. Generally, parents wish to know the diagnosis as soon as possible, and prefer to be told together; however, often their needs are not met (Quine and Pahl, 1987).

Parents' responses to the child may greatly influence decisions regarding future care, including whether they wish to take the child home with them. Any questions regarding developmental potential must be answered carefully by the nurse. Intelligence can vary from severe intellectual impairment to low normal intelligence (Sharav *et al*, 1985). There are also wide ranges in the achievement of developmental milestones. The nurse should make available any sources of assistance at this difficult time, including information about parent groups and organizations such as the Down's Syndrome Association.

Down's syndrome creates many physical problems for a child. Nurses can work closely with families to overcome these. This may involve advising on holding and handling children complicated by hypotonicity of muscles and hyperextensibility of joints. Children with DS are susceptible to upper respiratory infection which, when combined with the cardiac anomalies which affect 30–40%, are the chief cause of death (Editorial, 1990). Nurses can help parents with preventive measures.

FRAGILE X SYNDROME

Within the last two decades, fragile X syndrome has been identified as the most common inherited cause of learning disabilities, affecting approximately one in 1000 people. It is the second most common chromosomal cause of learning disabilities after Down's syndrome. Unlike Down's syndrome, it does not include obvious physical features. Diagnosis is not always made, therefore, and it is suggested that the true incidence of this syndrome remains unclear. Its name is taken from the 'fragile' appearance of the region on the lower end of the long arm of the X chromosome, which appears as an abnormal gap when magnified under a microscope.

The genetics of fragile X are unusual and do not reflect the classic X-linked recessive pattern. It affects mostly males, but also females, and both may be carriers. Although the syndrome generally manifests itself in a wide range of learning disabilities and behaviours, mental development is more obviously affected in males than in females. Some of the problems experienced by people with fragile X syndrome have little impact upon their lives. Others may lead to the complex needs that severe learning disabilities bring.

One particularly obvious way in which the syndrome may manifest is in the speech and language of affected people. It seems that understanding of words may be underestimated as a consequence of abnormalities of speech. These include skipping from subject to subject, pausing in conversation inappropriately, and repetition of words and phrases (Barnicoat *et al*, 1992). Similarly, particular cognitive difficulties, for example with numbers, may hinder overall intellectual development.

Children with fragile X are also likely to develop specific behavioural problems which present as an overall picture of hyperactivity. They may also have significant difficulties relating to other people, and may appear to have the condition known as autism.

It is also possible to identify some physical features which are associated specifically with the syndrome, including particular facial features, tendency towards shortsightedness, and 'glue ear'. Epilepsy is also commonly found in association with fragile X.

The possibility of extensive screening of the population has been made more likely with the identification, in 1991, of the molecular basis of the condition. As knowledge of the condition continues to develop and to disseminate among professionals, nurses will increasingly be involved in its diagnosis and will be able to offer specific interventions pertinent to the needs of children and adults with fragile X syndrome. The Fragile X Society is committed to this process.

KEY POINTS

◆ One in 50 people in the United Kingdom has some kind of learning disability. This term reflects intellectual impairment and associated difficulties in acquiring skills of independent living, which originate in childhood.

◆ Diagnosis of intellectual impairment is confirmed in several ways, including the use of IQ tests, and enables some degree of disability to be established. It often confirms parental and professional concerns over developmental delay.

◆ Learning disabilities can be caused by single or multiple factors. Mild learning disabilities fail to receive diagnosis more often than severe learning disabilities.

◆ Preventative strategies not only aim to reduce the incidences of learning disabilities but also the consequences of coexisting problems.

◆ Early diagnosis and intervention can enable a child's potential for development to be maximized.

◆ Nurses can help a child achieve independence in self-help skills ,such as feeding and dressing, and significantly improve the family's ability to cope.

◆ Integration is a lifelong process and nurses can increase opportunities for a child with learning disabilities to participate in ordinary experiences.

◆ A child with learning disabilities and their family may have additional needs when accessing ordinary services.

◆ Communication between the different agencies and professionals involved in providing services for children with learning disabilities is essential for effective care.

◆ Nursing practice is informed by ongoing research which identifies the causes and particular needs of people with learning disabilities. Fragile X syndrome has recently been identified as a major cause of learning disabilities.

REFERENCES

Ayer S, Alaszewski A: *Community care and the mentally handicapped: services for mothers and their mentally handicapped children*, London, 1986, Croom Helm.

Barnicoat A *et al.*: *Fragile X syndrome: an introduction*, Hastings, 1992, Fragile X Society.

Brigden P, Todd M: Behavioural approaches. In Todd M, Gilbert T, editors: *Learning disabilities — practice issues in health settings*, London, 1995, Routledge.

Bryne EA, Cunningham CC: The effects of mentally handicapped children on families — a conceptua review, *J Child Psychol Psychiatr* 36(6):847, 1985.

Chamberlain A *et al*: Issues in fertility control for mentally retarded female adolescents: (1) sexual activity, sexual abuse, and contraception, *Pediatrics* 73(4):445, 1984.

Committee on Child Health Services: *Fit for the future (Cmnd 6)*, London, 1976, HMSO.

Craft A, Hitching M: Keeping safe: sex education and assertiveness skills. In Brown H, Craft A, editors: *Thinking the unthinkable*, London, 1989, FPA Education Unit.

Cuckle HS, Wald NJ, Thompson SG: Estimating a woman's risk of having a pregnancy associated with Down's syndrome using her age and serum alpha fetoprotein level, *Br J Obstetr Gynaecol* 94:387, 1987.

Department of Health: *Learning disabilities*, Heywood, 1994, NHSME Health Publications Unit.

Department of Health: *Targeting practice: the contribution of nurses, midwives and health visitors*, Heywood, 1993, NHSME Health Publications Unit.

Department of Health and Human Services, Welsh Office: *Better services for the mentally handicapped (Cmnd 4683)*, London, 1971, HMSO.

Eayrs CB, Ellis N, Jones RSP: Which label? An investigation into the effects of terminology on public perceptions of and attitudes towards people with learning difficulties, *Disability Handicap Society* 8(2):114, 1993.

Editorial: Declining mortality from Down's syndrome — no cause for complacency, *Lancet* 335(8694):888, 1990.

Farmer R, Rohde J, Sacks B: *Changing services for people with learning disabilities*, London, 1993, Chapman & Hall.

Hall DMB: *The child with a handicap*, Boston, 1984, Blackwell Scientific.

Hogg J, Raynes NV, editors: *Assessment in mental handicap*, London, 1988, Croom Helm.

Lear R: *Play helps — toys and activities for children with special needs*, London, 1993, Heinemann Medical.

McConkey R: *Working with parents*, London, 1985, Croom Helm.

Middleton L: *Children first — working with children and disability*, Birmingham, 1992, Ventura Press.

Nicholson A, Alberman E: Prediction of numbers of Down's syndrome infants to be born in England and Wales up to the year 2000 and likely survival rates, *J Intellectual Disability Res* 36(6):505, 1992.

O'Brien J: A guide to life-style planning; using the activities catalog to integrate services and natural support systems. In Wilcox B, Bellamy GT, editors: *A comprehensive guide to the activities catalog: an alternative curriculum for youths and adults with severe learning difficulties*, Baltimore, 1987, Brooks.

Office of Home Economics (OHE/Mencap): *Mental handicap — partnership in the community?*, London, 1986, OHE.

Pueschel SM *et al*, editors: *New perspectives on Down's syndrome*, Baltimore, 1987, Paul H Brookes.

Quine L, Pahl J: First diagnosis of severe handicap — a study of parental reactions, *Devel Med Child Neurol* 29:232, 1987.

Sharav T, Collins R, Shlomo L: Effect of maternal education on prognosis of development in children with Down syndrome, *Pediatr* 76(3):387, 1985.

Smith GF, Berg JM: *Down's anomaly*, Edinburgh, 1976, Churchill Livingstone.

Spitz HH: Preventing and curing mental retardation by behavioural intervention — an evaluation of some claims, *Intelligence* 10:197, 1986.

Tymchuk A, Andron L: Rationale, approaches, results and resource implications of programmes to enhance parenting skills of people with learning disabilities. In Craft A, editor: *Sexuality and learning disabilities*, London, 1994, Routledge.

Wishart J: Education and training. In Fraser WI *et al*: *Hallas caring for people with mental handicaps*, Oxford, 1992, Butterworth Heinemann.

Wishart JG: The development of learning difficulties in children with Down's syndrome, *J Intellectual Disability Res* 37(4):389, 1993.

Wolfensberger W: *Normalisation: the principle of normalisation in human services*, Toronto, 1972, National Institute of Mental Retardation.

WHO (World Health Organization): *Organization of services for the mentally retarded —fifteenth report of the WHO Expert Committee on Mental Health*, Geneva, 1968, WHO Technical Report Series 392.

Yule W, Carr J: *Problem behaviour in people with severe learning disabilities: a practical guide to a constructional approach*, London, 1988, Croom Helm.

FURTHER READING

Ayer S, Alaszewski A: *Community care and the mentally handicapped: services for mothers and their mentally handicapped children*, London, 1986, Croom Helm.

Chasty H, Friel J: *Children with special needs, assessment, law and practice — caught in the act*, London, 1991, Jessica Kingsley.

Craft A, editor: *Practice issues in sexuality and learning disabilities*, London, 1994, Routledge.

Cunningham C: *Down's syndrome — an introduction for parents*, London, 1988, Souvenir Press.

Dykens EM, Hodapp RM, Leckman JF: *Behaviour and development in Fragile X syndrome*, London, 1993, Sage.

Hornby G: *Counselling in child disability, skills for working with parents*, London, 1994, Chapman & Hall.

Lear R: *Play helps: toys and activities for children with special needs*, London, 1993, Heinemann Medical.

Lindsay G, editor: *Screening for children with special needs, multidisciplinary approaches*, London, 1984, Croom Helm.

McCormack M: *Special children, special needs: families talk about mental handicap*, London, 1992, Thorsons.

Royal College of Nursing: *Nursing intervention for people with a mental handicap — a role model and framework*, Middlesex, 1988, Scutari.

Serfontein G: *The hidden handicap*, Sydney, 1994, Simon & Schuster.

Shanley E, Starrs TA, editors: *Learning disabilities, a handbook of care*, London, 1994, Churchill Livingstone.

Stow L, Selfe L: *Understanding children with special needs*, London, 1989, Unwin Hyman.

Yule W, Carr J: *Behaviour modification for people with mental handicap*, London, 1980, Croom Helm.

USEFUL ADDRESS

Fragile X Society, 53 Winchelsea Lane, Hastings, East Sussex, TN35 4LG.

Unit Four

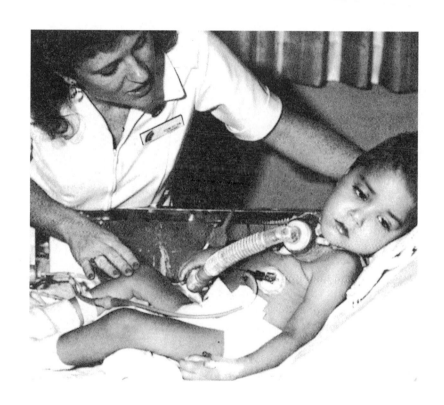

The Child with Dysfunction

Chapter 23

The Child with Sensory or Communication Impairment

LEARNING OUTCOMES

After studying this chapter you should be able to:

◆ Identify different types of sensory impairment.

◆ Discuss the problems associated with sensory and communication impairment.

◆ State the common causes of sensory impairment.

◆ Describe ways in which children with sensory or communication impairment, and their families, can be supported.

◆ Define the glossary terms.

GLOSSARY

agnosia Inability to interpret sound correctly

amblyopia Reduced visual acuity in one eye, despite appropriate optical correction, in the absence of any pathological defect

anisometropia Difference of refractive strength in each eye

aphasia Inability to express ideas in any form, either written or verbal

astigmatism Unequal curvatures in the cornea or lens

BSL British Sign Language

central auditory imperception Hearing loss that is not caused by defects in the conductive or sensorineural structures

conductive hearing loss Loss from interference of transmission of sound to the middle ear

ELM Early Language Milestone Scale

emmetropia A normal eye that does not require spectacle correction to focus correctly

light perception Vision limited to recognizing shades of light

mixed conductive-sensorineural hearing loss Loss from interference with transmission of sound in the middle ear and along neural pathways

myopia Nearsightedness; ability to see objects clearly at close range, but not at a distance

sensorineural hearing loss Nerve deafness from damage to the inner ear structures and/or the auditory nerve

tinnitus Ringing in the ears

Sensory impairments pose special threats to a child's developmental potential. Deprived of visual or auditory cues, the child must rely more heavily on other sensory experiences to learn about and relate to the environment. The child with a communication disorder may function well during early childhood, but be unable to achieve in an academic setting. Without assistance and rehabilitation, these children are vulnerable to the lifelong disadvantages of being an individual with a disability (Henderson, Barnett and Henderson, 1994).

Parents are the major rehabilitators of the child. However, they need guidance and support from specially trained professionals to help the child learn. The nurse is often in a strategic position to prevent and identify sensory or communication disorders, to support the family in adjusting to the disorder, and to assist them in learning methods of overcoming or compensating for the impairment. This chapter is primarily concerned with prevention, identification and rehabilitation.

HEARING IMPAIRMENT

Hearing impairment is a common problem in the United Kingdom. Approximately 1-2 in 1000 children have significant permanent sensorineural loss and will require specialist support. Temporary conductive hearing loss effects about 20% of children (Webster and Wood, 1991).

DEFINITION AND CLASSIFICATION

Several definitions exist regarding categories of hearing impairment, including terms such as *deaf and dumb*, *mute*, or *deaf mute*. However, these terms are unacceptable; hearing-impaired persons are not dumb and, if mute, have no physical speech defect other than that caused by the inability to hear.

Hearing defects may also be classified according to aetiology, pathology or symptom severity. Each is important in terms of treatment, possible prevention, and rehabilitation.

AETIOLOGY

Hearing loss may be caused by various antenatal and postnatal conditions. These include a family history of childhood hearing impairment, anatomical malformations of the head or neck, low birth weight, severe perinatal asphyxia, perinatal infection (cytomegalovirus, rubella, herpes, syphilis, toxoplasmosis, bacterial meningitis), chronic ear infection, cerebral palsy, Down's syndrome, or administration of ototoxic drugs.

In addition, high-risk neonates surviving formerly fatal antenatal or perinatal conditions may be susceptible to hearing loss from the disorder or its treatment. For example, sensorineural hearing loss may be the result of continuous humming noises or high noise levels associated with incubators, oxygen hoods, or intensive care units, especially when combined with the use of potentially ototoxic antibiotics.

In very-low-birth-weight infants, risk factors for sensorineural hearing loss may include ototoxic drugs (e.g., aminoglycosides), low pH, hypoxaemia, high bilirubin levels, and poorer overall medical status (Salamy, Eldredge and Tooley, 1989).

Environmental noise is a special concern. Sounds loud enough to damage sensitive hair cells of the inner ear can produce irreversible hearing loss. Very loud, brief noise, such as gunfire, can cause immediate, severe and permanent loss of hearing. Longer exposure to less intense, but still hazardous, sounds can also produce hearing loss (Consensus Conference, 1990). In addition to hearing loss, noise can also interfere with learning, can increase stress, and can provoke aggression (Bronzaft, 1989).

The exact sound level that produces hearing loss is unknown; duration of exposure and individual susceptibility to the sound influence the degree of risk. As a general rule, sound appreciably louder than conversational speech is potentially harmful if the sound persists for a sufficient time.

PATHOLOGY

Disorders of hearing are divided according to location of the defect. *Conductive* or middle-ear hearing loss results from interference of transmission of sound to the middle ear. It is the most common of all types of hearing loss and most frequently is a result of recurrent serous otitis media. Conductive hearing impairment mainly involves interference with loudness of sound.

Sensorineural hearing loss, also called perceptive or nerve deafness, involves damage to the inner ear structures and/or the auditory nerve. The most common causes are congenital defects of inner ear structures or the consequences of acquired conditions, such as kernicterus, infection, administration of ototoxic drugs, or exposure to excessive noise. Sensorineural hearing loss results in distortion of sound and problems in discrimination. Although children hear some of everything going on around them, the sounds are distorted, severely affecting discrimination and comprehension.

Mixed conductive–sensorineural hearing loss results from interference with transmission of sound in the middle ear and along neural pathways.

Central auditory imperception includes all hearing losses that do not demonstrate defects in the conductive or sensorineural structures. They are usually divided into organic or functional losses. In the *organic type* of central auditory imperception, the defect involves the reception of auditory stimuli along the central pathways and the expression of the message into meaningful communication. Examples are *aphasia*, an inability to express ideas in any form, either written or verbal; *agnosia*, the inability to interpret sound correctly; and *dysacusis*, difficulty in processing details or discrimination among sounds.

In the *functional type*, there is no organic lesion to explain a central auditory loss. Examples of functional hearing loss are conversion hysteria (an unconscious withdrawal from hearing to block remembrance of a traumatic event), infantile autism and childhood schizophrenia.

SYMPTOM SEVERITY

For clinical purposes, hearing impairment is described according to the degree or severity of loss. Hearing is expressed in decibels (dB), which are units of loudness; it is measured at various frequencies, such as 500, 1000, and 2000 cycles per second, the critical listening speech range. Calculation of the relationship between decibels and intensity of a noise involves logarithmic formulas, the discussion of which is beyond the scope of this book. An example is that the loudness of a noise at 40 dB is 31 times that of the noise at 10 dB. The same relationship applies to the loudness of noise for any fourfold change in decibels. For example, the loudness of a noise at 160 dB is also 31 times that of a noise at 40 dB.

The term *hearing-threshold level* refers to the measurement of an individual's hearing threshold by means of an audiometer. Hearing impairment can be classified according to hearing-threshold level and the degree of symptom severity as it affects speech.

Most deaf children have some perception of loud sounds, but no usable hearing. Their primary mode of communication is visual (lipreading or sign language). Children who are hard-of-hearing use auditory cues together with visual cues to communicate.

Infancy

At birth the nurse can observe the neonate's response to auditory stimuli as evidenced by the startle reflex head turning, eye blinking, and cessation of body movement. The infant may vary in the intensity of the response, depending on the state of alertness. However, a consistent absence of a reaction should lead to suspicion of hearing loss.

THERAPEUTIC MANAGEMENT

Treatment of hearing loss depends on the cause and type of hearing impairment. Many conductive hearing defects are amenable to medical or surgical treatment, such as antibiotic therapy for acute otitis media, or insertion of tympanostomy tubes (or 'grommets') for chronic otitis media. When the conductive loss is permanent, hearing can be improved with the use of a hearing aid to amplify sound.

Treatment for sensorineural hearing loss is much less satisfactory. Since the defect is not one of intensity of sound, hearing aids are of less value in this type of defect. The use of cochlear implants (a surgically implanted prosthetic device) is providing hope for some affected children (Freeland, 1989).

Disorders of central auditory imperception depend on the cause. Functional types, such as conversion hysteria, may require psychological intervention, but others, such as autism, may not respond to any therapy.

NURSING CARE OF THE CHILD WITH HEARING IMPAIRMENT

Nursing care of hearing-impaired children is often a specialized area, requiring additional training in auditory testing and rehabilitation. However, general nursing goals that focus on assessment, prevention and rehabilitation are every nurse's responsibility. In addition, nurses may have to care for a hearing-impaired child who is hospitalized and must know how to best meet the child's and family's special needs.

ASSESSMENT

Discovery of a hearing impairment within the first 12 months of life is essential to prevent social, physical and psychological damage to the child. Assessment involves: (1) identifying children whose history places them at risk, (2) observing for behaviours that indicate a hearing loss, and (3) screening all children for hearing loss. Neonatal screening may use one of the following methods: an automated behavioural method known as the auditory responce cradle (ARC), brain stem evoked response audiometry (BSRA) or measurement of cochlear emissions (Hall, 1991). There is currently debate as to whether this screening should be universal or offered only to 'high risk' neonates.

At approximately 8 months of age infants are universally screened with a behavioural test known as the 'distraction test'. This test is usually performed by the health visitor working in collaboration with another trained person. Between the ages of 18 months and five years children may have their hearing tested using cooperation methods. One example, used for children from about the age of three is the McCormick Toy test (Mccormick, 1988). This discussion focuses on developmental/behavioural indices associated with hearing impairment.

Since hearing-impaired children rely on vision to supplement communication skills, and since many have associated visual defects, a careful assessment of ocular impairments is also needed.

Infancy

At birth the nurse can observe the neonate's response to auditory stimuli as evidenced by the startle reflex, head turning, eye blinking, and cessation of body movement. The infant may vary in the intensity of the response, depending on the state of alertness. However, a consistent absence of reaction should lead to suspicion of hearing loss. Other clinical manifestations of hearing impairment in the infant are summarized in the box on p.

Childhood

The profoundly deaf child is much more likely to be diagnosed during infancy than is a less severely affected child. If the defect is not detected during early childhood, it probably will surface during entry to school, when the child has difficulty in learning. Unfortunately, some of these children are erroneously placed in special classes for students with learning disabilities.

Of primary importance is the effect of hearing impairment on speech development. A child with a mild conductive hearing loss may speak fairly clearly, but in a loud, monotone voice. A child with a sensorineural defect usually has difficulty in articulation. For example, inability to hear higher frequencies may result in the word *spoon* being pronounced *poon*. Children with articulation problems need to have their hearing tested (Kramer and Williams, 1993).

Once the goals are identified, specific interventions are carried out. The following discussion presents general interventions for most children with hearing impairment. Modifications are needed in specific situations, particularly if other physical or mental disabilities coexist.

Promote the communication process

The nurse's initial role in rehabilitation is to encourage the family to participate in an auditory training programme. Rehabilitation training consists of using a hearing aid and learning lipreading, sign language and verbal communication.

Hearing aids

The nurse should be familiar with the types, basic care, and handling of hearing aids, especially when the child is hospitalized. Types of aids include those worn in or behind the ear, models incorporated into an eyeglass frame, or types worn on the body with a wire connection to the ear.

Another option for sound amplification is the radio frequency (FM) system, which combines binaural ear-level instruments with an additional receiver worn on the child's body and an FM transmitter used by the speaker. With this system, the speaker can talk directly into the transmitter from a greater distance, and the background noise is minimized. When the FM transmitter is turned off, the device functions as a standard hearing aid (Roush, 1990).

One of the most common problems with a hearing aid, especially an ear-level device, is acoustic feedback, an annoying whistling sound usually caused by improper fit of the ear mould. Sometimes the whistling may be at a frequency that the child cannot hear, but that is annoying to others. In this case, if children are old enough, they are told of the noise and asked to readjust the aid.

As children grow older, they may be self-conscious about the device. Every effort is made to make the aid inconspicuous, such as an appropriate hairstyle to cover behind-the-ear or in-the-ear models, attractive frames for glasses, and placement of the on-the-body type where it is not seen, such as under a blouse or sweater. Children are given responsibility for the care of the device as soon as they are able, since fostering independence is a primary goal of rehabilitation.

Lipreading

Even though the child may become expert at lipreading, only about 40% of the spoken word is understood, and less if the speaker has an accent, moustache or beard. Exaggerating pronunciation or speaking in an altered rhythm further lessens comprehension. The child learns to supplement the spoken word with sensitivity to visual cues - primarily body language and facial expression.

Sign language

Sign language, such as the British Sign Language (BSL) or American Sign Language (ASL), is a visual-gestural language that uses hand signals which roughly correspond to specific words and concepts in the English language. Family members are encouraged to learn signing, because using or watching hands requires much less concentration than lipreading or talking. Also, a symbol method enables some deaf children to learn more and to learn faster.

Speech therapy

The most formidable task in the education of a deaf child is learning to speak. Speech is learned through a multisensory approach, using visual, tactile, kinaesthetic, and auditory stimulation. Since the usual mechanism for learning language (imitation and reinforcement) is not available to the deaf child, systematic formal education is required. Parents are encouraged to participate fully in the learning process.

Additional aids

Everyday activities present problems to the older child. For example, the child may not be able to hear the telephone, doorbell or alarm clock. Several commercial devices are available to help the deaf person adjust to these dilemmas. Special teletypewriters (TTY) or telecommunications devices for the deaf (TDD) help deaf people communicate with each other over the telephone; the typed message is conveyed via the telephone lines and displayed on a small screen.

As deaf children learn to compensate for their lack of hearing, they become extremely perceptive to visual and vibratory changes. They often know when another person wishes to talk to them because the person will walk close by, but not pass. They learn to be alert to other people approaching them, by seeing their shadows or feeling the vibrations of their footsteps. They are acutely aware of facial expressions and may comprehend the unspoken word more quickly than the spoken word.

Socialization

Since socialization is extremely important to the child's development, the nurse should discuss with the family methods of fostering social contact. If children attend a special school for the deaf, they are able to socialize with peers in that setting. Classmates become a potential source of close friendships because they communicate more easily among themselves. Parents are encouraged to promote these relationships whenever possible.

Children with a hearing impairment may need special help in school or social activities. For children who wear hearing aids, background noise should be kept to a minimum. Since many of these children are able to attend regular classes, the teacher may need assistance in adapting methods of teaching for the child's benefit. Since group projects and audiovisual teaching aids may hinder the deaf child's learning, these educational methods should be carefully evaluated.

Support the family

Once the diagnosis of hearing impairment is made, parents need extensive support to adjust to the shock of learning about their child's disability. This may be the first time they learn that the child's poor speech development and behaviour problems are the result of a hearing deficit, not because of difficulty with the tongue, refusal to talk, or disobedience. Parents may need time to deal with guilt feelings over previous attempts to teach the child to talk or past punishment for the child's misbehaviour.

Parents also need an opportunity to realize the extent of the hearing loss. Sometimes, parents benefit from a demonstration of what it is like to be deaf or hard-of-hearing. For example, showing them a moving film without sound helps them appreciate the profound effect of living in a world devoid of hearing and the great difficulty in comprehending the spoken word. If the child has a selective hearing loss, the parents can better understand the distortion of sound and difficulty with discrimination if they are placed in a soundproof room and allowed to hear only the frequencies the child hears. Central auditory imperception is similar to hearing a foreign language with no understanding of the meaning of the words. The parents gradually need to adjust to the idea that the child's major obstacle will be the development and use of language. The parents may benefit from being told that, with appropriate teaching, the child can learn receptive language skills. This step will precede attempts to use expressive language, because children need to know and understand what is being communicated to them before they can be expected to communicate expressively to others.

After the parents have been able to assimilate the magnitude of their child's loss, they may benefit from encouragement and support to set realistic goals for themselves and for their child. A hearing-impaired child's education cannot wait until the child is 4-5 years old. It must begin as early as possible and be continued in the home, where the parents play a significant role in teaching and reinforcing language skills.

Parents need to know how impaired hearing affects a child's normal development. For example, infants with a hearing loss, especially in the moderate or greater range, are unaware of parental verbal cues. Consequently, they are less likely to demonstrate the same degree of reciprocity in relating to the parents as a hearing child. However, they do acknowledge significant others by looking at them, nestling in their arms during holding, or quieting when their needs are met. These behaviours are stressed to help parents establish meaningful contact with the infant. Although the child is unable to hear, parents are encouraged to talk as they would to a hearing child, supplement stimulation needs with visual and tactile cues, and relate in the face-to-face position to help the child learn facial expressions.

Care for the child during hospitalization

The needs of hospitalized deaf children are the same as those of other hospitalized children, but the disability presents special challenges to the nurse. For example, verbal explanations as the primary method of preparation for admission or procedures must be supplemented with tactile and visual aids, such as books or actual demonstration and practice. When written materials are used, the reading level must be appropriate for the child. Although the acquired reading skill depends on the child's age and individual abilities, the average reading comprehension of deaf adults is often at a reduced level because sign language, not English, is their primary language.

Children's understanding of the explanation needs to be constantly reassessed. If their verbal skills are poorly developed, they can answer questions through drawing, writing or gesturing. When explaining procedures or conditions related to the body, the nurse needs to be very specific. Deaf children's perception of internal body parts is less clearly developed than hearing children's perception (Gibbons, 1985). For example, if the nurse is attempting to clarify where a lumbar puncture is done, the child is asked to point to where the needle is placed. Since deaf children often need more time to grasp the full meaning of an explanation, the nurse must be careful not to judge the slowness as a sign of a learning disability, and must allow ample time for the child to understand.

When communicating with the child, the nurse should use the same principles as those outlined for facilitating lipreading. The child's hearing aid is checked to ensure that it is working properly. The nurse always makes sure the child can see him or her before any procedures are performed, even routine ones such as changing a nappy or regulating an infusion. It is important to remember that the child may not be aware of one's presence until alerted through visual or tactile cues.

Ideally, parents are encouraged to remain with the child. Although the parents' aid can be enlisted in familiarizing the child with the hospital and explaining procedures, the nurse also talks directly to the child. Parents often can be helpful by explaining the child's usual speech habits/pronunciation.

Nonvocal communication devices that employ pictures or words that the child can point to are also available. Such boards can also be made up by drawing pictures or writing the words of common needs on cardboard, such as parent, food, water, or toilet.

The nurse has a special role as child advocate with deaf children and is in a strategic position to alert other health team members and other patients to the child's special needs regarding communication. Caregivers sometimes forget that the child has the ability to perceive and learn, despite a hearing loss, and consequently communicate only with the parents. As a result, the child's needs and feelings remain unrecognized and unmet.

Since deaf children often have difficulty forming social relationships with other children, the child is introduced to roommates and encouraged to engage in play activities. The hospital setting can provide growth-promoting opportunities for social relationships. With the assistance of a play specialist, the child can learn new recreational activities, experiment with group games, and engage in therapeutic play.

Measures to prevent hearing impairment

A primary nursing role is prevention of hearing loss. Since the most common cause of impaired hearing is chronic otitis media, it is essential that appropriate measures be instituted to treat existing infections and to prevent recurrences. Children with histories of ear or respiratory infections, or any other condition known to increase the risk of hearing impairment, should receive periodic auditory testing.

To prevent the causes of hearing loss that begin antenatally and perinatally, pregnant women need counselling regarding the necessity of early antenatal care, including genetic counselling for known familial disorders; avoidance of all ototoxic drugs, especially during the first trimester; tests to rule out syphilis, rubella, or blood incompatibility; medical management of maternal diabetes; control of alcoholism; and adequate dietary intake. During childhood, the necessity of routine immunization to eliminate the possibility of acquired sensorineural loss from rubella, mumps and measles (encephalitis) is stressed.

Exposure to excessive noise pollution is a well-established cause of sensorineural hearing loss. The nurse should routinely assess the possibility of environmental noise pollution, and advise children and parents of the potential danger. When individuals engage in activities associated with high-intensity noise, such as flying model aeroplanes, or target shooting, they should wear ear protection such as earmuffs or earplugs (not ordinary dry cotton). Even common household equipment can be hazardous, such as lawn mowers, power vacuum cleaners, and cordless telephones. The nurse should also be aware of potential problems in old buildings and noise which may occur with the transfer of patients, such as neonates in incubators (reference).

The effectiveness of nursing interventions for hearing impairment is determined by continual reassessment and evaluation of care. The following guidelines may be used:

1. Observe the techniques used to communicate with the child. Inquire if child is enrolled in an auditory training programme. Inquire about socialization opportunities for the child (i.e., who are child's friends, what are child's extracurricular activities).
2. Interview the family regarding their adjustment to the sensory impairment. Observe the family members' relationships with the child. Interview the child regarding feelings about the sensory impairment and its effect on activities of daily living (especially important if a recent impairment).
3. Observe types of preparation/communication used to prepare the child for hospitalization or procedures. Observe parents' involvement in child's care. Observe interaction of child and family with other patients.
4. Investigate community programmes aimed at preventing or detecting hearing loss and inquire about nursing involvement in these efforts.

VISION IMPAIRMENT

Visual impairment is a common problem during childhood. An estimated 21,000 children in the United Kingdom have some degree of visual impairment, even with corrective glasses. Of this group, 21% are registered as blind and 15% are registered as partially sighted; the remainder have varying degrees of visual impairment (Royal National Institute for the Blind, 1992). In some instances, a child may not be placed on the blind or partially sighted register, even though he or she may be eligible. A study by the Royal National Institute for the Blind (1992) suggested at least 10% of visually impaired children are not on either register, although their degree of impairment suggested they would be eligible for registration. In deciding when to place a child on the blind or partially sighted registers, consideration is given to how the child will benefit from this act, and whether there is any chance of vision improving. Fear of labelling may also contribute to the reluctance to place a child on the register.

DEFINITION AND CLASSIFICATION

Vision impairment is a general term referring to visual loss that cannot be corrected with regular prescriptive lenses. However, a more useful system for classifying visual impairments is based on the type of activity in which the child can be expected to engage, which may include the following categories (Helveston and Ellis, 1984):

- **Partially sighted** — visual acuity between 30/60 and 6/60. The child should be able to obtain an education in the usual school system with the use of normal-sized print. Near vision is almost always better than distance vision.
- **Registered blind** — visual acuity of 3/60 or less and/or a visual field of 20 degrees or less in the better eye. This is useful only as a legal definition, not as a medical diagnosis. It allows special consideration with regard to benefits provision.
- **Navigational vision** — visual acuity enabling counting of fingers only. This vision allows the child to travel in unfamiliar surroundings provided the child is otherwise healthy. The use of print may be possible, but difficult. Learning braille may be required.
- **Light perception** — this is primarily important for the child's sense of well-being and may be an aid in mobility, but it is not useful for other educational purposes.

AETIOLOGY

The aetiology of visual impairment can be classified according

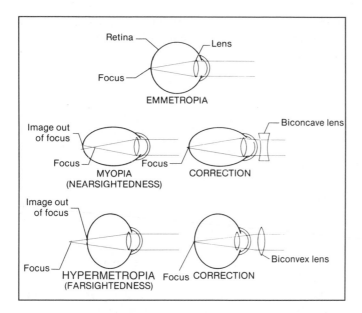

Fig. 23-1 Comparison of normal vision and refractive errors. Emmetropia (normal vision); myopia (nearsightedness); hypermetropia (farsightedness).

to several divisions. In addition, diseases such as cataracts, optic atrophy, or glaucoma may cause visual defects. Factors causing vision impairment include:

- **Familial factors** — genetic diseases associated with visual defects, such as Tay-Sachs disease, albinism, galactosaemia or retinoblastoma.
- **Antenatal/intrauterine factors** — especially maternal infections, such as rubella, syphilis, herpes simplex or toxoplasmosis.
- **Perinatal factors** — prematurity, maternal infection (ophthalmia neonatorum), and oxygen toxicity (retinopathy of prematurity).
- **Postnatal factors** — primarily trauma, infections (mumps, measles, rubella, poliomyelitis, chickenpox), and disorders such as juvenile rheumatoid arthritis, leukaemia and myasthenia gravis.

Refractive errors are the most common types of visual disorders in children. The term refraction means bending and refers to the bending of light rays as they pass through the different structures of the eye. Normally, light rays entering the eye focus on the retina (*emmetropia*). However, in refractive disorders the light rays either fall in front of the retina (*myopia*) or beyond it (*hypermetropia*) (Fig. 23-1). Other eye problems, such as strabismus, may or may not include refractive errors but are important because, if untreated, they may result in blindness from amblyopia.

Amblyopia, or 'lazy eye', is a reduced visual acuity in one eye despite appropriate optical correction. It can occur in the absence of any pathological defect in the affected eye. Misplaced, blurred or absent retinal images during early childhood cause loss of vision in the visually deprived eye. It does not occur after 9 years of age, when the retinal system is mature.

The most common types of amblyopia are secondary to strabismus and to unequal refractive errors *(anisometropia)*. Other causes include cataracts, corneal opacities, or prolonged occlusion of one or both eyes (a condition that can occur from prolonged therapeutic patching for strabismus) (Friendly, 1987).

Trauma is a common cause of blindness in children. The most common sources are balls, fists and sticks. Injuries to the eyeball and adnexa (supporting or accessory structures; e.g., eyelids, conjunctiva, lacrimal glands) can be classified as penetrating or nonpenetrating. In penetrating wounds, the globe is perforated, while in nonpenetrating it is not. Damage to structures within the eye can occur in either type of injury. Although most instances of eye trauma are unintentional, the possibility of child abuse should be considered, especially when marked facial trauma, bilateral corneal abrasions, unexplained hyphaemas, and cigarette burns are present (Frey, 1983).

THERAPEUTIC MANAGEMENT

Treatment of eye disorders depends on the specific problem. In all instances the goal is preservation of vision. Treatment in early childhood is necessary to prevent vision loss from amblyopia, especially resulting from strabismus; treatment must be instituted as soon as possible after serious trauma.

Treatment of strabismus may involve surgery of affected muscles, prescription lenses to correct refractive errors, and occlusion therapy. Occlusion therapy is a common procedure and involves patching the stronger eye to increase the visual stimulation to the weaker eye, to prevent amblyopia.

Treatment of ocular injury involves adequate examination of the injured eye (with the child sedated or anaesthetized in severe injuries), and appropriate immediate emergency treatment. Prognosis varies according to the type of injury. It is usually guarded in all cases of penetrating wounds, because of the high risk of serious complications, especially retinal detachment, panophthalmitis (infection of uvea, retina, vitreous body, and sclera), and sympathetic ophthalmia (autoimmune disease of the uveal tract occurring in the uninjured eye). Treatment of infections is usually with topical antibiotics. Severe infections may require systemic antibiotic therapy. Steroids are used cautiously, because they exacerbate viral infections such as herpes simplex, increasing the risk of damage to the involved structures.

NURSING CARE OF THE CHILD WITH VISION IMPAIRMENT

Nursing care of visually impaired children is often a specialized area, requiring additional training in vision testing and rehabilitation. However, general nursing goals that focus on assessment, prevention, and rehabilitation are every nurse's responsibility. In addition, nurses may have to care for a vision-impaired child who is hospitalized, and must know how best to meet the child's and family's special needs.

ASSESSMENT

Assessment of children for vision impairment is a critical nursing responsibility. Early discovery of a vision impairment is essential to prevent social, physical and psychological damage to the child. Assessment involves: (1) identifying children whose history places them at risk, (2) observing for behaviours that indicate a vision loss, and (3) screening all children for visual acuity and signs of other ocular disorders, such as strabismus.

Infancy

Of special importance in detecting visual impairment during infancy are the parents' concerns regarding visual responsiveness in their child. Their concerns must be taken seriously, such as lack of eye-to-eye contact from the infant. Lack of binocularity after four months of age is considered to be abnormal and must be treated to prevent amblyopia.

Childhood

Since the most common visual impairments during childhood are refractive errors, testing for visual acuity is essential (Walker, Tobin and McKennell, 1992). The school nurse usually assumes major responsibility for vision testing in school children. Besides refractive errors, the nurse should be aware of signs and symptoms that indicate other ocular problems.

Support the child and family

The shock of learning that their child is blind or partially sighted is an immense crisis for the family. Of all types of disabilities, many people fear loss of sight the most. Vision is involved in almost every activity of daily living. Parents need support during the initial phase of learning about the diagnosis and need help to gain a realistic understanding of their child's abilities. The family is encouraged to investigate appropriate stimulation and educational programmes for their child as soon as possible. Sources of information include the Royal National Institute for the Blind, the Association of Blind and Partially Sighted Teachers and Students, National Association for the Education of the Partially Sighted, and the Partially Sighted Society.

When blindness is not congenital, but acquired, newly blind children need much support to help them adjust to the disability (Conyers, 1992). They are usually frightened and confused by the sudden or progressive loss of sight, and benefit from an environment that provides security and familiarity.

Promote parent-child attachment

A crucial time in the life of blind infants is when they and their parents are getting acquainted with each other. Pleasurable patterns of interaction between the infant and parents may be lacking if there is not enough reciprocity. For example, if the parent gazes fondly at the infant's face and seeks eye contact, but the infant fails to respond because he or she cannot see the parent, a troubled cycle of responses may occur. The nurse can help parents learn to look for other cues that indicate the infant is responding to them, such as whether the eyelids blink; whether the activity level accelerates or slows; whether respiratory patterns change, such as faster or slower breathing when they come near; and whether the infant makes throaty sounds when they speak to the infant. With time, parents learn that the infant has unique ways of relating to them. They are encouraged to show affection using nonvisual methods, such as talking or reading, cuddling, and walking the child.

Promote the child's optimum development

Promoting the child's optimum development requires rehabilitation in several important areas. These include learning self-help skills and appropriate communication techniques to become independent. Although nurses may not be directly involved in such programmes, they can provide direction and guidance to families regarding the availability of programmes and the need to promote these activities in their child.

Development and independence

Motor development is almost as dependent on sight as verbal communication is on hearing. From earliest infancy, parents are encouraged to expose infants to as many visual-motor experiences as possible, such as sitting supported in an infant seat or swing, and being given opportunities for holding up the head, sitting unsupported, reaching for objects and crawling.

Despite visual impairment, children can become independent in all aspects of self-care. The same principles used for promoting independence in sighted children apply, with additional emphasis on nonvisual cues.

Play and socialization

Blind children do not learn to play automatically, because they cannot imitate others or actively explore the environment as sighted children do. They depend much more on others to stimulate and teach them how to play. Parents need help in selecting appropriate play materials, especially those that encourage fine and gross motor development and stimulate the senses of hearing, touch and smell. Toys with educational value are especially useful, such as dolls with various clothing closures.

Blind children have the same needs for socialization as sighted children. Since they have little difficulty learning verbal skills, they are able to communicate with age-mates and participate in suitable activities. The nurse discusses with parents opportunities for socialization outside of the home, especially regular nursery schools. The trend is to include these children with sighted children, to help them adjust to the outside world for eventual independence.

To compensate for inadequate stimulation, these children may develop blindisms, such as body rocking, finger flicking, or arm twirling. Such habits retard the child's social acceptance and should be discouraged. Behaviour modification is often successful in reducing or eliminating blindisms.

Education

The main obstacle to learning in blind children is their total dependence on nonvisual cues. Although they can learn via verbal lecturing, they are unable to read the written word or to write without special education. Therefore they must rely on braille, a system that uses raised dots to represent letters and numbers. The child can then read the braille with the fingers and can write a message using a braille writer. However, unless others read braille, this is not useful for communicating with them. A more portable system for written communication is the use of a braille slate and stylus or a microcassette tape recorder. A recorder is especially helpful for leaving messages for others and for taking notes during classroom lectures. Both the braille slate and stylus, and the tape recorder are as important to a blind person as paper and pencil are to a sighted individual. For mathematical calculations, portable calculators with voice synthesizers are available.

Braille is a complex language and is difficult to learn. This may be a particular problem for children of a lesser ability and those with learning disabilities. The moon language provides one alternative. It is simpler, but is less flexible and occupies more space than Braille. It is developments in computer technology which have really made a difference for the visually impaired (BBC, 1994). Text on computer screens can easily be enlarged to make it more readable, or add-on devices can be used to convert text to speech. Future developments in computer technology, such as speech recognition (Green, 1995), will bring with them increasing benefits for the visually impaired.

Records and tapes are significant sources of reading material, other than Braille books, which are large and cumbersome. The British Talking Book Service for the Blind has a wide range of talking books available on cassette. There is a small subscription fee, but postage of cassettes is free under the articles for the blind scheme. Recorded books are also available from most public libraries.

Learning to use a standard typewriter is another form of writing, but has the disadvantage of the blind person being unable to check the accuracy of the typing. Recent developments with computers have eliminated this drawback. A home computer with a voice synthesizer can be adapted to speak each letter or word that has been typed.

The partially sighted child benefits from specialized visual aids, which produce a magnified retinal image. The basic devices are accommodation, such as bringing the object closer, special plus lenses, hand-held and stand magnifiers, telescopes, video projection systems, and large print. Special equipment is available to enlarge print. Information about services for the partially sighted is available from the Royal National Institute for the Blind. Children with diminished vision often prefer to do close work without their glasses and compensate by bringing the object very near to their eyes. This should be allowed. The exception is the child with vision in only one eye, who should always wear glasses for protection.

Care for the child during hospitalization

Because nurses are more likely to care for children who are hospitalized for procedures that involve temporary loss of vision than for children who are blind, the following discussion concentrates primarily on the needs of such children. The nursing care objectives in either situation are to: (1) reassure the child and family throughout every phase of treatment, (2) orient the child to his or her surroundings, (3) provide a safe environment, and (4) encourage independence. Whenever possible, the same nurse should care for the child to ensure consistency in the approach. These same principles also apply to a blind child who requires hospitalization.

When sighted children temporarily lose their vision, almost every aspect of the environment becomes bewildering and frightening. Nurses have a major role in minimizing the effects of temporary loss of vision. They need to talk to the child about everything that is occurring, emphasizing aspects of procedures that are felt or heard. They should approach the child by always identifying themselves as soon as they enter the room. Since unfamiliar sounds are especially frightening, these are explained. Parents are encouraged to stay overnight with their child and participate in the care. Familiar objects, such as a teddy bear or doll, should be brought from home to help lessen the strangeness of the hospital. As soon as the child is able to be out of bed, he or she is oriented to the immediate surroundings. If the child is able to see on admission, this opportunity is taken to point out significant aspects of the room. The child is encouraged to practise ambulating with his or her eyes closed, to become accustomed to this experience.

The room is arranged with safety in mind. For example, a stool or chair is placed next to the bed to help the child climb in and out of bed. The furniture is always placed in the same position to prevent collisions. Domestic staff are reminded of the need to keep the room in order. If the child has difficulty navigating by feeling the walls, a rope can be attached from the bed to the point of destination, such as the bathroom. Attention to details such as well-fitting slippers or robes that do not hang on the floor is important in preventing tripping. Unlike the child who is blind, these children are not familiar with navigating with a cane.

The child is encouraged to be independent in self-care activities, especially if the visual loss may be prolonged or potentially permanent. For example, during bathing the nurse sets up all the equipment and encourages the child to participate. At mealtime the nurse explains where each food item is on the tray, opens any special containers, prepares cereal or toast, but encourages the child in self-feeding. Favourite finger foods, such as sandwiches, hamburgers, hot dogs or pizza, may be good selections. The child is praised for efforts at being cooperative and independent. Any improvements made in self-care, no matter how small, are stressed.

Appropriate recreational activities are provided, and if a play specialist is available, such planning is done jointly. Since children with temporary blindness have a wide variety of play experiences to draw on, they are encouraged to select activities. They should have familiar toys from home to play with, since familiar items are more easily manipulated than new ones.

If parents wish to bring presents, they should be objects that stimulate hearing and touch, such as a radio, music box, or stuffed animal.

Occasionally, children who are blind come to the hospital for procedures to restore their vision. Although this is an extremely happy time, it also requires intervention to help them adjust to sight. They need an opportunity to take in all that they see. They should not be bombarded with visual stimuli. They may need to concentrate on people's faces or their own to become accustomed to this experience. They often need to talk about what they see and to compare the visual images with their mental ones. The child may also go through a period of depression (Gregory, 1990), which must be respected and supported.

Newly sighted children also need time to adjust to the ability to engage in activities that were impossible before. For example, they may prefer to use braille to read, rather than learning a new 'visual approach', because of familiarity with the touch system. Eventually, as they learn to recognize letters and numbers, they will integrate these new skills into reading and writing. However, parents and teachers must be careful not to push them before they are ready. This applies to social relationships and physical activities, as well as to learning situations.

Assist in measures to prevent vision impairment

An essential nursing goal is to prevent visual impairment. This involves many of the same interventions discussed under hearing impairments, namely: (1) antenatal screening for pregnant women at risk, such as those with rubella or syphilis infection and family histories of genetic disorders associated with visual loss; (2) adequate antenatal and perinatal care to prevent prematurity and iatrogenic damage from excessive administration of oxygen; (3) periodic screening of all children, especially newborns through to preschool children, for congenital blindness and visual impairments caused by refractive errors, strabismus, etc.; (4) rubella immunization of all children; and (5) safety counselling regarding the common causes of ocular trauma.

Following the detection of eye problems, the nurse has a responsibility to prevent further ocular damage by ensuring that corrective treatment is employed. For the child with strabismus, this often necessitates occlusion patching of the stronger eye. Compliance with the procedure is greatest during the early preschool years. It is more difficult to encourage school-aged children to wear the occlusive patch, because the poor visual acuity of the uncovered weaker eye interferes with schoolwork and the patch sets them apart from their peers. In school, they benefit from being positioned favourably (closer to the chalkboard) and allowed extra time to read or complete an assignment. If treatment of the eye disorder requires instillation of ophthalmic medication, the family is taught the correct procedure (see Chapter 8).

The nurse helps children with refractive errors adjust to wearing glasses. Young children, who often pull glasses off, benefit from temporal pieces that wrap around the ears or an elastic strap attached to the frames and around the back of the head to hold them on securely. Once children appreciate the value of clear vision, they are more likely to wear the corrective lenses.

Glasses should not interfere with any activity. Special protective guards are available during contact sports to prevent accidental injury, and all corrective lenses should be made from safety glass, which is shatterproof. Often, corrective lenses improve visual acuity so dramatically that children are able to compete more effectively in sports.

Contact lenses are a popular alternative, especially for adolescents. Several types are available, such as hard lenses (including gas-permeable ones), and soft lenses, which may be designed for daily or extended wear. Contact lenses offer several advantages over glasses, such as greater visual acuity, total corrected field of vision, convenience (especially with the extended-wear type), and optimum cosmetic benefit. However, they require much more care than glasses, including learning techniques for insertion and removal. If they are prescribed, the nurse can be helpful in teaching parents and children how to care for the lenses. General guidelines for care include regular removal and cleaning (daily for both hard and soft lenses or every seven days or less for the extended-wear type), thorough handwashing before handling lenses, and the use of commercially prepared saline solutions only — not tap water or home-made saline solutions — for soft lenses. In addition, soft lenses require periodic disinfection.

The effectiveness of nursing interventions for vision impairment is determined by continual reassessment and evaluation of care. The following guidelines may be used:

1. Interview the family regarding their adjustment to the sensory impairment. Observe the family members' relationships with the child. Interview the child regarding feelings about the sensory impairment and its effect on activities of daily living.
2. Have parents identify cues that indicate the infant is responding to them. Observe nonvisual behaviours of parents as they respond to their infant.
3. Observe the techniques the child uses to read and navigate. Inquire if the child is enrolled in a visual training programme. Inquire about socialization opportunities for the child (i.e., who are the child's friends, what are the child's extracurricular activities).
4. Observe preparation of room and self-care activities that provide for the child's safety and independence during hospitalization.
5. Investigate community programmes aimed at preventing or detecting vision loss and inquire about nursing involvement in these efforts.

THE DEAF-BLIND CHILD

The most traumatic sensory impairment is loss of sight and hearing. One of the chief causes of deaf blindness was congenital rubella syndrome, but immunization has decreased its incidence. Other causes are usually the result of one congenital sensory impairment combined with an acquired impairment, such as congenital blindness and acquired deafness from meningitis. Most children with multisensory impairments have some residual hearing and vision to supplement the senses of touch, smell and taste.

Auditory and visual impairments have profound effects on the child's development. They interfere with the normal sequence of physical, intellectual and psychosocial growth. Although the child often achieves the usual motor milestones, they are delayed. Support for the deaf and blind is available from the National Association for Deaf/Blind and Rubella Handicapped Children and the National Deaf–Blind Helpers' League.

IMPLICATIONS FOR NURSING

Caring for children with multisensory impairments is an area in which few nurses have much experience. It involves an overwhelming adjustment for families, and the child's educational needs cannot be met in most school programmes. Most of the interventions discussed for the hearing or visually impaired child are applicable to the care of these children, such as activities to facilitate learning self-care and increased stimulation for motor development. The following paragraphs discuss some of the special problems encountered by these families and presents constructive interventions.

One of the major concerns of families with deaf-blind children is helping them to establish communication. The nurse is in a vital position to help parents with this goal. Since infants cannot laugh or make eye movements, they are limited in the cues they can send and receive. Therefore, initiating and maintaining communication is the caregiver's responsibility. The nurse discusses with parents behaviours that signal the infant's recognition of them, such as quieting behaviour, blinking and change in respiration. The parents are encouraged to find ways to increase stimulation for the child, especially cues that help the child identify each parent. For example, each person involved with the child should choose something that he or she, and only he or she, does, such as a kiss on the forehead or a stroke on the cheek. In this way, the infant learns to discriminate among people in the environment.

The infant should be held close to the adult with the child's hands placed on the face while the person talks or changes facial expression. Eventually this technique becomes structured to associate a certain facial vibration with a word. However, such associations take time, patience and effort from both the child and the parents.

As many sensory experiences as possible are provided, such as placing children in different positions during the day in relation to light, and providing variation in stimuli so that they will be motivated to move towards, reach, touch and explore the environment. Changing position also encourages muscle development and movement patterns. Sound vibra-

tions should be brought near and made interesting to these children. For example, they can participate in hearing by placing the hand on a radio or on a person's throat. Consistent tactile cues should be associated with a change of position and activities so that the movement is experienced as a positive, nonthreatening experience. The nurse encourages family members to urge the child to participate in games that require repositioning and body action, such as peekaboo and pat-a-cake.

Deaf-blind children need secure, safe experiences while learning to walk and while gaining confidence. Once ambulatory, they need help in exploring the environment on a gradual, planned basis. The environment should not be haphazard, since children may become fearful and may avoid growth-producing experiences. After they succeed in becoming well oriented to the environment, and can overcome any abnormal movement patterns, they are ready for a plan of locomotion. Sighted guide, trailing (movement directed by touching objects, such as the wall), and cane walking are three methods. An individually planned mobility programme is based on the child's age, needs and functional status, and is shared with the child's therapist, teachers, parents and siblings.

The future prospects for deaf-blind children are at best unpredictable. Sometimes, congenital blindness and/or deafness is accompanied by other physical or neurological handicaps, which further lessen the child's learning potential. The most favourable prognosis is often for children who have acquired deaf-blindness and have few, if any, associated disabilities. Their learning capacity is greatly potentiated by their developmental progress before the sensory impairments. Although total independence, including gainful vocational training, is the goal, some deaf-blind children are unable to develop to this level. They may require lifelong parental or residential care. The nurse working with such families helps them deal with future goals for the child, including possible alternatives to home care during the parents' advancing years. In this respect, much of the nurse's role is similar to that discussed in Chapter 18 for the child with learning disabilities.

COMMUNICATION IMPAIRMENT

One of the most outstanding differences between human beings and lower animals is the human ability to communicate by using verbal language. The profound effect of hearing loss on speech development, discussed earlier in this chapter, laid a foundation for understanding how inability to communicate affects a child's life. However, hearing impairment is only one of several reasons for communication disorders. Often, a child has language and speech, but is still unable to communicate effectively. This discussion focuses on types of communication disorders, guidelines for detecting children who require referral, and techniques to promote language/speech development and to prevent problems.

GENERAL CONCEPTS

Communication impairment is a broad term that refers to the inability to: (1) receive and/or process a symbol system, (2) represent concepts or symbol systems, and/or (3) transmit and use symbol systems (ASLHA, 1982). Although communication disorders are concerned with verbal symbols of the spoken word, other symbol systems include nonverbal methods, such as gestures, sign language and braille. With severe communication impairment, these methods may be needed to substitute for the spoken word.

Because of the complexity of communication, various classification systems are available and there is no universal agreement on one system. Basically, a communication impairment may occur in language, speech, or hearing or any combination of these. The problems encountered when hearing is affected are discussed earlier in this chapter. *Language* primarily refers to the symbol system used to convey thoughts or feelings to others. The two major types are *receptive* language, or understanding the spoken word, and *expressive* language, or speaking verbal symbols. *Speech* is the oral production of language, including articulation of sounds, rhythm, and tone.

Delayed development of language and speech is the most common manifestation of developmental delay in children and affects from 5-10% of all children (Coplan, 1985). Speech problems are more prevalent than language disorders, and both impairments decline as children grow older.

AETIOLOGY

The most common cause of communication impairment is learning disability, followed by hearing impairment. Other causes include: (1) central nervous system dysfunction, such as attention deficit disorders; (2) severe emotional disturbance, such as autism and schizophrenia; (3) organic problems, such as cerebral palsy, cleft palate, vocal cord injury, and paralysis or foreshortening of the soft palate and uvula; and (4) some genetic disorders, such as cri-du-chat syndrome and Gilles de la Tourette syndrome. In some instances, such as in stuttering, the cause is unknown or speculative. Although the exact influence of environmental factors is controversial, current opinion deemphasizes the importance of laziness, birth order or bilingualism on delayed language development (Coplan, 1985).

LANGUAGE IMPAIRMENT

Language disorders include an inability to:
1. Assign meaning to words (vocabulary).
2. Organize words into sentences.
3. Alter word forms to indicate tense, possession, and plurality.

Examples of language disorders are failure to develop vocabulary at the expected age, a reduced vocabulary for age, poor sentence structure, such as 'Me see dog', or omitting words from the sentence, such as 'Me fun'. Such short or 'telegraphic' phrases are normal during the first two years, but should be replaced by more complete statements during the preschool years.

SPEECH IMPAIRMENT

Speech impairments include differences from normal in articulation, fluency and voice production. *Articulation* errors refer to sounds a child makes incorrectly or inappropriately. For example, the child tends to distort or substitute a few consonants or blends, especially those that are learned last — s, l, r, and *th* — or the child omits many consonants, usually at the end of words, and substitutes the letters t, d, k, or y for them.

Dysfluencies, or rhythm disorders, usually consist of repetitions of sounds, words, or phrases. One of the most common and potentially serious dysfluencies is stuttering. *Stuttering* describes dysfluent speech characterized by tense repetition of sounds or complete blockages of sounds or words. A stutter is sometimes referred to as a *block* when no sound comes out when the person tries to speak (Guitar, 1989).

Voice disorders are characterized by differences in pitch, loudness, and/or quality.

NONSPEECH COMMUNICATION

Another category receiving increased attention is concerned with individuals who have severe disabilities, such as cerebral palsy, learning disability, or multiple physical impairments, that prevent acquisition of meaningful verbal speech. Many of these people comprehend language, but are unable to speak. Consequently, they benefit from communication methods that employ nonverbal symbols such as sign language. Besides the use of hand or body gestures, numerous other communication systems exist. For example, *Blissymbols* are a highly stylized system of graphic symbols that represent words, ideas, and concepts (Murray, 1984).

NURSING CARE OF THE CHILD WITH COMMUNICATION IMPAIRMENT

Nursing goals focus primarily on assessment of communication disorders and prevention of primary problems, or development of further difficulties, especially through parent education (Law and Pollard, 1994).

PREVENTION

The primary intervention for communication disorders is prevention. Much of prevention directly relates to factors that predispose to the causes of language and/or speech impairment; namely, mental retardation and hearing loss. Infants at risk for either condition should be referred for audiological evaluation before six months of age so that audiological and speech therapy can be initiated immediately.

One area that is particularly important in preventing communication impairment through appropriate parental guidance is stuttering. This hesitancy or dysfluency in speech pattern

---

◆ **BOX 23-1**

Guidelines for assessing communication impairment

Key Questions for Language Disorders

1. How old was your child when he or she began to speak his or her first words?
2. How old was your child when he or she began to put words into sentences?
3. Does your child have difficulty in learning new vocabulary words?
4. Does your child omit words from sentences (i.e. do sentences sound telegraphic?) or use short or incomplete sentences?
5. Does your child have trouble with grammar, such as the verbs 'is', 'am', 'are', 'was', and 'were'?
6. Can your child follow two to three directions given at once?
7. Do you have to repeat directions or questions?
8. Does your child respond appropriately to questions?
9. Does your child ask questions beginning with 'who', 'what', 'where', and 'why'?
10. Does it seem that your child has made little or no progress in speech and language in the last 6 to 12 months?

Key Questions for Speech Impairment

1. Does your child ever stammer or repeat sounds or words?
2. Does your child seem anxious or frustrated when trying to express an idea?
3. Have you noticed certain behaviours, such as blinking the eyes, jerking the head, or attempting to rephrase thoughts with different words, when your child stammers?
4. What do you do when any of these occur?
5. Does your child omit sounds from words?
6. Does it seem as if your child uses *t, d, k*, or *g* in place of most other words?
7. Does your child omit sounds from words or substitute the correct consonant with another one (such as 'rabbit' with 'wabbit')?
8. Do you have any difficulty in understanding your child's speech? How much of it is unintelligible?
9. Has anyone else ever remarked about having difficulty in understanding your child?
10. Has there been any recent change in the sound of your child's voice?

---

is a *normal* characteristic of language development during the preschool years. It occurs because children's advancing mental ability and level of comprehension exceed vocabulary acquisition. Children know what they want to say, but hesitate or repeat words or sounds as they try to find the vocabulary to express themselves. Eventually, their language skills parallel the other abilities, and speech becomes fluent.

However, when parents or other significant persons place undue emphasis or stress on this pattern of dysfluency, an abnormal speech pattern may result. Chances for reversal of stuttering are good until about five years of age. Therefore, prevention must begin early. The nurse discusses with parents the normal dysfluencies in children's speech. When stuttering does occur, parents are advised to use the suggestions listed under Parent Guidelines to prevent inadvertently reinforcing the dysfluent pattern. If excessive concern of the parent or frustration and struggling behaviour from the child are noted, the child is referred for language and speech evaluation.

ASSESSMENT

Communication disorders can occur at any age, but are most often found during childhood. The preschool period is considered critical to language development and therefore is a prime age for assessment and intervention. Failure to detect communication disorders during early childhood affects the development of social relationships and emotional interactions, increases difficulty in developing academic skills, and lessens the chances for successful correction of deficit skills.

Three methods are available for assessing speech and language development:
1. Direct observation of the child's verbal skills.
2. Questioning of the parents.
3. Testing.

Direct observation necessitates spontaneous language interaction between the child and the nurse. Suggestions for initiating conversation include showing children an object and asking them to describe it (asking children to name the object often results in one-word responses that are too limited for evaluation of speech, although appropriate for evaluation of language) or posing questions such as, 'If you could have three wishes, what would you want?'. The word-imitative procedure may also be used, by having children repeat sentences or words. This approach is valid because children are not able to reproduce statements using correct grammatical forms that they have not previously learned to use. Whenever possible, the child's conversation should be tape-recorded for serial documentation of progressive language and/or speech development and further evaluation by, or consultation with, a language or speech therapist.

Indirect assessment relies on parental information obtained through a history. Key questions that reflect problems in language or speech are listed in Box 23-1. Information obtained from the history is critically important, and parental comments such as, 'He doesn't say much' or 'Her use of words is so much slower than her older brother's was' must be taken seriously. However, caution must also be exercised in evaluating parental comments. Parents may be unaware of the child's difficulties, because of lack of comparison with normal language development. Also, they may not realize the degree of unintelligible speech because of familiarity with the child's approximation of words. Conversely, parents may have unrealistic expectations regarding verbal development and may exaggerate the degree of dysfluency, misarticulation, or word usage. Consequently, screening tests are a very important component of objective measurement of speech development.

Denver Articulation Screening Examination

The Denver Articulation Screening Examination (DASE) employs the word-imitative procedure and is one of the most frequently used tests. The child repeats 22 words but pronounces 30 different sound elements. The raw score, or the number of correctly pronounced sounds, is then compared with the percentile rank for children in that age group. The examiner must be careful to evaluate the specific sound rather than the quality of the entire word. For beginning examiners, it is helpful to validate the final score by comparing the results with a different examiner, ideally a speech therapist. The child is also scored on intelligibility, by selection of one of four possible categories: (1) easy to understand, (2) understandable half of the time, (3) not understandable, or (4) cannot evaluate. The DASE is a reliable, effective screening tool because it requires only ten minutes for the examiner to perform and is designed to discriminate between significant speech delay and normal variations in the acquisition of speech sounds. It also detects common abnormal physical conditions such as hyponasality, hypernasality, tongue thrust and lateral lisp.

Early Language Milestone Scale

The Early Language Milestone Scale (ELM) is a standardized screening instrument for assessing language development in children less than three years of age. The test focuses on expressive, receptive and visual language, and the revised form includes intelligibility (Coplan and Gleason, 1988; Coplan *et al*, 1982). The ELM relies primarily on the parent's report, with occasional direct testing of the child, and takes 1-4 minutes to administer. The best age range for the ELM is 25-36 months (Walker *et al*, 1989).

Other tests

Several other tests are available to screen children for impaired language development. The Denver II, a revision of the Denver Developmental Screening Test, includes an expanded section on language items, and delays in that area provide an early indication for those children who require further evaluation. For children 2.5 to 18 years, the *Peabody Picture Vocabulary Test—Revised* is a useful screening instrument for word comprehension (Dunn and Dunn, 1981).

Referral

Following assessment and detection of language or speech problems, the nurse must make a decision regarding appropriate referral. The all-too-frequent advice of 'let's wait and see what happens' or 'your child will grow out of it' is often to the detriment of the child's future development. Since children normally vary greatly in their development of verbal skills, the nurse needs some guidelines for determining which child's development is abnormal. Box 23-2 lists general recommendations for referring children for specialized audiological and language evaluations.

EDUCATION

When a child is delayed in language development, it becomes very important to try to structure the parents' communication to expand the child's language, including new words, new sentence construction and rules of grammar. The underlying principle is not to bombard children with words so that they

---

◆ BOX 23-2

Guidelines for referral regarding communication impairment

Age 2 Years
Failure to speak any meaningful words spontaneously
Consistent use of gestures rather than vocalizations
Difficulty in following verbal directions
Failure to respond consistently to sound

Age 3 Years
Speech largely unintelligible
Failure to use sentences of three or more words
Omission of initial consonants
Frequent omission of final consonants
Use of vowels rather than consonants

Age 5 Years
Stutters or has any other type of dysfluency
Sentence structure noticeably impaired
Substitutes easily produced sounds for more difficult ones
Omits word endings (plurals, tenses of verbs, etc.)

Over 5 Years
Poor voice quality (monotonous, loud, or barely audible)
Vocal pitch inappropriate for age
Any distortions, omissions, or substitutions of sounds after age 7 years
Connected speech characterized by use of unusual confusions or reversals

General
Any child with signs suggesting a hearing impairment
Any child who is embarrassed or disturbed by his or her speech
Parents who are excessively concerned or who pressure the child to speak at a level above that appropriate for the child's age

learn more language, but to plan what will be said to them, what responses will be expected, and how they will be reinforced. Suggestions to help parents foster their child's attainment of language skills are presented in the Parent Guidelines.

Parents should also be aware that children learn language through imitation. Therefore, serving as role models by speaking clearly, fluently and with proper grammar is essential to children's mastery of language and speech. Parents need guidance regarding normal language and speech development so that they expect neither too little nor too much from their child.

Parent Guidelines

Helping a Child Learn Language

Provide listening opportunities
  Select a small group of words connected to a specific activity (e.g. say 'open' each time a door is opened).
  Repeat the word with the activity several times, then repeat the word but wait for the child to initiate the activity.
  Choose vocabulary that is useful, easy to pronounce, and understandable to the child.
Encourage vocabulary by having the child say the word rather than gesture before fulfilling a request (e.g. expect the child to say all or part of the word 'drink' before giving a beverage).
Speak at a level slightly above the child's level (e.g. if the child speaks two words, use three or four-word phrases).
Expand the statement, preserving the child's intent*.
  Expand the statement using the same noun.
    CHILD: Kitty jump
    ADULT: The kitty is on the chair.

Replace the noun with a pronoun.
    CHILD: Kitty jump
    ADULT: She is jumping.
Expand the statement adding new information.
    CHILD: Kitty jump
    ADULT: The dog is jumping, too.
Respond by indicating the meaning of the child's utterance, rather than its linguistic accuracy (or inaccuracy).*
    CHILD: Kitty jump
    ADULT: Yes, the kitty is jumping.
Substitute questions with statements about an observed activity (e.g. rather than asking, 'What's that?' say, 'Look at the kitten').
Reinforce the child's attempt to use language with verbal praise and affection.

*Data from the US Department of Health and Human Services, Developmental speech and language disorders: hope through research, Pub No 188, Bethesda, MD, 1988, Public Health Service, National Institutes of Health.

KEY POINTS

- Hearing disorders may be classified according to the location of the defect: conductive, sensorineural, mixed conductive-sensorineural, and auditory imperception.
- Some of the effects of hearing loss on growth and development are impaired knowledge of objects, emotional behaviour, poor motor development, impaired academic learning, and decreased socialization.
- Visual impairments may vary in degree from total blindness to significant levels of residual vision.
- Visual impairment may result from familial factors, prenatal/intrauterine factors, perinatal factors, and postnatal factors.
- Common visual impairments in childhood are refractive errors, amblyopia, strabismus, cataracts, glaucoma, trauma, and infections.

- Effects of visual impairment on development include impaired motor function, lack of stimulation, and diminished academic learning.
- Nursing goals in visual rehabilitation are helping the family and child adjust to the child's visual impairment, promoting parent-child attachment, fostering optimum development and independence, providing for play and socialization, and being aware of educational facilities.
- Nursing interventions for the deaf-blind child are helping the family adjust to the child's impairment, choosing appropriate educational channels, facilitating self-care, promoting communication, and assisting with ambulation.
- Causes of impaired communication include mental retardation, hearing impairment, central nervous system dysfunction, severe emotional disturbances, and organic problems.

REFERENCES

ASLHA: Communicative disorders and variations, *Am Speech Lang Hear Assoc J* 24:949, 1982.

BBC: *The in-touch handbook*, London, 1994, Broadcasting Support Services.

Bronzaft AL: Noise is hazardous to child's health and well-being, *Child Behav Dev Lett* 5(10):1, 1989.

Consensus Conference: Noise and hearing loss, *JAMA* 263(23):3185, 1990.

Conyers M: *Vision for the future—meeting the challenge of sight loss*, 1992, Kingsway.

Coplan J et al: Validation of an early language milestone scale in a high-risk population, *Pediatr* 70(5):677, 1982.

Coplan J, Gleason J: Unclear speech: recognition and significance of unintelligible speech in preschool children, *Pediatr* 82(3, pt 2):447, 1988.

Coplan J: Evaluation of the child with delayed speech or language, *Pediatr Ann* 14(3):202, 1985.

Dunn L, Dunn L: *The Peabody Picture Vocabulary Test—revised*, Circle Pines, MN, 1981, American Guidance Service.

Freeland A: *Deafness: the facts*, Oxford, 1989, Oxford University Press.

Frey T: Pediatric eye trauma, *Pediatr Ann* 12(7):487, 1983.

Friendly DS: Amblyopia: definition, classification, diagnosis, and management considerations for pediatricians, family physicians, and general practitioners, *Pediatr Clin North Am* 34(6):1389, 1987.

Gibbons CL: Deaf children's perception of internal body parts, *Matern Child Nurs J* 4(1):37, 1985.

Green T: A word in your ear, *Personal Computer World* 18(4):364, 1995.

Gregory RL: *Eye and brain: the psychology of seeing*, ed 4, London, 1990, Weidenfeld & Nicolson.

Guitar B: Stuttering, *Feelings Med Signif* 31(3):9, 1989.

Hall DMB, editor: *Health for all children*, ed 2, Oxford, 1991, Oxford University Press.

Helveston E, Ellis F: *Pediatric ophthalmology practice*, ed 2, St Louis, 1984, Mosby–Year Book.

Henderson SE, Barnett A, Henderson L: Visuospatial difficulties and clumsiness: on the interpretation of conjoined deficits, *J Child Psychol Psychiatry* 35(5):961, 1994.

Kramer SJ, Williams DR: The hearing-impaired infant and toddler: identification, assessment and intervention, *Infants Young Children* 6(1):35, 1993.

Law J, Pollard C: Identifying speech and language delay, *Health Visitor* 67(2):59, 1994.

McCormick B: Screening for hearing impairment in young children, London, 1988, Croom Helm.

Murray F: Language for the handicapped, *Point of View* 21(3):8, 1984.

Roush J: Acoustic amplification for hearing-impaired infants and young children, *Inf Young Child* 2(4):59, 1990.

Royal National Institute for the Blind: *Blind and partially sighted children in Britain—the RNEB study*, vol 2, London, 1992, HMSO.

Salamy A, Eldredge L, Tooley WH: Neonatal status and hearing loss in high-risk infants, *J Pediatr* 114(5):847, 1989.

US Department of Health and Human Services: *Developmental speech and language disorders: hope through research*, Pub No. 188, Bethesda, MD, 1988, Public Health Service, National Institute of Health.

Walker D et al: Early Language Milestone Scale and language screening of young children, *Pediatr* 83(2):284, 1989.

Walker E, Tobin M, McKennell A: *Blind and partially sighted children in Britain: the RNIB survey*, vol 2, London, 1992, HMSO.

Webster A, Wood D: *Children with hearing difficulties*, London, 1991, Cassell.

FURTHER READING

Hearing Impairment

Coplan J: Deafness: ever heard of it? Delayed recognition of permanent hearing loss, *Pediatr* 79(2):206, 1987.

Hanawalt A, Troutman K: If your patient has a hearing aid, *AJN* 84(7):900, 1984.

Holder L: Hearing aids: handle with care, *Nurs '82* 12(4):64, 1982.

Kaplan SL et al.: Onset of hearing loss in children with bacterial meningitis, *Pediatr* 73(5):575, 1984.

McKerrow K: Minimal hearing loss may not be benign, *AJN* 87(7):904, 1987.

Northern J, Downs M: *Hearing in children*, ed 4, Baltimore, 1984, Williams & Wilkins.

Oberklaid F, Harris C, Keir E: Auditory dysfunction in children with school problems, *Clin Pediatr* 28(9):397, 1989.

Vision Impairment

Cromie BW: Superglue inadvertently used as eyedrops, *BMJ* 300(6725):680, 1990.

Ingram RM: Amblyopia, *BMJ* 298(6668):204, 1989.

Kodadek SM, Haylor MJ: Using interpretive methods to understand family care giving when a child is blind, *J Paed Nurs* 5(1):42, 1990.

Lyons C, Stevens J, Bloom J: Superglue inadvertently used as eyedrops, *BMJ* 300:328, 1990.

Perry J, Tullo A: *Care of the ophthalmic patient*, London, 1990, Chapman & Hall.

Phillips S, Hartley JT: Developmental differences and interventions for blind children, *Paed Nurs* 14(3):201, 1988.

Stollery R: Ophthalmic nursing, Oxford, 1987, Blackwell Scientific Publications.

Tumulty G, Resler MM: Eye trauma, *AJN* 84(6):740, 1984.

Vaughan D, Asbury T: *General ophthalmology*, ed 13, California, 1992, Lange Medical Publications.

Communication Impairment

Accardo P, Whitman B: Toe walking: a marker of language disorders, *Clin Pediatr* 28(8):347, 1989.

Casper J: Disorders of speech and voice, *Pediatr Ann* 14(3):220, 1985.

Cohen C: Augmentative communication: a perspective for pediatricians, *Pediatr Ann* 14(3):232, 1985.

Fischel J et al.: Language growth in children with expressive language delay, *Pediatr* 82(2):218, 1989.

Fuller CW: Speech and hearing problems. In Green M, Haggerty, RJ, editors: *Ambulatory pediatrics,* III, Philadelphia, 1984, WB Saunders.

Goldberg R: Identifying speech and language delays in children, *Pediatr Nurs* 15(4):252, 1984.

Graham JM, Bashir AS, Stark RE: Communicative disorders. In Levine MD *et al,* editors: *Developmental-behavioral pediatrics,* Philadelphia, 1983, WB Saunders.

Hall D: Delayed speech in children, *BMJ* 297(6659):1281, 1988.

Lombardino L, Stapell J, Gerhardt K: Evaluating communicative behaviors in infancy, *J Pediatr Health Care* 1(5):240, 1987.

Menyuk P: Language development in a social context, *J Pediatr* 109(1):217, 1986.

Resnick TJ, Allen DA, Rapin I: Disorders of language development diagnosis and intervention, *Pediatr Rev* 6(3):85, 1984.

Speech dysfluency, *Lancet* 8637(1):530, 1989.

USEFUL ADDRESSES

Royal National Institute for the Blind, the Association of Blind and Partially Sighted Teachers and Students, National Association for the Education of the Partially Sighted, and the Partially Sighted Society.

National Association for Deaf/Blind and Rubella Handicapped Children and the National Deaf–Blind Helpers' League.

Chapter 24

Balance and Imbalance of Body Fluids and Electrolytes

LEARNING OUTCOMES

After studying this chapter you should be able to:

- Outline the principles involved in the maintenance of water balance in children.
- List the fluid and electrolyte requirements for infants and children based on body weight.
- Describe the clinical manifestations of fluid and electrolyte disturbances in children.
- List the mechanisms involved in the formation of oedema in children.
- Discuss the nursing role in the assessment of children experiencing fluid and electrolyte disturbances.
- Describe the main conditions that produce fluid and electrolyte disturbances in children.
- Outline the aetiology of gastrointestinal disorders which predispose children to fluid and electrolyte disturbances.
- Outline the aetiology of shock — acute circulatory collapse — in children.
- Discuss the nursing care required to meet the needs of children with fluid and electrolyte disturbances.
- Discuss the specialist role of the nurse in caring for burn-injured children.
- Define the glossary terms.

GLOSSARY

acidosis Serum pH equal to or less than 7.35

alkalosis pH equal to or greater than 7.45

azotaemia Accumulation of excessive amounts of nitrogenous products in the blood

colitis Inflammation of the colon

dysentery Intestinal inflammation accompanied by cramping, abdominal pain, tenesmus, and watery stools containing blood and mucus

electrolyte An element or compound that, when dissolved in a liquid (e.g., water), dissociates into ions and is able to conduct an electric current

enteral By way of the alimentary tract

enteritis Inflammation of the intestine

gastritis Inflammation of stomach

gastroenteritis Inflammation of stomach and intestines

hypertonic Having a greater osmotic pressure than a reference solution

hypotonic Having a lesser osmotic pressure than a reference solution

insensible Loss of fluid from the body by evaporation and/or respiration

intraosseous infusion The injection of blood, medications or fluids into bone marrow rather than into a vein, the technique may be performed in emergency treatment of a child when IV infusion is not feasible

isotonic Having the same osmotic pressure as a reference solution

NBM Nil by mouth

osmolality Number of particles (proteins or electrolytes) suspended in fluid

parenteral By some means other than through the digestive tract

regurgitation Return of undigested food from the stomach

septic Relating to or caused by sepsis

solute a substance dissolved in a solution

The basic elements related to fluid and electrolyte balance — body water, electrolytes, and pH — are so closely interrelated that they rarely can be separated in clinical disorders; however, for simplicity, they will be reviewed separately. An understanding of the basic principles of fluid dynamics and acid-base balance is essential for the nurse to be able to interpret observations, correlate these findings with the course of the disease process, and comprehend the rationale behind therapy in order to participate intelligently in a treatment regimen.

DISTRIBUTION OF BODY FLUIDS

Water is the major constituent of body tissues. The total body water (TBW) in an individual ranges from 45-75% of total body weight. Its importance to body function is related not only to its abundance, but also to the fact that it is the medium in which body solutes are dissolved and all metabolic reactions take place. Since these metabolic processes are affected by even small alterations in fluid composition, precise regulation of the volume and composition of the fluid is essential. In healthy individuals, body water remains singularly constant, but marked alterations in either its volume or distribution that occur in many disease states can produce severely damaging physiological consequences.

WATER BALANCE

Under normal conditions, the amount of water ingested closely approximates the amount of urine excreted in a 24-hour period, and the water in food and from oxidation balances that lost in faeces and through evaporation. In this way, equilibrium is maintained.

MECHANISMS OF FLUID MOVEMENT

Water is retained in the body in a relatively constant amount and, with few exceptions, is freely exchangeable between all body fluid compartments. The proximity of the extravascular compartment to the cells allows for continual change in volume and distribution of fluids, largely determined by solutes (especially sodium) and physical forces. Transport mechanisms are the basis for all activity within the cells and, since they have limited ability to store materials, movement in and out of cells must be rapid. Internal control mechanisms are responsible for distribution and maintenance of fluid balance.

Maintaining water balance

Maintenance water requirement is the volume of water needed to replace insensible water loss (through the skin and respiratory tract), evaporative water loss and losses through urine and stool formation. The amount and type of these losses may be altered by disease states such as fever (with increased sweating), diarrhoea, gastric suction, and sequestration of body fluids in a body space.

Basal maintenance calculations are used for conditions in which a child is in a normal state of hydration; for example, preoperative preparation or in a coma. Requirements for a 24-hour period are: 100 ml/kg of body weight for the first 10 kg plus 50 ml/kg for next 10 kg plus 20 ml/kg for greater than 20 kg, or 1500 ml/m² (Abelson and Smith, 1987).

Maintenance fluids contain both water and electrolytes, and can be estimated from the child's age, body weight, degree of activity and body temperature. *Basal metabolic rate (BMR)* is derived from standard tables and adjusted for the child's activity, temperature and disease state. For example, for afebrile patients at rest, the maintenance water requirement is approximately 100 ml for each kilocalorie expended. Children with fluid losses or other alterations require adjustment of these basic needs to accommodate abnormal losses of both water and electrolytes as a result of a disease state. For example, insensible losses are increased when basal expenditure is increased by unusual activity in bed, fever and hypermetabolic states. Hypometabolic states, such as hypothyroidism and hypothermia, decrease the BMR.

CHANGES IN FLUID VOLUME RELATED TO GROWTH

The percentage of total body water varies among individuals. In adults and older children, it is related primarily to the amount of body fat.

In a child three years of age, total body water comprises 63% of body weight and decreases slowly until the age of 12, when it reaches approximately 58%. At maturity, the percentage of total body water is somewhat higher in the male than in the female and is probably a result of the differences in body composition, particularly fat and muscle content (Fig. 24-1).

WATER BALANCE IN INFANTS

During the first year, there is a sharp decrease in total body water when expressed as a percentage of body weight. The percentage of extracellular fluid (ECF) also decreases from approximately 45% to 27%. The gradual alteration in water distribution that accompanies growth and maturation is a result of several changes that occur from infancy to childhood. Muscle growth associated with expanding size of individual cells increases the actual and relative intracellular fluid (ICF) volume and decreases the relative ECF volume. In addition to muscle growth, other organs also increase in size; for example, the size of nerve cells grows with a corresponding decrease in ECF volume, and the fraction of total body water contained in the skin diminishes during growth. Furthermore, the daily volume of secretions into the gastrointestinal tract is relatively much higher in infants than in children. The net result of these changes is a decrease in the proportion of ECF as the infant grows older.

Surface area

The infant's relatively greater surface area allows larger quantities of fluid to be lost in insensible perspiration through the skin. The gastrointestinal tract, sometimes considered to be an extension of the body surface area, is also relatively larger in infancy and is a source of proportionately greater fluid loss, especially from diarrhoea. The large surface area is an important factor in metabolism and heat production, which also influence fluid loss.

Metabolic rate

The rate of metabolism in infancy is significantly higher than in adulthood, because of the larger surface area in relation to the mass of active tissue. Consequently, there is a greater production of metabolic wastes that must be excreted by the kidneys. Any condition that increases metabolism causes a rise in heat production, with its concomitant insensible fluid loss and growing need for water for excretion.

Kidney function

The kidneys of the infant are functionally immature at birth and are therefore inefficient in excreting waste products of metabolism. Of particular importance for fluid balance is the inability of the infant's kidneys to concentrate or dilute urine, to conserve or excrete sodium, and to acidify urine.

Fluid requirements

As a result of these characteristics, infants ingest and excrete a greater amount of fluid per kilogram of body weight than older children. Since electrolytes are excreted with water and the infant has limited ability for conservation, maintenance requirements include both water and electrolytes. The daily exchange of ECF in the infant is much greater than that in older children, which leaves little fluid volume reserve in dehydration states. Water requirements for infants and children at various ages are listed in Table 24-1.

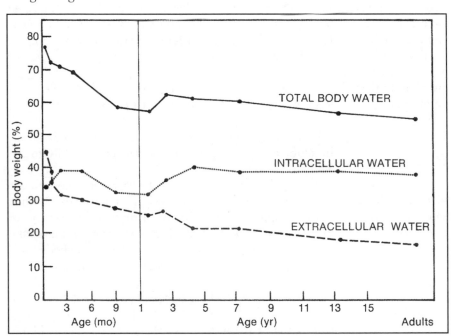

Fig. 24-1 Changes in total body water, extracellular water, and intracellular water in percentages of body weight (After Fris-Hansen B: *Pediatrics* 28:169, 1961.)

Body Weight (kg)	Surface Area (m²)	Body Water (ml/kg)	Cal/kg	Na⁺/kg (mmol)	K⁺/kg (mmol)
3	0.20	100	40-50	3-4	
5	0.27	90	50-70	3-4	3-4
10	0.45	75	40-60	2-3	2-3
15	0.64	65	40-50	2-3	2-3
30	1.10	55	35-45	2-3	1-2
50	1.50	45	25-40	1-2	1-2
70	1.75	40	15-20	1-2	1-2

From Barnes, 1986.

Requirements/m²: water 1500 ml; Na⁺ 60 mmol/l; K⁺ 45 mmol/l.

Table 24-1 Maintenance requirements.

DISTURBANCES OF FLUID AND ELECTROLYTE BALANCE

Disturbances of fluids and their solute concentration are closely interrelated. Alterations in fluid volume affect the electrolyte component, and changes in electrolyte concentration influence

fluid movement. Since intracellular water and electrolytes move to and from the ECF compartment, any imbalance in the ICF is reflected by an imbalance in the ECF. Disturbances in the ECF involve either an excess or a deficit of fluid and/or electrolytes; of these, fluid loss occurs more frequently. The major fluid disturbances and clinical manifestations are outlined in Table 24-2.

MECHANISMS/SITUATIONS	MANIFESTATIONS	MANAGEMENT/NURSING CARE
Water depletion	General symptoms:	Provide replacement of
Failure to absorb or reabsorb water	Thirst	fluid losses commensurate
Complete sudden cessation of intake	Variable temperature –	with volume depletion
or prolonged diminished intake:	increased (infection)	Provide maintenance fluids
Neglect of intake by self or caregiver –	Dry skin and mucous	Determine and correct
confused, psychotic, unconscious, or	membranes	and correct cause
helpless	Poor skin turgor	of water depletion
Loss from gastrointestinal tract –	Poor perfusion (decreased	Measure intake and output
vomiting, diarrhoea, nasogastric	pulse, slowed capillary refill	Monitor vital sign
suction, fistula	time)	
Disturbed body fluid chemistry:	Weight loss	
inappropriate ADH secretion	Fatigue	
Excessive renal excretion: glycosuria	Diminished urine output	
(diabetes)	Irritability and lethargy	
Loss through skin or lungs:	Tachycardia	
Excessive perspiration or vapourization –	Tachypnoea	
febrile states, hyperventilation,	Altered level of consciousness	
increased ambient temperature	Symptoms depend to some	
Impaired skin integrity - transudate	extent on proportion of	
from injuries	electrolytes lost with water	
Haemorrhage	Laboratory findings:	
Iatrogenic:	High urine specific gravity	
Overzealous use of diuretics	Increased haematocrit	
Improper postoperative fluid	Variable serum electrolytes	
replacement	Variable urine volume	
	Increased blood urea nitrogen	
	(BUN)	
	Increased osmolality	
Water excess	Oedema:	Limit fluid intake
Water intake in excess of output:	Generalized	Administer diuretics
Excessive oral intake	Pulmonary (moist rales)	Monitor vital signs
Hypertonic fluid overload	Intracutaneous (noted	Determine and treat cause
Plain water enemas	especially in loose areolar	of water excess
Failure to excrete water in presence	tissue)	Analyse laboratory
of normal intake:	Elevated venous pressure	electrolyte measurements
Kidney disease	Hepatomegaly	frequently
Congestive heart failure	Slow, bounding pulse	
Malnutrition	Weight gain	
	Lethargy	
		(cont.)

Table 24-2 Disturbances of fluid and electrolyte balance.

Increased spinal fluid pressure
Central nervous system
  manifestations (seizures, coma)
Laboratory findings:
  Low urine specific gravity
  Decreased serum electrolytes
  Decreased haematocrit
  Variable urine volume

Sodium depletion (hyponatraemia)

Prolonged low-sodium diet	Associated with water loss:	Determine and treat cause
Fever	Same as with water loss -	Administer IV fluids with
Excess sweating	dehydration, weakness,	appropriate saline
Tachypnoea (infants)	dizziness, nausea, abdominal	concentration
Cystic fibrosis	cramps. apprehension	
Burns and wounds	Mild - apathy, weakness,	
Vomiting, diarrhoea, nasogastric	nausea, soft pulse	
suction, fistulas	Moderate - decreased blood	
Adrenal insufficiency	pressure	
Renal disease	Laboratory findings:	
Diabetic acidosis	Sodium concentration <130	
	mmol/L (may be normal if	
	volume low)	
	Specific gravity depends on	
	water deficit or excess	

Sodium excess (hypernatraemia)

High salt intake - nasogastric or IV	Intense thirst	Determine and treat cause
Renal disease	Dry, sticky mucous membranes	Administer fluids as
	Flushed skin	prescribed
	Temperature may be increased	Measure intake and output
	Hoarseness	Monitor laboratory data
	Oliguria	
	Nausea and vomiting	
	Irritability and possible	
	progression to disorientation,	
	convulsions	
	Laboratory findings:	
	Serum sodium concentration	
	≥ 150 mmol/L	
	High plasma volume	
	Alkalosis	

Potassium depletion (hypokalaemia)

Starvation	Muscle weakness, cramping,	Determine and treat cause
Clinical conditions associated with	stiffness, paralysis,	Monitor vital signs, includ-
poor food intake	hyporeflexia	ing ECG
Malabsorption	Hypotension	Administer supplemental
IV fluid without added potassium	Cardiac arrhythmias, gallop	potassium
Diarrhoea, vomiting, fistulas,	rhythm	Assess for adequate renal
nasogastric suction	Tachycardia or brachycardia	output before
Diuresis	Ileus	administration
Administration of diuretics	Apathy, drowsiness	IV: administer slowly

Table 24-2 Disturbances of fluid and electrolyte balance (continued).

Administration of cortiocosteroids	Irritability	Oral: offer high-potassium
Diuretic phase of nephrotic syndrome	Fatigue	fluids and foods
Healing stage of burns	Laboratory findings:	
Potassium-losing nephritis	Decreased serum potassium	
Hyperglycaemic diuresis (e.g.,	concentration ≤ 3.5 mmol/L	
diabetes mellitus)	Abnormal ECG - flat, notched,	
Familial periodic paralysis	or inverted T waves,	
IV administration of insulin in	prolonged ST segment	
ketoacidosis		
Alkalosis		

Potassium excess (hyperkalaemia)

Renal disease	Muscle weakness, flaccid	Determine and treat cause
Renal shutdown	paralysis	Monitor vital signs,
Adrenal insufficiency (Addison	Twitching	including ECG
disease)	Hyperreflexia	Administer exchange resin,
Associated with metabolic acidosis	Bradycardia	if prescribed
Too rapid administration of IV	Ventricular fibrillation	Administer IV fluids as
potassium chloride	and cardiac arrest	prescribed
Transfusion with old donor blood	Oliguria	Administer insulin (if
Severe dehydration	Apnoea - respiratory	ordered) to facilitate
Crushing injuries	arrest	movement of potassium
Burns	Laboratory findings:	into cells
Haemolysis from sudden	High serum potassium	Monitor serum potassium
massive water intake	concentration ≥ 5.5 mmol/L	levels
Dehydration	Variable urine volume	
	Flat P wave on ECG, peaked	
	T waves	

Calcium depletion (hypocalcaemia)

Inadequate dietary calcium	Neuromuscular irritability	Determine and treat cause
Vitamin D deficiency	Tingling of nose, ears,	Administer calcium
Rapid transit through gastrointestinal	fingertips, toes	supplements as prescribed;
tract	Tetany	administer slowly
Advanced renal insufficiency	Laryngospasm	Monitor IV site; calcium
Administration of diuretics	Generalized convulsions	may cause vascular
Hypoparathyroidism	May be changes in clotting	irritation
Alkalosis	Positive Chvostek sign	Monitor serum calcium
Trapped in diseased tissues	Hypotension	levels
Increased serum protein (albumin)	Cardiac arrest	Monitor serum protein
Cow's milk formula - tetany of the	Laboratory findings:	levels
newborn	Decreased serum calcium	
Exchange transfusion with citrated	concentration (N = 8.8 - 10.8	
blood	mg/dl)	
	or	
	Increased serum protein	

Calcium excess (hypercalcaemia)

Acidosis	Few problems (ordinarily)	Determine and treat cause
Prolonged immobilization	Constipation	Monitor serum calcium
Conditions associated with increased	Anorexia	levels
bone catabolism	Dryness of mouth (thirst)	Monitor ECG
Hypoproteinaemia	Muscle hypotonicity	*(cont.)*

Table 24-2 Disturbances of fluid and electrolyte balance (continued).

Kidney disease	Bradycardia/cardiac arrest
Hypervitaminosis D	Increased calcium concentration
Hyperparathyroidism	in urine may cause formation of
	kidney stones
	Laboratory findings:
	Increased serum calcium levels,
	≥ 10.8 mg/dl
	or
	Decreased serum protein levels

Table 24-2 Disturbances of fluid and electrolyte balance (continued).

Problems of fluid and electrolyte disturbance always involve both water and electrolytes; therefore, replacement includes administration of both, calculated on the basis of ongoing processes and laboratory serum electrolyte values.

DEHYDRATION

Dehydration is a common body fluid disturbance encountered in the nursing of infants and children. It occurs whenever the total output of fluid exceeds the total intake, regardless of the underlying cause. Although dehydration can result from lack of oral intake (especially in elevated environmental temperatures), more often it is a result of abnormal losses, such as those that occur in vomiting or diarrhoea, when oral intake only partially compensates for the abnormal losses. Other significant causes of dehydration are diabetic ketoacidosis and extensive burns.

TYPES OF DEHYDRATION

Sodium is the primary osmotic force that controls fluid movement between the major fluid compartments. Other osmotic forces may play the dominant role in dehydration, such as glucose in diabetic dehydration and protein in nephrotic syndrome. Consequently, dehydration is conventionally classified as: (1) isotonic, (2) hypotonic, and (3) hypertonic.

Isotonic dehydration
Isotonic dehydration occurs in conditions in which electrolyte and water deficits are present in approximately balanced proportion. The observable fluid losses are not necessarily isotonic, but losses from other avenues make adjustments so that the sum of all losses, or the net loss, is isotonic. Since there is no osmotic force present to cause a redistribution of water between the ICF and ECF, the major loss is sustained from the ECF compartments. This significantly reduces the plasma volume and hence the circulating blood volume with its effect on skin, muscle and kidneys. Shock is the greatest threat to life in isotonic dehydration, and the child with isotonic dehydration displays symptoms characteristic of hypovolaemic shock. Plasma sodium remains within normal limits, between 130-150 mmol/L.

Hypotonic dehydration
Hypotonic dehydration occurs when the electrolyte deficit exceeds the water deficit. Since ICF is more concentrated than ECF in hypotonic dehydration, water transfers from the ECF to the ICF to establish osmotic equilibrium. This movement further increases the ECF volume loss, and shock is a frequent result. Because there is a greater proportional loss of ECF in hypotonic dehydration, the physical signs tend to be more severe with smaller fluid losses than isotonic or hypertonic dehydration. Plasma sodium concentration is less than 130 mmol/L.

Hypertonic dehydration

Hypertonic (hyperosmotic or hypernatraemic) dehydration results from water loss in excess of electrolyte loss and is usually caused by a proportionately larger loss of water and/or a larger intake of electrolytes. This sometimes occurs in infants with diarrhoea who are given fluids by mouth that contain large amounts of solute, or in children receiving high-protein nasogastric tube feedings that place an excessive solute load on the kidneys. In hypertonic dehydration, fluid shifts from the lesser concentration of the ICF to the ECF. Plasma sodium concentration is greater than 150 mmol/L.

Since the ECF volume is proportionately larger, hypertonic dehydration consists of a greater degree of water loss for the same intensity of physical signs. Hypodermic shock is less apparent in hypertonic dehydration. However, neurological disturbances, such as seizures, are more likely to occur. Cerebral changes are serious and may result in permanent damage. These include disturbance of consciousness, poor ability to focus attention, lethargy, increased muscle tone with hyperreflexia, and hyperirritability to stimuli (tactile, auditory, bright light).

DEGREE OF DEHYDRATION

Clinical signs provide clues to the extent of dehydration. The earliest detectable sign is usually tachycardia, followed by dry skin and mucous membranes, sunken fontanelle, signs of circulatory failure (coolness and mottling of extremities), loss of skin elasticity and delayed capillary filling time.

Hypodermic shock is a common manifestation of severe depletion of ECF volume accompanied by tachycardia and signs of poor perfusion. Peripheral circulation is poor as a result of reduced blood volume; therefore, the skin is cool and mottled, with poor capillary filling after blanching. Impaired kidney circulation often leads to oliguria and uraemia. While low blood pressure may accompany other symptoms of shock, in infants and young children it is usually a late sign and may herald the onset of cardiovascular collapse.

PROCESS OF DIAGNOSIS

To initiate a therapeutic plan, several factors must be determined: the degree of dehydration based on physical assessment; the type of dehydration based on the pathophysiology of the specific illness responsible for the dehydrated state; specific physical signs other than general signs; initial plasma sodium concentrations; and associated electrolyte (especially serum potassium) and acid-base imbalances. Initial and regular ongoing evaluations are carried out to assess the patient's progress towards equilibrium and the effectiveness of therapy.

WATER INTOXICATION

Water intoxication, or water overload, is observed less often than dehydration. However, it is important that nurses and others who care for children are aware that this can occur and are alert to the possibility in certain situations. Patients who ingest excessive amounts of fluid develop a concurrent decrease in serum sodium and central nervous system symptoms. There is a large urine output and, because water moves into the brain more rapidly than sodium moves out, the child also exhibits irritability, somnolence, headache, vomiting, diarrhoea and generalized seizures. The affected child usually appears well hydrated, but may be oedematous or even dehydrated.

Fluid intoxication can occur during acute IV water overloading, too rapid dialysis, or with too rapid reduction of glucose levels in diabetic ketoacidosis. Patients with central nervous system infections occasionally retain excessive amounts of water. Administration of inappropriate hypotonic solutions (e.g., 5% dextrose in water) may cause a rapid reduction in sodium and result in symptoms of water overload.

Infants are especially vulnerable to fluid overload. Their thirst mechanism is not well developed; therefore, they are unable to 'turn off' fluid intake appropriately. A decreased glomerular filtration rate does not allow for repeated excretion of a water load, and ADH levels may not be maximally reduced. Consequently, infants are unable to excrete a water overload effectively.

OEDEMA

Oedema is the presence of excess fluid in the interstitial spaces as a result of some defect in the normal circulation of body fluids that causes increased pressure in the interstitial spaces. Fluid removal from the interstitial spaces depends on venous hydrostatic pressure, oncotic pressure of intravascular and interstitial spaces, an intact semipermeable capillary wall, tissue tension and lymphatic flow.

MECHANISMS OF OEDEMA FORMATION

A defect in any of the homeostatic mechanisms maintaining fluid balance can cause accumulation of interstitial fluid. Disequilibrium results from anything that: (1) alters the retention of sodium, such as renal disease or hormonal influences; (2) affects the formation or destruction of plasma proteins, such as starvation or liver disease; or (3) alters membrane permeability, such as nephrotic syndrome or trauma.

Oedema may be localized to a small or large area, such as that occurring in urticaria, infection and pulmonary congestion, or it can be generalized, as in the hypoproteinaemia of the nephrotic syndrome and starvation.

Increased venous pressure

The colloidal osmotic pressure (COP) of the plasma proteins draws fluid back into the vascular system as long as this force is greater than the venous hydrostatic pressure. However, when the venous pressure is increased, fluid tends to be retained in the interstitial spaces. Constrictive dressings or restraints applied too tightly to extremities will obstruct venous return, increase venous and capillary pressure, and cause oedema. The most graphic pathological illustrations are pulmonary oedema caused by pulmonary circulation overload in cardiac defects with a left-to-right shunt and ascites caused by portal hypertension. Oedema from any cause is increased in dependent areas, because of this added factor of increased venous hydrostatic pressure and the gravitational effects in these areas.

Capillary permeability

Damage to capillary walls or alteration in their permeability permits exudation of plasma protein into the interstitial space. Most often this occurs as local oedema, such as manifested in inflammatory and hypersensitivity reactions. Capillary damage from burns allows extensive exudation of protein-rich fluid into the interstitial spaces to compound oedema formation.

Diminished plasma proteins

A decrease in plasma protein levels hampers the osmotic pull back into the vessels. Consequently, fluid remains in the interstitial spaces. Although other factors play a role, such as hydrostatic pressure of both the arterial vascular system and the tissues and Na^+ concentration, significantly low protein levels (below 4.5 mg/dl) are associated with oedema. Examples of this are the massive albumin losses of the nephrotic syndrome, diminished serum protein from insufficient dietary protein, and (sometimes) haemodilution of plasma proteins from IV fluid administration in chronic dehydration.

Lymphatic obstruction
Obstruction of lymph flow creates oedema high in protein content. This is uncommon in childhood, but can result from trauma to the lymphatic glands or removal of lymph nodes.

Tissue tension
Tissue hydrostatic pressure is ordinarily of little consequence. However, it plays a significant role in determining distribution of oedema fluid in certain pathological conditions. Loose tissues allow a greater amount of fluid accumulation than tissues that are tightly bound by dense fibrous bands in which tissue pressure rapidly increases to limit further extravasation of fluid. Oedema appears earlier and more readily in loose structures such as those in the periorbital and genital tissues. The alveolar structure of lung tissue is probably a contributing factor in pulmonary oedema, as well as in increased hydrostatic pressure in the pulmonary vessels.

Other factors in oedema formation
Any factor that causes Na^+ retention by the kidneys will produce or augment oedema formation. This includes stimulation of the renin-angiotensin-aldosterone mechanisms for Na^+ reabsorption created by the diminished plasma volume in oedema, which resulted from primary causes. The salt-retaining property of steroids is responsible for the oedema associated with their administration.

A particularly threatening form of oedema is cerebral oedema caused by trauma, infection or other aetiological factors, including vascular overload or injudicious IV administration of hypotonic solutions. The problems and assessment of cerebral oedema are always nursing considerations in fluid administration.

DISTURBANCES OF ACID-BASE BALANCE

The ability of the body to regulate the acid-base status is one of its most crucial physiological functions. Many disease states, such as diarrhoea, vomiting or febrile conditions, are complicated by disturbances in the acid-base balance, which are often more hazardous to the child's survival than the primary disease process. Sometimes, simply providing adequate hydration, replacing electrolytes and correcting acid-base disturbances are all that is needed to sustain an infant or child until the primary disorder has run its course.

ACID-BASE IMBALANCE

A disturbance of acid-base equilibrium in the direction of acidosis or alkalosis may come about in a variety of ways. However, very simply stated, *acidosis (acidaemia)* results either from accumulation of acid or from loss of base, and *alkalosis (alkalaemia)* results either from accumulation of base or from loss of acid.

HYDROGEN ION CONCENTRATION
The pH represents the concentration of H^+ in solution and indicates only whether the imbalance is acidic or alkaline. It does not reflect the nature of the imbalance; that is, whether it is metabolic or respiratory in origin.

In a simple pH disturbance, there is a single primary factor that affects one component of the acid-base pair. This is accompanied by a compensatory or secondary response which attempts to correct the deviation.

The laboratory tests of value in the assessment of acid-base status are outlined in Table 24-3. The three variables are serum pH, serum $PaCO_2$ (the respiratory component), and serum HCO_3^- (the metabolic component). A summary of the relationship between these variables and compensatory responses is outlined in Table 24-4.

The major signs and symptoms of H^+ imbalance, acidosis or alkalosis, reflect central nervous system involvement. In respiratory and metabolic acidosis, depression of the central nervous system manifests as lethargy, diminished mental capacity, delirium, stupor, and coma. Alkalosis, however, produces stimulation and excitement of the central nervous system, manifesting as excitability, nervousness, tingling sensations, and in extreme cases, tetany progressing to convulsions.

ASSOCIATED DISTURBANCES IN ACID-BASE BALANCE

Physiological functions of the body take place optimally when the pH is maintained within a normal range. In addition, electrolyte shifts that take place in response to changes in pH alter the electrolyte concentration in the fluid compartments to disturb the normal concentrations. For example, cell membrane permeability is affected by changes in pH. A lowered pH allows K^+ to move from the ICF to the ECF. Serum K^+ levels increase with acidosis and decrease with alkalosis.

Serum potassium
One of the disturbances that complicates both fluid losses and acid-base imbalance is an alteration in K^+ levels. During dehydration, fluid moves out of the ICF compartment into the ECF compartment in an attempt to balance the fluid losses. In doing so, K^+ also moves out, creating a total body K^+ depletion. Since renal function is drastically reduced in dehydration, normal excretion of K^+ does not take place. This causes elevated serum levels that can produce all the signs and symptoms of hyperkalaemia. During rapid rehydration therapy for gastrointestinal losses and diabetic ketoacidosis, the ECF K^+ moves back into the ICF compartment, thereby posing the risk of hypokalaemia unless there is an anticipated replacement. However, K^+ is not replaced until the ICF is sufficient to restore adequate renal function.

ABBREVIATION	TEST	NORMAL VALUES*	DESCRIPTION
pH	Partial pressure of hydrogen	Birth: 7.11-7.36 1 day: 7.29-7.45 Child: 7.35-7.45	Expression of hydrogen ion concentration
$PaCO_2$	Partial pressure of carbon dioxide or carbon dioxide tension	Newborn: 3.6-5.3kPa Infant: 3.6-5.5kPa Girls: 4.3-6.0kPa Boys: 4.7-6.4kPa	Measure of carbon dioxide tension: reflects carbonic acid (H_2CO_3) concentration of plasma
HCO_3 (serum) arterial	Carbon dioxide content or carbon dioxide combining power	Infant: 21-28 mmol/L	Concentration of base bicarbonate
BE	Base excess (whole blood)	Newborn: -2 to -10 Infant: -1 to -7 Child: +2 to -4 Thereafter: +3 to -3	Used to express extent of deviation from normal buffer base concentration; indicates quantity of blood buffers remaining after hydrogen ion is buffered

*Data from Behrman and Vaughan, III, 1987.

Table 24-3 Laboratory tests employed in assessment of acid-base status.

DISTURBANCE	PLASMA pH	PLASMA $PaCO_2$	PLASMA HCO_3
Respiratory acidosis	↓	↑	↑
Respiratory alkalosis	↑	↓	↓
Metabolic acidosis	↓	↓	↓
Metabolic alkalosis	↑	↑	↑

Table 24-4 Summary of simple acid-base disturbances (partially compensated).

Serum calcium

Disturbed ECF calcium (Ca^{2+}) levels may occur in various types of dehydration. Usually, the disturbance is in the form of reduced serum Ca^{2+} levels, especially where there is a concomitant potassium loss. Although hypocalcaemia is a common finding, it rarely reaches a point of tetany in current practice, which includes adequate replacement of potassium losses. Immediate effects of Ca^{2+} imbalance associated with acidosis or alkalosis are tetany of metabolic alkalosis; long-term effects of chronic acidosis are related to bone reabsorption from renal disturbances.

Oxygen combination

The capacity of oxygen (O_2) to combine with haemoglobin is also affected by changes in pH. The affinity of haemoglobin for O_2 decreases with a decrease in pH so that, in a state of acidosis, less O_2 will be picked up by the haemoglobin as blood travels through the lungs. However, O_2 is more easily released to the tissues when the pH is lowered. The opposite effects operate during an increase in pH.

Blood flow

Blood flow in various areas is altered by changes in pH. Pulmonary circulation constricts in acidosis, whereas decreased pH (acidosis) causes vasodilation in systemic vessels.

NURSING RESPONSIBILITIES IN FLUID AND ELECTROLYTE DISTURBANCES

Nursing observation and intervention are essential to the detection and therapeutic management of disturbances in fluid and electrolyte balance. There are a wide variety of circumstances in which imbalances may be precipitated, and the balance is so precarious, especially in infants, that changes can take place in a very short time. Therefore, an important nursing responsibility is perceptive observation for any signs of imbalance, particularly in situations and conditions in which imbalance is likely to occur.

Nurses need to be comfortable with equipment used to deliver fluids to infants and children, and should be familiar with the knowledge and techniques for assessment. An understanding of normal serum levels provides additional data on which to base assessments and interventions, and on which to validate observations. Data that are helpful in assessment related to fluid and electrolyte balance are the medical diagnosis, the treatment that the child is receiving (especially medications and fluid therapies), laboratory reports, history, and records of intake and output. An important nursing role in child care is teaching parents to recognize early signs of dehydration.

ASSESSMENT

Whether the child is at home, in the clinic or in the hospital, nursing assessment is an essential part of the nursing care plan. The assessment of suspected or potential fluid and electrolyte disturbance begins with the observation of general appearance. Ill children usually have drawn, flaccid expressions, and their eyes are lacklustre. Loss of appetite is one of the first behaviours observed in the majority of childhood illnesses, and the infant's or child's activity level is diminished. The cry of an ill infant is less vigorous, often whining, and higher pitched than usual. The child is irritable, seeks the comfort and attention of the parent, and displays purposeless movements and inappropriate responses to people and familiar things. As the child's illness becomes more severe, the irritability progresses to lethargy and even unconsciousness.

HISTORY

Much of the information regarding the child's behaviour can be elicited from the parent. In addition to initial observations, a good history is extremely valuable to the assessment. The amount and type of intake and output (especially abnormal output) are important. An accurate estimate of fluid losses is beyond the capacity of history givers, but rough estimates of excessive fluid losses or diminished output can usually be obtained from information such as the number and consistency of stools the child has passed in the past 24 hours, the number of times the child voided, and the type and amount of food and fluid ingested or vomited. Parents frequently omit this information from their discussion with the health professional. They tell how much has been taken, but not how much was excreted unless asked specifically for this information.

Both the type and the amount of intake provide valuable information. The quality and quantity can be determined, if intake is sustained, excessive or curtailed. Loss early in diarrhoeal illness progresses rapidly, and the water losses can exceed sodium losses, leading to hypernatraemia. Hypernatraemic dehydration indicates a significant interference with water intake. Also important is a history of normal or increased intake of an unusual fluid such as one containing sugar, tea, athletic hydration fluid or other solute-containing fluids, which can contribute to hyponatraemic dehydration in the face of abnormal losses (Finberg, 1990).

History of gradual weight gain and observations of any puffiness, especially in areas with less dense tissues (periorbital, scrotal), or 'clothes fitting tighter' offer early clues to oedema. History of excessive intake, especially when associated with diminished output, is important in assessing oedema and water intoxication.

CLINICAL OBSERVATIONS

Tachycardia, the earliest manifestation of dehydration, can also be produced by fever and infection; therefore, these are considered in the assessment of dehydration. Dry skin and mucous membranes usually appear early. A sunken fontanelle is a useful observation if the configuration of the fontanelle is known when the child is healthy. Signs of circulatory failure usually indicate severe dehydration, since compensatory mechanisms are able to sustain blood pressure in the low normal range for some time. Loss of skin elasticity, generally manifest in children less than two years of age, is measured by the length of time it takes for pinched abdominal skin to recoil. This sign is also observed in undernourished children. Also, in hypertonic dehydration the skin has a smooth, velvety feel before it develops disturbed elasticity.

Capillary filling time is assessed by pinching the abdominal skin, a toe, or a thumb and estimating the time that blood is observed to return. Capillary filling time in mild dehydration is less than two seconds, increasing to more than three seconds in severe dehydration. The technique is effective in children of all ages. However, it can be altered in the presence of heart failure, which affects circulation time, and hypertonic dehydration, in which fluid loss is primarily intracellular.

When caring for the ill child, vital signs are assessed as often as every 15-30 minutes, and weight is recorded frequently during the initial phase of therapy. It is important to use the same scale each time the child is weighed and to predetermine the weight of any equipment or devices that must remain attached during the weighing process, including arm boards and sandbags. Routine weights should be taken at the same time each day.

INTAKE AND OUTPUT MEASUREMENT

One of the most important roles of the nurse in fluid and electrolyte disturbance is related to intake and output (I & O). Accurate measurements are essential to the assessment of fluid balance. Measurements from all sources — including both gastrointestinal and parenteral intake and output from urine, stools, vomitus, fistulas, nasogastric suction, sweat, and drainage from wounds — must be taken and considered.

Infants or small children who are unable to use a bedpan or those who have bowel movements with every voiding will require the application of a collecting device. If collecting bags are not used, wet nappies or pads are carefully weighed to ascertain the amount of fluid lost. This includes liquid stool, vomitus and other losses. The volume of fluid in millilitres is approximately equivalent to the weight of the fluid measured in grams. The specific gravity as a measure of osmolality is determined with a urinometer and assists in assessing the degree of hydration.

Disadvantages of the weighed nappy method of fluid measurement include: (1) inability to differentiate one type of loss from another because of admixture; (2) loss of urine or liquid stool from leakage or evaporation, especially if the infant is under a radiant warmer; and (3) additional fluid in nappy (superabsorbent disposable type) from absorption of atmospheric moisture (high-humidity incubators) (Hermansen and Buches, 1987 and 1988). Evaporative losses render measurements inaccurate unless the nappy is weighed and measured for specific gravity at least every 30 minutes when critical values are needed. Evaporative losses are greater in infants under radiant warmers or being treated with phototherapy.

ORAL FLUID INTAKE

Under ordinary circumstances, an adequate oral intake is no problem in children who are able to respond to thirst cues. Hydration becomes a nursing problem when infants or children are unable to respond to the thirst mechanism and when fatigue or discomfort makes them reluctant to swallow. Children with elevated temperatures, those with continued gastrointestinal losses, and those with labile diabetes are especially prone to dehydration. Occasionally, dehydration caused by inadequate intake has been observed in breast-fed infants.

When an electrolyte formula is prescribed, it is advisable to have the parents demonstrate their ability to prepare it, because a mistake or misunderstanding of measurements (e.g., substitution of a tablespoon for the teaspoon measure, using heaped rather than level measurements, or adding other ingredients, such as milk) can significantly alter the electrolyte concentration.

Persuading a reluctant child to drink fluids can be a nursing challenge and is not uncommon in the care of infants and children. Older children will often respond to the challenge of meeting a specific goal for fluid intake (or deprivation) and can be active participants in planning an intake schedule. Contracts and rewards are effective strategies. However, young children require more creative tactics.

THE CHILD WHO IS NBM

Infants or children who are unable or not permitted to take fluids by mouth (NBM) have special needs. To ensure they do not receive fluids, a sign can be placed in some obvious place, such as over their beds or pinned to their shirts, to alert others to the NBM status. Fluids are removed from the bedside to reduce the temptation. Drinking fountains and wash basins are monitored.

Oral hygiene, a part of routine hygienic care, is especially important when fluids are restricted or withheld (see Chapter 8). For young children who cannot brush their teeth or rinse their mouths without swallowing fluid, the mouth and teeth can be cleaned and kept moist by swabbing with saline-moistened gauze or other appliance. Judicious administration of ice chips provides moist, cool relief (if permitted by the practitioner). A thin layer of petrolatum or other commercial lip aid helps to keep lips soft and prevents cracking and caking. To meet the need to suck, infants could be provided with a dummy.

The child on restricted fluids provides an equal challenge. Limiting fluids is often more difficult for the child than NBM, especially when IV fluids are also eliminated. To make certain the child does not drink the entire amount allowed early in the day, the daily allotment is calculated to provide fluids at periodic intervals throughout the child's waking hours. Serving the fluids in small containers gives the illusion of larger servings. No extra liquid is left at the bedside if compliance is a problem.

PARENTERAL FLUID THERAPY

Since most hospitalized infants and children with serious disturbance of fluid and electrolyte balance are maintained with IV fluids, monitoring IV fluid replacement is a major nursing responsibility. Most of the general principles of IV therapy apply to infants and children, but with several important variations. **N.B.:** In an emergency, an intraossseous infusion may be used.

INTRAVENOUS INFUSION

Before an IV infusion is started, several preparatory activities must take place. All needed equipment is gathered so that the operator can proceed without interruption. More importantly, the child and the family must be prepared for this universally stressful procedure.

Solution

The composition of IV solution is selected on the basis of tonicity (osmolality) and electrolyte content. A solution that is *isotonic* has the same osmolality, or tonicity, as body fluids such as plasma. A *hypertonic* solution is one that has a greater concentration of solutes than plasma; a *hypotonic* solution has a lower concentration. Examples of isotonic solutions are 0.9% saline solutions and 5% dextrose in water; 10% glucose in water is a hypertonic solution; plain water and 0.2% sodium are hypotonic solutions.

PREPARING THE CHILD AND PARENTS

Children of any age are anxious and fearful of injections, and unless the IV infusion is implemented as an emergency procedure, there will be time to prepare them. The use of emlacream is now commonplace.

PROCEDURE

The site selected for IV infusion depends on accessibility and convenience. In older children, any accessible vein may be used. Whenever possible, it is best to avoid the child's favoured hand in order to reduce the disability related to the procedure. A site is chosen that restricts the child's movements as little as possible — a site over a joint in an extremity is avoided. An older child can help to select the site and thereby maintain some measure of control. In small infants, a superficial vein of the wrist, hand, foot, arm or scalp is usually convenient and most easily stabilized.

Locating a vein may be difficult because the veins are smaller and children have a significant amount of subcutaneous fat. When veins are not readily visible, applying a warm compress to the site or, when using an extremity, holding the limb in a dependent position below body level will help fill the veins for better visualization. Gentle tapping sometimes causes the veins to stand out. A flashlight held against the skin below the intended site sometimes assists in locating vessels. If these measures do not help, a tourniquet applied with light pressure medially to the site may be needed. Although the tourniquet makes the veins more visible and provides a more rapid blood return, the added venous pressure may cause fragile veins to 'blow' when punctured, producing a haematoma.

Following insertion, the cannula is firmly secured at the puncture site with nonallergenic tape and protected from becoming dislodged by immobilization of the extremity. The insertion site and about one inch of skin beyond the site are left uncovered for early detection of infiltration. Clear plastic dressings are ideal, because they allow ready visualization of the insertion site. Some finger or toe areas are left unoccluded by dressings or tape to allow for assessment of circulation. The thumb is never immobilized, because of the danger of contractures with limited movement later on. A plastic or wax paper cup that is cut in half (with the rigid edges covered with tape) and applied directly over the cannula site will further protect the infusion. Some needle containers make excellent protective covers. A colourful and interesting sticker can be applied to the armboard or protecting device to add a positive note to the procedure.

Older children who are alert and cooperative can usually be trusted to protect the IV site. An IV infusion is not always a deterrent to mobility. When the child is feeling well and the insertion site is well secured, the child can be held or be walked, but precautions must be observed to preserve the integrity of the IV system.

Infants, small children, and uncooperative children require varying degrees of immobilization, and on rare occasions, complete restriction of movement may be needed to prevent removal of the IV infusion. The board is secured to the bed, and the remaining extremities that might be used to dislodge the needle are restrained. This includes feet as well as hands, since most infants will attempt to brush away the offending attachment by rubbing it against another extremity or body part.

Immobilization is intolerable to the naturally active child, and every effort should be extended to relieve the stress of immobilization (see Chapter 33).

When it comes time to discontinuing an IV infusion, many children are distressed by the thought of cannula removal. Therefore, they need a careful explanation of the process and suggestions for helping.

Complications

The same precautions regarding maintenance of asepsis, prevention of infection and observation for infiltration are carried out with patients of any age. However, infiltration is more difficult to detect in infants and small children than in adults. The increased amount of subcutaneous fat and the amount of tape used to secure the needle often obscure the signs of early infiltration. When the fluid appears to be infusing too slowly or ceases, the usual assessment for obstructions within the apparatus, that is, kinks, three-way taps, and positioning interference (e.g., a bent elbow), often locates the difficulty. When these actions fail to detect the problem, it may be necessary to carefully remove some of the tape and other material that obscure a clear view of the venepuncture site. Dependent areas, such as the palm and undersides of the extremity or the occiput and behind the ears, are examined.

Since IV therapy is often used in paediatrics and tends to be difficult to maintain, extravasation injuries are reported with relative frequency. Several drugs are toxic to subcutaneous tissues and can result in varying degrees of damage with extended hospitalization and treatment. The IV infusion is discontinued and the cannula removed as soon as extravasation is recognized. The affected limb is elevated to promote venous return, and the area is assessed every 15 minutes for approximately two hours. No heat is applied to the area.

Prevention of infection is a major nursing function during IV therapy. The infusion site is protected from trauma and entry of bacteria. When an IV infusion continues for several days or longer, the tubing and bottle are changed at regular intervals according to hospital policy. Frequency ranges from every 24-72 hours — most often every 48 hours. To ensure that the equipment is changed regularly, it is labelled with the date and time that the new bottle and tubing are attached. Any signs of inflammation, such as redness or pain, should be reported immediately. This usually requires removal of the infusion and restarting it at another site.

LONG-TERM VENOUS ACCESS

Even greater mobility is possible with the use of some form of venous access device (VAD). The heparin lock is used as an alternative for a keep-open infusion when extended access to a vein is required without the need for fluid. It is most frequently employed for intermittent infusion of medication into a peripheral venous route. A short, flexible catheter is used for the heparin lock device, and a site is selected where there will be minimum movement, such as the forearm. The needle is inserted and secured in the same manner as any IV infusion device, but the needle hub is occluded with a stopper.

The type of device used may vary among medical establishments, and the care and use of the heparin lock are carried out according to the specific protocol of the institution or unit. However, the general concept is the same. The catheter remains in place and is flushed with heparin following infusion of the medication. The heparin solution prevents blood from clotting in the device between infusions. Children may be discharged with a heparin lock in place, so they can continue receiving medications without hospitalization. Heparin locks are usually reserved for children who require medications on a short-term basis. Those who require long-term chemotherapy are best managed with a central VAD.

The children and parents are taught the procedure before discharge from hospital, including preparation and injection of the prescribed medication, the heparin flush, and dressing changes.

CENTRAL VENOUS CATHETERS

Other alternatives for long-term venous access include the indwelling central venous catheters (Broviac or Hickman catheters) and implanted infusion ports (Infus-A-Port, MediPort, Port-a-cath).

With the patient under local or general anaesthesia, the central venous catheter of choice is placed with aseptic technique. A vein, such as the jugular or subclavian, is entered through a small cutdown site, and the catheter is threaded to the junction of the superior vena cava and right atrium, confirmed by fluoroscopic dye injection, and then sutured in place. To stabilize the catheter and reduce the risk of infection, the remainder is tunnelled beneath the skin to exit through a small incision at a convenient location on the anterior aspect of the chest or upper abdomen (Fig. 24-2). One or two Dacron cuffs on the catheter remain in the subcutaneous tunnel; as tissue adheres to the cuff, the cuff provides a barrier to infection. The cutdown site is surgically closed, the catheter is sutured to the skin at the exit site, and a sterile dressing is applied.

INTRAVENOUS ALIMENTATION

Total parenteral nutrition (TPN), also known as intravenous alimentation or hyperalimentation, provides for the total nutritional needs of infants or children whose lives are threatened because feeding by way of the gastrointestinal tract is impossible, inadequate or hazardous. Common conditions for which TPN is used therapeutically include chronic intestinal obstruction from peritoneal sepsis or adhesions, bowel fistulae, inadequate intestinal length, chronic non-remitting severe diarrhoea, extensive body burns, and abdominal tumours treated by surgery, irradiation and chemotherapy. TPN may also be initiated prophylactically when prolonged starvation is expected.

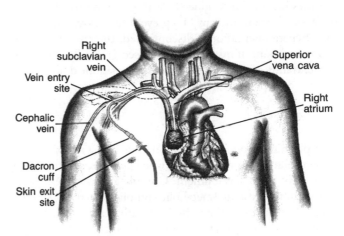

Fig. 24-2 Central venous catheter insertion and exit site.

The highly irritating nature of concentrated glucose precludes the use of the small peripheral veins in most instances. However, dilute glucose-protein hydrolysates that are appropriate for infusing into peripheral veins are being used with increasing frequency. When peripheral veins are used, intralipids become the major calorie source. This fat solution cannot be mixed with the glucose solutions; it requires administration through a multilumen catheter or a separate bottle and tubing that enters the circuit near the venous entry site, through a Y-type of injection adapter. **N.B.:** Now available is a combination solution for short-term peripheral feeding (e.g. Vitrimix).

The major nursing responsibilities are the same as for any IV therapy: control of sepsis, monitoring of infusion rate and continuous observations.

The infusion is maintained at a uniform rate by means of a constant infusion pump. This requires accurate calculation of the rate required to deliver a measured amount in a given length of time. Since alterations in flow rate are relatively common, the drip should be checked frequently to ensure an even, continuous infusion. If for some reason the infusion rate slows, the rate should not be increased to compensate for the uninfused amount.

General assessments such as vital signs, intake and output measurements, and checking results of laboratory tests facilitate early detection of infection or fluid and electrolyte imbalance. Additional amounts of K^+ and Na^+ are often required in hyperalimentation; therefore, observation for signs of K^+ or Na^+ deficit or excess is part of nursing care. This is rarely a problem, except in children with reduced renal function or metabolic defects.

Hyperglycaemia may occur during the first day or two as the child adapts to the high-glucose load of the hyperalimentation solution. Addition of insulin may be required to assist the body's adjustment to the hyperglycaemia. Nursing responsibilities include blood glucose testing to monitor the effectiveness of insulin therapy. To prevent hypoglycaemia at the time hyperalimentation is discontinued, the rate of infusion and the amount of insulin are decreased gradually. The high concentration of glucose may produce an osmotic diuresis with the risk of hypertonic dehydration.

COMPLICATIONS

Complications from TPN are numerous, and a major nursing responsibility is to prevent these, when possible, and to be alert to signs of their development. Complications either (1) are related to the infusate (metabolic complications) or (2) result from the presence of the indwelling catheter.

Metabolic complications are associated with the infant's or child's capacity for the various components of the hyperalimentation solution. Excessive intake of any of the components will create an imbalance, such as hyperglycaemia, azotaemia, acid-base disorders, anaemia, bone demineralization, vitamin and mineral deficiencies, hyperosmotic dehydration and coma, fluid overload and a variety of electrolyte imbalances.

Liver disease is the most important gastrointestinal complication in paediatric populations. The cause is obscure, but liver disease appears to be more prevalent in preterm infants who have minimum enteral feedings and who were begun on TPN at an early age. Affected children develop cholestasis, hepatocellular necrosis, and, in advanced disease, cirrhosis or hepatic failure. Manifestations include hepatomegaly; jaundice; and elevated serum transaminase, bilirubin, and alkaline phosphatase levels, which become evident approximately two weeks after initiation of TPN. Cholelithiasis is an uncommon but possible occurrence in paediatric patients. Therefore, children on TPN should be assessed periodically for signs and symptoms of cholelithiasis and/or cholecystitis.

Catheter-related complications include those involving catheter placement such as pneumothorax, haemothorax, perforation and catheter dislodgement. However, the major complication associated with the catheter is infection: infection at catheter entrance site, catheter 'seeding' sepsis, venous thrombosis with infection and embolization, and endocarditis.

CONDITIONS THAT PRODUCE FLUID AND ELECTROLYTE IMBALANCE

Fluid and electrolyte disturbances are common in the paediatric age group. Acute attacks of vomiting and diarrhoea are so common in this group that they can almost be regarded as part of normal life. However, the nature of the anatomical and physiological structure of the infant and small child renders them particularly vulnerable to imbalances when pathological changes affect the fluid compartments. The most serious disturbances involve the gastrointestinal tract or the cardiovascular system, and losses resulting from massive burn injury.

GASTROINTESTINAL DISORDERS

The numerous secretions of the gastrointestinal (GI) tract are produced in large amounts, but under ordinary conditions most fluid is reabsorbed in the lower bowel. Except for saliva, which is hypotonic, the total solute concentration in most of the GI secretions is similar to that of interstitial fluid, but there are marked differences in electrolyte composition among the secretions. Consequently, fluid lost from the GI tract depends largely on the composition of the fluid that is lost. Fluid losses from the GI tract in vomiting, diarrhoea or other routes (fistula, nasogastric tube) not only produce rapid and profound depletion of extracellular volume, but can cause marked distortion in the electrolyte composition as well. Most illnesses create some disturbance in body fluids or electrolytes, and in many children these disturbances are more threatening than the primary disorder. Replacement requires careful attention to both volume and solute composition.

DIARRHOEA

Diarrhoea is a symptom that can result from disorders involving digestive, absorptive and secretory functions. It is usually defined as an increase in the number of stools or a decrease in their consistency. However, there are wide variations in colonic function between individuals. For example, normally one infant may have one firm stool every second or third day, whereas another normally passes from five to eight small, soft stools daily. More important are: (1) a noticeable or sudden increase in number of stools, (2) a reduction in their consistency with an increase in fluid content, and (3) a tendency for the stools to be greenish in colour.

Diarrhoea may be acute or chronic, inflammatory or noninflammatory, and the physiological consequences vary considerably in relation to its severity, duration, associated symptoms, child's age and the child's nutritional status before the onset of diarrhoea. Diarrhoea related to inflammatory processes is usually described as *gastroenteritis*, and the terms are often used interchangeably.

AETIOLOGY

Diarrhoea can be attributed to many specific causes, mechanisms and predisposing factors. Several major mechanisms produce diarrhoea in infants or children who are susceptible or exposed to a causative agent, and more than one mechanism may be operative (Box 24-1). Some agents create their effect by direct invasion of the intestinal tract; others exert their effect through parenteral means.

Acute diarrhoea
Acute diarrhoea, a sudden change in frequency and consistency of stools, is often caused by an inflammatory process of infectious origin, but may also be the result of toxic reaction to ingestion of poisons, dietary indiscretions, or infection outside

the alimentary tract (Box 24-2). Most are self-limited and will ultimately subside without specific treatment if consequent dehydration does not create a serious complication.

Antibiotic therapy is a common cause of diarrhoea in children. Antibiotics such as ampicillin, neomycin and tetracyclines cause a decrease in glucose absorption and disaccharidase activity. They should be discontinued and a lactose-free diet implemented if diarrhoea occurs. Antibiotics can also cause diarrhoea by allowing an overgrowth of a bacterium responsible for pseudomembranous colitis.

Severe diarrhoea

Severe diarrhoea is largely a problem of infants and very young children. Regardless of the cause, successful management relies primarily on appropriate treatment of physiological disturbances and is only secondarily concerned with specific treatment of the aetiological agent. Severe diarrhoea warrants hospitalization, comprehensive evaluation, and parenteral fluid therapy. Intravenous fluid therapy is directed towards rapid replacement of: (1) the fluid deficit, (2) ongoing normal losses, and (3) abnormal ongoing losses. The magnitude of the deficit is determined from loss of body weight and ongoing losses by calculating the energy requirements of the child. The energy requirements include not only predicted caloric expenditure for age and size, but other factors that increase the use of energy, such as elevated temperature (metabolism increases by about 12% for each 1°C) and hyperventilation. Additional

replacement covers abnormal losses as determined by output measurement, weight and electrolyte determinations.

Once the severe effects of dehydration are under control, specific diagnostic and therapeutic measures are instigated to detect and to treat the cause of the diarrhoea.

The frequency and volume of stools will subside within 48 hours in fasted patients receiving intravenous fluids. The caloric intake is increased gradually until the usual dietary intake is re-established, usually within 7-8 days.

Chronic diarrhoea

Chronic diarrhoea, the passage of loose stools with increased frequency of more than two weeks' duration, is likely to be associated with disorders of malabsorption, anatomical defects, abnormal bowel motility, hypersensitivity (allergic) reaction or a long-term inflammatory response.

◆ **BOX 24-1**

Mechanisms known to produce diarrhoea

Osmotic factors Osmotic gradients cause water to passively cross intestinal mucosa in isotonic proportions. Unabsorbed solutes create an osmotic gradient that results in movement of sodium and water in the intestinal lumen (e.g., ingestion of nonabsorbable solutes and malabsorption of water-soluble nutrients).

Diminished absorption or increased secretion of water and electrolytes. Diminished absorption of solutes causes decreased absorption of water and electrolytes (e.g., mucosal disease). Increased secretion can result from passive secretion secondary to inflammation or active secretion secondary to stimulation of mucosal cells (e.g., toxin-producing bacteria).

Reduction in anatomical or functional surface area. The anatomically short bowel has reduced absorptive surfaces to absorb all ingested substances.

Altered motility. Both hypermotility and hypomotility reduce the amount of substance absorbed by the intestinal mucosa.

Data from Silverman and Roy, 1983.

◆ **BOX 24-2**

Causes of acute diarrhoea

Dietary
Overfeeding
Introduction of new foods
Unripe fruit
Reinstituting milk too soon after diarrhoeal episode
Osmotic diarrhoea from excess sugar or fat in formula
Toxic
Ingestion of:
• Heavy metals (arsenic, lead, mercury)
• Organic phosphates
• Ferrous sulphate
• Antibiotics
Enteropathological
Bacteria: *Escherichia coli, Shigella, Salmonella, Yersinia enterocolitica, Campylobacter, Staphylococcus aureus, Clostridium perfringens, Vibro cholerae, Vibro parahaemolyticus,* tuberculosis
Viruses: Adenoviruses, rotavirus, parvovirus-like organisms
Infestations: Amoebiasis, giardiasis, ascariasis, coccidioidosis
Parenteral Infection
Communicable diseases
Upper respiratory tract infections
Urinary tract infections
Otitis media
Inflammatory Bowel Disease
Necrotizing enterocolitis of the newborn
Enterocolitis secondary to Hirschsprung disease
Emotional
Episodes of nervous excitement
Periods of emotional tension
Fatigue
Psychogenic 'irritable colon syndrome' in hyperactive children

Intractable diarrhoea of infancy

Intractable diarrhoea of infancy is a syndrome defined as diarrhoea occurring in the first three months of life that persists for longer than two weeks with no recognized pathogens, and is refractory to treatment. It is classified as either primary, which is identified as nonspecific enterocolitis, or secondary, which is associated with disease entities such as allergy, bowel anomalies, or a variety of congenital diseases. The age of onset ranges from four days to three months.

The primary form, although the triggering factor is not well defined, may be secondary to such trivial causes as an infection or feeding difficulties, but in most cases no predisposing cause can be identified. The immediate concerns are dehydration and electrolyte imbalances, but these children universally suffer from malnutrition and its consequences. Because the diarrhoea occurs during a period of high caloric need, affected infants can quickly become severely ill.

The diarrhoea rapidly becomes self-perpetuating through a combination of secondary consequences: malnutrition deprives the infant of the elements protein, vitamins, calcium and magnesium needed for mucosal regeneration; the villi of the small intestine atrophy; the bowel wall becomes inflamed and irritated by undigested foodstuffs or microorganisms; and secondary digestive and absorptive disorders develop as a result of malnutrition, various patterns of motility, and overgrowth of bacteria caused by the infant's debilitated state.

CLINICAL MANIFESTATIONS

The most serious and immediate physiological disturbances associated with severe diarrhoeal disease are: (1) dehydration, (2) acid-base derangements with acidosis, and (3) shock that occurs when dehydration progresses to the point that circulatory status is seriously disturbed (see Dehydration). Mild diarrhoea is described as a few loose stools each day without other evidence of illness that terminates in a few days. With moderate diarrhoea the child is sicker, may have a fever, vomits, appears fretful and irritable, and passes several loose or watery stools daily. Although the child may not gain weight or may even show a slight loss, signs of dehydration are usually absent.

In severe diarrhoea, the child has numerous to continuous stools and evidence of moderate to severe diarrhoea; the child is drawn, flaccid, and expressionless; the eyes lack lustre; and the cry lacks vigour and is often whining and higher pitched than usual. The child is irritable, seeks the comfort and attention of the parents, and displays purposeless movements and inappropriate responses to people and familiar things. The child may become lethargic, moribund or comatosed.

Fluid losses and metabolic acidosis in severe diarrhoea contribute to rapid deterioration in diarrhoeal disease in infancy (Box 24-3), and although the fluid deficit cannot be stated precisely, it can be estimated from changes in body weight and objective clinical signs.

Alterations in body potassium occur in association with both fluid losses and acidosis. Potassium is continually lost in stools,

---

◆ **BOX 24-3**

Consequences of diarrhoea

Dehydration

Voluminous losses of fluid and electrolytes in frequent watery stools

Losses when there is frequent vomiting

Reduced fluid intake resulting from nausea or anorexia

Increased insensible losses from fever, hyperpnoea and, sometimes, high environmental temperature

Continued (although diminished) obligatory renal losses

Metabolic Acidosis

Losses of bicarbonate, sodium and potassium in diarrhoeal stools

Impaired renal function

Accumulation of lactic acid from tissue hypoxia secondary to hypovolaemia

Ketosis from fat metabolism when glycogen stores are depleted in untreated diarrhoeal dehydration or inadequate carbohydrate intake

---

cellular potassium leaves the cells in exchange for sodium and hydrogen ions entering the cells, and potassium is lost from cells damaged by hypoxia. Thus, the cellular potassium is seriously depleted. However, because renal excretion is impaired as a result of the circulatory adjustments, the serum levels of potassium are normal or even elevated. When circulatory volume and renal function are restored, potassium redistribution and excretion may produce a potassium deficit unless adequate amounts are restored during rehydration.

PROCESS OF DIAGNOSIS

The history provides valuable information regarding exposure to infectious agents, personal contact, travel, or probable contact with contaminated foods. Allergic and dietary history may indicate food sensitivities or allergies. Crowding and close person-to-person contact, as in institutions, make epidemics with any enteric pathogen more likely.

Most acute, inflammatory diarrhoeas are infectious, and the type of stools and symptoms associated with diarrhoea provide clues to the organism. For example, fever is not a symptom of *Escherichia coli* disease until late, whereas it is a common early feature even in mild cases of shigellosis. Abdominal cramps are also common in shigellosis. Explosive onset of diarrhoea accompanied by or preceded by vomiting suggests food poisoning. Although vomiting may occur in all infectious diarrhoeas, it is not a major feature.

Laboratory examination

The specimen obtained from evacuated stool should include mucus or tissue shreds, if present.

Rectal swabs for culture are indicated for a rotazyme test or whenever a bacterial agent is suspected. Serum electrolyte values are obtained in the young infant who is hospitalized with diarrhoea because of the likelihood of complicating dehydration and associated electrolyte imbalances, particularly in relation to sodium and potassium alterations. Dehydrated infants will have an elevated haematocrit as a result of volume loss, and elevated blood urea nitrogen will be found in the presence of reduced renal circulation.

THERAPEUTIC MANAGEMENT

Mild or moderate diarrhoea is usually managed by simple measures, and the child seldom requires hospitalization. When the moderate diarrhoea becomes worse or does not respond to simple measures, hospitalization is indicated. This provides the opportunity for closer observation and examination, and for a brief course of parenteral fluid therapy, which usually results in rapid improvement.

Rehydration
Orally administered rehydration solutions (ORS) are currently the therapy of choice in treatment of diarrhoea of any cause and in a wide range of age groups, except in severe dehydration or other complicating circumstances.

The usual approach is to administer ORS with initial fluid provided within 4-6 hours for mild or moderate dehydration. The amounts and rates are increased if the patient does not appear fully hydrated or continues to have diarrhoea. The amounts are decreased if the patient appears to be fully hydrated earlier than expected or if signs of overhydration (e.g., periorbital oedema) develop. Infants can be allowed to continue breast-feeding as desired after treatment has been started.

When oral rehydration is complete, maintenance therapy is begun. Most mild to moderate acute diarrhoea can be managed at home under careful health supervision. The volume of ORS ingested should equal the volume of stool losses.

The issue of continued or delayed feedings has not been resolved. Some advocate continuing the child's regular diet; others advise removing all milk for 24-36 hours. Research has indicated that infants recover from mild disease regardless of the carbohydrate ingested (Groothuis, Berman, and Chapman, 1986), and unrestricted diet does not appear to affect the course or symptoms in mild diarrhoea (Margolis *et al*, 1990). Breast milk is generally well tolerated by infants. The current trend is towards rapid resumption of the previous diet after oral or intravenous (IV) hydration.

Hypernatraemic diarrhoeal dehydration is usually managed by *slow* oral rehydration (over 12 hours) to avoid cerebral oedema with accompanying seizures (Pizarro, Posada and Levine, 1984).

Diluted fruit juices and soft drinks are not recommended for rehydration, especially in infants. The high carbohydrate content of these fluids aggravates the diarrhoea by an osmotic effect produced by nonabsorbable carbohydrate (Ghishan, 1988). Some antibiotics (such as ampicillin, which destroy

bacteria that normally break down and ferment carbohydrate) may increase the carbohydrate load in the colon. Cola soft drinks are deficient in electrolyte replacement, especially sodium and potassium (Ghishan, 1988; Weizman, 1986). Recently, observers have advocated cereals or rice as a source of glucose to reduce the osmolality of rehydration solution.

Lactose-free formulas are often substituted (Brown and MacLean, 1984), and investigators have found that introduction of a soy-based, lactose-free formula (usually diluted 50%) after the initial four hours of rehydration reduced stool output and duration of diarrhoea in most infants (Santosham *et al*, 1985). In some children, a secondary lactase deficiency may cause a temporary intolerance to milk and exacerbation of diarrhoea; therefore, reintroduction of lactose is attempted progressively. Milk is usually withheld until at least one week after the disappearance of symptoms, and the feeding consists of some type of hydrolysed lactose-free formula. Feeding lactose-containing formulas as a sole nutrient source can cause diarrhoea sufficient to increase the risk of dehydration in these children (Penny, Paredes and Brown, 1989).

Medications
Antimicrobial therapy is instituted in some types of diarrhoea. It significantly shortens the course of shigellosis and appears to be beneficial in *E. coli* infections, but does not affect the course of *Salmonella* disease. It is always indicated in bacteraemia, and parenteral infections are treated with appropriate drugs.

Antidiarrhoeal medications such as diphenoxylate hydrochloride with atropine sulphate are sometimes prescribed for older children, but are contraindicated in infants and children younger than two years of age, because of their narrow margin of safety.

Adsorbents, such as kaolin and pectin, alter consistency and cosmetic appearance of stools, and decrease the frequency of evacuation, but do not reduce the amount of fluid loss and may mask significant fluid losses.

ACUTE INFECTIOUS GASTROENTERITIS

When diarrhoea is presumed or established to be caused by a microorganism, the term infectious gastroenteritis or bacterial gastroenteritis is applied. In the paediatric age group, *infectious gastroenteritis* is second only to upper respiratory tract infections as a cause of illness (Silverman and Roy, 1983). Although ordinarily benign and self-limited, they are a major paediatric problem and account for a significant number of hospital admissions.

EPIDEMIOLOGY

A variety of organisms are responsible for GI tract disorders in infants and children, and most are spread by the faecal-oral route. Organisms can be transmitted by direct person-to-person contact (especially where sizeable groups are in direct contact, such as in daycare centres), animals (primarily family pets), foods (especially raw milk and poultry), and water (including swimming water). Most of the illnesses show seasonal variations. Viral gastroenteritis is seen more frequently in winter months; most bacterial disorders are more prevalent during the summer and autumn.

Although acute gastroenteritis affects all age groups, certain patterns are discernible. There is a greater frequency of diarrhoeal disease in younger children, and specific organisms are more prominent at different ages; for example, *E. coli* in the newborn, rotaviruses in children younger than two years of age, and *Giardia, Shigella, Yersinia* and *Campylobacter* in toddlers. The relative chance of a given illness being associated with *C. jejuni* is greater in older children. Adolescents who are sexually active are subject to enteric pathogens that are transmitted by sexual contact, as well as the traditional sexually transmitted organisms that present with diarrhoea or proctitis (e.g., *Neisseria gonorrhoeae, syphilis, Chlamydia* and herpes simplex).

Traveller's diarrhoea is a common problem for some persons travelling to other countries, especially developing countries. Daycare centres are a prime source of infection in younger children, especially in centres that care for children in nappies. Toddlers not only explore their environment with their mouths, but many are not toilet trained and engage in direct contact with other children and caregivers. Other persons at risk are children with immune system disorders.

CLINICAL MANIFESTATIONS

Infectious diarrhoeas have some features in common, such as vomiting, and there is frequently abdominal discomfort. Bacterial infections and some viral infections are accompanied by fever. The severity is variable among the various forms (Table 24-5).

PROCESS OF DIAGNOSIS

Laboratory confirmation of the specific organism confirms the diagnosis and serves as a guideline for appropriate medical therapy.

THERAPEUTIC MANAGEMENT

The primary concern in infectious gastroenteritis, as in all conditions in which fluid is lost in large amounts, is dehydration and the attendant deterioration. Fluid replacement and monitoring of electrolyte status with replacement are the same as for any diarrhoeal disorder. When the organism is identified, appropriate antibiotics are prescribed for those diarrhoeas for which specific therapy has been found to be effective.

IMPLICATIONS FOR NURSING

Basic nursing care for the infant or child with infectious gastroenteritis is the same as for any diarrhoeal disease. However, appropriate precautions are carried out to prevent the spread of the infection to others (see Infection Control, Chapter 8).

It may be necessary to obtain stool specimens from the child and other family members who are affected or suspected to be carriers of infectious organisms. The parents are provided with specimen containers and instructed in collection and disposition of stool samples.

VOMITING

Vomiting, a very common symptom in childhood, is usually of little concern. Often it is of a minor and temporary nature, but when vomiting is persistent and prolonged, the consequences to the infant or child can be rapid and serious. An associated hazard, especially in very young and debilitated infants and children, is the risk of aspiration with the possibility of asphyxiation, atelectasis or pneumonia.

The amount and character of the vomiting are important observations, and nurses should be able to distinguish between and describe the various forms this behaviour takes. *Vomiting* is the forcible ejection of stomach contents and is usually accompanied by nausea. In *projectile vomiting* vomitus is forcefully ejected as far as 0.6-1.2 m from the child. Projectile vomiting is not associated with nausea.

Vomiting in childhood can be caused by numerous intrinsic and extrinsic factors, but is usually caused by readily detected infections or psychological causes. Vomiting and diarrhoea are common manifestations of a variety of infectious disorders, responses to an allergen, or ingestion of drugs or other toxic substances, and symptoms associated with appendicitis or GI tract obstruction. Recurrent, prolonged, or persistent vomiting is also associated with encephalographic variations and results from increased intracranial pressure (ICP).

Many children are prone to motion sickness when riding in a car or aeroplane, or even when swinging in a swing. Some children, especially overly dependent children, maladjusted children or children who react to environmental stress (e.g., a high-anxiety home environment) with somatic symptoms, respond to tension or stress with stomach upset and vomiting.

ASSESSMENT

Vomiting is the first symptom of a variety of common infections, as well as a manifestation of more serious conditions. It is a relatively frequent symptom during the neonatal period, usually caused by simple regurgitation from overfeeding or insufficient winding, and has little clinical significance. However, it can indicate the presence of GI tract disorders or increased ICP. The following nursing observations can provide valuable information for evaluating the nature and importance of vomiting.

Character of vomitus
Oesophageal vomitus contains unchanged food and no gastric juice. A relaxed cardiac sphincter or rumination (habitual regurgitation) will produce frequent small amounts of vomitus emitted with little force. The presence of sour milk curds with

ORGANISM	PATHOLOGY	CHARACTERISTICS	COMMENTS
Viral agents			

Rotavirus
  Incubation period:
  1-3 days
	Remains unexplained
	Severely distorted
	  mucosal architecture
	  with atrophic mucosa
	  and severe inflammatory
	  changes
		Abrupt onset
		Fever (38°C or above)
		  lasting approxi-
		  mately 48 hours
		Associated upper
		  respiratory tract
		  infection
		Diarrhoea may persist
		  for more than a week
			Incidence higher in cool
			  weather (80% in winter)
			Affects all age groups; 6 to
			  24-month-old infants
			more vulnerable
			Usually mild and self-
			  limited
			Important cause of
			  nosocomial infections in
			  hospitals and
			  gastroenteritis in children
			  attending daycare centres

Norwalk-like
  organisms
Incubation period:
  1-3 days
	Mechanism of effect
	  unknown
	Blunting of villi and
	  inflammatory changes
	  in lamina propria
	Reduced enzymes
		Fever
		Loss of appetite
		Nausea/vomiting
		Abdominal pain
		Diarrhoea
		Malaise
			Source of infection: drink-
			  ing water, recreation
			  water, food (including
			  shellfish)
			Affects all ages
			Benign, seldom lasts more
			  than 3 days
			Self-limited (2-3 days)

Bacterial agents			

Pathogenic
  Escherichia coli
Incubation period:
  highly variable;
  depends on strain
	Usually caused by
	  enterotoxin production
	  (small bowel)
	Reduces absorption
	  and increases secretion
	  of fluids and
	  electrolytes
		Onset gradual or
		  abrupt
		Variable clinical
		  manifestations
		Most - green, watery
		  diarrhoea with mucus;
		  becomes explosive
		Vomiting may be
		  present from onset
		Abdominal distension
		Diarrhoea
		Fever; appears toxic
			Incidence higher in summer
			Usually interpersonal
			  transmission but may
			  transmit via inanimate
			  objects
			A cause of nursery
			  epidemics
			With symptomatic treat-
			  ment only, may continue for
			  weeks
			Full breast-feeding has a
			  protective effect
			Symptoms generally
			  subside in 3-7 days
			Relapse rate
			  approximately 20%

Salmonella groups
  (nontyphoidal)
  gram-negative, non-
  encapsulated, non
sporulating Incubation
  period: 6-72 hours for
  gastroenteritis (usu-
  ally less than 24); 3-
  60 days for enteric
  fever (usually 7-14)
	Penetration of lamina
	  propria (small bowel
	  and colon)
	Local inflammation –
	  no extensive
	  destruction
	Stimulation of intes –
	  tinal fluid excretion
	Systemic invasion of
	  other sites
		Rapid onset
		Variable symptoms –
		  mild to severe
		Nausea, vomiting, and
		  colicky abdominal
		  pain followed by
		  diarrhoea,
		  occasionally with
		  blood and mucus
		Chills may occur
			Two-thirds of patients are
			  younger than 20 years of
			  age; highest incidence in
			  children younger than
			  9 years, especially infants
			Highest incidence occurs
			  July through October,
			  lowest from January
			  through April
			Transmission primarily

(cont.)

Table 24-5 Enteropathological causes of acute gastroenteritis.

		Hyperactive peri-stalsis and mild abdominal tenderness Symptoms usually subside within 5 days May have fever, headache, and cerebral manifestations, e.g., drowsiness, confusion, meningismus, or seizures Infants may be afebrile and non-toxic May result in life-threatening septicaemia and meningitis	via contaminated food and drink - most from animal sources, including fowl, mammals, reptiles, and insects Most common sources are poultry and eggs In children - pets, e.g., dogs, cats, hamsters, and especially pet turtles Communicable as long as organisms are excreted
Salmonella typhimutium	Rapid invasion of bloodstream from minor sites of inflammation Marked inflammation and necrosis of intestinal mucosa and lymphatics	Variable in infants Older children - irregular fever, headache, malaise, lethargy Diarrhoea occurs in 50% at early stage Cough is common In a few days, fever rises and is consistent; fatigue, cough, abdominal pain, anorexia, and weight loss develop; diarrhoea begins	Decreased incidence in last decade Acute symptoms may persist for a week or more Transmitted by contaminated food or water (primary), infected animals (e.g., pet turtles)
Shigella groups - gram negative, nonmotile, anaerobic bacilli Incubation period: 1-7 days, usually 2-4	Enterotoxin Stimulates loss of fluids and electrolytes Invasion of epithelium with superficial mucosal ulcerations *S. dysenteriae* forms exotoxin	Onset variable but usually abrupt Fever and cramping abdominal pain initially Fever - may reach 40.5°C Convulsions in 10% - usually associated with fever Patients appears sick Headache, nuchal rigidity, delirium Watery diarrhoea with mucus and pus starts about 12-48 hours after onset Stools preceded by abdominal cramps; tenesmus and straining follow Symptoms usually subside in 5-10 days	Approximately 60% of cases in children younger than age 9 years with more than one third between ages 1 and 4 years Peak incidence late summer Transmitted directly or indirectly from infected persons Communicable for 1-4 weeks Self-limited disease Treat with antibiotics Severe dehydration and collapse can affect all patients Acute symptoms may persist 1 week or more

Table 24-5 Enteropathological causes of acute gastroenteritis (continued).

Yersinia enterocolitica Incubation period: dose dependent; 1-3 weeks		Diarrhoea - may be bloody Fever(>38.7°C) Abdominal pain right lower quadrant (RLQ) Vomiting, diarrhoea	Seen more frequently in winter Majority in first 3 years of life Transmitted by food and pets Can resemble appendicitis May be relapsing and last for months
Campylobacter jejuni Incubation period: 1-7 days or longer	Precise mechanism unclear Jejunum and ileum involvement Extensive ulceration with haemorrhagic ileitis Broadening and flattening of mucosa	Fever Abdominal pain - often severe, cramping, periumbilical Watery, profuse, foul-smelling diarrhoea Vomiting	Person-to-person transmission; may be transmitted by pets (e.g., cat, dog, hamster) Food (especially chicken) and water-borne transmission Relapse possible Most patients recover spontaneously Antibiotics advocated to speed recovery Peak incidence in summer
Vibrio cholerae (cholera) groups Incubation period: usually 2-3 days; range from few hours to 5 days	Enterotoxin causes increased secretion of chloride and possibly bicarbonate Intestinal mucosa congested with enlarged lymph follicles Intact mucosal surface	Sudden onset of profuse, watery diarrhoea without cramping, tenesmus, or anal irritation, although children may complain of cramping Stools are intermittent at first, then almost continuous Stools are whitish, almost clear, with flecks of mucus - 'rice water stools'	Rare in infants younger than 1 year old Mortality high in both treated and untreated infants and small children Transmitted via contaminated food and Endemic in Bengal Attack confers immunity

Food poisoning

Staphylococcus Incubation period: 4-6 hours	Produce heat-stable enterotoxin	Nausea, vomiting Severe abdominal cramps Profuse diarrhoea Shock may occur in severe cases May be a mild fever	Transferred via contaminated food - inadequately cooked or refrigerated, e.g. custards, mayonnaise, cream-filled or -topped desserts Self-limited; improvement apparent within 24 hours Excellent prognosis

(cont.)

Table 24-5 Enteropathological causes of acute gastroenteritis. (continued).

Clostridium perfringens Incubation period: 8-24 hours, usually 8-12	Produces heat- resistant and heat- sensitive toxins	Moderate to severe crampy, midepigas- tric pain	Self-limited illness Transmission by commer- cial food products, most often meat and poultry
Closrtidium botulinum Incubation period: 12-26 hours (range, 6 hours to 8 days)	Highly potent neuro- toxin	Nausea, vomiting Diarrhoea Central nervous sys- tem (CNS) symptoms with curare-like effect Dry mouth, dysphagia	Transmitted by contaminat- ed food products Variable severity - mild symptoms to rapidly fatal within a few hours Antitoxin administration

Table 24-5 Enteropathological causes of acute gastroenteritis (continued).

no green or brown colour indicates vomitus from the stomach and excludes an oesophageal cause. Uncurdled milk may also be vomited during or shortly after feedings. Vomitus containing greenish material indicating the presence of bile pigment is most likely to occur when an obstruction is situated below the ampulla of Vater; bile in the vomitus almost always excludes pyloric stenosis. Vomitus with a faecal odour suggests a lower intestinal obstruction or peritonitis.

Blood in the vomitus may appear as bright red, bloody streaks or brown coffee grounds **emesis** and may be insignificant or of major importance. Haematemesis is sometimes observed in the immediate neonatal period in infants who have swallowed maternal blood during delivery or occasionally from a cracked nipple. Other causes of haematemesis in early infancy include haemorrhagic disease of the newborn or other defects of coagulation and early oesophageal erosion associated with regurgitation of gastric juice related to reflux (see Chapter 27). Trauma from nasogastric tubes or tracheal catheters may cause bleeding followed by vomiting of swallowed blood.

In older children, haematemesis may be caused by swallowed blood from epistaxis or after nose or throat surgery. Rupture of oesophageal varices and peptic ulcer can cause profuse haematemesis. Coagulation defects or vascular damage may cause bloody vomiting in many diseases.

Frequency and persistence
Frequent or persistent vomiting indicates that the causative factor is still operating. The primary danger is loss of fluids and electrolytes, which increases with the frequency and duration of vomiting. In early infancy, the most frequent causes of persistent vomiting are pylorospasm, pyloric stenosis, adrenocortical insufficiency, and urinary tract infections. Recurrent vomiting suggests GI allergy, an epileptic equivalent ('abdominal epilepsy'), a childhood form of migraine, or intermittent intestinal obstruction, as might occur with malrotation of the colon. It is frequently associated with the onset of a febrile illness or a period of increased emotional tension.

Amount
The amount of the **emesis** should be measured and recorded, because it often furnishes information regarding the amount of fluid lost in relation to intake. This provides a clue to the extent of dehydration. Overfeeding or too rapid feeding may cause the child to vomit part of the feeding.

Force of vomiting
Repeated regurgitation is most often related to rumination or gastro-oesophageal reflux. Forceful vomiting during or after a meal is usually caused by overdistention with milk and air. Repeated forceful vomiting of a projectile nature is one of the cardinal signs of pyloric stenosis in early infancy and can be a result of increased ICP at any age. When combined with abdominal distention, it suggests intestinal obstruction.

Relationship to feeding
Vomiting in infants may be related to the nature of their formula. Highly diluted formula may cause hungry infants to consume so much that they vomit from overdistention. High-fat or acidified formulas may cause others to vomit. Food that is contaminated by bacteria or food that is inappropriate for the child, such as unripe fruits or rich, highly seasoned foods, may cause a child to vomit.

Vomiting soon after eating may be a symptom of food allergy or acute, febrile illness. More often, vomiting is initiated by gastric distention by milk and air, which is caused by such feeding practices as failure to wind the infant during and immediately after feedings, feeding formula through teats with holes so small that the infant takes in air while sucking for milk, improper positioning of the bottle so that air instead of milk enters the teat, feeding too rapidly, and swallowing air from prolonged sucking on an empty breast. Underfeeding leads to hunger, causing the infant to swallow air while sucking on fingers or fists. Cold formula may cause a few infants to vomit, and hurried eating at any age may precipitate vomiting, particularly when the child is excited or overly tired.

History

Sometimes, the cause of vomiting is readily apparent from the history. Vomiting associated with diarrhoea is usually caused by gastroenteritis; vomiting that occurs suddenly in a previously healthy child suggests the early stages of an infection. When several children or members of a family who have eaten together vomit, food poisoning is the most likely possibility. Vomiting accompanied by fever, abdominal pain, and tenderness is a common symptom of appendicitis or other abdominal conditions requiring surgical repair. Vomiting is not an uncommon reaction to toxins or drugs taken as prescribed or ingested accidentally.

PROCESS OF DIAGNOSIS

When vomiting is persistent and cannot be attributed to an obvious and temporary condition, a more comprehensive evaluation is warranted. It may be the child's only symptom or, more often, only one clinical feature of a variety of disorders. The importance of vomiting also varies. It may be a minor manifestation or the dominant feature of a serious illness. Vomiting that is not associated with feeding may be an indication of increased ICP.

Diagnostic tests

Physical examination and routine tests of blood and urine are performed, but special laboratory tests are seldom employed. Radiological studies can detect anomalies of the alimentary tract. If vomiting has persisted to the degree that dehydration and electrolyte imbalance are present, the child's weight and serum electrolyte, blood urea nitrogen, and carbon dioxide content of the blood are determined to assess the state of hydration and to serve as the basis for therapy.

THERAPEUTIC MANAGEMENT

Management is directed towards detection and treatment of the cause of the vomiting and prevention of complications of the vomiting. Vomiting that results in fluid loss of considerable degree may require parenteral fluid therapy. Fluids are administered in the same manner and in a similar electrolyte composition to those administered in diarrhoea. This includes both parenteral and oral fluids.

Although most children respond well to these measures, centrally acting antiemetic drugs may be prescribed when the cause of the vomiting is known, and the vomiting is predictable and of limited duration. Antiemetics can exert their effect on neural labyrinth pathways, depress the chemoreceptor trigger zone and the vomiting centre, or act on the aural vestibular apparatus.

IMPLICATIONS FOR NURSING

The major emphasis of nursing care of the vomiting infant or child is on observation and reporting of vomiting behaviour and associated symptoms, and the implementation of measures to reduce the vomiting. Accurate assessment of the type of vomiting, the appearance of the vomitus and the child's behaviour associated with the vomiting greatly aids in establishing a diagnosis of disorders that have vomiting as a clinical manifestation.

Nursing interventions will be determined by the cause of the vomiting. The thirst mechanism is the most sensitive guide to fluid needs, and *ad libitum* administration of a glucose-electrolyte solution to an alert child will restore water and electrolytes satisfactorily. It is important to include carbohydrate to spare body protein and to avoid ketosis resulting from exhaustion of glycogen reserves. Once vomiting has abated, more liberal amounts can be offered, followed by simple foods such as plain biscuits, clear soup, and buttered toast in small amounts, when the child desires, followed by gradual resumption of the regular diet.

The vomiting infant or child is positioned to prevent aspiration and observed for evidence of dehydration. It is important to emphasize the need for the child to brush the teeth or rinse the mouth after vomiting, to dilute hydrochloric acid that comes in contact with the teeth. A flavoured mouthwash or brushing also helps freshen the mouth. Careful monitoring of fluid and electrolyte status must be exercised to avoid the possibility of hyperelectrolytaemia.

SHOCK STATES

Several conditions constitute medical and nursing emergencies; severe shock is one of these conditions. Nurses should be prepared for this possibility and intervene early and appropriately when patients display signs that indicate circulatory impairment.

SHOCK

Shock, or acute circulatory failure, is a clinical syndrome characterized by prostration and tissue perfusion that is inadequate to meet the metabolic demands of the body, resulting in depressed vital cell function. Although the causes are different, the physiological consequences are the same: hypotension, tissue hypoxia and metabolic acidosis.

AETIOLOGY

Circulatory failure in children is the result of hypovolaemia, altered peripheral vascular resistance, pump failure or obstruction. The most common type of circulatory failure in children is hypovolaemia, or *hypovolaemic shock*, which follows a reduction in circulating blood volume related to blood, plasma or extracellular fluid losses beyond the child's physical ability to compensate. *Cardiogenic shock* resulting from decreased output is not common in children. The types of shock and their most frequent causes are listed in Box 24-4.

◆ **BOX 24-4**

Types of shock

Hypovolaemic Shock

Characteristics

Reduction in size of vascular compartment

Falling blood pressure

Poor capillary filling

Low central venous pressure (CVP)

Most frequent causes

Blood loss (haemorrhagic shock) — trauma, GI bleeding, intracranial haemorrhage

Plasma loss — increased capillary permeability associated with sepsis and acidosis, hypoproteinaemia, burns, peritonitis

Extracellular fluid loss — vomiting, diarrhoea, glycosuric diuresis, sunstroke

Distributive Shock

Characteristics

Reduction in peripheral vascular resistance

Profound inadequacies in tissue perfusion

Increased venous capacity and pooling

Acute reduction in return blood flow to the heart

Diminished cardiac output

Most frequent causes

Anaphylaxis (anaphylactic shock) — extreme allergy or hypersensitivity to a foreign substance

Sepsis (septic shock, bacteraemic shock, endotoxic shock) — overwhelming sepsis and circulating bacterial toxins

Loss of neuronal control (neurogenic shock) — interruption of neuronal transmission (spinal cord injury)

Myocardial depression and peripheral dilation — exposure to anaesthesia or ingestion of barbiturates, tranquilizers, narcotics, antihypertensive agents or ganglionic blocking agents

Obstructive Shock

Characteristic

Inflow or outflow obstruction of main bloodstream

Most frequent sites of obstruction and probable causes

Vena cava — compression

Pericardium — tamponade, pneumopericardium

Cardiac chambers — ball-valve thrombus, anatomical obstruction (atresia)

Pulmonary circuit — embolism, pulmonic stenosis, tension pneumothorax, pleural effusion

Aorta — coarctation

Cardiogenic Shock

Characteristic

Decreased cardiac output

Most frequent causes

Congenital heart disease in infancy — usually systemic-to-pulmonary shunting

Primary pump failure — myocarditis, myocardial trauma, biochemical derangements

Dysrhythmias — paroxysmal atrial tachycardia, atrioventricular block, and ventricular dysrhythmias; secondary to myocarditis or biochemical abnormalities (occasionally)

CLINICAL MANIFESTATIONS

Shock can be regarded as a form of compensation for circulatory failure and, because of its progressive nature, can be divided into three stages or phases: *compensated, uncompensated* and *irreversible*. At all stages, the principal differentiating signs are observed in degree of: (1) tachycardia and perfusion to extremities, (2) level of consciousness, and (3) blood pressure. Additional signs or modifications of these more universal signs may be present depending on the type and cause of the shock.

Compensated shock

When vital organ function is maintained by intrinsic mechanisms and the child's ability to compensate is effective, cardiac output and systemic arterial blood pressure are usually normal or increased, but blood flow is generally uneven or maldistributed in the microcirculation. Early clinical signs are subtle, including apprehension, irritability, normal blood pressure, narrowing pulse pressure, thirst, pallor and diminished urinary output.

Decompensated shock

As shock progresses, perfusion in the microcirculation becomes marginal despite compensatory adjustments, and signs are more obvious and indicate early decompensation. These signs are tachypnoea, moderate metabolic acidosis, oliguria, and cool, pale extremities with decreased skin turgor and poor capillary filling. The outcomes of circulatory failure that progress beyond the limits of compensation are tissue hypoxia, metabolic acidosis and eventual dysfunction of all organ systems.

Irreversible shock

Irreversible, or terminal, shock implies damage to vital organs such as the heart or brain of such magnitude that the entire organism will be disrupted regardless of therapeutic intervention. There is pronounced systemic vasoconstriction and hypoxia of visceral and cutaneous circulations, with hypotension, acidosis, lethargy or coma, and oliguria or anuria. The child is totally obtunded. Thready, weak pulse; hypotension; periodic breathing or apnoea; anuria; and stupor or coma are signs of impending cardiopulmonary arrest. Death occurs even if cardiovascular measurements return to normal levels with therapy.

PROCESS OF DIAGNOSIS

The cause of shock can be discerned from the history and the physical examination. The extent of the shock is determined by measurement of vital signs, including CVP and capillary filling. Laboratory tests that assist in assessment are blood gas measurements, pH, and sometimes various liver function tests such as serum glutamic oxaloacetic transaminase (SGOT), bilirubin, and total serum protein (TSP). Coagulation status (prothrombin time [PT], partial thromboplastin time [PTT], platelet count, fibrinogen, fibrin) is evaluated when there is evidence of bleeding, such as oozing from a venepuncture site, bleeding from any orifice, or petechiae. Cultures of blood and other sites are indicated when there is a high suspicion of sepsis. Renal function tests are performed when impaired renal function is evident.

THERAPEUTIC MANAGEMENT

Treatment of shock consists of three major thrusts: (1) mechanical ventilation, (2) fluid administration, and (3) improvement of the pumping action of the heart (vasopressor support). The first priority is to establish an airway and administer oxygen. Once the airway is assured, circulatory stabilization is the major concern. Placement of an intravenous catheter for rapid volume replacement is the most important action for re-establishment of circulation. Where individuals are familiar with and skilled in the technique, percutaneous cannulation of the internal jugular or subclavian veins is preferred.

Ventilatory support

The decreased or redistribution of blood flow to respiratory muscles plus the increased work of breathing can rapidly lead to respiratory failure. Critically ill patients are unable to maintain an adequate airway. Tracheal intubation is initiated early with positive-pressure ventilation and supplemental oxygen. Blood gases and pH are monitored frequently.

Increased extravascular lung water caused by oedema — both hydrostatic and permeable — contributes to the development of respiratory complications. Hydrostatic oedema occurs from elevation of pulmonary microvascular pressure as a result of left ventricular dysfunction; permeable oedema occurs when damage to alveolar cell and pulmonary capillary epithelium causes fluid to leak into the interstitial space resulting in the so-called adult respiratory distress syndrome (ARDS) or shock lung. Therapy is directed towards maintaining normal arterial blood gas measurements, normal acid-base balance, and circulation.

Cardiovascular support

In the majority of cases, rapid restoration of blood volume is all that is needed for resuscitation of the child in shock. The nature of the fluid depends primarily on the availability of the appropriate fluid and the kind of fluid loss incurred. It may be a crystalloid solution such as 5% Dextrose, a colloid in the form of fresh frozen plasma, or blood. Successful resus-

citation will be reflected by an increase in blood pressure and a reduction in heart rate. An increased cardiac output will result in improved capillary circulation and skin colour. For these children effective monitoring includes accurate measurements and recording of vital signs and objective observations. Urinary output measurement is an important indicator of adequacy of circulation.

For the critically ill child with shock and multisystem dysfunction, more aggressive monitoring is needed. Central venous measurements of right atrial pressure or pulmonary wedge pressure help guide fluid therapy. In children with persistent shock, a Swan-Ganz catheter should be placed for more accurate monitoring. Determination of arterial blood gases, haematocrit, serum electrolytes, glucose, and calcium concentrations provides additional information concerning composition of circulating blood. Correction of acidosis, hypoxaemia, and any metabolic derangements is mandatory.

Vasopressor support

Temporary pharmacological support may be required to enhance myocardial contractility, to reverse metabolic or respiratory acidosis and to maintain arterial pressure. The principal agents used to improve cardiac output and circulation are the sympathetic amines administered by continuous infusion. Dopamine is the preferred drug in most situations because it also improves renal perfusion. Other agents used to improve cardiac output (e.g., dobutamine, adrenaline) may be used as appropriate, depending on the situation. Digoxin may be given to augment myocardial contractility in a failing heart.

Metabolic acidosis is usually corrected with adequate tissue perfusion and improved renal function. This is accomplished with adequate ventilatory support, including oxygen, and restoration of blood volume and peripheral circulation. The administration of sodium bicarbonate may be associated with complications; therefore, it is used only to partially correct the pH to levels that do not pose a threat to life.

Calcium chloride may be administered to improve cardiac function and to offset the reduced ionized calcium associated with large amounts of albumin, whole blood or fresh-frozen plasma. Diuretics, such as frusemide, cause a reduction in the ventricular filling pressures without changing cardiac output or heart rate and promote sodium and water excretion by the kidney in cases where pulmonary congestion is a problem.

Other therapies

Peritoneal dialysis may be necessary if hyperkalaemia, acidosis, hypervolaemia or altered mental status occurs. Nutritional support is provided by both enteral and parenteral routes. Prevention of infection is a primary concern, because host resistance is depressed in patients in shock. Other complicating disorders, for example, disseminated intravascular coagulation and gastrointestinal problems (e.g., paralytic ileus, stress ulceration), are managed appropriately.

The intra-aortic balloon pump (IABP) may be employed for the child with low cardiac output who is refractory to conventional medical management (Webster and Veasy, 1985).

Extracorporeal membrane oxygenation (ECMO) is used occasionally as a last resort where this therapy is available.

SEPTIC SHOCK

Septic shock occurs frequently and is associated with high mortality rates in children and differs in pathology from other forms of shock (Perkin and Anas, 1986). The mechanisms producing septic (bacteraemic) shock are not clear, but appear to be the result of many interrelated factors. Multiple vasoactive substances, released in response to endotoxin exposure, produce a marked reduction in systemic vascular resistance (Zimmerman and Dietrich, 1987). Uneven blood flow and inadequate tissue oxygenation result in progressive decompensation of the capillary circulation and tissue cells.

Three stages have been identified in septic shock (Box 24-5). In early septic shock there are chills, fever and vasodilation with increased cardiac output that results in the warm, flushed skin reflecting vascular tone abnormalities and *hyperdynamic*, or hyperdynamic-compensated, responses. The patient has the best chance for survival from this stage. The *normodynamic*, cool, or hyperdynamic-uncompensated stage lasts for only a few hours. With advancing disease, signs progress through decompensatory manifestations, which deteriorate to signs of circulatory collapse indistinguishable from late shock of any cause. In *hypodynamic* shock, cardiovascular function progressively deteriorates even with aggressive therapy. This is the most dangerous stage of shock. A later and ominous development is disseminated intravascular coagulation (the major haematological complication of septic shock), which is evidenced by petechiae or purpura fulminans, a severe form of subcutaneous haemorrhage.

ANAPHYLAXIS

Anaphylaxis is the acute clinical syndrome resulting from the interaction of an allergen and a patient who is hypersensitive. Severe reactions are immediate in onset, are often life threatening, and frequently involve multiple systems, primarily the cardiovascular, respiratory, gastrointestinal, and integumentary. Exposure to the antigen can be by ingestion, inhalation, or injection. The most common allergens are listed in Box 24-6.

Prevention of a reaction is the primary goal of anaphylaxis. Preventing exposure is more easily accomplished in children known to be at risk, including those with: (1) a history of previous allergic reaction to specific antigen, (2) a history of atopy, (3) a history of severe reactions in immediate family members, and (4) a reaction to a skin test, although skin tests are not available for all allergens.

CLINICAL MANIFESTATIONS

The onset of clinical symptoms usually occurs within seconds or minutes of exposure to the antigen, and the rapidity of the reaction is directly related to its intensity — the sooner the onset, the more severe the reaction. Typically, the reaction is preceded by one or more prodromal signs and symptoms, including vague complaints of uneasiness or impending doom, restlessness, irritability, severe anxiety, headache, dizziness, paraesthesia and disorientation. The patient may lose consciousness. Cutaneous signs are the most common initial sign, and the child may complain of feeling warm. Angio-oedema is most noticeable in the eyelids, lips, tongue, hands, feet and genitalia. Any or all of several reactions may affect one or more organ systems, as outlined in Box 24-7.

Cutaneous manifestations are often followed by bronchiolar constriction. Bronchiolar constriction causes a narrowing of the airway, dilated pulmonary circulation produces pulmonary oedema and haemorrhages, and there is often life-threatening laryngeal oedema. Shock occurs as a result of mediator-induced vasodilation and sudden inadequacy of the

---

◆ **BOX 24-5**

Stages of septic shock

Hyperdynamic Stage (Warm Shock, Pink Shock)
Tachycardia
Tachypnoea
Chills and fever
Skin flushed, warm
Warm extremities
Bounding pulse
Normal or elevated systemic blood pressure
Wide pulse pressure
Normal urine output or polyuria
Mental confusion
Normodynamic Stage (Cool Shock)
Tachycardia
Hyperventilation
Normal temperature
Skin cool
Cool extremities
Normal pulse
Normal or slightly elevated systemic blood pressure
Normal to slightly narrow pulse pressure
Oliguria
Depressed sensorium
Hypodynamic Stage (Cold Shock)
Tachycardia
Respiratory distress
Profound hypothermia
Skin cold, clammy
Cold, pale extremities
Weak, thready pulse
Severe hypotension
Narrow pulse pressure
Severe oliguria or anuria
Lethargy or coma

◆ **B O X 2 4 - 6**

Common allergens associated with anaphylaxis

Drugs

Antibiotics (penicillin, cephalosporins, tetracycline, aminoglycosides, streptomycin, amphotericin B)

Analgesics (aspirin, indomethacin, codeine, phenylbutazone)

Local anaesthetics (lignocaine, procaine, bupivacaine, tetracaine)

Chemotherapeutic agents (adriamycin, bleomycin, cisplatin, cyclophosphamide, L-asparaginase, melphalan)

Diagnostic contrast media (sulphobromophthalein sodium [BSP] dye, dehydrocholic acid, iodinated contrast media, iopanoic acid)

Foods

Eggs

Seafood (fish, shellfish)

Milk and milk products

Chocolate

Nuts and seeds

Berries

Legumes (soybeans, beans, lentils, peanuts)

Wheat

Citrus fruits

Venoms

Hymenoptera (bee, yellow jacket, hornet, wasp, fire ant)

Snake

Jellyfish

Spider

Biological agents

Allergen extracts

Antisera (snake, tetanus, diphtheria)

Enzymes

Hormones

Immune globulin (gammaglobulin, cryoprecipitate, blood, plasma)

◆ **B O X 2 4 - 7**

Possible manifestations of anaphylactic reaction

Cardiovascular

Tachycardia

Dysrhythmia

Hypotension

Relative hypovolaemia

Respiratory

Rhinitis - sneezing, nasal itching, rhinorrhoea

Laryngeal oedema - stridor

Bronchospasm - cough, wheezing

Gastrointestinal

Nausea and vomiting

Abdominal pain

Diarrhoea

Skin

Diffuse flushing

Urticaria

Angiooedema - periorbital, perioral

Central Nervous System

Seizures

Loss of consciousness

THERAPEUTIC MANAGEMENT

Successful outcome of anaphylactic reactions depends on rapid recognition and institution of treatment. The goals of treatment are to provide ventilation, restore adequate circulation, and prevent further exposure by identifying and removing the cause, when possible.

A mild reaction with no evidence of respiratory distress or cardiovascular compromise can be managed with antihistamines and adrenaline. Moderate or severe distress presents a potentially life-threatening emergency and requires immediate intervention. Severely unresponsive patients are transferred to hospital intensive care units, when possible.

BURNS

Minor thermal injuries are experienced by everyone in day-to-day living and are relatively commonplace in nursing practice. Extensive burns, on the other hand, are relatively uncommon; however, they account for some of the most difficult nursing problems encountered in the paediatric age group. Serious burn injury accounts for a very large number of children who must undergo prolonged, painful and restrictive hospitalization, and many of whom emerge from the experience with scars to both body and personality that profoundly affect their social and emotional development. It is tragic, too, that the great majority (75%) of burn injuries are preventable.

OVERVIEW

Although severe burns are manifest primarily in damage to the skin, they produce a complex illness that requires the utmost

circulation. The hypovolaemia is further enhanced by increased capillary permeability and loss of intravascular fluid into the interstitial space. Laryngeal oedema with its acute upper airway obstruction and related hypovolaemic shock carries a more ominous prognosis.

in nursing skill and care. Every organ system becomes involved, and sometimes the treatment even creates additional problems. Nursing care of patients with extensive burns involves an understanding of a variety of specialized areas, including surgical principles and techniques, respiratory physiology, fluid and electrolyte physiology, nutrition, bacteriology, growth and development, occupational therapy, physiotherapy and principles of psychiatric nursing.

EPIDEMIOLOGY

In the United Kingdom, approximately 900 deaths per year occur as a result of injury by fire. Each year, 150,000 people attend UK accident and emergency departments with burn injuries, of which 15,000 are admitted to hospital (Harvey-Kemble and Lamb, 1987) (Fig. 24-3). Approximately 50% of all major burn victims are children (Fig. 24-4).

Children are more prone to accidental injury and 75% of burn accidents occur in the home. Most of these injuries are scalds, frequently less deep and less extreme than fire burns. However, scalds account for 7,000 hospital admissions per year for children.

Severity of burn illness is determined by the percentage of body surface burned. Children have a comparatively larger body surface area in proportion to body weight; therefore, the child will be more acutely affected by what might appear to be

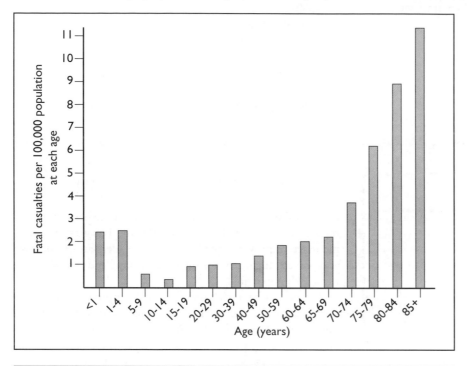

Fig. 24-3 Fire burn casualties per 100,000 population by age. (From Harvey–Kemble JV, Lamb BE: *Practical burns management*, London, 1987, Hodder & Stoughton)

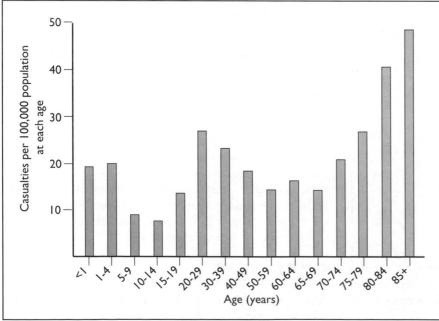

Fig. 24-4 Fatal fire casualties per 100,000 population by age. (From *Fire statistics, United Kingdom,* London, 1983, Home Office)

a relatively minor burn in an adult. Fig. 24-5 outlines the predicted mortality rates associated with different percentages of body area burned. Additional factors which may affect outcome are the inhalation of noxious gases or smoke, and the presence of serious wound contamination and infection.

AETIOLOGY

Burns can be caused by thermal, chemical, electrical or radioactive agents. Most burn injuries are caused by thermal agents, principally flame, direct contact (stove, heater), and hot water (scalding water, steam), and to a lesser extent by friction and frostbite. Chemical burns can be caused by either acids or alkalis, and radiation burns by either x-rays or ultraviolet radiation. The extent of tissue destruction is determined by the intensity of the heat source, the duration of contact or exposure, and the speed with which the heat energy is dissipated by the burned surface. For example, a brief exposure to high-intensity heat, such as a flame, or a longer exposure to low-intensity heat, such as hot water, can produce similar burn injuries. Burns caused by boiling oil or liquid fat tend to cause deep partial-thickness burns. Prolonged exposure to the sun's rays or to a heated object, such as a pavement, is also capable of producing significant burns.

Full-thickness destruction frequently occurs when clothing is ignited. Cotton and nylon clothing burns most easily, whereas clothing made from wool or other animal fibres burns less readily. Synthetic fabrics melt and stick to the skin surface. Contact burns from heated metal or liquids (e.g., tar) at extreme temperatures, prolonged immersion in hot water, chemical burns without rinsing with water, and electric burns are all significant in the cause of severe burn trauma. Chemical agents continue to cauterize the tissues until the injurious agent is chemically united with tissue elements, neutralized, or removed by washing with running water.

Electric burns are especially deceptive, because they are characterized by a more extensive thrombosis that is not evident until 24-36 hours after injury. Electricity is converted to thermal energy as it encounters resistance. Inasmuch as body tissues vary in the degree of resistance they offer, the type of tissue through which an electric current passes plays a role in the extent of the burn injury. Bone offers the greatest amount of resistance. Other tissues in descending order of resistance are fat, tendon, skin, muscle, blood and nerves. Although blood offers less resistance than most tissues, it is an extremely good conductor of electric current. All other things being equal, the greater the skin resistance, the more severe is the local burn; the less the skin resistance, the greater are the systemic effects. The extensive destruction of an electric burn has been described as resembling a crush injury.

BURN WOUND CHARACTERISTICS

The physiological responses, therapy, prognosis and disposition of the injured child are all directly related to the *amount of tissue destroyed*; therefore, the severity of the burn injury is assessed on the basis of percentage of body surface burned, depth of the burn and location of the burn(s) (Fig. 24-6).

Also important in determining the seriousness of the injury are age of the child, aetiological agent, extent of respiratory tract involvement, general health of the child, and presence of any associated injury or condition. Suspected or confirmed child abuse is significant because of the associated impact on long-term progress and additional risk (see Table 24-6).

EXTENT OF INJURY

The extent of a burn is usually expressed as a percentage of total body surface area, which is most accurately estimated by using

Statistical values of mortality with age and percentage area of body burned (0.1 = 10% mortality, 0.9 = 90% mortality).									
Area of body burned %	Age (years)								
	0-4	5-14	15-24	25-34	35-44	45-54	55-64	65-74	75+
93+	1	1	1	1	1	1	1	1	1
83-92	0.9	0.9	0.9	0.9	1	1	1	1	1
73-82	0.7	0.8	0.8	0.9	0.9	1	1	1	1
63-72	0.5	0.6	0.6	0.7	0.8	0.9	1	1	1
53-62	0.3	0.3	0.4	0.5	0.7	0.8	0.9	1	1
43-52	0.2	0.2	0.2	0.3	0.5	0.6	0.8	1	1
33-42	0.1	0.1	0.1	0.2	0.3	0.4	0.6	0.9	1
23-32	0	0	0	0.1	0.1	0.2	0.4	0.7	1
13-22	0	0	0	0	0	0.1	0.2	0.4	0.7
3-12	0	0	0	0	0	0	0.1	0.2	0.4
0-2	0	0	0	0	0	0	0	0.1	0.3

Source: Adapted from Bull, (1971)

Fig. 24-5 Statistical values of mortality with age and percentage area of body burned (0.1 = 10% mortality, 0.9 = 90% mortality). (Adapted from Bull JP: Revised analysis of mortality due to burns, *Lancet* II:1133, 1971)

specially designed age-related charts (Fig. 24-7). Because of the body proportions, especially the head and lower extremities, the standard 'rule of nines' charts used for adults are not applicable to small children (Fig. 24-8).

DEPTH OF INJURY

A thermal injury is a three-dimensional wound and therefore is also assessed in relation to depth of injury. Traditionally the terms *first-*, *second-*, and *third-degree* have been used to describe the depth of tissue injury. However, with the current emphasis on burn healing, these are gradually being replaced by more descriptive terms based on the extent of destruction to the epithelializing elements of the skin. Partial-thickness burns heal in time; full-thickness burns require skin grafting for closure. Partial-thickness injury is further categorized by many as superficial or deep dermal burns, depending on how rapidly they heal. Because both terminologies are used, often inter-

changeably, both are presented in describing the characteristics of burn wounds (Fig. 24-9).

Superficial (first-degree) burns are usually of minor significance. There is frequently a latent period followed by erythema. Tissue damage is minimal, protective functions remain intact, and systemic effects are rare. Pain is the predominant symptom.

Partial-thickness (second-degree) burns are deeper and involve not only the epithelium, but also a minimal to substantial portion of the corium. The severity of the injury and the rate of healing are directly related to the amount of undamaged corium from which new tissue can regenerate. Superficial burns are often classified with first-degree burns and heal uneventfully. Deep dermal burns, although classified as second-degree or partial-thickness burns, in many respects resemble third-degree burns. There is hyperaemia in areas with less heat, and leakage of protein in areas with the most heat. Systemic effects are similar to those that occur with deeper

Age in years	Birth	1	5	10	15	Adult
Head and neck	21%	19%	15%	12%	11%	9%
Thigh	5%	6%	8%	9%	9%	9%
Calf	5%	5%	5%	6%	6%	7%
Foot	3%	3%	3%	3%	3%	3%
Arm	7%	7%	7%	7%	7%	7%
Hand	3%	3%	3%ß	3%	3%	3%
Chest	7%	7%	7%	7%	7%	7%
Abdomen	7%	7%	7%	7%	7%	7%
Back and Buttocks	18%	18%	18%	18%	18%	18%

Modified from Lund and Browder, 1987.

Table 24-6 Relative percentages of different parts of the body at different ages.

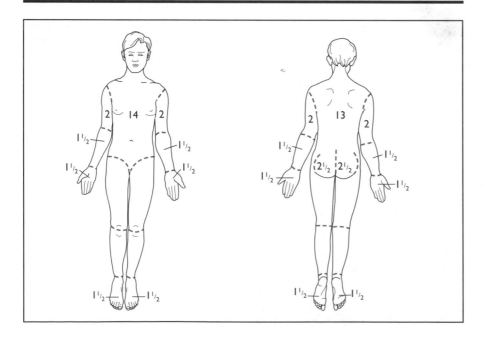

Fig. 24-6 Relative percentages of different parts of the body at all ages. (Modified from Lund, Browder. From Harvey Kemble JV, Lamb BE: *Practical burns management*, London, 1987, Hodder & Stoughton)

burns. Whereas first-degree and superficial partial-thickness burns are painful, deep dermal burns are often anaesthetic for the first one or two days after injury.

Full-thickness (third-degree) burns are serious injuries in which all layers of the skin are destroyed, may involve underlying tissues as well, and are usually combined with extensive partial-thickness damage. Presence of visible thrombosed veins in the burn wound is pathognomonic of a full-thickness burn. Systemic effects can be life threatening and involve every organ system in the body. Although a notable characteristic of third-degree burns is lack of sensation at the wound surface, this is misleading. Superficial nerve endings are destroyed in the full-thickness areas, but nerve endings are hypersensitive on wound edges. In addition, deep somatic pain is present in the full-thickness area as a result of inflammation and ischaemia (LaMotte, Thalhammer, 1982).

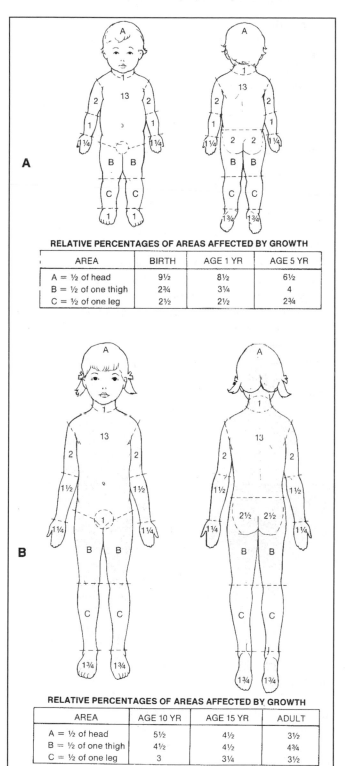

RELATIVE PERCENTAGES OF AREAS AFFECTED BY GROWTH

AREA	BIRTH	AGE 1 YR	AGE 5 YR
A = ½ of head	9½	8½	6½
B = ½ of one thigh	2¾	3¼	4
C = ½ of one leg	2½	2½	2¾

RELATIVE PERCENTAGES OF AREAS AFFECTED BY GROWTH

AREA	AGE 10 YR	AGE 15 YR	ADULT
A = ½ of head	5½	4½	3½
B = ½ of one thigh	4½	4½	4¾
C = ½ of one leg	3	3¼	3½

Fig. 24-7 Estimation of distribution of burns in children. **A,** Children from birth to age 5 years. **B,** Older children.

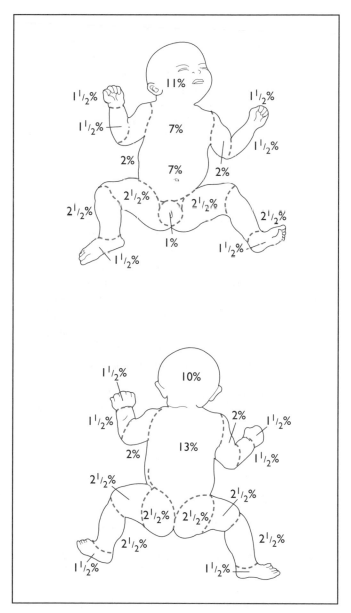

Fig. 24-8 Relative percentages of different parts of the body of a newborn baby. (Modified from Lund, Browder. From Harvey Kemble JV, Lamb BE: Practical burns management, London, 1987, Hodder & Stoughton.)

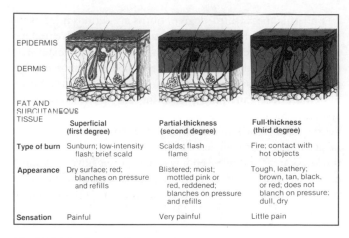

	Superficial (first degree)	Partial-thickness (second degree)	Full-thickness (third degree)
Type of burn	Sunburn; low-intensity flash; brief scald	Scalds; flash flame	Fire; contact with hot objects
Appearance	Dry surface; red; blanches on pressure and refills	Blistered; moist; mottled pink or red, reddened; blanches on pressure and refills	Tough, leathery; brown, tan, black, or red; does not blanch on pressure; dull, dry
Sensation	Painful	Very painful	Little pain

Fig. 24-9 Classification of burn depth.

Sometimes, additional categories are used to further describe full-thickness burns. Fourth-degree burns involve fat and are difficult to prepare for grafting. Burns involving muscle may be designated as fifth-degree burns. Because of the myoglobin released from muscle destruction, burns involving muscle may lead to kidney damage. Burns that destroy bone are sixth-degree burns, are usually hard and dry, and lead to amputation of the affected part (Jacoby, 1984).

SEVERITY OF INJURY

Burns are also appraised on the basis of their severity. This is useful in determining the disposition of the patient for treatment. Burned patients can usually be distinguished as: (1) those with a critical burn who require the services and equipment of a special burn facility, (2) those with moderate burns who may be treated in any hospital unit, and (3) those with minor burns who are able to be treated on an outpatient basis. Although each burn unit and specialist in the field of burn management has criteria for admission to special units, there are several factors that influence the effects of the injury, the probability of recovery, and response to therapy.

Children younger than two years of age have a significantly higher mortality than older children with burns of similar magnitude. They are subject to rapid fluid shifts, which places them in jeopardy in the early hours, and their immune competence is not well developed; therefore, sepsis is a frequent complication. The classification of burns according to severity is outlined in Box 24-8.

LOCAL RESPONSES

Local changes at the site of the burn injury begin to occur at approximately 45°C; tissues die at 65°C and higher because of coagulation necrosis.

The burn wound consists basically of three distinct layers (Fig. 24-10), as described in Box 24-9. It is within the two outer zones that significant changes take place, and these zones are involved in the pathophysiology of the burn wound and the systemic responses to the initial burn injury.

◆ BOX 24-8
Burn severity criteria

Minor Burns
Partial-thickness burns of less than 10% of body surface area (BSA)
Full-thickness burns of less than 2% of BSA

Moderate Burns
Partial-thickness burns of 15-25% of BSA (age related; see Major or Critical Burns)
Full-thickness burns of less than 10% of BSA, except in small children and when the burns involve critical areas, such as the face, hands, feet or genitalia

Major or Critical Burns
Burns complicated by respiratory tract injury
Partial-thickness burns of 25% of BSA or greater
Burns of face, hands, feet or genitalia, even if they appear to be partial thickness
Full-thickness burns of 10% of BSA or greater
Any child younger than two years of age, unless the burn is very small and very superficial (20% of BSA or greater considered critical in child less than two years of age)
Electric burns that penetrate
Deep chemical burns
Respiratory tract damage
Burns complicated by fractures or soft tissue injury
Burns complicated by concurrent illness, such as obesity, diabetes, epilepsy, and cardiac and renal diseases

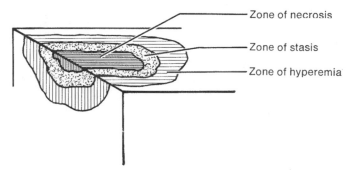

Zone of necrosis
Zone of stasis
Zone of hyperemia

Fig. 24-10 Zones of injury in burn.(After Zawacki B: *Ann Surg* 180:98, 1974.)

Oedema formation
Thermal injury to the vessels in the two outer zones causes increased capillary permeability. At the same time, vasodilation results in increased hydrostatic pressure within the capillaries. The increased hydrostatic pressure plus the increased capillary permeability cause loss of water, protein, and electrolytes from the intravascular compartment into the interstitial spaces. This shift is further enhanced by a diminishing intravascular oncotic pressure, as protein and sodium are lost to the interstitial spaces. Although the oedema involves both burned and nonburned areas, at the site of injury the accu-

mulation of oedema fluid beneath and around the burn can reach tremendous proportions until the extravasation of fluid is limited by tissue tension.

In addition, there are also changes in the permeability of tissue cells in and around the burned area that allow an abnormal exchange of electrolytes between the cells and the interstitial fluid; that is, sodium enters the cells in exchange for potassium, causing further depletion of intravascular sodium.

Fluid loss

Without the protective skin, fluid loss at the air-wound interface can be extremely high. These losses reach a maximum about the fourth day after the burn occurs but continue to pose problems until the denuded surfaces are debrided and grafted.

Circulatory stasis

Significant circulatory alterations take place in the zone of stasis located around the coagulated dead tissue. Heated red blood cells become spherical in shape when heated. These heat-damaged cells, together with haemoconcentration from fluid loss, depressed cardiac output, and tissue oedema, reduce the blood flow in the burn area, causing capillary stasis. Thrombi develop that further impede circulation, producing tissue ischaemia and eventual necrosis, which may also prolong the oedema phase. Further hyperviscosity and impaired blood flow are attributed to the release of substances from damaged cells, such as thromboplastin and clot-activating factors, that cause the production of microthrombi, platelet adhesiveness and aggregation, and increased pain and swelling.

Circulation in the area around partial-thickness burns ceases immediately after injury but is rapidly restored within 24-48 hours. In full-thickness burns, however, the vascular supply is completely occluded, and no appreciable circulation is reestablished until granulation takes place at the interface between burned and unburned tissue.

SYSTEMIC RESPONSES

Along with and subsequent to the pathophysiological response at the site of thermal injury, several systemic responses occur.

Circulation

The immediate postburn period is marked by dramatic alterations in circulation, known as *burn shock*. There is a precipitous drop in cardiac output (about 50% of normal resting values) that precedes any changes in circulating blood or plasma volume. With the large fluid losses through denuded skin, vasodilation, and oedema formation, the blood volume decreases rapidly and cardiac output is reduced even further, usually levelling off at 20% of normal resting values. Cardiac output returns to normal spontaneously in 24-36 hours, although the plasma volume lags far behind.

The initial decrease in cardiac output is attributed to a circulating myocardial depressant factor, associated with severe burn injury, that affects the contractility of the heart muscle directly. The blood volume deficit, although slower in onset, can be profound and appears to be directly proportional to the extent and depth of the burn.

Capillary permeability with leakage of fluid takes place in noninjured areas including bowels, brain and other organs, as well as in the outer zones of the burn wound. Oedema fluid accumulates rapidly in the first 18 hours after injury to reach a maximum in about 48 hours. Capillary permeability returns to normal and fluid is reabsorbed, chiefly by way of the lymphatics. Reabsorption usually proceeds at the rate of fluid accumulation, although it may persist longer. Redistribution of fluid is often complex and unpredictable. After a time, the lymphatics become incompetent and inapparent lymph accumulation may take place in compartments within the trunk or extremities.

In most children, the cardiovascular system is able to withstand the demands placed on it, although shock is a prominent feature of large thermal injuries and many children are prone to congestive heart failure and pulmonary oedema. In addition, peripheral circulation in the infant is less efficient and more labile, which complicates burn response and therapy in children in this age group.

Anaemia

Initially red blood cell destruction is reflected by an increased haematocrit. A significant loss of circulating red cell mass is associated predominantly with deep burns. The anaemia characteristic of thermal injury is attributed to several factors - red blood cells are damaged or destroyed by heat; circulating red blood cells are lost in the zone of stasis; there is direct bleeding from the wound; bone marrow is depressed as a result of sepsis; and (later) loss from bleeding during repeated debridement of the wound surface occurs.

Renal

Loss of fluid from the intravascular compartment causes renal vasoconstriction that in turn leads to reduced renal plasma flow and depressed glomerular filtration. When adequate fluids are provided, the glomerular filtration rate returns to normal, and by the third or fourth day of fluid therapy, urine output increases as oedema fluid is mobilized and eliminated. In the first few days oliguria is more commonly the result of inadequate fluid replacement than of acute renal failure. If the patient does not respond to treatment or if there is inadequate fluid resuscitation, acute renal failure may develop with permanent kidney damage. Children with a history of a prior kidney disorder are at increased risk.

Blood urea nitrogen and creatinine levels are elevated from tissue breakdown and oliguria. Haematuria may also be evident from haemolysis of red blood cells, and oliguria may develop as a consequence of the increased pigment load the kidneys must handle, especially myoglobin from extensive electric burn destruction, which blocks the kidney tubules. Except for electric burns, renal failure is uncommon in burns involving less than 20% of the body surface. Cell destruction following electric burns releases large amounts of myoglobin, which places the victim at high risk for renal failure. Renal failure also occurs more frequently following flame burns sustained indoors than after scalds.

Metabolism

The metabolic rate in burned patients is greatly accelerated, and the nitrogen losses are far in excess of those seen in other types of injuries. The magnitude of energy requirements of a burned child frequently exceeds the requirements of a normal active child, and when the burned area is extensive, may approach twice the normal requirements.

Many of the metabolic consequences of extensive burn injuries are attributed to the amount of energy needed for the energy-consuming process of evaporation of water from the damaged skin surface. Infants or young children are especially vulnerable because of the large surface area relative to metabolically active tissue. Burning destroys a lipid layer and converts skin that is normally virtually impermeable to water to a freely water-permeable state that transmits water vapour at least four times as rapidly as normal skin. In partial-thickness burns this loss is greatest the day of injury; in full-thickness areas it rises slowly at first and then rapidly increases to reach a peak about the fourth day after the burn occurs. Evaporative losses are maintained until partial-thickness burns are healed and full-thickness injuries are grafted. Thus body stores of energy are rapidly depleted unless sufficient replacement is provided or losses are reduced.

Neuroendocrine system

As a response to stress of any origin, the hypothalamic-hypophyseal mechanism restores equilibrium by secreting trophic hormones, which stimulate various target organs of the neuroendocrine system. Adrenal activity is stimulated maximally. The medulla responds by secreting increased amounts of the catecholamines adrenalin and noradrenalin, which appear to have a sustained elevation. Adrenocortical hormones are elevated and reach a peak immediately after injury, but remain high for some time. Aldosterone secretion is elevated and sustained at a high level throughout hospitalization, and there is release of antidiuretic hormone. Despite this increased adrenal activity, adrenal insufficiency is a rare complication.

Acidosis

Most burned patients exhibit some degree of metabolic acidosis. Reduced blood volume and cardiac output result in diminished tissue perfusion with resultant tissue hypoxia, which causes a shift to anaerobic metabolism with formation of metabolic acids. However, this is usually sufficiently compensated by increased ventilation as a result of pulmonary irritation or an independent respiratory alkalosis. Renal compensatory mechanisms are impaired by the decreased blood flow.

Growth changes

Changes in the growth pattern are frequently observed, particularly in older children who have burns covering large areas of their body. As in any severely burned individual, nail and hair growth essentially cease during the catabolic phase of burn response. It is believed that bone growth is also affected; weight loss is marked. During convalescence following full recovery, there is a catch-up spurt in bone growth and weight recovery. Prepubertal children who suffer thermal injury frequently experience a rapid acceleration of pubertal changes, with development of secondary sex characteristics, which may occur 2-3 years before usual. It is believed that these changes are probably caused by a prolonged and heavy production of growth hormone.

COMPLICATIONS

Thermally injured children are subject to several serious complications, both from the wound and from systemic alterations resulting from the wound. The immediate threat to life is asphyxia resulting from irritation and oedema of the lungs and respiratory passages. In the first 48-72 hours, the greatest hazard is unremitting shock with its associated complications. During healing, infection — both local and generalized sepsis — is the primary complication. Mortality associated with thermal injury in children decreases with the age of the child and increases with the extent of the burn. In children older than age three years, the fatality rate is similar to that in adults; below this age, resistance to the burn or its complications is considerably lessened. Although the cause for this is unknown, it may be a function of physiological immaturity.

THERAPEUTIC MANAGEMENT

The treatment of burns is commonly divided into phases, because of the nature of the pathological processes. The phases are described and titled differently by various authorities. However, for the purpose of this discussion, the emergency care is discussed first, followed by the medical management for minor and major burns. No phases are delineated.

EMERGENCY CARE

The aims of immediate treatment of thermal injury are to stop the burning process, cover the burn, transport the child to medical aid and provide reassurance.

Stop burning process

The chief aim of rescue in flame burns is to smother the fire, not to fan it. Children tend to panic and run, which only serves to fan the flames and make assistance more difficult. The victim should not run and should not remain standing. The injured child should be placed in a horizontal position and rolled in a blanket, rug or similar article, being careful not to cover the head and face because of the danger that the child might inhale the toxic fumes.

Spontaneous cooling of burns by slow immersion in cool water or any nonflammable liquid helps to relieve the pain, inhibit oedema formation, and slow the process of heat damage, especially in the zone of stasis. However, if a large amount of skin surface is denuded, immersion may precipitate hypothermia. Ice water or ice packs are contraindicated, because the resulting vasoconstriction interferes with capillary perfusion and carries the risk of further damage from cold burn. Burned clothing and jewelry are removed.

Emergency procedures

As soon as the flames are extinguished, the condition of the victim is assessed. Airway, breathing and circulation are the priority concerns. Cardiopulmonary or cerebral emergencies are always a possibility following a severe injury. Cardiopulmonary resuscitation is begun if indicated from the assessment. Cardiopulmonary complications may result from hypovolaemic (or electric) shock and seizures may be caused by lack of oxygen to the brain, inhalation of noxious fumes, or aggravation of a pre-existing tendency to convulsions by stress of the injury.

Cover burn

The burn wound should be covered with a clean cloth or cling film to prevent contamination and to alleviate pain by avoiding air contact. The child with extensive burns is covered to prevent hypothermia and to help ease pain from contact with the air. No attempt should be made to treat the burn. Application of topical ointments, oils or other home remedies is avoided.

Transport child to medical aid

The child with an extensive burn should not be given anything by mouth, because of the risk of aspiration. The child is transported to the nearest place where medical aid is available.

Provide reassurance

Providing reassurance and psychological support to both the parents and the child helps immeasurably during postinjury crisis. Reducing anxiety helps to conserve energy needed to cope with the physiological and emotional stress of a traumatic injury.

MANAGEMENT OF MINOR BURNS

Treatment of burns classified as minor usually can be managed adequately on an outpatient basis when it is determined that the *caregivers can be relied on to carry out instructions for care and observation*. Children with burns of the hands and most children with burns of the feet are admitted to the hospital so that they can receive careful local wound care and proper splinting to prevent deformity. In addition, children with burns of the face should be observed for airway obstruction and cosmetic reasons.

If there is a high probablity of infection or other complication, parents may be directed to return daily for dressing change and inspection or a nurse may be assigned to make a home visit for that purpose.

A tetanus history is obtained on admission. When there is no history of immunization, human tetanus antitoxin should be administered. Administration of antibiotics for minor burns is controversial. Most mild burns heal with little difficulty, but if the wound margin becomes erythematous, gross purulence is noted, or the child develops evidence of systemic reaction, such as fever or tachycardia, hospitalization is indicated. A mild analgesic is usually sufficient to relieve any discomfort, and the antipyretic effect of the drug helps alleviate the sensation of heat.

MANAGEMENT OF MAJOR BURNS

When a child with serious burns is admitted to the hospital for treatment, a variety of assessments are made and therapies initiated. Of these, the priority concerns are:
- establish and maintain an adequate airway
- establish a lifeline for fluid resuscitation
- care for the burn wound.

Other needs and therapies, including nutritional support, splinting to prevent contractures, treatment of anaemia and hypoproteinaemia, psychological support, and rehabilitative aspects of burn management, are initiated as appropriate throughout the course of treatment.

Establishment of adequate airway

The first priority of care is airway maintenance. Thermal injuries to the face, nares or upper torso; history of fire in an enclosed area; or examination of the oral and nasal membranes that reveals oedema of these membranes, hyperaemia, burns of mucous membranes, or evidence of trauma to upper respiratory passages all suggest inhalation of noxious agents or presence of respiratory burn. Oxygen is administered and blood gases, including carbon monoxide, are quickly determined. If the child exhibits changes in sensorium, air hunger, or otherwise appears in a critical condition, an endotracheal tube is inserted to maintain the airway. The usual practice is to place a tube if there is any question regarding the possibility of respiratory problems. Pharyngeal oedema may make delayed intubation difficult, and the child will become restless from hypoxia.

Tracheostomy is rarely employed, because it has been associated with serious complications and significant mortality in childhood burn injuries, such as a high incidence of infection, tracheobronchitis, delayed haemorrhage, and cannula obstruction from secretions and granulations. Inasmuch as early oedema subsides within 24-48 hours and many have been managed successfully for longer periods without significant damage, nasotracheal intubation is the safer and preferred approach. It allows for the delivery of humidified air with oxygen, the easy removal of secretions from respiratory passages, and the use of a pressure ventilator if needed.

Frequently, placing the child in semi-Fowler position inside a tent or under an oxygen hood with a high flow of oxygen and maximum humidity is sufficient to reduce reflex bronchospasm produced by trauma to the bronchial mucosa.

Fluid replacement therapy

The objectives of fluid therapy are to:
* compensate for water and sodium lost to traumatized areas and interstitial spaces
* replenish sodium deficits
* restore plasma volume
* obtain adequate perfusion
* correct acidosis
* improve renal function.

Fluid and electrolyte therapy for children in the first 24 hours after a burn is still controversial. This controversy is centred primarily around whether colloid solution, usually albumin, dextran or plasma, should be part of the resuscitation phase of fluid therapy.

The composition of the fluid selected varies with the philosophy of the individual practitioner. Needs are determined by several parameters, such as vital signs, including blood pressure, urine volume and character, pulse, adequacy of capillary filling and state of sensorium. In complicated cases arterial, central venous and pulmonary artery pressures are monitored. These criteria, based on individual needs, are more effective for fluid resuscitation. Periodic monitoring of potassium, chloride, carbon dioxide, blood urea nitrogen, and osmolality helps determine the adequacy of fluid therapy and evidence of acidosis (Herndon *et al*, 1985).

After diuresis, in 48-72 hours when capillary permeability is restored, fluid requirements decrease to a constant that remains so long as the burn wound is open. Sometimes, colloid solutions such as albumin or plasma are used in maintaining plasma volume. During this phase, interstitial fluid is returning rapidly to the vascular compartment, and increasing intake to match urine output may cause circulatory overload. Early enteral feeding is the rule and may begin within the first 24 hours postburn (Guzzetta and Holihan, 1988). Fluid balance may continue to be a problem throughout the course of treatment, especially during the periods in which there may be considerable evaporative loss from the wound.

Nutrition

The high metabolic requirements and catabolism in severe burns make nutritional needs of paramount importance and often difficult to provide. Hypermetabolism, increased glucose flow, and severe protein and fat wasting are characteristic of the response to major trauma and infection. Children with multiple trauma and who are respiratory dependent can have metabolic requirements 30-75% above normal. The metabolic rate of those with burns greater than 40% total body surface is 100% greater than normal (Herndon *et al*, 1985) and may reach 200% of normal resting energy expenditure (Harmel, Vane and King, 1986).

The diet must provide sufficient protein to prevent negative nitrogen balance and extra calories to utilize the proteins, sustain the adaptive hypermetabolism, and spare protein breakdown. Normal protein requirements may be three times the standard adult intake and increase proportionately as a result of trauma and stress. The child's proportionately less body fat and substantially smaller muscle mass predispose to the rapid development of protein-calorie malnutrition (Harmel, Vane and King, 1986). Extra calories should be derived from carbohydrates, because fat, although higher in total calories, will not spare protein. The normal energy stores of glycogen are depleted; therefore, exogenous glucose must be provided early. Intravenous 5% glucose can supply minimum requirements, but these are inadequate to meet added needs.

Most burn patients are able to eat, and the child is given oral feedings as soon as possible.

Nasogastric feedings may be needed to supplement oral intake, and peripheral parenteral alimentation has been used to provide a large amount of concentrated glucose and amino acids, especially in infants. The anorexia, delayed gastric emptying, and osmotic diarrhoea secondary to high-solute tube feedings lead to this mode of nutrition, despite difficulties encountered in placement of the catheter and the increased risk of sepsis.

To facilitate growth and proliferation of epithelial cells, administration of vitamins A and C is begun early in the postburn period. Zinc sulphate is also administered by some practitioners, because zinc stores are depleted during catabolism and it appears to facilitate wound healing and epithelialization.

MANAGEMENT OF BURN WOUND

After the initial period of shock and restoration of fluid balance, the primary concern is the burn wound. The objectives of management for epidermal and superficial (first- and second-degree) burns is to prevent infection by providing an environment as aseptic as possible. Occlusive dressings help to reduce pain by minimizing exposure to air. The exposure method allows the wound to dry and is used primarily for mild to moderate face wounds. All methods employ topical antibacterial applications, or daily hydrotherapy, or both, to remove loose tissue and debris and to allow inspection of the wound. The objectives for management of full-thickness wounds are prevention of invasive infection, removal of dead tissue, protection from mechanical trauma and closure of the wound.

Debridement

The use of hydrotherapy has reduced the need for surgical debridement under general anaesthesia. Debridement is painful and requires some type of analgesic before the procedure (Fig. 24-11). Morphine and fentanyl are drugs of choice in most units. Ketamine hydrochloride in subanaesthetic doses has proved highly effective in children, and nitrous oxide inhalation is employed in a number of burn units. The child will require instruction in how to breathe the gas at the appropriate time and coaching during its use.

Topical antimicrobial agents

Several methods are used for covering the burn wound (Box 24-10). All meet the objective of preparation for permanent wound coverage and all employ some type of topical agent. Before the development of effective topical agents for reducing the incidence of invasive organisms, wound sepsis was the major cause of mortality from burn injury. Successful burn therapy relies on both topical antibacterial applications and thorough cleansing and debridement to reduce the amounts of necrotic material on which the bacteria grow. To be effective,

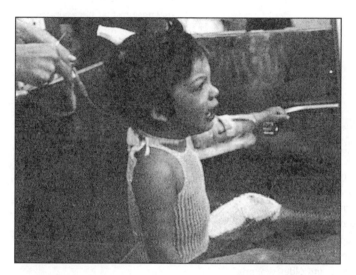

Fig. 24-11 An analgesic is administered before removal of dressings and debridement. In this instance analgesic is injected directly into intravenous line at time of hydrotherapy.

a topical application must be nontoxic, capable of diffusing through eschar, harmless to viable tissue, inexpensive, and easy to apply. It should not cause an increase in resistant strains and should produce minimum electrolyte derangements.

Several topical agents are employed, but those used most frequently are 0.5% silver nitrate solution, 10% mafenide acetate, and 1% silver sulfadiazine. All three are effective bacteriostatic agents, but each has advantages and disadvantages. The significant aspects of each are summarized in Table 24-7.

BIOLOGICAL SKIN COVERINGS

Biological dressings are used during the acute phase of therapy to cover wound surfaces, protect the wound from bacterial invasion, limit fluid and protein loss, reduce pain and increase rate of epithelialization (Herndon *et al*, 1985) (Box 24-11).

The type of graft particularly suitable and used most frequently for temporary covering in children is the porcine xenograft (Fig. 24-12). The split-thickness pigskin is available commercially and is an effective covering agent after eschar separation. Changed regularly, it reduces evaporative loss,

---

◆ BOX 24-10

Methods of burn wound management

Exposure — wounds are left open to the air; crust forms on partial-thickness wounds, and eschar forms on full-thickness wounds.

Open — topical antimicrobial ointment is applied directly to wound surface, but wound is left uncovered.

Modified — ointment is applied directly to wound or impregnated into thin gauze and applied to wound; a stretched gauze or net covering secures the area.

Occlusive — ointment-impregnated gauze or ointment covered with gauze layer is placed on the burn wound; multiple layers of bulky gauze are placed over the primary layer and secured with stretched gauze or net.

◆ BOX 24-11

Types of skin grafts
Temporary Grafts

Allografts (homografts) — skin is obtained from genetically different members of the same species, living or dead, usually cadavers, that are free from disease.

Xenografts (heterografts) — skin is obtained from members of a different species, primarily pigskin, either fresh or frozen.

Permanent Grafts

Autografts — tissues are obtained from undamaged areas of the patient's own body.

Isografts — histocompatible tissue is obtained from genetically identical individuals, that is, the patient's identical twin.

Methods of Applying Split-Thickness Grafts

Full-cover graft — a sheet of skin, removed from the donor site, is placed intact over the recipient site and sutured in place or maintained in place by pressure dressings.

Postage-stamp graft — a sheet of skin from the donor site is cut into postage-stamp pieces and placed on the recipient bed; may be covered with a dressing or left exposed for inspection and rolling serum from beneath the graft.

Mesh, lace, or slit graft — a sheet of skin is removed from donor site with multiple slits so that, when stretched, it expands to cover from one-and-one-half to nine times (usually three times) the area of a full-cover graft; requires suturing to maintain tension; may be exposed or covered with occlusive dressing for about 48 hours; effective for large areas.

AGENT	DRESSINGS	ADVANTAGES	DISADVANTAGES
Silver nitrate, 0.5% (AgNO₃)	Exposure, modified or occlusive Impedes joint movement Dressings changed twice daily	Greatly reduces evaporative losses, thus lower metabolic rate and lower weight loss Does not interfere with wound healing Nonallergenic Inexpensive Effective against major burn flora, including *Pseudomonas* and *Staphylococcus*	Cannot allow dressings to become dry; requires frequent wetting (at least every 2 hours) Difficult to use Ineffective on established burn wound infections Does not penetrate eschar; therefore, should be applied before bacterial growth established Hypotonicity pulls electrolytes from wound, causing depletion of sodium, chloride, potassium, and magnesium that necessitates continuous monitoring and replacement Little effect on *Klebsiella* and *Aerobacter* groups Stains skin, linens, clothes
Mafenide acetate 10%	Usually exposure Occasionally with dressings Reapplied twice daily	Diffuses rapidly into burn wound and underlying tissues Rapidly excreted Easily applied Penetrates through eschar and deeply into burn wound; therefore effective in deep flame, electric, and older wounds Effective against many gram-positive and gram-negative organisms, including *Pseudomonas* and *Clostridium*	Mild acidosis caused by inhibition of carbonic anhydrase in kidney Hypersensitivity reaction in many children Causes discomfort during application Inhibits wound healing
Silver sulfadiazine, 1% (AgSD)	Occlusive Motion of joints maintained Applied once or twice daily	Nontoxic Combines advantages of silver nitrate and mafenide acetate Painless (relatively) Easy to apply Absorbs slowly Bactericidal for up to 48 hours Effective against gram-positive and gram-negative bacteria and *Candida albicans*	Does not penetrate eschar as well as mafenide acetate or gentamicin sulfate Children complain that the application feels 'cold', may be interpreted as pain May cause neutropenia; usually reverses in 48 hours

(cont.)

Table 24-7 Comparison of common topical preparations.

| Gentamicin sulfate, 0.1% | Exposure, modified or occlusive | No pain associated with use
Relatively nontoxic
Penetrates burn wound quickly
Especially effective against *Klebsiella* and *Enterobacter* | 40% of pseudomonal organisms have become resistant
Occasionally nephrotoxicity and ototoxicity |
| Povidone-iodine ointment | Exposure, modified or occlusive
Impedes joint movement | Apparently nontoxic
Effective against broad spectrum of organisms | Elevation of protein-bound iodine (PBI)
Use associated with considerable pain
Causes eschar to 'tan' and become very stiff, making debridement and evaluation of burn wound difficult
May cause acidosis |

Table 24-7 Comparison of common topical preparations. (continued).

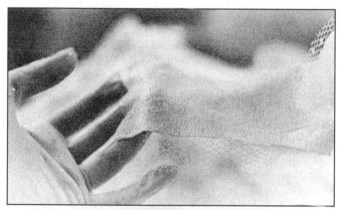

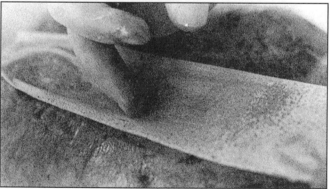

Fig. 24-12 Porcine dressing. Removed from net backing (above). Applied to wound (below).

protects the wound bed, and is believed to protect the wound from infection and trauma. The grafts usually adhere within a few hours, and dressings are not needed. They are particu-larly effective in children with second-degree scald burns of hands and face, because they allow relatively pain-free movement, which reduces contracture and has the added benefit of improved appetite and morale. Pigskin dressings are replaced daily or at least every 3-4 days; as a result acceptance of the graft is minimal. When left in place for longer periods, antibody development causes increasingly rapid rejection.

Other allografts that are used are from human cadavers, when available. Rejection of these grafts occurs in about 14 days. Skin allografts from closely histocompatible living related donors, used in conjunction with immunosuppression therapy, maintain wound coverage continuously over a longer period of time. Short-term coverage can be accomplished with human amnion (obtained by stripping the amniotic membrane from the placenta).

Combined biological and synthetic skin substitutes have been developed for covering burns and skin graft sites. This is the collagen wound dressing and contains a porous collagen fibrillous 'dermal' layer combined with an impermeable 'epi-dermal' layer of Silastic. The synthetic skin is gradually replaced with normal vascularized connective tissue elements as it is slowly biodegraded. This new tissue is then ready to support a standard split-thickness skin graft, which is placed as the Silastic is removed (Burke *et al*, 1981).

Permanent skin covering

Permanent skin grafting is part of the rehabilitative stage to restore cosmetic appearance and to achieve maximum functional capacity. Permanent grafting of full-thickness burns is usually accomplished with a split-thickness skin graft, which can be obtained from only two sources: autograft from the patient's own tissue or isografts from an identical twin (see Box 24-12).

◆ BOX 24-12

Requirements for a successful graft

Sufficient nourishment until new blood supply grows in from the base of the recipient bed

Primary tissue contact, that is, actual contact between cut surface of the graft and the recipient bed

Avoidance of bleeding; the possibility of even the slightest bleeding must be controlled with light pressure

Prevention of infection, especially in full-cover grafts; postage-stamp grafts will often 'take' in contaminated areas

IMPLICATIONS FOR NURSING

Nursing care is the most important aspect of burn therapy. Because the care of severely burned children encompasses such a broad range of skills and foci, it is divided into segments that correspond with the major phases of burn treatment: the *acute phase* (also referred to as the resuscitative, emergent, or metabolic phase), which involves the first 24-48 hours; the *management phase,* which extends from the time a child has been adequately resuscitated until the major rehabilitative aspects of care are initiated; and the *rehabilitative phase,* which begins with permanent grafting. This phase continues until all full-thickness injuries are covered and reconstructive procedures and corrective measures have been accomplished. This often extends over a period of months or years.

ACUTE PHASE

The primary emphasis during the initial phases of burn care is prevention of burn shock and management of pulmonary status. Checking vital signs, monitoring the intravenous infusion line, and measuring urinary output are ongoing nursing activities in the hours immediately after injury. The intravenous infusion is started immediately and is regulated according to urine output and specific gravity, laboratory data, and objective signs of adequate hydration. Urine volume, measured at least every hour, should be 1-2 ml/kg of body weight/hour.

Children are observed for all parameters. They require constant observation and assessment with special attention to signs of complications. Respiratory, cardiac and renal complications may appear early in the postburn period.

Care of the burn wound is secondary to the more critical problems of circulatory or respiratory failure. The burn wound is treated according to the protocol of the specific burn facility. When inhalation injury is suspected, the nurse observes the child for evidence of pulmonary involvement. Activities include listening for inspiratory wheezing and detecting increasing hoarseness.

Throughout the acute phase of care, children's emotional needs must not be overlooked. They are frightened, uncomfortable and often confused. Children are isolated from familiar persons and surroundings, and the often overwhelming physical needs at this time are the primary focus of staff and parents. Children need to be reassured that they are all right and that they will get better.

MANAGEMENT AND REHABILITATIVE PHASES

After the patient's condition is stabilized, the lengthy management phase begins. During this phase, the major goal is care of the wound to facilitate healing and prepare for permanent closure. The rehabilitative phase begins when permanent closure of the wound begins, although rehabilitation essentially begins with initiation of care.

The management phase of burn care involves intensive nursing care, which can be arduous for patient, family, and nursing staff. Except for minor burns, care usually takes place in a burn unit.

The burn pain is overwhelming, engulfing and irrepressible. Consequently, the pain causes anxiety and a feeling of profound helplessness in a child and can produce reactions of confusion, fear and panic. Compounding the pain is a child's interpretation of it and of the procedures; this is closely related to the developmental level of a child. Many burned children believe their pain is punishment for past misdeeds and therefore deserved. There are often feelings of anger, guilt, and depression, and, as in all illness, regressive behaviour. When children appear to accept their pain and show little or no aggressive behaviour, psychological consultation is usually in order.

It is always difficult to deal with children in pain, and to inflict pain on helpless children is contrary to the empathetic nature of nursing. Adequate management of pain is essential to reduce discomfort of the burn and the necessary therapeutic procedures. Management of pain consists of choosing the: (1) correct analgesic (opioids are needed for severe pain), (2) adequate dosage, and (3) appropriate timing. Relaxation techniques, distraction therapy and cutaneous stimulation by touching may be helpful.

Care of burn wound

The nurse has the major responsibility for cleansing, debriding, and applying topical medication and dressings to the burn wound. Because dressing removal is a painful procedure, children should receive adequate analgesia and the peak effect of the drug should coincide with the procedure.

Research has demonstrated that children are more cooperative and demonstrate less anxiety and depression when they are allowed to be active participants in their care (Kavanagh and Freeman, 1984). Predictability and controllability are promoted during dressing changes. Predictability is increased by providing cues (nurses wearing specific clothing for dressing changes), focusing the patient on the procedure, and providing children with information about physical sensations they are likely to experience (e.g., pulling, stinging, pressure) before they experience them. Controllability is enhanced by providing the children with as many choices as possible during the burn care and encouraging active participation. These strategies are unlike the traditional approaches of distraction and passivity. 'Learned helplessness' is most intense when the outcomes are unpleasant and the situation is perceived to be unchangeable (Murphy, 1982). See suggestions for reducing the stress of burn wound management outlined in Box 24-13.

There are some psychological implications that may influence a child's reaction to the hydrotherapy and application of medication. Children who acquired the burn from hot water are particularly fearful, especially if the injury was inflicted as a punishment (non-accidental injury). Application of the medication also can be a painful experience, when mafenide cream is the agent employed. Both the nurse and the children must understand that there is a painful sensation often described as 'burning' that may have special significance for these children, who must be reassured that the medication is not inflicting further injury.

When occlusive dressings are applied, elastic bandages are worn over dressings to prevent epithelial breakdown, to stimulate circulation, and to make mobility easier. The bandage is applied in a figure eight to promote optimum circulation. A stable dressing is especially important when the children are ambulatory.

There are other aspects of burn care of which nurses should be aware. Universal precautions are followed. Many children are placed in protective isolation, which severely limits their contact with others. Complete coverings on all who enter their presence, including most of the face, serve to further isolate these children. Children who are accustomed to having someone nearby continuously, as in the intensive care burn

unit, may become anxious and uneasy when transferred to a transitional unit or a regular unit where staff members are available only intermittently or when summoned.

Nutrition

After the initial phase of care, children are usually allowed oral feedings (unless paralytic ileus persists). If they will not eat, tube feeding is necessary, but every effort should be made to encourage oral intake without a power struggle.

Because children frequently lack appetite and their caloric needs and protein needs are markedly increased, a great deal of encouragement, help, and patience is required on the part of the nursing staff. Consultation with the parents and the dietitian is arranged to determine the best way to provide needed nutrients in foods the child will be more likely to eat. Children who are old enough to participate should be included in the planning.

Many children eat better when they can feed themselves and when they can eat in an atmosphere more nearly like that they are accustomed to at home. Even if they are unable to feed themselves (e.g., if their arms are bandaged), they do better if they can sit up or at least see the tray of food so that they can instruct the person feeding them how they prefer their food and what they want to be fed next. When their condition allows, children enjoy sitting at a table for their meals, especially with other children. Parents are encouraged to bring a child's favourite dish from home.

Prevent complications: acute care

Attempts should be made to decrease the excess metabolic expenditures of burned children. This means avoiding overheating and underheating. The hypermetabolic response is temperature sensitive, but not temperature dependent. Environmental temperatures greater than skin temperature cause the metabolic rate of patients with burns in excess of 40% to increase at twice the normal rate. Therefore, the environmental temperature in the child's room should be maintained between 28-33°C to minimize metabolic expenditure and maximize comfort (Herndon *et al*, 1985).

Hypothermia is also a threat, and a means must be provided to prevent heat loss, such as expeditious dressing changes to avoid prolonged exposure and intermittent hypothermia that result in 'cold stress'. An overhead warming unit may be provided to maintain body heat.

The chief danger in this phase of burn care is infection — wound infection, generalized sepsis, and bacterial pneumonia. All burn patients are treated in a protected environment. It is important to make accurate ongoing assessments of all parameters that provide clues for diagnosis. For example, wound cultures are done at least three times weekly, and a blood culture is indicated in any child with a rectal temperature of 39.5°C or higher.

Antacids are usually administered prophylactically to prevent or minimize the effect of Curling ulcer, but nurses must be alert for any signs of bleeding.

◆ **BOX 24-13**

Guidelines for easing distress of dressing changes in burn management

Have all materials ready before beginning

Administer appropriate analgesics

Remind child of impending procedure to provide sufficient time for child to prepare for the ordeal

Allow child to test and approve the temperature of the water for hydrotherapy

Allow child to state on which area of the body to begin

Allow child to request *one* short rest period during procedure

Allow child to remove dressings if desired

Provide something constructive for child to do during procedure (e.g., holding a package of dressings, holding someone's hand)

Inform child when the procedure is near completion

Praise child for cooperation

Continued observations are made to detect any indication of other complications associated with burns and their management. Rashes are not uncommon in children and may be of viral origin or a reaction to medications. They should be evaluated. The nurse must be alert to the possibility of any of the complications described previously — hypertension, renal disorders and convulsion disorders.

Because children are reluctant to move, because doing so causes pain or discomfort, stiffness and joint contracture develop easily. In an effort to prevent this complication, they are encouraged to move whenever feasible and active physiotherapy is included as an essential aspect of burn care. When children are resting or sleeping, contracture is prevented by proper splinting. Children's natural tendency is to be active, and they will usually move spontaneously unless the pain is severe.

Prevent complications: long-term care

The rehabilitative phase of burn care begins when permanent closure of the wound is implemented. The primary focus of this phase is to obtain functional use of burned areas and cosmetic results as nearly normal as possible. Efforts in the care of children with skin grafts are directed towards facilitating a 'take'. Trauma, infection, and bleeding must be avoided for a successful transplantation to occur. When the grafted area is left exposed, children must be immobilized to prevent the graft from becoming dislodged. Flat surfaces usually pose few problems, but grafts over irregular or mobile areas may require special techniques such as splints or skeletal traction. Small children usually need to be restrained, and sedation is sometimes needed for very restless or uncooperative children for the first two or three days after surgery.

The exposed method allows for easier inspection of the grafts, and collection of fluid under the graft can be removed by gently rolling the fluid out with a sterile applicator. This should be attempted with collections of fluid 1.25 cm or less from the edge of the graft. For those further toward the middle, a tiny slit is made in the graft tissue through which the fluid can be rolled. The less disturbance to any fibrous attachments, the better.

Some plastic surgeons prefer to use occlusive pressure dressings over the grafted tissue or secured with sutures attached to normal surrounding skin and tied over the grafted skin to hold it in place.

Wound contraction and scar tissue formation are normal parts of wound healing (Fig. 24-13). Scar tissue is metabolically active tissue that continually rearranges itself; as a result, disabling contractures, deformity and disfigurement are ever-present possibilities. Splints and other methods are employed to minimize these long-term effects. Pressure splints and elastic bandages or pressure garments help reduce scar hypertrophy and are sometimes worn for months after hospitalization.

Scar tissue has some properties that are significant, particularly for growing children. Intense itching occurs in healing burn wounds and scar tissue until the scar is no longer oedematous and raised. Scar tissue does not grow as do normal

tissues, which may create difficulties, especially in areas such as hands. Additional surgery is sometimes needed to maintain function in contracted areas.

Severely burned children must return to the hospital periodically for additional skin grafts and scar revisions, especially to release contractures over joint spaces and for cosmetic considerations. Achievement of optimum results frequently requires years. In the meantime, burn scars are unsightly, and although improvements can be made, hope should not be extended to the parents and child for complete cosmetic and functional repair.

The psychological pain and sequelae of severe burn trauma are as intense as the physical trauma. All burned children have a tremendous amount of pain, often continuous for varying periods, and are separated from the family for extended periods. During the painful ordeal of hospitalization, children develop coping mechanisms for dealing with the acute and ever-present pain. Self-induced hypnosis is not uncommon.

Life becomes a struggle for children after burn trauma. They are puzzled, confused and bombarded by a new way of life in a frightening world of strange people, things and language. They wonder why this has happened to *them* — what they have done that they should be punished so. Past experiences cannot serve them in this crisis. They do not understand the 'ugliness'

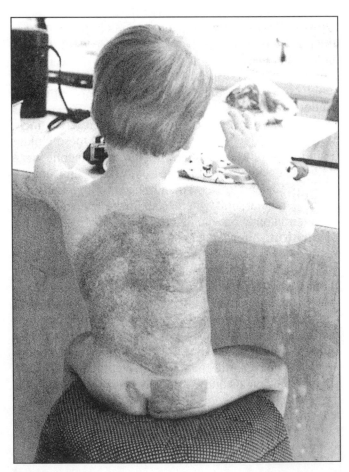

Fig. 24-13 Extensive scars from flame burn. Note donor graft site on right buttock.

and disfigurement they see as their bodies. They wonder, "Am I going to die?".

Preparation for facing friends and classmates may be more than they are able to cope with; some severely burned children are ashamed to show their bodies in the hospital. In addition, pressure garments and other therapeutic measures greatly intensify the feeling of being different. It is not difficult to imagine how children dread facing a world of stares or imagined stares. Undressing at school can be a painful experience. It is not surprising that many children withdraw from contacts with others, even at a very early age. In time, as understanding and acceptance increase, they may feel more comfortable with themselves, and the emotional scars may fade somewhat.

The impact of such severe injury taxes the capabilities of children at all ages, but young children, who suffer acutely from separation anxiety, and adolescents, who are developing an identity, are probably most affected psychologically.

Child support

One of the most difficult aspects of burn care, especially in children, is the impact it has on nurses. The appearance and smell of the burn and the necessary discomfort that must be inflicted on the child as a part of the therapy are often beyond the nurse's ability to cope and remain therapeutic. Throughout the entire process of burn management, nurses must deal with their own feelings and anxieties regarding their therapeutic role in burn care.

Children should begin early to do as much for themselves as possible and to be active participants in their care. It takes a great deal of warm firmness and fortitude on the part of the nurse to force these children to do this. Moving hurts. Many children are able to move and help themselves. Others need considerable help and encouragement. If children are unable to move, they should be told firmly but gently that it must be done, that the nurses will help them, and that it will be done as quickly as possible. They should be told how they can help to make it easier.

Children should be encouraged to participate in as many aspects of their care as possible. With illness, children always regress to the developmental level that allows them to deal with the stress. As their condition permits, children can be expected to do things that they were capable of doing for themselves before they were burned, such as oral hygiene, face washing, feeding themselves, and playing. Allowing children to make choices and to help make decisions about the time of their care and recreational activities makes them feel a part of the team and provides them with a small measure of control. They will probably require assistance; however, as children see themselves contributing to their care, they gain confidence and self-esteem. Fears and anxieties diminish with accomplishment and self-confidence.

Activities are selected and encouraged according to each child's level of development and interest, but, as with any ill child, they should be somewhat simpler and less challenging than would be expected in a state of health. Otherwise their already taxed energies may be further depleted and self-esteem

threatened. Quiet games and activities such as reading, colouring, drawing, games, and puzzles are always appropriate. Television is a satisfactory diversion but should not replace active participation and should not substitute for contacts with others. Play that encourages the expression of feelings of guilt, frustration, and anger is especially therapeutic. Contacts should also include those that help children to understand what can be expected, their role, and what the nurse will do. During the acute, resuscitative phase, children are frequently isolated, but they should be moved to where they have contact with others, especially other children, as soon as their physical condition allows. School-aged children should continue with schoolwork.

Children need to be bolstered in other ways. They like to look and smell nice, and the unattractive burns, dressings, and assorted paraphernalia do little to foster a positive self-image. They know how they appear to others, and small things such as careful hair combing and a bright ribbon, colourful nightgown or pyjamas (when possible), slippers, or any decoration (a flower, pin, necklace, badge) will help make them feel that they look better and are worthwhile to others.

All hospitalized children, especially those who must undergo painful procedures, must be allowed to express their anger and frustration appropriately through verbalization or play. They need to know that their injury and the treatments are not punishment for specific or general, real or imagined transgressions and to know that nurses understand their fears, anger and discomfort. They also need body contact. This is often difficult to arrange for the child with massive injury. The discomfort associated with moving and the bulky, messy dressings or the bare open wound are deterrents and frequently provide justification for the nurse to avoid such action because of fear or repulsion. Even older children enjoy sitting on the nurse's or parent's lap and being cuddled and hugged. This can be a comfort in times of stress or used as a reward, but most of all it should be kept in mind that it is a natural part of childhood.

Family support

Members of the family as well as the child feel the impact of severe burn injury. They are concerned about the child's survival, recovery, and future appearance. Because they, too, have overwhelming anxieties, fears, frustrations and feelings of guilt, their needs must be met in order that they, in turn, can provide the support and encouragement so desperately needed by the child. It is the family, particularly the parents, who are the most significant persons in the child's life.

Nurses are in the most opportune position to assist parents to cope with the stresses of the child's illness and their own feelings of guilt and helplessness. The parents need to be informed of the child's progress and helped in their efforts to cope with their feelings while providing support to the child. The nurse is the person who can help them understand that it is not selfish to look after themselves and their own needs in order that they can better meet the needs of the child. For parents whose response to the illness is too severe or whose response to stress is manifest in destructive behaviour, professional help may be needed.

KEY POINTS

◆ Infants are subject to fluid depletion because of their relatively greater surface area, their high rate of metabolism and their immature kidney function.

◆ Management of fluid volume disturbances focuses on the following areas: volume of body fluids, osmolality, hydrogen ion status, electrolyte deficits, and disturbances in mineral skeleton and body fluid equilibrium.

◆ Parenteral fluid therapy is initiated to meet ongoing daily physiological losses, restore previous deficits, and replace ongoing abnormal losses.

◆ Oedema formation is caused by increased venous pressure, capillary permeability, diminished plasma proteins, lymphatic obstruction, or decreased tissue tension.

◆ Nursing assessment off fluid and electrolyte disturbances entails observation of general appearance, vital signs, intake and output measurement, and review of relevant laboratory results.

◆ Intravenous alimentation provides total nutritional needs when feeding via the gastrointestinal tract is impossible, inadequate or hazardous.

◆ Acute infectious gastroenteritis is caused by enterotoxin production, invasion and destruction of epithelial cells, penetration and system invasion, or adherence without destruction of mucosa and without enterotoxin production.

◆ Vomiting may result from infectious disorders, responses to an allergen or ingestion of drugs or other toxic substances, symptoms associated with appendicitis or gastrointestinal obstruction, motion sickness, environmental stress and oral-defence mechanisms.

◆ Nurses should observe character, frequency, amount and force of vomitus.

◆ People at risk for anaphylaxis may be identified by a history of previous allergic reaction, history of atopy, history of severe reactions in family, and positive skin test to the allergen.

◆ Burns are assesed on the basis of percentage of body surface burned, depth, location, age, aetiological agent, respiratory involvement, general health and presence of associated injury or condition.

◆ Emergency measures for severe burns include stopping the burning process; assessing for airway, breathing, and circulation; covering the burn; transporting the child to medical aid; and providing reassurance to child and family..

REFERENCES

Ableson WH, Smith RG: *Residents handbook of paediatrics,* ed 7, Toronto, 1987, BC Decker.

Barnes LA: Fluid and electrode therapy. In Glisss SS, Kagan BM, editots: *Current paediatric therapy 12*, Philadelphia, 1986, WB Saunders Co.

Behrman RE, Vaaughan VC, III, editors: *Nelson textbook of pediatrics*, ed. 13, Philadelphia, 1987, WB Saunders Co.

Brown KH, MacLean WC: Nutritional management of acute diarrhea: an appraisal of the alternatives, *Pediatr* 73:119, 1984.

Bull JP: Revised analysis of mortality due to burns, *Lancet* II:1133, 1971.

Burke JF *et al*: Successful use of a physiologicallly acceptable artificial skin in the treatment of extensive burn injury, *Ann Surg* 194:413, 1981.

Finberg L: Assessing the clinical clues to dehydration, *Contemp Paediatr* 7(4):45, 1990.

Fire Statistics, United Kingdom, London, 1983, Home Office.

Ghishan FK: The transport of electrolytes in the gut and the use of oral rehydration solutions, *Pediatr Clin N Am* 35:3, 1988.

Ghishan FK: The transport of electrolytes in the gut and the use of oral rehydration solutions, *Pediatr Clin North Am* 35:35, 1988.

Groothuis JR, Berman S, Chapman J: Effect of carbohydrate injested on outcome in infants with mild gastroenteritis, *J Pediatr* 108:903, 1986.

Guzzetta P, Holihan J: Burns. In Eichelberger M, Pratsch G, editors: *Pediatric trauma care*, Rockville, MD, 1988, Aspen.

Harmel RP, Vane DW, King DR: Burn care in children—special considerations, *Clin Plast Surg* 13:95, 1986.

Harvey–Kemble JV, Lamb BE: *Practical burns management,* London, 1987, Hodder and Stoughton.

Hermansen MC, Buches M: Super diapers and premature infants, *Pediatr* 79:1056, 1987.

Hermansen MC, Buches M: Urine output determination from superabsorbant and regular diapers under radiant heat, *Paediatr* 81:428, 1988.

Herndon DN *et al*: Treatment of burns in children, *Pediatr Clin N Am* 32:1311, 1985.

Jacoby F: Care of the massive burn wound, *Crit Care Q* 7(3):44, 1984.

Kavanagh CK, Freeman R: Burn care and the pediatric patient: a preliminary report, *PRN Forum* 3(2):1, 1984.

Kempe CH, Silver HK and O'Brien D: *Current pediatric diagnosis and treatment*, ed 9, Los Altos, Calif, 1986, Lange Medical Publications.

LaMotte R, Thalhammer J: Peripheral neural mechanisms of cutaneous hyperalgesia following mild injury by heat, *Neuroscience* 2:765, 1982.

Lund, Browder. In Harvey–Kemble JV, Lamb BE: *Practical burns management*, London, 1987, Hodder & Stoughton.

Margolis PA *et al*: Effects of unrestricted diet on mild infantile diarrhea, *Am J Dis Child* 144:162, 1990.

Murphy SA: Learned helplessness: from concept to comprehension, *Perspect Psychiatr Care* 20(2):27, 1982.

Penny ME, Paredes P, Brown KH: Clinical and nutritional consequences of lactose feeding during persistent postenteritis diarrhea, *Pediatr* 84:835, 1989.

Perkin RM, Anas NG: Cardiovascular evaluation on support in the critically ill child, *Pediatr Ann* 15(1):30, 1986.

Pizarro D, Posada G, Levine MM: Hypernatremic diarrhea dehydration treated with slow oral rehydration therapy: a preliminary report, *J Pediatr* 104:316, 1984.

Santosham M *et al*: Role of soy-based, lactose-free formula during treatment of acute diarrhea, *Pediatr* 76:292, 1985.

Silverman A, Roy CC: Pediatric clinical gastroenterology, ed 3, St Louis, 1983, Mosby–Year Book.

Webster H, Veasy LG: Intra-aortic balloon pumping in children, *Heart Lung J Crit Care* 14:548, 1985.

Weizman Z: Cola drinks and rehydration in acute diarrhea (letter), *N Engl J Med* 315:768, 1986.

Zimmerman JJ, Dietrich KA: Current perspectives on septic shock, *Pediatr Clin North Am* 34:131, 1987.

FURTHER READING

General

Campbell AGM, McIntosh N, editors: *Forfar and Arneil's textbook of paediatrics*, ed 4, Edinburgh, 1992, Churchill Livingstone.

Chenevey B: Overview of fluid and electrolytes, *Nurs Clin North Am* 22:749, 1987.

Lancaster LE: Renal and endocrine regulation of water and electrolyte balance, *Nurs Clin North Am* 22:761, 1987.

Scratcherd T: *Aids to physiology*, Edinburgh, 1988, Churchill Livingstone.

Shock

Hinds CJ: *Intensive care: a concise textbook*, London, 1987, Baillière Tindall.

Long-Term Venous Access

Brown G, Husband JE: Mediastinal widening—a valuable radiographic sign of superior vena cava thrombosis, *Clin Radiol* 47(6):415, 1993.

Dann A: Central venous sepsis in children with gastrointestinal disorders, *Gastroenterol Nurs* 16(6):259, 1994.

Keegan-Wells D, Stewart JL: The use of venous access devices in pediatric oncology nursing practice, *J Pediatr Oncol Nurs* 9(4):159, 1992.

Schultz S, Kerlan RK: Managing Hickman catheter problems without surgery, *Western J Med* 160(5):457, 1994.

Parenteral Nutrition

Collier S *et al*: Use of cyclic parenteral nutrition in infants less than 6 months of age, *Nutr Clin Pract* 9(2):65, 1994.

Intravenous Therapy

Blough LD: Starting intravenous lines in children: a different perspective (letter), *J Emerg Nurs* 18(5):374, 1992.

Seigler RS, Tecklenburg FW, Shealy R: Prehospital intraosseous infusion by emergency medical services personnel: a prospective study, *Pediatr* 84:173, 1989.

Diarrhoea

Candy CE: Recent advances in the care of children with acute diarrhoea: giving responsibility to the nurse and patient, *J Adv Nurs* 12(1):95, 1987.

Walker-Smith JA: Intractable diarrhoea in infancy: a continuing challenge for the paediatric gastroenterologist (review), *Acta Paediatr Supple* 83(395):6, 1994.

Infectious Gastroenteritis

Buzby M: Infectious gastroenteritis in infants and children, *Gastroenterol Nurs* 14(6):302, 1992.

Burns

Chapman JC, Sarhadi NS, Watson ACH: Declining incidence of paediatric burns in Scotland: a review of 1114 children with burns treated as inpatients and outpatients in a regional centre, *Burns* 20(2):106, 1994. Child Accident Prevention Trust: *Fact sheets on burns to children*, London, 1987, Child Accident Prevention Trust.

Kelly H: Initial nursing assessment and management of burn-injured children, *BJN* 3(2):54, 1994.

Locke G: A & E: care and transfer of the burns patient, *Nurs Standard* 7(3):5, 1992.

Lowry M: Taking the heat out of burns: nursing management of burns, *Prof Nurse* 8(1):26, 1992.

Raeside F: Physiotherapy management of burned children: a pilot study, *Physiotherapy* 78(12):891, 1992.

Sheridan RL, Tompkins RG: Prognostic significance of prehospital cardiac or pulmonary resuscitation in paediatric burns patients, *Burns* 20(3):265, 1994.

Wallace E: Nursing a teenager with burns, *Nurs* 2(5):278, 1993.

Witchell M: Dressing burns in children, *Nurs Times* 87(36):63, 1991.

Chapter 25

The Child with Genitourinary Dysfunction

LEARNING OUTCOMES

After studying this chapter you should be able to:

◆ Understand and describe the two types of dialysis available.
◆ Define nephrotic syndrome and describe the nursing needs of a child with this illness.
◆ Recognize the effect of chronic renal failure on other systems of the body.
◆ Understand the importance of investigating a child with a proven urinary tract infection.
◆ Describe the objectives of treating a child with urinary tract infection.
◆ Define the glossary terms.

GLOSSARY

azotaemia Excessive amounts of nitrogenous compounds in the blood

bacteriuria Growth of bacteria in uncontaminated urine

cystitis Inflammation of the bladder

dialysis Process of separating colloids and crystalline substances in solution by the difference in their rate of diffusion through a semipermeable membrane

haemodialysis Dialysis in which blood is circulated outside the body through artificial membranes

hyperkalaemia Abnormal potassium concentration in the blood

oliguria Diminished output of urine

osteodystrophy Defective bone formation

peritoneal dialysis Dialysis in which the peritoneum serves as a semipermeable membrane

tubular Involving renal tubules

uraemia Presence of excessive amounts of urea and other nitrogenous waste in the blood

urethritis Inflammation of the urethra

Diseases involving the kidneys are relatively common in childhood and are caused by a variety of aetiological factors. To better understand the way in which the pathological processes produce an effect, the basic kidney structure and function are briefly reviewed, and the most frequently used tests of renal function are outlined to help the reader understand the relationship of these studies to renal physiology and pathology.

Discussion of the common disorders of renal function is followed by discussion of the critical therapies of dialysis and renal transplant.

RENAL STRUCTURE AND FUNCTION

The primary responsibility of the kidney is to maintain the composition and volume of the body fluids. This is accomplished by the formation of urine. The structural and functional unit of the kidney is the nephron, which is composed of a complex system of tubules, arterioles, venules and capillaries.

The kidney also produces erythropoietin stimulating factor which acts on plasma globulin to form erythropoietin, which stimulates erythropoiesis in the bone marrow. Renin is secreted by the kidney and plays a part in the maintenance of blood pressure.

ASSESSMENT OF RENAL FUNCTION

Assessment of kidney and urinary tract integrity, and the diagnosis of renal or urinary tract disease, are based on several evaluative tools. Physical examination, history and observation of symptoms are the initial procedures. In suspected urinary tract diseases or disorders, further assessment by laboratory, radiological, and other evaluative methods is carried out.

CLINICAL MANIFESTATIONS

As in most disorders of childhood, the incidence and type of kidney or urinary tract dysfunction change with the age and maturation of the child. In addition, the presenting complaints and the significance of these complaints vary with maturation. For example, a complaint of enuresis has greater significance at age eight years than at age four. In the newborn, urinary tract disorders are associated with several obvious malformations of other body systems, including the unexplained but frequent association between malformed or low-set ears and urinary tract anomalies.

Many of the clinical manifestations are common to a variety of childhood disorders, but their presence is an indication to obtain further information from past history, family history and laboratory studies as part of a complete physical examination. Suspected renal disease can be further evaluated through radiological studies and renal biopsy.

LABORATORY TESTS

Both urine and blood studies contribute vital information for detection of renal problems. The single most important test is probably the routine urinalysis. Glomerular filtration rate is a measure of the amount of plasma from which a given substance is totally cleared in one minute. Clearance is calculated from the ratio of substance excreted to the concentration of that substance in the plasma. Any significant degree of renal disease can diminish the glomerular filtration rate, but diseases of the glomerulus and renal vascular disease have the most immediate effect.

IMPLICATIONS FOR NURSING

Nursing responsibilities in assessment of genitourinary disorders and/or diseases begins with observation of the child for any manifestations that might indicate dysfunction. In addition to the general manifestations, many conditions have specific characteristics that distinguish them from other disorders.

Nurses maintain careful intake and output measurements on most children with genitourinary dysfunction and those who might be at risk to develop renal complications (e.g., children in shock, postoperative patients). Nurses observe the characteristics of urine collected, often perform tests on urine specimens (e.g., urine specific gravity, protein, blood, glucose, ketones), and assist with more complex diagnostic tests (e.g., radiography, cystoscopy)

GENITOURINARY TRACT DISORDERS

Urinary tract anomalies and disorders may adversely affect urinary excretion by producing inflammation, tissue damage, and scarring of tissue components. Infection of the genitourinary tract is one of the most common conditions in childhood. In many cases, the predisposing cause is obstruction within the kidneys and within the urinary drainage and storage structures. Obstructive uropathy has been discussed in relation to congenital anomalies. This section is devoted to infections in the genitourinary tract and a common aetiological condition, vesicoureteric reflux.

URINARY TRACT INFECTION

Urinary tract infection (UTI) is the term used to describe a clinical condition that may involve the urethra, bladder (lower urinary tract), and/or the ureters, renal pelvis, calyces and renal parenchyma (upper urinary tract). Because it is often impossible to localize the infection, the broad designation, UTI, is applied to the presence of significant numbers of micro-organisms anywhere within the urinary tract (except the distal one-third of the urethra, which is usually colonized with bacteria).

Infection of the urinary tract may be present with or without clinical symptoms. As a result, the site of infection is often difficult to pinpoint with accuracy. Various terms used to describe urinary tract disorders are listed in Box 25-1.

Classification of urinary tract infection or inflammation

Bacteriuria — growth of bacteria in uncontaminated urine (greater than 100,000 colonies/ml)

Asymptomatic bacteriuria — significant bacteriuria with no clinical evidence of active infection

Symptomatic bacteriuria — significant bacteriuria accompanied by physical symptoms

Recurrent UTI — repeated symptomatic episodes, usually caused by entry of new organisms from the perineal-faecal flora (sometimes termed *reinfection*)

Relapse of UTI — persistence of the same organism despite appropriate antibiotic therapy

Urethritis — inflammation of the urethra

Cystitis — inflammation of the bladder

Ureteritis — inflammation of the ureters

Pyelonephritis — inflammation of the kidney and upper tract (may be acute or chronic)

The peak incidence of UTI not caused by structural anomalies occurs between two and six years of age. Except for the neonatal period, females have a 10-30 times greater risk for developing UTI than males. Approximately 3-5% of girls will have one or more episodes of UTI prior to puberty (Jodal and Winberg, 1987). The likelihood of recurrence is 50% or greater in girls; the recurrence rate is lower in boys (Edelmann, 1988).

UTI in newborns differs in some respects from infections occurring in older children. In this group, males outnumber females. At all ages asymptomatic bacteriuria is more common than symptomatic disease, and recurrence is not uncommon, especially in girls. Rate of recurrence of UTI in neonates is estimated at 25% (Cepero-Akselrod Ranirez, Seijas and Castaneda, 1993). An increased incidence of UTI is observed in adolescents, especially those with evidence of sexual activity. Overall recurrence rate in older children is estimated at 30% (Cepero-Akselrod Ranirez, Seijas and Castaneda, 1993).

AETIOLOGY

A variety of organisms can be responsible for UTI. *Escherichia coli* (80% of cases) and other gram-negative enteric organisms are most frequently implicated; all are common to the anal, perineal, and perianal region. Other organisms associated with UTI include *Proteus, Pseudomonas, Klebsiella, Staphylococcus aureus, Haemophilus,* and coagulase-negative *Staphylococcus*. Several factors contribute to the development of UTI. These include anatomical, physical, and chemical conditions or properties of the host urinary tract.

Anatomical and physical factors

The structure of the lower urinary tract is believed to account for the increased incidence of bacteriuria in females. The short urethra, which measures about 2 cm in young females and 4 cm in mature women, provides a ready pathway for invasion of organisms. In addition, the closure of the urethra at the end of micturition may return contaminated bacteria to the bladder. The longer male urethra (as long as 20 cm in an adult) and the antibacterial properties of prostatic secretions inhibit the entry and growth of pathogens. Reports indicate an increased incidence of UTI in infants less than one year of age who are not circumcised when compared to infants who are circumcised (Herzog, 1989; Roberts, 1988; Wiswell and Geschke, 1989; Wiswell and Roscelli, 1986). The presence of a foreskin is associated with a greater quantity of periurethral bacteria that can ascend the urethra easily (Wiswell *et al*, 1988). The incidence of renal scarring is greatest in patients whose first infection occurs during infancy.

The single most important host factor influencing the occurrence of UTI is urinary stasis. Ordinarily urine is sterile, but at 37°C it provides an excellent culture medium. Under normal conditions, the act of completely and repeatedly emptying the bladder flushes away any organisms before they multiply and invade surrounding tissue. However, urine that remains in the bladder allows bacteria from the urethra to rapidly become established in the rich medium.

Incomplete bladder emptying (stasis) may result from reflux, anatomical abnormalities, dysfunction of the voiding mechanism, or extrinsic ureteral or bladder compression. Pressure of overdistention within the bladder may increase the risk of infection by decreasing host resistance, probably as a result of lessened blood flow to the mucosa. This frequently occurs in neurogenic bladder or as a consequence of voluntarily holding back urine despite the urge to void.

Extrinsic factors that may be responsible for *functional* bladder neck obstruction are chronic and intermittent constipation, and pregnancy. In both conditions, the full rectum or uterus displaces the bladder and posterior urethra in the fixed and limited space of the bony pelvis, causing obstruction, incomplete micturition, and urinary stasis. Treating constipation along with antibiotic therapy for UTI reduces the recurrence of infection, whereas failure to relieve the faecal retention despite adequate treatment of the UTI may result in recurrence.

Other extrinsic factors that can contribute to UTI include catheters, especially short-term indwelling catheters, and administration of antimicrobial agents. Antimicrobials alter the host's normal perineal flora, allowing easier colonization with uropathogens. Tight clothing or nappies, poor hygiene, and local inflammation, such as from vaginitis, masturbation, or pinworm infestation, may also increase the risk of ascending infection. The essential oils in bubble baths and shampoos have been found to irritate the urethra of both boys and girls, causing painful and frequent urination (Rogers, 1985). Sexual intercourse may produce transient bacteriuria in females and is associated with an increased risk of UTI.

Altered urine and bladder chemistry

Several chemical characteristics of the urine and bladder mucosa help maintain urinary sterility. An increased fluid intake promotes flushing of the normal bladder and lowers the concentration of organisms in the infected bladder. Water diuresis also seems to enhance the antibacterial properties of the renal medulla. One effect of water diuresis is increased blood flow to the medulla (where it is normally low), thereby increasing the availability of white cells at the site of inflammation.

Most pathogens favour an alkaline medium. Normally urine is slightly acidic, but it can be made more acidic by diet (e.g., apple or cranberry juices, large amounts of ascorbic acid, animal protein) or by acid-forming drugs. When the urine pH is about 5, bacterial multiplication is hampered, although the acidification rarely eliminates the bacteriuria. However, it may enhance the therapeutic effectiveness of drugs and of the natural defence mechanisms, as well as help relieve some of the symptoms.

CLINICAL MANIFESTATIONS

The clinical manifestations of UTIs depend on the age of the child. In newborn infants and children less than two years of age, the signs are characteristically nonspecific. They more nearly resemble gastrointestinal tract disorders: failure to thrive, feeding problems, vomiting, diarrhoea and abdominal distention. Newborns may have fever or hypothermia and/or sepsis. Other evidence that may be observed includes frequent or infrequent voiding, constant squirming and irritability, strong smelling urine and abnormal stream.

The classic symptoms of UTI are often observed in children over two years of age. These include enuresis or daytime incontinence in the child who has been toilet trained, fever, strong or foul-smelling urine, increased frequency of urination, dysuria or urgency. They may also complain of abdominal pain or costovertebral angle tenderness (flank pain). Some will present with haematuria; some young children may vomit. There is a high frequency of obstructive uropathy in young infants and boys that is characterized by dribbling of urine, straining with urination, or a decrease in the force and size of the urinary stream. High fever and rigors accompanied by flank pain, severe abdominal pain, and leukocytosis suggest pyelonephritis. However, flank pain and tenderness may be the only indication of pyelonephritis on physical examination.

Manifestations in adolescents are more specific. Symptoms of lower tract infections include frequency and painful urination of a small amount of turbulent urine that may be grossly bloody. Fever is usually absent. Upper tract infection is characterized by fever, rigors, flank pain, and lower tract symptoms, which may appear one or two days after the upper tract symptoms.

Many UTIs in children are asymptomatic or atypical in clinical presentation, and many complaints may be unrelated to the urinary tract. Many are treated as respiratory or gastrointestinal infections. It is important that these children be identified so that treatment can be initiated. Significant scarring can take place, especially in infants and very young children.

PROCESS OF DIAGNOSIS

The diagnosis of UTI depends on evaluation of history and physical examination, and urinalysis and culture. Urine characteristic of possible infection appears cloudy, hazy, or thick with noticeable strands of mucus and pus; it may also smell fishy and unpleasant even when fresh. Presumptive UTI diagnosis can be made on the basis of microscopic examination of the urine, which often reveals pyuria (5-8 white blood cells/ml of uncentrifuged urine) and the presence of at least one bacterium in a Gram stain. However, a normal urinalysis may also be present in conditions of asymptomatic bacteriuria.

Diagnosis of UTI is confirmed by detection of bacteriuria in urine culture, but urine collection is often difficult, especially in infants and very small children. Several factors may alter a urine specimen. Contamination of a specimen by organisms from sources other than the urine is the most frequent cause of false-positive results. Bag urine specimens are frequently contaminated by perineal and perianal flora.

More accurate estimates of bacterial content are obtained from suprapubic aspiration (children less than two years of age) and properly performed bladder catheterization (as long as the first few millilitres are excluded from collection).

Micturating cystogram (MCUG), intravenous pyelogram (IVP), and DSMA (dimercaptosuccinic acid) scan may be performed after the infection subsides, to identify anatomical abnormalities contributing to the development of infection and existing kidney changes from recurrent infection.

THERAPEUTIC MANAGEMENT

The objectives of treatment of children with UTI are: (1) to eliminate the infection, (2) to detect and correct functional or anatomical abnormalities, (3) to prevent recurrences and (4) to preserve renal function (Rushton, 1992). Antibiotic therapy should be initiated based on identification of the pathogen, the child's history of antibiotic use, and the location of the infection. A variety of antimicrobial drugs are available for treating UTI, but all of them can occasionally be ineffective because of resistance of organisms. Antibacterial compounds used in the management of UTI include: (1) systemic penicillins and sulfonamides, which are used for a short, intensive course of therapy; and (2) antiseptic preparations, which are often continued over longer periods to maintain urinary sterility, especially in children with long-term susceptibility to infection, such as those with neurogenic bladder.

Children with suspected pyelonephritis and fever are admitted to hospital and given appropriate antibiotics intravenously for a minimum of 48 hours. Blood and urine cultures are obtained on admission and following therapy.

All children with a documented UTI warrant ultrasound or radiological evaluation (Royal College of Physicians, 1991). If anatomical defects such as primary reflux or bladder neck obstruction are present, surgical correction of these abnormalities may be necessary to prevent recurrent infection. Follow-up study is an important component of medical management, since the relapse rate is high and recurrent infection tends to occur 1-2 months after termination of treatment. Even with recurrent infections, renal damage is rare if no anatomical abnormalities complicate the condition. The aim of therapy and careful follow-up in such cases is to prevent morbidity rather than reduce the chance of renal failure.

Prognosis

With prompt and adequate treatment at the time of diagnosis, the long-term prognosis for UTIs is usually excellent. However, the hazard of progressive renal injury is greatest when infection occurs in young children (especially under two years of age) and is associated with congenital renal malformations and reflux. Therefore, early diagnosis of children at risk is particularly important during infancy and toddlerhood.

NURSING CONSIDERATIONS

When infection is suspected, collecting an appropriate specimen is essential.

Frequently, other tests are performed to detect anatomical defects. Children are prepared for these tests as appropriate for their age. Children who are old enough to understand need an explanation of the procedure, its purpose, and what they will experience.

Since antibacterial drugs are indicated in UTI, the nurse advises parents of proper dosage and administration. When antiseptics such as nitrofurantoin or prophylactic antibiotics are used for prolonged therapy to maintain urine sterility, parents need an explanation of their continued necessity when no signs of infection are present. For all children, an adequate or increased fluid intake is encouraged.

Prevention

Prevention is the most important goal in both primary and recurrent infection, and most preventive measures are simple, ordinary hygienic habits that should be a routine part of daily care. Any signs of intestinal parasites (e.g., scratching between the legs and around anal area) should be investigated and treated appropriately. Sexually active adolescent females are advised to urinate as soon as possible after intercourse to flush out bacteria introduced during sex play. Parents and older children are taught health practices that prevent UTI (Box 25-2).

VESICOURETERAL REFLUX

Vesicoureteral reflux (VUR) refers to the retrograde flow of bladder urine into the ureters. Reflux increases the chance for and perpetuates infection, since with each void urine is swept up the ureters and then allowed to empty after voiding. Therefore, the residual urine from the ureters remains in the bladder until the next void (Fig. 25-1). The International Classification System describes the degree of reflux from the bladder into upper genitourinary tract structures (Box 25-3).

Primary reflux results from the congenitally abnormal insertion of the ureters into the bladder and predisposes to development of infection. A familial incidence of VUR is sometimes observed. *Secondary reflux* occurs as a result of infection. Normally, the ureters enter the bladder wall in such a manner that the accumulating urine compresses the submucosal segment of the ureter, preventing reflux. However, the oedema caused by bladder infection renders this mechanism at the ureterovesicular junction incompetent. In addition, in infants and young children the shortness of the submucosal portion of the ureter decreases the effectiveness of this antireflux mechanism. Other causes of secondary reflux are neurogenic bladder from either chronic obstruction or neural dysfunction, or as an iatrogenic result from progressive dilation of the ureters following surgical urinary diversion.

Reflux with infection can lead to kidney damage, since refluxed urine ascending into the collecting tubules of the nephrons allows the micro-organisms to gain access to the renal parenchyma, initiating renal scarring. Most renal scars associated with reflux occur at a very young age and are present at the

---

◆ BOX 25-2

Guidelines for prevention of urinary tract infection

Factors Predisposing to Development	Measures of Prevention
Short female urethra close to vagina and anus	Perineal hygiene — wipe from front to back Avoid tight clothing or nappies; wear cotton panties rather than nylon Check for vaginitis or pinworms, especially if child scratches between legs
Incomplete emptying (reflux) and overdistention of bladder	Avoid 'holding' urine; encourage child to void frequently, especially before a long trip or other circumstances where toilet facilities are not available Empty bladder completely with each void
Concentrated and alkaline urine	Avoid straining at stool Encourage generous fluid intake Acidify urine with juices, such as apple, and a diet high in animal protein

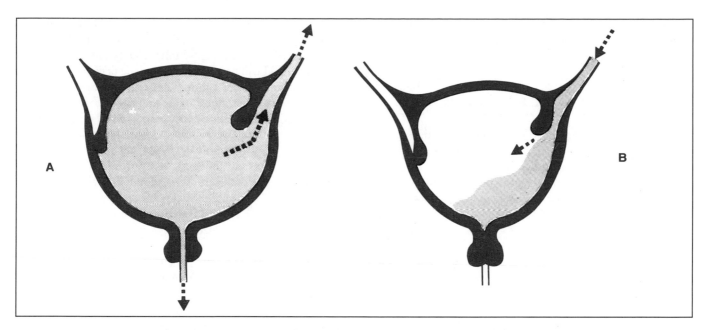

Fig. 25-1 Mechanisms of vesicoureteral reflux. **A,** During voiding, urine refluxes into ureter. **B,** After voiding, residual urine from ureter remains in bladder.

◆ **BOX 25-3**

Vesicoureteral reflux grading system

Grade I: VUR into the lower ureter only
Grade II: Ureteral and pelvic filling without calyceal dilation
Grade III: Ureteral and pelvic filling with mild calyceal blunting
Grade IV: Marked distention of pelvis, calyces, and ureter
Grade V: Massive VUR associated with severe hydronephrosis

time of diagnosis; few develop after five years of age. However, between 30% and 60% of children with VUR have evidence of renal scarring, and scarring is almost always found in association with reflux (Smellie, 1994). Therefore UVR is an important cause of renal damage, and careful examination for its presence is indicated. Careful routine follow-up is a critical part of management of children with urinary tract infection (UTI), and children with reflux, documented by voiding cystoureterography, are assessed repeatedly during ensuing years.

THERAPEUTIC MANAGEMENT

Conservative, nonoperative therapy is effective in controlling infection in most cases of VUR. There is a high incidence of spontaneous resolution over time — approximately 20-30% for each two-year period throughout childhood. A 90% probability of remission may occur in Grades I and II reflux when managed medically (Smellie, 1994). Therapy consists of continuous low-dose antibacterial therapy with frequent urine cultures. This long-term therapy requires medical supervision

and reliable, cooperative parents. Surgical correction of reflux may be required for Grades IV and V reflux. Grade III is managed conservatively unless complications interfere.

The major indications for surgical intervention include significant anatomical abnormality at the ureterovesical junction, recurrent UTI, high grades of VUR, noncompliance with medical therapy, intolerance to antibiotics, and VUR after puberty in females (Hensle and Burbige, 1986). Antireflux surgery consists of reimplantation of the ureters. Postsurgical antibiotic therapy is continued until a micturating cystogram demonstrates no further VUR. Micturating cystogram is performed three months postoperatively to check reflux is no longer present, at which time prophylactic antibodies can be discontinued. There is an argument that definitive surgery is preferable to years of antibiotic therapy and medical follow-up. Accelerated renal growth is observed in some children after surgery.

IMPLICATIONS FOR NURSING

The primary nursing goal in children on medical therapy is encouraging compliance. The medications prescribed are usually well tolerated by children, but parents may need help in encouraging children to take the medication.

GLOMERULAR DISEASE

The glomerulus is responsible for the initial step in formation of urine, by separating a fraction of the water and dissolved solutes from the formed elements and macromolecules of the blood flowing through the glomerular capillaries. The rate of filtration is determined by physical forces previously described; the efficiency of filtration depends on an intact glomerular membrane. The permeability of the membrane far exceeds that of capillaries in skeletal muscle, due to the increased number of pores through which filtration takes place. Anything that alters the rate of flow or the filtrating capacity can disturb the body equilibrium.

ACUTE GLOMERULONEPHRITIS

Acute glomerulonephritis (AGN) as a classification includes several distinct entities. It may be a primary event or a manifestation of a systemic disorder. The disease can range from minimal to severe. Common features include oliguria, oedema, hypertension and circulatory congestion, haematuria, and proteinuria. Most are postinfectious and have been associated with pneumococcal, streptococcal, and viral infections. All postinfectious diseases are presumed to result from immune complex formation and glomerular deposition, and the clinical presentations may be indistinguishable.

Acute post-streptococcal glomerulonephritis (APSGN) is the most common of the noninfectious renal diseases in childhood and the one for which a cause can be established in the majority of cases. APSGN can occur at any age, but affects primarily early school-aged children with a peak age of onset of six to seven years. It is uncommon in children younger than two years of age, and males outnumber females 2:1.

AETIOLOGY

It is now generally accepted that APSGN is an immune-complex disease; that is, a reaction that occurs as a by-product of an antecedent streptococcal infection with certain strains of the group A ß-haemolytic streptococcus. Most streptococcal infections do not cause APSGN. A latent period of 10-14 days occurs between the streptococcal infection and the onset of clinical manifestations. The peak incidence of disease corresponds to the incidence of streptococcal infections.

CLINICAL MANIFESTATIONS

Typically, affected children are in good health until they experience the antecedent infection. In some instances there is no history of an infection, or it is only described as a mild cold. The onset of nephritis appears after an average latent period of about ten days. Since the child appears well during this time, the association is not recognized by parents.

Initial signs of nephrotic reaction include puffiness of the face, especially around the eyes (periorbital oedema), anorexia and passage of dark-coloured urine. The oedema is more prominent in the face in the morning, but spreads during the day to involve the extremities and abdomen. The oedema is only moderate and may not be appreciated by someone unfamiliar with the child's normal appearance. The urine is cloudy, smoky brown, or what parents describe as resembling tea or cola, and severely reduced in volume.

The child is pale, irritable and lethargic. He or she appears unwell, but seldom expresses specific complaints. Older children may complain of headaches, abdominal discomfort and dysuria. Vomiting is not uncommon. On examination there is usually a mild-to-moderate elevation in blood pressure (diastolic, 80-120 mm-Hg; systolic, 120-180 mm-Hg). Occasionally a child will have an atypical mode of onset with severe symptoms such as convulsions (secondary to cerebral ischaemia and/or hypertension), pulmonary and circulatory congestion, minimal urine findings, or haematuria in the absence of hypertension and oedema.

Clinical course

The acute oedematous phase of glomerulonephritis usually persists from 4-10 days, but may persist for two or three weeks, during which time the child remains listless, anorexic and apathetic. The weight fluctuates, the urine remains smoky brown in colour, and the blood pressure may suddenly reach dangerously high levels at any time during this phase.

The first sign of improvement is a small increase in urine output with a corresponding decrease in body weight, followed in one or two days by copious diuresis. With diuresis the child begins to feel better, the appetite improves, and the blood pressure decreases to normal with the reduction of oedema. Gross haematuria diminishes, in part because of dilution of the red blood cells in the more dilute urine, but microscopic haematuria may persist for weeks or months. The blood urea level decreases during diuresis, but it, along with a slight to moderate proteinuria, may persist for several weeks.

Prognosis

Almost all children correctly diagnosed as having APSGN recover completely, and specific immunity is conferred so that subsequent recurrences are uncommon. Deaths from complications still occur but are, fortunately, rare.

Complications

The major complications that may develop during the acute phase of glomerulonephritis are hypertensive encephalopathy, acute cardiac decompensation, and acute renal failure. Normally, cerebral blood flow responds to acute arterial hypertension by vasoconstriction. However, acute and severe hypertension may cause this protective autoregulation of cerebral blood flow to fail, leading to hyperperfusion of the brain and cerebral oedema. The premonitory signs of encephalopathy are headache, dizziness, abdominal discomfort and vomiting. If the condition progresses there may be transient loss of vision and/or hemiparesis, disorientation, and generalized convulsions of the grand mal type.

Cardiac decompensation during the acute oedematous phase of nephritis is caused by hypervolaemia and not by cardiac failure. Signs of circulatory congestion are evident, however. The heart is enlarged, and increased pulmonary vascular markings are evident on x-ray. Increased pulmonary capillary permeability is also believed to be an important factor in the development of pulmonary oedema.

Acute renal failure with persistent oliguria or anuria is an uncommon complication, but one that requires an appropriate treatment regimen.

PROCESS OF DIAGNOSIS

Urinalysis during the acute phase characteristically shows haematuria, proteinuria, and increased specific gravity. The specific gravity is moderately elevated and seldom exceeds 1.020. Proteinuria generally parallels the haematuria, and the content usually shows 3+ or 4+ but is not the massive proteinuria seen in nephrotic syndrome. Gross discolouration of urine reflects its red blood cell and haemoglobin content.

Blood examination reveals normal electrolyte levels (sodium, potassium and chloride ions) and carbon dioxide levels, unless the disease has progressed to renal failure. Uraemia resulting from impaired glomerular filtration is reflected in elevated blood urea and creatinine levels in at least 50% of cases. When proteinuria is heavy, there may be changes associated with nephrotic syndrome; that is, transient hypoproteinaemia and hyperlipidaemia.

Some serological tests may help in diagnosis. Antibody responses to the extracellular products of the streptococci provide indirect evidence of previous streptococcal infection. These include antistreptolysin O (ASO), antistreptokinase (ASKase), antihyaluronidase (AHase), antideoxyribonuclease-B (ADNase-B), and antinicotyladenine dinucleotidase (ANADase). The ASO titre is the most familiar and readily available test for streptococcal antibodies. ASO appears in the serum about ten days after the initial infection and persists for 4-6 weeks; however, there is no correlation between the degree of elevation and its duration, and the severity or prognosis of the glomerulonephritis. It is a useful diagnostic tool when nephritis follows a pharyngeal infection, but is of less value after pyoderma. An ASO titre of 250 Todd units or higher is of diagnostic significance, as is a rising titre in two samples taken one week apart. More consistent and reliable antibody tests following streptococcal skin infections are elevated AHase and ADNase-B titres.

Nonspecific acute-phase reactants that reflect acute inflammatory processes, such as the erythrocyte sedimentation rate (ESR), C-reactive protein (CRP), and serum mucoprotein tests are elevated during the early stages of acute disease and then gradually return to normal as healing takes place. The ESR is sometimes used as a guide to the progress of the nephritis.

Since glomerulonephritis is an immune-complex disease, there is reduced total serum complement activity in the early stages of acute disease. The simpler measurements of the C3 complement component (beta$_1$ C globulin) are used as an index of total complement activity. The test is most useful in children with no oedema or minimal urine findings. Renal biopsy for diagnostic purposes is seldom required, but may be useful in the diagnosis of atypical cases.

Correlations between laboratory and morphological findings indicate a significant relationship between creatinine clearance and severity of glomerular damage. Greater damage is reflected in a reduced creatinine clearance and is also associated with a higher blood urea nitrogen level. An increased excretion of cellular protein is associated with increasing glomerular capillary obliteration. There appears to be no correlation between the extent of glomerular damage and ASO titre, oliguria or blood pressure.

THERAPEUTIC MANAGEMENT

No specific treatment is available for acute glomerulonephritis, but recovery is spontaneous and uneventful in most cases. Children who have normal blood pressure and a satisfactory urine output can generally be treated at home. Those with substantial oedema, hypertension, gross haematuria, and/or significant oliguria should be hospitalized because of the unpredictability of complications. Short hospitalization is the rule in uncomplicated cases.

Fluid balance

Regular measurement of vital signs, body weight, and intake and output is essential in order to monitor the progress of the disease and to detect complications that may appear at any time during the course of the disease. A record of daily weight is the most useful means to assess fluid balance. Water restriction is seldom necessary, unless the output is significantly reduced and the child is fluid overloaded. In these children, the water allowed is equivalent to the calculated insensible loss plus the volume of urine excreted. Children on restricted fluids, especially those who are severely oedematous or those who have lost weight, should be observed for signs of dehydration.

Rarely, children with acute glomerulonephritis develop acute renal failure with oliguria that significantly alters the fluid and electrolyte balance. These children require careful management that may include peritoneal dialysis or haemodialysis.

Loss of glomerular filtration may produce electrolyte imbalances in children with severe forms of APSGN, especially hyperkalaemia, acidosis, hypocalcaemia and hyperphosphataemia.

Hypertension

Acute hypertension must be anticipated and identified early. Blood pressure measurements are taken every 4-6 hours. Significant but not severe hypertension is controlled with hydralazine or nifedepine, usually in conjunction with a diuretic.

Nutrition

Dietary restrictions depend on the stage and severity of the disease, especially the extent of oedema. A normal diet is permitted in uncomplicated cases, but the intake of sodium is usually limited (no salt is added to foods). Moderate sodium restriction is usually instituted for children with hypertension or oedema. Foods with substantial amounts of potassium are generally restricted during the period of oliguria.

Antibiotics

Antibiotic therapy is indicated only for children with evidence of persistent streptococcal infections.

IMPLICATIONS FOR NURSING

Nursing care of children with glomerulonephritis involves careful assessment of the disease status and regular monitoring of vital signs (including frequent measurement of blood pressure), fluid balance, and behaviour. Vital signs provide clues to the severity of the disease and early signs of complications. They are carefully measured, and any abnormalities reported and recorded. The volume and character of urine are noted, and the child is weighed daily. The child with oedema, hypertension, and gross haematuria may be subject to complications. Control of hypertension should be regarded as an emergency measure.

For most children a normal diet is allowed, but it should contain no added salt. Salted treats and other foods high in sodium should be eliminated, and parents and friends should be advised not to bring items, such as crisps, to the child in hospital. However, the total amount of salt ingested is usually less than prescribed, because of poor appetite. Fluid restriction, if prescribed, is more difficult, and the amount permitted should be evenly divided throughout the waking hours, and served in small cups to give the illusion of larger servings.

During the acute phase, children are generally quite content to lie in bed, but should be encouraged to sit up and potter around to prevent complications associated with prolonged bed rest. A good play specialist is invaluable to interest the child.

CHRONIC OR PROGRESSIVE GLOMERULONEPHRITIS

The majority of cases of renal glomerular disease are acute glomerulonephritis, minimal change nephrotic syndrome, and glomerulonephritis associated with systemic diseases. These pose relatively few problems of diagnosis, and their natural course is fairly predictable. A few cases present a prolonged course and a poor ultimate prognosis. They are a rather heterogeneous group, defined by correlating the clinical manifestations, pathological conditions, and natural course of the individual diseases.

Persistent glomerulonephritis is used to describe cases of glomerulonephritis that have no specific histological picture, but fail to show the rapid recovery expected in acute nephritis. *Chronic glomerulonephritis (CGN)* describes advanced glomerular disease, which includes a variety of different disease processes. *Rapidly progressive glomerulonephritis* describes acute illness with severe, acute onset resembling acute poststreptococcal glomerulonephritis, but causes rapidly progressive deterioration of renal function within weeks or months.

PROCESS OF DIAGNOSIS

Laboratory findings may include proteinuria, with casts, and red and white blood cells. Failing renal function is evidenced by elevated blood urea, creatinine, and uric acid levels. Electrolyte alterations include metabolic acidosis, decreased sodium from the chronic salt-losing state, elevated potassium, elevated phosphate, and decreased calcium levels. As the disease progresses, urine specific gravity eventually stabilizes at an isotonic state (about 1.012) as a result of the inability of the kidney to reabsorb solutes or respond to antidiuretic hormone. The renal insufficiency may extend from 5-15 years and even longer, or rapid deterioration may progress to end-stage renal disease (ESRD).

THERAPEUTIC MANAGEMENT

Early in the course of the disease, treatment is appropriate to the underlying disease and is largely symptomatic in most cases. As few restrictions as feasible are imposed, and the child is allowed to live as normal a life as possible for as long as possible. Marked hypertension is controlled with antihypertensive agents, and anaemia may require erythropoietin injections. Salt is only moderately restricted. Ultimately, dialysis and transplantation may restore relatively good health; however, these are usually not available alternatives until renal failure is far advanced. Children with rapidly progressive glomerulonephritis should always be referred to a centre specializing in renal disease.

NEPHROTIC SYNDROME

Nephrotic syndrome is the most common presentation of glomerular injury in children. It is defined as massive proteinuria, hypoalbuminaemia, hyperlipaemia and oedema, but the disorder is a clinical manifestation of many distinct glomerular disorders in which increased glomerular permeability to plasma protein results in massive urinary protein loss. Following a brief description of the three major forms of nephrotic syndrome, the remainder of the discussion is devoted to minimal change nephrotic syndrome.

TYPES OF NEPHROTIC SYNDROME

Nephrotic syndrome can be classified as *primary,* when the syndrome is restricted to glomerular injury, or *secondary,* when it develops as part of a systemic illness. Although it may have several different histological variations, the most common form of the primary disease is *minimal change nephrotic syndrome.* A congenital form is also recognized.

Minimal change nephrotic syndrome (MCNS)

Approximately 80% of cases of nephrotic syndrome in children occur in the absence of recognizable systemic disease or pre-existing renal disease, and are categorized as idiopathic. MCNS can present at any age, but is predominantly a disease of the preschool child. In 74% of children, the onset of the disease occurs between the ages of two and seven years (McEnery and Strife, 1982). The disease is rare in children younger than six months of age, uncommon in infants younger than one year of age, and unusual after the age of eight.

The cause of MCNS remains obscure. Often, a nonspecific illness, usually a viral upper respiratory infection, precedes the manifestations by 4-8 days, but is considered to be a precipitating factor rather than a cause.

Secondary nephrotic syndrome

Nephrotic syndrome may occur after or in association with glomerular damage of known or presumed aetiology. Prominent among causes of glomerular damage is acute or chronic glomerulonephritis. Less commonly, secondary nephrotic syndrome occurs during the course of collagen diseases (such as disseminated lupus erythematosus and Henoch-Schönlein purpura) or as the result of toxicity to drugs (such as trimethadione and heavy metals), stings, or venom. Nephrotic syndrome is the major presenting symptom of renal disease in paediatric patients with acquired immune deficiency syndrome (AIDS).

Congenital nephrotic syndrome

The hereditary form of nephrotic syndrome is caused by a recessive gene on an autosome. The disease does not respond to the usual therapy, and death in the first year or two of life is the rule if the infant does not receive a successful renal transplant or maintenance on dialysis.

PATHOPHYSIOLOGY

The glomerular membrane, which is normally impermeable to albumin and other large proteins, becomes permeable to proteins, especially albumin, which leak through the membrane and are lost in urine (hyperalbuminuria). This reduces the serum albumin level (hypoalbuminaemia), which decreases the colloidal osmotic pressure in the capillaries. Consequently, the hydrostatic pressure exceeds the pull of the colloidal osmotic pressure, and fluid accumulates in the interstitial spaces and body cavities, particularly the abdominal cavity (ascites). The shift of fluid from the plasma to the interstitial spaces reduces the vascular fluid volume (hypovolaemia), which in turn stimulates the renin-angiotensin system and the secretion of antidiuretic hormone and aldosterone. Tubular reabsorption of sodium and water is increased in an attempt to increase intravascular volume. The elevation of serum cholesterol, phospholipids, and triglycerides is unexplained.

CLINICAL MANIFESTATIONS

A previously well child begins to gain weight, which progresses insidiously over several days or weeks. Puffiness of the face, especially around the eyes, is apparent on arising in the morning but subsides during the day, when swelling of the abdomen and lower extremities is more prominent. The generalized oedema develops so slowly that parents may consider it to be a sign of healthy growth. Although an acute infection may precipitate severe generalized oedema, the usual course is one of progressive weight gain until either rapid or gradual increase in oedema prompts the family to seek medical evaluation. Usually present are periorbital oedema, abdominal swelling from ascites, and labial or scrotal swelling (Fig. 25-2). Oedema of the intestinal mucosa may cause diarrhoea, loss

of appetite, and poor intestinal absorption. The volume of urine is decreased, and it appears darkly opalescent and frothy. Extreme skin pallor is often present, and the child has a tendency towards skin breakdown during periods of oedema. Weight loss from poor appetite and loss of protein is not uncommon, although it is frequently obscured by oedema. The blood pressure is usually normal or slightly decreased. The child is more susceptible to infection, especially cellulitis, pneumonia, peritonitis, or septicaemia.

In rare instances, children with MCNS have significant or persistent hypertension, and gross or persistent haematuria.

PROCESS OF DIAGNOSIS

The diagnosis of MCNS is made on the basis of history and clinical manifestations (oedema, proteinuria and hypoalbuminaemia and hypercholesterolaemia in the absence of haematuria and hypertension) in children presenting between the ages of two and four years. Massive proteinuria is reflected in urine excretion of protein that frequently reaches levels in excess of 2 g/m^2/day of body surface with relatively greater clearance of low-molecular-weight proteins. If hypovolaemia is not significant and the child is well hydrated, the glomerular filtration rate is usually normal.

Total serum protein concentrations are reduced, with the albumin fractions significantly reduced (less than 2 g/dl) and plasma lipids elevated. Serum cholesterol may be as high as 450-1500 mg/dl. Haemoglobin and haematocrit are usually normal or elevated, and the platelet count is high (500,000-1,000,000) due to haemoconcentration. Serum sodium concentration is usually low, about 130-135 mEq/l.

If renal biopsy is performed, it provides information regarding the glomerular status and type of nephrotic syndrome, response to drugs, and probable course of the disease. Under the microscope, the foot processes of the basement membrane appear fused. The major focuses in differential diagnosis are to establish the oedema as renal in origin and to distinguish minimum change nephrotic syndrome from other glomerulopathies with nephrotic syndrome as a manifestation.

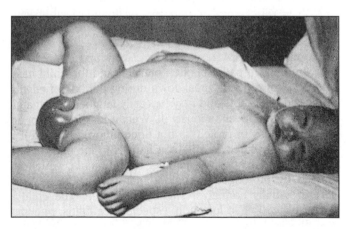

Fig. 25-2 Two-year-old child with nephrosis. (From Shirkey HC, editor: *Pediatric therapy*, ed 6, St Louis, 1980, Mosby–Year Book)

THERAPEUTIC MANAGEMENT

Medical management consists of general and specific measures. The primary objective is to reduce the excretion of urinary protein and to maintain a protein-free urine.

General measures

General treatment is principally supportive. Children can be remarkably active with no evidence that restriction affects the ultimate outcome. Acute and intercurrent infections are treated with appropriate antibiotics.

Diet

The child who is in remission is allowed a normal diet; however, during periods of massive oedema, salt is restricted in the form of no added salt at the table and excluding foods with very high salt content. Although oedema cannot be removed by a low-sodium diet, its rate of increase may be reduced.

Corticosteroid therapy

The response of most affected children to corticosteroids has established these drugs as prime therapeutic agents in management of nephrotic syndrome. Corticosteroid therapy is begun as soon as the diagnosis has been determined. The medication is administered orally in a dosage of 2 mg/kg of body weight or 60 mg/m^2/day in evenly divided doses. Prednisone, the safest and least expensive drug, is the steroid of choice. The drug is continued until the urine is free from protein and remains normal for ten days to two weeks.

The course of the disease is fairly predictable. There is little change during the first few days of therapy. In most patients, diuresis occurs as the urine protein excretion diminishes within 7-21 days after the initiation of steroid therapy. Other clinical manifestations stabilize or return to normal shortly thereafter. Almost 95% of patients between one and ten years of age with no hypertension, haematuria, or renal insufficiency and who have satisfactory laboratory measurements of C3 complement and a renal clearance of IgG will have complete resolution of proteinuria with therapy.

If the child has not responded to therapy within 28 days of daily steroid administration, the likelihood of subsequent response diminishes rapidly. When the child is free of proteinuria and oedema, the total daily dose of prednisone is usually given for a time as a single daily dose every 48 hours. The dose is gradually tapered to discontinuation over a variable period, from several weeks to months. Once a satisfactory response is achieved, steroid therapy is reduced to every other day (q.o.d.). This dosage is less likely to depress pituitary-adrenal function and produces fewer side effects during prolonged therapy. If a tendency to relapse is demonstrated, the number of relapses can be reduced with administration of a low-dose, q.o.d. schedule of prednisone therapy that continues for six months to one year (provided remission is achieved and successful tapering to low-dose q.o.d. therapy occurs).

Children with MCNS are often described according to their response to corticosteroid therapy (Box 25-4). Children with MCNS typically relapse one to three times per year. Children who are steroid-dependent tend to have frequent relapses over many years and receive large amounts of steroids, which results in cushingoid features and growth retardation. They also require supportive treatment (diuretics, diet). The prognosis for children who are steroid-unresponsive is less predictable than for those who are steroid-responsive (McEnery and Strife, 1982).

Children who require frequent courses of steroid therapy are highly susceptible to complications of steroids, such as growth retardation, cataracts, obesity, hypertension, gastrointestinal bleeding, bone demineralization, infections and hyperglycaemia. Children who do not respond to steroid therapy, those who have frequent relapses, and those in whom the side effects threaten their growth and general health, may be considered for a course of therapy using other immunosuppressive medications.

Immunosuppressant therapy

It is often possible to reduce the relapse rate and induce long-term remission with administration of an oral alkylating agent (usually cyclophosphamide) alternating with prednisone. Both drugs are administered for up to 2-3 months, after which cyclophosphamide is discontinued abruptly, and the prednisone is decreased by decrements. Chlorambucil has also proved to be effective when given with corticosteroids.

Significant side effects of cyclophosphamide must be considered and discussed with parents of children for whom this drug is contemplated. Leucopenia must be anticipated, and evidence suggests that cyclophosphamide may cause azoospermia with potential sterility in males treated for more than 2-3 months and variable effects on gonadal function in females. Cyclosoprin A is now also being used to treat nephrotic syndrome with some success.

Diuretics

One characteristic of the oedema of nephrotic syndrome is its usual lack of responsiveness to diuretic agents. However, in

---

◆ **BOX 25-4**

Classification of nephrotic syndrome according to steroid response

1. 'Steroid-sensitive' (20-40%)—response to a single short course of steroids without evidence of relapse after cessation of therapy.
2. 'Frequent relapsers' or 'steroid-dependent' (60-80%) — respond to steroids and can be tapered off completely; have three or more relapses in a 6- to 12-month period; remit when placed on steroids but tend to relapse on lowered dosage.
3. 'Steroid-unresponsive' or 'steroid-resistant' — never respond to steroids or become resistant to steroids at some point during the course of disease.

Modified from McEnery and Strife, 1982.

cases in which oedema interferes with respiration or if there is hypotension, hyponatraemia, or evidence of skin breakdown, loop diuretics are sometimes useful; usually frusemide in combination with metolazone. In addition, plasma expanders such as salt-poor human albumin may be administered to severely oedematous children requiring prompt control; however, they must be administered frequently, since the glomeruli are readily permeable to albumin in the acute stage (Haws and Baum, 1993).

Prognosis

The prognosis for ultimate recovery in most cases is good. It is a self-limiting disease and, in children who respond to steroid therapy, the tendency to relapse decreases with time. With early detection and prompt implementation of therapy to eradicate proteinuria, progressive basement membrane damage is minimized, so when the tendency to exacerbations is past, renal function is usually normal or near normal. It is estimated that approximately 80% of nephrotic children have this favourable prognosis, although 50% of children have relapses even after five years, and 20% after 10 years (Kim and Grupe, 1986).

IMPLICATIONS FOR NURSING

Planning

The goals of nursing care for children with nephrotic syndrome are:
1. Reduce the excretion of urinary protein and maintain a protein-free urine.
2. Prevent skin breakdown and infection.
3. Establish and maintain good nutrition.
4. Support and educate child and family.

Implementation

An oedematous child may find movement difficult, but should be encouraged to sit up and participate in some activity to prevent complications such as chest infections or skin breakdown. Skin must be kept clean and dry.

Although they are easily fatigued, children are usually able to adjust activities according to their individual tolerance but may require guidance in selection of play activities. Suitable recreational and diversional activities are an important part of their care. Once oedema fluid has been lost, children are able to resume their usual activities with discretion. Irritability and mood swings accompanying the inactivity, disease process, and steroid therapy are not unusual manifestations in these children.

Family support and home care

The prolonged course of the relapsing form of nephrotic syndrome is taxing to both the child and the family. The up-and-down course of remissions and exacerbations with periodic disruption of family life by hospitalization places a severe strain on the child and the family, both psychologically and financially. Parents and children over five or six years of age need reassurance regarding this characteristic of the course of the disease, so they will not become discouraged with the frequent relapses.

Evaluation

The effectiveness of nursing interventions is determined by continual reassessment and evaluation of care based on the following observational guidelines and expected outcomes:
1. Measure intake and output, and examine urine for albumin.
2. Monitor vital signs and assess skin for evidence of breakdown or infection.
3. Assess appetite and eating behaviours.
4. Observe and interview child and family regarding their understanding of the disease, therapies, and compliance with prescribed regimen.

RENAL TUBULAR DISORDERS

Disorders of renal tubular function include a variety of conditions in which there are one or more abnormalities in specific mechanisms of tubular transport or reabsorption, whereas initially glomerular function is normal or comparatively less impaired. Eventually, there may be more widespread kidney destruction with renal failure. In some cases the dysfunction has little, if any, effect on renal function. These disorders may be permanent or transient and may originate as primary defects or arise as a secondary effect of metabolic disease or exogenous toxins. Renal tubular disorders may be congenital (usually displaying characteristic patterns of genetic transmission), may appear without evidence of hereditary transmission, or may be acquired as a result of known or unknown causes.

Unlike the classic manifestations of glomerular diseases, oedema and hypertension are absent and the blood urea level and routine urinalysis are usually normal. Proteinuria may be demonstrated, but only by elaborate tests. Manifestations of tubular disorders are primarily metabolic disturbances or deficiencies, such as failure to thrive, metabolic bone disease or persistent acidosis. The variety of these disorders is extensive and the incidence rare.

RENAL TUBULAR ACIDOSIS

Renal tubular acidosis (RTA) is a syndrome of sustained metabolic acidosis in which there is impaired reabsorption of bicarbonate and/or excretion of net hydrogen ion, but in which glomerular function is normal or comparatively less impaired. On the basis of underlying pathophysiology, renal tubular acidosis is divided into *proximal renal tubular acidosis*, which results from a defect in bicarbonate absorption, and *distal renal tubular acidosis*, which results from inability to establish an adequate gradient of pH between blood and tubular fluid.

PROXIMAL TUBULAR ACIDOSIS (TYPE II)

Proximal tubular acidosis is caused by impaired bicarbonate reabsorption in the proximal tubule. It may occur as an isolated defect (primary); however, more often it appears in association with other proximal tubular disorders (secondary). As a result of a depressed renal threshold, bicarbonate reabsorption in the proximal tubule is incomplete, causing the plasma concentration of bicarbonate to stabilize at a lower level than normal. This results in a hyperchloraemic metabolic acidosis. There is no impairment of distal tubular integrity nor, in most cases, of the distal acidifying mechanism. A more complex abnormality in the proximal tubules is the *Fanconi syndrome* in which transport mechanisms are damaged by the accumulation of toxic metabolites or the tubular epithelium is damaged by heavy metals, such as lead or arsenic.

The cause of the primary disorder is unknown, but it appears to be almost entirely restricted to male infants. The major clinical manifestation and presenting symptom is growth failure. Tachypnoea from hyperchloraemic metabolic acidosis is also evident. Dehydration, vomiting, episodic fever, nephrolithiasis secondary to hypercalciuria, muscle weakness or paralysis as a result of hypokalaemia, and episodes of severe, life-threatening acidosis (sometimes triggered by a concurrent infection) may also be seen.

Complications are rare. The disorder appears to be transient and resolves spontaneously in time.

DISTAL TUBULAR ACIDOSIS (TYPE I)

Distal tubular acidosis is caused by the inability of the kidney to establish a normal pH gradient between tubular cells and tubular contents. Its most characteristic feature is the inability to produce a urinary pH below 6.0, despite the presence of severe metabolic acidosis.

Distal renal tubular acidosis may occur as a primary, isolated defect or in association with other diseases or disorders. Most secondary causes are rare. The primary disorder is usually considered to be a hereditary defect with a variable degree of expression and a greater penetrance in females. After the age of two years, the child usually has growth failure, although there is often a history of vomiting, polyuria, dehydration, anorexia, and failure to thrive. Evidence of bone demineralization (see *Calcium and phosphorous disturbances*) may be present along with, occasionally, the formation of urinary calculi (urolithiasis) in older children.

The inability to secrete hydrogen ion causes an accumulation of the ion in the body, which soon depletes the available hydrogen buffer, producing a sustained acidosis. Acidosis retards normal somatic growth, and demineralization of bone occurs as bone salts are mobilized to buffer the excessive hydrogen ions. Increased serum levels of both calcium and phosphorus contribute to the development of stones within the renal system. Both sodium and potassium are secreted in larger amounts. Serum potassium levels are depleted as the distal tubules excrete large amounts of potassium ions in an attempt to conserve sodium, since hydrogen ions are unable to participate in the exchange. Hyponatraemia stimulates increased aldosterone secretion, which further aggravates the hypokalaemia. With the depletion of bicarbonate ions, more chloride is reabsorbed in the proximal tubule to create a hyperchloraemia.

Prognosis

The primary disorder is usually permanent, but with early diagnosis and therapy, secondary effects on growth and stone formation can be avoided. When it occurs as a secondary complication and renal damage is prevented, the prognosis is good.

THERAPEUTIC MANAGEMENT

Treatment of both proximal and distal disorders consists of administration of sufficient bicarbonate or citrate to balance metabolically produced hydrogen ions and maintain the plasma bicarbonate level within normal range, and to correct associated electrolyte disorders, especially hypokalaemia. Proximal disorders require large volumes of bicarbonate to compensate for urinary losses; in distal disorders, the alkali required to maintain a normal plasma concentration is low. Most authorities favour a mixture of sodium and potassium bicarbonate (or citrate) in order to prevent deficiencies of either cation.

IMPLICATIONS FOR NURSING

Nursing goals include recognizing the possibility of RTA in children who fail to thrive or who display other symptoms suggestive of the disorders, and referring these children for medical evaluation. Helping parents understand the importance of compliance in administration of medications on a long-term basis is a primary goal of nursing management. Children who must continue the medication indefinitely are taught the importance of taking the medications as soon as they are old enough to assume responsibility for their own care.

NEPHROGENIC DIABETES INSIPIDUS

Nephrogenic diabetes insipidus (NDI) is the major disorder associated with a defect in the ability to concentrate urine. In this disorder, the distal tubules and collecting ducts are insensitive to the action of antidiuretic hormone or its exogenous counterpart, vasopressin. The nature of the defect is unknown, but it occurs primarily in males, which supports X-linked recessive inheritance. The disease is more variable in female carriers of the defective gene who may exhibit only a mild defect in urine-concentrating ability. The differential diagnosis for NDI should include chronic obstructive renal disorders, sickle cell disease, renal tuberculosis, and other renal disorders, which may cause high urine output with failure of the kidney to respond to vasopressin.

CLINICAL MANIFESTATIONS

The disease is manifest in newborns by vomiting, unexplained fever, failure to thrive, and severe recurrent dehydration with hypernatraemia. The passage of copious amounts of dilute urine, which produces severe dehydration and hypoelectroly-taemia, is a serious threat to life during this period and may be responsible for the high incidence of mental and motor retardation found in affected persons. Growth retardation is probably related to diminished food intake and poor general health because of uncontrolled polydipsia. Diagnosis is confirmed by a urine osmolality value consistently below that of plasma. Lack of response to vasopressin administration rules out other causes.

THERAPEUTIC MANAGEMENT

Therapy involves providing adequate volumes of water to compensate for urinary losses. As a result of an insatiable thirst, most of the child's time is spent drinking and voiding, with little time for activity and stimulation. A low-sodium/low-solute diet and the use of chlorothiazide or ethacrynic acid diuretics to increase the reabsorption of sodium and water in the proximal tubule, help reduce the amount of tubular fluid delivered to the distal tubules and help diminish the volume of water excreted. If the disease is recognized early and treatment instituted and maintained, normal growth can be expected, and a normal life span anticipated.

IMPLICATIONS FOR NURSING

Nursing goals for children and families with NDI are to recognize signs of the disorder early and assist them in coping with the long-term inconvenience of the continual thirst and elimination problems. The problem of ensuring adequate hydration is lifelong, and families need to adapt to away-from-home fluid needs and to avoid activities that contribute to dehydration when fluids may not be available. Genetic counselling is recommended.

OTHER RENAL DISORDERS

Renal damage occurs as a major or minor complication in many systemic diseases and with varying degrees of severity. In some cases, the renal complication may be the principal cause of death or one of several complications with fatal consequences.

There are a wide variety of hereditary disorders of renal function. It is estimated that 15% of renal diseases are genetically determined. In addition, there are several miscellaneous renal conditions for which a cause is unknown.

HAEMOLYTIC-URAEMIC SYNDROME

Haemolytic-uraemic syndrome (HUS) is an uncommon acute renal disease that is characterized by a triad of manifestations: acute renal failure, haemolytic anaemia and thrombocytopenia. HUS occurs primarily in infants and small children

between the ages of six months and five years. There have also been reports of increased incidence in families. HUS represents the main cause of acute renal failure in early childhood (Rizzoni *et al*, 1988).

AETIOLOGY

A strong association has been found between HUS and enteric infection with verocytotoxin-producing *E. coli*, specifically the O157:H7 serotype (Karmali *et al*, 1985). The disease usually follows an acute gastrointestinal or upper respiratory infection and tends to occur in scattered outbreaks in small geographic areas. HUS is clinically and pathologically similar to thrombocytopenic purpura, except for the hypertension that is associated with HUS. Some have speculated that thrombocytopenic purpura may be the adult version of the haemolytic-uraemic syndrome of infancy and early childhood.

PATHOPHYSIOLOGY

The primary site of injury appears to be the endothelial lining of the small glomerular arterioles, although other organs and tissues may be involved (e.g., the liver, brain, heart, pancreatic islet cells, and muscles). The endothelium becomes swollen and occluded with deposition of platelets and fibrin clots (intravascular coagulation). Red blood cells are damaged as they move through the partially occluded blood vessels. These fragmented red blood cells are removed by the spleen, causing acute haemolytic anaemia. Fibrinolytic action on the precipitated fibrin causes these fibrin-split products to appear in the serum and urine. The platelet aggregation within damaged blood vessels or the damage and removal of platelets produce the characteristic thrombocytopenia.

CLINICAL MANIFESTATIONS

The disease is preceded by a prodromal period during which there is an episode of diarrhoea and vomiting. Less often, the illness is an upper respiratory infection and occasionally varicella, measles or urinary tract infection.

The haemolytic process persists for several days to two weeks. During this time the child is anorexic, irritable and lethargic. There is marked and rapid onset of pallor, accompanied by haemorrhagic manifestations such as bruising, purpura, or rectal bleeding. Severely affected patients are anuric and are frequently hypertensive. Convulsions and stupor suggest central nervous system involvement, and there may be signs of acute heart failure. Mild cases demonstrate anaemia, thrombocytopenia and uraemia; urine output may be reduced or increased.

PROCESS OF DIAGNOSIS

The triad of anaemia, thrombocytopenia and renal failure is sufficient for diagnosis. Renal involvement is evidenced by proteinuria, haematuria and presence of urinary casts; blood urea nitrogen and serum creatinine levels are elevated. A low haemoglobin and haematocrit, and a high reticulocyte count confirm the haemolytic nature of the anaemia.

THERAPEUTIC MANAGEMENT

The initial supportive measures for most children are those used in managing renal failure — fluid replacement (calculated with great care), treatment of hypertension, and correction of acidosis and electrolyte disorders. The most consistently effective treatment is early and repeated haemodialysis or peritoneal dialysis. Blood transfusions with fresh, washed, packed cells are administered for severe anaemia, but are used with caution to prevent circulatory overload from added volume.

Once vomiting and diarrhoea have resolved, the child is restarted on enteral nutrition. Sometimes parenteral nutrition is required for children with severe persistent colitis and for children in whom tissue catabolism is marked.

Prognosis
With prompt treatment, the recovery rate is about 95%, but residual renal impairment ranges from 10-50% in various areas. Death is usually caused by residual renal impairment or central nervous system injury.

RENAL FAILURE

Renal failure is the inability of the kidneys to excrete waste material, concentrate urine and conserve electrolytes. The disorder can be acute or chronic and affects most of the systems in the body.

ACUTE RENAL FAILURE

Acute renal failure (ARF) is said to exist when the kidneys suddenly are unable to regulate the volume and composition of urine appropriately in response to food and fluid intake and the needs of the organism.

AETIOLOGY

ARF can develop as a result of many related or unrelated clinical conditions — poor renal perfusion, acute renal injury, or the final expression of chronic, irreversible renal disease. The most common cause in children is transient renal failure resulting from dehydration or other causes of poor perfusion that respond to restoration of fluid volume. Causes of ARF are usually classified as *prerenal, intrinsic renal* and *postrenal* causes. This implies that only intrinsic renal causes are characterized by damage to the renal parenchyma, whereas prerenal and postrenal causes can be more easily remedied. However, severe or long-standing prerenal or postrenal aetiologies can produce severe secondary renal damage.

Prerenal causes
Prerenal causes of ARF are most common in children and are always related to reduction of renal perfusion in an anatomically and physiologically normal kidney and collecting system. Dehydration secondary to diarrhoeal illness or persistent vomiting is the most frequent cause of prerenal failure in infants and children. Surgical shock and trauma (including burns) are also common causes.

Intrinsic renal causes
Intrinsic renal causes of ARF comprise the largest group that requires extended management. These include diseases and nephrotoxic agents that damage the glomeruli, tubules or renal vasculature. Glomerular disease is the most common cause of glomerular damage, whereas tubular destruction is more often caused by ischaemia or nephrotoxins. Vascular damage is an uncommon cause of renal failure in childhood. The type and extent of damage determine the degree and duration of renal insufficiency.

Postrenal causes
ARF resulting from obstructive uropathy is uncommon in children, except during the first year of life. However, renal function can be restored by relief of the obstruction. The degree of recovery depends on the duration of the renal failure.

Clinical course
The clinical course of the child with ARF is variable and depends on the cause. In reversible ARF there is a period of severe oliguria, or the low-output phase, followed by an abrupt onset of diuresis, or a high-output phase, followed by a gradual return to, or towards, normal urine volumes.

CLINICAL MANIFESTATIONS

In many instances of ARF the infant or child is already critically ill with the precipitating disorder, and the explanation for development of oliguria may or may not be readily apparent. Often, the underlying illness overshadows the renal failure and frequently assumes the priority of care — for example, the patient who is in shock from endotoxaemia, or the infant who is severely dehydrated from gastroenteritis.

The primary manifestation of ARF is oliguria. Other symptoms related to ARF include oedema, drowsiness, circulatory congestion, and cardiac arrhythmia from hyperkalaemia. Seizures may be caused by hyponatraemia or hypocalcaemia and tachypnoea from metabolic acidosis. With continued oliguria, biochemical abnormalities can develop rapidly, and circulatory and central nervous system manifestations appear.

PROCESS OF DIAGNOSIS

When a previously well child develops ARF without obvious cause, a careful history is taken to reveal symptoms that may be related to glomerulonephritis, to obstructive uropathy, or regarding exposure to nephrotoxic chemicals, such as ingestion of heavy metals or inhalation of carbon tetrachloride, or other organic solvents or drugs, such as methicillin, sulfonamides, neomycin, polymixin and kanamycin.

THERAPEUTIC MANAGEMENT

The most effective management of ARF is prevention. The development of ARF is a known risk in certain situations. This should be anticipated and recognized, and adequate therapy should be implemented; for example, fluid therapy for children with hypovolaemia in such conditions as dehydration, burns and haemorrhage. Nephrotoxic drugs should be used with caution or avoided in children with renal disease.

The treatment of ARF is directed towards: (1) treatment of the underlying cause, (2) management of the complications of renal failure, and (3) provision of supportive therapy within the constraints imposed by the renal failure. Treatment of poor perfusion resulting from dehydration consists of volume restoration, as described in the treatment of dehydration. If oliguria persists after restoration of fluid volume or if the renal failure is caused by intrinsic renal damage, the physiological and biochemical abnormalities that have resulted from kidney dysfunction must be corrected or controlled.

Oliguria
When there is persistent oliguria in the presence of adequate hydration and no lower tract obstruction, mannitol or frusemide, or both, may be administered as a test to provoke a flow of urine.

Fluid and calories
The child with ARF has a tendency to develop water intoxication and hyponatraemia, which make it difficult to provide calories in sufficient amounts to meet the needs of the child and reduce the tissue catabolism, metabolic acidosis, hyperkalaemia and uraemia. If the child is able to tolerate oral foods, concentrated food sources high in carbohydrate and fat but low in protein, potassium, and sodium may be provided. However, many children have functional disturbances of the gastrointestinal tract, such as nausea and vomiting; therefore, the intravenous route may be necessary and usually consists of essential amino acids or a combination of essential and nonessential amino acids administered by the central venous route.

Control of water balance in these patients requires careful monitoring of feedback information, such as accurate intake and output, body weight and electrolyte measurements. In general during the oliguric phase no sodium, chloride or potassium is given unless there are other large ongoing losses.

Hyperkalaemia
Elevated serum potassium is the most immediate threat to the life of the child with ARF. Potassium ions are not being excreted, whereas at the same time release of potassium from cells is accelerated by acidosis, stress, and tissue breakdown in cases associated with internal bleeding or trauma.

NURSING ALERT

Any of the following signs of hyperkalaemia constitute an emergency situation and should be reported immediately:
Serum potassium concentrations in excess of 7 mEq/l
Presence of ECG abnormalities, such as prolonged QRS complex, depressed ST segment, high peaked T waves, bradycardia, or heart block

Several measures are available to reduce the serum potassium concentration, and the priority of implementation is usually based on the rapidity with which the measures are effective. Temporary measures that produce a rapid, but transient, effect are:
1. Calcium gluconate, 0.5 ml/kg, administered intravenously over 2-4 minutes, with continuous ECG monitoring, exerts a protective effect on cardiac conduction.
2. Sodium bicarbonate, 2-3 mEq/kg, administered intravenously over 30-60 minutes, elevates the serum pH to cause a transient shift of extracellular fluid potassium into the intracellular fluid. However, there is risk of hypocalcaemia, tetany, and fluid overload.
3. Glucose, 50%, and insulin, 1 U/kg, administered intravenously, accelerate glycogen synthesis, causing glucose and potassium to move into the cells. Insulin facilitates the entry of glucose into cells.

These effects produce only transient protection by redistributing existing potassium stores; they do not remove potassium from the body. However, they provide relief while more definitive but slower-acting measures are being implemented. Potassium can be removed by:
1. Administration of an ion-exchange resin calcium resonium, 1 g/kg, administered orally or rectally, to bind potassium and remove it from the body. This requires time to be effective, and a calcium ion is exchanged for each potassium ion.
2. Dialysis. Haemodialysis is efficient, but requires specialized facilities. Peritoneal dialysis is simpler and can be carried out in almost any hospital setting. Indications for dialysis in ARF are continued oliguria associated with any of the following:

Severe, persistent acidosis
Inability to reduce serum potassium levels to a safe range with other methods
Clinical uraemic syndrome, consisting of nausea and vomiting, drowsiness, and progression to coma
Circulatory overload, hypertension, and evidence of cardiac failure

A popular philosophy is to institute dialysis after 24-48 hours of oliguria, regardless of other symptoms. Supporters of this approach believe that early and frequent dialysis is associated with reduced morbidity and mortality, and that it permits improved nutrition with relaxed diet restrictions. The combination of dialysis and nutrition tends to reduce the complications of ARF.

Hypertension

Hypertension is a frequent and serious complication of ARF and, to detect it early, blood pressure readings are taken every 1–2 hours. The most common cause of hypertension in ARF is overexpansion of the extracellular fluid and plasma volume together with activation of the renin-angiotensin system. The goal of therapy is to prevent hypertensive encephalopathy and to avoid overtaxing the cardiovascular system.

Other complications

Other complications that may occur with ARF are anaemia, convulsions and coma, cardiac failure and pulmonary oedema. *Anaemia* is frequently associated with ARF. Transfusions consist of fresh, packed red blood cells given slowly to reduce the likelihood of increasing blood volume, hypertension and hyperkalaemia. If dialysis is required, transfusions should be given only on dialysis.

Cardiac failure with pulmonary oedema is almost always associated with hypervolaemia. Treatment is directed towards reduction of fluid volume, with water and sodium restriction, and administration of diuretics. Digitalis is ineffective and can be hazardous.

Diuretic, or high-output, phase

When the output begins to increase, either spontaneously or in response to diuretic therapy, the intake of fluid, potassium and sodium must be monitored, and adequate replacement provided to prevent depletion and its consequences. In some cases the high-output phase is mild and lasts only a few days; in others enormous amounts of electrolyte-rich urine are passed.

Prognosis

The prognosis of ARF depends largely on the nature and severity of the causative factor or precipitating event and the promptness and competence of management. The mortality rate is less than 20%. The outcome is least favourable in children with rapidly progressive nephritis and cortical necrosis. Children in whom ARF is a result of haemolytic-uraemic syndrome or acute glomerulitis may recover completely, but residual renal impairment or hypertension may occur. Complete recovery is usually expected in children whose renal failure is a result of dehydration, nephrotoxins, or ischaemia. ARF following cardiac surgery is less favourable.

IMPLICATIONS FOR NURSING

Nursing care of the infant or child with ARF involves care of the underlying cause, plus careful observation and management of the renal status. The major goal is re-establishment of renal function, with emphasis on providing an adequate caloric intake to minimize reduction of protein stores, prevention of complications, and monitoring of fluid balance, laboratory data and physical manifestations. Because the child requires intensive observation and often specialized equipment, it is preferable to admit the child to an intensive care unit or a renal unit where equipment and personnel trained in its use are available.

Planning

Major goals in the care of the child with ARF are:
1. Monitor laboratory data and physical manifestations.
2. Provide an adequate caloric intake to minimize reduction of protein stores.
3. Prevent and/or manage complications.
4. Support and educate child and family.

Evaluation

The effectiveness of nursing interventions is determined by continual reassessment and evaluation of care based on the following observational guidelines and expected outcomes:
1. Carry out frequent assessment of vital signs and behaviours.
2. Observe eating behaviours and energy expenditure; monitor intake of protein and calories; carefully monitor intake and output, weigh daily or more often as prescribed.
3. Monitor vital signs, sensorium and other neurological signs; evaluate laboratory results and observe for signs of electrolyte imbalance.
4. Observe and interview child and family regarding their understanding of the disease and therapies; encourage child and family to express their feelings and concerns.

CHRONIC RENAL FAILURE

The kidneys are able to maintain the chemical composition of fluids within normal limits until more than 50% of functional renal capacity is destroyed by disease or injury. Chronic renal failure (CRF) or insufficiency begins when diseased kidneys can no longer maintain the normal chemical structure of body fluids under normal conditions. Progressive deterioration over months or years produces a variety of clinical and biochemical disturbances that eventually culminate in the clinical syndrome known as *uraemia*. When the kidneys can no longer function, even with medical intervention, and the patient must resort to dialysis for clearing wastes, the term *end-stage renal disease (ESRD)* is applied.

Retention of waste products

Moderate decrease in renal function is not associated with a rise in fasting blood urea concentration. With progressive nephron destruction and diminished function, the serum level of these end products of protein metabolism increases. However, the blood urea nitrogen level is affected by protein intake, whereas the creatinine concentration is not; therefore, creatinine is a more reliable index of renal failure.

Water and sodium retention

The damaged kidneys are able to maintain sodium and water balance under normal circumstances, although the few remaining functional nephrons are required to increase their rate of filtration and reabsorption in proportion to their numbers. The limitations of this capacity become apparent under stress. The nature of abnormalities in adjustment depends on the underlying renal disease: infants and small children with kidney dysplasia or urinary obstructive disease tend to excrete large volumes of dilute urine low in sodium content, children with glomerular disease tend to retain both sodium and water as a result of a greater reduction in glomerular filtration than of tubular reabsorption, and children with defective sodium reabsorption from tubular disease tend to lose sodium with a corresponding osmotic water loss. Consequently, sodium excesses may cause oedema and hypertension, whereas sodium deprivation can result in hypovolaemia and circulatory failure. Only in end-stage renal disease is markedly reduced glomerular filtration inadequate to handle normal amounts of sodium and water. Retention of these substances leads to oedema and vascular congestion.

Hyperkalaemia
Dangerous hyperkalaemia is an infrequent occurrence in CRF until the terminal stages. However, the kidneys are unable to adjust readily to increased ingestion of potassium, and they require a longer period of time to rid the body of this excess.

Acidosis
A sustained metabolic acidosis is characteristic of CRF; it results from the inability of the damaged kidney to excrete a normal load of metabolic acids generated by normal metabolic processes. There is reduced capacity of the distal tubules to produce ammonia and impaired reabsorption of bicarbonate. Although there is continual hydrogen ion retention and bicarbonate loss, the plasma pH is maintained at a level compatible with life by other buffering mechanisms, particularly the bone salt (see following sections).

Calcium and phosphorus disturbances
One of the distressing features of CRF is its effect on calcium and phosphorus homeostasis. Profound and complex disturbances in the metabolism of these substances result in significant bone demineralization and impaired growth (Box 25-5). The result of these complex disturbances in calcium, phosphorus and bone metabolism produces growth arrest or retardation, bone pain and deformities known as *renal osteodystrophy*, sometimes called *renal rickets*, since the disorganization of bone growth and demineralization is similar to that caused by vitamin D-resistant rickets.

Anaemia
A consistent feature of chronic renal insufficiency is anaemia that appears to result from several factors (Box 25-6).

Growth disturbance
One of the most striking effects of CRF in childhood, and one that can have profound psychological and social consequences for the developing child, is retarded growth. The cause is poorly understood but may be related to nutritional and biochemical factors (Box 25-7).

Sexual maturation may be delayed or may not occur in children with CRF, and secondary amenorrhoea frequently develops in girls past puberty. CRF can also cause sexual dysfunction by creating imbalances in gonadal hormone levels.

Other disturbances
Children with CRF are more susceptible to infection, especially pneumonia, urinary tract infection, and septicaemia, although the reason for this is not entirely clear.

CLINICAL MANIFESTATIONS

The first evidence of difficulty is usually loss of normal energy and increased fatigue on exertion. The child is usually somewhat pale, but it is often so inconspicuous that the change may not be evident to parents or others. Sometimes, blood pressure is elevated.

As the disease progresses, other manifestations may appear. The child eats less well (especially breakfast), shows less interest in normal activities, such as schoolwork or play, and has a decreased or increased urinary output and a compensatory intake of fluid. The child may complain of headache, muscle cramps and nausea. Other signs and symptoms include weight loss, facial puffiness, malaise, bone or joint pain, growth retardation, dryness or itching of the skin, bruised skin and, sometimes, sensory or motor loss. Amenorrhoea is common in adolescent girls.

Therapy is generally instigated before the appearance of the *uraemic syndrome*, although there are occasions in which the symptoms may be observed. Manifestations of untreated uraemia reflect the progressive nature of the homeostatic disturbances and general toxicity. Gastrointestinal symptoms include loss of appetite, nausea and vomiting. Bleeding tendencies are apparent in bruises, bloody diarrhoeal stools, stom-

---

◆ **BOX 25-5**

Factors related to bone demineralization in chronic renail failure

1. In a state of acidosis there is dissolution of the alkaline salts of bone, which serve as buffers, and the release of phosphorus and calcium into the bloodstream.
2. Reduced glomerular filtration and excretion of inorganic phosphate lead to an elevation of plasma phosphate with a concomitant decrease in serum calcium.
3. Decreased serum calcium concentration stimulates the secretion of parathyroid hormone (PTH), which results in resorption of calcium from bones. Under normal circumstances parathyroid hormone inhibits the tubular reabsorption of phosphates.
4. Diseased kidneys are unable to complete the synthesis of vitamin D to its most active form, 1,25-dihydroxycholecalciferol, which is necessary for the absorption of calcium from the gastrointestinal tract and deposition of calcium in bone. This acquired resistance to vitamin D decreases calcium absorption, permits retention of phosphorus, and contributes to secondary hyperparathyroidism.

◆ BOX 25-6

Causes of anaemia in chronic renal failure

1. Shortened life span of red blood cells caused by some extracorpuscular factor associated with the uraemic state
2. Impaired red blood cell production resulting from decreased production of erythropoietin
3. Increased tendency to bleed, associated with a prolonged bleeding time, probably related to impaired platelet function
4. Superimposed nutritional anaemia

◆ BOX 25-7

Probable causes of growth failure in chronic renal failure

1. Renal osteodystrophy
2. Poor nutrition associated with dietary restrictions (especially protein) and loss of appetite
3. Biochemical abnormalities associated with renal failure, such as sustained acidosis, hyperkalaemia, chronic hyposmolarity secondary to hyposthenuria (secretion of urine with low specific gravity), and phosphorus depletion

---

atitis, and bleeding from lips and mouth. There is intractable itching, probably related to hyperparathyroidism, and deposits of urea crystals appear on the skin as 'uraemic frost'. There may be an unpleasant 'uraemic' odour to the breath. Respirations become deeper as a result of metabolic acidosis, and circulatory overload is manifest by hypertension, congestive heart failure, and pulmonary oedema. Neurological involvement is reflected by progressive confusion, dulling of sensorium, and, ultimately, coma. Other signs may include tremors, muscular twitching, and seizures.

THERAPEUTIC MANAGEMENT

In irreversible renal failure, the goals of medical management are to promote effective renal function, to maintain body fluid and electrolyte balance within acceptable limits, to treat systemic complications, and to promote as active and normal a life as possible for the child for as long as possible.

Diet

Regulation of diet is the most effective means, short of dialysis, for reducing the quantity of materials that require renal excretion. The goal of the diet in renal failure is to provide sufficient calories and protein for growth while limiting the excretory demands made on the kidney, to minimize metabolic bone disease (osteodystrophy), and to minimize fluid and electrolyte disturbances. Dietary phosphate, principally the intake of cow's milk, is restricted.

Bottle-fed infants are placed on a low-protein, low-electrolyte formula with additional caloric supplements. When given with meals, substances that bind phosphate in the intestines prevent its absorption and allow a more liberal intake of phosphate-containing protein. Sodium and water are not usually limited, unless there is evidence of oedema or hypertension.

Potassium is not restricted as long as creatinine clearance remains at acceptable limits (greater than or equal to 30-35 ml/min). Restrictions are instituted for patients with oliguria or anuria, however.

Because of modified dietary intake, altered metabolism, and poor appetite, some dietary supplementation is usually needed. Because fat-soluble vitamins can accumulate in patients with CRF, vitamins A, E, and K are not supplemented beyond normal dietary intake. Vitamin D is prescribed, and water-soluble vitamin supplementation may be required if diet is inadequate.

Osteodystrophy

Measures directed at prevention or correction of the calcium/phosphorus imbalance are reduction of dietary phosphate, administration of a phosphate-binding agent, provision of supplemental calcium, control of acidosis, and administration of vitamin D.

Dietary phosphate is controlled by the reduction of protein and milk. Phosphate levels can be further reduced by the oral administration of calcium carbonate or tablets that combine with the phosphate to decrease gastrointestinal absorption and thus the serum levels of phosphate.

When serum phosphate levels are within a normal range, appropriate vitamin D therapy is instituted. The serum calcium level is monitored weekly during periods when the drugs are being changed or regulated. Parathyroid hormone levels are measured every 2-3 months.

Osseous deformities that result from renal osteodystrophy, especially those related to ambulation, are troublesome and require correction as soon as feasible. It has been found that noticeable deformities develop in one third of patients with osteodystrophy despite medical therapy (Hsu *et al*, 1982).

Acidosis

Pharmacological treatment of acidosis is initiated early in children who have chronic renal insufficiency. Acidosis is alleviated by alkalizing agents such as sodium bicarbonate. Correction of acidosis is best attempted after calcium levels are elevated, since rapid correction may precipitate tetany in a hypocalcaemic child.

Anaemia

Because the anaemia associated with renal failure is related to decreased production of erythropoietin, it usually cannot be successfully managed with haematinic agents. However, sufficient sources of folic acid and iron should be provided in the diet, although this is difficult when protein sources are restricted. Inadequate intake and iron losses that may occur are managed by supplemental iron, usually ferrous sulphate.

Recombinant human erythropoietin (rHuEPO), corrects anaemia (improving energy level and general well-being) and eliminates the need for frequent blood transfusions in patients with CRF (Rigden *et al*, 1990).

Hypertension

Hypertension of advanced renal disease may be managed initially by cautious use of a low-sodium diet, fluid restriction, and perhaps diuretics such as frusemide. Strict restriction of sodium intake may be necessary in oliguric patients. Severe hypertension may require the use of a combination of a beta blocker and a vasodilator (propranolol and hydralazine). Other drugs that may be used include nifedipine, atenolol, minoxidil, prazosin, captopril or labetatol singly or in combination.

Growth retardation

One major consequence of CRF is growth retardation, especially in preadolescents. These children grow poorly both before and after initiation of haemodialysis. Depletion of body protein is characteristic of children with CRF, in addition to a number of metabolic abnormalities. Studies are now being conducted in various paediatric centres to evaluate the use of recombinant human growth hormone to accelerate growth in children with growth retardation secondary to CRF or following renal transplant. Evidence indicates marked acceleration in growth velocity in children treated with growth hormone (Rees *et al*, 1990).

Miscellaneous complications

Intercurrent infections are treated with appropriate antimicrobials at the first sign of infection. Most of these drugs are excreted through the kidneys; therefore, the dosage is usually reduced in proportion to the decrease in renal function and the interval between doses extended in these children to avoid possible toxic effects from accumulation.

Once evidence of ESRD appears in a child, the disease runs its relentless course and terminates in death in a few weeks, unless waste products and toxins are removed from body fluids by dialysis and/or kidney transplantation. Since these techniques have been adapted for infants and small children, the outlook for them has improved remarkably.

IMPLICATIONS FOR NURSING

The child with CRF is a prime example of an individual whose life is maintained by drugs and artificial means, and the multiple stresses placed on these children and their families are often overwhelming. There is no means to prevent the irreversible progress of renal insufficiency, nor is there any known cure. As the affected child progresses from renal insufficiency to uraemia and then to haemodialysis and transplantation with a need for intensification of therapy, the need for supportive nursing care is also intensified.

Progressive disease places several stresses on the child and family. There is continuing need for repeated examinations that often entail painful procedures, side effects, and frequent hospitalizations. Diet becomes progressively more restricted and intense, and parents may need help in learning to select appropriate foods, reading labels carefully for sodium and potassium content. The child is required to take a variety of medications. Compliance is difficult when long-term therapies are involved.

One of the first and most noticeable changes is the alteration in physical appearance — fluctuations in weight, anaemia, and failure to grow. Children must adjust to the fact that they will always be different from their peers in some ways. They will be shorter, often more tired, and unable to participate in all the activities that are attractive to young people.

In some families, illness and stressful experiences act as a unifying force; in others, stress aggravates pre-existing problems and contributes to family disharmony. The relentless nature of the disease and its therapies not only place physical and emotional stresses on the family, but are also a chronic drain on family finances. Hidden costs abound, such as transportation to special treatment centres, meals and sometimes lodging away from home. The involvement of a social worker can be invaluable in providing assistance to these families. The British Kidney Patients' Association is an organization which provides help and information to patients with renal failure.

TECHNOLOGICAL MANAGEMENT OF RENAL FAILURE

Technological advances in the care of children with acute and chronic renal failure have provided a means for maintaining excretory function in acute disease and for prolonging life in those with ESRD. The primary modalities are haemodialysis, peritoneal dialysis, haemofiltration and transplantation.

Dialysis is the process of separating colloids and crystalline substances in solution by the difference in their rate of diffusion through a semipermeable membrane. This movement across the membrane is accomplished by three processes: osmosis, diffusion, and utrafiltration.

Methods of dialysis currently available for clinical management of renal failure are:

1. **Haemodialysis,** in which blood is circulated outside the body through artificial cellophane membranes that permit a similar passage of water and solutes
2. **Peritoneal dialysis,** wherein the abdominal cavity acts as a semipermeable membrane through which water and solutes of small molecular size move by osmosis and diffusion according to their respective concentrations on either side of the membrane
3. **Haemofiltration,** in which blood filtrate is circulated outside the body by hydrostatic pressure exerted across a semipermeable membrane and replaced (simultaneously) by electrolyte solution

All these treatments can be used for acute renal failure. For chronic renal failure, the choice is influenced by patient preference. In the UK, peritoneal dialysis is becoming more widely used as the treatment of choice for children, because it can be done at home by either the child or parents, allowing full-time school attendance.

Although each child is assessed on an individual basis, indications for instituting dialysis in CRF are biochemical abnormalities including elevated urea, acidosis, severe hyperphosphataemia, elevated potassium, and anaemia requiring transfusion (placing child at risk for fluid overload).

Most children show rapid clinical improvement with the implementation of dialysis. Growth rate and skeletal maturation improve, but recovery of normal growth is uncommon. In many cases sexual development, although delayed, has progressed to completion.

HAEMODIALYSIS

Haemodialysis is a very efficient form of dialysis. It has three major disadvantages, however:
1. It is usually hospital based.
2. It is intermittent; therefore, there are swings in fluid and electrolyte status.
3. Access to the circulation is needed.

Over the last ten years, peritoneal dialysis has become the treatment of choice for the majority of children in the UK and home haemodialysis has diminished (though it is still an important form of treatment for adults).

There are some occasions when haemodialysis would be the preferred treatment, such as in cases of severe poisoning; abdominal injury or major surgery; repeated peritonitis; where peritoneal dialysis has failed; or if hospital haemodialysis is socially preferable to the child and family. Before haemodialysis is undertaken, access to the circulation allowing blood to be cycled at a rate of 200 ml/min must be available. Many types of vascular access are currently available for long- or short-term use.

To haemodialyse a child requires skilled paediatric renal staff and expensive equipment (Fig. 25-3). The fluid volume required to fill the dialyser and circuit must be less than 8–10% of the child's corporeal blood volume. Most paediatric dialysis regimens are 3–5 hours, three times a week. This means a child on dialysis often misses important schooling .

Dietary restrictions are necessary for the child on dialysis. A high calorie diet is important to achieve growth and prevent fluid overload. It is impossible for the patient to stick to a fluid restriction diet if salt is not also restricted.

Potassium is restricted to prevent hypokalaemia. Phosphate restriction, together with active vitamin D supplementation, helps to prevent bone disease.

PERITONEAL DIALYSIS

For *acute* conditions peritoneal dialysis (PD) is quick, relatively easy to learn, and safe to perform. PD is a slow gentle process, which decreases the stress on body organs that can occur with the rapid chemical and volume changes of haemodialysis. The procedure is indicated for neonates, children with severe cardiovascular disease, or those with bleeding abnormalities who are poor risks for vascular access and heparinization.

Chronic PD is the preferred form of dialysis for children/parents who are independent, families who live a long distance from the hospital, infants, school-aged children, and children who prefer fewer dietary restrictions and a gentler form of dialysis. Chronic peritoneal dialysis is most often performed at home.

Contraindications for use of PD include recent abdominal surgery, peritoneal adhesions and scarring.

PROCEDURE

In acute situations, PD catheter insertion may be accomplished at the bedside; catheters for long-term use are placed surgically in the operating room under anaesthesia. A catheter is inserted through the anterior abdominal wall, and the catheter cuff sutured into place. At the time of dialysis, a commercially prepared dialysis solution (dialysate) is allowed to flow by gravity through the catheter into the peritoneal cavity, where it remains while equilibrium between plasma and dialysis fluid takes place. Approximately 30-50 ml/kg of dialysate is instilled at each treatment. The fluid is then allowed to flow by gravity drainage into a receptacle, and fresh dialysate is again instilled.

In acute PD, each cycle generally takes about 30 minutes: 5 minutes for the fluid to flow into the peritoneal cavity, 20 minutes for equilibration, and 5-10 minutes for removal. The procedure is usually continued until renal function is restored, poisons are reduced, or (in prolonged need) the patient is placed on a form of chronic PD—*continuous ambulatory peritoneal dialysis (CAPD)* or *continuous cycling peritoneal dialysis (CCPD)*.

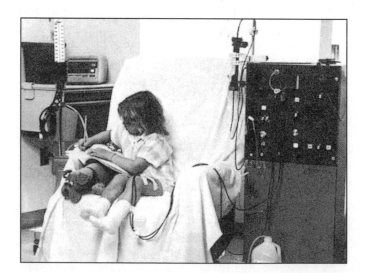

Fig. 25-3 Child undergoing haemodialysis.

HOME DIALYSIS

The development of satisfactory methods for CAPD and its alternative, CCPD, has provided additional means for managing ESRD at home. In both methods, commercially available sterile dialysate solution is instilled into the peritoneal cavity through the surgically implanted indwelling catheter. The warmed solution is allowed to enter the peritoneal cavity by gravity and remains a variable length of time according to the procedure used.

In CAPD the dialysate is instilled, the line clamped off, and the giving set disconnected. The solution is allowed to remain in the peritoneum for 4-6 hours. A new bag is attached, the line is unclamped, and the fluid is drained into the bag by gravity. Another heated bag is instilled, and the process is repeated so that there is fluid in the abdomen continuously. The procedure is performed three times during the day and once at night. For an active child, CAPD has proved to be a satisfactory alternative to haemodialysis that can be continued for an indefinite time.

CCPD is a modification of CAPD and intermittent peritoneal dialysis. The dialysis exchange is performed only at night using an automatic dialysis machine, which controls the timed cycles of inflow and outflow of dialysate. The catheter is opened only at night rather than four times per day, although an additional exchange may be prescribed during the day. The night-time dialysis allows the child more freedom during the day and relieves parents from having to perform multiple exchanges (Alliapoulos *et al*, 1984).

Complications

CAPD and CCPD are presently considered to be the methods of choice for most children who require dialysis, because they are easier to initiate and maintain than haemodialysis. Peritonitis is the major complication of home peritoneal dialysis. The patients are treated intraperitoneally with antibiotics, and some may require catheter replacement. Although the risk of infection is continuously present, most practitioners believe it is not great enough to discourage the use of these methods (Fine *et al*, 1983).

However, other complications have been noted in patients on home peritoneal dialysis. Tunnel infections are evidenced by swelling, warmth, and tenderness along the subcutaneous catheter tract; however, they can be managed with administration of antibiotics. Peritoneal leaks and ventral hernias caused by the sustained hydraulic pressure that develops within the peritoneum have also been found in a significant number of children. Most of these patients respond to reduction in dialysate volume or surgical intervention.

IMPLICATIONS FOR NURSING

The availability of home dialysis has offered a greater degree of freedom for those undergoing long-term dialysis. The need for a residence convenient to a dialysis unit and the necessity for frequent trips to the unit are eliminated, except for monthly evaluations. The nurse is responsible for teaching the family. Education focuses on: (1) the disease, its implications, and the therapeutic plan; (2) the possible psychological effects of the disease and the treatment; and (3) the technical aspects of the procedure.

The family must learn how to take vital signs before and after the dialysis, and how to interpret the significance of blood pressure and temperature variations. They need to know how to vary the composition of the dialysate to compensate for variations in the vital signs, and how to maintain an accurate record of all aspects of the treatment.

CONTINUOUS ARTERIOVENOUS HAEMOFILTRATION

A third type of dialysis used primarily in acute care settings is continuous arteriovenous haemofiltration (CAVH), a gentle form of dialysis that employs specialized equipment (filter, pump, tubing connected to a vascular access) to ultrafiltrate blood continuously at a very slow rate. With this procedure, fluid balance may be achieved within 24-48 hours after initiation. CAVH is a procedure used to remove excess fluid from patients with severe oliguric fluid overload.

CAVH is an ideal form of dialysis for children with fluid overload from surgical procedures (such as cardiovascular surgery) who do not have severe biochemical abnormalities. It is frequently used for critically ill children who require volume-expanding fluids such as hyperalimentation solution, albumin, or packed red cells. It creates space for the infusion of these replacement solutions in fluid-sensitive patients. CAVH has proven to be a highly successful alternative form of dialysis for critically ill children who might not survive the rapid volume changes that occur with haemodialysis and peritoneal dialysis.

TRANSPLANTATION

Renal transplantation is now an acceptable and effective therapy in children. Although peritoneal dialysis and haemodialysis are life-preserving and are able to be carried out in the home in many cases, neither method is compatible with a normal lifestyle. Transplantation, on the other hand, offers the opportunity for a relatively normal life. It is presently regarded as the preferred form of treatment for many children with chronic renal failure.

Kidneys for transplant are available from two sources: a living related donor (LRD), usually a parent, and cadaver donor (CD), wherein the family of a dead or brain-dead patient consent to donation of a healthy kidney. The criteria for selection of kidney recipients are quite liberal, but uniform criteria have not been established among the various centres that specialize in the procedure. There is a high incidence of recurrent disease in the donor kidney in children who receive a transplant for rapidly progressive glomerulonephritis or focal segmental glomerulonephritis.

PROCEDURE

The kidney graft is placed in the extraperitoneal space, usually the anterior iliac fossa, the renal artery is anastomosed to the internal iliac or hypogastric artery, the renal vein is anastomosed to the hypogastric vein, and the ureter is implanted into the bladder or anastomosed to the recipient's ureter. Small children receiving a large donor kidney may require placement within the abdomen with vessel anastomoses to the aorta and inferior vena cava. Unless there is medical contraindication, the recipient's failed kidneys are left in place. Severe hypertension, neoplasm, obstructive uropathy, and repeated urinary tract infections are the usual reasons for nephrectomy.

The primary goal in transplantation is the long-term survival of the grafted tissue. The means by which this is attempted is: (1) securing tissues that are antigenically similar to that of the recipient and (2) suppressing the recipient's immune mechanism.

SELECTION OF DONOR TISSUE

The source of a donor kidney is either a live person or a cadaver soon after death. The closer the genetic relationship between the donor and recipient, the better the possibility of long-term survival. The only truly compatible tissue match is that between identical twin siblings. The next best possible match is a sibling, then a parent, and finally an uncle or aunt. In the United Kingdom, a sibling would not be used as a donor until over the age of consent. Unrelated donors are least likely to be compatible. Careful immunological studies are carried out to determine the donor whose kidney is least likely to be rejected by the recipient.

SUPPRESSION OF THE IMMUNE RESPONSE

After the best possible tissue match is obtained for a transplant, the survival time can be significantly lengthened by suppressing the immune response of the recipient. The immunosuppressant therapy of choice in kidney transplantation is corticosteroids (prednisone) in conjunction with cyclosporine and azathioprine. Other therapies include antilymphoblast globulin or monoclonal antibodies, administered intravenously for 14 days after transplant.

The administration of these drugs is not without hazard. The major problem encountered with nonspecific immunosuppression is that it not only suppresses the immune response to the grafted tissue, but also suppresses the body's capacity to respond to other antigenic stimuli. Consequently, the child is vulnerable to overwhelming infections.

Prednisone is a powerful immunosuppressant and anti-inflammatory agent that acts to stabilize cell walls, reduce migration of white blood cells into the inflamed area, and inhibit deposition of fibrin and collagen. It also depresses T-cells, B-cells, and phagocytes. Several complications that are directly attributable to corticosteroid therapy are cause for concern for children on steroid therapy. Interference with calcium absorption retards linear growth, and in most units alternate-day administration is being used in an effort to improve growth rates and to decrease other long-term side effects. Other corticosteroid-induced side effects may include the characteristic cushingoid facies, cataracts, fluid and sodium retention, gastric ulcer and obesity.

Cyclosporine is a powerful immunosuppressant that acts to decrease production of T-cells. Side effects of this drug are arterial hypertension, which may appear within three weeks of transplant; hirsutism; and nephrotoxicity, a major concern in renal transplantation. Maintenance doses of cyclosporine are determined by serum blood levels. Low therapeutic cyclosporine levels usually prevent untoward side effects, as well as rejection. After the initial intravenous therapy immediately following transplant, the drug is administered orally.

Azathioprine is a powerful immunosuppressant that interferes with cellular protein synthesis. The problem related to the toxic effect of azathioprine is mainly neutropenia, which is usually managed by reduced dosage.

REJECTION

Rejection of a transplanted kidney is the most frequent cause of transplant failure. Rejection can be one of three types — hyperacute, acute, or chronic. Hyperacute rejection is irreversible, develops immediately or within a few hours after revascularization, and is related to circulating antibodies preformed in the recipient against the donor tissue antigens. These are seen in second transplants or in persons sensitized from blood transfusions.

Acute rejection usually occurs between the first few days and six months after transplantation but may occur as late as one or two years later. Rejection is evidenced by both biochemical and clinical abnormalities. The most frequent finding is fever, which is usually accompanied by swelling and tenderness over the graft, hypertension, and diminished urine output. A severe reaction may cause oliguria. Increases in serum blood urea and creatinine levels are laboratory evidence of decreased transplant function. Most acute rejection episodes respond to intravenous administration of methylprednisolone sodium succinate, antilymphoblast globulin, or monoclonal antibodies.

Chronic rejection is characterized by slow, gradual deterioration of renal function that typically begins six months or more after transplantation. Evidence of rejection may be heralded by proteinuria and/or haematuria, and the rejection may have symptomatology indistinguishable from the original kidney disease. No present therapy can halt the progressive process, which inevitably leads to loss of the implanted kidney.

PROGNOSIS

The overall graft survival rate for kidneys from living related donors is 89% at one year and 80% at three years. For cadaver kidneys the graft survival rate is 74% at one year and 62% at three years (McEnery *et al*, 1992). Posttransplant complications include infection, hypertension, steroid toxicity, hyperlipidaemia, aseptic necrosis, malignancy, and growth retardation (Ettenger and Fine, 1987). Long-term graft survival is not guaranteed, and many children require a second or third transplant. Successful renal transplantation does improve rehabilitation of children with CRF, both educationally and psychologically.

IMPLICATIONS FOR NURSING

The possibility of renal transplantation often comes as a hope for relief from the rigors of haemodialysis and the hated diet restrictions. Except for children with pre-existing personality problems or residual physical disabilities, most children and families respond well to kidney transplant, and the majority return to normal life within a year after surgery. The dynamics related to accepting and donating kidneys are fraught with emotional overtones, caused in part by the issues related to the child's receiving an organ from another person.

Corticosteroid therapy, necessary in kidney transplants, creates undesirable side effects - for example, growth failure, obesity, characteristics of Cushing syndrome, acne, and hirsutism - that are frequently a source of emotional and social problems for older children. Characteristic facial changes (coarseness, thickened nares, puffy cheeks, prominent supraorbital ridges, and mandibular prognathism) have also been reported in children on cyclosporine (Reznik *et al*, 1987).

The most frequent reason for noncompliance in childhood renal transplant recipients is dislike of undesirable side effects. The cosmetic implications of the side effects can be overwhelming, especially to adolescent girls. Deliberate discontinuation of the drugs is most commonly observed in teenage girls. Noncompliance is also seen frequently in children from poorly communicating families who are not very supportive.

Working with children and their families during the various stages of renal failure, dialysis, and transplantation is a difficult and challenging experience.

KEY POINTS

◆ Common inflammatory disorders of the genitourinary tract include urinary tract infection, nephrotic syndrome and acute glomerulonephritis.

◆ Management of UTIs is directed at eliminating infection, detecting and correcting functional or anatomical abnormalities, preventing recurrences and preserving renal function.

◆ Vesicoureteral reflux is the retrograde flow of bladder urine into the ureters.

◆ Common features of acute glomerulonephritis are oliguria, oedema, hypertension, circulatory congestion, haematuria, and proteinuria.

◆ Therapeutic management of acute glomerulonephritis is maintenance of fluid balance, treatment of hypertension, and antibiotic therapy.

◆ Nephrotic syndrome is characterized by increased glomerular permeability to protein.

◆ The most common renal tubular disorders are renal tubular acidosis and nephrogenic diabetes insipidus.

◆ Management of haemolytic-uraemic syndrome is aimed at control of complications and haematological manifestations of renal failure.

◆ In acute renal failure, management is directed at determining treatment of underlying cause, management of complications of renal failure, and supportive therapy.

◆ When the child will need home dialysis, the nurse educates the family about the disease, its implications, the therapeutic plan, possible psychological effects of the disease, and the treatment and technical aspects of the procedure.

◆ The major concerns in renal transplantation are tissue matching and prevention of rejection; psychological concerns involve self-image as related to possible body changes as a result of the effects of corticosteroid therapy.

REFERENCES

Edelmann CM: Urinary tract infection and vesicoureteral reflux, *Pediatr Ann* 17:568, 1988.

Ettenger RB, Fine RN: Renal transplantation. In Holiday, MA, Barratt TM, Vernmier RL, editors: *Pediatric nephrology,* Baltimore, 1987, Williams & Wilkins.

Fine RN *et al*: Peritonitis in children undergoing continuous ambulatory peritoneal dialysis, *Pediatr* 71:806, 1983.

Haws RM, Baum M: Efficacy of albumin and diuretic therapy in children with nephrotic syndrome, *Pediatrics* 91(6):1142, 1993.

Hensle TW, Burbige KA: Vesicoureteral reflux. In Gellis SS, Kagan BM, editors: *Current paediatric therapy 12,* Philadelphia, 1986, WB Saunders.

Herzog LW: Urinary tract infections and circumcision: a case-control study, *Am J Dis Child* 143:348, 1989.

Hsu AC *et al*: Renal osteodystrophy in children with chronic renal failure: an unexpectedly common and incapacitating complication, *Pediatr* 70:742, 1982.

Jodal IU, Winberg J: Management of children with unobstructed urinary tract infection, *Pediatr Nephrol* 1:647, 1987.

Karmali MA *et al*: The association between idiopathic hemolytic uremic syndrome and infection by verotoxin-producing Escherichia coli, *J Infect Dis* 151:775, 1985.

McEnery PT, Strife CF: Nephrotic syndrome in childhood, *Pediatr Clin North Am* 89:875, 1982.

McEnery et al: *Renal Transplantation in children, N Engl J Med* 326(26):1727, 1992

Rees et al: Treatment of short stature in renal disease with recombinant human growth hormone, *Arch Dis Child* 65:856, 1990.

Reznik VM et al. Changes in facial appearance during cyclosporin treatment, *Lancet* 1:1405, 1987.

Rigden SPA et al: Recombinant human erythropoitin therapy in children maintained by haemodialysis, *Paed Nephrol* 4:618, 1990.

Rizzoni G. et al.: Plasma infusion for hemolytic-uremic syndrome in children: results of a multicenter controlled trial, *J Pediatr* 112:284-290, 1988.

Roberts JA: URI: an argument for circumcision, *Comtemp Pediatr* 5(8):42, 1988.

Rogers WB: Shampoo urethritis, *Am J Dis Child* 139:748, 1985.

Royal College of Physicians: Guidelines for the management of acute urinary tract infection in childhood. Report of the Working Group of the Research Unit, *RCP J Royal College Physicians, London* 25:36, 1991

Rushton HG: Nonspecific infections. In Kelalis PP, King LR, Belman AB, editors: *Clinical pediatric urology,* Philadelphia, 1992, WB Saunders.

Smellie JM: Clinical medical nephrology, ed 2, Oxford, 1994, Butterworth-Heinemann.

Wiswell TE et al: Effect of circumcision status on periurethral bacterial flora during the first year of life, *J Pediatr* 113:442, 1988.

Wiswell TE, Gescheke DW: Risks from circumcision during the first month of life compared with those for uncircumcised boys, *Paediatrics* 83:1011, 1989.

Wiswell TE, Roscelli JD: Corroborative evidence for the decreased incidence of urinary tract infections in cirumcised male infants, *Paediatrics* 78:96, 1986.

FURTHER READING

General

Barratt TM, Vernier RL: *Paediatric nephrology,* ed 2, Baltimore, 1987, Williams & Wilkins.

Dillon MJ: Drug treatment of hypertension. In Holiday MA, Barratt TM, Vernmier RL, editors: *Pediatric nephrology,* Baltimore, 1987, Williams & Wilkins.

Gabriel R: A patient's guide to dialysis and transplantation, ed 3, London, 1987, Butler & Tanner.

Postlethwaite RJ: *Clinical paediatric nephrology,* Oxford, 1994, Butterworth-Heinemann.

Rizzoni G et al: Plasma infusion for hemolytic-uremic syndrome in children: results of a multicenter controlled trial, *J Pediatr* 112:284, 1988.

Urinary Tract Infection/Reflux

Conti MT, Euthropius L: Preventing UTI's: What works? *Am J Nurs* 87:307, 1987.

Edelmann CM: Urinary tract infection and vesicoureteral reflux, *Pediatr Ann* 17:568, 1988.

Heldrich FJ: Pinning down the diagnosis of UTI, *Contemp Pediatr* 5:52, 1988.

Glomerular Diseases

Brodehl J, Ehrich JHH: Short versus standard prednisone therapy for initial treatment of idiopathic nephrotic syndrome in children, *Lancet* 1:380, 1988.

Schnaper HW: The immune system in minimal change nephrotic syndrome, *Pediatr Nephrol* 3:101, 1989

Tejani A et al: Cyclosporin A–induced remission in relapsing nephrotic syndrome in children, *Kidney Int* 33:729, 1988.

Haemolytic-Uraemic Syndrome

Havens PL et al: Laboratory and clinical variables to predict outcome in hemolytic-uremic syndrome, *Am J Dis Child* 142:961, 1988.

Kavi J, Wise R: Causes of the haemolytic uraemic syndrome, *Br Med J* 298:65, 1989.

Siegler RL: Management of hemolytic-uremic syndrome, *J Pediatr* 112:1014, 1988.

Acute Renal Failure

Gaudio KM, Siegel NJ: Pathogenesis and treatment of acute renal failure, *Pediatr Clin North Am* 34:771, 1987.

Hahn K: The many signs of renal failure, *Nurs '87* 17:34, 1987.

Ruley EJ, Bock GH: Acute renal failure in infants and children. In Shoemaker WC et al, editors: *Textbook of critical care,* ed 2, Philadelphia, 1989, WB Saunders.

Chronic Renal Failure

Bock GH et al: Disturbances of brain maturation and neurodevelopment during chronic renal failure in infancy, *J Pediatr* 114:231, 1989.

Crittenden MR, Holaday B: Physical growth and behavioral adaptations of children with renal insufficiency, *ANNA J* 16:87-92+, 1989.

Foreman JW, Chan JCM: Chronic renal failure in infants and children, *J Pediatr* 113:793, 1988.

Quinlan M: Nursing assessment and management of malnutrition in uremic infants, *ANNA J* 15:19, 1988.

Dialysis

Bell S: CAVH in pediatrics: Meeting the challenge, *ANNA J* 15:25, 1988.

Gharbieh PA: Renal transplant: surgical and psychologic hazards, *Crit Care Nurse* 8(6):58, 1988.

Moskop JC: Organ transplantation in children: ethical issues, *J Pediatr* 110:175, 1987.

Neff EJ: Nursing the child undergoing dialysis, *Issues Compr Pediatr Nurs* 10:173, 1987.

Suddaby EC, Bell SB, and Murphy KJ: Continuous hemofiltration in infants and children, *Pediatr Nurs* 16:79, 1990.

Transplantation

Frauman AC, Miles MS: Parental willingness to donate the organs of a child, *ANNA J* 14:401, 1987.

Morris PJ: Therapeutic strategies in immunosuppression after transplantation, *J Pediatr* 111(6):1004, 1987.

USEFUL ADDRESS

British Kidney Patient Association, Bordon, Hants, GU35 9J.

Chapter 26

The Child with Disturbance of Oxygen and Carbon Dioxide Exchange

LEARNING OUTCOMES

After studying this chapter you should be able to:

◆ Describe the anatomical differences between the adult and child that influence the way in which infants and children respond to respiratory infection.
◆ Identify objective and subjective elements of respiratory assessment in infants and children.
◆ Describe specific respiratory therapies that support the infant and child with respiratory failure.
◆ Describe the objective and subjective features of respiratory failure.
◆ Delineate specific cardiopulmonary resuscitation measures in infants and children.
◆ Name at least six childhood respiratory infections.
◆ Describe the major features of respiratory infection in the infant and child.
◆ Describe the major features of inhalation of substances injurious to the respiratory system.
◆ Discuss the features of childhood asthma and cystic fibrosis, and related nursing management.
◆ Identify the major nursing responsibilities in looking after the child with respiratory disease.
◆ Define the glossary terms.

GLOSSARY

ALS Advanced life support

apnoea Absence of airflow (breathing)

atelectasis A collapsed or airless state of all or part of the lung

bronchiolitis Inflammation of the bronchioles

bronchitis Inflammation of the bronchi

CF Cystic fibrosis

COPD Chronic obstructive pulmonary disease

coryza Acute nasal congestion

CPAP Continuous positive airway pressure

dyspnoea Difficulty breathing

epiglottitis Inflammation of the epiglottis

hyperpnoea Deep, rapid, or laboured respiration

hypopnoea Slow or shallow respirations

hypoxaemia Deficiency of oxygen in the arterial blood

hypoxia Inadequate, reduced tension of cellular oxygen

laryngitis Inflammation of the larynx

MDI Metered-dose inhaler

respiratory failure Inability of the respiratory apparatus to maintain adequate oxygenation

respiratory insufficiency Increased work of breathing or inability to maintain normal blood gas tensions

stridor (laryngeal) A shrill, harsh respiratory sound, often described as a 'crowing' sound, which is particularly marked during inspiration

tachypnoea Abnormally rapid rate of breathing

TV Tidal volume (amount of air inhaled and exhaled during any respiratory cycle)

ventilation Process by which gases are moved into and out of the lungs

Disorders involving the respiratory tract, many of which can be life threatening, occur frequently in childhood. Various factors influence the development of respiratory disease during these periods. Gas exchange, oxygen (O_2) and carbon dioxide (CO_2) tension, and the activity of chemoreceptors are much the same in children and adults. Anatomically, however, there are several differences that influence the way in which children, particularly infants, respond to respiratory disturbances. This chapter will first review some of these differences, before examining factors involved in respiratory assessment, and general respiratory therapy. It will then review respiratory dysfunction and pulmonary resuscitation before focusing on specific infections and conditions involving the respiratory system.

RESPIRATORY TRACT STRUCTURE AND FUNCTION

The respiratory tract consists of a complex of structures that function under neural and hormonal control. The primary responsibility of these structures is to distribute air and exchange gases so that cells are supplied with O_2, and CO_2 is removed. The nose, pharynx, larynx, trachea, bronchi and lungs provide the means whereby gases enter the body; the circulatory system distributes gases to and from the millions of cells throughout the body. It is within the alveoli that the gas exchange takes place.

STRUCTURE

The thoracic cavity is lined by the smooth parietal pleura, which adheres to the ribs and superior surface of the diaphragm. Each lung is encased in a separate visceral pleural sac that, when inflated, lies against the parietal pleura. Normally, the two pleural membranes are separated by only enough fluid to lubricate the surface for painless movement during filling and emptying of the lungs. In disease states, this space may contain air *(pneumothorax)* or fluid *(pleural effusion)*, more specifically serum *(hydrothorax)*, blood *(haemothorax)*, or pus *(pyothorax, also known as empyema)*. Inflammation of the pleura causes the painful friction of pleurisy during respiratory movements.

CHEST

The chest has a relatively round configuration at birth, but changes gradually to one that is more or less flattened in the anteroposterior diameter in adulthood (Fig. 26-1). In certain lung diseases, chronic overinflation causes changes in these measurements. For example, in severe obstructive lung disease (e.g., asthma, cystic fibrosis) the anteroposterior measurement approaches the transverse measurement to produce the so-called 'barrel' chest. Periodic measurements provide clues to the course of lung disease or the efficacy of therapy.

The shape of the ribs and the angle at which they are attached to the spine allow the thorax to change size during respiration. Contraction of the intercostal muscles lifts the ribs from a downward angle to a more horizontal angle, which increases the dimensions of the chest. This also changes the diameter of the bronchi. The diameter increases during inspiration and decreases during expiration, an important factor when the bronchi are narrowed as a result of obstruction or inflammation. Contraction and relaxation of the diaphragm cause the chest cavity to lengthen and shorten, which also increases the volume of the chest cavity during inspiration.

An adult's ribs articulate with the vertebrae and sternum from a downward and lateral angle. Contraction of the intercostal muscles raises the ribs to a horizontal position in a 'bucket-handle' type of respiratory motion, causing the chest

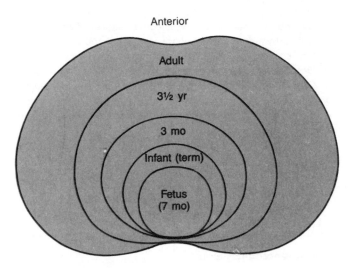

Fig. 26-1 Changes in chest shape with age.

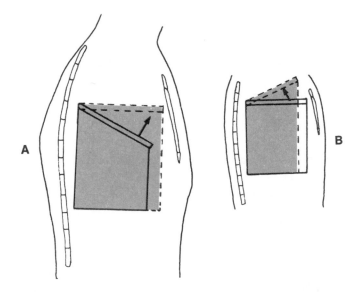

Fig. 26-2 Mechanisms of respiratory excursion. **A,** Downward and lateral position of rib in adult and expansion of lung capacity on thoracic inspiration. **B,** More horizontal position of rib in infant and decreased expansion of lung capacity of thoracic inspiration.

cavity to enlarge. In the newborn infant, the ribs articulate with the spine at a horizontal rather than a downward slope and, if raised further, decrease the diameter of the chest (Fig. 26-2). Therefore, the infant relies almost entirely on diaphragmatic-abdominal breathing. During inspiration, the diaphragm is forced downward, increasing the available space for lung expansion. The intercostal muscles serve primarily as stabilizing forces.

The elastic properties of lung tissue (compliance) also change with age. Compliance represents the relative ease with which the chest wall and lungs expand with increasing volume. The increased compliance in the newborn causes the rib cage to be easily distorted and can be observed in the infant with lung disease. Inspiration causes an inward movement of the rib cage as the abdomen moves outward, because the greater negative pleural pressure required to move the lungs pulls in the soft, compliant, and easily distorted rib cage. The two major factors determining compliance are: 1) alveolar surface tension, which is maintained by surfactant, a lipoprotein at the air-fluid interface that allows expansion and prevents alveolar collapse; and 2) elastic recoil, the tendency of the lung to return to the resting state after inspiration, a passive process that requires no muscular effort. Other factors influencing compliance include: degree of tissue hydration, lung blood volume, surface forces at the air/fluid interface, and chest and lung tissue pathology (i.e. fibres of elastin or collagen). Factors that interfere with compliance and recoil increase the work of breathing.

As the child grows, chest wall compliance decreases and elastic recoil increases; therefore, ventilation becomes progressively more efficient.

In pathological states an increase in compliance indicates that the lungs or chest wall are abnormally easy to inflate and have lost some elastic recoil, such as in asthma. A decrease in compliance indicates that the lungs or chest wall are abnormally stiff or difficult to inflate, such as in respiratory distress syndrome (McCance and Huether, 1994).

In the newborn, the diaphragm is attached higher in front and consequently is longer. Therefore, this already stretched diaphragm is unable to contract as far or as forcefully as that of the older infant or child. Also, young infants are less able to withstand diaphragmatic fatigue because of fewer energy-producing components. Abdominal distention from gas or fluid can impede diaphragmatic excursion significantly.

AIRWAYS

The nasal structures warm, moisten and filter air of impurities and destroy microorganisms that come into contact with immune defences in the mucosa. In infancy, the nasal passages are narrow, and infants are primarily nose-breathers, which substantially increases airway resistance. Any factor that decreases the size of the passages and further increases airway resistance, such as nasal mucosal swelling and mucous accumulation, hampers infants' breathing and feeding.

The pharynx is a passageway for the entry and exit of air, and plays a role in phonation by helping produce vowel sounds. It contains the palatine and lingual tonsils, which are involved in infection control.

The larynx, situated at the upper end of the trachea, is constructed of a rigid circular framework of cartilage and contains the epiglottis and the glottis (vocal cords). These structures prevent solids or liquids from entering the airway during swallowing. In infancy, the glottis is located higher in the neck than in later childhood. The epiglottis is longer and projects further posteriorly in infants. The narrowest portion of the larynx is at the level of the cricoid cartilage. In the infant and young child, the tissue below the vocal cords is more susceptible to oedema formation. Swelling of the glottis and epiglottis produces hoarseness and often life-threatening airway obstruction.

The trachea is composed of smooth muscle supported by C-shaped rings of cartilage that ensure an open airway to the bronchi and lungs. The trachea divides into two primary bronchi. Each bronchus enters the lung on its respective side, where it divides into secondary bronchi that continue to branch and divide into progressively smaller bronchioles. As the bronchioles become smaller, the cartilaginous rings become increasingly irregular and then disappear completely in the smallest bronchioles. There is a range of 23–26 levels of branches divided into the conducting airways and the terminal respiratory units. The different levels, called generations, are divided into five types (Thomson *et al*, 1993) (Fig. 26-3).

All the structures are subject to obstruction from oedema or foreign objects, but the degree of obstruction from constriction of smooth muscle differs. The relatively rigid upper airway is less subject to constriction than the lower airways, which contain very little cartilaginous support. The highly reactive bronchiolar smooth muscle of the lower airways can cause life-threatening obstruction during bronchoconstriction. The airway cartilage in young infants is very soft and compressible; therefore, the intrathoracic airways are highly reactive to stimuli.

The airways of the newborn have very little smooth muscle, but in children 4-5 months of age they contain sufficient muscle to cause narrowing in response to irritating stimuli. By one year of age, smooth muscle development and reactivity are comparable to those in the adult. The infant's airways grow faster than the thoracic and cervical portions of the vertebral column. Consequently, the larynx and trachea descend in relation to the upper spine. For example, the bifurcation of the trachea that lies opposite the third thoracic vertebra in the infant descends to a position opposite the fourth in adulthood (Fig. 26-4). Likewise, the cricoid cartilage descends from a position opposite the fourth cervical vertebra in the infant to opposite the sixth cervical vertebra in the adult. These anatomical changes produce differences in the angle of access to the trachea at various ages and must be considered when the infant or child is to be positioned for resuscitation and airway clearance.

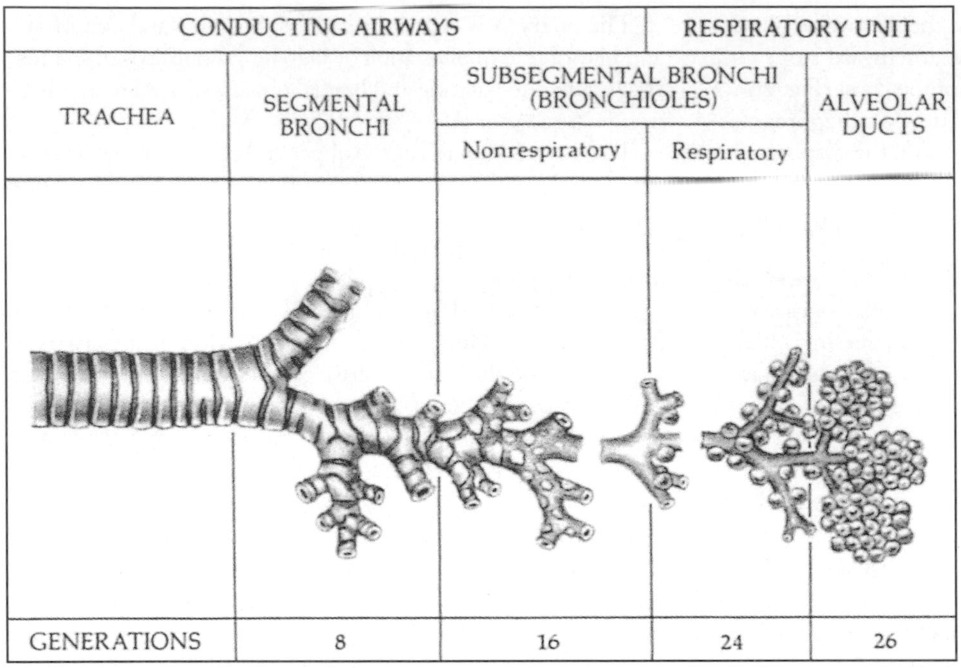

CONDUCTING AIRWAYS				RESPIRATORY UNIT
TRACHEA	SEGMENTAL BRONCHI	SUBSEGMENTAL BRONCHI (BRONCHIOLES)		ALVEOLAR DUCTS
		Nonrespiratory	Respiratory	
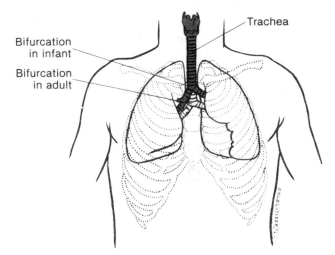				
GENERATIONS	8	16	24	26

Fig. 26-3 Structures of the lower airway. (From Thompson JM *et al: Mosby's clinical nursing*, ed 3, St Louis, 1993, Mosby)

Trachea

Bifurcation in infant

Bifurcation in adult

Fig. 26-4 Difference in level of bifurcation of trachea in infant and adult.

RESPIRATORY UNITS

The two cone-shaped lungs consist of the bronchi, bronchioles and innumerable small air sacs, or alveoli. Through these thin-walled structures, gas exchange occurs between the inspired air and the bloodstream.

With age, changes take place in the air passages that increase respiratory surface area. The major changes are in the number and size of alveoli and in the increased branching of terminal bronchioles. Whereas the number of conducting airways is complete early in fetal life, the air sacs are shallow with wide necks, but have few septa at birth. This promotes patency, but limits surface area for gas exchange. The alveoli are large with thick septa that have little elastic recoil. During the first year, bronchioles continue to branch and the alveoli

rapidly increase in number. These alveoli partition and divide to form smaller lobular units separated by thinner septa, thus enlarging the area available for gas exchange.

Alveoli increase steadily in number, so that approximately nine times as many alveoli are present at age 12 years than at birth. In addition, collateral pathways of ventilation develop, including pores through alveolar walls and possibly pathways between bronchioles.

These factors are significant to respiratory disorders in young children. Infants and young children have less alveolar surface area for gas exchange, the narrowly branching peripheral airways become easily obstructed, and lack of collateral pathways inhibits ventilation beyond obstructed units. Consequently, young children are more readily subject to obstruction and atelectasis.

GAS EXCHANGE

Ventilation occurs as air moves in and out of the lungs. The alveoli are surrounded by pulmonary capilliaries, and in most areas of the lung the membranes that separate these structures are exceedingly thin. Gas exchange takes place by simple diffusion in the alveoli.

GAS TRANSPORT

Once O_2 has diffused from the alveolus to the pulmonary capillary, it is transported throughout the body, either dissolved in plasma (approx. 3%) or attached to haemoglobin (approx. 97%). Since each gram of haemoglobin can combine with 1.34 ml of oxygen, the transport capacity is largely determined by the amount of haemoglobin present. Increasing the amount of oxygen delivered to the alveoli can increase the oxygen carried by the blood only in proportion to the available haemoglobin.

CO_2 is carried by the blood in several ways. A small amount is transported in the plasma and the water of red blood cells. More than one-half is carried as bicarbonate and hydrogen ions. The remaining CO_2 combines with certain plasma proteins and haemoglobin. The diffusion of CO_2 into the alveoli is very rapid, thus the equilibrium between the CO_2 in the pulmonary capillaries and the alveoli is achieved promptly.

DEFENCES OF THE RESPIRATORY TRACT

The respiratory tract has several anatomical and biochemical characteristics that provide natural defences against the many biological and inanimate agents that can damage respiratory tissues. Intact defences help to repel and resist the impact of injurious agents; factors that reduce the integrity of these mechanisms increase the vulnerability of these tissues to invasion and disease. Respiratory tract defences include lymphoid tissues, viscid secretions, cough epiglottis, lymphatics and humoral defences (phagocytes, immunoglobulins, etc.).

ASSESSMENT OF RESPIRATORY FUNCTION

A variety of procedures relating to respiratory function can assist in diagnosis and therapy. Some can be performed by most health professionals; others require specialized skills or equipment. This section discusses only the ones used more frequently.

PHYSICAL ASSESSMENT

The nurse can obtain initial information about the child's respiratory status from simple observations of physical signs and behaviour.

RESPIRATION

Much can be determined from the configuration of the chest and the pattern of respiratory movement, including rate, regularity, symmetry of movements, depth, effort, and use of accessory muscles of respiration. To assess deviations from the usual, the observer must know the normal type and rate of respiration in relation to the child's size and age. Respirations are best determined when the child is sleeping or quietly awake and before touching the child.

Tachypnoea is observed with anxiety, elevated temperature, severe anaemia and as the result of metabolic acidosis. The progress of disorders such as pneumonia, pulmonary oedema, and pleural effusion, can be followed and evaluated by observing changes in respiratory rate.

ASSOCIATED OBSERVATIONS

Associated observations also contribute to assessment. *Recession*, or a sinking in of soft tissues relative to the cartilaginous and bony thorax, may be noted in some pulmonary disorders. Although slight intercostal recession is normal, in disease states (particularly in severe airway obstruction) recession becomes extreme. Subcostal recession indicates a flattened diaphragm. In severe obstruction, recessions extend to the supraclavicular areas and the suprasternal notch. (See Fig. 26-5 for location of recession.)

Nasal flaring is a sign of increased work of breathing. The enlargement of the nostrils helps reduce nasal resistance and maintain airway patency. Nasal flaring may be intermittent or continuous and should be described as minimal or marked.

Head bobbing in a sleeping or exhausted infant is a sign of dyspnoea. The head, supported on the caregiver's arm only at the suboccipital area, will bob forward with each inspiration. This is caused by neck flexion resulting from contraction of the scalene and sternocleidomastoid muscles.

Grunting is produced by exhalation against a partially closed glottis and serves to increase end-expiratory pressure and thus prolong the period of O_2 and CO_2 exchange across the alveolocapillary membrane.

Colour changes of the skin, especially mottling, pallor and cyanosis, are noted. Except for the peripheral bluish discolouration resulting from circulatory stasis in the newborn, cyanosis is significant and usually indicates cardiopulmonary disease.

Chest pain may be caused by disease of any of the chest structures — oesophagus, pericardium, diaphragm, pleura or chest wall. Parietal pleural pain is usually localized over the affected area and is aggravated by respiratory movements. The pain of diaphragmatic pleural irritation may be referred to the base of the neck posteriorly and anteriorly, or to the abdomen. Most pleural pain is related to respiration; therefore respiratory movements are shallow and rapid.

Clubbing, or proliferation of tissue about the terminal phalanges, accompanies a variety of conditions, frequently those associated with chronic hypoxia, primarily cardiac defects and chronic pulmonary disease.

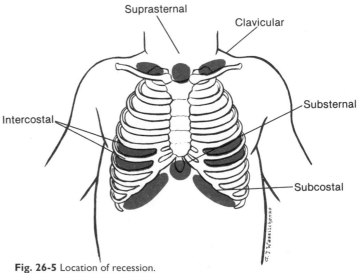

Fig. 26-5 Location of recession.

Inflammation or infection almost anywhere in the upper or lower respiratory tract may produce coughing. Some types of cough are characteristic of specific diseases. For example, severe cough is associated with measles and cystic fibrosis, and the paroxysmal cough accompanied by an inspiratory 'whoop' is pathognomonic of pertussis. A brassy cough is part of the symptomatology of croup and foreign body aspiration. Because there are no cough receptors in the alveoli, a cough may be absent in a child with lobar pneumonia in the early stages of the disease.

DIAGNOSTIC PROCEDURES

Various procedures are available for assessing respiratory function and diagnosing respiratory disease. For nurses caring for the child with respiratory disorders, understanding how the tests are carried out helps devise the best strategies for preparing children for the tests, gaining their cooperation, and supporting them during the procedure.

PULMONARY FUNCTION TESTS

Noninvasive pulmonary mechanics can easily be measured with new technology at the bedside of infants and children with the use of pneumotachography. This information is sometimes limited in diagnosis, since the same functional abnormality may occur in different diseases. These tests are useful to evaluate the severity and course of a disease and to study the effects of treatment. Examples of these include vital capacity/peak flow, forced expiratory volume and tidal volume.

RADIOLOGY AND OTHER DIAGNOSTIC PROCEDURES

Radiology is used frequently in diagnostic evaluation of children. Careful protection of the immature gonads of the infant or child with lead shields is essential. Other sensitive areas are the thyroid gland, ocular lens and bone marrow.

Nurses can make certain that the infant or child receives proper protection from possible hazards. Play can be used effectively to reduce the trauma sometimes associated with the procedure and to gain the child's cooperation.

BLOOD GAS DETERMINATION

Blood gas measurements are sensitive indicators of change in respiratory status in acutely ill patients. They provide valuable information regarding lung function, lung adequacy, and tissue perfusion and are essential for monitoring conditions involving hypoxaemia, CO_2 retention and pH. This information provides cues for decision making regarding therapeutic interventions, such as adjusting the ventilator, increasing chest physiotherapy, administering O_2, or positioning the child for maximum ventilation.

Noninvasive monitoring

For continuous monitoring of blood gases, noninvasive measurements are used whenever possible.

Transcutaneous monitoring (TCM) provides continual monitoring of transcutaneous partial pressure of O_2 in arterial blood ($tcPaO_2$) and CO_2 in arterial blood ($tcPaCO_2$). An electrode is attached to the warmed skin to facilitate arterialization of cutaneous capillaries. The site of the electrode must be changed every 3-4 hours to prevent burning the skin, and the machine must be calibrated with every site change. This monitoring is used in neonatal intensive care units, but it may not reflect PaO_2 (arterial oxygen pressure) in infants with impaired local circulation or in older infants whose skin is thicker.

Pulse oximetry measures the amount of light absorbed by oxyhaemoglobin and uses this information to calculate oxygen saturation (SaO_2). A sensor with a bright light is taped to a finger or toe. The sensor must identify every pulse beat to calculate an accurate SaO_2. Since movement can interfere with sensing, false alarms occur when the patient is active. However, some devices synchronize the arterial saturation reading with the heartbeat, thereby reducing the interference caused by motion.

Oximetry offers several advantages over TCM. Oximetry: (1) does not require heating the skin, thus reducing the risk of burns; (2) eliminates a delay period for transducer equilibration; and (3) maintains an accurate measurement regardless of the patient's age or skin characteristics or the presence of lung disease. However, oximetry is insensitive to hyperoxia because haemoglobin approaches 100% saturation for all PaO_2 readings above approximately 100 mmHg (13.3 kPa) (Lough and Carlo, 1988). This can be dangerous for the premature infant at risk for developing retinopathy of prematurity (see Chapter 13). Therefore, the premature infant being monitored with oximetry should have upper limits identified and a protocol established for decreasing O_2 when saturations are high (Harbold, 1989). Hypoxia cannot be detected reliably when SaO_2 is 95-100%.

Arterial blood sampling

Some controversy surrounds the collection of capillary blood for blood gas measurements; however, many believe it to be a safe, convenient and relatively accurate method.

Arterial blood samples are obtained through an indwelling catheter or by arteriopuncture. The artery most frequently used is the radial artery. The posterior tibial, and umbilical arteries can be used effectively in the newborn. The femoral and brachial arteries may also be used. The radial and posterior tibial arteries are the first choice for intermittent arterial blood sampling because of the collateral circulation present.

The PO_2 of the neonate tends to be slightly lower than that of older babies and children. Otherwise, normal arterial blood gas (ABG) values are much the same for all ages and depend on the concentration of O_2 the child is breathing. When one is assessing the significance of ABG values, it is essential to know the percentage of O_2 administered. Of further interest is the child's body temperature, since as little as 0.5°C may alter

COMPONENT	DEFINITION	NORMAL VALUE	ACIDOSIS	ALKALOSIS
pH	Indicates acid-base status of body	7.40	Less than 7.40 indicates an excess of acid	Greater than 7.40 indicates an exces of base
PCO_2	Pressure exerted by dissolved CO_2 in blood Under control of lungs Respiratory component	7.36-7.44 kPa 4.7-60 kPa	Greater than 5.4 kPa Causes: obstructive lung disease, hypo-ventilation of any cause	Less than 5.4 kPa Causes: hypoxia, pulmonary embol-ism, hypervent-ilation of any cause
HCO_3	Buffers effect of acid in blood Under control of kidneys Metabolic component	24 mEq/L 22-28 mEq/L	Less than 24 mEq/L Causes: diarrhoea, lactic acidosis, renal failure, shock, thera-py with acetazola-mide, diabetic keto-acidosis, drainage of pancreatic juice	Greater than 24 mEq/L Causes: fluid loss from upper gastro-intestinal tract, diuretics, cortico-steroid therapy
Base excess (BE)	Reflects status of all bases in the blood	0-2 mm/L	Negative	Positive
PO_2	Pressure exerted by dissolved O_2 In blood Indicates effectiveness of oxygenation by the lungs	10.6-13.3 kPa (lower in neonates)	Less than 10.6 kPa hypoxia Causes: obstructive lung disease, high CO_2 levels, low FIO_2, hypoventilation	Greater than 13.3 kPa hyperoxy-genation Causes: high FIO_2, hyperventilation

Based on *Quick Reference to Pediatric Intensive Care Nursing* by P.A. Brown et al., p. 92, with permission of Aspen Publishers, Inc. © 1989.

NOTE: The SaO_2 printed with blood gas reports cannot be used as a standard to confirm oximetry readings. Blood gas analysers provide only approximate blood O_2 saturations based on calculations using measured blood gases, pH, and PaO_2.

Table 26-1 Blood gas analysis.

the blood gas values by 5-8%, and the presence of anxiety, which causes many children to hyperventilate and blow off extra CO_2. Crying can cause breath-holding and apnoea, which can decrease PaO_2.

Table 26-1 lists normal ABG and pH measurements in patients breathing room air at sea level.

The significance of ABG determination is related primarily to the relationships among these three determinations: pH, PO_2, and PCO_2. Any change in a blood gas value must be compared with the other values and with previous readings as well as with the child's clinical appearance and behaviour, medical history, and associated physiological factors.

Nurses within critical care areas need to be skilled in the techniques of drawing blood from an arterial catheter and flushing the line. The nurse must ensure that the sample site is frequently checked for signs of bleeding or infection and that the distal to the site is well perfused.

The results of the gas analysis provide the nurse with information on which to base further nursing action. Nurses must be able to understand the report's significance and to implement nursing activities; for example, adjusting the concentration of O_2 the patient is receiving, changing the position, performing suction, administering prescribed drugs, or notifying medical staff, according to the interpretation of the gas analysis.

RESPIRATORY THERAPY

Respiratory care is an all-inclusive term that encompasses a variety of therapies that involve changing the composition, volume or pressure of inspired gases. This includes primarily increasing the O_2 concentration of inspired gas (*oxygen therapy*), increasing the water vapour content of inspired gas (*humidification*), adding airborne particles with beneficial properties (*nebulizer therapy*), and employing various means for controlling or assisting respiration (e.g., *artificial ventilation*).

OXYGEN THERAPY

The indication for administration of O_2 is *hypoxaemia*, as evidenced by reduced PaO_2 and cyanosis. O_2 is administered by mask, head box, nasal cannula, O_2 tent or ventilator. The mode of delivery is selected on the basis of the concentration needed and the child's ability to cooperate in its use. Since O_2 is dry, it is always humidified in some manner.

O_2 therapy is primarily carried out in hospital, although increasing numbers of children are receiving O_2 in the home. It is the responsibility of the nurse to ensure uninterrupted delivery of the appropriate O_2 concentration and monitoring of the child's response to the therapy.

OXYGEN ADMINISTRATION

Oxygen delivered to infants is best tolerated using a head box. Low and high concentrations of O_2 can be easily maintained in this head box, and most nursing procedures can be continued without interrupting the O_2 delivery. At least 4-5 L/minute of flow is needed to maintain O_2 concentrations and remove the exhaled CO_2.

The gas should not be allowed to blow directly into the face of an infant in a head box. Cold fluid or air applied to the face stimulates receptors that trigger the diving reflex, which causes bradycardia and shunting of blood from peripheral to central circulation. Older infants and children can use nasal prongs, which can supply a concentration of about 50%. Masks are not well tolerated by children. A nasal cannula allows for more freedom for infant and caregiver and facilitates breast-feeding because the upper lip is not restricted.

OXYGEN TOXICITY

Oxygen is essential to life and a valuable therapeutic aid. However, prolonged exposure to high O_2 tensions can be damaging to lung tissue. Although the exact pathogenesis of the pulmonary changes is unclear, evidence indicates damage to lung capillaries, which causes diffuse microhaemorrhagic changes, diminished mucus flow, inactivation of surfactant, and altered ciliary function. The total effect appears to be the direct result of 'lung burn' and is therefore a result of PAO_2 (alveolar oxygen pressure) and not PaO_2. The result of these changes is a gradual impairment of alveolar ventilation.

Oxygen-induced CO_2 narcosis is a physiological hazard of O_2 therapy that may occur in persons with chronic pulmonary disease. It is seldom encountered in children except those with cystic fibrosis where the respiratory centre has adapted to the continuously higher $PaCO_2$ levels, and hypoxia has become the more powerful stimulus to respiration. When the PaO_2 is elevated during O_2 administration, the hypoxic drive is removed, causing progressive hypoventilation and increased $PaCO_2$ levels, and the child rapidly becomes unconscious. CO_2 narcosis can also be induced by the administration of sedation in these patients

SUPPORTIVE THERAPIES

Several therapies are carried out in the management of respiratory dysfunction. Some are administered as an isolated therapy; others are performed in conjunction with O_2 administration.

AEROSOL THERAPY

Aerosol therapy can be effective in depositing medication directly into the airway, thus avoiding side effects of certain drugs. Bronchodilators, steroids and antibiotics, suspended in particulate form, can be inhaled so that the medication reaches the small airways.

Medications can be aerosolized with air or with O_2-enriched gas. Hand-held nebulizers are the most frequently used equipment. To avoid particle deposition in the nose and pharynx, the child is instructed to take slow, deep breaths through an open mouth during treatment. Young children in particular can be extremely frightened by the noise of a nebulizer in use and having a mask held on or near their face. It may be helpful for the nurse or parent to give the child's teddy or doll a nebulizer first. The child should be enabled to hold the mask when possible.

The metered dose inhaler (MDI) is a self-contained, hand-held device that allows for intermittent delivery of a specified amount of medication. Many bronchodilators are available in this form and are used successfully by children with asthma. For children younger than five or six years of age, a 'spacer' device attached to the MDI can help coordinate breathing and aerosol delivery and allows the aerosolized particles to remain in suspension for a longer time.

A major nursing responsibility during aerosol therapy is to assess the effectiveness of the treatment and the child's tolerance of the procedure. Small children who become upset with a mask held close to the face may become fatigued from fighting the procedure and may appear worse during and immediately after the therapy. It may be necessary to take time to calm the child after the therapy, allowing vital signs to return to baseline levels, in order to assess accurately changes in breath sound and work of breathing.

Continuous administration of mist, or aerosolized water, for the treatment of inflammatory conditions of the airways has no proven benefit (Alderson and Warren, 1984), but improvement has been noted in some cases. For example, a very humid environment (e.g., a steamy bathroom) for treatment of croup is a common practice, but generally there is a lack of information on the use of humidified air in croup

(Skolnik, 1989). For other pathologies, mist therapy can be detrimental. For example, bronchoconstriction in children with asthma can be exacerbated by mist therapy. Contrary to popular belief, inhaled mist does not affect the water content of expectorated mucus.

BRONCHIAL (POSTURAL) DRAINAGE

Bronchial drainage is indicated whenever excessive fluid or mucus in the bronchi is not being removed by normal ciliary activity and cough. The techniques of segmental drainage, percussion, and vibration assist the normal cleansing mechanisms of the lung. Positioning the child to take maximum advantage of gravity further facilitates removal of secretions. The effect is sometimes dramatic in children with chronic lung disease (e.g., asthma, cystic fibrosis) characterized by thick mucous secretions.

Postural drainage is carried out three to four times daily and is more effective when it follows other respiratory therapy, such as bronchodilator and/or nebulization medication. Bronchial drainage is generally performed before meals (or 1-1.5 hours after meals) to minimize the chance of vomiting and is repeated at bedtime. The length and duration of treatment depend on the child's tolerance level — usually 20-30 minutes.

The positions used and the frequency and duration of treatment are individualized.

CHEST PHYSIOTHERAPY

Chest physiotherapy usually means the use of postural drainage in combination with adjunctive techniques that are thought to enhance the clearance of mucus from the airway. These techniques include manual percussion, vibration, and squeezing of the chest; cough; forceful expiration; and breathing exercises. However, the efficacies of such techniques, both individually and combined, are controversial (Kyff, 1987). Postural drainage in combination with forced expiration has been shown to be beneficial, but the benefit of other techniques has yet to be demonstrated. Because of controversy surrounding the various types of physiotherapy, nurses should be guided by the physiotherapist on the frequency and type of physiotherapy to be performed.

The most common technique used in association with postural drainage is manual *percussion* of the chest wall. The child is placed in the postural drainage position with his or her chest protected with a towel. The practitioner then gently but firmly strikes the chest wall with a cupped hand. A 'popping', hollow sound should be the result, not a slapping sound. Percussion should be done over the rib cage only and should be painless. Percussion can also be performed with a soft circular mask.

Chest physiotherapy is contraindicated when patients have pulmonary haemorrhage, pulmonary embolism, end-stage renal disease, increased intracranial pressure, osteogenesis imperfecta, or minimum cardiac reserves. Chest physiother-

apy is a time-consuming procedure and effective for only certain patients. After an exhaustive review of the literature, Sutton (1988) has offered the guidelines for performing chest physiotherapy (see Box 26-1).

Squeezing is sometimes a useful manoeuvre while the child is in the drainage position. The child is directed to take a deep breath and then to exhale through the mouth rapidly and as completely as possible. The depth of the expiratory effort is increased by brief, firm pressure from the practitioner's hands compressing the sides of the chest. The inspiration after the activity often stimulates a deep, productive cough.

Deep breathing is often encouraged when the child is relaxed in the desired position for drainage. The child is directed to take several deep breaths using diaphragmatic breathing. Expirations after these deep breaths often carry secretions and may stimulate a cough. Other methods that can be employed to stimulate deep breathing are blow bottles of various types, incentive spirometers, and incorporation of play that extends the expiratory time and increases expiratory pressure. Such play may include using items such as pinwheel toys, moving small items by blowing through a straw, blowing cotton wool balls or a table tennis ball on a table, preventing a tissue from falling by blowing it against a wall, blowing up balloons (under supervision), and singing loudly (especially songs with a lot of words between breaths).

With or without stimulation, children are encouraged to *cough*, not to suppress a cough, and not to waste strength and energy with repeated weak and ineffective coughs. One or two hard coughs after a deep breath are more efficient. Children should be encouraged to sit up while they cough.

ARTIFICIAL VENTILATION

A variety of methods are available for controlling or assisting ventilation. Temporary assistance can be provided by a hand-operated self-inflating ventilation bag with a mask and a non-

---

◆ **BOX 26-1**

Guidelines for performing chest physiotherapy

Chest physiotherapy should be used for patients who have increased sputum production. It is probably of no value to the uncomplicated postoperative patient or the patient with pneumonia.

Forced expiration combined with postural drainage is more effective than cough alone.

Percussion and vibration have no proven value.

Appropriate use of bronchodilators before chest physiotherapy will enhance mucus clearance.

returnable valve to prevent rebreathing. With the mask placed on the nose and mouth, the bag is rhythmically compressed, forcing gas from the bag into the patient's airways. The bag should be supplied with 100% O_2 and should have a reservoir so that 100% O_2 is delivered to the patient. An open airway is established by correct positioning with the child's chin directed forward and the neck extended to the 'sniffing' position, unless the patient is an infant, in which case the chin should be left in the neutral position (BMJ, 1993). It is important not to hyperextend an infant's neck, because this can occlude the airway.

For more prolonged assistance, mechanical ventilation is used to replace the function of the diaphragm and thoracic chest wall muscles. The lungs are inflated by application of either positive or negative pressure. A positive-pressure machine inflates the lung by increasing airway pressure above atmospheric pressure, and a negative-pressure ventilator creates a subatmospheric pressure around the chest wall and inside the chest, thus allowing air to move into the chest. Application of positive pressure by mechanical means usually improves gas distribution within the lung and often reinflates partially collapsed lung segments. The overall effect is improvement of gas exchange.

CARE OF THE PATIENT

Before nurses care for a child being artificially ventilated, they should understand the function of the ventilator being used and be able to detect signs of malfunction and deviations from the desired settings. The nurse also promotes the effectiveness of ventilation by suctioning, positioning, and providing support and reassurance to the child and family.

Weaning the child from a ventilator involves gradual physical and psychological withdrawal from dependence on the mechanical device. Criteria for beginning the weaning process varies with the primary disease and unit policy.

Sedation or other respiratory depressants are contraindicated so that the child can be observed for respiratory activity. Resuscitation and reintubation equipment is available at the bedside. Often, suction is performed just before tube removal. Post extubation, the child is monitored for respiratory distress, and ABG measurements are observed. The most common complications are airway oedema, fatigue and atelectasis.

ENDOTRACHEAL AIRWAYS

In children with upper airway obstruction, endotracheal intubation can be accomplished by the nasal (nasotracheal), oral (orotracheal), or direct tracheal (tracheostomy) routes. Oral intubation is usually the method of choice for emergency situations, but for prolonged intubation a nasotracheal tube is more often used. Although it is more difficult to place technically, nasotracheal intubation is preferred to orotracheal intubation, because it facilitates oral hygiene and provides more stable fixation, which reduces the complication of tracheal erosion and the danger of accidental extubation.

Complications

The most severe complication related to immediate intubation is hypoxia with accompanying bradycardia. Patients must be closely monitored during intubation attempts and, if hypoxia occurs, the procedure is discontinued until vital signs are stable. Ventilation with bag mask and O_2 is reinstituted. Other complications include trauma to mouth and teeth, epistaxis, creation of air leaks, traumatic laryngitis, infection, glottic oedema, and mucosal lesions of the larynx secondary to pressure exerted by the rigid ET tube. The most severe sequela of intubation is laryngeal stenosis secondary to fibrosis.

TRACHEOSTOMY

Tracheostomy consists of a surgical opening in the trachea between the second and fourth tracheal rings (Fig. 26-6). It is usually performed in children to: (1) bypass upper airway obstruction caused by conditions (e.g., congenital or acquired subglottic stenosis) or infectious processes (e.g., croup, epiglottitis) or (2) provide access to the airway for long-term ventilatory support.

Paediatric tracheostomy tubes are usually made of plastic or Silastic. These tubes are constructed with a more acute angle than adult tubes, and they soften at body temperature, conforming to the contours of the trachea. Since these materials resist the formation of crusted respiratory secretions, they are made without an inner cannula. However, some children require a metal tracheostomy tube, which contains an inner cannula.

TRACHEOSTOMY CARE

Before the tracheostomy is performed, it is important to prepare the child and family. Preoperative teaching should include communication methods that will be used with the

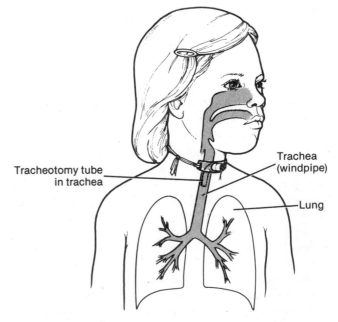

Fig. 26-6 Tracheostomy tube in trachea and securely tied with tape.

child, preparation for the appearance of the stoma and routine postoperative management.

Children who have undergone tracheostomy must be monitored continually for the first few days after surgery. The focus of postoperative nursing care is that of maintaining a patent airway, facilitating removal of pulmonary secretions and preventing complications.

Some bleeding from the surgical site can be expected, but profuse bleeding is unusual and medical staff should be notified immediately if this occurs.

Suction equipment, scissors, an extra tracheostomy tube of the same size with ties already attached, and another tracheostomy tube (one size smaller), and tracheal dilators are kept at the bedside. A source of humidification is provided to the tracheostomy, since the normal humidification and filtering functions of the airway have been bypassed.

Suctioning

The airway must remain patent and requires frequent suctioning during the first few hours after tracheostomy. Vacuum pressure should range from 80-100 mmHg. Unless secretions are thick and tenacious, the lower range of negative pressure is recommended. The catheter selected should have a diameter one half the diameter of the tracheostomy tube (Kleiber *et al*, 1988). The catheter is inserted 0.5 cm beyond or just to the end of the tracheostomy tube. A small amount of sterile isotonic saline (a few drops to 0.5-2 ml, depending on the child's size) injected into the tube may help loosen secretions and crusts for easier aspiration although the value of this practice is unproven.

Hyperventilating the child with 100% O_2 before and after suctioning is usually performed to prevent hypoxia, using a bag-valve mask or by increasing the FIO_2 ventilator setting. Closed-tracheal suctioning systems that allow for uninterrupted O_2 delivery may also be used (Hart and Mahutte, 1992).

Suctioning is carried out at frequent intervals to prevent build up of crusts and, as often as needed, for signs of mucus in the airway, such as bubbling, noisy breathing, or coughing. The cough is ineffectual because the glottis, which normally closes and releases suddenly to effect a cough, is bypassed by the tracheostomy. Suctioning should take no longer than 5 seconds. The child is allowed to rest for 30-60 seconds after each aspiration to allow O_2 tension to return to normal; then the process is repeated until the trachea is clear. Oximetry is an effective feedback tool to monitor suctioning and to prevent hypoxia.

Aseptic technique is essential during care of the tracheostomy. Secondary infection is a major concern, since the air entering the lower airway bypasses the natural defences of the upper airway. A new tube, gloves and sterile saline solution are used each time.

Routine care

Assessments of the stoma area include observations for signs of infection and breakdown of the skin. The skin is kept clean and dry. Special sterile dressings made of nonshredding

material can be placed under the flanges of the tracheostomy tube if desired. These should be changed frequently, however, since a soiled dressing may be a reservoir for bacteria (Sigler, 1985).

The tracheostomy tube is held in place with tracheostomy ties which are changed daily and when soiled. New ties are looped through the flanges and tied snugly in a triple knot at the side of the neck *before* the soiled ties are cut and removed. Some nurses have found that threading the ties through a piece of foam tubing cushions the ties; others have found the tubing to be irritating to the skin. The ties should be tight enough to allow just a fingertip to be inserted between the ties and the neck.

Routine tracheostomy tube changes are carried out at least weekly after a tract has been formed to minimize formation of granulation tissue. The first change is usually performed by the surgeon; subsequent changes are performed by the nurse. Ideally, two caregivers participate in the procedure to assist with positioning the child and to reassure and comfort the child. Parental presence will be of further comfort.

The inner cannula, if used, should be removed with each suctioning, cleaned with sterile saline and pipe cleaners to remove crusted material, and reinserted.

Accidental decannulation requires immediate tube replacement. Some children have a fairly rigid trachea, so that the airway remains partially open when the tube is removed. However, others have malformed or flexible tracheal cartilage, which causes the airway to collapse when the tube is removed or dislodged. Since many infants and children with upper airway problems have little airway reserve, if replacement of the dislodged tube is impossible, a smaller-sized tube should be inserted. If the stoma cannot be cannulated with another tracheostomy tube, oral intubation should be performed.

DECANNULATION

The tracheostomy tube is removed as soon as it is no longer needed. The usual procedure is to wean the child to the smallest possible tracheostomy tube. Once this has been accomplished and the child's respiratory status is unimpaired for 24 hours, the tube is occluded, with removal within the next 24 hours. The procedure is carried out where continuous observation is available and emergency reintubation can be accomplished if necessary. Following successful decannulation, the child remains under close observation for an additional 48 hours (Blumer, 1991).

RESPIRATORY DYSFUNCTION

Disorders of respiratory structure and function that may result in ventilatory failure are a significant cause of childhood illness. They may have a variety of causes, both pulmonary and nonpulmonary, and the pulmonary dysfunction can result in disturbances in other organs and systems. Inadequacy of the O_2-supplying role results in *hypoxaemia* and tissue *hypoxia*;

inadequate CO_2 removal causes *hypercapnia*. Often, both gases may be insufficiently exchanged.

RESPIRATORY FAILURE

In general, the term *respiratory insufficiency* is applied to two conditions: (1) children with increased work of breathing while preserving gas exchange function near normal and (2) children who are unable to maintain normal blood gas tensions and develop hypoxaemia and acidosis secondary to CO_2 retention.

Respiratory failure is defined as the inability of the respiratory apparatus to maintain adequate oxygenation of the blood, with or without CO_2 retention. *Respiratory arrest* is the cessation of respiration.

Apnoea is absence of airflow (breathing). Apnoea can be: (1) central, in which respiratory efforts are absent; (2) obstructive, in which respiratory efforts are present; and (3) mixed, in which both central and obstructive components are present.

Effective pulmonary gas exchange requires clear airways, normal lungs and chest wall, and adequate pulmonary circulation. This functional pulmonary unit plus normal respiratory control mechanisms ensures adequate total alveolar ventilation and perfusion, which are reflected in O_2 and CO_2 tensions in arterial blood leaving the lung. Anything that affects these functions or their relationships can compromise respiration.

Respiratory failure can occur as an emergency situation or may be preceded by gradual and progressive deterioration of respiratory function.

CONDITIONS THAT PREDISPOSE TO RESPIRATORY FAILURE

1. *Obstructive lung disease,* in which there is increased resistance to airflow in either the upper or the lower respiratory tract (e.g., choanal atresia, tracheal/bronchostenosis, croup, epiglottitis, foreign bodies, tumours, pneumonia, bronchiolitis, asthma).
2. *Restrictive lung disease,* in which there is impaired lung expansion resulting from loss of lung volume, decreased distensibility, or chest wall disturbance (e.g., hyaline membrane disease, pneumonia, pneumothorax, pulmonary oedema or haemorrhage, diaphragmatic hernia, kyphoscoliosis, obesity).
3. *Primary inefficient gas transfer,* in which there is insufficient alveolar ventilation for CO_2 removal or impaired oxygenation of pulmonary capillary blood as a result of dysfunction of the respiratory control mechanism or a pulmonary diffusion defect (e.g., decreased alveolar capillary surface area [pulmonary emboli/hypertension], inadequate erythrocytes [anaemia, haemorrhage], increased CSF pressure [meningitis], CNS depression [drug overdose—opioids, barbiturates, diazepam]).

RECOGNITION OF RESPIRATORY FAILURE

Respiratory failure that occurs as a result of acute obstruction of a major airway or cardiac arrest is sudden and readily apparent. Gradual and more covert development of signs and symptoms is less easily recognized. Situations occur in which severe respiratory distress may be present without significant CO_2 retention, and hypoxaemia may occur without clinically detectable cyanosis. Therefore, evaluation of respiratory adequacy is based on both clinical assessment and laboratory studies. Nursing observation and judgement are vital to successful management of respiratory failure.

Unless respiratory arrest occurs suddenly, signs of hypoxaemia and hypercapnia are usually subtle in their development and become more obvious as respiratory failure progresses. The unknowing observer may attribute early signs such as mood changes and restlessness to other causes, and some signs can be altered by other factors, for example, anaemia. Haemoglobin is needed to show some cyanosis; therefore, it may not be observed in the child with a haemoglobin level of less than 6 g/dl. Cyanosis is usually apparent at a PaO_2 of 5.4–6.7 kPa. The signs of respiratory failure are outlined in Box 26-2.

MANAGEMENT AND RELATED IMPLICATIONS FOR NURSING

If respiratory arrest occurs, the primary objectives are to recognize the situation and initiate resuscitative measures within moments. When the situation is not an arrest, the suspicion of respiratory failure is confirmed by assessment and the severity defined by ABG analysis. When severity is established, an attempt is made to determine the underlying cause by thorough evaluation.

The principles of management are to: (1) treat the underlying cause, (2) correct hypoxaemia/hypercapnia, (3) minimize ventilation and maximize oxygen delivery, (4) minimize extrapulmonary organ failure, (5) apply specific and non-specific therapy to control oxygen demands, and (6) anticipate complications.

OBSERVATION AND MONITORING

The child is monitored to evaluate the cause of the failure, to help determine a course of action, and to assess the child's response to treatment. If close continuous monitoring is required, the child is transferred to an intensive care unit.

The child's cardiac and respiratory status are monitored by observation and by electronic means. However, no monitoring equipment can replace conscientious nursing observations (Box 26-3).

Optimum temperature is maintained, since fever increases the need for O_2 and increases respiratory efforts.

◆ BOX 26-2

Signs of respiratory failure

Cardinal Signs
Restlessness
Tachypnoea
Tachycardia
Diaphoresis

Early but Less Obvious Signs
Mood changes, such as euphoria or depression
Headache
Altered depth and pattern of respirations
Hypertension
Exertional dyspnoea
Anorexia
Increased cardiac output and renal output
Central nervous system symptoms (decreased efficiency, impaired judgement, anxiety, confusion, restlessness, irritability)
Flaring nares
Chest wall recession
Expiratory grunt
Wheezing and/or prolonged expiration

Signs of More Severe Hypoxia
Hypotension or hypertension
Dyspnoea
Depressed respirations
Dimness of vision
Bradycardia
Somnolence
Stupor
Coma
Cyanosis, peripheral or central

◆ BOX 26-3

Nursing observations for the child with respiratory failure

Visual inspection of skin colour to estimate level of arterial O_2 saturation

Observation of respiratory effort or distress—nasal flaring, grunting, gasping, retraction

Observation of diaphragmatic movement, lung expansion, and use of accessory muscles—depth, symmetry, inspiration/expiration ratio

Auscultation of thorax to assess:
 Breath sounds—presence, intensity, quality, symmetry
 Tube placement and need for endotracheal suction when child is intubated

---

FAMILY SUPPORT

Children who are fatigued and in distress before a procedure will probably fall into a restful sleep after establishment of an airway. However, unless they remain unconscious or semiconscious, they will probably be anxious and frightened when they are unable to communicate. Children who are old enough to write and who are not too fatigued can use a pad of paper and a pencil or spelling board to express their needs and concerns. Other alternative means for communication are pictures illustrating various items and activities. Simple sign language has proved to be an effective and easily learned communication medium.

It is often a terrifying experience for young children to discover that they are unable to make vocal sounds, including crying. It is also stressful to parents to watch their children plead with frightened eyes and cry noiselessly. It is important to talk to children and reassure them that their voices will return when they are able to breathe again.

Parents have numerous concerns relative to tracheostomies, endotracheal tubes and ventilators. If time allows before a tracheostomy, the reasons for the decision to implement the therapy, the expected results and the appropriate length of time it will remain in place, should be discussed with them.

Parental concern is centred around the (often) life-threatening implications generated by the need for the procedure and the possible long-term effects on the child, both physiological and psychological. Parents are concerned about the visible wound and the scar. Parents who must face the possibility of caring for the child with a tracheostomy at home have additional worries regarding their ability to assume this responsibility.

Before discharge, the parents will need careful instruction and practice in the care and management of the tracheostomy, including basic life support (cardiopulmonary resuscitation [CPR]). During hospitalization, the parents should be involved in the child's care as much as possible in anticipation of home care. The more comfortable they are with all aspects of tracheostomy care, the more confident and less anxious they will be when faced with total care of the child at home. It sometimes requires weeks before they feel comfortable with suctioning, cleaning and changing the tube. Instructions should be detailed and explicit.

Ideally, a community children's nurse should be available to the family and should periodically assess the family's ability to carry out the activities needed in care of the child. The parents may find it helpful to talk to other parents of children with tracheostomies. They also need to know whom to call and where they can obtain help and support in times of uncertainty or in an emergency.

The child has a need to understand what has happened. Any misconceptions the child may hold should be identified and corrected as early as possible. However, nurses also need to recognize when a child is tired and wishes to use denial and withdrawal as a protection device to prevent information overload.

Parents are encouraged to provide as normal a life as possible for their child and other family members. The child can usually be allowed to engage in most activities appropriate to their age and ability. Both parents and child must be informed about safety precautions regarding play near water; for example, a swimming pool, stream, or bath. The child should not be exposed to noxious fumes (e.g., paint, hairspray, baby powder). Young children who may spill food near the stoma should wear a fabric bib (without a plastic lining) to prevent dribbled food from being aspirated.

CARDIOPULMONARY RESUSCITATION

Cardiac arrest in the paediatric population is less often of cardiac origin than from prolonged hypoxaemia secondary to inadequate oxygenation, ventilation, and circulation (shock). Some causes include injuries, suffocation (e.g., foreign body aspiration), smoke inhalation, sudden infant death syndrome (SIDS), or infection. Respiratory is associated with a better survival than cardiac arrest. Once cardiac arrest occurs, the outcome of resuscitative efforts is poor (Innes, Summers *et al*, 1993). Most children either die or survive with significant neurologic morbidity, especially if the cardiac arrest occurred outside of a hospital (Zaritsky, 1993).

Complete apnoea signals the need for rapid and vigorous action to prevent cardiac arrest. Regardless of the cause of the arrest, some very basic procedures are carried out, modified according to the child's size.

Outside the hospital situation, the first action in an emergency is to assess quickly the extent of any injury and determine whether the child is unconscious. A child who is struggling to breathe, but is conscious, should be transported immediately to an advanced life support (ALS) facility. Transport by emergency medical services is preferable.

An unconscious child is managed with care to prevent additional trauma if a head or spinal cord injury has been sustained. The child should be turned as a unit with firm support to the head and neck to prevent rolling, twisting, or tilting backward or forward.

RESUSCITATION PROCEDURE— BASIC LIFE SUPPORT (BLS)

Help should be summoned immediately and the situation assessed for danger either to the rescuer or continuing danger for the child. Where danger exists, the situation should be made safe before BLS is continued. The child's airway and breathing are then assessed.

Airway patency

With loss of consciousness, the tongue, which is attached to the lower jaw, relaxes and falls back, obstructing the airway. To open the airway, the head is positioned with either head tilt/chin lift or jaw thrust. Head tilt is accomplished by placing one hand on the victim's forehead and applying firm, backward pressure with the palm to tilt the head back. The fingers of the free hand are placed underneath the chin to lift and bring the chin forward (chin lift). This supports the jaw and helps tilt the head back. The desirable degree of tilt are: (1) neutral in the infant, and (2) sniffing in the child (see Figs 26-7 and 26-8) (BMJ, 1993). The jaw thrust position should be used where there is suspicion of spinal injury. The position is accomplished by grasping the angles of the victim's lower jaw and lifting with both hands, one on each side, displacing the mandible forward (Fig. 26-9A).

The patency of the airway should then be assessed by: (1) *looking* for chest movement, (2) *listening* for breath sounds, and (3) *feeling* for breath (BMJ, 1993). After restoration of the airway using these methods, rescue breathing is initiated if the child has not resumed breathing.

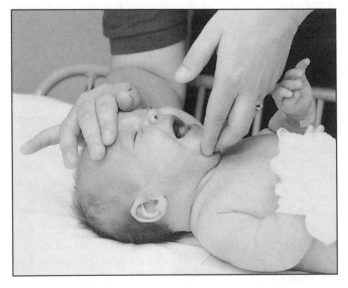

Fig. 26-7 Chin lift in infants.

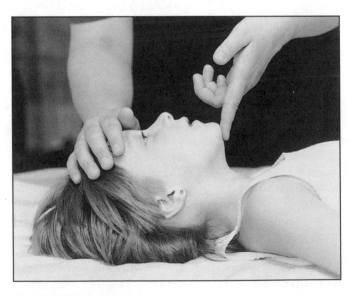

Fig. 26-8 Chin lift in children.

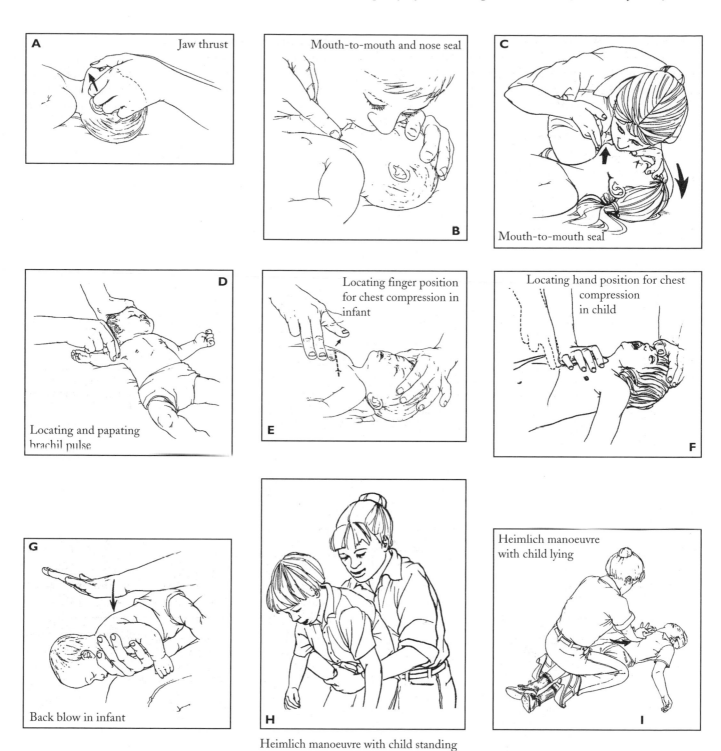

Fig. 26-9 Procedures for cardiopulmonary resuscitation, **A** to **H,** and airway obstruction, **I**

Note that finger sweeping of the mouth is *not* recommended in children, as it may cause damage to the soft palate and exacerbate the situation, particularly if material is pushed further down the airway. Standard ventilation procedures are as follows:

1. To ventilate the lungs of an infant (approximately birth to one year) — the rescuer's mouth is placed over both the mouth and nostrils (Fig. 26-9B) (BMJ, 1993).
2. Children (over one year) — ventilation is through the mouth while the nostrils are firmly pinched for airtight contact (Fig. 26-9C).

Since the differences are relative and vary according to the child's size, the correct volume of air and force of the resistance cannot be stated with certainty. If air enters freely and the chest rises, the airway is assumed to be clear. Breaths should be given slowly. Gastric distension, which interferes with diaphragmatic excursion, can be minimized by avoiding large, rapid inflation breaths. An initial five rescue breaths are delivered.

Circulation

After an initial five rescue breaths, a peripheral pulse is palpated to ascertain the presence of a heartbeat. The carotid is the most central and accessible artery. However, the very short and often fat neck of the infant renders the carotid pulse difficult to find and palpate. It is preferable to use the brachial pulse, located on the inner side of the upper arm, midway between the elbow and shoulder (Fig. 26-9D).

Absence of carotid or brachial pulse or inadequate output (<60 beats/min in infants) is considered sufficient indication to commence external cardiac massage (BMJ, 1993).

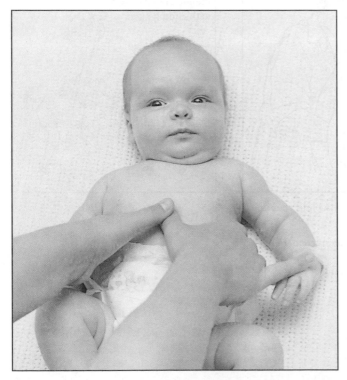

Fig. 26-10 Infant chest compression: hand-encircling technique.

Chest compressions

External chest compressions consist of serial, rhythmic compressions of the chest to maintain circulation to vital organs until the child achieves spontaneous vital signs or ALS can be provided. Chest compressions are always accompanied by simultaneous ventilation of the lungs. For optimal compressions, it is essential that the child's spine is supported on a firm surface during compressions of the sternum, and sternal pressure must be forceful, but not traumatic. In general, infants younger than one year old require a different technique from small and larger children (BMJ, 1993).

Landmarking

The site for placement of the fingers for compression in infants is one fingerbreadth below the intersection of the sternum and an imaginary line drawn between the nipples (Fig. 26-9E). Sternal compression to infants is applied with two fingers on the sternum exerting a downward thrust to a depth of approximately 1.5–2.5 cm. The hands encircling the infant's chest technique may also be used (Fig. 26-10) (BMJ, 1993), but it should be noted that checking landmarking during compressions is more convenient in the former.

Compressions on the small child (aged 1-8 years) are applied to the lower sternum, one fingerbreadth above the sternal notch. Pressure is applied with the heel of one hand and compression is approximately to a depth of 2.5-3.5 cm.

The location of compressions for children over eight years of age is the same as for adults — two fingerbreadths above the sternal notch, to a depth of approximately 3.0-4.5 cm, with appropriate modification to allow for size. The heels of both hands are used (Fig. 26-9F).

Compression rate

Compressions are delivered at a rate of 100/min. Ventilation and compressions are continued by the mouth-to-mouth method or bag and mask, at a rate of one breath for five compressions, whatever the number of rescuers, until signs of recovery appear or until 20 full CPR cycles have been delivered. At this point, emergency services must be contacted if not already organized and CPR resumed. Signs of recovery are evidenced by palpable peripheral pulses, return of pupils to normal size, the disappearance of mottling and cyanosis and possibly return of spontaneous respiration. A summary of BLS techniques is shown in Table 26-2.

Medications

Medications are an important adjunct to resuscitation, especially cardiac arrest, and are used during and following resuscitation. Medications are used to:

- Correct hypoxaemia.
- Increase perfusion pressure during chest compression.
- Stimulate spontaneous or more forceful myocardial contraction.
- Accelerate cardiac rate.
- Correct metabolic acidosis.
- Suppress ventricular ectopy.

	OBJECTIVES	LARGE CHILD (OVER 8 YR)	CHILD (1 TO 8 YR)	INFANT (UNDER 1 YR)
A.AIRWAY	1. Assessment: Determine unresponsiveness.	Tap or gently shake shoulder.		
		Say. "Are you okay?"		Observe.
	2. Get help.	Call out "Help!"		
	3. Position the victim.	Turn on back as a unit, supporting head and neck if necessary (4-10 seconds).		
	4. Open the airway.	Head-tilt/chin-lift/jaw thrust		
B.BREATHING	5. Assessment: Determine breathlessness.	Maintain open airway. Place ear over mouth, observing chest. Look, listen, feel for breathing. (3-5 seconds).		
	6. Give 5 rescue breaths.	Maintain open airway. Seal mouth to mouth. Give 5 rescue breaths, 1 to 1½ seconds each. Observe chest rise. Allow lung deflation between breaths.		Mouth to nose/mouth.
	7. Option for obstructed airway.	a. Reposition victim's head. Try again to give rescue breaths.		
		b. Activate the EMS system.		
		c. Give 10 subdiaphragmatic abdominal thrusts (the Heimlich manoeuvre) unless object isexpelled before then.		Give 5 back blows. Give 5 chest thrusts
C.CIRCULATION	8. Assessment: Determine pulselessness.	Feel for carotid pulse with one hand; maintain head-tilt with the other (5-10 seconds).		Feel for brachial pulse, keep head-tilt
	9. Activate EMS system.	If someone responded to call for help, send them to activate the EMS system		
	Begin chest compressions: 10. Landmark check.	Run middle finger along bottom edge of rib cage to notch at centre (tip of sternum).		Imagine a line drawn between the nipples.
	11. Hand position.	Place 2 fingers next to 1 finger on notch:		Place 2 fingers on sternum, 1 finger's width below line. Depress 1.5-2.5 cm.
		Two hands next to fingers. Depress 3-4.5 cm.	Heel of one hand next to index finger. Depress 2.5-3.5 cm.	
	12. Compression rate.	100 per minute.		
CPR CYCLES	13. Compressions to breaths.	1 breath to every 5 compressions.		
	14. Number of cycles.	20		

Reproduced with permission. Copyright, *Healthcare Provider's Manual for Basic Life Support*, American Heart Association, 1988, p.107

Table 26-2 One-rescuer CPR.

Three main drugs used in paediatric resuscitation (adrenaline, sodium bicarbonate and atropine) and their action are shown in Table 26-3.

AIRWAY OBSTRUCTION

Attempts at clearing the airway should be considered for: (1) children in whom aspiration is witnessed or strongly suspected and in whom dyspnoea is increasing and (2) unconscious, nonbreathing children whose airways remain obstructed despite the usual manoeuvres to open them.

When a child is obviously choking, the initial step is to open the mouth and attempt to visualize and dislodge the object. The methods currently recommended are a combination of *back blows* and *chest thrusts* for infants younger than one year of age and the *Heimlich manoeuvre* for children older than one year of age. Because of the risk of injury to abdominal organs, abdominal thrusts are not recommended for infants one year of age or younger.

INFANTS

A choking infant is placed face down over the rescuer's arm with the head lower than the trunk and the head supported (Fig. 26-9, G). Additional support can be achieved if the rescuer supports the arm firmly against the thigh. Five quick, sharp, back blows are delivered between the infant's shoulder blades with the heel of the rescuer's hand. Less force is required than would be applied to an adult. After delivery of the back blows, the rescuer's free hand is placed flat on the infant's back so that the infant is 'sandwiched' between the two hands, making certain the neck and chin are well supported. While the rescuer maintains support with the infant's head lower than the trunk, the infant is turned and placed supine on the rescuer's thigh, where five chest thrusts are applied in succession in the same manner as external chest compressions described for CPR but slower (BMJ, 1993). Five back blows and five chest thrusts are continued until the object is removed or the infant becomes unconscious.

CHILDREN

Back blows can be used for children as in infants. The Heimlich manoeuvre is recommended for children over 1 year of age. The manoeuvre creates an artificial cough that forces air, and with it the foreign body, out of the airway. The procedure is carried out with the child in a standing, sitting, or lying position (Fig. 26-9H and I). In the conscious choking child, upward thrusts are delivered to the upper abdomen with the fisted hand at a point just below the rib cage. To prevent damage to the internal organs, the rescuer's hands should not touch the xiphoid process of the sternum or the lower margins of the ribs. The thrusts are repeated in rapid succession until the foreign body is expelled.

RESPIRATORY INFECTION

Acute infection of the respiratory tract is the most common cause of illness in infancy and childhood. Young children ordinarily have four or five such infections each year, which manifest a wide range of severity from trivial to severe or even fatal illness. The type of illness and the physical response are also related to a variety of factors, including the type of infectious agent, the age of the child, and the integrity of the child's defence mechanisms.

GENERAL ASPECTS OF RESPIRATORY INFECTIONS

Infections of the respiratory tract are described in several different ways, according to the general areas of involvement in the more common infections. The upper respiratory tract consists

DRUG/DOSE	ACTION	IMPLICATIONS
Adrenaline 10 µg/kg (initial dose) 100 µg/kg (subsequent dose)	Adrenergic Acts on both alpha- and beta-receptor sites, especially heart and vascular and other smooth muscle	Most useful drug in cardiac arrest Disappears rapidly from bloodstream after injection May produce renal vessel constriction and decreased urine formation
Sodium bicarbonate 0.5–1 mmol/kg	Alkalinizer Buffers pH	Infuse slowly and only when ventilation is adequate
Atropine sulphate 20 µg/kg	Anticholinergic-parasympatholytic Increases cardiac output, heart rate by blocking vagal stimulation in heart	Used to treat brachycardia after ventilatory assessment Maximum dose: infants and children, 1.0mg; adolescents, 2.0 mg

Table 26-3 Drugs for paediatrics cardiopulmonary resuscitation.

primarily of the nose and pharynx. The lower respiratory tract consists of the bronchi and bronchioles and the alveoli. The trachea is considered with lower tract disorders, and infections of the epiglottis and larynx are categorized as croup syndromes.

Infections tend to spread from one structure to another. Consequently, infections of the respiratory tract involve several areas rather than a single structure, although the effect on one may predominate in any given illness.

AETIOLOGY AND CHARACTERISTICS

The aetiology and course of respiratory infections are influenced by several factors, including the age of the child, the season, living conditions, and pre-existing medical problems.

Infectious agents
The largest percentage of infections are caused by viruses, particularly in the upper respiratory passages. Other agents that may be involved in primary or secondary invasion include group A β-haemolytic streptococci, staphylococci, *Haemophilus influenzae*, *Chlamydia trachomatis*, *Mycoplasma* and pneumococci.

Age
The pattern of respiratory infection varies considerably with the age of the child. Infants younger than three months have a lower infection rate, presumably because of the protective function of maternal antibodies. The infection rate soars from age 3-6 months, the time between the disappearance of maternal antibodies and the infant's own antibody production. The viral infection rate continues to be high during the toddler and preschool years, but drops steadily. By the time the child reaches five years of age, viral respiratory infections are much less frequent, but the incidence of *Mycoplasma pneumoniae* and group A β-streptococcal infections increases.

Some of the viral agents produce a mild illness in older children, but cause severe lower respiratory tract illness and croup in infants. The amount of lymphoid tissue increases throughout middle childhood, and repeated exposure to organisms confers increasing immunity as the child grows older; thus older children have a greater resistance to most organisms. Whooping cough is a relatively harmless tracheobronchitis in childhood, but a serious disease in infancy.

Resistance
The ability to resist invading organisms depends on several factors. The general conditions that appear to decrease resistance to infection are malnutrition, anaemia, fatigue and chilling of the body. Conditions affecting the respiratory tract that weaken its defences and predispose to infection include allergies such as allergic rhinitis and asthma, cardiac anomalies that have the tendency to develop pulmonary congestion, and cystic fibrosis. Day care attendance, especially if the caregivers smoke, also increases the likelihood of infection (Holberg, Wright, and Martinez, 1993; Hurwitz *et al*, 1991).

Seasonal variations
The most common respiratory tract pathogens appear in epidemics during the winter and spring months, but mycoplasma infections occur more often in autumn and early winter. Infection-related asthma occurs more frequently during cold weather.

CLINICAL MANIFESTATIONS

Infants and young children, especially those between six months and three years of age, react more severely to acute respiratory tract infection than older children, and they appear to be much more ill than their local manifestations would indicate. Young children display a number of generalized signs and symptoms, as well as local manifestations, that differ from those seen in older children and adults. An infant or child may display any or all of the signs and symptoms listed in Box 26-4.

IMPLICATIONS FOR NURSING

Assessment
The general assessment of the respiratory system follows the guidelines described earlier in this chapter and is summarized in Box 26-5.

Planning
The nursing goals for care of the child with an acute respiratory infection are as follows:
1. Facilitate respiratory efforts.
2. Promote rest.
3. Promote comfort.
4. Prevent spread of primary infection to others.
5. Reduce temperature if significantly elevated.
6. Prevent dehydration and provide nourishment.
7. Prevent complications.
8. Educate and support family.

Implementation
Since most children with upper respiratory tract infections are treated at home, most of the nursing care is directed towards education and guidance of parents in caring for their child and serving as resources for problem solving.

Ease respiratory efforts
Most acute respiratory infections are mild and cause few distressing symptoms. Although children may feel uncomfortable and suffer from a 'stuffy' nose and some mucosal swelling, respiratory distress is uncommon. However, children with croup or epiglottitis may develop sufficient swelling to obstruct the airway. These children are hospitalized for observation and therapy (see discussions of specific disorders). Positioning for optimum respiration and observation for signs of respiratory distress are primary nursing functions.

The atmosphere in homes heated during the winter months is often very dry. Warm mist has traditionally been a common therapeutic measure for symptomatic relief of respiratory discomfort. The moisture seems to be beneficial when there is hoarseness or any laryngeal involvement. In the past, mist tents were frequently used in hospital for humidifying the air and relieving discomfort. Their use, however, is controversial and they are used rarely within UK hospitals.

Promote rest

Children who have an acute febrile illness should be helped to rest. This is not usually a problem while the temperature is elevated, but may be more difficult when the child feels fairly well. Often, children are more likely to comply if they are allowed to lie on a couch where they can watch television or participate in quiet activity.

Promote comfort

Older children are usually able to manage nasal secretions with little difficulty. For very young infants instillation of 0.9% saline drops may help clear nasal passages and promote feeding (Hable, 1993).

For children over three months old nose drops may be administered 15–20 minutes before feeding and at bedtime.

◆ BOX 26-4

Signs and symptoms associated with respiratory infections in infants and small children

Fever
May be absent in newborn infants
Greatest at ages 6 months to 3 years
Temperature may reach 39.5° to 40.5°C even with mild infections
Often appears as first sign of infection
May be listless and irritable or somewhat euphoric and more active than normal, temporarily; some children talk with unaccustomed rapidity
Tendency to develop high temperatures with infection in certain families
May precipitate febrile seizures (sudden temperature rise to 40° C [104° F])
More gradual temperature rise will not elicit a seizure
Febrile seizures uncommon after 3 or 4 years of age
Meningismus
Meningeal signs without infection of the meninges
Occurs with abrupt onset of fever
Accompanied by:
Headache
Pain and stiffness in the back and neck
Presence of Kernig and Brudzinski signs
Subsides as the temperature drops
Anorexia
Common to most childhood illnesses
Almost invariably accompanies acute infections in small children
Frequently the initial evidence of illness
Persists to a greater or lesser degree throughout febrile stage of illness; often extends into convalescence
Vomiting
Small children vomit readily with illness
A clue to the onset of infection
May precede other signs by several hours
Usually short lived, but may persist during the illness
Diarrhoea
Mild transient diarrhoea
Often accompanies respiratory infections, especially viral infections
May be severe

Abdominal Pain
Common complaint
Sometimes indistinguishable from pain of appendicitis
Mesenteric lymphadenitis may be cause
Muscle spasms from vomiting may be a factor, especially in nervous, tense children
Nasal Blockage
Small nasal passages of infants easily blocked by mucosal swelling and exudation
Can interfere with respiration and feeding in infants
Contributes to the development of otitis media and sinusitis
Nasal Discharge
Frequently accompanies respiratory infections
May be thin and watery (rhinorrhoea) or thick and purulent
Depends on the type and/or stage of infection
Associated with itching
May irritate upper lip and skin surrounding the nose
Cough
Common feature of respiratory disease
May be evident only during the acute phase
May persist several months after a disease
Respiratory Sounds
Sounds associated with respiratory disease:
Cough
Hoarseness
Grunting
Stridor
Wheezing
Auscultation:
Wheezing
Crackles
Hyperresonance
Absence of sound
Sore Throat
Frequent complaint of older children
Young children (unable to describe symptoms) may not complain even when highly inflamed but will refuse fluids/food
Elastic nature of the tissues in young children may cause less pressure on nerve endings

---

◆ BOX 26-5

Guidelines for assessment of respiratory function

Respirations

The pattern of respirations is observed for rate, depth, ease, and rhythm of breathing:

Rate—rapid (tachypnoea), normal, or slow for the particular child

Depth—normal depth, too shallow (hypopnoea), too deep (hyperpnoea); usually estimated from the amplitude of thoracic and abdominal excursion

Ease—effortless, laboured (dyspnoea), orthopnoea, associated with intercostal recessions, pulsus paradoxus (blood pressure falls with inspiration and rises with expiration), flaring nares, head bobbing, grunting, or wheezing

Laboured breathing—continuous, intermittent, becoming steadily worsening, sudden onset, at rest or on exertion, associated with wheezing, grunting, associated with pain

Rhythm—variation in rate and depth of respirations

Other Observations

In addition to respirations, particular attention is addressed to the following:

Evidence of infection—check for elevated temperature, enlarged cervical lymph nodes, inflamed mucous membranes, and purulent discharges from the nose, ears or lungs (sputum)

Cough—observe the characteristics of the cough (if present); for example, under what circumstances the cough is heard (e.g. night only, on arising), the nature of the cough (paroxysmal with or without wheeze, 'croupy' or 'brassy'), frequency of cough, associated with swallowing or other activity

Wheeze—expiratory or inspiratory, high-pitched or musical, prolonged, slowly progressive or sudden, associated with laboured breathing

Cyanosis—note distribution (peripheral, perioral, facial, trunk as well as face), degree, duration, associated with activity

Chest pain—note location and circumstances: localized or generalized, referred to base of neck or abdomen, dull or sharp, deep or superficial, associated with rapid, shallow respirations or grunting

Sputum—supervised older children may provide sputum sample. Note volume, colour, viscosity, and odour

Bad breath—may be associated with some lung infections

Xylometazole 0.05% is the only preparation recommended for children. Bottles of nose drops should be used for one child only and only for one illness, since they become easily contaminated with bacteria. Nose drops or sprays should not be administered for more than three days, to avoid rebound congestion.

Prevent spread of infection

Careful handwashing should be carried out when caring for children with respiratory infections. Children and families are encouraged to use a tissue or their hand to cover their nose and mouth when they cough or sneeze and to dispose of the tissues properly.

Reduce temperature

If the child has a significantly elevated temperature, controlling the fever becomes a major nursing task. The parent should know how to take a child's temperature and to read the thermometer accurately. Those who cannot will require instruction in use of the thermometer.

If paracetamol has been prescribed, parents may need help administering the drug. It is important to emphasize accuracy in both the amount of drug given and the time intervals at which the drug is administered in order to avoid accumulation effects.

Promote hydration

Dehydration is always a hazard when children are febrile or anorexic, especially when vomiting or diarrhoea is also present. Adequate fluid intake should be encouraged by offering small amounts of favourite fluids at frequent intervals. High-calorie liquids, such as colas and fruit juices, help prevent catabolism and dehydration. Forcing fluids may create the same difficulties as urging unwanted food.

Parents are advised to observe the frequency of voiding and notify the practitioner if there appears to be insufficient voiding.

Provide nutrition

Loss of appetite is characteristic of children with acute infections, and in most cases, children can be permitted to determine their own need for food. Since the illness is relatively short, the nutritional state is seldom compromised. In fact, urging foods on anorexic children may precipitate nausea and vomiting.

Family-centred care

Small children with respiratory infections are irritable and often difficult to comfort. Therefore, the family needs support, encouragement and practical suggestions for care. Since most care involves comfort measures and administration of medication, a primary goal of education is related to these activities.

In addition to antipyretics and nose drops, the child may require antibiotic therapy. Parents need to understand the importance of regular administration and of continuing the drug for the prescribed length of time, regardless of whether the child appears to be ill.

It should be emphasized that some drugs interact with others to produce serious side effects and therefore parents should not give any other drugs without consultation with their doctor.

Evaluation

The effectiveness of nursing interventions is determined by

continual reassessment and evaluation of care based on the following observational guidelines and expected outcomes:

1. Observe individual child's respiratory behaviour and movement.
2. Observe signs and symptoms for progress towards pre-illness status.
3. Observe child's behaviour and activity.
4. Observe other family members and contacts for evidence of infection.
5. Take temperature.
6. Observe for signs of adequate hydration.
7. Observe eating behaviour.
8. Assess child for evidence of complications, such as dehydration, weight loss, or spread of infection to other areas of the body.
9. Observe family's behaviour and interview members regarding their feelings and concerns.

UPPER RESPIRATORY TRACT INFECTIONS

Upper respiratory infections (URIs) include infectious processes involving any or all of the structures in the upper respiratory tract. Most are caused by viruses and are self-limited. Most URIs have a viral aetiology and need only symptomatic treatment and support. However, secondary infection or extension of URIs can cause serious or long-lasting effects, especially in infants and very young children. A primary site for extension is the middle ear.

ACUTE VIRAL NASOPHARYNGITIS

Acute nasopharyngitis (the equivalent of the 'common cold' in adults) is caused by any of a number of different viruses, usually rhinoviruses, respiratory syncytial virus (RSV), adenovirus, influenza virus or parainfluenza virus.

CLINICAL MANIFESTATIONS

Symptoms of nasopharyngitis are more severe in infants and children than in adults. Fever is common, especially in young children. Older children have low-grade fevers, which appear early and suddenly in children three months to three years of age and are associated with irritability, restlessness, and decreased appetite and activity. Nasal inflammation may lead to obstruction of passages, producing open-mouth breathing. Other symptoms (e.g., vomiting and diarrhoea) may be evident in some children.

The initial symptoms in older children are dryness and irritation of nasal passages and sometimes the pharynx, followed in a few hours by sneezing, chilly sensations, muscular aches, an irritating nasal discharge and sometimes cough. Nasal inflammation may lead to obstruction, and continual wiping away of secretions causes skin irritation to nares.

The disease usually resolves within 4-10 days without complications. The most common complication is otitis media, especially in infants, and this should be suspected if fever recurs. Pneumonia is a less frequent complication and observed more often in infants.

THERAPEUTIC MANAGEMENT

Children with nasopharyngitis are managed at home. Antipyretics are usually prescribed for mild fever and discomfort (see Chapter 8 for management of fever). Decongestants may be prescribed for children and infants older than three months of age, though there is little evidence they are of value in the young child (Dinwiddie, 1990). Decongestants exert their effect by vasoconstriction and since these drugs affect all vascular beds they should be given with caution to children with diabetes.

There is no support for the usefulness of expectorants, and antibiotics are usually contraindicated because they can sensitize a child who may need the drugs in a severe illness. Administration of vitamin C has not been shown to have significant therapeutic or prophylactic value (Goldbloom, 1986).

Prevention

Nasopharyngitis is so widespread in the general population that it is impossible to prevent. Very young infants are subject to relatively serious complications; therefore, some attempt should be made to protect them from exposure.

IMPLICATIONS FOR NURSING

A cold is often the parents' first introduction to an illness in their infants. Parents are assisted in managing the infant or child as described for general care. Most of the distress of nasopharyngitis is related to the nasal obstruction, especially in small infants. Placing the child in a sitting position and giving gentle nasal suction, particularly before feeding, is sometimes useful. The infant should never be laid in a prone position.

Maintaining adequate fluid intake is essential during any infectious process. Although a child's appetite for solid foods is usually diminished for several days, it is important to offer favourite fluids to prevent dehydration.

Family-centred care

Because URIs are so frequent in children younger than three years of age, families may feel they are on an endless rollercoaster of illness. They can be reassured that frequent colds are a normal part of childhood and that by five years of age their children will have developed immunity to many viruses. If the children are cared for routinely in daycare centres, the infection rate will be higher than if they were being cared for in the home. Parents should know the signs of respiratory complications and be counselled to notify a health professional if any signs of complications appear or if the child does not improve within 2-3 days.

ACUTE STREPTOCOCCAL PHARYNGITIS

Group A β-haemolytic streptococci (GABHS) infection of the upper airway (strep throat) is not in itself a serious disease, but affected children are at risk for a serious sequela — acute rheumatic fever (ARF) and acute glomerulonephritis.

CLINICAL MANIFESTATIONS

GABHS is generally a relatively brief illness that varies markedly in severity from subclinical (no symptoms) to comparatively severe toxicity. The onset is generally abrupt and characterized by pharyngitis, headache, fever and (especially in small children) abdominal pain. The tonsils and pharynx may be inflamed and covered with exudate, which usually appears by the second day of illness. Anterior cervical lymphadenopathy (30-50% of cases) usually occurs early, and the nodes are often tender. Pain can be relatively mild to severe enough to make swallowing difficult. Clinical manifestations usually subside in 3-5 days unless complicated by sinusitis or parapharyngeal, peritonsillar, or retropharyngeal abscess. Nonsuppurative complications may appear after the onset of GABHS—acute nephritis in about 10 days and rheumatic fever in an average of 18 days (Feigin, 1990).

PROCESS OF DIAGNOSIS

Clinical diagnosis of GABHS infection can present difficulties. Although 80-90% of all cases of acute pharyngitis are viral, a throat culture should be performed to rule out GABHS and (in some cases) *Corynebacterium diphtheriae*. Because some children normally harbour streptococci in their throats, a positive culture is not always conclusive evidence of active disease. Since most streptococcal infections are short-term illnesses, antibody (antistreptolysin O) responses do not appear until relatively late and are useful only for retrospective diagnosis.

THERAPEUTIC MANAGEMENT

Virtually all children presenting with the symptoms of a GABHS infection are prescribed penicillin as it is not possible to differentiate a viral infection from a streptococcal infection on clinical grounds alone (Dinwiddie, 1990). Penicillin does not appear to prevent the development of acute glomerulonephritis in susceptible children. It may, however, prevent the spread of a nephrogenic strain of GABHS to other family members.

IMPLICATIONS FOR NURSING

Most children prefer to remain in bed during the acute phase of the illness. Cold or warm compresses to the neck may provide relief. Pain may interfere with oral intake, and the child should not be forced to eat. Cool liquids or are usually more acceptable than solids and are encouraged.

Prevention

The organism is spread by close contact with affected persons — direct projection of large droplets or physical transfer of respiratory secretions containing the organism. As a result, spread of infection is common in families, classrooms and daycare centres. Children with streptococcal infection are noninfectious to others within a few hours after initiation of penicillin therapy.

It is important to know when the organism is epidemic in the community so that families can be on the alert for symptoms. Managers of daycare centres and school officials should share infectious disease information with parents. Obtaining throat cultures from children who are close family contacts of patients with streptococcal infection is advised. Penicillin administration before the onset of symptoms prevents most cases of streptococcal disease.

TONSILLITIS

The tonsils are masses of lymphoid tissue located in the pharyngeal cavity. Their function is to filter and protect the respiratory and alimentary tracts from invasion by pathogenic organisms. They also may have a role in antibody formation. Children generally have much larger tonsils than adolescents or adults. This difference is thought to be a protective mechanism at a time when young children are especially susceptible to upper respiratory infection.

AETIOLOGY

Tonsillitis usually occurs in association with pharyngitis. Because of the abundant lymphoid tissue and the frequency of URIs, tonsillitis is a very common cause of morbidity in young children. The causative agent may be viral or bacterial.

CLINICAL MANIFESTATIONS

The manifestations of tonsillitis are chiefly caused by inflammation. As the palatine tonsils enlarge from oedema, they may meet in the midline, obstructing the passage of air or food. The child has difficulty swallowing and breathing. Enlargement of the adenoids blocks the space behind the posterior nares, making it difficult or impossible for air to pass from the nose to the throat. As a result, the child breathes through the mouth.

If mouth breathing is continuous, the mucous membranes of the oropharynx become dry and irritated. There may be an offensive mouth odour and impaired senses of taste and smell. Because air cannot be trapped for proper speech sounds, the voice has a nasal and muffled quality. A persistent, harassing cough is also common. Because of the proximity of the adenoids to the eustachian tubes, this passageway is frequently blocked by swollen adenoids, interfering with normal drainage and frequently resulting in otitis media and/or difficulty hearing.

THERAPEUTIC MANAGEMENT

The diagnosis is established from visual examination of the throat. The majority of children with tonsillitis respond to medical treatment. However, a significant number undergo surgical intervention, although the exact criteria for this common procedure are controversial.

Medical

Since the illness is self-limiting, treatment of viral pharyngitis is symptomatic. Throat cultures positive for GABHS infection warrant antibiotic treatment. In general, viral tonsillitis has been found to be more common in children younger than three years of age and GABHS more common in children six years or older (Putto, 1987).

Surgical

Many authorities believe that the majority of tonsillectomies are unwarranted. Others, who have seen children improve measurably after tonsillectomy and adenoidectomy, continue to recommend it for selected patients.

Tonsillectomy is indicated for massive hypertrophy that results in difficulty breathing or eating. Absolute indications are malignancy and obstruction of the airway that result in cor pulmonale. *Adenoidectomy* (removal of the adenoids) is recommended for children with recurrent otitis media, especially when associated with hearing loss, and in those children where hypertrophied adenoids obstruct nasal breathing. Follow-up after adenoidectomy should include assessment of hearing, smell and taste for expected improvement. Contraindications to either tonsillectomy or adenoidectomy are: (1) cleft palate, since both tonsils help minimize escape of air during speech; (2) acute infections at the time of surgery, since the locally inflamed tissues increase the risk of bleeding; and (3) uncontrolled systemic diseases or blood dyscrasias.

IMPLICATIONS FOR NURSING

Nursing care of the child with tonsillitis mainly involves providing comfort. A soft to liquid diet is generally preferred. A cool-mist vaporizer helps keep the mucous membranes moist during periods of mouth breathing. Warm salt-water gargles, throat lozenges, and analgesic/antipyretic drugs such as paracetamol are useful to promote comfort.

If surgery is needed, the child requires the same psychological preparation and physical care as for any other operation (see Chapters 5 and 8). The following discussion focuses on specific nursing care for tonsillectomy and adenoidectomy (T & A).

Assessment

A complete history is taken, with special notation of any bleeding tendencies, since the operative site is highly vascular. Baseline vital signs are important for postoperative monitoring and observation. Signs of any URI are noted and reported, and bleeding and clotting times are included in the usual laboratory work requests.

Planning

The nursing goals for postoperative care of the child with a T & A are as follows:
1. Facilitate drainage of secretions.
2. Promote comfort and relieve pain.
3. Observe for evidence of bleeding.
4. Prevent complications.
5. Provide fluids and nutrition.
6. Instruct family for home care.
7. Support child and family.

Implementation

Until they are fully awake, children are placed on the abdomen or side to facilitate drainage of secretions, and any needed suctioning is performed carefully to avoid trauma to the oropharynx. When alert, children may prefer sitting up, although they should remain in bed for the remainder of the day. They are discouraged from coughing frequently or clearing the throat, which may aggravate the operative site.

Some secretions are common, particularly dried blood from surgery. All secretions and vomitus are inspected for evidence of fresh bleeding. Dark brown (old) blood is usually present in the vomit, as well as in the nose and between the teeth. If parents do not expect this, they may be frightened at a time when they need to be calm and reassuring for their children.

The throat is very sore after surgery. Most children experience moderate pain after a T&A and should receive pain medication for at least the first 24 hours (Rauen and Holman, 1989). Analgesics are ordered, but may need to be given rectally or intravenously to avoid the oral route. Pain control should be continuous.

Food and fluid are restricted until children are fully alert and there are no signs of haemorrhage. Cool water, crushed ice, iced lollies or dilute fruit juice is given first, although fluids with a red or brown colour are avoided to distinguish fresh or old blood in vomit from the ingested liquid. Citrus juice may cause discomfort and is usually poorly tolerated. Milk, ice cream or custard are not offered until clear fluids are retained, because milk products coat the mouth and throat, causing the child to clear the throat more often, which may initiate bleeding. Soft foods are started as the child tolerates feeding.

Postoperative haemorrhage is unusual, but can occur. Therefore, the nurse observes the throat directly for evidence of bleeding, using a good source of light. Other signs of haemorrhage are increased pulse (above 120 beats per minute), pallor, frequent clearing of the throat, and vomiting of bright red blood. Restlessness, an indication of haemorrhage, may be difficult to differentiate from general discomfort after surgery. Decreasing blood pressure is a later sign and signals impending shock.

NURSING ALERT

The most obvious early sign is the child's continuous swallowing of the trickling blood. While the child is sleeping, the frequency of swallowing is noted.

If continuous bleeding is suspected, the surgeon is notified immediately. Surgery may be required to ligate a bleeding vessel. Airway obstruction may occur as a result of oedema or accumulated secretions.

Family-centred care

Discharge instructions include: (1) avoiding foods that are irritating or highly seasoned, (2) avoiding the use of gargles or vigorous toothbrushing, (3) discouraging the child from coughing or clearing the throat or putting objects in the mouth, and (4) using mild analgesics. Haemorrhage may occur 5-10 days after surgery as a result of tissue sloughing from the healing process. Any sign of bleeding warrants immediate medical attention. Objectionable mouth odour and slight ear pain with a low-grade fever are common for a few days postoperatively. However, persistent severe earache, fever or cough requires medical evaluation. Most children are ready to resume normal activity within 1-2 weeks of the operation.

A tonsillectomy and adenoidectomy often represents the first hospitalization experience for the child and family. Since the surgery is usually an elective procedure, there is ample opportunity to prepare both children and parents for this event. Both need reassurance about what to expect at the time of admission, before and after surgery, and at discharge. Parents are encouraged to visit often or be resident if possible and participate in their child's care if they wish. Children are honestly appraised of postoperative discomfort and reassured that they will be able to talk. Sometimes, children believe that the operation will immediately 'make the throat all better' and are dismayed to find that it still hurts after the surgery. Children should have an opportunity to discuss the experiences to gain a feeling of mastery and to overcome any fears or misconceptions.

Evaluation

The effectiveness of nursing interventions is determined by continual reassessment and evaluation of care based on the following observational guidelines and expected outcomes:

1. Monitor the child's vital signs and behaviour.
2. Observe for evidence of bleeding.
3. Observe and interview family about their understanding of the child's condition.
4. Have family demonstrate an understanding of home care.
5. Encourage family to discuss concerns that provide some insight into their ability to comply with instructions.

INFLUENZA

Influenza, or 'flu', one of the most common disorders, has been overused in diagnosis of relatively nondescript respiratory infections. Influenza is caused by three of the orthomyxoviruses, which are antigenically distinct: types A and B, which cause epidemic disease, and type C, which is unimportant epidemiologically. The viruses may undergo significant changes from time to time.

The disease is spread from one individual to another by direct contact (large-droplet infection) or by articles recently contaminated by nasopharyngeal secretions. Attack rates are highest in young children who have not had previous contact with a strain. It is frequently most severe in infants. Influenza is more common during the winter months.

The disease has a 1- to 3-day incubation period, and affected persons are most infectious for 24 hours before and after onset of symptoms.

CLINICAL MANIFESTATIONS

The manifestations of influenza may be subclinical, mild, moderate or severe. In most cases of overt illness, the throat and nasal mucosa are dry, there is a dry cough, and a tendency towards hoarseness. There is a sudden onset of fever and chills accompanied by flushed face, photophobia, myalgia, hyperaesthesia and sometimes prostration. Subglottal croup is common, especially in infants. The symptoms last for 4-5 days. Complications include severe viral pneumonia, encephalitis, and secondary bacterial infections, such as otitis media, sinusitis or pneumonia. Reye's syndrome can be a serious complication of influenza A or B at any age, but occurs most often in the UK in school-aged children. Because of the strong correlation with Reye's syndrome, in 1986 the Committee on Safety of Medicines recommended that aspirin should not be prescribed to children under 12 years of age except for those with rheumatic disease. Nurses should keep parents aware of the dangers of giving aspirin preparations to children with feverish illnesses (Newton and Hall, 1993).

THERAPEUTIC MANAGEMENT

Uncomplicated influenza in children usually requires only symptomatic treatment — paracetamol for fever, and sufficient fluids to maintain hydration.

Prevention

Inactivated influenza viral vaccines are safe and effective for prevention of influenza provided the antigens in the vaccine correlate with circulating influenza viruses.

IMPLICATIONS FOR NURSING

Nursing care is the same as for any child with a URI, including helping the family to implement measures to relieve symptoms. The greatest danger to affected children is development of a secondary infection.

OTITIS MEDIA

Otitis media is one of the most prevalent diseases of early childhood. It has been determined that two of every three children have been affected by the age of three years. The peak incidence is from 6–36 months of age, declining after six years (Habel, 1993). The incidence of acute otitis media is highest in the winter months. Children living in households with many members (especially smokers) are more likely to have otitis media than those living with fewer persons, and children with siblings or parents who had a history of chronic otitis media have a higher incidence than those who do not (McFadden *et al*, 1985).

Otitis media has been defined in a variety of ways. The acute, more severe, disease has been known as 'suppurative', 'purulent', or 'bacterial' otitis media and otitis media with effusion as 'serous', 'secretory', 'nonsuppurative', and 'glue ear'. The standard terminology that has been established to describe otitis media is outlined in Box 26-6.

AETIOLOGY

Acute otitis media is most frequently caused by *Streptococcus pneumoniae* and *H. influenzae*. The aetiology of the noninfectious type is unknown, although it is frequently the result of blocked eustachian tubes from the oedema of upper respiratory infections, allergic rhinitis or hypertrophic adenoids. Chronic otitis media is frequently an extension of an acute episode.

It has been suggested that smoke inhalation via passive smoking increases the risk of a blocked eustachian tube by impairing mucociliary function, causing congestion of soft nasopharyngeal tissues, or predisposing patients to upper respiratory infection (Strachan, Jarvis, and Feyerabend, 1989). Day care attendance is also a risk factor for otitis media (Alho *et al*, 1993).

A relationship has been observed between the incidence of otitis media and the feeding methods in early infancy. Infants fed breast milk have a lower incidence of otitis media compared with formula-fed infants, while other studies indicate that the average number of episodes decreases significantly with an increased duration and exclusivity of breast feeding (Duncan *et al*, 1993). Breast feeding protects infants against respiratory viruses and allergy and limits the exposure of the eustachian tube and middle ear mucosa to microbial pathogens and foreign proteins.

CLINICAL MANIFESTATIONS

As purulent fluid accumulates in the small space of the middle ear chamber, pain results from the pressure on surrounding structures. Infants become irritable and indicate their discomfort by holding or pulling at their ears and rolling their head from side to side. Young children will usually verbally complain of the pain. A temperature as high as 40°C is common, and postauricular and cervical lymph glands may be enlarged. Rhinorrhoea, vomiting, and diarrhoea, as well as signs of concurrent respiratory or pharyngeal infection, may also be present. Loss of appetite is common, and sucking or chewing tends to aggravate the pain. As the exudate accumulates and pressure increases, the tympanic membrane may rupture spontaneously, resulting in immediate relief of pain.

Severe pain or fever is usually absent in otitis media with effusion, and the child may not appear ill. Instead, there is a feeling of 'fullness' in the ear, a popping sensation during swallowing, and a feeling of 'motion' in the ear if air is present above the level of fluid. Audiometry may reveal deficient hearing.

PROCESS OF DIAGNOSIS

In acute otitis media, otoscopy reveals an intact membrane that appears bright red and bulging, with no visible landmarks or light reflex. The usual landmarks of the bony prominence from the long and the short process of the malleus are obscured by the outwardly bulging membrane. In otitis media with effusion, otoscopic findings may include a slightly injected, dull grey membrane, obscured landmarks, and a visible fluid level or meniscus behind the eardrum if air is present above the fluid.

THERAPEUTIC MANAGEMENT: ACUTE OTITIS MEDIA

In treating acute otitis media, administration of antibiotics is the mainstay of therapy. A variety of antibiotics may be prescribed individually or in combination, with amoxicillin the antibiotic of choice due to its ease of use, relatively inexpensive cost, and availability.

In addition to amoxicillin, other oral antibiotics frequently prescribed include sulphonamides, trimethoprim-sulphamethoxazole, erythromycin-sulphisoxazole, and the cephalosporins, which, in many settings, are becoming the first-line drugs due to their broad spectrum, activity, dosage schedule, decreased side effects, and bactericidal activity against beta-lactamase producing pathogens. Many of these antibiotics may be effective in treating symptoms (e.g., pain) and in returning fluid to a sterile state, but may not be effective in eliminating the eustachian tube blockage.

Other measures include the use of analgesic/antipyretic drugs such as paracetamol to reduce the pain and/or fever. The efficacy of oral decongestants is questioned, but they may provide relief from symptoms of associated upper respiratory infection or allergy. Myringotomy (incision of the eardrum) may be required to relieve the symptoms in some children, especially those with acute suppuration who are in severe pain.

Children with acute otitis media should be seen following antibiotic therapy to evaluate the effectiveness of the treatment and to identify potential complications, such as effusion or hearing impairment. Hearing loss may not be noticed by parents but should be determined by audiometric testing.

THERAPEUTIC MANAGEMENT: RECURRENT OTITIS MEDIA

Therapies have been examined including chemoprophylaxis with long-term antibiotic therapy, steroid utilization, immunotherapy, and surgery. For children on long term dosing, an evaluation once a month is usually done to detect any evidence of effusion, and any acute infection during prophylaxis is treated with an alternative antibiotic regimen. The use of corticosteroids has also been considered, with evidence suggesting that a brief course of a steroid and concurrent antimicrobial therapy is efficacious for the short-term cure of otitis media with effusion (Rosenfield, 1992). It is important to note, however, that the suggestion was that antibiotics should be the first therapy to be tried and that the routine use of steroid therapy in unselected children with otitis media with effusion is not warranted. Further, while a short course of antibiotics appears to be effective in short-term clearance, the effect tends to be limited and is of relatively short duration (Williams *et al*, 1993).

From a surgical standpoint, myringotomy with tubes (grommets) is very effective in eliminating fluid, pain, and hearing loss secondary to the presence of recurrent and chronic otitis media where there is no spontaneous perforation of the tympanic membrane. Myringotomy alone is effective in relieving fluid, pain, and hearing loss temporarily in cases not responding to medical treatment. If, however, a eustachian tube remains blocked, fluid will return following a fairly rapid spontaneous healing of the myringotomy. Adenoidectomy may be successful in treating recurrent otitis media if a blocked eustachian tube secondary to hypertrophy of adenoids is the cause, while tonsillectomy in not generally considered a beneficial treatment (Maw and Bawden, 1993). Mastoidectomy may be performed when antibiotic therapy has failed and the child's life is threatened by infection, with tympanoplasty (middle ear reconstructive surgery) possibly being done following surgery.

THERAPEUTIC MANAGEMENT: OTITIS MEDIA WITH EFFUSION

Many children have fluid that persists in the middle ear for weeks or months; there is usually some impairment of hearing. The major goal of therapy, therefore, is to establish and maintain an aerated middle ear that is free of fluid with a normal mucosa and to ultimately achieve normal hearing. The medical management of recurrent as well as otitis media with effusion is often open-ended and seemingly uncertain (Williams *et al*, 1993) with regard to antimicrobial and surgical management. As indicated above with otitis media and recurrent otitis media, there are many preventive, prophylactic and active treatment modalities.

When medical interventions are unsuccessful in achieving the goals of therapy, then surgical management is often considered. Myringotomy tubes facilitate continued drainage of fluid, as well as allowing ventilation of the middle ear. The primary objective is to allow the eustachian tube a period of recovery while the tubes perform their functions. While the surgery is relatively benign, it is important to remember that tubes may tend to become plugged and often require reinsertion. Complications of repeated or long-term tube placement are tympanosclerosis, localized or diffuse atrophy of the membrane, persistent perforation, or, rarely, cholesteatoma. It has also been shown that adenoidectomy and tube insertion for children with otitis media with effusion and hearing loss is beneficial, and that children in households where there was no smoking also did considerably better and were free of symptoms for longer (Maw and Bawden, 1993).

IMPLICATIONS FOR NURSING

Since otitis media is such a common aftermath of URIs, nurses should be continually alert to this possibility when caring for a child with such infections.

Assessment
Nurses should be able to detect manifestations that indicate possible middle ear infection or dysfunction.

Planning
Nursing objectives for the child with acute otitis media include the following:
1. Relieve pain.
2. Facilitate drainage when possible.
3. Prevent complications or recurrence.
4. Educate family in care of the child.
5. Provide emotional support to child and family.

Implementation
Analgesics are often very helpful to reduce severe earache. High fever, particularly in infants, should be reduced with antipyretic drugs to avoid febrile convulsions. The application of heat may reduce pain in some children, but may aggravate discomfort in others. Local heat should be placed over the ear while the child lies on the affected side. This position also facilitates drainage of the exudate if the eardrum has ruptured or if myringotomy was performed. An ice compress placed over the affected ear may also provide comfort, since it reduces oedema. If the child is cooperative, either procedure can be tried to determine which offers maximum relief.

◆ **BOX 26-6**

Standard terminology for otitis media

Otitis media—an inflammation of the middle ear without reference to aetiology or pathogenesis

Acute otitis media—a rapid and short onset of signs and symptoms lasting approximately 3 weeks

Otitis media with effusion—an inflammation of the middle ear in which a collection of fluid is present in the middle ear space

Subacute otitis media—middle ear effusion lasting from 3 weeks to 3 months

Chronic otitis media with effusion—middle ear effusion

If the ear is draining, the external canal may be cleansed with sterile cotton swabs soaked in normal saline. If ear wicks or lightly rolled sterile gauze packs are placed in the ear after surgical treatment, they should be loose enough to allow accumulated drainage to flow out of the ear; otherwise the infection may be transferred to the mastoid process. Parents should be told to keep these wicks dry during shampoos or baths.

Parents require some anticipatory guidance regarding temporary hearing loss that accompanies otitis media. For example, they may need to speak louder, at closer proximity, and while facing the child. Persistent difficulty in hearing beyond the acute stage should be evaluated.

With antibiotics, symptoms of pain and fever usually subside within 24-48 hours, but nurses must emphasize that although the child looks well in a couple of days, the infection is not completely eradicated until all of the prescribed medication is taken. At the risk of alarming parents, it is important to stress the potential complications of otitis media, especially hearing loss.

A concern presented by the use of grommets is the possibility of water entering the middle ear. Several studies indicate that small amounts of water pose little hazard and that even swimming without earplugs or occlusive bathing caps carries no higher risk for an increased incidence of otitis media. However, diving, jumping and submerging may be forbidden by some doctors. Wearing earplugs, although not watertight, prevents total flooding of the external canal and provides sufficient protection. Parents should be aware of the appearance of a grommet (usually a tiny, white plastic, spool-shaped tube) so that they can observe if it falls out. They should reassured that this is normal and requires no immediate intervention (Isaacson and Rosenfeld, 1994).

Reducing the chances of otitis media is possible with some simple measures, such as sitting or holding an infant upright for feeding. Gentle nose blowing, rather than sniffing, should be encouraged, as negative middle ear pressure is induced in the latter (Habel, 1993). Early detection of possible middle ear effusion is a primary nursing goal in the prevention of complications. Infants and preschool children should be screened for effusion. Frequent audiological evaluations are advised when middle ear effusion is detected.

Evaluation

The effectiveness of nursing interventions is determined by continual reassessment and evaluation of care based on the following observational guidelines and expected outcomes:
1. Observe behaviours that indicate pain relief; seek verbal confirmation.
2. Observe skin in and around external auditory canal.
3. Interview family regarding practices that prevent recurrence of infection, especially instructions regarding administration of prescribed medications.
4. Observe and interview family regarding their understanding of otitis media and therapies.
5. Interview family regarding their feelings and concerns.

OTITIS EXTERNA

Infections of the external ear may result from normal ear flora (*Staphylococcus epidermidis* and *Corynebacterium,* primarily) that assume pathogenic characteristics under conditions of excessive wetness or dryness. Inflammation occurs when the external ear environment is altered by swimming, bathing or increased environmental humidity *(swimmer's ear);* by infection, dermatoses or insufficient cerumen; or by trauma from a foreign body or a finger.

Secondary invasion of foreign pathogens also occurs. In addition to the resident flora, the offending agents can be *Pseudomonas aeruginosa* (most commonly), *Enterobacter aerogenes, Proteus mirabilis, Klebsiella pneumoniae,* streptococci, and fungi such as *Candida* and *Aspergillus.* The ear canal becomes irritated, and maceration takes place.

The predominant symptom of external ear infection is ear pain accentuated by manipulation of the pinna, especially pressure on the tragus. The pain often appears to be out of proportion to the degree of inflammation. Conductive hearing loss may be present as a result of the oedema, secretions, and accumulation of debris within the canal. Oedema, erythema, and a cheesy green-blue-grey discharge and tenderness appear as the infection progresses. The external canal may be so tender and swollen that visualization is difficult. There may be fever.

Therapeutic objectives include relief of pain, oedema, and itching and restoration of normal flora, cerumen, and canal epithelium. Analgesics are prescribed for pain. Debris is gently swabbed out and antibiotic and steroid drops are instilled in the canal. A gauze wick is usually inserted to facilitate the medication reaching the site of inflammation. The wick is removed after swelling and pain have subsided, but the drops are continued for at least three days after relief of pain.

IMPLICATIONS FOR NURSING

Nurses can teach parents or patients to apply simple measures to prevent recurrent infections. Children are advised to limit their stay in the water to less than an hour, if possible, and ears should dry completely (1-2 hours) before children enter the water again. Placing a combination of white vinegar and rubbing alcohol (50/50) in both ear canals upon arising, at bedtime, and at the end of each swim (the most common cause of otitis externa) is effective in preventing recurrence. The solution must remain in the canal for five minutes (Marcy, 1989).

CROUP SYNDROMES

Croup is a general term applied to a symptom complex characterized by hoarseness, a resonant cough described as 'barking' or 'brassy' (croupy), varying degrees of inspiratory stridor, and varying degrees of respiratory distress resulting from swelling or obstruction in the region of the larynx. Acute infections of the larynx are of greater importance in infants and small children than they are in older children, in part because of the increased incidence in children in this age group and the smaller diameter of the airway, which renders it subject to significantly greater narrowing with the same degree of inflammation (Fig. 26-11).

Acute respiratory infections of the nonreactive airway are seldom restricted to one area and affect to varying degrees the larynx, trachea and bronchi. However, laryngeal involvement often dominates the clinical picture because of the severe effects on the voice and breathing. Croup is usually described according to the primary anatomical area affected, that is, epiglottitis, laryngitis, laryngotracheobronchitis (LTB), and tracheitis. In general, LTB tends to occur in very young children, whereas epiglottitis is more characteristic of older children (see Table 26-4 for a comparison of croup syndromes).

ACUTE EPIGLOTTITIS

Acute epiglottitis, or acute supraglottitis, is a serious obstructive inflammatory process that occurs principally in children between 6–12 months and six years of age, with peak incidence between 2-4 years of age (Dinwiddie, 1990). The disorder requires immediate attention. The obstruction is supraglottic as opposed to the subglottic obstruction of laryngitis. The responsible organism is usually *H. influenzae;* LTB and epiglottitis do not occur together.

CLINICAL MANIFESTATIONS

The onset of epiglottitis is abrupt and rapidly progressive to severe respiratory distress. The child usually goes to bed asymptomatic to awaken later complaining of sore throat and pain on swallowing. The child has a fever, appears sicker than clinical findings would suggest, and presents a classic picture. The child generally insists on sitting upright, leaning forward, with chin thrust out, mouth open, and tongue protruding. Drooling of saliva is common because of the difficulty or pain on swallowing and excessive secretions.

NURSING ALERT

Three clinical observations that have been found to be predictive of epiglottitis are absence of spontaneous cough, presence of drooling, and agitation (Mauro et al, 1988).

The child is irritable and markedly restless, and has an anxious, apprehensive and frightened expression. The voice is thick and muffled, with a froglike croaking sound on inspiration. The child is not hoarse. Suprasternal and substernal recessions may be visible. The child seldom struggles to breathe, and slow quiet breathing provides better air exchange. The sallow colour of mild hypoxia may progress to frank cyanosis. The throat is red and inflamed, and a distinctive large, cherry-red, oedematous epiglottis is visible on careful throat inspection.

The child suspected of epiglottitis should be examined where facilities are available for coping with this type of emergency. The child is best transported while sitting in a parent's lap to reduce distress. Examination of the throat with a tongue blade is contraindicated until properly experienced personnel and equipment are at hand to proceed with immediate intubation in the event that the examination precipitates further or complete obstruction.

THERAPEUTIC MANAGEMENT

Progressive obstruction leads to hypoxia, hypercapnia, and acidosis followed by decreased muscular tone, reduced level of consciousness, and, when obstruction becomes more or less complete, a rather sudden death. A presumptive diagnosis of epiglottitis constitutes an emergency.

Endotracheal intubation is usually considered for *H. influenzae* epiglottitis with severe respiratory distress. Whether or not there is an artificial airway, the child requires intensive observation by experienced personnel. The epiglottal swelling usually decreases after 24 hours of antibiotic therapy, and the epiglottis is near normal by the third day. Intubated children are generally extubated at this time.

Children with suspected bacterial epiglottitis are given antibiotics intravenously, followed by oral administration to complete a 7- to 10-day course. The use of corticosteroids for reducing oedema is controversial.

Prevention
As administration of the haemophilius influenzae type B (HIB) vaccine becomes a routine part of the regular UK immunization schedule, a decline in the incidence of epiglottitis can be anticipated.

IMPLICATIONS FOR NURSING

Epiglottitis is a serious and frightening disease for child, family and health professionals. It is important to act quickly but calmly and to provide support without unduly increasing anxiety. The child is allowed to remain in the position that provides the most comfort and security, and parents are reassured that everything possible is being done to obtain relief for their child.

NURSING ALERT

Nurses who suspect epiglottitis should not attempt to visualize the epiglottis directly with a tongue depressor or take a throat culture, but should refer the child to a paediatric anaesthetist immediately.

Acute care of the child is that earlier described for the child with acute respiratory distress and artificial airways. Continuous monitoring of respiratory status, including blood gases, is part of the nursing observations, and the intravenous infusion is maintained as necessary.

ACUTE LARYNGITIS

Acute infectious laryngitis is a common illness in older children and adolescents. Viruses are the usual causative agents and the principal complaint is hoarseness, which may be accompanied by other upper respiratory symptoms (e.g., coryza, sore throat, nasal congestion) and systemic manifestations (e.g., fever, headache, myalgia, malaise).

ACUTE LARYNGOTRACHEOBRONCHITIS

Viral laryngotracheobronchitis (LTB) (viral croup) primarily affects children younger than five years of age. Organisms usually responsible for LTB are the parainfluenza and influenza viruses RSV and rhinovirus (Dinwiddie, 1990).

Inflammation of the mucosa lining the larynx and trachea causes a narrowing of the airway. When the airway is significantly narrowed, the child struggles to inhale air past the obstruction and into the lungs, producing the characteristic inspiratory stridor and suprasternal recessions. When the child is unable to inhale a sufficient volume of air, symptoms of hypoxia become evident. Obstruction severe enough to prevent adequate exhalation of carbon dioxide causes respiratory acidosis, and, eventually, the child experiences respiratory failure.

THERAPEUTIC MANAGEMENT

The major objective in medical management of infectious LTB is maintaining an airway and providing for adequate respiratory exchange. Children with mild croup (no stridor at rest) are managed at home. Parents are taught the signs of respiratory distress so that professional help can be summoned early if needed.

Children who develop a continuous respiratory stridor using accessory muscles of respiration should receive medical attention, usually with hospitalization.

Though often administered, high humidity with cool mist is of no proven value. In the hospital setting, humidified oxygen for hypoxia can be delivered via a face mask or nasal prongs as tolerated.

In North America, racemic epinephrine (nebulized adrenaline) is frequently administered, but is less commonly used in the United Kingdom. Racemic epinephrine causes vasoconstriction and reduces swelling of the airway. Because the effects of epinephrine are temporary, airway obstruction can return to its original severity in a few hours. For this reason, the drug should not be used for outpatient therapy, and children receiving it are monitored continuously.

If intubation is required, the procedure should be performed in a controlled environment (preferably an intensive care unit), and the swollen airway necessitates a smaller than normal endotracheal (ET) tube. When the swelling begins to subside, an air leak usually forms around the ET tube, indicating that the obstruction has reversed and extubation can be attempted.

The use of corticosteroids for acute LTB is now less controversial, with several research studies supporting the practice (Kairys, Olmstead, and O'Connor, 1989; Kunkel and Baker, 1992; Tibballs, Shann, and Landau, 1992). The onset of action is clinically detectable as early as six hours after administration with continued improvement over 12–24 hours (Kairys, Olmstead, and O'Connor, 1989). Antibiotics are not indicated unless a bacterial infection is detected.

IMPLICATIONS FOR NURSING

The most important nursing function in the care of children with croup is continuous, vigilant observation and accurate assessment of respiratory status. Changes in therapy are frequently based on nurses' observations and assessment of a child's status, response to therapy, and tolerance of procedures. The trend away from early intubation of children with LTB emphasizes the importance of nursing observation and the ability to recognize impending respiratory failure so that intubation can be implemented without delay.

To conserve energy, children are given every opportunity to rest. Infants or small children find that being enclosed within a cot, coughing, laryngeal spasms and intravenous therapy are additional sources of distress. Infants and small children prefer sitting upright, and most want to be held. Children need the security of the parent's presence. Since crying increases respiratory distress and hypoxia, a child may do better when held in the parent's lap.

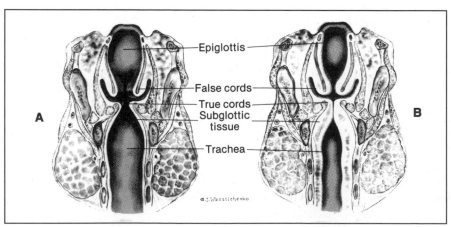

Fig. 26-11A, Normal larynx. **B,** Obstruction and narrowing resulting from oedema of croup.

Epiglottis

False cords

True cords
Subglottic tissue

Trachea

A

B

The rapid progression of croup, the alarming sound of the cough and stridor, and the child's apprehensive behaviour and ill appearance combine to create a very frightening experience for the parents. They need reassurance regarding the child's progress and an explanation of treatments. They may feel guilty for not having suspected the seriousness of the condition sooner. The family should be allowed to remain with their child as much as possible, especially when this decreases the child's distress.

The nurse can provide them with an opportunity to express their feelings, thus minimizing any blame or guilt. They need frequent reassurance provided in a calm, quiet manner and education regarding what they can do to make their child more comfortable. Fortunately, as the crisis subsides and the child responds to therapy, breathing becomes easier and recovery is generally prompt.

ACUTE SPASMODIC LARYNGITIS

Acute spasmodic laryngitis (spasmodic croup) is distinct from laryngitis and LTB and characterized by paroxysmal attacks of laryngeal obstruction that occur chiefly at night. Signs of inflammation are absent or mild, and there is frequently a history of previous attacks lasting for 2-5 days followed by uneventful recovery. It usually affects children of ages 1-3 years.

The child goes to bed well or with some very mild respiratory symptoms but awakes suddenly with characteristic barking, metallic cough, hoarseness, noisy inspirations, and restlessness. The child appears anxious, frightened, and prostrated. Dyspnoea is aggravated by excitement; but there is no fever, the attack subsides in a few hours, and the child appears well the next day.

IMPLICATIONS FOR NURSING

Children with spasmodic croup are managed at home. Those with moderately severe symptoms may be hospitalized for observation. The disease is usually self-limited.

BACTERIAL TRACHEITIS

Bacterial tracheitis, an infection of the mucosa of the upper trachea, is a distinct entity with features of both croup and epiglottitis. The disease is seen in children of ages one month to six years and may be a serious cause of airway obstruction — severe enough to cause respiratory arrest. It is believed to be a complication of LTB, and although *Staphylococcus aureus* is the most frequent organism responsible, group A β-haemolytic streptococci and *H. influenzae* have also been implicated.

Many of the manifestations of bacterial tracheitis are similar to those of LTB, but are unresponsive to LTB therapy. There is a history of previous upper respiratory infection with croupy cough, stridor unaffected by position, toxicity and high fever. A prominent manifestation is the production of thick, purulent tracheal secretions. Respiratory difficulties are secondary to these copious secretions.

IMPLICATIONS FOR NURSING

Bacterial tracheitis requires vigorous management. Humidified oxygen, antipyretics and antibiotics are prescribed. Most children require endotracheal intubation and frequent tracheal suctioning to prevent airway obstruction. The emphasis in this disorder is early recognition in order to prevent catastrophic airway obstruction.

INFECTIONS OF THE LOWER AIRWAYS

The reactive portion of the lower respiratory tract includes the bronchi and bronchioles in children. Cartilaginous support of the large airway is not fully developed until adolescence. Consequently, the smooth muscle in these structures represents a major factor in the constriction of the airway, particularly in the bronchioles.

The infectious disorders involving the reactive portion of the airway are diverse in nature and aetiology. Bronchial inflammation is usually seen as tracheobronchitis or laryngotracheobronchitis. Infection of the bronchioles (bronchiolitis, or capillary bronchitis) is an entirely different illness that is more closely related to interstitial pneumonia. The major portion of the following discussion is focused on bronchiolitis.

BRONCHITIS

Bronchitis describes inflammation of large airways (trachea and bronchi), which is almost invariably associated with an upper respiratory infection. Viral agents are the primary cause of the disease, although *M. pneumoniae* is a common cause in children older than six years of age. The condition is characterized by a dry, hacking and nonproductive cough that is worse at night and becomes productive in 2-3 days.

Bronchitis is a self-limiting disease that requires only symptomatic treatment, including analgesics, antipyretics and humidity. Cough suppressants may be useful to allow rest, but can interfere with cough clearance of secretions (Neddenriep, Taussig, and Mietens, 1989). Most patients recover uneventfully in 5-10 days.

BRONCHIOLITIS

Bronchiolitis is an acute viral infection. The infection occurs primarily in winter and spring and is rare in children over two years of age. Although few children with bronchiolitis require hospitalization, it can be a serious disease (McIntosh, 1987). Respiratory syncytial virus (RSV) is responsible for over half of all episodes of bronchiolitis (80% during epidemics) (Guerra, Kemp, and Shearer, 1990; Neddenriep, Taussig, and Mietens, 1989). Adenoviruses and parainfluenza viruses may also cause acute bronchiolitis. The virus becomes epidemic in communities during the late autumn and winter months and is easily spread by hand-to-nose transmission.

CLINICAL MANIFESTATIONS

Bronchiolitis begins as a simple upper respiratory infection with serous nasal discharge that may be accompanied by mild fever. The child gradually develops increasing respiratory distress with tachypnoea, paroxysmal cough and irritability. There may be wheezing. Chest x rays show hyperaeration and areas of consolidation that are difficult to differentiate from bacterial pneumonia.

The chest may appear barrel shaped from overinflation, and respirations are usually shallow and rapid, with flaring nares and suprasternal and subcostal recessions. Apnoea may be the first recognized indicator of RSV infection in very young infants.

Severe disease may be followed by a rise in arterial carbon dioxide tension ($PaCO_2$) (hypercapnia), leading to respiratory acidosis.

PROCESS OF DIAGNOSIS

Diagnosis of bronchiolitis is made on the basis of clinical findings, child's age, the season and the epidemiology of the community. Positive identification of RSV is accomplished by immunofluorescence of nasopharyngeal secretions. The most difficult distinction to make in infants is between bronchiolitis and asthma. Diagnosis of asthma is favoured in repeat attacks, where there is a history of atopy, and if the child responds favourably to the administration of bronchodilators. Chest radiography helps rule out pneumonia.

THERAPEUTIC MANAGEMENT

Bronchiolitis is treated symptomatically with adequate fluid intake and rest. Hospitalization is usually recommended for children with complicating conditions, such as underlying lung or heart disease, associated debilitated states, or questionable adequacy of the caregiver. The child should also be admitted who is tachypnoeic, has marked recessions, seems listless, or has a history of poor fluid intake (Guerra, Kemp, and Shearer, 1990). Oxygen is given in concentrations sufficient to alleviate dyspnoea and hypoxia. Fluids by mouth may be contraindicated because of tachypnoea, weakness, and fatigue; therefore, intravenous fluids are preferred until the crisis of the disease has passed.

Clinical assessments, noninvasive oxygen monitoring, and blood gas values guide therapy. Bronchodilators, corticosteroids, cough suppressants and antibiotics have not proved to be effective in uncomplicated disease and are not recommended for routine use.

Ribavirin, an antiviral agent recently approved for aerosol, is the first specific therapy available for RSV infection. The drug is delivered via a head box. Infants receiving the drug have demonstrated improvement (Hall, 1993; Jury, 1993).

Prognosis
The disease lasts about 3-10 days, and the prognosis is generally good. Although most infants with RSV bronchiolitis appear to recover completely, severe disease is associated with recurrent pulmonary infection and bronchospasm.

	ACUTE EPIGLOTTITIS (SUPRAGLOTTITIS)	ACUTE LARYNGOTRACHEO-BRONCHITIS	ACUTE SPASMODIC LARYNGITIS (SPASMODIC CROUP)	ACUTE TRACHEITIS
Age-group affected	1–8 years	3 months–8 years	3 months–3 years	1 month–6 years
Aetiological agent	Bacterial, usually *H. influenzae*	Viral	Viral with allergic component	Bacterial, usually *S. aureus*
Onset	Rapidly progressive	Slowly progressive	Sudden; at night	Moderately progressive
Major symptoms	Dysphagia	URI	URI	URI
	Stridor aggravated when supine	Stridor	Croupy cough	Croupy cough
	Drooling	Brassy cough	Stridor	Stridor
	High fever	Hoarseness	Hoarseness	Purulent secretions
	Toxic	Dyspnea	Dyspnea	High fever
	Rapid pulse and respirations	Restlessness	Restlessness	No response to LTB therapy
		Irritability	Symptoms waken child	
		Low-grade fever	Symptoms disappear during day	
		Nontoxic	Tends to recur	
Treatment	Antibiotics	Humidity	Humidity	Antibiotics
	Airway protection	Racemic epinephrine		

Table 26-4 Comparison of croup symptoms.

IMPLICATIONS FOR NURSING

The child is placed in a bed away from others, frequently in a small, segregated area used only for children with respiratory infections. Because RSV has been found to be readily transmitted by close contact, precautions against cross-infection are especially important. The primary routes of inoculation for the organisms are the nose and eyes; therefore, infection control should stress handwashing of all persons caring for affected children and keeping their hands away from faces. There has also been controversy over the possible toxicity of ribaviran, as it produced teratogenic effects on laboratory rodents from studies done in the late 70s and early 1980s: to date, all the studies done have indicated not only its efficacy but also its safety in both patients and in health care personnel taking care of children receiving the drug (Englund, 1992).

PNEUMONIA

Pneumonia is common in childhood but occurs more frequently in infancy and early childhood. Morphologically, pneumonias are recognized as lobar pneumonia, bronchopneumonia and interstitial pneumonia (Box 26-7).

In general, pneumonia is caused by four aetiological processes: viruses, bacteria, mycoplasmas and aspiration of foreign substances. The clinical manifestations of pneumonia vary greatly depending on the aetiologic agent, the age of the child, the child's systemic reaction to the infection, the extent of the lesions, and the degree of bronchial and bronchiolar obstruction. The aetiologic agent is identified largely from the clinical history, the child's age, the general health history, the physical examination, radiology, and the laboratory examination.

◆ BOX 26-7

Types of pneumonia

Lobar pneumonia—all or a large segment of one or more pulmonary lobes is involved. When both lungs are affected, it is known as bilateral or 'double' pneumonia.

Bronchopneumonia—begins in the terminal bronchioles, which become clogged with mucopurulent exudate to form consolidated patches in nearby lobules; also called lobular pneumonia.

Interstitial pneumonia—the inflammatory process is more or less confined within the alveolar walls (interstitium) and the peribronchial and interlobular tissues.

VIRAL PNEUMONIA

Viral pneumonias occur more frequently than bacterial pneumonia and are seen in children in all age groups. They are often associated with viral upper respiratory infections, and involve interstitial pneumonitis with inflammation of the mucosa and the walls of bronchi and bronchioles. Of the many viruses that produce pneumonia in children, RSV accounts for the largest percentage. Others are the influenza virus, parainfluenza virus, psittacosis, rhinovirus and adenovirus.

CLINICAL MANIFESTATIONS

The onset may be acute or insidious, and symptoms are variable, ranging from mild fever, slight cough, and malaise to high fever, severe cough, and prostration. Early in the course of the illness the cough is likely to be unproductive or productive of small amounts of whitish sputum.

THERAPEUTIC MANAGEMENT AND IMPLICATIONS FOR NURSING

The prognosis is generally good, although viral infections of the respiratory tract render the affected child more susceptible to secondary bacterial invasion. Treatment is usually symptomatic. Antibiotic therapy is usually reserved for cases in which the presence of infection is demonstrated by appropriate cultures.

PRIMARY ATYPICAL PNEUMONIA

Mycoplasma *(M. pneumoniae)* is the most common cause of pneumonia in children between the ages of 5 and 12 years of age (Moffet, 1989). It occurs principally in autumn and winter months and is more prevalent in crowded living conditions.

CLINICAL MANIFESTATIONS

The onset may be sudden or insidious and is usually manifest first by general systemic symptoms, including fever, chills (in older children), headache, malaise, anorexia and muscle pain (myalgia). Rhinitis, sore throat and a dry, hacking cough may follow. The cough, initially nonproductive, produces seromucoid sputum that later becomes mucopurulent or blood streaked. The duration and degree of fever may last from several days to two weeks. Dyspnoea is uncommon.

THERAPEUTIC MANAGEMENT AND IMPLICATIONS FOR NURSING

Most affected persons recover from acute illness in 7-10 days with symptomatic treatment, followed by a week of convalescence. Hospitalization is rarely necessary. Erythromycin for 2–3 weeks may be effective (Habel, 1993).

BACTERIAL PNEUMONIA

AETIOLOGY AND EPIDEMIOLOGY

Aetiology of pneumonia varies with the age of the child. *S. pneumoniae* (pneumococcus), group A streptococcus, staphylococcus, or enteric bacilli are the most likely agents in infants under three months of age. Chlamydial infection is also a cause of pneumonia in this age group. In the three-month to five-year age group, pneumococcal infection and *H. influenzae* type b are common causes. Pneumococcus accounts for 90% of all bacterial infections in children over age five years (Rao, 1988).

CLINICAL MANIFESTATIONS

Clinical manifestations of bacterial pneumonia in normal children usually appear acutely with fever and toxic appearance. Older children may complain of headache, abdominal pain, or chest pain. Respiratory distress may or may not be present. Initially, cough is usually hacking and nonproductive.

Lack of specific signs indicating infection makes diagnosis in infancy particularly difficult. First evidence of infection is often irritability or lethargy and poor feeding. Abrupt fever may be accompanied by seizures. Respiratory distress is evident with air hunger, tachypnoea, and circumoral cyanosis.

PROCESS OF DIAGNOSIS

Laboratory examination shows elevated white blood cell counts (may be normal in infants with staphylococcal disease) and positive blood cultures in several patients. Children with staphylococcal disease have an elevated antistreptolysin O titre.

THERAPEUTIC MANAGEMENT

Antibiotic therapy has significantly reduced the morbidity and mortality from bacterial pneumonia. Penicillin G is effective in treatment of pneumococcal and streptococcal pneumonia and is implemented as soon as the diagnosis is suspected. Other antibiotics may be used, however. Because staphylococcal infections are caused by penicillin G-resistant staphylococci, semisynthetic penicillins are administered. In hospital, medications are given parenterally for rapid action and maximum effect.

The majority of older children with pneumococcal pneumonia can be treated at home, especially if the condition is recognized and treatment initiated early. Hospitalization is indicated when pleural effusion or empyema accompanies the disease, and is mandatory for children with staphylococcal pneumonia. Pneumonia in the infant or young child is best treated in the hospital, since the course of illness is more variable and complications are more common in very young patients. In addition, intravenous fluid administration is frequently necessary, and oxygen may be required if the child is in respiratory distress.

Prognosis

The prognosis for pneumococcal infections is generally good, with rapid recovery when they are recognized and treated early. The course of staphylococcal pneumonia is generally prolonged.

Complications

At present, the classic features and clinical course of pneumonia are rarely seen because of early and vigorous antibiotic and supportive therapy. However, a large number of children, especially infants, with staphylococcal pneumonia develop empyema, pyopneumothorax or tension pneumothorax. Pleural effusion is not uncommon in children with lobar (pneumococcal) pneumonia. Nonpurulent effusions, such as occur in pneumococcal pneumonia, do not require surgical drainage.

Continuous closed chest drainage is instituted when purulent fluid is aspirated, a frequent finding in staphylococcal infections, and is continued until drainage fluid is free of pathogens - rarely more than 5-7 days.

IMPLICATIONS FOR NURSING

Nursing care of the child with a lower respiratory tract infection is primarily supportive and symptomatic to meet the needs of each child. Rest and conservation of energy are encouraged by relief of physical and psychological stress. The child is disturbed as little as possible by clustering care to encourage the child's regular sleep cycle. Fluids may be administered intravenously during the acute phase. Oral fluids are given cautiously to avoid aspiration and to decrease the possibility of aggravating a fatiguing cough.

Oxygen is administered via a tent, head box, mask or nasal prongs, according to the child's tolerance and age. Children are usually more comfortable in a semi-erect position but should be allowed to determine the position of comfort. Lying on the affected side (if pneumonia is unilateral) splints the chest on that side and reduces the pleural rubbing that often causes discomfort. Fever is usually controlled by a cool environment and administration of antipyretic drugs as prescribed. Temperature is monitored regularly to detect a rapid increase that might trigger a febrile seizure.

Vital signs and chest sounds are monitored to assess the progress of the disease and to detect early signs of complications. Children with ineffectual cough or those with difficulty handling secretions, especially infants, will require suctioning to maintain a patent airway. Postural drainage and chest physiotherapy are generally prescribed every four hours or more often, depending on the child's condition.

Reducing anxiety and apprehension reduces psychological distress in the child and, when the child is more relaxed, the respiratory efforts are lessened. Easing respiratory efforts makes the child less apprehensive, and encouraging the presence of the caregiver provides the child with a customary source of comfort and support.

OTHER INFECTIONS OF THE RESPIRATORY TRACT

Although less common than the previously described illnesses, several infectious disorders are capable of causing significant morbidity, especially in the infant and very young child.

PERTUSSIS (WHOOPING COUGH)

Pertussis, or whooping cough, is an acute respiratory infection caused by *Bordetella pertussis* that occurs chiefly in children younger than four years of age who have not been immunized. It is highly contagious and is particularly threatening in young infants, in whom there is a higher morbidity and mortality rate. The incidence is highest in winter, occurring in cycles with intervals of four years. Pertussis vaccine is effective, but the immunity diminishes with time after the initial infection or immunization. A small number of immunized adolescents and adults develop an asymptomatic type of pertussis (Cromer, Goydos and Hackell, 1993).

TUBERCULOSIS

Tuberculosis (TB) is an ancient disease and, although controlled in most developed countries, still remains a health hazard and a leading cause of death throughout many parts of the world (Murray, 1990). TB in children in the UK is still a problem. Reported cases in 1983 numbered 2.4:100,000 for Caucasian children, 32:100,000 in Indian children, and 52:100,000 in Bangladeshi and Pakistani children (MRC report, 1988). An examination of reported cases in 1988 found that a marked difference in the occurrence of the disease in different ethnic groups remained. The report highlighted the need for improvement in the prevention and control of tuberculosis in children known to be at increased risk (MRC, 1994). Small increases in the total number of notifications were observed in 1988 and 1989 (Joseph, Watson, and Fern, 1992).

AETIOLOGY

TB is caused by *Mycobacterium tuberculosis,* an acid-fast bacillus (i.e., the organism is not readily decolourized by acids after staining). The main types of tubercle bacilli that cause disease in humans are the human *(M. tuberculosis)* and the bovine *(M. bovis).* Children are susceptible to both varieties, but bovine TB has now been eradicated in the UK.

Although the causative agent is the tubercle bacillus, other factors influence the degree to which the organism is able to produce an altered state in the host. Resistance to the bacillus can be modified by several factors (Box 26-8).

CLINICAL MANIFESTATIONS

The disease may be asymptomatic or produce a broad range of symptoms, including general responses such as fever, malaise, anorexia and weight loss or more specific symptoms related to the site of infection (e.g., lungs, bone, brain, kidneys). Lung disease may or may not include cough (which progresses slowly over weeks to months), aching pain and tightness in the chest, and (rarely) haemoptysis.

In children (usually infants) who are unable to contain the spread of infection, the fever persists; the generalized symptoms are manifest; and they develop pallor, anaemia, weakness and weight loss.

PROCESS OF DIAGNOSIS

Several tests and procedures are used to establish a diagnosis. Diagnosis is based on information derived from physical examination, history, reaction to tuberculin tests, radiological examinations, and organism cultures. In addition, it must be determined whether or not the lesion is in the active, quiescent or healed stage.

◆ **BOX 26-8**

Factors affecting resistance to tuberculosis

Heredity
No positive evidence to indicate hereditary tendency
Evidence that resistance to infection may be genetically transmitted

Sex
Early years: no sex differences in incidence
Later childhood and adolescence: morbidity and mortality higher in girls than in boys

Age
Diminished resistance to infection in infancy
  Delay in development of acquired immunity
  Diminished capacity to resist extension of infective process
Increased tendency to develop disease during puberty and adolescence
  New infection superimposed on an old one
  Increased contacts
  Indigenous reinfection stimulated by metabolic changes or suboptimal diets during a period of rapid growth

Stress States
Temporary stressful circumstances (e.g. injury or illness, undernutrition, emotional distress, or chronic fatigue) may increase susceptibility to infection
Increased secretion of adrenal steroids suppresses protective inflammatory response and permits infection to spread
Therapeutic administration of corticosteroids (similar effect)

Nutrition
Active disease inversely proportional to state of nutrition
Excellent nutrition is essential to young children's recovery from disease

Intercurrent Infection
Infectious diseases (especially measles and pertussis) may activate latent tuberculosis

---

History

Symptoms generally do not contribute significantly to a diagnosis. History of possible contact with a person known to be infected or subsequently found to be infected is helpful. All contacts of an affected child are examined for the disease.

Tuberculin test

The tuberculin test is the single most important test to determine whether a child has been infected with the tubercle bacillus. A primary infection initiates a hypersensitivity reaction to the protein fraction of the tubercle bacillus, which can be detected 2-10 weeks after the infection.

The tests most frequently used are the Mantoux and Heaf tests. The Mantoux test contains purified protein derivative (PPD), which is injected intradermally. The Heaf test consists of a multiple puncture skin test, with needles primed with tuberculosis.

A positive reaction indicates that the person has been infected and has developed a sensitivity to the protein of the tubercle bacillus; it does not confirm the presence of active disease. Once individuals react positively, they will continue to do so. A positive reaction in a previously negative reactor indicates the person has been infected since the last test.

A negative reaction will usually mean that the child has never been infected with the organism. However, circumstances may produce a false-negative reaction, e.g., severe malnutrition, intercurrent disease (measles, rubella, mumps), corticosteroids and faulty technique.

Bacteriological examination

A definitive diagnosis is made by demonstrating the presence of mycobacteria in culture. The organism is identified from microscopic examination of properly prepared and stained smears from early morning gastric washings, spinal fluid, draining lymph nodes, and other body fluids.

THERAPEUTIC MANAGEMENT

Medical management consists of adequate nutrition, chemotherapy, general supportive measures, avoidance of exposure to other infections that further compromise the body's defences, prevention of reinfection and sometimes surgical procedures. The child is helped to rest in order to conserve energy, avoid fatigue and decrease metabolic demands. Bed rest is continued until the child is free of fever, exhibits evidence of returning strength, has no manifestations that limit ambulation, and desires to be up and about.

Chemotherapy is the single most important therapeutic modality available for management of TB. A variety of chemical agents can be used, and a regimen involving two or more drugs simultaneously has been found to be effective. Preventative therapy is intended to keep latent infection from progressing to clinically active tuberculosis, as well as being used for primary prevention to prevent initial infection in persons in high risk exposure situations. The most common drug used for this is isoniazid (INH) for 9 months and up to 12 months for the HIV-infected child. The drug has no effect on the child's reaction to tuberculin; therefore, the test continues to be useful in detecting acquired infection. For the child with clinically active tuberculosis, the goal is to achieve sterilization of the tuberculous lesion. Treatment consists of INH, rifampicin and pyrazinamide over 6–12 months. Additional medications used less frequently include streptomycin and ethambutol.

The optimum duration of therapy is unknown, but it is important to treat patients for the shortest period of time. This practice reduces the cost of treatment, diminishes the exposure to toxic effects from the drugs, and increases the likelihood of compliance.

Surgical procedures

Surgical procedures may be required to remove the source of infection in tissues that are inaccessible to chemotherapy or that are destroyed by the disease. Orthopaedic operations for correction of bone deformities, bronchoscopy for removal of a tuberculous granulomatous polyp, or resection of a portion of a diseased lung may also be performed.

Prognosis

Most children recover from primary tuberculosis infection and are often unaware of its presence. However, very young children have a higher incidence of disseminated disease. It is a serious disease during the first two years of life, during adolescence, and in children infected with HIV. Except in cases of tuberculous meningitis, death seldom occurs in treated children.

Prevention

The only certain means to prevent TB is to avoid contact with the tubercle bacillus. Maintaining an optimum state of health with adequate nutrition and avoidance of fatigue and debilitating infections promotes natural resistance, but does not prevent infection. There is no means to induce reliable immunity.

Pasteurization of milk and routine testing and elimination of diseased cattle have helped reduce the incidence of bovine tuberculosis. Infants and children should be given only pasteurized milk from TB-free cattle.

Of concern to hospital personnel is that infected family members may spread the disease when visiting a child in the hospital. The child and all visitors may be restricted to the child's room until the family can be screened for evidence of the disease.

Limited immunity can be produced by administration of the only successful vaccine to date, BCG (bacillus Calmette-Guérin) vaccine containing bovine bacilli with reduced virulence. The freshly prepared vaccine, injected intradermally, produces definite although incomplete protection against tuberculosis. In 1995, the Joint Committee on Vaccination and Immunization is to review its current recommendation that all school children receive the BCG vaccination, in the light of the 1993 notification survey results (Habel, 1993). In spite of government advice, some health authorities have ceased immunizing school children, and others have no policy for the immunization of neonates (Joseph et al, 1992). Given that many children in the UK are now growing up in poverty, notification figures for the 1990s will be particularly significant.

IMPLICATIONS FOR NURSING

Only children with the more serious forms of tuberculosis are placed in the hospital for therapy; others are managed satisfactorily at home. Most children with tuberculosis are nursed within the community.

Asymptomatic children are able to lead an essentially unrestricted life. They can and should attend school (or nursery school), but older children are restricted from vigourous activities such as competitive games and contact sports during the active stage of primary TB. The regular immunization schedule should be continued. Care should be exerted to maintain an optimum health status with proper diet, adequate rest and avoidance of infection.

Diagnosis

Nurses assume several important roles in management of the disease, including assisting with radiological examinations, performing skin tests, and obtaining specimens for laboratory examination. Skin tests, whether used as screening tools or diagnostic aids, must be carried out correctly in order for the results to be accurate. A wheal 6-10 mm in diameter is formed in the skin when the solution is injected. If a wheal is not formed, the procedure is repeated.

Sputum specimens are difficult or impossible to obtain in an infant or young child. Therefore the best means for obtaining material for smears or culture is by aspiration of lavaged contents from the fasting stomach. The procedure is carried out and the specimen obtained early in the morning before the customary breakfast time.

Community care

Since children usually acquire the disease from an adult in the home, parents often feel guilty. Historically, the disease has been regarded with fear, and numerous misconceptions need to be clarified. Reducing parental anxieties helps them to deal with the illness more constructively and to collaborate more effectively in planning for the child's continued care. The success of therapy depends on the acceptance and cooperation of the family. The nurse can help the family to understand the rationale of diagnostic procedures and therapy, and the importance of maintaining the therapeutic plan over the extended period needed for recovery.

Case finding

Every case of tuberculosis identified in the community involves the community health service in follow-up of known contacts — contacts from which the affected person may have acquired the disease and persons who may have been exposed to the diseased individual.

PULMONARY DISTURBANCE CAUSED BY NONINFECTIOUS IRRITANTS

FOREIGN BODY ASPIRATION

Small children characteristically explore matter with their mouths and are therefore particularly prone to aspirate foreign bodies into the air passages. Aspiration of foreign bodies is most commonly seen in children of ages 1-3 years. Dry vegetable matter, such as a seed, nut or piece of carrot or popcorn, that does not dissolve and that may swell when wet creates a particularly difficult problem. The high fat content of potato crisps and peanuts may cause the added risk of lipoid pneumonia. 'Fun foods' of any kind are among the worst offenders.

The types of food items are significant. Aspiration of a foreign body presents a serious and sometimes fatal condition. Severity is determined by the location, type of object aspirated, and extent of obstruction. More than 90% of deaths from food-related asphyxiation occur in children younger than five years of age and 65% in infants. Hot dogs and other meat products, raw apple and carrot, round sweets, nuts, biscuits and grapes comprise more than 40% of all aspirated food items.

A sharp or irritating object produces irritation and oedema. A round, pliable object that does not readily break apart is more likely to occlude an airway than an object with a different shape. Balloons are especially hazardous. A small object may cause little if any pathological change, whereas an object of sufficient size to obstruct a passage can produce various changes, including atelectasis, emphysema, inflammation and abscess.

CLINICAL MANIFESTATIONS

Initially a foreign body in the air passages produces choking, gagging, wheezing or cough. The child's face may become livid and sometimes the child falls unconscious and dies of asphyxiation if the object is not removed. If obstruction is partial, there is often an interval of hours, days, or even weeks without symptoms after the initial period. Secondary symptoms are related to the anatomical area in which the foreign body is lodged and are usually caused by a persistent respiratory infection focused distally to the obstruction. A history of recurrent intractable pneumonia is reason to consider a foreign body in an airway. Often, by the time secondary symptoms appear, the parents have forgotten the initial episode of coughing and gagging. The most common symptoms observed in children brought to medical attention are stridor, wheezing, sternal recession and cough (Esclamado and Richardson, 1987).

PROCESS OF DIAGNOSIS

The diagnosis of a foreign body is usually suspected on the basis of history and physical signs. Radiological examination reveals opaque foreign bodies, but may be of limited use in localizing vegetable matter. Bronchoscopy is usually required for a definitive diagnosis of foreign bodies in the larynx and trachea. Fluoroscopic examination is a valuable aid in detecting and localizing foreign bodies in the bronchi.

THERAPEUTIC MANAGEMENT

Foreign bodies rarely are coughed up spontaneously; therefore, they must be removed instrumentally by direct laryngoscopy or bronchoscopy. After removal of the foreign body, any secondary infection is treated with appropriate antibiotics.

IMPLICATIONS FOR NURSING

A major role of nurses caring for a child who has aspirated a foreign body is to keep the child as quiet as possible while waiting for surgical removal of the object as an agitated child can cause a foreign body to descend and lodge further down in the respiratory tree.

Prevention

Small children should not be allowed access to enticing small objects that they might place in their mouth. Rubber balloons are high-risk items for children; Mylar balloons are the only safe variety for children. Unlikely items (foil tabs from soft drink containers, elastoplasts applied to fingers of infants or very small children, and plastic tabs from price tags on clothing) can be hazardous. Peanut butter should never be given to a child unless it is spread on bread or a cracker. A spoonful of peanut butter can obstruct the airway and stick to mucous membranes, becoming difficult or impossible for the child to dislodge.

Nurses, as child advocates, are in a position to teach prevention in a variety of settings. They can educate parents about hazards of aspiration in relation to the developmental level of their children and encourage them to teach their children safety.

FOREIGN BODY IN THE NOSE

Children will sometimes introduce a foreign object into the nose. This includes such items as food, crayons, small toys, pieces of plastic, beans, beads, erasers, wads of paper, and small stones. A foreign body can be suspected when there is evidence of local obstruction with sneezing, mild discomfort, and (rarely) pain. The irritation produces local mucosal swelling and, with items that increase in size as they absorb moisture (hygroscopic), the signs of obstruction and discomfort increase with time. Infection usually follows, as evidenced by foul breath and a purulent or bloody discharge from one nostril.

Removal is carried out as soon as possible to prevent the risk of aspiration and to prevent local tissue necrosis. Removal can usually be accomplished with topical anaesthesia and either forceps or suction. Infection and irritation usually disappear promptly after removal.

FOREIGN BODY IN THE EAR

A variety of objects can be inserted in the external ear canal by children. First an attempt should be made to remove the object by straightening the ear canal by pulling on the pinna and gently shaking the child's head.

A smooth object (such as a bead) can often be removed by applying a cotton-tipped applicator with warmed dental wax or collodion against the object for 1-2 minutes, then withdrawing the applicator. The object remains attached to the wax or collodion. Irregularly shaped objects might be removed with bayonet forceps, and steel objects (e.g., a ball bearing) can sometimes be removed with a magnetic probe. A right-angle hook or ear curette can be inserted behind the object and the hook withdrawn, pushing the object ahead of it. A simple suction catheter can remove objects that are not firmly embedded.

However, if the object is large, wedged in place, cannot be removed on the first attempt, or the child is uncooperative, referral to an otolaryngologist for removal is necessary to avoid the risk of damage to the tympanic membrane or ossicles.

ASPIRATION PNEUMONIA

Aspiration of fluid or food substances is a particular hazard in the child who has difficulty with swallowing or is unable to swallow because of paralysis, weakness, debility, congenital anomalies such as cleft palate or tracheo-oesophageal fistula, or absent cough reflex (unconscious) or who is force fed, especially while crying or breathing rapidly. The newborn may develop a severe pneumonia from aspirating amniotic fluid and debris during the process of birth. Rarely, aspiration causes immediate death from asphyxia; more often the irritated mucous membrane becomes a site for secondary bacterial infection. In addition to fluids, food, vomitus and nasopharyngeal secretions, other substances that cause pneumonia are hydrocarbons, lipids or powder.

HYDROCARBON PNEUMONIA

Children frequently develop pneumonia secondary to the ingestion of various forms of hydrocarbons, such as petrol, paraffin, solvents, and lighter fluid. Petroleum distillates are generally impure substances and contaminated with heavy metals or other toxic chemicals that can cause systemic as well as local effects. Many, but not all, hydrocarbons are made from petroleum (e.g., turpentine is made from pine oil), and many are found in the home or garage.

On average, children will swallow less than 30 ml (often about 3-4 ml). They begin coughing severely and swallow no more. Although central nervous system abnormalities, gastrointestinal irritation, myocardiopathy, and renal toxicity can all occur, the most serious complication is pneumonitis.

Inducing the child to vomit is contraindicated, because of the renewed danger of aspiration. Hydrocarbons are readily absorbed by the gastrointestinal tract and excreted by the lungs. Bronchitis or pneumonia usually develops early (within the first 24 hours) but may be delayed. Recovery from pulmonary involvement occurs in most instances, despite a severe clinical course. Death, if it occurs, is generally the result of hepatic failure complicated by pulmonary factors. Treatment is the same as for any lower respiratory tract inflammation and consists of oxygen, hydration and treatment of any secondary infection.

LIPOID PNEUMONIA

Oily substances aspirated into the respiratory passages cause progressive changes in lung tissues. First, an interstitial proliferative inflammation occurs that may include an exudative pneumonia. The next stage involves a diffuse, chronic, proliferative fibrosis that is often complicated by acute bronchopneumonia. The final stage features multiple localized nodules or tumour-like paraffinomas. There are no characteristic manifestations. Cough is usually present, and dyspnoea is seen in severe cases. Secondary bronchopneumonia infections are common. The outcome depends on the extent of pulmonary damage, the general condition of the child, and discontinuing the oily inhalation. There is no specific treatment.

POWDER

The use of powder has been discouraged for infants; however, although the incidence has decreased, a significant number of infants suffer talcum powder aspiration. The true incidence of powder inhalation is unknown, but of those with respiratory distress serious enough to be brought to medical attention, the mortality is high.

IMPLICATIONS FOR NURSING

Care of the child with aspiration is the same as that described for the child with pneumonia from other causes. However, the major thrust of nursing care is aimed at prevention of aspiration. Proper feeding techniques should be carried out for weak, debilitated and uncooperative children; and preventive measures are used to prevent aspiration of any material that might enter the nasopharynx.

ADULT RESPIRATORY DISTRESS SYNDROME

Adult respiratory distress syndrome (ARDS) was first described in adults and is now recognized as occurring in children. It has been associated with a large number of clinical conditions and injuries such as sepsis, aspiration, near-drowning, pulmonary contusion and long bone fractures, immune deficiency, metabolic derangements, infections, drug overdose, and multisystem trauma (Sarnaik and Lieh-Lai, 1994). It is characterized by respiratory distress and hypoxaemia that occur within 72 hours from any of the above, and may be described as shock lung, wet lung, stiff lung, congestive atelectasis, and post-traumatic lung.

The hallmark of ARDS is increased permeability of the alveolar-capillary membrane that results in pulmonary oedema. There are essentially three stages of injury: acute phase developing into a latent period, followed by the development of acute respiratory failure, with the final stage involving a recuperative period usually characterized by severe pulmonary abnormalities. During the acute phase, the alveolar capillary membrane is damaged, with an increasing pulmonary capillary permeability with resultant interstitial oedema occurring. The later stages are characterized by pneumoctye and fibrine infiltration of the alveoli, with the start of either the healing process or fibrosis occurring. When the latter occurs, the child may demonstrate respiratory distress and the need for mechanical ventilation.

With ARDS, the lungs become stiff, gas diffusion is impaired, and eventually there is bronchiolar mucosal swelling and congestive ateletasis. The net effect is decreased functional residual capacity and increased pulmonary right-to-left shunting of pulmonary circulation. Surfactant secretion is reduced, and the atelectasis and fluid-filled alveoli provide an excellent medium for bacterial growth.

The child entering into ARDS may first demonstrate only symptoms caused by the injury or infection, but, as the condition deteriorates will manifest with hyperventilation, tachypnoea, increasing respiratory effort, cyanosis and a decreasing oxygen saturation. At times, the developing hypoxaemia is not responsive to oxygen administration.

THERAPEUTIC MANAGEMENT

Based on these symptoms, it is vitally important to begin and continue with careful monitoring and provision of oxygenation and ventilatory function. The majority of treatment modalities is supportive.

Treatment involves general supportive measures such as prevention of infection, maintenance of vascular pressure, adequate nutrition, comfort measures, positioning to improve functional residual capacity, and psychological support. Surfactant therapy that has been successful in infant respiratory distress syndrome may be a definitive therapy for ARDS.

Nursing care involves careful monitoring of pulse, heart rate, perfusion, capillary filling, and urine output, as well as assessment of respiratory status. Respiratory distress is a frightening situation for both the child and the parents, and attention to their psychological needs is a major element in the care of these children.

Recent developments in the treatment of ARDS include: 1) medications to interrupt the formation or activation of mediators contributing to progression of intrapulmonary shunting and lung injury such as nonsteroidal agents; 2) immunotherapy, with monoclonal antibodies that work against the specific toxins causing the lung injury; and 3) human and artificial surfactant to reduce the severity of and sequalae from ARDS, and may be useful in treating lung disease associated with ARDS and near-drowning (Hazinski, 1992).

SMOKE INHALATION INJURY

Several noxious substances that may be inhaled are toxic to humans. They are primarily products of incomplete combustion and cause more deaths from fires than do flame injuries. The severity of the injury depends on the nature of the substances generated by the material being burned, whether the victim is confined in a closed space, and the duration of contact with the smoke.

GENERAL ASPECTS

Possible inhalation injury is suspected when there is a history of flames in a closed space whether or not burns are present. Sooty material around the nose or in the sputum, singed nasal hairs, or mucosal burns of the nose, lips, mouth, or throat are all signs that the affected person demands observation for possible pulmonary injury from inhalants. A hoarse voice and cough are further evidence of airway involvement, and increased inspiratory and expiratory stridor indicates severe damage to the upper passages. Smoke inhalation causes three different types of injury: heat, local chemical and systemic.

Heat injury

Heat causes thermal injury to the upper airways, but since air has low specific heat, the injury goes no further than the upper airway. Reflex closure of the glottis prevents injury to lower airways. Heat may reach the middle airway occasionally but it rarely penetrates to the lungs.

Chemical injury.

A wide variety of gases may be generated during the combustion of materials such as clothing, furniture, and floor coverings. Acids, alkalis, and their precursors in smoke can produce chemical burns. These substances can be carried deep into the respiratory tract, including the lower respiratory tract, in the form of insoluble gases. Soluble gases tend to dissolve in the upper respiratory tract.

Inhalation of small amounts of noxious irritants produces alveolar and bronchiolar damage that can lead to obstructive bronchiolitis. Severe exposure causes further injury, including alveolar-capillary damage with haemorrhage, necrotizing bronchiolitis, inhibited secretion of surfactant, and formation of hyaline membranes — manifestations of ARDS described in the previous section.

Systemic injury

Gases that are nontoxic to the airways (e.g., carbon monoxide [CO] and hydrogen cyanide) can cause injury and death by interfering with or inhibiting cellular respiration. When it enters the bloodstream, CO readily binds reversibly with haemoglobin to form carboxyhaemoglobin (COHb). Because it combines more readily and is released less readily, very low levels of tissue oxygen levels must be reached before appreciable amounts of oxygen are released from the haemoglobin. Therefore, tissue hypoxia reaches dangerous levels before oxygen is available to meet tissue needs.

The signs and symptoms of CO poisoning are secondary to tissue hypoxia and vary with the level of COHb. Mild manifestations include headache, visual disturbances, irritability, and nausea, whereas more severe intoxication causes confusion, hallucinations, ataxia and coma. CO may increase cerebral blood flow, increase cerebral capillary permeability, and increase cerebrospinal fluid pressure, all of which contribute to the central nervous system (CNS) signs observed. The bright, cherry-red lips and skin often described are less often observed; more frequently pallor and cyanosis are seen.

THERAPEUTIC MANAGEMENT

When inhalation injury is suspected, the patient is given humidified 100% oxygen by mask. If CO poisoning is confirmed, 100% oxygen is continued until COHb levels fall to the nontoxic range of about 10%, and artificial ventilation may be implemented in selected cases. Where a hyperbaric oxygen chamber is available, the breakdown of the CO-haemoglobin bond is greatly accelerated. Other therapies that may be used but that remain controversial are transfusion with washed red blood cells to increase the oxygen carried to tissues, and hypothermia to reduce the tissue demand for oxygen and to prevent CNS complications.

Respiratory distress may occur early in the course of smoke inhalation as a result of hypoxia, or patients who are breathing well on admission may later develop sudden respiratory distress. Intubation is often necessary when: (1) severe burns in the area of the nose, mouth, and face increase the likelihood of developing oropharyngeal oedema and obstruction; (2) vocal cord oedema causes obstruction; (3) the patient has difficulty handling secretions; and (4) progressive respiratory distress requires artificial ventilation.

Use of corticosteroids, although controversial, may be of value in reducing oedema, and bronchodilators are often given intravenously or by nebulizer. A broad-spectrum antibiotic is sometimes administered prophylactically, but this too is controversial.

IMPLICATIONS FOR NURSING

Nursing care of the child with inhalation injury is the same as that for any child with respiratory distress. Vital signs and other respiratory assessments are performed frequently, and the pulmonary status is carefully observed and maintained. Pulmonary physiotherapy is usually performed.

In addition to the observation and management of the physical aspects of inhalation injury, the nurse also deals with the psychological needs of a frightened child and distraught parents. As with any accidental injury, the parents feel overwhelming guilt, even when the injury occurred through no fault of their own. More often, however, the injury could have been prevented, which compounds their guilt feelings. They need a great deal of support and reassurance, as well as information about the child's condition, treatment and progress.

PASSIVE SMOKING

Numerous researchers have investigated the effects of environmental pollution on children's health and have determined that the worst pollutant is parental smoking, especially maternal smoking. It has been found that children in passive smoking situations have an increased number of respiratory illnesses when compared with children of nonsmoking parents and that the number of illnesses is positively correlated with the number of cigarettes smoked (Neuspiel *et al*, 1989; Chen, Li, and Yu, 1986; Ogston, 1985, Pedreira *et al*, 1985). Parental smoking may have a deleterious effect on children's growth (Rona *et al*, 1981). In the UK, 50% of children live in a house where at least one adult smokes (Couriel, 1993).

IMPLICATIONS FOR NURSING

Passive smoking during childhood may well be the most important precursor of chronic lung disease in the adult. Nurses could play a stronger role in ridding children's environments of tobacco smoke by informing parents; setting an example for children and families; and becoming advocates for 'no smoking' ordinances in public places and prohibition of advertising tobacco products in the media. Where smokers are unable to stop, home rules could be established for reducing smoke in the child's environment; for example, not smoking when the child is in the room or in those rooms they most often occupy.

LONG-TERM RESPIRATORY DYSFUNCTION

Respiratory disorders that assume a long-term aspect are not uncommon in childhood. They are responsible for significant morbidity and school absenteeism, as well as altering the quality of life and physical and social development of children. Bronchial asthma is prominent among these, and cystic fibrosis is the most common inherited disease of children.

ALLERGIC RHINITIS

Allergic rhinitis is the most common of all allergic disorders and, although not life-threatening, is a significant cause of morbidity in all age groups. The manifestations may be episodic or perennial. Seasonal allergic rhinitis, also known as 'hay fever', occurs during certain months of the year and does not develop until the individual has been sensitized by two or more pollen seasons.

CLINICAL MANIFESTATIONS

Symptoms of allergic rhinitis may include paroxysms of sneezing; itching of the nose, eyes, palate, pharynx, and conjunctiva; nasal stuffiness progressing to partial or total obstruction of air flow; and mucus secretion, frequently accompanied by postnasal drainage. Classic facial features often exhibited by affected children include an open mouth caused by chronic nasal obstruction ('allergic gape'), discoloration and oedema around the eyes from chronic nasal obstruction, transverse nasal crease from the 'allergic salute' (rubbing of the nose), and radiating lines in the lower orbitopalpebral grooves (*Dennies lines*).

Other symptoms may appear during peak symptom periods, including tearing and soreness of the eyes and gelatinous conjunctival discharge in the morning, irritability, fatigue, depression, and loss of appetite. Chronic rhinitis leading to significant nasal obstruction can lead to various abnormalities in growth and development and in psychosocial and intellectual development (Pearlman, 1988).

PROCESS OF DIAGNOSIS

Diagnosis of allergic rhinitis is based on a thorough history and physical examination. Since allergic rhinitis is often associated with atopic dermatitis or asthma, examination of the skin and chest is indicated (Simons, 1988). Other tests that may be used include mucus examination for eosinophils, superficial biopsy of nasal mucosa, fibreoptic rhinoscopy, blood examination for elevated eosinophils, and various challenge tests.

Sensitization testing

Tests for sensitization to specific allergens include skin tests, the radioallergosorbent test (RAST) and related tests (David, 1994). Skin testing involves injection of specific allergens and remains the most commonly used diagnostic test for allergy. After a suitable time period (10-30 seconds) the size of the resultant wheal and flare reaction is measured to assess the patient's sensitivity. The magnitude of the wheal and flare response correlates roughly with the severity of symptoms produced by natural exposure to the same allergen; however, a positive skin test does not always indicate the presence of clinical reactivity (Wood and Sampson, 1987).

Skin testing and immunotherapy are generally safe procedures, but they are not without risk. Severe and even fatal reactions can occur within a short period of time, depending on the type of extract used and sensitivity of the individual. To minimize the risk of severe reactions the child should remain under observation for at least two hours.

The RAST test, which measures the specific immunoglobulin E (IgE), requires only one serum sample. Allergists are divided in their preferences between skin and RAST tests. All agree that the tests should be used as supplemental procedures for history and physical examination and not as screening tools.

THERAPEUTIC MANAGEMENT

Therapy is directed towards avoidance of offending allergens, medication, and immunotherapy (hyposensitization or desensitization). Avoidance measures involve removing allergens from the environment and are usually effective for allergy to foods, drugs, and animals.

If a patient is unable to avoid the allergens, symptoms can be controlled with drugs in many cases. However, treatment should be highly individualized. Four main classes of drugs are used: H_1-receptor antagonists (antihistamines), adrenergic and anticholinergic drugs, disodium cromoglycate, and topical corticosteroids.

Antihistamines are the preferred medications, and any of a variety of these drugs are effective. If nasal obstruction is a prominent feature, relief can often be obtained from an α-adrenergic decongestant given singly or in combination with an antihistamine. Disodium cromoglycate is used prophylactically on a regular basis and is effective in preventing both the early and late responses to antigen. For cases that cannot be controlled with the previous therapies, some suggest the use of topical (nasal) corticosteroids.

Immunotherapy may be necessary if drug therapy and avoidance of allergens are ineffective in controlling symptoms or if drugs evoke undesirable side effects. Skin tests are performed to determine the offending antigens and desensitization injections are carried out. About 80-90% of patients achieve significant clinical improvement, but the duration of immunotherapy injections depends on the patient's overall clinical response.

IMPLICATIONS FOR NURSING

Nurses can help affected children by recognizing the existence of rhinitis and referring them for diagnosis and therapy.

The major nursing goal in care of the child with allergic rhinitis is preparation for skin tests and desensitization injections, which are the source of greatest stress to children. It is difficult to make them understand how inflicting discomfort regularly over a long time is going to make them better.

To help allay children's fears of skin tests, they need a careful and thorough explanation of what is to be done. The skin is pricked with a stylet, then a drop of allergen is placed on the pierced skin.

BRONCHIAL ASTHMA

Asthma is an obstructive disease of the airways characterized by reversible hyperreactivity of the bronchi and trachea to a variety of stimuli. All triggers produce the same response in the airways - constriction of the smooth muscles of the airway, inflammation and oedema of the bronchial mucosa, and increased production of bronchial mucus. Manifestations most frequently associated with asthma are coughing and wheezing.

The incidence, severity, and mortality associated with asthma have risen steadily throughout the world (Williams, 1989). Asthma is the most common cause of school absences and is responsible for a major proportion of paediatric admissions to casualty departments and hospitals (Eggleston, 1990). Although the onset of asthma may be at any age, 80% of children have their first symptoms before five years of age

(Habel, 1993). Boys are affected more frequently than girls until adolescence when the incidence is approximately equal (Avery and First, 1989).

Asthma can be classified as *intermittent,* in which the child is symptom-free for extended periods without medication, and *chronic,* which describes the child who requires frequent or continuous medical therapy. Both intermittent and chronic disease are variable in intensity, and the choice of therapy depends on both the classification and the severity.

AETIOLOGY

While the exact aetiology of asthma remains equivocal, evidence suggests that the disease occurs from hypersensitivity to environmental substances which trigger an allergic reaction. A strong relationship exists between viral infections and asthma induction in infants, with allergens playing a less important role in this age group because it takes time for allergic sensitivity to develop. While there tends to be a family predisposition toward hyperactivity of the airways, this relationship remains just one variable as a potential cause of asthma.

The allergic reaction in the airways is significant for two reasons: 1) it can cause an immediate reaction, with obstruction occurring, and 2) it can precipitate a late bronchial obstructive reaction several hours after the initial exposure. This delayed bronchial response is associated with an increase in the airway hyperresponsiveness to nonimmunological stimuli and can persist for several weeks or more after a single allergen exposure (National Heart, 1991).

While allergy does provide an explanation for triggering asthma, there are instances where no allergic process can be detected. Asthma is an extremely complex disorder involving biochemical, immunological, infectious, endocrine, and psychological factors.

Numerous stimuli have been found to provoke an asthma attack, including viruses, allergens, smoking (both active and passive), cold air, exercise and inhaled irritants. Of these, viral infection of the airways is the most common trigger of asthma in children, with RSV and parainfluenza viruses the most frequent offenders. Bacterial infection is rarely associated with triggering a hyperreactive airway response. Psychological stress has been named as a trigger in the past, but there is no evidence to indicate that this contributes to asthma in early childhood (Weinberger, 1989). Less frequently, sulphites in food and non-steroidal anti-inflammatory drugs are the responsible triggers.

CLINICAL MANIFESTATIONS

Timing of symptoms varies markedly among patients. Bronchoconstriction in response to an allergen can have an immediate, histamine-type pattern or a late response with airway hypersensitivity lasting for days, weeks, or months. Since a second wave of symptoms sometimes appears 6-8 hours after the initial antigen exposure, patients should have sufficient medicine to control late response symptoms if they occur.

It has been observed that children may experience a pro-dromal itching localized at the front of the neck or over the upper part of the back. An asthmatic episode begins with a hacking, paroxysmal, irritative and nonproductive cough caused by bronchial oedema. Accumulated secretions, acting as a foreign body, stimulate the cough. As the secretions become more profuse, the cough becomes rattling and pro-ductive of frothy, clear, gelatinous sputum. Bronchial spasm and mucosal oedema reduce the size of the bronchial lumen, which is, as a result, more easily occluded by mucous plugs.

A common symptom of asthma is coughing in the absence of respiratory infection, especially at night. This may disrupt sleep, leading to excessive fatigue during the day and poor school performance. Wheezing may be mild or discernible only on auscultation at the end of expiration, or severe enough to be audible. The child is frequently short of breath.

The child with a more severe attack is short of breath and tries to breathe more deeply; the expiratory phase becomes pro-longed and is accompanied by an audible wheezing. The child often appears pale, but may have a malar flush and red ears. The lips assume a deep, dark red colour that may progress to cyanosis observed in the nail beds and skin, especially around the mouth. The child is restless and apprehensive with an anxious facial expression. Sweating may be prominent as the attack progresses. Older children have a tendency to sit upright with shoulders in a hunched-over position, hands on the bed or chair, and arms braced to facilitate the use of accessory muscles of respiration. The child speaks with short, panting, broken phrases. Infants and small children are restless, irrita-ble and difficult to make comfortable.

The prolonged expiratory phase is less apparent in infants and young children, because of a more pliable chest and the normal rapid respiratory rate. Wheezing can be heard, becoming more high pitched as obstruction progresses. With minimal obstruction, wheezing may be only mild or even absent, but can be accentuated by rapid, deep breathing.

With severe spasm or obstruction, air flow may be so limited there is no wheezing and may be misinterpreted as improve-ment by unknowing examiners. Cough is ineffective despite repeated, hacking manoeuvres.

Children with chronic asthma develop generalized vascu-larization, mucosal thickening, and hypertrophy of the mucous glands and fibres of the bronchial musculature. With repeated episodes, the thoracic cavity becomes fixed in a hyperventilat-ed state (barrel chest) with depressed diaphragm, elevated shoulders, and use of accessory muscles of respiration.

PROCESS OF DIAGNOSIS

A diagnosis of asthma is most often made on the basis of history of symptoms and physical examination.

Generally, chronic cough in the absence of infection or diffuse wheezing during the expiratory phase of respiration is sufficient to establish a diagnosis, particularly if the child has a persistent night-time cough. Most children with asthma are well nourished and do not display signs of chronic hypoxia.

Diagnostic tests

The anteroposterior (AP) diameter may be increased (barrel chest), and chest radiographs show hyperexpansion of airways. Pulmonary function tests reveal air trapping and decreased expi-ratory flow and are helpful in diagnosis and follow-up of patients with asthma. Measurements of forced expiratory volume at one second (FEV_1), forced respiratory capacity (FRC), respiratory volume (RV), and total lung capacity (TLC) provide some indication of the degree of obstruction and are used for both diagnosis and as guidelines for management.

THERAPEUTIC MANAGEMENT: GENERAL

The overall goal of asthma management is to prevent disabil-ity and to minimize physical and psychological morbidity — to assist the child in living as normal and happy a life as possible (Box 26-9). This includes facilitating the child's social adjustments in the family, school and community, and normal participation in recreational activities and sports. To accom-plish these goals, efforts are directed towards recognizing acute episodes early and implementing appropriate therapy, iden-tifying and eliminating irritant and allergic factors from the child's environment, educating parents to the long-term nature of the disease and how to manage exacerbations, and helping the child to deal constructively with the disease. Adherence to the prescribed regimen is essential to successful management. Since asthma is a chronic condition with acute exacerbations, treatment requires a continuous care approach to prevent an episode and to control symptoms.

Allergen control

Basic to any therapeutic plan is an evaluation of the child's general health and an assessment of the specific allergenic factors and the nonspecific factors that precipitate symptoms. House dust mites and other components of house dust are the agents identified most often in children allergic to inhalants. Other causes are animal dander (especially cats and dogs), fungi, and allergenic pollens. Irritants that can cause bron-choconstriction in individuals with asthma, whether or not there is allergy, are cigarette smoking — especially parental smoking — paraffin stoves and open fires.

Often, simply removing the offending environmental factors will decrease the frequency of attacks; for example, removal of a dog or cat from the home of a child sensitive to animal dander.

Drug therapy

The goal is to control the acute attack; therefore, early recog-nition and treatment at the onset are most important. Provid-ing rapid relief of the bronchospasm reduces the need for drastic measures and increases the likelihood that relief will be complete.

Pharmacological therapy is used to treat reversible airflow obstruction and airway hyperresponsiveness. Consensus reports have indicated the need to use anti-inflammatory drugs as the primary agents to control chronic childhood asthma, as well as to consider the use of cromolyn sodium as a first-line agent (Larsen, 1992; Murphy and Kelly, 1992, 1993). Medications available include the following categories:

1. Anti-inflammatory agents, such as corticosteroids, cromolyn sodium or cromolyn-like compounds, and other agents.
2. Brochodilators, such as β-adrenergic agonists and methyl xanthines
3. Anticholinergic agents.

β-Adrenergic agents

β-Adrenergic agonists (primarily salbutamol, terbutaline and salmeterol) are the medications of choice for treatment of acute exacerbations of asthma and for the prevention of exercise-induced asthma. Most β-adrenergics used in asthma therapy affect only beta-2 receptors, which help eliminate bronchospasm. Beta-1 effects, which are reflected in increased heart rate and gastrointestinal disturbances, have been minimized. β-Adrenergic agonists can be given via inhalation or as oral or parenteral preparations. The inhaled drug, administered by metered-dose inhaler (MDI), rotahaler, diskhaler, turbohaler or nebulizer, has a more rapid onset of action than the oral form but is more costly. The MDI may have a spacing unit or reservoir attached, which makes it easier for small children to use. Inhalation also reduces troublesome systemic side effects — irritability, tremor, nervousness and insomnia.

Inhaled β-adrenergics can be taken two to four times daily for acute symptoms. Children with exercise-induced bronchospasm are advised to use the drug prophylactically 10-15 minutes before exercise. Small children who have difficulty using the MDI can get effective relief with nebulization.

Methylxanthines

The methylxanthine drugs, principally theophylline, have been used for decades to relieve symptoms and prevent asthma attacks and are prepared for oral or rectal administration. Theophylline, however, is now considered a third line agent and perhaps even unnecessary for treating asthma exacerbations (Weinberger, 1993; Murphy and Kelly, 1993). The drug is available in sustained-release form so it can be taken once or twice daily. The rectal form is rarely used because of its variable and unpredictable absorption. Theophylline is given by injection as ammophylline (a combination of theophylline and ethylenediamine), which is more soluble than theophylline. In addition to its potent bronchodilator effect, theophylline is also a central respiratory stimulant and increases respiratory muscle contractility (Galant, 1987).

The dose of theophylline varies with age. Children over 12 months of age metabolize the drug faster than adults, so the dose per kilogram must be higher. Because absorption also varies among individuals, it is important to follow serum levels of the drug until a therapeutic dose is achieved. Symptoms of toxicity include nausea, tachycardia and irritability; and rarely, seizures and dysrhythmias. Questions surrounding theophylline have largely focused on safety issues rather than efficacy (Murphy and Kelly, 1993). The most recent review of 125 patients' intoxications over five years suggests a more severe outcome at lower concentrations for chronic toxicity (Shannon and Lovejoy, 1992).

Recent reports suggest that theophylline causes behaviour problems and poor school performance in children (Gutstadt *et al*, 1989; Rachelefsky *et al*, 1986) and depression and anxiety (Furukawa *et al*, 1988). Other researchers challenge these findings (Rappaport *et al*, 1989; Weinberger *et al*, 1987). Further and more definitive studies need to be conducted to confirm or deny these observations.

Corticosteroids

Corticosteroids are the most potent drugs available for treatment of asthma. They diminish the inflammatory cell responses and restore β-adrenergic sensitivity. The drugs can be given intravenously, orally, or topically by aerosol, diskhaler, or rotahaler. Metabolism is slow; therefore results are delayed for up to six hours, and one daily dose is usually sufficient. Inhaled corticosteroids are not effective for acute attacks. Intravenous administration is warranted during acute, severe exacerbations. Oral steroids can be taken without risk of adrenal suppression if given every other day or daily administration is limited to seven days (Goldenhersh and Rachelefsky, 1989). Tapering must be planned if the hormone is prescribed for an extended period. Patients who are steroid dependent may require increased dosage for periods of stress or exacerbation of respiratory illness. Corticosteroids are life-saving in status asthmaticus.

Sodium cromoglycate

Cromoglycate is neither a bronchodilator nor an anti-inflammatory agent, but acts superficially to inhibit mast cell degranulation in both early and late phases of asthma. The action is essentially prophylactic and is of no value when administered after the allergic reaction; it cannot reverse bronchospasm.

◆ BOX 26-9

Goals of asthma therapy

1. Control symptoms to the maximum possible with a minimum number of the safest medications.
2. Relieve airway obstruction and normalize pulmonary function.
3. Prevent acute episodes that require emergency treatment.
4. Reduce the number and frequency of hospitalizations.
5. Educate the patient and family to understand, accept, and manage asthma within the context of the family's life-style.
6. Participate in normal daily activities and sports without restrictions or with minimum and specific restrictions.
7. Improve the long-term prognosis.
8. Achieve normal growth and development.
9. Minimize school absenteeism.

Modified from Hen J: An overview of pediatric asthma, *Pediatr Ann* 15:92, 1985.

Cromoglycate is administered via nebulizer, MDI or spinhaler, and a single dose inhibits allergen-, exercise-, and sulphur dioxide-induced asthma. It has virtually no toxicity and few side effects (Eggleston, 1990), although it may produce airway irritation and aggravation of cough in some patients.

Anticholinergics

Anticholinergic therapy, the oldest form of bronchodilator therapy for asthma, works by reducing the intrinsic vagal tone to the airways and blocking reflex bronchoconstriction caused by inhaled irritants. The principle reasons these agents are not favoured is due to the length of time for onset of action, as well as adverse side effects such as drying of respiratory secretions, blurred vision, and cardiac and central nervous system stimulation. The primary drugs used are atropine or its derivative ipratropium, which does not cross the blood–brain barrier and therefore elicits no CNS effects. Ipratropium has been shown to be effective during status asthmaticus when used in nebulized form in combination with adrenergics (National Heart, 1991).

Chest physiotherapy

Chest physiotherapy (CPT) is a standard adjunct to treatment of chronic asthma. This includes breathing exercises, physical training and inhalation therapy. These therapies help produce physical and mental relaxation, improve posture, strengthen respiratory musculature and develop more efficient patterns of breathing.

Hyposensitization

The role of hyposensitization in childhood asthma has not been clarified. In many cases, the child demonstrates multiple sensitivities, which makes such therapy impractical. Moreover, the injections can be expensive and uncomfortable. Currently, within the UK, hypersensitization is not part of widespread practice.

Exercise

Airway obstruction often develops in children with asthma. *Exercise induced asthma (EIA),* does not represent a unique syndrome, but rather an example of the airway hyperactivity common to all persons with asthma. EIA is defined as an acute, reversible, usually self-terminating airway obstruction that develops 5-15 minutes after strenuous exercise and lasts 15-60 minutes after the onset (Pierson, 1988). Usually, the episode subsides spontaneously in 0.5-1 hour.

Pretreatment with a bronchodilator provides relief through the exercise period. Inhaled β-adrenergic agonists or sodium cromoglycate provide protection in the majority of cases.

Children with asthma are sometimes excluded from exercise by parents and teachers. Children themselves may also avoid exertion from reluctance to provoke an attack. This can seriously hamper peer interaction. It has been found that moderate or even strenuous exercise is advantageous for children with asthma.

Participation in sports is encouraged, but should be evaluated on an individual basis in terms of tolerance for duration and intensity of effort.

Prognosis

The outlook for children with asthma varies widely. An impressive number of children become asymptomatic at puberty, but there is no factor that can predict which children will 'outgrow' their asthma. Some develop other forms of allergy in adulthood. It has been postulated that just as the skin manifestations of infancy (eczema) shift to the bronchi in childhood, there may be another shift in the susceptible tissues (shock organ) at adulthood — most frequently to the nose.

The prognosis for control or disappearance of symptoms will differ from children who have rare and infrequent attacks to those who are constantly wheezing or are subject to status asthmaticus. In general, the more severe and numerous the symptoms, the longer they have been present, and a family history of allergy increases the likelihood of a poor prognosis. Many who outgrow their attacks are subject to exercise-induced asthma as adults.

Deaths from asthma have been relatively uncommon, especially in young age groups, but increases have been reported from various regions worldwide (McFadden and Gilbert, 1992). Adolescents appear to be the most vulnerable, with the greatest increase occurring in the ages between 10-14 years. To reduce the risk of mortality, it is essential that hospitals should permit free access and have a clear protocol for the management of children with severe asthmatic attacks (Fletcher *et al*, 1990).

THERAPEUTIC MANAGEMENT: SPECIFIC

Children are subject to asthmatic exacerbations at varying intervals, with severity ranging from wheezing to life-threatening status asthmaticus. The modes of management vary according to the frequency and severity of the disease.

Intermittent (mild) asthma

Children with intermittent asthma have extended symptom-free periods, and their symptoms are usually relieved promptly with medical intervention. A variety of drug therapies are available for management, most commonly a short course of inhaled or oral bronchodilators. When symptoms have disappeared for several days, the drugs are discontinued. Occasionally, children with intermittent asthma have severe episodes requiring a short course of corticosteroids for control.

Status asthmaticus

Children who continue to display respiratory distress, despite vigorous therapeutic measures, are considered to be in *status asthmaticus*. The condition may develop gradually or rapidly, often coincident with complicating conditions such as pneumonia that can influence the duration and treatment of the attack. Status asthmaticus is a medical emergency that can result in respiratory failure and death if untreated.

Persistent hypoventilation leads to accumulation of carbon dioxide, with a decrease in arterial pH and respiratory acidosis. As a result, compensatory buffering mechanisms become overtaxed and the pH may drop to dangerous levels. Vomiting and dehydration cause further reduction of arterial pH by promoting retention of metabolic acids. Therapy of status asthmaticus is directed towards correction of dehydration and acidosis, improvement of ventilation, and treatment of any concurrent infection.

A child suspected of status asthmaticus is usually admitted to a paediatric intensive care unit for close observation and continuous cardiorespiratory monitoring.

The child is given intravenous fluids and nothing by mouth except liquids if the condition permits. Correction of dehydration, acidosis, hypoxia and electrolyte derangements is guided by frequent determination of arterial pH, blood gases and serum electrolytes.

Bronchospasm is relieved by constant intravenous infusion of aminophylline and β-adrenergic agents via nebulizer, regulated by continual monitoring. Corticosteroids are given for any child with severe asthma who does not improve immediately, who has been taking steroids chronically, or who does not respond to other therapy (Eggleston, 1990).

Humidified oxygen is administered to maintain saturation at 90-95% to avoid the danger of oxygen narcosis. Controlled ventilation with endotracheal intubation may be needed when the condition progresses to respiratory failure, but it is rarely needed for more than 12 hours.

Sodium bicarbonate is administered to correct acidosis, since pH less than 7.25 impairs systemic, pulmonary and coronary blood flow; normal pH enhances the response of bronchial smooth muscle to bronchodilator therapy (Galant, 1987). Antibiotics are frequently prescribed, since infection may be masked or may not always be evident and is always a threatening complication. As the attack subsides, fluids and medication are given orally (adrenergic agonists may be administered by MDI, diskhaler, or spinhaler) and discharge plans are begun, especially follow-up care. Administration of steroids is withdrawn as soon as possible.

IMPLICATIONS FOR NURSING—ACUTE CARE

Children who are admitted to the hospital with acute asthma are ill, anxious, and uncomfortable. In most instances, children are admitted as an emergency with status asthmaticus and are in acute distress. The importance of continual observation and assessment cannot be overemphasized.

An intravenous infusion is begun immediately, and medication, usually corticosteroids and aminophylline, is administered to relieve bronchospasm. The child is monitored closely and continuously during aminophylline administration for relief of respiratory distress and signs of side effects or toxicity.

Side effects from aminophylline include nausea, headache, irritability and insomnia. Early signs of toxicity are nausea, tachycardia and irritability; seizures and dysrhythmias.

If aerosol medications are administered, the β-adrenergics are administered first to open the airways before administration of anti-inflammatory agents.

It is especially important that the child receives sufficient fluid either orally or intravenously to replace losses through diaphoresis and hyperventilation. Liquids are best tolerated if they are warm or at room temperature. Cold liquids can trigger reflex bronchospasm and should be avoided (Seaman-Bates, 1980). Nourishment is provided in small, frequent feedings to avoid abdominal distention that might interfere with diaphragm excursion.

Children usually prefer the high-Fowler position, although they may be more comfortable sitting upright or leaning slightly forward. When possible, the nurse communicates in such a way that a child need only reply in a few words to avoid fatigue. Shortness of breath makes talking difficult. Oxygen is indicated for relief of dyspnoea and cyanosis, and is regulated according to the blood gas analysis and objective observation of colour, respiratory effort and sensorium.

Children in status asthmaticus are apprehensive and anxious. Moreover, they are usually tired from respiratory efforts and loss of sleep. The calm, efficient presence of a nurse helps to reassure them that they are safe and will be cared for during this stressful period. It is important to assure children that they will not be left alone and that their parents are allowed to be near and available when needed.

Parents need reassurance, too. They want to be informed of their child's condition and therapies. They are upset and apprehensive about the child's condition. Often, they feel that they may have in some way contributed to the child's condition or could have prevented the attack. They may even feel, consciously or unconsciously, anger towards the child for continuing to display symptoms despite their efforts to prevent or control the attack. Reassurance about their efforts expended on the child's behalf and their parenting capabilities can help alleviate their stress. All efforts to reduce parental apprehension will, in turn, help reduce the child's distress. Anxiety is easily communicated to the child from parents and members of the staff.

IMPLICATIONS FOR NURSING — GENERAL CARE

Nursing care of children with asthma involves both acute and long-term care. Nurses who are involved with children in the home, clinic or general practice play an important role in helping the child and family to learn to live with the condition. The disease can be tolerated if it does not interfere with family life, physical activity or school attendance, or if it does not require hospitalization.

Assessment

A respiratory assessment as described earlier is necessary. Physical characteristics of chronic respiratory involvement are noted and evaluated, including chest configuration (such as barrel chest), posturing and type of breathing. A history of current and previous attacks and precipitating factors is important. An assessment is made of: (1) the degree to which the disorder interferes with everyday activities; (2) alteration in the child's self-concept; and (3) the extent to which the family and child feel in control of the disorder and able to comply with the prescribed regimen.

Planning

The plan of care for a child with asthma includes the following:

1. Eliminate or avoid proven or suspicious irritants and allergens.
2. Relieve bronchospasm.
3. Maintain optimum health.
4. Prevent complications.
5. Promote normal activities.
6. Support and educate child and family regarding the disease and its management.

Implementation

The major emphasis of nursing care is directed towards outpatient management by the family. Parents are even able to manage acute attacks if they maintain contact with the practitioner and know how to observe for the expected response and signs of probable toxicity.

Allergen avoidance

The primary goal of asthma management is avoidance of an attack. Parents need to know the nature of the disease and, when the allergens are determined, how they can avoid and/or relieve asthmatic attacks. The nurse assists the parent in modifying the environment to reduce contact with the offending allergen(s). The parents are cautioned to avoid exposing a sensitive child to excessive cold, wind or other extremes of weather, smoke, sprays or other irritants. Passive smoking has been associated with exacerbation of symptoms in children with hyperresponsive airways, especially in boys and older children (Murray and Morrison, 1989).

Foods known to provoke symptoms should be eliminated from the diet. Food additives (especially monosodium glutamate [MSG]), sulphites, and dyes) have been reported to produce allergic responses in sensitive people. Families are taught to read labels carefully for the presence of these substances.

Paracetamol is recommended as the analgesic of choice. Children with aspirin-induced asthma may also be sensitive to nonsteroidal anti-inflammatory drugs and tartrazine (yellow dye number 5, a common food colouring) (Tan and Collins-Williams, 1982). In the UK, aspirin is not recommended for children under 12 years (unless they have rheumatic disease) because of a strong correlation with Reye's syndrome. In theory, therefore, children should not present with aspirin-induced asthma, but it is important for nurses to ensure that parents are cautioned against the use of aspirin in any child with asthma. Other drugs that should be avoided by children with asthma are antihistamines (dry airway secretions, making expectoration difficult), cough suppressants (impair clearance of secretions), and sedatives (depress respirations and aggravate hypoventilation).

Relieve bronchospasm

The parents and older children need to learn how to use the medications prescribed to relieve bronchospasm. They are taught to recognize early signs and symptoms of an impending attack so that it can be controlled before symptoms become distressing. Most children can recognize prodromal symptoms well before an attack (about six hours) so that preventive therapy can be implemented. Some objective signs that parents may observe include rhinorrhoea, cough, low-grade fever, irritability, itching (especially in front of neck and chest), apathy, anxiety, sleep disturbance, abdominal discomfort and loss of appetite. A simple, inexpensive peak expiratory flowmeter is available for use in the home to help the parents and child assess the extent of the symptoms.

Children who use a nebulizer or aerosol device to deliver drugs need to learn how to use the device correctly. It is important that the child learns to breathe slowly and deeply for better distribution to narrowed airways. Rapid inspiration causes the drugs to move through unobstructed bronchioles to patent airways where they are less needed. Controversy exists regarding the amount of time to wait between puffs. Recommendations range from 2–10 minutes.

Young children and those who are otherwise unable to manipulate the device or coordinate breathing with activation of the MDI are able to use special chambers called spacers. These permit an operator to deliver the medication from the MDI into the spacer from which the child inhales. Children aged from 3–4 years should be able to use a rotahaler or diskhaler, which deliver their medication in the form of a dry powder.

Parents and child are taught to report any changing reaction to a drug or if the drug appears to be losing its effectiveness, as evidenced by more frequent need for the drug.

Maintain health and prevent complications

The child should be protected from a respiratory infection that can trigger an attack or aggravate the asthmatic state, especially in young children. The equipment used for the child, such as nebulizers, must be kept absolutely clean to decrease the chances of contamination with bacteria and fungi. Oral candidiasis is a major complication of aerosolized steroids; therefore children with severe asthma who are taking steroids by this route are taught to rinse the mouth thoroughly with water after each treatment to minimize the risk of infection.

Breathing exercises and controlled breathing are taught and encouraged for the motivated youngster, and the nurse can help to select activities suitable to the child's capacity. Anything that promotes proper diaphragmatic breathing, side expansion, and generally improved mobility of the chest wall is encouraged.

Promote normal activities

Self-care is the hallmark of effective asthma management, and self-management programmes are important in helping the child and family to learn as much as possible about the factors that precipitate an asthma attack and the most effective means of bringing the disease under control.

Asthma is a very common disease, and to have asthma is annoying but not disgraceful. Even though emotions have been implicated in asthma, psychological aspects are primarily a response to it rather than a cause.

People with asthma are able to live full and active lives. Learning about others who have accomplished their goals and meeting children of the same age who are dealing effectively with their disease, including engaging in age-related activities, such as sports, provide positive examples of what is possible.

It is much easier to prevent than to treat an asthmatic attack. The importance of compliance to a therapeutic programme and learning the activities or factors that trigger an attack are emphasized. Sustained-release medications and appropriate drug administration before exercise or with a respiratory infection have made it possible for children with asthma to avoid an attack.

Asthma education and awareness are an important aspect of asthma management. Although the principles of self-management are very general, each child and family have their own special needs that require individualized care and attention. Families may also obtain information from organizations such as the Asthma Training Society.

Child and family support

The nurse working with children with asthma can provide them with support in several ways. Many asthmatic children voice frustration about the ways their attacks interfere with their goal achievements and social lives. They need education about their disease, and they need to realize that it is not as bad as they might think. Children, their families, and their peers need to know what to do to prevent an attack and what to do during an attack. These children need reassurance from the health team and reinforcement of their coping mechanisms.

Both short- and long-term adaptation of affected children to the disease depends to a great extent on the family's acceptance of the disorder. The task of living day-to-day with affected children involves the family continually. There are periodic crises and the ever-present threat of a crisis, requiring parental vigilance, sleepless nights, and frequent emergency trips to the hospital, involving expense. Throughout these stresses, parents are expected and encouraged to promote as normal a life as possible for their children without neglecting the needs of siblings. Nurses can contribute to family coping by helping families set up support groups (Swallow and Thompson, 1992).

Evaluation

The effectiveness of nursing interventions is determined by continual reassessment and evaluation of care based on the following observational guidelines and expected outcomes:
1. Interview family about removal or avoidance of known allergens.
2. Observe child for evidence of respiratory symptoms.
3. Assess child's general health.
4. Observe child and interview family about any infections or other complications.
5. Interview child about daily activities.
6. Determine the degree to which the family and child understand the child's condition and the extent to which the therapies are carried out.

CYSTIC FIBROSIS

Cystic fibrosis (CF) is the most common serious pulmonary and genetic disease of children. CF, a multisymptom disorder, primarily affects the exocrine (mucus-producing) glands of white children. In the early 1950s, life expectancy for children with CF was very short. It is estimated that individuals born with CF in the 1990s can be expected to survive into their forties; the outlook appears even better when one considers the advances in new therapies, impact of protein and gene therapy, continued aggressive chest physiotherapy, aerosolized antibiotic therapy and nutritional education (Collins, 1992; Elborn, Shale and Britton, 1991).

AETIOLOGY

CF is inherited as an autosomal recessive trait, with the affected child inheriting the defective gene from both parents with an overall incidence of 1:4. In 1989, researchers discovered that the mutated gene responsible for CF was located on the long arm of chromosome seven (Kerem *et al*, 1989). Since that time, almost 300 alterations that diverge from the original sequence of the gene have been reported; at least 230 of these are associated with disease. Among them, the ΔF508 is the most common alteration, found in about 70% of all known CF chromosomes (Tizzano and Buchwald, 1993). Variance in the mutation does result in some phenotypic variation, but concordance for ΔF508 leads to both pancreatic deficiency and pulmonary disease (Fulginiti and Lewy, 1993). Although both sodium and chloride are affected, the defect appears to be primarily a result of abnormal chloride movement (Quinton, 1989).

CLINICAL MANIFESTATIONS

The clinical manifestations vary widely among children with CF and change as the disease progresses. The usual pattern is one of failure to thrive, with an increased weight loss despite an increased appetite, and gradual deterioration of the respiratory system. The diagnosis is not readily apparent in most cases, especially when there is no familial evidence of disease. Some children display symptoms at birth; others may not develop symptoms for weeks, months, or years. Some show only mild forms of the disease with limited impairment of digestion and respiratory problems, whereas others have severe malabsorption and life-threatening pulmonary complications. Although most affected children display both pulmonary and GI symptoms, a few have only enzyme deficiency without pulmonary disease; and a few have only pulmonary disease without pancreatic insufficiency.

Respiratory tract

Initial pulmonary manifestations are often wheezing respirations and a dry, nonproductive cough. Eventually, diffuse bronchial and bronchiolar obstruction leads to irregular aeration with progressive pulmonary disturbance and secondary infection. Dyspnoea increases, the cough often becomes paroxysmal, and the mucoid impactions within the small air passages cause a generalized obstructive emphysema and patchy areas of atelectasis.

Progressive pulmonary involvement with hyperaeration of functioning alveoli produces an overinflated, barrel-shaped chest. When ventilation is significantly impaired, cyanosis and clubbing of fingers and toes occur. The child suffers repeated episodes of bronchitis and bronchopneumonia, and is subject to chronic sinusitis and nasal polyps. Respiratory symptoms mimic diseases such as pneumonia, bronchitis, asthma, whooping cough, tuberculosis and bronchiectasis.

Gastrointestinal tract

The earliest postnatal manifestation of CF is *meconium ileus,* which occurs in 7-10% of newborns with the disease (McMullen, 1992). Thick, puttylike, tenacious, mucilaginous meconium blocks the lumen of the small intestine, which gives rise to signs of intestinal obstruction, including abdominal distention, vomiting, failure to pass stools, and rapid development of dehydration with associated electrolyte imbalance.

As the disease progresses, obstruction of pancreatic ducts prevents digestive enzymes (trypsin, chymotrypsin, amylase, lipase) from being released into the duodenum, which prevents conversion of ingested food into compounds that can be absorbed by the intestinal mucosa. Consequently, the nondigested food is excreted (chiefly unabsorbed fats and proteins), increasing the bulk of faeces to two or three times the normal amount. The bulky nature of the stools may go unnoticed at first, but usually by six months of age the child passes large, loose stools with normal frequency or a chronic diarrhoea of unformed stools. As solid foods are added to the diet, the excessively large stools become frothy and extremely foul smelling.

Because so little is absorbed from the intestine, affected children have difficulty maintaining weight, despite a healthy appetite and diet. The impaired ability to absorb fats results in a deficiency of the fat-soluble vitamins A, D, E, and K (which causes easy bruising); and anaemia is a common complication. These GI symptoms are similar to those seen in children with coeliac disease, and failure to thrive is a frequent initial diagnosis in young children with CF. When the child is ill with an infection, especially *Pseudomonas,* the appetite usually decreases with subsequent weight loss. Sometimes hospitalization is necessary.

Affected children of all ages are subject to peptic ulcers, pancreatic insufficiency, and intestinal obstruction from inspissated or impacted faeces. Abdominal distention is common, abdominal cramps may be excessive, and foul-smelling flatus is a common complaint. Malnutrition is another commonly associated problem.

Reproductive system

Reproductive systems of both males and females with CF are affected. Females with CF have normal fallopian tubes and ovaries, but fertility can be inhibited by highly viscous cervical secretions, which act as a plug, blocking sperm entry. With few exceptions, males are sterile, which may be caused by blockage of the vas deferens with abnormal secretions or by failure of normal development of the wolffian duct structures (vas deferens, epididymis, and seminal vesicles), resulting in decreased or absent sperm production.

Integumentary system

The consistent finding of abnormally high sodium and chloride concentrations in the sweat is a unique characteristic of CF. Parents frequently observe that their infants taste 'salty' when they kiss them. The chloride channel defect in sweat glands prevents reabsorption of sodium and chloride, which leaves the affected person at risk for abnormal salt loss, dehydration, and hypochloraemic and hyponatraemic alkalosis during hyperthermic conditions. This is especially important to the infant, because of limited fluid stores and the potential for inadequate sodium intake with most commercially prepared infant formulas.

PROCESS OF DIAGNOSIS

An initial evaluation is conducted with general appraisal in the areas of general activity, physical findings, nutritional status, and findings on chest x-rays. The diagnosis of CF is suspected in the child who fails to thrive or has frequent upper respiratory infections and is established on the basis of duplicate sweat chloride tests. Diagnosis of CF requires a positive sweat test result in the presence of either clinical symptoms consistent with CF or a family history of CF.

The quantitative sweat chloride test (pilocarpine iontophoresis) involves stimulating the production of sweat, collecting the sweat, and measuring the sweat electrolytes. The quantitative analysis requires a minimum of 50 mg of sweat; 75-100 mg is preferable. Two separate samples are collected to assure the reliability of the test for any individual. Because newborns do not have active sweat glands, it is often difficult to obtain an adequate sample for analysis. Therefore, if results are questionable, the test is repeated at a later date. Sodium of >70 mmol/kg on a sample weighing 100 mg is indicative of CF.

Chest x-ray reveals characteristic patchy atelectasis and obstructive emphysema. Pulmonary function tests are sensitive indexes of lung function, providing evidence of abnormal small airway function in CF. Other diagnostic tools that may aid in diagnosis include stool fat and/or enzyme analysis. Stool analysis requires a 72-hour sample with accurate recording of food intake during that time. Radiographs, including barium enema, are used for diagnosis of meconium ileus.

SCREENING FOR CYSTIC FIBROSIS

The impact of genetic discoveries on understanding aetiology and treatment is only beginning to unfold at the same time that approaches to detection are changing to reflect new technologies. The standard methods of diagnosis rely on either detection of abnormal chloride secretion in sweat or, in newborns, on elevated immunoreactive trypsinogen (Fulginiti and Lewy, 1993). Carrier screening is available and reliable for siblings and family members of a child with CF (Beaudet *et al*, 1989). Development of DNA probes, however, has enabled the identification of the disease in families in which there is an individual affected with CF. The tests detect the major gene defect (ΔF508) for CF, which is located in about 70% of white and 30% of black cases. Heterozygote screening and prenatal testing will continue to be studied and researched during the 1990s.

THERAPEUTIC MANAGEMENT

The improved survival rate of patients with CF during the past two decades is attributable largely to antibiotic therapy and improved nutritional management. Goals of therapy, therefore, include: 1) to prevent or minimize pulmonary complication; 2) to assure adequate nutrition for growth; and 3) to assist the child and family in adapting to a chronic disorder. In attempting to attain these, there is a multi-system approach to treatment. Current and future technologies are examining the methods of lessening the effects of the CFTR and are gearing up for direct attacks on the defect rather than reliance on management of the end results, i.e., traditional treatment for pulmonary and gastrointestinal complications. Some of these new modalities include (Fulginiti and Lewy, 1993; Tizzano and Buchwald, 1993; McMullen, 1992):

1. Blockade of the 'sodium pump' by the aerosolized drug amiloride hydrochloride (changes transmembrane chloride transport in respiratory epithelia and inhibits sodium and thus water reabsorption)
2. Use of various substances intended to alter the characteristically abnormal mucus in the airways (e.g., DNase I)
3. Aerosolized agents such as α1-antitrypsin to inhibit neutrophil elastase (a powerful enzyme that causes inflammation)
4. Drugs that promote chloride secretion
5. Replacement gene therapy.

Management of pulmonary problems

Management of pulmonary problems is directed towards prevention and treatment of pulmonary infection by improving aeration, removing mucopurulent secretions, and administering antibiotics. Most children will develop respiratory symptoms by three years of age. Young children normally have small airways and are predisposed to frequent viral infections. The large amounts and viscosity of respiratory secretions in children with CF contribute to the likelihood of infection. Once infection becomes established in relatively defenceless lungs, it is difficult to eradicate.

Prevention of infection involves a daily routine of chest physiotherapy. In theory, postural drainage and percussion of the lungs loosen and move secretions towards the glottis to facilitate expectoration. Numerous studies have been conducted to evaluate the efficacy of the procedure. Several researchers have pursued the concept that exercise, deep breathing, and directed coughing are just as effective in preventing pulmonary deterioration. However, patients have been found to regress when conventional chest physiotherapy (CPT) is discontinued (Reisman *et al*, 1988). Therefore, although it is time-consuming for the child and family, conventional physiotherapy remains the cornerstone of pulmonary therapy.

Physiotherapy is usually performed twice daily (on rising and in the evening) and more frequently if needed, especially during pulmonary infection. Bronchodilator medication delivered in an aerosol helps open bronchi for easier expectoration and is administered before physiotherapy when the patient exhibits evidence of reactive airway disease. No effective agents are available to decrease viscosity of secretions or break up mucus secretions. Mist therapy is of little proven value.

Another form of aerosolized medication is *recombinant human deoxyribonuclease (DNase)*, a drug developed from the original DNA medications which were found to decrease the viscosity of mucus. The dosing schedule may involve inhalation three times a day, five days a week, for two weeks; it is well tolerated and has no major adverse effects (minor reactions are all typical of the patients' underlying disease prior to treatment). In addition, improvements in spirometry, pulmonary function tests and dyspnoea scores have been seen, as well as the reduction in viscosity of sputum (Aitken *et al*, 1992).

Forced expiration, or 'huffing', with the glottis partially closed helps move secretions from small airways so that subsequent coughing can move secretions forcefully from large airways (Sutton, 1988). Several studies indicate this manoeuvre enhances the pulmonary function of patients with CF (Bain, Bishop and Olinsky, 1988).

Physical exercise is an important adjunct to daily conventional physiotherapy. Exercise not only stimulates mucus secretion, it also provides a sense of well-being and increased self-esteem. In some instances, exercise can be substituted for CPT.

Pulmonary infections are treated as soon as they are recognized. Some practitioners prefer to prescribe oral antistaphylococcal drugs prophylactically at the time of diagnosis; others begin therapy when pulmonary symptoms arise. Sputum culture and sensitivity guide the choice of antibiotic. The trend is toward aggressive therapy even for milder disease.

Colonization with *P. aeruginosa* signals progressive involvement. Although the bacteria are impossible to eradicate, they can be successfully controlled for many years. Once the organism has become established, antibiotic therapy is most effective when given intravenously. Patients with CF metabolize antibiotics more rapidly than normal; therefore, drug dosage is often higher than would be expected. Duration of therapy depends on the patient's response, measured with clinical indicators including cough, fatigue, and exercise intolerance in addition to tests such as pulmonary function tests (PFTs), chest radiograph, and O_2 and CO_2 measurements.

Intravenous antibiotics can be administered at home as an alternative to hospitalization as long as the family agrees and regular monitoring for toxicity can be accomplished. Legal and ethical implications of home administration of antibiotics should be fully explored before decisions on care are made.

Oxygen administration is usually recommended for children with acute episodes where O_2 saturations are low, but since many of these children have chronic CO_2 retention, the unsupervised use of oxygen can be harmful.

Haemoptysis occurs frequently in older children with CF, but is usually mild and often associated with exacerbation of bacterial infection of the airway. Bronchoscopy may be performed to determine the bleeding site, and bronchial artery embolization or lobectomy may be necessary.

Cor pulmonale is right ventricle hypertrophy in response to increased resistance in the pulmonary vascular bed. Low-flow O_2 therapy can reverse some of the pulmonary hypertension induced by alveolar hypoxia. O_2 is usually begun when arterial saturation is below 90% for extended periods and is often administered at nighttime only, so that the patient can be up and about unhindered during the daytime (Wheeler and Colton, 1988). Diuretics, digitalis, and salt restriction can be helpful in decreasing the vascular load on the right heart. In advanced disease, the right heart decompensates and congestive heart failure becomes evident.

Lung transplantation is a final therapeutic option for children with advanced pulmonary vascular disease who are severely disabled by dyspnoea and hypoxia. The obstacles surrounding this technique are availability of donated organs and complications from surgery (Fiel, 1993).

Management of gastrointestinal problems

The principal treatment for pancreatic insufficiency is replacement pancreatic enzymes, which are administered with meals and snacks to ensure that digestive enzymes are mixed with food in the duodenum. Enteric-coated products prevent the neutralization of enzymes by gastric acids, thus allowing activation to occur in the alkaline environment of the small bowel. The amount of enzymes depends on the severity of the insufficiency and the response of the child to enzyme replacement. Usually 1-5 capsules are administered with a meal, and a smaller amount is taken with snacks. The amount of enzyme is adjusted to achieve normal growth and a decrease in the number of stools to two or three per day.

Children with CF require a well balanced, high-protein and high-calorie diet (the latter due to the impaired intestinal absorption). They often require up to 150% of the recommended daily allowances in order to meet their needs for growth. Breastfeeding with enzyme supplementation should be continued whenever possible for parents who prefer this method and, when necessary, supplementation of higher calorie per ounce formula. For formula-fed infants, cow's milk formulas are usually adequate, though frequently a hydrolysate formula with medium-chain triglycerides (such as Pregestimil or Alimentum) may be recommended. Enzymes are mixed into cereal or fruit. Since the uptake of fat-soluble vitamins is decreased, water-miscible forms of these vitamins (A, D, E, K) are given, along with multivitamins and the enzymes. While fat restriction is not necessary (Luder *et al*, 1989) one concern is that other nutrients might not be provided from a diet with increased fats. When high-fat foods are eaten, the child is encouraged to add extra enzymes. Pancreatic enzymes should not be taken within 30 minutes of eating, and the beads should not be chewed or crushed: by destroying the enteric coating, inactivation of the enzymes and excoriation of oral mucosa can occur.

Children with CF should thrive with adequate replacement therapy and calorie intake. Failure to thrive despite adequate nutritional support usually indicates deterioration of pulmonary status. Occasionally, patients will be placed on supplemental tube feedings of parenteral alimentation in an effort to build up nutritional reserves. This therapy may result in short-term improvement; however, long-term benefits have not been demonstrated (Stern, 1986).

Salt depletion through sweating can be a problem during hot weather or physical exertion. Most children are able to adjust salt to their needs, and older children often exhibit a preference for salty foods. Salt supplementation is often needed during hot weather or febrile periods.

Prognosis

Despite over 40 years of progress and a recent surge in new treatment modalities, cystic fibrosis remains a progressive and incurable disease. It is the pulmonary involvement that ultimately determines the patient's outcome, since pancreatic enzyme deficiency is less of a problem if adequate nutrition is ensured. With the advances in technology, parents and adolescents are now being challenged to set future goals that may include college, careers, social relationships, and marriage. Concurrently, they are faced with the increasing morbidity and higher rates of CF complications as they grow older.

IMPLICATIONS FOR NURSING

Nursing care of infants and children with CF involves both acute and chronic management. These children require regular observation and medical supervision, including ongoing assessment of general health and nutritional and pulmonary status. The nurse's contact with an affected child usually begins when the child is brought to the hospital or clinic for confirmation of the diagnosis. Perhaps the reason for hospitalization is failure to thrive or recurrent respiratory infections. Later, during recurrent admission to the hospital or during ongoing follow-up in the clinic or at home, the nurse, child and family develop a sustained relationship.

Assessment

Assessment of the child with CF involves both pulmonary and GI observations. Pulmonary assessment is the same as that described for bronchial asthma, with special attention to lung sounds, observation of cough, and evidence or degree of finger clubbing. GI assessment primarily involves observing the frequency and nature of the stools and abdominal distention. The observer is also alert to evidence of failure to thrive (e.g., weight loss, wasting, pallor and fatigue). Family members are interviewed to determine the child's eating and eliminating habits, to observe salty perspiration, and to confirm a history of frequent respiratory infections or bowel obstruction in infancy.

Planning

Nursing objectives for the child with CF include the following:
1. Promote pulmonary function, especially improve aeration and facilitate lung clearance.
2. Promote intake and absorption of nutrients.
3. Prevent or manage complications.
4. Facilitate growth and maintain optimum health.
5. Promote normal activities.
6. Support and educate child and family.

Implementation

On the initial contact, nurses are involved in assisting with diagnostic tests, primarily sweat for laboratory analysis of chloride content and, less often, stool specimens for trypsin and fat. The child, usually an infant, needs comfort during the procedures; young children need distraction while they are confined during iontophoresis. Children need an explanation of the strange, and sometimes painful, procedures and the equipment used for tests and treatments.

Parents are anxious and puzzled. Few of them have any understanding of the disease process and the long-term implications it has for their family. They need patient and careful explanations of the disease, how it might affect their family, and what they can do to provide the best possible care for their child.

Hospital care

When the child is hospitalized for confirmation of pulmonary complications, aerosol therapy is instituted or continued. Respiratory therapy is usually initiated and supervised by a physiotherapist. Occasionally, it may be the responsibility of the nurse to perform the prescribed aerosol therapy. Chest physiotherapy should not be performed before or immediately after meals.

Oxygen is cautiously administered to children in respiratory distress, but the child requires frequent assessment. The hazard of oxygen narcosis is a constant threat in children with long-standing disease who receive oxygen. The child requires close observation to assist with cough and expectoration.

The diet is implemented for the newly diagnosed child or continued for the child who is hospitalized for pulmonary disease. Children in the early stages of the disease maintain a good appetite, and some will eat excessively. With infection and increased lung involvement, the appetite diminishes, however. Some children may object to the extra fluids that are encouraged to prevent dehydration. Food is considered therapy for these patients. The caloric intake should be increased significantly. Pancreatic enzymes are supplied for each meal or snack, and adequate salt is provided, especially for febrile children.

Intravenous fluids and blood tests are almost always a part of the treatment, and the child soon associates hospitalization with these stress-provoking procedures.

Support to both child and family is a vital part of nursing care. The progressive nature of the disease makes each illness requiring hospitalization a potentially life-threatening event. Skilled nursing care and sympathetic attention to the emotional needs of the child and family help them cope with the stresses associated with repeated respiratory infections and hospitalization.

When discussing the nature of the illness and the genetic aetiology, families should have access to counselling. It is important that the family fully understands the 1:4 likelihood of an affected child with each pregnancy.

Home care

After the diagnosis is confirmed and a treatment programme determined, preparation for home care is implemented. A plan of care should be flexible enough so that family activities are disrupted as infrequently as possible. They will need opportunities to learn about and practice the use of the equipment, as well as some of the problems they may encounter.

They need to learn about the preferred diet of nutritious meals with tolerated fat and ample protein and carbohydrate, and the administration of pancreatic enzymes. It is important to stress to parents that the enzymes, in the amount regulated to the child's needs, should be administered with all meals and snacks, excluding most fruits and fruit sweets. They are cautioned about not restricting salt, especially during hot weather, and ensuring an adequate fluid intake, since dehydration aggravates the thick mucus secretions. Oral hygiene is important because of interference with salivation and the increased susceptibility to oral infections.

One of the most important aspects of educating parents for home care is teaching chest physiotherapy and breathing exercises. The number of times these therapies are performed each day is determined on an individual basis, based on severity of disease and amount of mucus produced each day.

For children up to the age of 2–3 years, physiotherapy consists of postural drainage and percussion, and can be delivered whilst the child is on their parent's knee. A wedge is used for postural drainage in children aged 3–7 years. From about two years of age, the physiotherapist may introduce breathing exercises and, eventually, the "active cycle of breathing technique" (Webber, 1994). From the age of seven, tippling frames are more frequently used. By the age of 16, children can be totally independent in their physiotherapy, as clapping is now considered to be less important than tipping and breathing exercises.

Other physiotherapy treatments have been shown to be effective. These include positive expiratory pressure (PEP) mask therapy (Falk *et al*, 1984; Oberwaldener *et al*, 1986).

Other techniques rely only on breathing techniques to move secretions. The method is chosen which is found to be most effective and convenient for the child.

For pulmonary infection, home intravenous antibiotics may be prescribed. Home intravenous care is preferred for willing and competent families who have access to good support services.

The nurse can assist the family in contacting resources that provide help to families with affected children, such as the Cystic Fibrosis Trust in the UK. The Trust raises money to fund vital hospital and university research into improved treatment and prevention of CF. It also provides a network of support and advice groups for people with CF and their families.

Family support

One of the most important and difficult aspects of providing care for the family of a child with CF is coping with the emotional needs of the child and family. The diagnosis, treatment, and prognosis are fraught with many problems, frustrations, and feelings. The diagnosis with all its implications evokes feelings of guilt and self-recrimination in parents. These feelings may be particularly marked if the newly diagnosed child is the second affected child in the family, and the parents had been counselled about the 1:4 risk of such an event occurring.

Both the child and the family must make many adjustments, the success of which depends on their ability to cope and also on the quality and quantity of support they receive from outside sources. Combined efforts of a variety of health professionals offer the most comprehensive services to families. It is often the responsibility of the nurse to organize and coordinate these services, to assess the home situation, and to collect the data needed to evaluate the effectiveness of the services in meeting the family's needs.

For the family, the illness means modification of numerous family activities. CPT must be continued wherever the child may be. In addition, members of the family hesitate to take the child too far from familiar and trusted medical care.

The persistent need for treatment several times daily also places a strain on the family. When possible, occasional trusted respite care should be made available to the parent or parents to allow them the opportunity to leave the situation for short periods without undue anxiety about the child's welfare.

The affected child also may become resentful about the disease, its relentless routine of therapy, and the necessary curtailment it places on activities and relationships. The child's activities are interrupted or built around treatment, medications, and diet that impose hardships (such as carrying medication to school and other places where the child may eat away from home), and growth retardation may be trying. Any of these aspects of the disease may be the cause of ridicule from other children. However, the child should be encouraged to attend school and join age-appropriate groups, such as scouting, to foster a life that is as normal and productive as possible.

A constant source of anxiety for both parents and child is the ever-present fear of death. However, despite the prognosis of a shortened life span, numerous hospitalizations and unpleasant complications, children with CF have been found to be amazingly well adjusted (Cowen, 1986). Patients and their siblings show generally healthy self-esteem, and family functioning is normal.

As the disease progresses, however, family stress should be expected, and the patient may become angry and noncompliant. It is important for the nurse to recognize the changing needs of the family. Families should be made aware of sources for counselling as stressful setbacks occur. Patients need to be guided into activities that enable them to express anger, sorrow and fear without guilt.

As life expectancy continues to rise for children with CF, issues related to marriage, childbearing and career choice become more pressing. Men must be informed at some point that they will be unable to produce offspring. It is important that the distinction be made between sterility and impotence. Normal sexual relationships can be expected. Some female patients may be able to bear children, but must be made aware of the possible deleterious effects on the respiratory system created by the burden of pregnancy. They need to know that their children will be carriers of the CF gene.

Life as an independent adult, the goal that most families have for their children, should be encouraged for children with CF. From the time that children can take partial responsibility for their own care (e.g., CPT and taking enzymes), independence and accountability should be fostered. Although the prognosis for these children has improved, many do not survive through the second decade. Anticipatory grieving and other aspects related to care of a child with a terminal illness are part of nursing care.

Evaluation

The effectiveness of nursing interventions is determined by continual reassessment and evaluation of care based on the following observational guidelines and expected outcomes:

1. Monitor vital signs (especially respiratory parameters), chest physiotherapy, and exercise to assess the expected outcomes (e.g., expectoration of secretions, increased lung expansion).

2. Observe nutritional intake and enzyme administration. For the child at home, interview family about child's intake or have the child maintain a log of nutritional intake. Obtain regular measurements of growth.

3. Monitor child for evidence of respiratory infection, GI dysfunction, and other complications. Interview family about prophylactic medications, procedures, and activities.

4. Perform regular physical assessments. Interview family about the child's health status and maintenance (e.g., dental care).

5. Observe child and activities selected for participation. Interview child and family about school attendance, interaction with peers, and participation in sports and other activities.

6. Explore family's understanding of the disease and its therapies and their ability to carry out the treatment plan. Maintain contact with family (if feasible) at follow-up evaluations and home care. Observe for readmissions. Interview child and family about involvement with agencies and services for children with CF.

KEY POINTS

◆ Several anatomical features predispose infants and young children to airway obstruction and atelectasis: there is less alveolar surface for gas exchange, narrowly branching peripheral airways become easily obstructed, and lack of collateral pathways inhibits ventilation beyond obstructed units.

◆ Pulse oximetry is a noninvasive method of determining the O_2 saturation in the blood. One limitation of the technology is that it does not identify dangerously high O_2 levels.

◆ Chest physiotherapy is useful for patients with increased sputum production, but is contraindicated for some.

◆ Occlusion of the tracheostomy tube is life-threatening; therefore, equipment for replacing a tube must always be at hand.

◆ Symptoms of respiratory tract infections include fever, febrile convulsions, meningismus, anorexia, vomiting, diarrhoea, abdominal pain, nasal blockage and discharge, cough, respiratory sounds and presence or absence of sore throat.

◆ Severe bleeding from the tonsil site can occur within six hours after surgery or 5-10 days after tonsillectomy.

◆ Epiglottitis is a medical emergency and is characterized by high fever, toxic appearance, and difficulty swallowing.

◆ Inducing a child to vomit is contraindicated in the event of hydrocarbon ingestion because of the danger of hydrocarbon aspiration.

◆ Bronchial asthma can be triggered by a variety of agents and is characterized by bronchospasm, oedema of the bronchial mucosa, and increased bronchial mucus secretion.

◆ Diagnosis of cystic fibrosis is based on family history, absence of pancreatic enzymes, chronic pulmonary involvement, and an abnormally high sweat chloride concentration.

REFERENCES

Aitken M et al: Recombinant human DNase inhalation in normal and cystic fibrosis subjects: a phase 1 study, *JAMA* 267(14):1947, 1992.

Alderson SH, Warren RH: Pediatric aerosol therapy guidelines, *Clin Pediatr* 23:553, 1984.

Alho OP et al: Control of the temporal aspect when considering risk factors for acute otitis media, *Arch Otolaryngol Head Neck Surg* 119:444, 1993.

Avery ME, First LR, editors: *Pediatric medicine,* Baltimore, 1989, Williams & Wilkins.

Bain J, Bishop J, Olinsky A: Evaluation of directed coughing in cystic fibrosis, *Br J Dis Chest* 82:138, 1988.

Beaudet A et al: Linkage disequilibrum, cystic fibrosis, and genetic counselling, *Am J Hum Genet* 44:319, 1989.

Blumer JL: *A practical guide to pediatric intensive care,* ed 3, St Louis, 1991, Mosby.

British Medical Journal: *Advanced paediatric life support: the practical support,* London, 1993, BMJ.

Calvi A: Care of the child requiring long-term mechanical ventilation, *Pediatr Nurs Update* 1(6):1, 1985.

Centers for Disease Control: Assessing exposures of health care personnel to aerosols of ribavirin—California, *MMWR* 37:560, 1988.

Chandra NC, Hazinski MF, editors: *Textbook of basic life support for healthcare providers,* 1994, American Heart Association.

Chen Y, Li W, Yu S: Influence of passive smoking on admissions for respiratory illness in early childhood, *BMJ* 293:303, 1986.

Collins F: Cystic fibrosis: molecular biology and therapeutic implications, *Science* 256:774, 1992.

Conrad DA et al: Aerosolized ribovarin treatment of respiratory syncytial virus infection in infants hospitalized during an epidemic, *Pediatr Infect Dis* 6:152, 1987.

Cowen L et al: Psychologic adjustment of the family with a member who has cystic fibrosis, *Pediatr* 77:745, 1986.

Cunningham DG et al: Unprescribed use of antibiotics in common childhood infections, *J Pediatr* 103:747, 1983.

Cromer BA, Goydos J, Hackell J: Unrecognized pertussis infection in adolescents, *Am J Dis Child* 147:575, 1993.

Dinwiddie R: *The diagnosis and management of paediatric respiratory disease,* London , 1990, Churchill Livingstone.

Dodge JA, Goodall J, Geddes D: Cystic fibrosis in the United Kingdom 1977–85: an improving picture, *BMJ* 297(6633):1599, 1988.

Duncan B et al: Exclusive breast-feeding for at least 4 months protects against otitis media, *Pediatrics* 91(5):867, 1993.

Eggleston PA: Asthma. In Oski FA et al, editors: *Principles and practice of pediatrics,* Philadelphia, 1990, JB Lippincott.

Elborn J, Shale D, Britton J: Cystic fibrosis: current survival and population estimates to the year 2000, *Thorax* 46:881, 1991.

Ellis EF: Allergic disorders. In Behrman RE, Vaughan VC: *Nelson textbook of pediatrics,* ed 13, Philadelphia, 1987, WB Saunders.

Englund J et al: High-dose, short duration ribavirin aerosol therapy in children with suspected RSV infection, *J Pediatr* 117:313, 1990

Esclamado RM, Richardson MA: Laryngotracheal foreign bodies in children, *Am J Dis Child* 141:259, 1987.

European Resuscitation Council: Guidelines for paediatric life support, *BMJ*, 305:1345, 1993

Falk M et al: Improving the ketchup bottle method with positive expiratory pressure (PEP): a controlled study with CF, *Europ J Resp Dis* 65(6), 1984.

Feigin RD: Group A streptococcal infections. In Oski FA et al, editors: *Principles and practice of pediatrics,* Philadelphia, 1990, JB Lippincott.

Fiel S: Clinical management of pulmonary disease in cystic fibrosis, *Lancet* 341(8852):1070, 1993.

Fletcher HD, Ibrahim SA, Speight N: Survey of asthma deaths in the Northern region 1970–83, *Arch Dis Child* 65(2):163, 1990.

Fulginiti V, Lewy J: Pediatrics: update on cystic fibrosis, *JAMA* 270(2):246, 1993.

Furukawa CT et al: Cognitive and behavioral findings in children taking theophylline, *J Allergy Clin Immunol* 81:83, 1988.

Galant SP: Therapeutic approach to acute asthma in children. In Tinkelman DG, Falliers CJ, Naspitz CK, editors: *Childhood asthma pathophysiology and treatment,* New York, 1987, Marcel Dekker.

Goldbloom RB: Nasopharyngitis. In Gellis SS, Kagan BM, editors: *Current pediatric therapy 12,* Philadelphia, 1986, WB Saunders.

Goldenhersh MJ, Rachelefsky GS: Childhood asthma: management, *Pediatr Rev* 10:259, 1989.

Guerra IC, Kemp JS, Shearer WT: Bronchiolitis. In Oski FA*et al,* editors: *Principles and practice of pediatrics,* Philadelphia, 1990, JB Lippincott.

Gutstadt LB *et al:* Determinants of school performance in children with chronic asthma, *Am J Dis Child* 143:471, 1989.

Habel A: *Synopsis of paediatrics,* London, 1993, Butterworth Heinemann.

Harbold LA: A protocol for neonatal use of pulse oximetry, *Neonatal Network* 8(1):41, 1989.

Hall C: Respiratory syncytial virus: what we know now, *Contemp Pediatr* 10(1): 92, 1993

Hart TP, Mahutte CK: Evaluation of a closed-system, directional-tip suction catheter, Respir Care 37(11):1260, 1992.

Hazinski MF: *Nursing care of the critically ill child,* ed 2, St Louis, 1992, Mosby.

Holberg CJ, Wright AL, Martinez FD: Child day care, smoking by caregivers, and lower respiratory tract illness in the first 3 years of life, Pediatrics 91:885, 1993.

Hurwitz ES *et al:* Risk of respiratory illness associated with day-care attendance: a nationwide study, *Pediatrics* 87:62, 1991.

Jury D: More on RSV and ribavirin, *Pediatr Nurs* 19(1):89, 1993.

Isaacson G, Rosenfeld RM: Care of the child with tympanostomy tubes: a visual guide for the pediatrician, *Pediatrics* 93(6):924, 1994

Joseph C, Watson J, Fern K: BCG immunisation in England and Wales: a survey of policy and practice in schoolchildren and neonates, *BMJ* 305(6852):495, 1992.

Kairys SW, Olmstead EM, O'Connor GT: Steroid treatment of laryngotracheobronchitis: a meta-analysis of the evidence from randomized trials, *Pediatr* 83:683, 1989.

Katz JN *et al:* Clinical features as predictors of functional status in children with cystic fibrosis, *J Pediatr* 108:352, 1986.

Kerem B *et al:* Identification of the cystic fibrosis gene: genetic analysis, *Science* 245:1073, 1989.

Kleiber C, Krutzfield N, Rose EF: Acute histologic changes in tracheobronchial tree associated with different suction catheter insertion techniques, *Heart Lung* 17:10, 1987.

Kunkel N, Baker M: Aerosolized epinephrine use in treatment of croup, *Am J Dis Child* 146:470, 1992.

Kyff JV: Current thoughts on chest physical therapy, *Respir Manage* 17(6):70, 1987.

Lough, Carlo WA: In Carlo WA, Chatburn RL: *Neonatal respiratory care,* ed 2, St Louis, 1988, Mosby–Year Book.

Luder E *et al:* Efficacy of a nonrestricted fat diet in patients with cystic fibrosis, *Am J Dis Child* 143:458, 1989.

Marcy SM: A summer refresher: swimmer's ear, *Contemp Pediatr* 6(5):90, 1989.

Maw R, Bawden R: Spontaneous resolution of severe chronic glue ear in children and the effect of adenoidectomy, tonsillectomy, and insertion of ventilation tubes (grommets), *BMJ* 306:756, 1993.

Mauro RD *et al:* Differentiation of epiglottitis and laryngotracheobronchitis in the child with stridor, *Am J Dis Child* 142:679, 1988.

McCance KL, Huether SE: *Pathophysiology: the biological basis for disease in adults and children,* ed 2, St Louis, 1994, Mosby.

McFadden E, Gilbert I: Asthma, *N Engl J Med* 327(27): 1928, 1992.

McFadden DM *et al:* Age-specific patterns of diagnosis of acute otitis media, *Clin Pediatr* 24:571, 1985.

McIntosh K: Respiratory syncytial virus infections in infants and children: diagnosis and treatment, *Pediatr Rev* 9:191, 1987.

McMullen A: Cystic fibrosis. In Jackson PL, Vessey JA: *Primary care of the child with a chronic condition,* St Louis, 1992, Mosby.

Medical Research Council Tuberculosis and Chest Disease Unit: Tuberculosis in children: a national survey of notification in England and Wales, *Arch Dis Child* 63(3):266, 1988.

Medical Research Council Cardiothoracic Epidemiology Group: Tuberculosis in children: a national survey of notification in England and Wales in 1988, *Arch Dis Child* 70(6):497, 1994.

Mertsola J *et al:* Intrafamilial spread of pertussis, *J Pediatr* 103:359, 1983.

Miller BD, Strunk RC: Circumstances surrounding the deaths of children due to asthma, *Am J Dis Child* 143:1294, 1989.

Moffet H: *Pediatric infectious disease,* ed 3, Philadelphia, 1989, JB Lippincott.

Murphy S, Kelly W: Asthma, inflammation, and airway hyperresponsiveness in children, *Curr Opin Pediatr* 5:255, 1993.

Murray AB, Morrision BJ: Passive smoking by asthmatics: its greater effect on boys than on girls and on older than on younger children, *Pediatr* 84:451, 1989.

Murray C: World tuberculosis burden (letter), *Lancet* 335(8696):1043, 1990.

National Heart, Lung, and Blood Institute, National Institutes of Health: *Guidelines for the diagnosis and management of asthma,* 91:3042, Bethesda, MD, Aug 1991.

Neddenriep D, Taussig LM, Mietens C: Infections of the lower respiratory tract. In Eichenwald HF, Ströder J, editors: *Current therapy in pediatrics-2,* Philadelphia, 1989, BC Decker.

Neuspiel DR *et al:* Parental smoking and post-infancy wheezing in children: a prospective cohort study, *Am J Publ Health* 79:168, 1989.

Oberwaldner *et al:* Forced expiration against a variable resistance: a new chest physiotherapy method in cystic fibrosis, *Paed Pulmonology* 2(6):358, 1986.

Ogston SA: The Tayside infant morbidity and mortality study: effect on health of using gas for cooking, *BMJ* 290:957, 1985.

Paradise JL: Otitis media during early life: how hazardous to development? A critical review of the evidence, *Pediatr* 68:869, 1981.

Paradise JL, Elster BA: Evidence that breast milk protects against otitis media with effusion in infants with cleft palate, *Pediatr Res* 18:283A, 1984.

Paradise JL, Rogers KD: On otitis media, child development, and tympanostomy tubes: new answers or old questions? *Pediatr* 77:88, 1986.

Pearlman D: Chronic rhinitis in children, *J Allergy Clin Immunol* 81:962, 1988.

Pedreira FA *et al:* Involuntary smoking and incidence of respiratory illness during the first year of life, *Pediatr* 75:594, 1985.

Pierson WE: Exercise-induced bronchospasm in children and adolescents, *Pediatr Clin North Am* 35:1031, 1988.

Putto A: Febrile exudative tonsillitis: viral or streptococcal? *Pediatr* 80:6, 1987.

Quinton P: Defective epithelial ion transport in cystic fibrosis, *Clin Chem* 35:726, 1989.

Rachelefsky GS *et al:* Behavior abnormalities and poor school performance due to oral theophylline use, *Pediatr* 78:1133, 1986.

Rao M: Chest diseases. In Rajkumar S, Toback C, editors: *Principles and practice of ambulatory pediatrics,* New York, 1988, Plenum Medical.

Rappaport L *et al:* Effects of theophylline on behavior and learning in children with asthma, *Am J Dis Child* 143:368, 1989.

Rauen KK, Holman JB: Pain control in children following tonsillectomies: a retrospective study, *J Nurs Qual Assur* 3(3):45, 1989.

Reisman J *et al:* Role of conventional physiotherapy in cystic fibrosis, *J Pediatr* 113:632, 1988.

Rodriguez WJ *et al:* Aerosolized ribavirin in the treatment of patients with respiratory syncytial virus disease, *Pediatr Infect Dis* 6:159, 1987.

Rona RJ *et al:* Parental smoking at home and the height of children, *BMJ* 283:1363, 1981.

Rosenfield R: New concepts for steroid use in otitis media with effusion, *Clin Pediatr* 31:615, 1992.

Sarnaik AP, Lieh-Lai M: Adult respiratory distress syndrome in children, *Pediatr Clin North Am* 41(2):337, 1994.

Shannon M, Lovejoy F: Effect of acute versus chronic intoxication on clinical features of theophylline poisoning in children, *J Pediatr* 121:125, 1992.

Schoni HH: Autogenic damage: a modern approach to physiotherapy in cystic fibrosis, *J Royal Soc Med* 82 (suppl.16):32, 1989.

Skolnik N: Treatment of croup: a critical review, *Am J Dis Child* 143:1945, 1989.

Seaman-Bates NJ: Emergency management of status asthmaticus, *J Emerg Nurs* 6(5):9, 1980.

Simons FER: Allergic rhinitis: recent advances, *Pediatr Clin North Am* 35:1053, 1988.

Starke JR: Tuberculosis. In Oski FA *et al,* editors: *Principles and practice of pediatrics,* Philadelphia, 1990, JB Lippincott.

Stern R: Cystic fibrosis: recent development in diagnosis and treatment, *Pediatr Rev* 7:276, 1986.

Stickler GB: The attack on the tympanic membrane, *Pediatr* 74:291, 1984.

Strachan DP, Jarvis MJ, Feyerabend BT: Passive smoking, salivary cotinine concentrations and middle ear effusion in 7 year old children, *BMJ* 298:1549, 1989.

Super DM *et al:* A prospective randomized double-blind study to evaluate the effect of dexamethasone in acute laryngotracheitis, *J Pediatr* 115:323, 1989.

Sutton P: Chest physiotherapy: time for reappraisal, *Br J Dis Chest* 82:127, 1988.

Swallow V, Thompson L: A parents support group, *Paed Nurs* 4(1):23, 1992.

Tan Y, Collins-Williams C: Aspirin-induced asthma in children, *Ann Allergy* 48:1, 1982.

Teele DW *et al:* Otitis media with effusion during the first three years of life and development of speech and language, *Pediatr* 74:282, 1984.

Thomson JM *et al: Mosby's clinical nursing,* ed 3, St Louis, 1993, Mosby.

Tibballs J, Shann F, Landau L: Placebo-controlled trial of prednisolone in children intubated for croup, *Lancet* 340:8822, 745, 1992.

Tizzano E, Buchwald M: Recent advances in cystic fibrosis research, *J Pediatr* 122(6):985, 1993.

Webber B: *The physical treatment of cystic fibrosis,* Bromley, 1994 , Bromley CF Trust.

Weinberger M: *Managing asthma,* Baltimore, 1989, Williams & Wilkins.

Weinberger M *et al:* Effects of theophylline on learning and behavior: reason for concern or concern without reason? *J Pediatr* 111:471, 1987.

Weinberger M: Theophylline: when should it be used? *J Pediatr* 112(3):403, 1993.

Wheeler WB, Colten HR: Cystic fibrosis: current approach to diagnosis and management, *Pediatr Rev* 9:241, 1988.

Williams MH: Increasing severity of asthma from 1960 to 1987 (letter), *N Engl J Med* 320:1015, 1989.

Williams R *et al:* Use of antibiotics in preventing recurrent acute otitis media and in treating otitis media with effusion, *JAMA,* 1993.

Wood RA, Sampson HA: A practical guide to allergy testing, *Contemp Pediatr* 4(special issue):8, 1987.

Zaritsky A: Outcome of pediatric cardiopulmonary rescutitation, *Crit Care Med* 21 (9 suppl):S325, 1993.

FURTHER READING

General

Dudell G, Cornish JD, Bartlett RH: What constitutes adequate oxygenation? *Pediatr* 85:39, 1990.

McConnell EA: Giving intradermal injections, *Nurs '90* 20(3):70, 1990.

Pulmonary Assessment

Dobson F, Dobson MJ: Shedding light on pulse oximetry, *Nurs Standard* 7(46):4, 1993.

Gunderson LP, Cusson RM: Biological measures for nursing research: pulse oximetry, *Neonatal Network—J Neonatal Nurs* 12(8):71, 1993.

Levene S, McKenzie SA: Trancutaneous oxygen saturation in sleeping infants: prone and supine, *Arch Dis Child* 65(5):524, 1990.

MacDonald PD, Yu VY: Simultaneous measurement of preductal and postductal oxygen saturation by pulse oximetry, *Arch Dis Child* 67(10):1166, 1992.

Respiratory Failure

Heckmatt JZ: Chronic respiratory failure in childhood, *Care Crit Ill* 5(4):159, 1993.

Curley MAQ, Vaughan SM: Assessment and resuscitation of the pediatric patient, *Crit Care Nurs* 7(3):26, 1987.

Airway Obstruction

Kilhman H, Gillis J, Benjamin B: Severe upper airway obstruction, *Pediatr Clin North Am* 34:1, 1987.

Asthma

Anderson HR: Is asthma really increasing? *Paed Resp Med* 1(2):6, 1993.

Carruthers P: Asthma and the school age child, *Primary Health Care* 3(3):16, 1993.

Carrieri VK, Kiecklefer G, Janson-Bjerklie S, Souza J: The sensation of pulmonary dyspnoea in school age children, *Nurs Res* 40(2):81, 1991.

Gajos M: Asthma: putting the child in charge, *Prof Care Mother Child* 2(4):10, 1992.

Lloyd BW: How useful do parents find home peak flow monitoring for children with asthma? *BMJ* 305(6862):1128, 1992.

Powell CVE: Asthma in childhood, *Br J Hosp Med* 49(2):127, 1993.

Silverman M: Reducing childhood asthma deaths: what should we be doing? *Matern Child Health* 17(11):326, 1992.

Sutherns S, Rebgetz P, Smith S: The paediatric asthma management plan: a guide for nursing, *Aust Nurses J* 21(8):14, 1992.

Wooler E: Asthma in children, *Paediatr Nurs* 5(6):22, 1993.

Therapeutic Procedures

Childs HJ, Dezateux CA: A national survey of nebuliser use, *Arch Dis Child* 66(11):1, 1991.

Moler FW, Bandy KP, Guster JR: Ribavarin therapy for acute bronchiolitis: need for appropriate controls (letter), *J Pediatr* 119(3):509, 1991.

Cystic Fibrosis

Cowley G: Closing in on cystic fibrosis, *Newsweek* 121(18)15, 1993.

Dryor JA: Physiotherapy for cystic fibrosis—which technique? *Physiotherapy* 78(2):105, 1992.

Ferguson K: *Physical treatment of cystic fibrosis,* Bromley, 1994, Cystic Fibrosis Trust.

Gill S: Home administration of IV antibiotics to children with cystic fibrosis, *Br J Nurs* 2(15):767, 1993.

Glew J: One of the family... cystic fibrosis... specialist cystic fibrosis nurses, *Nurs Times* 89(15):46, 1993.

Hill CM, Rolles CJ, Keegan P, Chand R: Pancreatic enzymes in cystic fibrosis, *Arch Dis Child* 68(1):150, 1993.

Mortensen J, Falk M, Groth S, Jenson C: The effects of postural drainage and PEP physiotherapy on tracheobronchial clearance in cystic fibrosis, *Chest* 100(5):1350, 1991.

Sawer EM: Family functioning when children have cystic fibrosis, *J Ped Nurs* 7(5):304, 1992.

Respiratory Infection

Cogswell J: Bronchiolitis—long term sequelac, *Paed Res Med* 2(1):9, 1994.

Green J: Recognising epiglottitis: how to identify and respond to this pediatric crisis, *Nurs* 22(8):33, 1992.

Sanchez I *et al*: Effects of racemic epinephrine and salbutamol on clinical score and pulmonary mechanics in infants with bronchiolitis, *J Pediatr* 122(1):145, 1993.

Tuberculosis

Rodriques LC, Gill N, Smith PG: BCG vaccination in the first year of life protects children of Indian sub continent ethnic origin against tuberculosis in England, *J Epidemiol Comm Health* 45(1):78, 1991.

Sadler C: Risky complacency, *Nurs Times* 88(39):16, 1992.

Endotracheal Airways and Ventilatory Support

Clancy M, Jones E: Care of the child with respiratory problems. In Carter B, editor: *Manual of paediatric intensive care nursing,* London, 1993, Chapman & Hall.

Helms P: Factors affecting lung growth and development, *Paediatr Resp Med* 1(2):11, 1993.

Knox AM: Performing endotracheal suction on children: a literature review and implications for nursing practice, *Intensive Crit Care Nurs* 9(1):48, 1993.

Paton JY: Factors affecting respiratory control, *Paediatr Resp Med* 1(2):15, 1993.

Russel RIR: Complications of mechanical ventilation in children, *Paed Resp Med* 1(1):17, 1993.

Cardiopulmonary Resuscitation

Anon: Guidelines for paediatric life support—Paediatric Life Support Working Party of the European Resuscitation Council, *BMJ* 308(6940):1349, 1994.

Chellel A: Outcomes, ethics and accountability, *Nurs Times* 17(7):37, 1993.

European Resuscitation Council: Guidelines for paediatric life support, *BMJ* 305:1345, 1992.

Matthews J: Insignificant others: family presence during resuscitation, *Nurs Times* 89(13):42, 1993.

Simpson S: Paediatric basic life support: an update, *Nurs Times* 90(21):40, 1994.

Woodward S: A guide to paediatric resuscitation, *Paediatr Nurs* 6(2):16, 1994.

Chapter 27

The Child with Gastrointestinal Dysfunction

LEARNING OUTCOMES

After studying this chapter you should be able to:

◆ Identify the functions of the gastrointestinal tract.
◆ Identify the clinical manifestations of gastrointestinal dysfunction in children.
◆ Discuss potential nursing interventions for children with constipation.
◆ Discuss potential nursing interventions for children with Hirschsprung's disease.
◆ Discuss potential nursing interventions for children with irritable bowel syndrome.
◆ Discuss potential nursing interventions for children with acute appendicitis.
◆ Discuss potential nursing interventions for children with pyloric stenosis.
◆ Discuss potential nursing interventions for children with intussusception.
◆ Discuss potential nursing interventions for children with short bowel syndrome.
◆ Discuss potential nursing interventions for children with acute hepatitis.
◆ Define the glossary terms.

GLOSSARY

diarrhoea Increased frequency or decreased consistency of stools

GOR Gastro-oesophageal reflux

Hep A Hepatitis A virus

Hep B Hepatitis B virus

HPS Hypertrophic pyloric stenosis

IBD Inflammatory bowel disease

IBS Irritable bowel syndrome

jaundice Yellowish discolouration of the skin and sclera

NG Nasogastric

PUD Peptic ulcer disease

SBS Short bowel syndrome

UC Ulcerative colitis

isorders of the gastrointestinal tract are very common and constitute one of the largest categories of illnesses that occur in infancy and childhood. Structural and obstructive defects interfere with the ingestion and transport of foodstuffs, and inflammatory, malabsorptive and maldigestive disturbances impair the functional integrity of the gastrointestinal tract. Furthermore, in most of the disorders, the primary defect can produce additional complications. For example, obstructive or inflammatory conditions affect digestion and absorption because bowel motility, mucosal functioning, enzymatic activity and bacterial flora are altered. This chapter is concerned with conditions that interfere with normal digestion and absorption of nutrients.

GASTROINTESTINAL STRUCTURE AND FUNCTION

Knowledge of the essential structure and function of the gastrointestinal tract is key to understanding problems of the gut (Box 27-1). In addition, the developmental aspects of structure and function, such as the change in stomach capacity with age, impinge on this understanding (Table 27-1).

ASSESSMENT OF GASTROINTESTINAL FUNCTION

Some GI disorders (e.g., vomiting and/or diarrhoea) occur as primary and isolated disturbances, but are also among the manifestations often associated with a variety of childhood illnesses. Structural and obstructive defects interfere with the ingestion and transport of ingested foodstuffs, and inflammatory, malabsorptive and maldigestive disturbances impair the functional integrity of the GI tract. Furthermore, in most of the disorders, the primary defect can produce additional complications. For example, loss of GI contents causes significant

AGE	CAPACITY (ml)
Newborn	10-20
1 week	30-90
2-3 weeks	75-100
1 month	90-150
3 months	150-200
1 year	210-360
2 years	500
10 years	750-900
16 years	1500
Adult	2000-3000

Table 27.1 Stomach capacity (approximate) at various stages of development.

alterations in fluid and electrolytes, and obstructive or inflammatory conditions affect digestion and absorption because bowel motility, mucosal functioning, enzymatic activity and bacterial flora are altered.

Numerous general observations provide possible clues to specific GI problems (Box 27-2). In some cases, only one manifestation may be observed; others may involve several signs and symptoms as part of the disease complex. In many disorders that involve GI losses, particularly large amounts of fluid, dehydration poses a serious threat to life and often dominates the clinical picture (see Chapter 24).

INGESTION OF FOREIGN BODIES

Children ingest a variety of foreign objects. Most ingested foreign bodies, such as marbles, coins, beads and small safety pins, pass through the alimentary tract without difficulty once they reach the stomach. Larger items and straight or sharp objects, such as hairpins, ring pulls on beverage cans, needles and large safety pins, may become lodged in the oesophagus or duodenal loop.

Once an ingested object passes the pylorus, its progress may be followed by x-rays, and the stools are examined for its presence. The child is fed the customary diet. If serial x-rays indicate that the object remains stationary, it is removed by an endoscope or in rare cases by laparotomy. Surgical removal is indicated in instances of perforation, bleeding or obstruction and when large or long objects have not cleared the stomach within 3-5 days (Webb, McDaniel and Jones, 1984).

Foreign bodies that become lodged in the oesophagus require immediate attention, since they may adhere to the oesophageal wall, where they cause erosion of the epithelium. Of particular concern is the increasing incidence of ingestion of 'button' batteries commonly found in watches, hearing aids, cameras and calculators. Some have been found to leak their alkaline electrolytes and other corrosive substances, or have been acted on by stomach and intestinal secretions (Brady, 1991). While many button battery ingestions are benign, the most difficulty arises from the larger-diameter batteries, which

---

◆ **BOX 27-1**

Functions of gastrointestinal tract
Process and absorb nutrients necessary to maintain metabolic processes and to support growth and development

Perform an excretory function for both digestive residue and other waste products that pour into the intestine from the blood or are excreted in the bile

Provide detoxification while other routes of elimination (kidneys, liver, skin) are still immature

Participate in maintaining fluid and electrolyte balance in infancy

---

◆ BOX 27-2

Clinical manifestations of gastrointestinal dysfunction in children

Failure to thrive, as evidenced by deceleration from established growth pattern or consistently below the 5th percentile for height and weight on standard growth charts.

Regurgitation, characteristic of infants, are discussed in Chapter 15.

Vomiting, the forceful ejection of stomach contents, involves a complex reflex that is associated with widespread autonomic discharge that causes salivation, pallor, sweating, and tachycardia. Vomiting is ordinarily accompanied by nausea.

Projectile vomiting, in which the vomitus is forcefully ejected as far as 0.6-1.2 m from the child, is not associated with nausea.

Haematemesis, the vomiting of blood, may result from swallowing blood from the oropharynx or from bleeding in the upper GI tract.

Nausea is an unpleasant sensation vaguely referred to the epigastrium, with an inclination to vomit.

Stools, the number, type, consistency, presence or absence of blood, and associated signs and symptoms provide clues to the aetiology of gastrointestinal dysfunction.

Constipation is the regular passage of firm or hard stools or of small, hard masses with associated symptoms such as difficulty expelling the stools, blood-streaked bowel movements, and abdominal discomfort. The apparent difficulty in passing stools is not a reliable sign, especially in infancy.

Diarrhoea is an increase in the number of stools or a decrease in their consistency as a result of alterations of water and electrolyte transport by the alimentary tract. Diarrhoea may be acute or chronic.

Abdominal pain, specific or nonspecific, is associated with several GI disorders.

Abdominal enlargement or distention is a common observation in a child with GI dysfunction.

Dysphagia, difficulty in swallowing, can be the result of structural abnormalities or neurological or neuromuscular impairment.

Bowel sounds, or their absence, can provide information about some GI disorders.

Jaundice is the yellow discolouration of the skin associated with liver dysfunction.

Fever is a common manifestation of illness in children. In GI disorders, it is usually associated with dehydration or infection.

---

become impacted in the oesophagus. Recommendations for treating battery ingestions include: (1) confirming the location by x-ray examination, (2) removing immediately those lodged in the oesophagus, (3) observing those beyond the oesophagus on an outpatient basis, (4) repeating x-ray after 48 hours if the ingested battery is larger than button size and removing those that still remain in the stomach, and (5) repeating x-ray if a small battery has not passed in the stool within 4-7 days (Litovitz, 1985).

Coins are the most frequently swallowed items and account for most oesophageal foreign bodies. If a coin passes into the stomach, it generally passes through the remainder of the GI tract without problems. If it remains in the oesophagus, it can be symptomatic or asymptomatic. Usual symptoms are refusal to take foods, increased salivation, pain or discomfort on swallowing, or vomiting. Symptomatic oesophageal coin ingestion is managed the same as battery ingestion. Therapeutic management of asymptomatic coin ingestion is controversial. Some advocate immediate x-ray evaluation to determine placement, regardless of symptoms (Gracia, Frey and Balaz, 1984; Schunk, Corneli and Bolte, 1989). Others recommend that asymptomatic patients be allowed a 24-hour period in which to pass the coin without x-ray or intervention (Caravati, Bennett, and McElwee, 1989; Joseph, 1990). An alternative to removal involves advancing the coin carefully into the stomach for continued travel through the GI tract (Bonadio *et al*, 1988).

IMPLICATIONS FOR NURSING

The primary nursing intervention is prevention of foreign body ingestion through family teaching. All children who are old enough to understand should be taught not to put anything in their mouths before asking permission. Infants and young children who cannot follow such advice must have their environment protected for them. Small objects are placed out of their reach or properly discarded. It is advisable to search the floor carefully on hands and knees, and remove small objects that are accessible to inquisitive young children. Nursing education regarding the dangers of pica, especially lead (see Chapter 16), and assistance in helping families remove the substance are important aspects of care.

Once an object is swallowed, parents need guidelines on seeking treatment (see Emergency Treatment). When no treatment is instituted, parents should examine the stool for verification that the object has passed safely through the GI tract, usually within 3-4 days. For children in nappies, this is easily accomplished by squeezing the stool between the nappy to locate the object, but in toilet-trained children it requires more effort. A piece of plastic wrap placed across the toilet bowl to collect the stool makes it easier to examine the faeces, although a spatula or some other disposable object may be needed to break up the stool.

◆ Emergency Treatment

Foreign Body Ingestion

1. Seek medical treatment *immediately* if:

a. Any sharp or large object or a battery was ingested.

b. There are signs that the object may have been aspirated (i.e., coughing, choking, inability to speak, or difficulty in breathing) (see Chapter 26 for emergency treatment of airway obstruction).

c. There are signs that the object may be lodged in the oesophagus (i.e., increased salivation, drooling, gagging or difficulty with swallowing).

d. There are signs that the object may be lodged in the pharynx (i.e., discomfort in the throat or chest [more likely with a fish or chicken bone]).

2. Seek medical advice if the object is smooth and small (usually less than the size of a ten pence piece).

3. If no treatment is required, check the stool for passage of the object; do not give laxatives.

DISORDERS OF MOTILITY

Several GI disorders are caused by disturbances in motility. Some, such as Hirschsprung's disease and gastro-oesophageal reflux, are seen primarily in infancy and cause problems in elimination or feeding. Others, such as constipation, can occur at any age and produce few serious effects, unless the primary disorder can lead to obstruction.

CONSTIPATION

Constipation is the regular passage of firm or hard stools or of small, hard masses with associated symptoms such as difficulty in expulsion of the stools, blood-streaked bowel movements and abdominal discomfort. The frequency of bowel movements is not considered a diagnostic criterion, because it varies widely among children (Clayden, 1991). However, less frequent bowel movements may be normal. Having extremely long intervals between defaecation is termed *obstipation*. Constipation with faecal soiling is *encopresis*. The following discussion is concerned primarily with causes of constipation in different age groups and the treatment of simple constipation during childhood.

Constipation can be a symptom of several abdominal disorders, primarily those that cause an obstruction in the lower intestinal tract, such as Hirschsprung's disease. Physical and mental disorders are often associated with defaecation problems; for example, neurological disorders, hypothyroidism and hypercalcaemia. However, the development and course of constipation can also be influenced by familial, cultural and social factors. Psychological factors play an important role in bowel habits, as well as toilet-training techniques, diet, overuse of laxatives and enemas (Lennard-Jones, 1993). The most common cause of constipation in children is environmental

change, such as change in feeding habits, using a new toilet, birth of a sibling, and relocation of housing or school (Johns, 1985).

NEWBORN

Normally, the newborn passes a first meconium stool within 24-36 hours of birth. Any infant who does not do so should be assessed for evidence of intestinal atresia or stenosis, Hirschsprung's disease, hypothyroidism, meconium plugs or meconium ileus. Meconium plugs are caused by meconium that has reduced water content; they are usually evacuated following digital examination, but they may require irrigations of normal saline or the iodinated contrast medium *diatrizoate meglumine (Gastrografin)*.

Meconium ileus, the initial manifestation of cystic fibrosis, is the presence of thick, mucilaginous meconium that clings to the abdominal wall, making it difficult, if not impossible, to pass. Treatment is the same as for a meconium plug. Rarely, surgical intervention may be necessary.

INFANCY

True constipation is relatively rare in infants, but normal stool patterns can vary markedly from infant to infant. Hard, painful bowel movements are mild to moderate problems, but distention associated with constipation requires further evaluation (Rappaport and Levine, 1986). Medical causes such as Hirschsprung's disease, hypothyroidism and strictures must be ruled out in chronic cases of constipation. The assessment history should always include frequency of bowel movements, the composition of the diet, and whether the constipation is recent or has been present since birth.

The most frequent cause of constipation in infancy is dietary mismanagement. It is almost unknown in breast-fed infants, who typically have more stools than bottle-fed infants. Constipation may accompany the change from human milk or modified cow's milk formula to whole cow's milk, presumably because of the greater protein-to-carbohydrate ratio of whole cow's milk. Some bottle-fed infants pass hard stools and develop anal fissures. To avoid the pain in defaecation, these infants voluntarily withhold stool. The infant's behaviour during withholding of stools is often misinterpreted by parents as constipation. The infant grunts and appears to be straining, displaying a red face and with legs drawn up on the abdomen. However, a red face and straining are normal behaviour in infancy.

Simple measures ordinarily correct the problem, e.g. offering supplementary clear fluids, or increasing the amount of cereal, vegetables and fruit in the diet of older infants. If the child has anal fissures, the temporary use of stool softeners, glycerine suppositories or mineral oil is usually sufficient to break the painful defaecation cycle.

EARLY CHILDHOOD

Children between 1-3 years of age are most likely to have constipation (Abrahamian and Lloyd-Still, 1984). Most constipation is due to environmental changes or is related to normal development when a child begins to attain control over bodily functions. A child who has experienced discomfort during bowel movements may deliberately try to avoid them. The rectum accommodates the stool accumulation, and the urge to defaecate passes. When bowel contents are ultimately evacuated, the result is that accumulated faeces are passed with even greater pain, reinforcing the desire to withhold. This generates a self-perpetuating cycle of further retention and discomfort (Pettei, 1987; Rappaport and Levine, 1986).

SCHOOL-AGED CHILDREN

School entrance often exacerbates bowel difficulties that were experienced earlier in life, and some children who never had constipation develop retentive tendencies at this time (Rappaport and Levine, 1986). Before school entry, children have ample opportunity for toileting in the home setting. Early and hurried departure for school immediately after breakfast is not conducive to leisurely bathroom use. Also, school and after-school activities are often rigidly scheduled and regimented. The most common cause of new-onset constipation at school entry is fear of using school lavatories, which are noted for their lack of privacy. Most schools will liberalize lavatory rules for individual children who have been identified and will ask a parent or health professional to intervene on the child's behalf (Hill, 1991).

THERAPEUTIC MANAGEMENT

If constipation is associated with manifestations such as vomiting, abdominal distention or pain, and evidence of growth failure, the condition merits further investigation. Constipation may result from some medications, such as iron preparations, diuretics, antacids and anticonvulsant agents. Constipation frequently accompanies enuresis, and treatment of the constipation often results in resolution of the enuresis (O'Regan *et al*, 1986).

The management of simple constipation is based on a plan to keep the bowel relatively empty of stool and dietary management, to prevent further constipation. The initial treatment of constipation may include the use of aperients or suppositories. Enemas and rectal washouts will be used only as a last resort. Ongoing dietary management is then discussed with the family, generally recommending a high-fibre diet. When high-fibre foods are added, additional sources of fluid must be given to the child to prevent the fibre from having a binding effect. One of the major functions of fibre is to absorb water to soften the stool. Other regimens may include a stool softener to keep the stool of a consistency that is more easily evacuated.

IMPLICATIONS FOR NURSING

Constipation, unfortunately, tends to be self-perpetuating. A child who has difficulty or discomfort when attempting to evacuate the bowels has a tendency to retain the bowel contents and thus begins a vicious cycle. Nursing assessment begins with an accurate history of bowel habits, diet, events that may be associated with the onset of constipation, drugs or other substances that the child may be taking, and the consistency, colour, frequency and other characteristics of the stool. If there is no evidence of a pathological condition that requires further investigation, the major task of the nurse is to educate the family regarding normal stool patterns and to relieve the cause of the constipation (Benninga, Buller and Taminiau, 1993).

Dietary modifications are usually essential in preventing constipation. During infancy, simply increasing the carbohydrate (sugar or syrup) in an infant formula will often relieve the problem. During childhood, the diet should contain increased amounts of fibre and fluid. Parents will benefit from guidance in dietary planning, especially regarding foods that facilitate bowel movements. If bran is added to the diet, creative ways to disguise the consistency are needed. For example, it can be added to cereal, mashed potatoes or milk shakes.

An excellent food for providing a high-fibre intake is popcorn. It is readily accepted by children, inexpensive and easy to prepare, and safe for children beyond the age when foreign body aspiration is a hazard. Popcorn has sufficient bulk and can be purchased in a variety of different tastes and forms.

Parents also need reassurance concerning the benign nature of the condition. It is important to discuss with them their attitudes and expectations regarding toilet habits and to discourage the use of stool softeners, laxatives and enemas. If such measures have been prescribed by a doctor, parents should understand that these are merely temporary and not to be continued beyond the current need.

HIRSCHSPRUNG'S DISEASE (CONGENITAL AGANGLIONIC MEGACOLON)

Hirschsprung's disease is a congenital anomaly that results in mechanical obstruction from inadequate motility in part of the intestine (Fig. 27-1). It accounts for about one-quarter of all cases of neonatal obstruction, although it may not be diagnosed until later in infancy or childhood. It is four times more common in males than females, follows a familial pattern in a small number of cases, and has a higher incidence in children with Down's syndrome. Depending on its presentation, it may be an acute, life-threatening condition or a chronic disorder.

CLINICAL MANIFESTATIONS

Clinical manifestations vary according to the age when symptoms are recognized and according to the occurrence of complications, such as enterocolitis. In the newborn, the chief signs and symptoms are failure to pass meconium within 24-48 hours after birth, reluctance to ingest fluids, bile-stained vomitus and abdominal distention. If the disorder is allowed to progress, other signs of intestinal obstruction develop, such as respiratory distress and shock.

During infancy, the child does not thrive and has constipation,

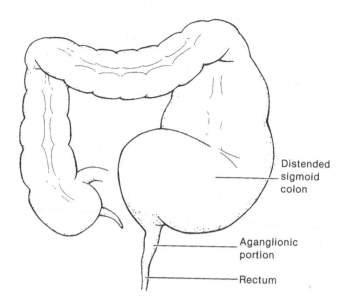

Distended
sigmoid
colon

Aganglionic
portion

Rectum

Fig. 27-1 Hirschsprung's disease.

abdominal distention, and episodes of diarrhoea and vomiting. Explosive, watery diarrhoea, fever, and severe prostration are ominous signs because they often signify the presence of enterocolitis (inflammation of the small bowel and colon), which greatly increases the risk of fatality. Enterocolitis may also be present without diarrhoea and is first evidenced with unexplained fever and poor feeding (Doig, 1994).

During childhood, the symptoms become chronic and include constipation; passage of ribbon-like, foul-smelling stools; abdominal distention and visible peristalsis. Faecal masses are easily palpable. The child is usually poorly nourished, anaemic and hypoproteinaemic from malabsorption of nutrients.

PROCESS OF DIAGNOSIS

In the neonate, diagnosis is suspected on clinical signs of intestinal obstruction and failure to pass meconium. In infants and children, the history is an important part of diagnosis and typically details a chronic pattern of constipation. On examination, the rectum is empty of faeces, the internal sphincter is tight, and there is leakage of liquid, offensive, pale stool and accumulated gas. X-ray studies using a barium enema often demonstrate the transition zone between the dilated proximal colon (megacolon) and the aganglionic distal segment. However, this typical megacolon and narrow distal segment may not develop until 3-4 weeks or even months after birth in some children.

To confirm the diagnosis, rectal biopsy is performed either surgically, to obtain a full-thickness biopsy for histological evidence of aganglionic cells, or by suction biopsy (i.e. Noblett biopsy), performed without anaesthesia, to detect the presence of ganglia in the submucosa.

THERAPEUTIC MANAGEMENT

Treatment is primarily surgical removal of the aganglionic bowel, to ensure continence. A very small number of children with chronic, but not severe, symptoms of megacolon are treated conservatively with occasional enemas to establish a regular pattern of defaecation. However, these children represent a distinct exception and may be at continued risk for the development of fatal enterocolitis (Martin and Torres, 1985). Surgical correction usually involves a two- or three-stage approach. In most cases, a temporary colostomy is created in part of the bowel with normal innervation (usually the sigmoid or transverse colon) and at a site that permits the corrective operation to be performed. The colostomy allows the bowel a period of rest in order to resume its normal calibre and tonicity, and provides an opportunity for the child to gain weight before the more extensive repair is undertaken.

Definitive correction is usually performed when the child is eight months to one year of age. The type of surgical procedure for reanastomosis involves 'pulling' the end of the intact bowel down to a point near the rectum. The most common surgical techniques are the Swenson, the Soave (endorectal pull-through), and the Duhamel operations, which usually require both an abdominal and a perineal incision.

Although a one-stage approach is now common, a third stage (if required) is closure of the colostomy, normally performed within a few (usually three) months of the definitive repair. Prognosis after complete surgical repair depends on the child's ability to adjust to a normal diet and to learn bowel control, and varies depending on the type of surgery. However, most children are able to attain satisfactory defaecatory function (Martin and Torres, 1985; Polley, Coran and Wesley, 1985).

IMPLICATIONS FOR NURSING

Many of the nursing concerns depend on the child's age and the type of treatment. Nursing observation in the neonatal period is most important as a factor in early diagnosis. In a retrospective study, all infants who were diagnosed by biopsy at a later date had onset of constipation in the neonatal period (Landman, 1987). If the disorder is diagnosed during the neonatal period, the main objectives are helping the parents adjust to a congenital defect in their child, fostering infant-parent bonding, preparing them for the medical/surgical intervention, and assisting them in caring for the colostomy after discharge.

When the disorder is not discovered during this period, the nurse can facilitate establishing a diagnosis by carefully listening to the parents' history, with special emphasis on bowel habits. In Hirschsprung's disease several areas must be investigated: (1) onset of constipation, especially if present since birth; (2) character of stools, particularly ribbon-like and foul smelling; and (3) frequency of bowel movements. Other clues in the history and physical examination include poor feeding habits, fussiness and irritability, a distended abdomen, and signs of undernutrition, such as thin extremities, pallor, muscle weakness and fatigue.

Preoperative care

Much of the child's preoperative care depends on the age and clinical condition. Physical preoperative preparation entails the same measures that are common to any surgery (see Chapter 7). In the newborn, whose bowel is sterile, no additional preparation is required. However, children beyond the newborn period need bowel emptying with saline rectal washouts. A nasogastric (NG) tube may be inserted to prevent abdominal distention. Increasingly a nasogastric tube administering bowel cleansing solution (e.g. Kleanprep) is used to completely clear the GI tract. This procedure continues until the bowel exudate is clear. The child requires close observation during this procedure. All intake and output of irrigant and drainage are noted, particularly any marked discrepancy in retention or loss of fluid.

Children need to be prepared for a colostomy fused (see Ostomies, Chapter 8). Parents also need preparation before surgery. Since a colostomy represents a change in body function and appearance, the nurse should investigate parents' previous knowledge of this procedure. It is not uncommon for parents to have some knowledge about a colostomy. For example, one mother related that a friend's father had a permanent colostomy because of cancer. As soon as the mother heard that her child needed this procedure, she was convinced that the mass in her child's abdomen was a cancerous tumour.

It is best not to assume that parents understand a verbal explanation of a colostomy. Drawing a picture or using a doll is excellent for parents, as well as children. During this teaching session, the nurse should briefly mention methods of care, since presenting too much information can overwhelm the parents.

It is important to stress to parents and older children that the colostomy for Hirschsprung's disease is temporary. The nurse should also keep in mind that although a temporary colostomy is favourable in terms of future health and adjustment, it also necessitates additional surgery, which may be very stressful to parents and children.

Since feeding and related behavioural problems are frequently associated with a chronic pattern of megacolon, the nurse should inform parents that although the defect can be corrected, it will take some time for the child's physical status and feeding practices to improve. Although the benefit of surgery should not be minimized, it is necessary to avoid implying that surgical correction is a panacea to all physical and behavioural complaints.

Postoperative care

Physical postoperative care usually includes: (1) nothing by mouth until bowel sounds return and the colostomy and/or anastomosed bowel are ready for feedings, (2) intravenous fluid to maintain hydration and replace lost electrolytes, (3) NG suctioning to prevent abdominal distention, (4) semipermeable dressing, (5) perineal dressing changes and (6) appropriate analgesia for use in infants.

To prevent contamination of the abdominal wound with urine, the nappy should be placed below the dressing. Sometimes a Foley catheter is used in the immediate postoperative period to divert the flow of urine away from the abdomen. Drainage from the NG tube and the colostomy is measured, since fluid and electrolyte replacement is partially calculated on these losses.

When parents initially visit their child postoperatively, they are frequently unprepared for the numerous tubes and intravenous lines attached to various body parts. Even when all the procedures are explained beforehand, the actual visual shock can be great. The nurse should explain the function of each piece of equipment, stressing safety features that permit the child to be safely moved and handled, such as length of tubing, use of splints at intravenous sites, and tape to secure the NG tube to the nose. In this way, parents are encouraged and assisted in holding and stimulating their child.

The nurse emphasizes the expected changes in the appearance of the stoma, which initially is large, protruding, red and raw looking. Since the stomal site appears painful, it is also important to stress that bowel mucosa is nonsensitive but that the surrounding abdominal skin must be protected.

NB: Hirschsprung's enterocolitis may not be eradicated by surgery and remains an ongoing risk through infancy and childhood.

GASTRO-OESOPHAGEAL REFLUX

Gastro-oesophageal reflux (chalasia, cardiochalasia) is relaxation or incompetence of the lower oesophageal sphincter, causing frequent return of stomach contents into the oesophagus. In newborns, this is considered a normal phenomenon because of immature neuromuscular control of the gastro-oesophageal sphincter. However, in a small percentage of infants reflux continues, producing symptoms that warrant investigation. The exact cause is not known, although it is thought to result from delayed maturation of lower oesophageal neuromuscular function or impaired local hormonal control mechanisms. Gastro-oesophageal reflux (GOR) is also more common in premature infants, children with neurological impairment (such as cerebral palsy or head injury), and in children after some kinds of oesophageal surgery. With improved diagnosis, gastro-oesophageal reflux is rapidly becoming one of the more common diagnoses in young children.

CLINICAL MANIFESTATIONS

The most common symptoms of gastro-oesophageal reflux are vomiting, weight loss, increased appetite, respiratory problems and bleeding. Vomiting is the most common symptom and in infants is quite forceful. It is frequently so severe that there is a loss of calories sufficient to cause weight loss and failure to thrive.

Reflux of stomach contents to the pharynx predisposes to aspiration and the development of respiratory symptoms, especially pneumonia, cyanotic episodes, reactive airway disease and apnoea. Repeated irritation of the oesophageal lining with gastric acid can lead to oesophagitis and consequently bleeding. Blood loss, in turn, causes anaemia and is seen as haematemesis or melaena (blood in stools). Heartburn is also a frequent symptom in older children, who can describe it, but it may go unrecognized in infants.

PROCESS OF DIAGNOSIS

The history is an important part of the process of diagnosis, including observation of the child's feeding habits. Several tests are available to evaluate the presence of reflux. Generally, the initial test is the barium oesophagram. Reflux of barium from the stomach to the oesophagus can be seen by fluoroscopy, although it may be missed because of the intermittent nature of the disorder. Other tests include manometry to measure oesophageal sphincter pressure; 24-hour intraoesophageal pH monitoring, which uses a probe to directly measure the pH of the distal oesophagus; and gastro-oesophageal nuclear medicine studies, which scans the oesophagus after a feeding of a radioactive compound to detect reflux or aspiration. Each of these diagnostic tests must be performed accurately to ensure a correct diagnosis.

THERAPEUTIC MANAGEMENT

Therapeutic management of GOR depends on its severity. Infants who are thriving ordinarily require no therapy other than parental reassurance that the child will outgrow the condition, although most infants benefit from appropriate positioning during and after feedings. For the symptomatic child, modification of feeding with small, frequent feedings of thickened formula, as well as positioning, may be helpful to minimize the symptoms of the reflux until the child grows and a normal physiological barrier to reflux develops (Orenstein, Shalaby and Putnam, 1992).

There is considerable controversy regarding the most advantageous position. Traditionally, the upright position (usually in an infant seat) has been recommended, but this position has been shown to increase intra-abdominal pressure and may cause the reflux to become worse. Research in infants less than six months of age demonstrated that positioning the child prone with the body inclined at about a 30-degree angle following feeds was more effective (Orenstein and Whitington, 1983). Medical practitioners will need to consider the risk of sudden infant death associated with the prone position against the clinical advantage of the position in GOR.

Drugs that promote gastric emptying and/or relax the pyloric sphincter have been used with some success, including bethanechol (a cholinergic agent), metoclopramide (a dopamine blocker), and domperidone (a benzimidazole derivative with peripheral dopamine antagonist properties). Cisapride, a recently approved prokinetic drug, increases LES pressure, promotes gastric emptying, and has fewer CNS side effects than metoclopromide. It could supercede other agents as the preferred medication for GOR (Oranstein, 1992). In some cases, antacids and H_2 blocking agents, such as cimetidine, have been used to reduce gastric acidity, although there is no evidence to support their value (Carcassonne *et al*, 1985).

Surgical intervention is selected for children with severe complications. However, a trial of medical management generally precedes surgical intervention, which creates an artificial sphincter by wrapping the fundus of the stomach around the distal oesophagus. The procedure involves an abdominal incision and generally insertion of a gastrostomy tube. Other antireflux procedures may be used in some centres.

Prognosis

Most infants achieve normal gastro-oesophageal function in the first 2-3 years of life without the need for surgical intervention; 90% will have complete resolution by 18 months of age (Belknap, 1990).

IMPLICATIONS FOR NURSING

Nursing care is directed at: (1) identifying children with symptoms suggestive of gastro-oesophageal reflux, (2) helping parents with home care of feeding and positioning when indicated, and (3) if appropriate, caring for the child undergoing surgical intervention. For the majority of infants, parental reassurance of the benign nature of the condition and its relationship to physiological maturity is the most important intervention. To help parents cope with the inconvenience of vomiting, simple measures such as using bibs and protective cloths during feeding, and upright positioning after feeding, are beneficial.

Feeding modification may require some rescheduling of the family's routine to accommodate more frequent feeding times. Formula is thickened with an artificial thickening agent (e.g. Carobel), and the teat opening may need to be enlarged for easier sucking. If the mother is breast-feeding her infant, a decision regarding the benefit of feeding modification must be made; she can express the milk if thickening is recommended. Alternatively, a more concentrated formula may be given to reduce volume or, in severe cases, NG or nasojejunal feedings may be necessary.

Non-nutritive sucking tends to hasten clearance of refluxed material from the oesophagus. In infants with GOR, non-nutritive sucking was found to affect the frequency of reflux episodes—increasing reflux in prone infants and decreasing it in seated infants (Orenstein, 1988). Non-nutritive sucking also reduces crying behaviour.

Infants receiving antacids should be given the medication at the same time as the feeding to improve its buffering (Sutphen, Dillard and Pipan, 1986). The older child should avoid caffeine-containing foods and beverages (e.g., cola drinks) to reduce gastric acid production. A low-fat diet, avoiding eating 2-4 hours before bedtime, and sleeping on a wedge are often beneficial.

Postoperative nursing care is similar to that for other types of abdominal surgery (see Chapter 8). Gastric decompression by NG tube or gastrostomy must be maintained to avoid distention. The nasogastric tube should be of a large bore to minimise the risk of 'gas bloat', which is a severe potential consequence of this surgery and may cause severe respiratory embarrassement. When postoperative ileus resolves, the NG tube is removed, or the gastrostomy tube is elevated in preparation for feeding. When feedings are initiated through the gastrostomy, the tube should remain vented for several days or longer to avoid gastric distention from swallowed air. Oedema surrounding the surgical site and compression of gastric wrap may prohibit the infant from expelling air through the oesophagus. Some infants benefit from clamping of the tube for increasingly longer intervals until they are able to tolerate continuous clamping between feedings. During this time, if the infant displays increasing irritability and evidence of cramping, some relief may be provided by venting the tube.

INFLAMMATORY CONDITIONS

Inflammatory conditions involving large or small segments of the gastrointestinal tract are not uncommon in childhood. They may be acute or chronic, and some are more likely to affect one age group more than another. For example, necrotizing enterocolitis is seen in the newborn, Meckel's diverticulum primarily affects children under age two years, ulcerative colitis occurs most frequently in the prepubescent and adolescent child, and acute appendicitis appears at any age.

ACUTE APPENDICITIS

Appendicitis, inflammation of the vermiform appendix, or blind sac, at the end of the caecum, is the most common reason for abdominal surgery during childhood. Although rare in children younger than two years of age, it is associated with increased complications and mortality in this age group. Primarily an acute disorder, appendicitis rapidly progresses to perforation and peritonitis if it remains undiagnosed. It is a significant problem, because early diagnosis is frequently delayed as a result of children's inability to verbalize symptoms and failure of health professionals (not parents) to interpret behavioural cues correctly.

While mortality has decreased greatly since the advent of antibiotics, the incidence of appendiceal rupture has still remained high, occurring in about 28% of patients (Berry and Malt, 1984). Other contributing factors are young age, lower social class, presence of faecaliths, absence of family history, and advice given by the first health professional the family contacted, especially the advice to observe the child at home (Brender *et al*, 1985a).

CLINICAL MANIFESTATIONS

The most common signs and symptoms of appendicitis are colicky abdominal pain, tenderness and fever. Initially, the pain is generalized or periumbilical; however, it usually descends to the lower right quadrant. The most intense site of pain may be at the McBurney point, located midway between the anterior superior iliac crest and the umbilicus. Other important signs are a rigid abdomen, decreased or absent bowel sounds, and rebound tenderness (the sudden pain at the point of tenderness elicited by pressing firmly over a part of the abdomen distal to the area of tenderness). Jumping or riding over bumps in a car or on a trolley aggravates the pain.

Vomiting commonly follows the onset of pain, especially in younger children, and constipation or diarrhoea may be present. Anorexia is a constant feature. Low-grade fever is typically seen early in the disease, but can rise sharply once peritonitis has begun. Probably the most significant clinical manifestation is a change in the child's behaviour. The younger, nonverbal child will assume a rigid, motionless, side-lying posture with the knees flexed on the abdomen. The older child may exhibit all of these behaviours while complaining of abdominal pain. The child walks very carefully with decreased range of motion in the right hip and usually lies with the hip flexed.

PROCESS OF DIAGNOSIS

Diagnosis is based primarily on history and examination. The chief clues that should alert the practitioner to appendicitis are the progression of abdominal pain, location of abdominal tenderness, decreased peristalsis, pain on rectal examination, and absence of any other symptoms or findings suggesting another disorder, such as pneumonia.

Laboratory evaluation includes a white blood cell count, which is usually elevated. X-ray studies of the abdomen are not very helpful, but may reveal possible contributing causes of appendicitis, such as faecaliths or a foreign body in the appendix. Ultrasound may be used to locate an abscess before surgery.

Diagnosis is not always straightforward. Numerous infectious processes have features in common. For example, fever, vomiting, abdominal pain, and elevated blood count are associated with inflammatory bowel disease, gastroenteritis, pelvic inflammatory disease, urinary tract infection, right lower lobe pneumonia, constipation, mesenteric adenitis, Meckel's diverticulum, and intussusception. Also, diagnosis may be delayed in infants and small children because they do not localize infections well and can become sick more rapidly than older children. Consequently, the risk of perforation is greater. Therefore, practitioners must have a high degree of suspicion for appendicitis in the differential diagnosis.

THERAPEUTIC MANAGEMENT

Treatment of appendicitis before perforation is surgical removal of the appendix (appendectomy). Recovery is rapid and generally uneventful, unless peritonitis has occurred. The following discussion is concerned with the special care of the child with a ruptured appendix.

Ruptured appendix
Management of the child diagnosed with peritonitis caused by a ruptured appendix often begins preoperatively with intra-

venous administration of fluid and electrolytes, systemic antibiotics and NG suction. Postoperative management includes fluid and electrolyte balance maintenance, continued administration of antibiotics, and NG suction for abdominal decompression until intestinal activity returns.

Most surgeons provide for external drainage when abscess formation has occurred, when there is necrotic or severely damaged tissue, or when there are purulent collections within the peritoneum. This is accomplished by wound drainage and wound irrigations.

IMPLICATIONS FOR NURSING

Because successful treatment of appendicitis is based on prompt recognition of the disorder, a primary nursing objective is assisting in establishing a diagnosis. Since the treatment is universally surgical, preoperative and postoperative care are major nursing functions. Although in many instances nurses may not perform the complete history and examination, they are often in a strategic position to make judgements regarding the child's care.

When the child with an *acute abdomen* (a general term used to describe conditions associated with acute abdominal pain) is admitted to the paediatric unit, staff nurses usually decide where to place the child, and how much observation and assessment of the child are required and by whom. Without an appreciation of the signs and symptoms suggestive of appendicitis, these nurses may not make decisions that facilitate rapid diagnosis.

MECKEL'S DIVERTICULUM

Meckel's diverticulum results when the omphalomesenteric or vitelline duct, which connects the midgut to the yolk sac during embryonic development, fails to completely obliterate. Although several different types of malformations can result, such as cysts, fistulas, or fibrotic cords, Meckel's diverticulum consists of an outpouching of the ileum, most commonly in proximity to the ileocaecal valve. It may vary in size from a small appendiceal process to a segment of bowel several inches long and wide. At times, it may be connected to the umbilicus by a cord.

Meckel's diverticulum is more common in males than in females, and complications are several times more frequent in males. Often, it exists without causing symptoms. Most symptomatic cases are seen in the first two years of life.

CLINICAL MANIFESTATIONS

Signs and symptoms are based on the specific pathological process, such as diverticulitis or intestinal obstruction. Rectal bleeding, however, is the chief presenting sign in more than half of the cases. Bright red or dark red rectal bleeding is much more common than black, tarry stools, and represents acute haemorrhage. Usually, there is no evidence of abdominal pain. Severe anaemia and shock are consequences of the haemorrhage.

PROCESS OF DIAGNOSIS

Diagnosis is usually based on the history. Barium enema, and in some cases radioisotope scan, confirm the diagnoses. Radiological studies are not helpful in confirming the diagnosis, because the diverticulum may be too small to be visualized or may fail to fill with barium. Blood studies are usually part of the general laboratory workup to rule out any bleeding disorder and to evaluate the severity of the anaemia.

THERAPEUTIC MANAGEMENT

Treatment is surgical removal of the diverticulum. In instances in which severe haemorrhage increases the surgical risk, medical intervention to correct hypovolaemic shock (e.g., blood replacement, intravenous fluids and oxygen) may be necessary. In diverticulitis, antibiotics may be used preoperatively to control infection. If intestinal obstruction has occurred, appropriate preoperative measures are used to reverse electrolyte imbalances and prevent abdominal distention.

IMPLICATIONS FOR NURSING

Nursing objectives are the same as for any child undergoing surgery (see Chapter 7). Since the onset is usually rapid, psychological support parallels that for other conditions, such as appendicitis. It is important to remember that massive rectal bleeding is most often traumatic to both the child and the parents, and may significantly affect their emotional reaction to hospitalization and surgery.

Specific preoperative considerations when rectal bleeding is present include: (1) frequent monitoring of vital signs and blood pressure for shock, (2) keeping the child on bed rest, and (3) recording the approximate amount of blood lost in stools. In the absence of rectal haemorrhage, the nurse tests the stools for occult blood.

INFLAMMATORY BOWEL DISEASE

Inflammatory bowel disease (IBD) is a general term used to designate two chronic intestinal disorders — *ulcerative colitis (UC)* and *Crohn's disease (CD)*. The term should not be confused with *irritable bowel syndrome (IBS)*, which refers to a functional disorder. Although these two diseases are grouped under the classification of IBD because they have similar epidemiological, immunological and clinical features, they are two distinct conditions with very significant differences, primarily in the intestinal features. The most important reason for differentiating between the two is prognosis. CD is considered the more serious and disabling disorder, and medical/surgical treatment is much less effective than in UC. Unfortunately, the incidence of CD is increasing in the population, although the reason for this change is not known.

CLINICAL MANIFESTATIONS

Clinical features are similar in both UC and CD, especially systemic and extraintestinal manifestations. Clinical presentations of intestinal signs and symptoms are different (Table 27-2). The diseases occur in both sexes with equal frequency, and both are primarily diseases of adolescence and young adulthood.

Intestinal manifestations

The most common feature of UC is persistent or recurring diarrhoea. In the acute, fulminating disease there is bloody diarrhoea preceded by cramping abdominal pain, and followed by abdominal distention. Diarrhoea may be severe, with marked urgency and frequency (20-30 stools daily). X-ray reveals characteristic pouches that give the normal colon a scalloped appearance, shortening of its length, and uniform reduction in diameter, all of which give the picture of the *lead-pipe colon*. Nocturnal diarrhoea is common and is associated with more extensive involvement. Children are usually healthy before the onset of the disease (Jackson and Grand, 1991).

The onset of CD is usually insidious. Diarrhoea and intermittent, cramping pain often resemble that of acute appendicitis. The pain is often triggered by eating. As the disease progresses, however, the abdominal pain becomes a constant aching or soreness. The diarrhoea may contain blood, but it is a less frequent finding in children. Malabsorption is more common in CD.

PROCESS OF DIAGNOSIS

Diagnosis is usually based on a combination of findings from history, physical examination and laboratory testing. Specific diagnostic tests to confirm the diagnosis and rule out other possibilities such as anal fissures, GI infections and diverticulitis include: (1) x-ray studies of the colon, especially barium enema, (2) endoscopy, and (3) mucosal biopsy for histological evidence of the inflammatory process (especially in CD). Stool samples may be obtained to rule out the presence of pathological organisms and malabsorptive defects. Blood

CHARACTERISTICS	ULCERATIVE COLITIS	CROHN'S DISEASE
Pathological changes		
Extent of involvement	Diffuse, mucosal	Focal, transmural (entire wall)
Ulceration	Superficial, extensive	Deep
Distribution of lesions	Contiguous, symmetric	Segmental, asymmetric with
Lymph nodes	Normal	'skip' areas
		Affected
Primary areas of involvement	Colon, rectum	Ileum, colon, rectum
Clinical features		
Rectal bleeding	Common	Uncommon
Diarrhoea	Often severe	Moderate to absent
Pain	Less frequent	Common
Anorexia	Mild or moderate	Can be severe
Weight loss	Moderate	Severe
Growth retardation	Usually mild	Often marked
Anal and perianal lesions	Rare	Common
Fistulas and strictures	Rare	Common
Surgical resection of affected bowel	Curative	Unsatisfactory because of frequent recurrence
Risk of carcinoma	Related to duration of disease Prevented by surgery	Occurs less frequently Not prevented by surgery

Table 27.2 Comparison of inflammatory bowel diseases - ulcerative colitis and Crohn's disease.

studies are done to determine severity of anaemia, extent of albumin loss, and immunoglobulin levels. Erythrocyte sedimentation rate and C-reactive protein are more likely to be elevated in CD. Diagnosis is established by endoscopy examination and, in CD, biopsy. Endoscopic features considered most useful in discriminating CD and UC include intermittent colonic involvement, perianal lesions, and cobblestoning of mucosa with CD, whereas erosions and mucosal granularity are more suggestive of UC (Bines and Walker, 1989).

THERAPEUTIC MANAGEMENT

The goals of therapy are: (1) to control the inflammatory process in order to reduce or eliminate the symptoms, (2) to maintain long-term remission, and (3) to allow as normal a lifestyle as possible. Treatment must be individualized and managed according to the severity of the disease, location of lesions and response to therapy.

Conservative treatment

The medical management of children with inflammatory bowel disease uses sulphasalazine and/or corticosteroid therapy. The nurse should be vigilant in maintaining the effects of steroid treatment.

Dietary management is often vigorous because of the child's poorly nourished state. The goals are: (1) to replace nutrient losses associated with the inflammatory processes, (2) to correct body deficits, and (3) to provide sufficient nutrients to promote energy and nitrogen balance for normal metabolic function (Motil and Grand, 1985). These goals can be accomplished by enteral and/or parenteral routes. The therapeutic diet consists of high protein, high calorie, normal to low fat, and low fibre. Vitamin and mineral supplements are usually provided to correct anaemia and other deficiencies.

During the acute stage, supplemental nutrition by way of intermittent or continuous drip gastric feedings, intravenous fluids to correct dehydration and associated electrolyte imbalances, and/or parenteral alimentation may be required.

Surgical treatment

In some instances, surgery may be performed to allow the bowel a period of rest. To arrest the disease process, the entire section of ulcerated bowel is removed, in which case total colectomy and ileostomy are usually required. Advances in surgical techniques over the incontinent abdominal stoma now provide options for some children. Surgical alternatives include a *continent (Koch) ileostomy* in which an intra-abdominal pouch or reservoir is created to allow continence, or an *ileoanal anastomosis,* which preserves the normal pathway for defaecation and eliminates the abdominal stoma.

Removal of the diseased bowel is a permanent remedy for UC and prevents possible development of carcinoma. However, in CD, surgical removal of the affected bowel is not curative. The disease tends to recur, and the risk of cancer of the bowel is not affected and requires appropriate screening for early detection.

IMPLICATIONS FOR NURSING

Many of the implications for nursing relate directly to the therapeutic management in treating colitis. However, the scope of nursing responsibilities extends beyond the immediate period of hospitalization and involves: (1) continued guidance of families in terms of dietary management and drug compliance, (2) adjusting to a disease of remissions and exacerbations or one of chronic ill health, and (3) when indicated, preparing the child and parents for the possibility of diversionary bowel surgery.

Since diet therapy is a very important component of therapy, encouraging the anorexic child to consume sufficient quantities of this diet is of primary importance and is frequently a nursing challenge. An approach that is more likely to meet with success involves including the child in meal planning; encouraging small, frequent meals or snacks rather than three large meals a day; serving meals around medication schedules when diarrhoea, mouth pain, and intestinal spasm are controlled; and preparing high-protein, high-calorie foods, such as milk shakes, cream soups, puddings or custard (if lactose is tolerated) (see also Feeding the Sick Child, Chapter 8).

Foods that are known to aggravate the condition are avoided, as are high-fibre foods. Since the best sources of folic acid and iron are found in high-fibre foods, such as fresh fruits and vegetables, the child is at risk for vitamin deficiency. Also, sulphasalazine inhibits folate absorption. It is important to emphasize the need to make up for these deficiencies with supplements. Occasionally, stomatitis further complicates adherence to dietary management. Good mouth care before eating and the selection of bland foods help relieve the discomfort of mouth sores.

The importance of continued drug therapy, despite remission of symptoms, must be stressed to the parents and child. Failure to adhere to the pharmacological regimen can result in exacerbation of the disease process.

Attending to the emotional components of a chronic disease requires a thorough assessment of stress factors that are disease related. Frequently, the nurse can be instrumental in helping these children adjust to the problems of growth retardation, delayed sexual maturation, dietary restrictions, feelings of being 'different' or 'sickly', inability to compete with peers, and necessary absence from school during exacerbations of the illness.

If a permanent colectomy/ileostomy is required, the nurse can assist the child and family in accepting and adjusting to the change by teaching them how to care for the ileostomy, by emphasizing the positive aspects of surgery (particularly accelerated growth and sexual development, permanent recovery, and eliminated risk of colonic cancer), and by stressing the normality of life despite bowel diversion. Introducing the child and parents to other ostomy patients, especially those of the child's age, can be the greatest therapeutic measure in fostering eventual acceptance. Whenever possible, the newer continent ostomies should be offered as options to the child, although they are not performed in all centres throughout the United Kingdom.

OBSTRUCTIVE DISORDERS

Obstruction of the bowel occurs when the passage of intestinal contents is mechanically impeded by a constricted or occluded lumen, or when there is interference with normal muscular contraction. Intestinal obstruction from any cause is characterized by similar signs and symptoms, although the progression may vary greatly.

Classically, acute mechanical intestinal obstruction is characterized by colicky abdominal pain, nausea and vomiting, abdominal distention and constipation. *Pain* is caused by severe, intermittent muscular contractions proximal to the obstruction as the bowel attempts to move luminal contents along the normal path. *Abdominal distention* is the result of accumulation of gas and fluid above the level of the obstruction. As these secretions continue to accumulate, the gut becomes excessively irritated and stimulates the vomiting centre in the medulla to rid itself of the irritants with or without nausea. *Vomiting* is often the earliest sign of a high obstruction and a later sign in lower obstructions. Conversely, *constipation* and *obstipation* are early signs of low obstructions and later signs of higher obstructions. For example, a child with a high obstruction can have normal stools for 1-2 days as the bowel evacuates itself distal to the defect.

In acute conditions, such as intussusception, the clinical manifestations are apparent within a few hours of the onset of the disorder. In other conditions, such as pyloric stenosis, the signs and symptoms may be more gradual and may be missed during early stages of the disorder. If the obstruction is below the stomach, reflux from the small intestine causes intestinal secretions to flow back into the stomach, where they are vomited along with stomach contents. As this progresses, large quantities of fluid and electrolytes are lost, causing *dehydration*.

As distention progresses, the abdomen may be rigid and board-like, with moderate to severe *tenderness*. *Bowel sounds* gradually diminish and cease. *Respiratory distress* occurs as the diaphragm is pushed up into the pleural cavity. As proteins are lost from the bloodstream into the intestinal lumen, the plasma volume diminishes and *shock* may occur (Stringer, Pablot and Brereton, 1992).

HYPERTROPHIC PYLORIC STENOSIS

Obstruction at the pyloric sphincter by hypertrophy of the circular muscle of the pylorus is one of the most common surgical disorders of early infancy. This functional anomaly is seen soon after birth, with vomiting that becomes progressively more severe and projectile. It is five times more common in male than in female infants, affecting approximately 5 of 1000 males and only 1 of 1000 females (Cohen, 1984). Hypertrophic pyloric stenosis (HPS) is seen less frequently in black and Oriental than in white infants. It is more likely to affect a full-term than a premature infant.

The cause of the increased size of the pyloric musculature is unknown. A higher incidence in first-degree relatives and in monozygotic as opposed to dizygotic twins implicates heredity in the aetiology, although the nature of the hereditary factors is only speculative.

CLINICAL MANIFESTATIONS

The age of onset and pattern of vomiting are variable. Typically, infants with pyloric hypertrophy are well during the first weeks of life. Initially, there is only regurgitation or occasional nonprojectile vomiting that begins about the second to the fourth week after birth, although in a few infants symptoms begin at birth. Others do well for the first few weeks and then suddenly develop projectile vomiting that rapidly leads to dehydration. The projectile vomiting usually develops within a week and may lead to complete obstruction by 4-6 weeks. The vomitus may be ejected 0.6-1.2 m (2-4 feet) from the child in a side-lying position, and 0.3 m (1 foot) or more when the infant is lying on the back.

Vomiting occurs most often shortly after a feeding, although it may occur as long as several hours later. In some instances, the vomiting may follow each feeding; in others, it appears intermittently. The infant is hungry and an avid nurser who eagerly accepts a second feeding after a vomiting episode. The vomitus is nonbilious, containing only gastric contents, but may be blood tinged. The infant does not appear to be in pain, other than the discomfort of chronic hunger.

The infant fails to gain weight or may lose weight, the stools diminish in number and size from the reduced intake, and evidence of dehydration becomes increasingly obvious. There is decreased elasticity of the skin, loss of subcutaneous tissue, and sunken eyeballs and depression of the fontanel. The upper abdomen is distended, and diagnosis can be established on the basis of: (1) a readily palpable olive-shaped tumour in the epigastrium just to the right of the umbilicus, which can best felt during a 'test feed', and (2) visible gastric peristaltic waves that move from left to right across the epigastrium. The pyloric tumour is most easily felt when the abdominal muscles are relaxed during a feeding or immediately after vomiting. Positive identification of these physical signs is sufficient evidence to establish a diagnosis.

Difficulty in diagnosis is related to children with feeding difficulties associated with disturbed parent-child relationships or hyperkinetic infants, who are exceptionally reactive to external stimuli and vomit more frequently than usual in the early weeks of life.

NB: The use of the term 'tumour' in this condition can be misleading since there is no suggestion of malignant disease. It is vital that this term is clarified to parents when used.

PROCESS OF DIAGNOSIS

If diagnosis is inconclusive from the history and physical signs, upper GI x-ray studies will reveal delayed gastric emptying and an elongated, thread-like pyloric channel. Ultrasound evaluation is as accurate as an x-ray, is less traumatic, and there is less risk of aspiration of contrast medium. The hazard of aspiration is increased with gastric outlet obstruction.

THERAPEUTIC MANAGEMENT

Surgical relief of the pyloric obstruction by pyloromyotomy is simple, safe and effective and is, with few exceptions, the standard treatment for this disorder. Inasmuch as the surgery is not an emergency procedure, the initial efforts are directed towards rehydration of the infant, replenishment of body potassium stores, and correction of alkalosis with parenteral fluid and electrolyte administration. In well-hydrated infants with no evidence of electrolyte imbalance, surgery is performed without delay. Replacement fluid therapy usually delays surgery for 24-48 hours. Most surgeons prefer the stomach to be empty during surgery to diminish postoperative vomiting from gastric irritation; some centres advocate saline gastric washouts preoperatively. The stomach is decompressed with an NG tube. The tube is often left in place during the surgical procedure to keep the stomach empty of fluid, air, or barium from x-ray procedures (Mu-tagh *et al*, 1992).

The surgical procedure is performed through a right upper quadrant incision and consists of a longitudinal incision through the circular muscle fibres of the pylorus down to, but not including, the submucosa (Fredet-Ramstedt operation). The procedure has a very high success rate when infants receive careful preoperative preparation to correct fluid and electrolyte imbalances. It may take up to 12 weeks for the pylorus to return to normal size (Okorie *et al*, 1988), hence vomiting may persist initially but will gradually diminish. Post-operative reintroduction of feeds varies according to local practice but is usually fully re-established within 24 hours.

The infant is ready to be discharged from the hospital by about the second to sixth postoperative day. The prognosis is excellent, and the mortality is low.

IMPLICATIONS FOR NURSING

Nursing care of the infant with HPS involves primarily observation for physical signs and behaviours that help establish the diagnosis, careful regulation of fluid therapy, and re-establishment of normal feeding behaviours. Nurses are in a position to recognize signs of the disorder in infants and to refer them for medical evaluation.

Preoperatively, emphasis is placed on restoring hydration and electrolyte balance, and beginning replacement of depleted body fat and protein stores. Some infants may require 24–48 hours of correction of electrolyte imbalance before surgery can be performed. These infants are allowed nothing by mouth and are given intravenous fluids of glucose and electrolytes based on laboratory serum electrolyte values; usually sodium chloride solution with added potassium (when there is adequate urine output). Depleted calcium must also be replaced. Careful monitoring of the intravenous infusion and assiduous attention to intake, output, and urine specific gravity measurements are important to the success of fluid replacement. Accurate description of any vomiting, as well as the number and character of stools, is recorded.

Observations include assessment of vital signs, particularly those that might indicate fluid or electrolyte imbalances, including glucose levels, because glycogen stores may be depleted from prolonged vomiting. These infants are especially prone to metabolic alkalosis from loss of hydrogen ions and to potassium, sodium and chloride depletion, all of which are contained in gastric secretions. The skin and mucous membranes are assessed for alterations in hydration status, and daily weight measurement provides added clues to water gain or loss.

It is the responsibility of the nurse to ensure that the NG tube is patent and functioning properly, and to measure and record the type and amount of drainage. The infant is usually positioned with the head slightly elevated.

General hygienic care, with particular attention to skin and mouth in dehydrated infants, is an important part of care. Protection from infection is also important, because infants with impaired nutritional status are even more susceptible than normal newborn infants. As with any child in the hospital, parents are encouraged to visit and to become involved in the child's care. Vomiting of a projectile nature is frightening to parents, and they often believe that they may have done something wrong. Most parents need support and reassurance that the condition is caused by a structural problem and is in no way a reflection of their parenting skills and capacities.

INTUSSUSCEPTION

Intussusception is a telescoping of one portion of the intestine into another. It most commonly occurs at the ileocaecal valve where the ileum telescopes into the caecum, and may go further, into the colon (see Fig. 27-2). Intussusception is one of the most frequent causes of intestinal obstruction during infancy. One-half of the cases occur in children younger than one year, more commonly between 3-12 months of age, and most of the others occur in children during the second year. However, several cases have been reported in infants under four months of age and children 5-15 years of age (Newman and Schuh, 1987; Reijnin, 1987). Intussusception is three times more common in males than in females. Although specific intestinal lesions can be found in a small percentage of the children, generally the cause is not known. The occurrence of intussusception is increased in children with cystic fibrosis and coeliac disease.

CLINICAL MANIFESTATIONS

Classic presentation of intussusception is a healthy, thriving child, usually between 3-12 months of age, who suddenly has an episode of acute abdominal pain. Typical behaviour includes screaming and drawing the knees up to the chest. These episodes of severe pain are characterized by intervals in which the child appears normal and comfortable.

During this initial period, vomiting usually occurs, and the child passes one normal brown stool. However, as the condition worsens, the vomiting increases and becomes bile stained, the child becomes apathetic, and subsequent stools may resemble red currant jelly due to the passage of stool mixed with blood and mucus.

The abdomen becomes tender and distended. A sausage-shaped mass may be felt in the upper right quadrant. In contrast, the lower right quadrant usually feels empty (Dance sign) as the bowel distal to the obstruction is less involved and free of contents. If treatment is not sought, the child becomes acutely ill with fever, prostration, and signs of peritonitis.

Manifestations in older children

Although the classic signs and symptoms of intussusception are paroxysmal abdominal pain, vomiting, palpable abdominal mass, and currant jelly stools, a more chronic picture may occur, characterized by diarrhoea, constipation, occasional vomiting and periodic colic. Since this condition is potentially life-threatening, the nurse must recognize such signs and closely observe and refer these children for further medical investigation.

PROCESS OF DIAGNOSIS

Frequently, the diagnosis can be made on subjective findings alone. However, diagnosis is usually based on a plain abdominal X-ray. A rectal examination reveals mucus, blood, and occasionally a low intussusception itself.

THERAPEUTIC MANAGEMENT

On admission, the child is likely to appear shocked, dehydrated and in need of urgent fluid resuscitation.

In most cases, the initial treatment of choice is nonsurgical hydrostatic reduction by air enema. Usually, correction of the invagination is carried out at the same time as the diagnostic testing. The principle behind this procedure is that the force exerted by the flowing barium will be sufficient to push the invaginated portion of the bowel into its original position, similar to pushing an inverted 'finger' out of a glove. Occasionally, barium enema may be used.

Since this procedure is only successful in 75%–80% of cases) and is not recommended if there are clinical signs of shock or perforation, the child is also prepared for surgery before the attempted reduction. Surgical intervention involves manually reducing the invagination and, where indicated, resecting any nonviable intestine.

IMPLICATIONS FOR NURSING

The nurse can assist in establishing a diagnosis by carefully listening to the parents' history of the child's physical and behavioural symptoms relating to the complaint. Although parents may not know the medical problem, they are astute diagnosticians in detecting that something is wrong.

As soon as a possible diagnosis of intussusception is made, the nurse begins to prepare the parents for the immediate need for hospitalization, the usual nonsurgical techniques, and the possibility of surgery. It is important at this time to explain the basic defect of intussusception, which can be easily demonstrated by pushing the end of a finger on a rubber glove back into itself or using the example of a telescoping rod. The principle of reduction by hydrostatic pressure can be simulated by filling the glove with water or blowing into it like a balloon, which pushes the 'finger' into a fully extended position. By using such demonstrations, the parents are aware of why surgery is sometimes necessary. Without this preparation, they may be left with the feeling that the doctor 'failed' or that their child had 'complications'.

Physical care of the child with intussusception differs little from that for any child undergoing abdominal surgery (see Chapter 8). Even though nonsurgical intervention may be successful, usual preoperative procedures are performed. For the child with signs of electrolyte imbalance, haemorrhage or peritonitis, additional medical preparation such as replacement fluids, whole blood or plasma, and NG suctioning may be included. All stools are monitored before surgery.

Postprocedural care includes the usual postoperative observations (see Chapter 7) with special observation of stool passage and return of bowel sounds. In the case of hydrostatic reduction or autoreduction, the nurse observes for passage of barium and the stool patterns, since recurrences of the intussusception are most likely to occur within the first 36 hours after reduction. For this reason, the child is kept in the hospital for 2-3 days. Overall recurrence of intussusception after nonsurgical or operative reduction is between 4-10% (Silverman and Roy, 1983).

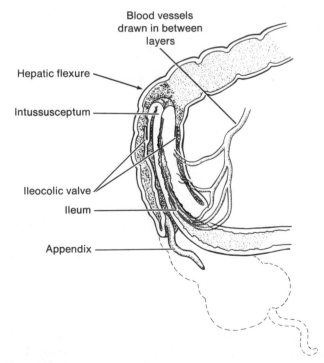

Fig. 27-2 Ileocaecal intussusception.

MALABSORPTION SYNDROMES

The term *malabsorption syndrome* is applied to a long list of disorders associated with some degree of impaired digestion and/or absorption. Most are classified according to the locations of the supposed anatomical and/or biochemical defect.

CLASSIFICATION AND MANIFESTATIONS

Malabsorption can be classified as: (1) failure of digestion (intraluminal), (2) failure of absorption (mucosal), and (3) lymphatic obstruction. Only digestive and absorptive dysfunctions are discussed here.

MANIFESTATIONS

Several manifestations are common to chronic malabsorption/maldigestion. Nutritional state is the most important aspect of assessment of chronic diarrhoea. Wasting of subcutaneous fat (especially noticeable in the gluteal area) is characteristic of failure to thrive. Oedema is observed in children with protein deficiency, and easy bruising often results from inadequate absorption of vitamin C and fat-soluble vitamin K. Coeliac syndrome is a primary manifestation of some major malabsorption diseases.

Coeliac syndrome

Coeliac syndrome and *malabsorption syndrome* are terms used to describe a symptom complex associated with several different diseases that have four characteristics in common: (1) steatorrhoea (fat, foul, frothy, bulky stools), (2) general malnutrition, (3) abdominal distention, and (4) secondary vitamin deficiencies. Two diseases with coeliac syndrome as manifestations are coeliac disease and cystic fibrosis. Coeliac disease, which, in adults, is often referred to as 'nontropical sprue', is discussed in the next section. Cystic fibrosis is the most common genetic disorder with coeliac syndrome as a feature.

COELIAC DISEASE (GLUTEN ENTEROPATHY)

Coeliac disease (CD), also known as *gluten enteropathy (GE)*, *gluten-sensitive enteropathy (GSE)*, and *coeliac sprue*, is infrequent in the paediatric population in the United Kingdom (Hull, Johnston, 1994). Although the exact reason is not known, there is an association between changes in feeding practices — specifically, delayed introduction of solid foods and encouragement of breast-feeding — and the declining incidence of coeliac disease.

Evidence of a link between the disease and genetic factors is the incidence of histocompatibility antigen HLA-B8 in 60-90% of affected individuals, which is a fourfold increase over that found in the general population (Savilahi *et al*, 1986; Silverman and Roy, 1983).

CLINICAL MANIFESTATIONS

The gliadin fraction of gluten damages the villi of the gastrointestinal tract, leading to the well-known symptoms. These symptoms, those of coeliac syndrome, are first noted about 3-6 months following introduction of gluten-containing grains into the diet, typically at 9-12 months of age, although it may not be evident until early childhood. Symptoms are usually insidious and chronic. The first evidence of the disease may be failure to regain weight or appetite after a bout of diarrhoea. Constipation, vomiting and abdominal pain may also be initial presenting signs. Behavioural changes, such as irritability, fretfulness, uncooperativeness or apathy, are common. As the disease progresses, signs of general wasting become evident.

PROCESS OF DIAGNOSIS

A definitive diagnosis is based on a peroral jejunal biopsy, which demonstrates the atrophic changes in the architecture of the mucosal wall. This procedure is performed by passing a polyethylene tube through the mouth along the alimentary tract to the jejunum of the small bowel. Measuring serum antigliadin and antireticulin antibodies aids in diagnosis.

The other essential criterion of diagnosis is dramatic clinical improvement after adherence to a gluten-restricted diet. Within a day or two after instituting the diet, most children with CD demonstrate a favourable personality change. Weight gain, improved appetite, and disappearance of diarrhoea and steatorrhoea usually do not occur for several days. Return of symptoms after reintroduction of gluten is positive evidence of gluten sensitivity.

THERAPEUTIC MANAGEMENT

Treatment of chronic coeliac disease is primarily dietary management. Although the prescribed diet is called 'gluten free', it is in reality low in gluten, since it is impossible to remove every source of this protein. Also, most patients are able to tolerate restricted amounts of gluten. Since gluten is found mainly in the grains of wheat and rye, but also in smaller quantities in barley and oats, these four foods are eliminated. Corn, rice and millet are substitute grain foods.

In children with severe malnutrition, specific deficiencies are treated with supplemental vitamins, iron and calories. Because absorption of fat-soluble vitamins is impaired, these are supplied in a water-miscible form.

Most patients with CD have a permanent sensitivity to gluten, which requires lifelong maintenance of a gluten-free diet. A small group of infants exhibit transient gluten sensitivity and are able to digest gluten safely after a period of time.

A coeliac crisis may be precipitated by a mild respiratory infection and is caused by vomiting and large, watery stools. This is a rare event, but requires prompt medical intervention to correct the dehydration and metabolic acidosis. Treatment involves intermittent NG decompression, intravenous fluids with appropriate electrolyte replacement, and intravenous steroid administration to decrease bowel inflammation. The prompt improvement in response to steroids is believed to support the immunological theory that gluten acts as an antigen to the mucosal cells.

IMPLICATIONS FOR NURSING

The main implication for nursing is helping the parents and child adhere to diet therapy. This involves considerable time explaining the disease process to the parents, the specific role of gluten in aggravating the disorder, and foods that must be restricted. It is especially difficult to maintain a diet indefinitely when the child has no symptoms and temporary transgressions result in no difficulties. Although the chief source of grain is cereal, grains are frequently added to processed foods as thickeners or fillers. To compound the difficulty, gluten is added to many foods, but obscurely listed on the label as 'hydrolyzed vegetable protein'. The nurse must advise parents of the necessity of reading all label ingredients carefully to avoid hidden sources of gluten. Health visitors provide invaluable support in case of these children.

Some of children's favourite foods contain these ingredients, including bread, cake, crackers, doughnuts, pies, spaghetti, pizza, prepared soups, some processed ice cream, many types of chocolate, some milk preparations, luncheon meats, meat gravy and some hamburgers. Many of these products can be eliminated from the infant's or young child's diet fairly easily, but monitoring the diet of a school-aged child or adolescent is a much more difficult situation. Luncheon preparation away from home is particularly difficult, since bread, luncheon meats and instant soups are not allowed. For families on restricted food budgets, adhering to the diet adds an additional financial burden, since many inexpensive or convenience foods cannot be used. It may be more economical for these families to buy rice or corn flour directly from the milling company.

Another deterrent to adherence is the recommendation that the child continue the diet indefinitely. This is especially difficult for parents and children to understand when there have been no symptoms of the disease for an extended time and occasional dietary indiscretions have not caused untoward effects. However, evidence demonstrates that the majority of individuals who relax their diet experience a relapse. There is also evidence that terminating the diet predisposes to development of malignant lymphoma of the small intestine, oesophageal cancer, and other gastrointestinal cancers in adulthood.

It is important to stress long-term complications, as well as to remind parents of the child's physical status before dietary treatment and dramatic improvement after it was begun. For the child, however, these arguments may not be as convincing, because the future is less significant than the present and the past has little meaning. The nurse can be instrumental in allowing the child to express these feelings, while focusing on ways in which the child can still be 'normal'. For example, the usual prepared foods, such as beefburgers, may be restricted, but tacos and others such as tortilla chips

are acceptable. Many children complain that the diet is boring because the parent prepares the same food all the time. The child can be encouraged to find new recipes using suitable ingredients. With the present emphasis on natural health foods, the nurse can encourage the child to investigate new foods, such as sesame seeds and rice flour, to enhance his or her choices, while still being in vogue with peer interests. In some children, permanent growth retardation presents another emotional crisis.

SHORT BOWEL SYNDROME

The short bowel syndrome (SBS) refers to a condition in which loss of intestine results in diminished ability to normally digest and absorb a regular diet. It occurs most often in infants or children following intestinal resection for inflammatory conditions, such as necrotizing enterocolitis or IBD, or congenital bowel anomalies, such as small intestine atresias, gastroschisis, exomphalus or volvulus (twisting of a large section of bowel).

Both the extent and location of the loss, especially the ileum, are important factors in determining the severity of the condition. As much as 50% of the intestine can be lost without affecting the health of the child, unless it includes the distal ileum. A loss of greater than 75% of the small bowel results in malabsorption. However, the remaining intestine and stomach can adapt to the loss provided the child is kept alive through nutritional support. Adaptation occurs in a compensatory growth of all coats of the bowel wall with increased length and diameter of the remaining gut (Klish and Putnam, 1981).

THERAPEUTIC MANAGEMENT

The goals of treatment are: (1) to preserve as much length of bowel surgically as possible and (2) to maintain the child's nutritional status until adaptation of the bowel occurs. Small amounts of dilute formula should be started as soon as possible, since the bowel must be challenged with formula for it to develop enzymes to tolerate feedings. This necessitates a planned schedule of gradually increased concentration of formula; enteral feedings may be prescribed, and severely affected children require total parenteral feeding to provide sufficient nutrition.

IMPLICATIONS FOR NURSING

Nursing care is directed towards maintaining the child's nutritional state, and prescribed orders for oral or enteral feedings must be followed exactly. If parenteral alimentation is required, every effort is made to preserve the intravenous line and to prevent complications such as infection. When longterm parenteral nutrition is required, preparing the family for home care of the child is a major nursing responsibility (see Chapter 24). Since hospitalization may be prolonged, the child's developmental and emotional needs must be attended to as well.

HEPATIC DISORDERS

The liver is the largest internal organ in the body and one of the most vital. It performs more than 400 functions that broadly include: (1) blood storage and filtration; (2) secretion of bile and bilirubin; (3) metabolism of fat, protein, and carbohydrate and synthesis of blood-clotting components; (4) detoxification of hormones, drugs and other substances; and (5) storage for glycogen, iron and vitamins A, D, E and B_{12}. Inflammatory, obstructive, or degenerative disorders that affect the liver will affect all or some of these functions. The following discussion is concerned with two disorders that affect the liver during childhood — hepatitis and cirrhosis. Biliary atresia, a congenital anomaly, is discussed in Chapter 14.

ACUTE HEPATITIS

Hepatitis, or inflammation of the liver, is rapidly emerging as one of the major causes of morbidity and a significant cause of mortality in children. The discussion that follows is primarily concerned with acute hepatitis, although the chronic form of the disease may involve many of the same mechanisms.

CLINICAL MANIFESTATIONS

The clinical manifestations for hepatitis A virus (HAV) and hepatitis B virus (HBV) are similar, except for a more rapid, acute onset in type A and a slower, more insidious onset in type B. Both types may have flu-like symptoms and may never be recognized as actual cases of hepatitis.

The initial anicteric (absence of jaundice) phase symptoms include nausea and vomiting, extreme anorexia, malaise, easy fatigability and slight to moderate fever. The child may have abdominal pain (especially epigastric or upper right quadrant), usually acts ill, preferring to rest in bed, and is fretful or irritable. The most significant finding, on physical examination, is liver tenderness with or without enlargement. This phase usually lasts 5-7 days.

The icteric (jaundice) phase begins with darkening of the urine and the presence of light-coloured stools, followed by yellowing of the sclera and skin. As jaundice worsens, the child usually begins to feel better, with improved appetite and behaviour, and the absence of nausea, vomiting and fever. This opposing course of rising bilirubin and improved clinical signs is regarded as a significant diagnostic and prognostic sign of benign viral hepatitis.

The appearance of jaundice with worsening constitutional symptoms is regarded as a poorer prognostic sign. A majority of these children develop fulminant, subacute, or chronic active hepatitis. Some children never develop jaundice; however, although their course is usually milder, they are still infectious.

The icteric phase commonly lasts less than four weeks. Complete recovery with return of normal liver function and a feeling of well-being with absence of fatigue or malaise may take 1-3 months. Generally, children recover promptly. However, it is not unusual for the child to experience a short relapse of slight jaundice and clinical symptoms 10-12 weeks after the illness. Unless the symptoms persist and continue to worsen, this relapse is considered benign.

Not all affected children exhibit signs of disease. Because the manifestations of hepatitis are the body's response to the viral antigen, individuals who are unable to muster an adequate defence will develop few, if any, symptoms. However, they may still harbour the virus as carriers. Newborn infants of mothers with HBV who have been exposed to the virus during antenatal life do not recognize the virus as a foreign protein and thus become chronic carriers.

PROCESS OF DIAGNOSIS

Diagnosis is based on history, physical examination, laboratory evidence of the virus, and liver function tests. Other assessment factors include evidence of: (1) contact with a person known to have hepatitis, especially a family member; (2) questionable sanitation practices, such as impure drinking water; (3) eating certain foods, such as clams or oysters (especially from polluted water); (4) recent immunizations or blood transfusions; (5) ingestion of hepatotoxic drugs, such as salicylates, sulphonamides, several antineoplastic agents, and many other medications; and (6) parenteral administration of illicit drugs or sexual contact with a person who uses these drugs. The last event is especially important when hepatitis B is suspected in an adolescent and should be coupled with a careful examination for signs of needle marks, especially in the antecubital fossa.

Diagnosis is confirmed by detection of antibodies or antigens produced in response to the specific virus, such as HBsAg (hepatitis B surface antigen). Clinical improvement is usually associated with a decrease and disappearance of antigens, followed by the appearance of their antibodies. Since the antibodies persist indefinitely, they are used to identify the carrier state (individuals with the HBV who have no clinical disease but are able to transmit the organism).

THERAPEUTIC MANAGEMENT

There is no specific treatment for hepatitis. Management is primarily treatment of symptoms. For example, antiemetics may be helpful to reduce the nausea or vomiting. The value of bed rest in promoting overall recovery is controversial. The child who feels ill and tired in the anicteric phase usually chooses to stay in bed. However, once improvement of physical complaints begins, the child prefers to resume normal activity gradually. The best approach is probably to allow the child to regulate his or her own pace. Hospitalization is rarely necessary, although proper isolation precautions at home are imperative.

The child is allowed preferred foods, especially during the initial stage, when anorexia is severe. Generally, low-fat foods cause less stomach distention and are better tolerated than foods high in fat content. Carbohydrates should be encouraged to ensure an adequate caloric intake to spare proteins for cell growth. Vitamin K is administered if prothrombin time is prolonged.

Prevention

Isolation or quarantine of the infected child is not necessary as long as measures are employed to prevent spread of the virus. An attack of either virus confers long-lasting immunity to that virus; however, there is no crossover protection to the other virus. Prophylactic use of immune serum globulin (ISG) is effective in preventing hepatitis virus A in situations of pre-exposure (such as anticipated travel to areas where Hep A is prevalent) or in situations of postexposure during the early part of the incubation period and, to a lesser extent, before the onset of the disease. It is of inconsistent benefit in preventing type B virus.

Passive immunity to Hep B can be achieved with hyperimmune gamma globulin (hepatitis B immune serum globulin, HBIG), but it is very expensive. However, it is used for post-exposure prophylaxis in the following situations: (1) newborn infants born to HBsAg-positive mothers, (2) accidental needle stick or mucosal exposure to HBsAg-positive blood, or (3) sexual contact with an HBsAg-positive person. The hepatitis B vaccine is highly effective in providing protection against Hep B and may be used alone or with HBIG. At present the vaccine is recommended for people at risk, including haemodialysis patients, recipients of certain blood products (e.g., people with haemophilia or thalassaemia), and health care workers with frequent exposure to blood.

More recently, a hepatitis A vaccine (Harvix) has become available although it is primarily used as protection prior to foreign travel, etc.

IMPLICATIONS FOR NURSING

Nursing objectives depend largely on the severity of the hepatitis, the rigidity of medical treatment, and factors influencing the control and transmission of the disease. Since children with benign viral hepatitis are frequently cared for at home, the responsibility of explaining any medical therapies and control measures is frequently left to the clinic or children's nurse. In instances in which further assistance is needed for parents to comply with such instructions, a public health nursing referral may be necessary.

The emphasis is on encouraging a well-balanced diet and a realistic schedule of rest and activity adjusted to the child's condition. Since hepatitis type A is not infectious within a week or so after onset of jaundice, the child may feel well enough to resume school shortly thereafter. The parents are also cautioned about administering any medication to the child without the practitioner's knowledge, since normal doses of many drugs may become dangerous because of the liver's inability to detoxify and excrete them. Common drugs that are affected by hepatic failure include acetaminophen, ferrous sulphate (oral iron), and propoxyphene hydrochloride.

Handwashing is the single most effective measure in prevention and control of hepatitis in any setting. Parents and children need an explanation of the usual ways in which hepatitis A virus (oral-faecal route) and hepatitis B virus (parenteral route) are spread; they may benefit from receiving written instructions.

Hospitalized children are not usually isolated in a separate room unless they are faecally unreliable or incontinent, or if their toys and other items might become contaminated with faeces. They are discouraged from sharing their toys.

For children who have type B virus and a known or suspected history of illicit drug use, the nurse has the additional responsibility of helping them realize the associated dangers of drug abuse, stressing the parenteral mode of transmission, and encouraging them to seek counselling from a drug programme.

KEY POINTS

- ◆ Constipation is usually managed by diet management and bowel training.
- ◆ Hirschsprung's disease requires surgical removal of aganglionic segments of bowel.
- ◆ Nursing care of gastro-oesophageal reflux is aimed at identifying children with suggestive symptoms, helping parents with home care feeding and positioning, and caring for the child undergoing surgical intervention.
- ◆ Although the cause of appendicitis is poorly understood, it is commonly a result of obstruction of the lumen, usually by a faecalith. Common signs and symptoms are colicky abdominal pain, tenderness and fever.
- ◆ Meckel's diverticulum is a congenital malformation of the GI tract characterized by rectal bleeding.
- ◆ Management of IBD includes high-protein diet, vitamin/mineral supplements, suphasalazine and/or corticosteroids, antibiotics, and general supportive therapy. Surgical removal of inflamed bowel may be necessary.

- ◆ Hypertrophic pyloric stenosis is detected by observation of projectile vomiting without loss of appetite. Therapy is surgical pyloromyotomy.
- ◆ Intussusception is a cause of intestinal obstruction during infancy. Treatment is either nonsurgical hydrostatic reduction or surgical reduction.
- ◆ Coeliac disease, the second leading cause of malabsorption in children, is characterized by an intolerance for gluten. The major role of the nurse in the management of coeliac disease is helping parents and child adhere to diet therapy and preventing infections.
- ◆ Viral hepatitis is caused by at least four types of virus — hepatitis A virus, hepatitis B virus, hepatitis D virus, and non-A, non-B virus.
- ◆ Hepatitis A virus is spread by the faecal-oral route, whereas hepatitis B virus is transmitted primarily by the parenteral route. The single most effective measure in prevention and control of hepatitis in any setting is handwashing.

REFERENCES

Abrahamian FP, Lloyd-Still JD: Chronic constipation in childhood: longitudinal study of 186 patients, *J Pediatr Gastroenterol Nutr* 3:460, 1984.

Belknap WM: Sucking and swallowing disorders and gastroesophageal reflux. In Aski FA et al, editors: *Principles and practice of pediatrics*, Philadelphia, 1990, JB Lippincott.

Benninga MA, Buller HA, Taminiau JA: Biofeedback training in chronic constipation, *Arch Dis Child* 68(1):126, 1993

Berry J, Malt RA: Appendicitis near its centenary, *Ann Surg* 200:567, 1984.

Bines JE, Walker WA: Advances in inflammatory bowel disease, *Curr Opin Pediatr* 1:48, 1989.

Bonadio WA *et al:* Esophageal bougienage technique for coin ingestion in children, *J Pediatr Surg* 23:917, 1988.

Brady P: Esophageal foreign bodies, *Gastroenterol Clin North Am* 20(4):691, 1991.

Brender JD *et al:* Childhood appendicitis: factors associated with perforation, *Pediatr* 76(2):301, 1985a.

Caravati EM, Bennett DL, McElwee NE: Pediatric coin ingestion: a prospective study on the utility of routine roentgenograms, *Am J Dis Child* 143:549, 1989.

Carcassonne M *et al:* Surgery of gastroesophageal reflux, *World J Surg* 9:269, 1985.

Clayden G: Managing the child with constipation, *Prof Care Mother Child* 1(2):64, 1991.

Cohen FL: *Clinical genetics in nursing practice*, Philadelphia, 1984, JB Lippincott.

Doig CM: Hirschsprung's disease and mimicking conditions, *Digestive Diseases* 12(2):106, 1994.

Gracia C, Frey CF, Balaz IB: Diagnosis and management of ingested foreign bodies: a ten-year experience, *Ann Emerg Med* 13:30, 1984.

Hill P: Assessing faecal soiling in children, *Nurs Times* 87(14):61, 1991

Hull D, Johnston D: Essential paediatrics, 3 ed, London, 1994, Churchill Livingstone.

Jackson W, Grand R: Crohn's disease. In Walker W *et al*, editors: *Pediatric gastrointestinal disease*, Philadelphia, 1991, BC Decker.

Johns C: Encopresis, *Am J Nurs* 85(2):153, 1985.

Joseph PR: Management of coin ingestion, *Am J Dis Child* 143:449, 1990.

Klish WJ, Putnam TC: The short gut, *Am J Dis Child* 135:1056, 1981.

Landman GB: A five-year chart review of children biopsied to rule out Hirschsprung's disease, *Clin Pediatr* 26:288, 1987.

Lennard-Jones: Clinical management of constipation, *Pharmacol* 47(1):216, 1993.

Litovitz TL: Battery ingestions: product accessibility and clinical course, *Pediatr* 75(3):469, 1985.

Martin LW, Torres AM: Hirschsprung's disease, *Surg Clin North Am* 65(5):1171, 1985.

Motil KJ, Grand RJ: Nutritional management of inflammatory bowel disease, *Pediatr Clin North Am* 32 (2):447, 1985.

Mu-tagh K *et al:* Infantile hypertropic pyloric stenosis, *Digestive Diseases* 10(4):190, 1992.

Newman J, Schuh S: Intussusception in babies under 4 months of age, *Can Med Assoc J* 136:266, 1987.

Okorie NM *et al:* What happens to the pylorus after pyloromyotomy? *Arch Dis Child* 63:1339, 1988.

O'Regan S *et al:* Constipation a commonly unrecognized cause of enuresis, *Am J Dis Child* 140(3):260, 1986.

Orenstein SR: Effect of nonnutritive sucking on infant gastroesophageal reflux, *Pediatr Res* 24:38, 1988.

Oranstein SR: Gastroesophageal reflux, *Pediatr Rev* 13(5):174, 1992.

Orenstein SR, Shalaby T, Putnam P: Thickening of infant feedings as a cause of increased coughing when used as therapy for gastroesophageal reflux in infants, *J Pediatr* 121(6):913, 1992.

Orenstein SR, Whitington PF: Positioning for prevention of infant gastroesophageal reflux, *Pediatrics* 103(4):534, 1982.

Pettei MJ: Chronic constipation, *Pediatr Ann* 16:796, 1987.

Polley TZ, Coran AG, Wesley JR: A ten-year experience with ninety-two cases of Hirschsprung's disease, *Ann Surg* 202(3):349-354, 1985

Rappaport LA, Levine MD: The prevention of constipation and encopresis: a developmental model approach, *Pediatr Clin North Am* 33:859, 1986.

Reijnin JAM *et al:* Intussusception in older children, *Br J Surg* 74:692, 1987.

Savilahti E *et al:* Celiac disease in insulin-dependent diabetes mellitus, *J Pediatr* 108(1):690, 1986.

Schunk JE, Corneli H, Bolte R: Pediatric coin ingestions: a prospective study of coin location and symptoms, *Am J Dis Child* 143:546, 1989.

Silverman A, Roy CC: *Pediatric clinical gastroenterology*, ed 3, St Louis, 1983, Mosby–Year Book, 1983.

Stringer MD, Pablot SM, Brereton RJ: Paediatric intussusception, *Br J Surg* 79(9):867, 1992.

Sutphen JL, Dillard VL, Pipan ME: Antacid and formula effects on gastric acidity in infants with gastroesophagal reflux, *Pediatr* 78:55, 1986.

Turgeon D, Barnett J: Meckel's diverticulum, *Am J Gastroenterol* 14(4):359, 1991.

Webb WA, McDaniel L, Jones L: Foreign bodies of the upper gastrointestinal tract: current management, *South Med J* 77:1083, 1984.

FURTHER READING

General

Cady C, Yoshioka RS: Using a learning contract to successfully discharge an infant on home total parenteral nutrition, *Pediatr Nurs* 17(1):67, 1991.

Coleman Stadtler A: Preventing encopresis, *Pediatr Nurs* 15(3):282, 1989.

Ellett MA: Constipation/encopresis—a nursing perspective, *J Pediatr Health Care* 4:141, 1990.

Ellett ML, Fitzgerald JF, Winchester M: Dietary management of chronic diarrhoea, *Soc Gastroenterol Nurses Assoc* 15(4):170, 1990.

Evans K: Pediatric management problems, *Pediatr Nurs* 16(6):590, 1990.

Finelli L: Evaluation of the child with acute abdominal pain, *J Pediatr Health Care* 5(5):251, 1991.

Fry T: Charting growth, *Child Health* 1(3):104, 1993.

Gartner JC, Novak D, Schwartz R: When abdominal pain strikes a child, *Patient Care* 26(14):121, 1992.

Heubi JE: Evaluating persistent diarrhoea in kids, *Patient Care* 26(12):179, 1992.

Joachum G, Hassal E: Familial bowel disease in a pediatric population, *J Adv Nurs* 17(11):1310, 1992.

MacDonald CA: Biliary atresia, *J Pediatr Nurs* 6(6):374, 1991.

McWade LJ: Irritable bowel syndrome: diagnosis and management in school-aged children and adolescents, *J Pediatr Health Care* 6(2):82, 1992.

Milla PJ: Gastrointestinal motility disorders in children, *Pediatr Clin North Am* 35:311, 1988.

Peck SN: Paediatric pseudo-obstruction: a case study, *Soc Gastroenterol Nurses Assoc* 14(5).272, 1992.

Sharrer VW, Ryan Wegner NM: Measurement of stress—coping among school aged children with and without recurrent abdominal pain, *J School Health* 61(2):89, 1991.

Smith DP: Common day-care diseases: pattern and prevention, *Pediatr Nurs* 12(3):175, 1986.

Smith LG: Home treatment of mild, acute diarrhoea and secondary dehydration of infants and small children: an educational programme for parents in a shelter for the homeless, *J Prof Nurs* 4(1):60, 1988.

Statler AC: Preventing encopresis, *Pediatr Nurs* 15(3):282, 1989.

Sutton MM: Nutritional needs of children with inflammatory bowel disease, *Comprehensive Therapy* 18(10):21, 1992.

Tucker JA, Sussman-Karter K: Treating acute diarrhoea and dehydration with an oral rehydration solution, *Pediatr Nurs* 13(3):169, 1987.

Winch AE, Ouverson C: Nursing interventions for thromboembolic complications of chronic ulcerative colitis in children, *Am J Matern Child Nurs* 17(2):86, 1992.

Assessment of Gastrointestinal Function

Ament ME *et al:* Fiberoptic upper intestinal endoscopy in infants and children, *Pediatr Clin North Am* 35:141, 1988.

Caulfield M *et al:* Upper gastrointestinal tract endoscopy in the pediatric patient, *J Pediatr* 115:339, 1989.

Kane NM *et al:* Pediatric abdominal trauma: evaluation by computed tomography, *Pediatr* 82:11, 1988.

Riddlesberger MM: Evaluation of the gastrointestinal tract in the child: CT, MRI, and isotopic studies, *Pediatr Clin North Am* 35:281, 1988.

Smith CE: Assessing bowel sounds, *Nurs '88* 18(2):42, 1988.

Steffen RM *et al:* Colonoscopy in the pediatric patient, *J Pediatr* 115:507, 1989.

Disorders of Motility

Bailey DJ *et al:* Lack of efficacy of thickened feedings as treatment for gastroesophageal reflux, *J Pediatr* 110:187, 1987.

Kurer M, Lowson J, Pambakian H: Techniques for diagnosing suction biopsy of Hirschsprung's disease, *Arch Dis Child* 61(1):83, 1986.

Lynn MR: Use of infant seats for gastroesophageal reflux, *J Pediatr Nurs* 1(2):127, 1986.

Milla PJ: Gastrointestinal motility disorders in children, *Pediatr Clin North Am* 35:311, 1988.

Orenstein SR, Orenstein DM: Gastroesophageal reflux and respiratory disease in children, *J Pediatr* 112:847, 1988.

Petersen M: Esophageal pH monitoring, *J Pediatr Nurs* 1:354, 1986.

Sondheimer JM: Gastroesophageal reflux: update on pathogenesis and diagnosis, *Pediatr Clin North Am* 35:103, 1988.

Inflammatory Conditions

Edwinson M, Arnbjörnsson E, Ekman R: Psychologic preparation program for children undergoing acute appendectomy, *Pediatr* 82:30, 1988.

Ellett ML, Schibler K: Adolescent psychosocial adaptation to inflammatory bowel disease, *J Pediatr Health Care* 2:57, 1988.

Farley J: Facts and myths about gastrointestinal bleeding, *Nurs '88* 18(3).23, 1988.

Lessman M: Painful chronicle, *Am J Nurs* 85(5):551, 1985.

Soll AH: Pathogenesis of peptic ulcer and implications for therapy, *N Engl J Med* 322:909, 1990.

Obstruction

Breaux CW *et al:* Changing patterns in the diagnosis of hypertrophic pyloric stenosis, *Pediatr* 81:213, 1988.

Foley LC *et al:* Evaluation of the vomiting infant, *Am J Dis Child* 143:660, 1989.

Jedd MB *et al:* Factors associated with infantile hypertrophic pyloric stenosis, *Am J Dis Child* 142:334, 1988.

McConnell EA: Meeting the challenge of intestinal obstruction, *Nurs '87* 17(7):34, 1987.

Rollins MD *et al:* Pyloric stenosis: congenital or acquired? *Arch Dis Child* 64:138, 1989.

Touloukian RJ *et al:* Analgesic premedication in the management of ileocolic intussusception, *Pediatr* 79:432, 1987.

Malabsorption Syndromes

Anson O, Weizman Z, Zeevi N: Celiac disease: parental knowledge and attitudes of dietary compliance, *Pediatr* 85:98, 1990.

Cacciari E *et al:* Can antigliadin antibody detect symptomless celiac disease in children with short stature? *Lancet* 1(8444):1469, 1985.

Chuan-Hao L *et al:* Nutritional assessment of children with short-bowel syndrome receiving home parenteral nutrition, *Am J Dis Child* 141:1093, 1987.

Hepatic Disorders

Balisteri WF: Viral hepatitis, *Pediatr Clin North Am* 35:637, 1988.

Edwards MS: Hepatitis B serology—help in interpretation, *Pediatr Clin North Am* 35:503, 1988.

Gurevich I: Viral hepatitis, *Am J Nurs* 83:572, 1983.

Kirkman-Liff B, Dandoy S: Hepatitis B: what price exposure? *Am J Nurs* 84(4):988, 1984.

Pachter A: Should nurses receive the hepatitis B vaccination? *Nurs '88* 18(6):51, 1988.

West DJ, Calandra GB, Ellis RW: Vaccination of infants and children against hepatitis B, *Pediatr Clin North Am* 37:585, 1990.

Withers J, Bradshaw E: Preventing neonatal hepatitis-B infection, *MCN* 11:270, 1986.

Chapter 28

The Child with Cardiovascular Dysfunction

LEARNING OUTCOMES

After studying this chapter you should be able to:

◆ Identify the more common congenital cardiac defects.
◆ Outline the electrical pathways and activity of the heart, including the normal paediatric ECG and common arrhythmias.
◆ Describe the effects of congenital heart disease on the health of infants and children.
◆ Discuss the importance of giving adequate family support, including preparing parents for their child's surgery.
◆ Identify the signs and symptoms of congestive cardiac failure in infants and children.
◆ Describe the nursing management of a child following cardiac catheterization.
◆ Describe the specific nursing management of infants and children following cardiac surgery.
◆ Define the glossary terms.

GLOSSARY

afterload Pressure that heart must pump against

bradyarrhythmia Abnormally slow heart rate: may have irregular rhythm

bradycardia Abnormally slow heart rate

cardiac cycle Sequential contraction (systole) and dilatation (diastole) of heart chambers

cardiac output Blood volume ejected by heart in 1 minute

cardiomegaly Enlargement of heart muscle

contractility Ability of heart muscle to pump

corrective procedure Surgical intervention that restores normal circulatory patterns, but does not necessarily create a normal heart

cyanosis Bluish colour in skin from reduced oxygen saturation

diastole Period of dilatation of heart, especially of ventricles

haemodynamic Pertaining to movements involved in circulation of blood

hypercyanotic spells Presence of acute cyanosis and hyperpnoea (also called 'blue' spells)

hypoxaemia Arterial oxygen tension less than normal

hypoxic Reduction in tissue oxygenation

palliative procedure Intervention, such as creating a shunt, that temporarily improves haemodynamic functioning until corrective repair can be performed

polycythaemia Increased number of red blood cells

preload Circulating blood volume returning to heart

pulmonary hypertension Increased arterial pressure in pulmonary vessels

pulmonary vascular resistance (PVR) Pressure exerted by blood vessels in lungs

stroke volume Volume of blood ejected by heart during one contraction

systemic perfusion Circulation of blood to tissues throughout body

systole Period of contraction of heart, especially of ventricles

tachyarrhythmia Abnormally rapid heart rate

Cardiovascular disorders in children are divided into two major groups: congenital cardiac defects and acquired heart disorders. *Congenital heart defects* are anatomical abnormalities present at birth that result in abnormal cardiac function. The clinical consequences of congenital heart defects fall into two broad categories: congestive heart failure and hypoxaemia. *Acquired cardiac disorders* refers to disease processes or abnormalities that occur after birth. They result from various factors, including infection, autoimmune responses, environmental factors, and familial tendencies.

CARDIAC FUNCTION

Understanding the effects of congenital and acquired heart defects requires knowledge of the normal structure and function of the heart, including embryological development, fetal circulation, and changes occurring with postnatal growth.

ASSESSMENT OF CARDIAC FUNCTION

Assessment of congenital or acquired heart disease is aided by a comprehensive history and physical examination to determine cardiac output status.

HISTORY

Parents of children with congenital or acquired heart disease will often report one or more of the following:
- Poor weight gain, poor feeding habits, and fatigue during feeding.
- Frequent respiratory infections and difficulties (tachypnoea, dyspnoea, shortness of breath).
- Cyanosis.
- Evidence of exercise intolerance.

A history of previous cardiac defects in a sibling, maternal rubella infection during pregnancy, the use of medications or chemicals during pregnancy, or chronic illness in the mother can be important clues to the diagnosis of congenital heart disease. Children with chromosomal abnormalities, such as Turner or Down's syndromes, are likely to have associated congenital heart defects, and the history is essential in evaluating their overall health.

In evaluating acquired heart disease, a history of a viral infection or toxic exposure is important if myocarditis is suspected. A history of previous streptococcal infection is essential in rheumatic form.

PHYSICAL EXAMINATION

During inspection, a general examination of overall nutritional status, skin colour (particularly the presence of cyanosis with or without clubbing), and position of comfort is performed. During palpation and percussion, the quality of chest activity, quality and symmetry of all pulses, warmth of extremities, and presence or absence of oedema are assessed. Locating the hepatic and splenic borders for evidence of organ enlargement is also important. An essential aspect of heart auscultation is recognition of the heart's position within the chest cavity and determining the overall flow of blood through the heart.

Auscultation of lung sounds and respiratory rate also provides valuable clues to heart function. Lung sounds may appear coarse from excess fluid within the interstitial spaces. This fluid may remain within the lungs because of the heart's inability to circulate blood adequately.

Murmurs
Although many murmurs are benign, they can also be an important sign of cardiac defects. The most frequent cause of murmurs is an abnormal shunting of blood between two heart chambers or between vessels. However, murmurs can also be produced by disturbing the flow of fluid through a vessel as a result of: (1) increasing the rate of flow, (2) constricting or dilating the lumen, and (3) creating some type of irregularity on the vessel wall, such as an aneurysm, which vibrates as fluid flows past. Murmurs are classified according to their timing within the Fdiac cycle.

TESTS OF CARDIAC FUNCTION

A variety of invasive and noninvasive tests may be employed in the diagnosis of heart disease. Table 28-1 briefly outlines cardiac diagnostic procedures. The more frequently conducted tests are described here.

RADIOGRAPHY

A chest x-ray examination is the most frequently ordered radiological test for children with suspected cardiac problems. A chest film provides a permanent record of: (1) the heart's size and configuration, its chambers, and the great vessels, and (2) the pattern of blood flow, especially in the pulmonary vessels.

ELECTROCARDIOGRAPHY

An electrocardiogram (ECG) measures the electrical activity of the heart and records it on graph paper. This allows the evaluation of the sequence and magnitude of the electrical impulses generated by the heart (Fig. 28-1). The normal ECG consists of the P wave, P-R interval, QRS complex, T wave, Q-T interval, and ST segment:
- **P-wave** — represents the spread of the impulse over the atria (atrial depolarization). The sinus node's electrical activity is not represented in the ECG.
- **P-R interval** — represents the time that elapses from the beginning of atrial depolarization to the beginning of ventricular depolarization.

PROCEDURE	DESCRIPTION
Electrocardiography	Measures electrical potential generated from heart muscle
Echocardiography	Short pulses of ultrasound transmitted through the heart bounce off heart structures: reflected on a screen
Ultrasonography	Similar to echocardiography; it is synchronized with ECG to provide a three-dimensional recording of heart structures
Roentgenography	
Fluoroscopy	Provides direct observation of heart size, position, contour, and relationships
Radiography	Provides permanent record of heart size and configuration
Angiocardiography	Opaque medium injected into circulatory system outlines blood flow through the heart and vessels; performed in conjunction with cardiac catheterization
Cardiac catheterization	Opaque catheter introduced into the heart chambers via large peripheral vessels is observed by fluoroscopy or image intensification; pressure measurements and blood samples provide additional source of information
Digital subtraction angiography (DSA)	Opaque media injected into circulatory system Provides computed images of vessels and tissues contianing dye - 'subtracts' all tissue not containing dye

Table 28-1 Procedures for cardiac diagnosis.

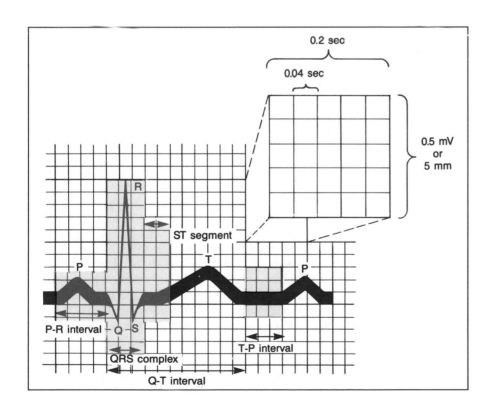

Fig. 28-1 Normal electrocardiogram pattern. Inset *(upper right)* shows conventional time and voltage or amplitude (height) calibrations.

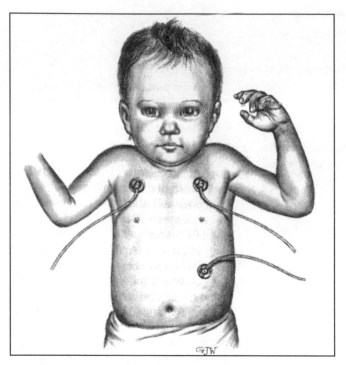

Fig. 28-2 Electrode placement for standard chest lead II in ECG monitoring.

- **QRS complex** — represents ventricular depolarization. It is actually composed of three separate waves (the Q, the R, and the S) that result from the currents generated when the ventricles depolarize before their contraction.
- **T wave** — represents ventricular repolarization.
- **Q-T interval** — represents ventricular depolarization and repolarization. This interval varies with heart rate - the faster the rate, the shorter the Q-T interval. Therefore, in children, this interval is normally shorter than in adults.
- **ST segment** — represents the time that the ventricles are in absolute refractory period, the period between ventricular depolarization and repolarization.

Information supplied by an ECG includes heart rate and rhythm, abnormalities of conduction, muscular damage (ischaemia), hypertrophy, effects of electrolyte imbalance, influence of various drugs, and pericardial disease.

Chest leads must be positioned correctly, because even minor misplacement can cause considerable inaccuracy in the recording. One common chest lead placement is illustrated in Fig. 28-2.

ECHOCARDIOGRAPHY

Recent improvements in echocardiographic techniques have made it increasingly possible to confirm the diagnosis without resorting to cardiac catheterization. A prenatal diagnosis of congenital heart disease can be made by fetal echocardiography.

Echocardiography involves the use of ultra-high-frequency sound waves to produce an image of the heart's structure. A transducer placed directly on the chest wall delivers repetitive pulses of ultrasound and processes the returned signals (echoes).

The test is noninvasive, painless, and associated with no known side effects. The child must lie quietly; therefore, infants and young children may need a mild sedative. Older children benefit from psychological preparation for the test.

CARDIAC CATHETERIZATION

The most invasive diagnostic procedure is cardiac catheterization, in which a radiopaque catheter is inserted through a peripheral blood vessel into the heart. It is usually combined with angiography (angiocardiography), in which a radiopaque contrast material is injected through the catheter into the circulation. Cardiac catheterization provides information regarding:

- Oxygen saturation of blood within the chambers and great vessels.
- Pressure changes within these structures.
- Changes in cardiac output or stroke volume (the amount of blood pumped out of the LV into the aorta with each contraction).
- Anatomical abnormalities, such as septal defects or obstruction to flow.

Interventional, or therapeutic, cardiac catheterization has become an alternative to surgery in some congenital heart defects, such as isolated valvular pulmonary stenosis and patent ductus arteriosus (Table 28-2).

Electrophysiological studies are increasingly being used to evaluate arrhythmias. These diagnostic catheterizations employ catheters with tiny electrodes that record the heart's electrical impulses directly from the conduction system.

IMPLICATIONS FOR NURSING

Cardiac catheterization has become a routine diagnostic procedure. Catheterization is not, however, without risks. Typical reactions include acute haemorrhage from the entry site (more likely with interventional procedures because larger catheters are used), low-grade fever, nausea, vomiting, loss of pulse in the catheterized extremity (usually transient, resulting from a clot, haematoma, or intimal tear), and transient arrhythmias (generally catheter induced).

Preprocedural care

A complete nursing assessment is necessary to ensure a safe procedure with minimum complications. This assessment should include an accurate height and weight. Specific attention to signs and symptoms of infection is crucial. Severe nappy rash may be a reason to cancel the procedure if femoral access is required. Since assessment of pedal pulses is important after catheterization, the nurse should assess and mark pulses (dorsalis pedis, posterior tibial) before the child goes to the catheterization room. The presence and quality of pulses in both feet are clearly documented. Baseline oxygen saturation in children with cyanosis is recorded using pulse oximetry.

DIAGNOSIS	INTERVENTION/STATUS
Transposition of the great arteries	Balloon atrioseptostomy Well established
Valvular pulmonary stenosis Distal pulmonary artery stenosis Recurrent coarctation of aorta Rheumatic mitral valve	Balloon dilatation; accept alternative to surgery
Patent ductus arteriosus	Transcatheter closure Routine in some institutions; requires further follow-up
Atrial septal defect	Transcatheter closure; clinical trials
Valvular aortic stenosis	Balloon dilatation routine in some institutions; requires further follow-up

Table 28.2 Current interventional cardiac catheterization procedures for children.

It is important to describe the catheterization room to the child and parents, because the x-ray machinery can appear frightening. Some institutions routinely take children on a brief tour of the area before the test. This has been shown to help decrease children's anxiety.

Prior to the test, the child may be sedated with several different drugs. A frequently prescribed regimen is chloral hydrate or temazepam, with or without atropine. General anaesthesia is usually unnecessary, except in selected interventional procedures. The child is allowed nothing by mouth for four hours before catheterization, although polycythaemic infants and children may require intravenous fluids to prevent dehydration, and neonates may need dextrose solution up to 2-3 hours before the procedure to prevent hypoglycaemia.

Postprocedural care

Essentially, the care following cardiac catheterization is the same as general postoperative care. The most important nursing responsibility is observation of the following for signs of complications:

- Pulses (especially below the catheterization site) for equality and symmetry (pulse distal to the site may be weaker for the first few hours after catheterization, but should gradually increase in strength).
- Temperature and colour of the affected extremity, since coolness or blanching may indicate arterial obstruction
- Vital signs, which are taken as frequently as every 15 minutes, with special emphasis on heart rate, evidence of arrhythmias or bradycardia.
- Blood pressure, especially for hypotension, which may indicate haemorrhage from cardiac perforation or bleeding at the site of initial catheterization.
- Dressing, for evidence of bleeding or haematoma formation in the femoral area.

The child may be kept in bed, overnight if possible, to facilitate healing of the cannulated vessel. If younger children have difficulty complying, they can be held in their parent's lap. The child is encouraged to void, to clear the contrast material from the blood. Generally, there is only slight discomfort at the percutaneous site. To prevent infection, the catheterization area is protected from possible contamination.

CONGENITAL HEART DISEASE

The incidence of congenital heart disease (CHD) in children is generally reported to be 4 to 10:1000 live births (Hoffman, 1990). CHD is the major cause of death in the first year of life. There are more than 35 well-recognized defects: the most common is ventricular septal defect (VSD).

The aetiological factor in CHD is not known in more than 90% of cases. However, several factors are associated with a higher-than-expected incidence of the defect. These include prenatal factors such as: (1) maternal rubella during pregnancy, (2) maternal alcoholism, (3) maternal age over 40 years, and (4) maternal insulin-dependent diabetes. Children with CHD are also more likely to have extracardiac defects, such as tracheo-oesophageal fistula, renal agenesis, and diaphragmatic hernias.

Several genetic factors are also implicated in CHD, although the influence is multifactorial. The risk of recurrence in families with an affected parent is 4-12%, especially if the mother has the defect (Hazinski, 1992). The rising recurrence rates may be the result of more children with previously fatal heart defects surviving to adulthood and having offspring. Certain chromosomal defects, such as Down's syndrome, are associated with increased risk of cardiac defects.

CLASSIFICATION AND CLINICAL CONSEQUENCES

Congenital heart defects have been divided into two categories. Traditionally, a physical characteristic, cyanosis, has been used as the distinguishing feature, dividing the anomalies into *acyanotic* and *cyanotic defects*. Because of the complexity of many defects and the variability of their clinical manifestations, the cyanotic-acyanotic classification system has proved inadequate and misleading.

Another classification system, based on *haemodynamic characteristics*, or movements involved in circulation of blood, is more frequently used. The defining characteristic is blood flow patterns.

With the haemodynamic classification system, the clinical manifestations of each group are more uniform and predictable. Defects that allow blood flow from the high-pressure left side of the heart to the lower-pressure right side (left-to-right shunt) result in increased pulmonary blood flow and cause CHF. Obstructive defects impede blood flow out of the ventricles; obstruction on the left side of the heart results in CHF, whereas severe obstruction on the right side causes cyanosis. Defects that cause decreased pulmonary blood flow result in cyanosis. Mixed lesions present a variable clinical picture based on degree of mixing and amount of pulmonary blood flow; hypoxaemia (with or without cyanosis) and CHF usually occur together.

CONGESTIVE HEART FAILURE

Congestive heart failure is inability of the heart to pump an adequate amount of blood to the systemic circulation to meet the body's metabolic demands.

CLINICAL MANIFESTATIONS

The signs and symptoms of CHF can be divided into three groups: (1) impaired myocardial function, (2) pulmonary congestion, and (3) systemic venous congestion.

Impaired myocardial function
One of the earliest signs of CHF is *tachycardia*, as a direct result of sympathetic stimulation. It is elevated, even during rest, but becomes extremely rapid with the slightest exertion. Ventricular dilatation and excess preload result in extra heart sounds S_3 and S_4, referred to as *gallop rhythm*. *Sweating* is often seen, especially on the head during exertion. Children are easily fatigued, have poor exercise tolerance, and are often irritable. Decreased cardiac output results in *poor perfusion*, manifested by cold extremities, weak pulses, low blood pressure and mottled skin. Extreme pallor and duskiness are ominous signs.

Pulmonary congestion
Tachypnoea occurs in response to decreased lung compliance. Tachypnoea can lead to hypoxaemia because oxygen does not reach the alveoli for gas exchange in adequate amounts with fast breathing rates. *Mild cyanosis* results from impaired gas exchange and is relieved with oxygen administration. *Dyspnoea*

is caused by a decrease in the compliance of the lungs. Inability to feed, with resultant poor weight gain, is primarily a result of tachypnoea and dyspnoea on exertion. *Costal recession* occurs as the pliable chest wall in the infant is drawn inward during attempts to ventilate the noncompliant lungs. Initially, dyspnoea may be evident only on exertion, but it may progress to the point that even slight activity results in laboured breathing. In infants, dyspnoea at rest is a prominent sign and may be accompanied by flaring nares.

As the LV fails, blood volume and pressure increase in the LA, pulmonary veins and lungs. Eventually, the pulmonary capillary pressure exceeds the plasma osmotic pressure, forcing fluid into the interstitial space and finally causing *pulmonary oedema*. Increased interstitial lung fluid also decreases compliance of the lungs and increases the work of breathing.

Orthopnoea (dyspnoea in the recumbent position) is caused by increased blood flow to the heart and lungs from the extremities. It is relieved by sitting up, because blood pools in the lower extremities, decreasing venous return. In addition, this position decreases pressure from the abdominal organs on the diaphragm. In infants, orthopnoea may be evident in their inability to lie supine and their desire to be held upright.

Oedema of the bronchial mucosa may produce *cardiac wheezing* from obstruction to airflow. Mucosal swelling and irritation result in a persistent, dry, hacking *cough*. As pulmonary oedema increases, the cough may be productive from increased secretions. Pressure on the laryngeal nerve results in *hoarseness*. A late sign of heart failure is *gasping* and *grunting respirations*.

Infants with CHF have an increased metabolic rate and require additional calories to grow. The work of the heart and breathing demands all the infant's energy, leaving little for normal activity. As a result of poor weight gain and activity intolerance, infants with CHF demonstrate *developmental delay*. Following surgical correction, most children will catch up to their peers with time. Older children with severe CHF will have decreased exercise tolerance and persistent developmental delay.

Systemic venous congestion
Systemic venous congestion from right-sided failure results in increased pressure and pooling of blood in the venous circulation. *Hepatomegaly* occurs from pooling of blood in the portal circulation and collection of fluid in the hepatic tissues. The liver may be tender on palpation, and its size is an indication of the course of heart failure.

Oedema forms as the sodium and water retention causes systemic vascular pressure to increase. The earliest sign is *weight gain*. However, as additional fluid accumulates, it leads to swelling of soft tissue, such as the sacrum and scrotum (when recumbent) and loose periorbital tissues, that is dependent and favours the flow of gravity. In infants, oedema is usually generalized and difficult to detect. Gross fluid accumulation may produce *ascites* and *pleural effusions*.

Distended neck and *peripheral veins* result from a consistently elevated central venous pressure. Increased venous pressure slows venous return, causing the veins to remain distended.

PROCESS OF DIAGNOSIS

Diagnosis is made on the basis of clinical symptoms such as tachypnoea and tachycardia at rest, dyspnoea, recession, activity intolerance (especially during feeding in infants), weight gain caused by fluid retention, and hepatomegaly. A chest x-ray demonstrates cardiomegaly and increased pulmonary vascular markings due to increased pulmonary blood flow. Ventricular hypertrophy appears on the ECG.

THERAPEUTIC MANAGEMENT

The goals of treatment are to: (1) improve cardiac function (increase contractility and decrease afterload), (2) remove accumulated fluid and sodium (decrease preload), (3) decrease cardiac demands and (4) improve tissue oxygenation and decrease oxygen consumption.

Improve cardiac function

Two types of drugs are used to enhance myocardial performance in CHF: (1) digoxin, which improves contractility and (2) angiotensin-converting enzyme inhibitors, which reduce the afterload on the heart, making it easier for the heart to pump.

The beneficial effects are increased cardiac output, decreased heart size, decreased venous pressure and relief of oedema.

During digitalization, the child is monitored with an ECG to observe for the desired effects (prolonged P-R interval and reduced ventricular rate) and detect side effects, especially arrhythmias. A decrease in serum potassium level of digoxin increases the risk of digoxin toxicity. Therefore, serum potassium levels must be carefully monitored.

Digoxin is the only oral inotropic agent generally available for infants and children, although other oral inotropic agents are in clinical trials in adults. For patients in severe CHF, intravenous inotropic agents such as dopamine, dobutamine, or amrinone are used to improve contractility. They are generally given in ICU settings.

A newer group of drugs that has proved beneficial in the treatment of CHF are the angiotensin-converting enzyme (ACE) inhibitors. Normal production of renin triggers the production of angiotensin I and angiotensin II, which cause vasoconstriction and aldosterone secretion. The ACE inhibitors block the conversion of angiotensin I to angiotensin II so that instead of vasoconstriction, vasodilatation occurs. Vasodilatation results in decreased pulmonary and systemic vascular resistance, decreased blood pressure, a reduction in afterload, and decreased right and left atrial pressures. It also reduces the secretion of aldosterone, which reduces preload by preventing volume expansion from fluid retention and decreases the risk of hypokalaemia. Renal blood flow is improved, which enhances diuresis. Two ACE inhibitors currently used in paediatrics are captopril and enalopril.

Remove accumulated fluid and sodium

Treatment consists of diuretics, possible fluid restriction and possible sodium restriction. Diuretics are the mainstay of therapy to eliminate excess water and salt to prevent re-accumulation. The most commonly used agents include frusemide, spironalactone and chlorothiazide. Since frusemide and the thiazides cause loss of potassium, potassium supplements and rich dietary sources of the electrolyte are given.

Fluid restriction may be required in the acute states of CHF and must be carefully calculated to avoid dehydrating the child, especially if cyanotic CHD and significant polycythaemia are present.

Decrease cardiac demands

To lessen the workload on the heart, metabolic needs are minimized by: (1) providing a thermoneutral environment to prevent cold stress in infants, (2) treating any existing infections, (3) reducing the effort of breathing and (4) using medication to sedate an irritable child.

Improve tissue oxygenation

All the preceding measures increase tissue oxygenation either by improving myocardial function or by lessening tissue oxygen demands. However, supplemental humidified oxygen may also be administered to increase the amount of available oxygen during inspiration.

Assist in measures to improve cardiac function

The child's apical pulse is always checked before administering digoxin, to observe for digoxin toxicity. As a general rule, the drug is not given if the pulse is below 90-110 beats/minute in infants and young children or below 70 beats/minute in older children.

The apical rate is taken because a pulse deficit (radial pulse rate lower than apical) may be present with decreased cardiac output. It is auscultated for one minute to evaluate alterations in rhythm. If the child is monitored by means of an ECG, a rhythm strip is obtained for analysis.

If digoxin toxicity occurs, especially as a result of a drug overdose, all subsequent doses are withheld. The child is closely monitored for arrhythmias, which are treated appropriately if they occur. Because of the long half-life of digoxin (1.5 days), it may be several days before the blood level returns to normal.

Afterload reduction

For patients receiving ACE inhibitors for afterload reduction, the nurse should carefully monitor blood pressure before and after dose administration, and should observe for symptoms of hypotension. Serum electrolytes should be monitored. Because ACE inhibitors also block the action of aldosterone, they act as potassium-sparing agents. Most patients do not need potassium supplements or spironolactone (Aldactone) while receiving these medications.

Decrease cardiac demands

The infant requires rest and conservation of energy for feeding. Every effort is made to organize nursing activities to allow for uninterrupted periods of sleep, minimizing stress.

Temperature is carefully monitored for pyrexia (a sign of infection) or hypothermia (loss of heat to ambient air). Infection must be promptly treated. Pyrexia increases oxygen demands and is poorly tolerated. Maintaining body temperature is very important for the child who is receiving humidified oxygen and for one who tends to sweat, losing heat via evaporation.

Skin breakdown from oedema is minimized or prevented by the use of pressure-relieving aids, meticulous observation of pressure areas, and risk assessment. Respiratory infections can exacerbate CHF and should be appropriately treated. Exposure to infection should be minimized.

Reduce respiratory distress

Careful assessment, positioning, and oxygen administration can reduce respiratory distress. Any evidence of increased respiratory distress should be reported, since this may indicate worsening heart failure.

Infants should be positioned to encourage maximum chest expansion and comfort, with the head of the bed elevated.

The child's response to oxygen therapy should be carefully evaluated by noting respiratory rate, ease of respiration, colour, and especially oxygen saturations, as measured by oximetry.

Maintain nutritional status

Attention to nutrition is essential, because of the fatigue associated with CHF. The infant may be fed by nasogastric/nasojejunal tube, if oral feeding is too exhausting.

Assist in measures to promote fluid loss

When diuretics are given, the nurse records fluid intake and output and monitors body weight at the same time each day to evaluate benefit from the drug. Diuretics should be given early in the day to children who are toilet trained, to avoid the need to urinate at night. If potassium-losing diuretics are given, the nurse encourages foods high in potassium, such as bananas, oranges, whole grains, legumes, and leafy vegetables, and administers prescribed supplements.

The effectiveness of nursing interventions for the family and the child with CHF is determined by continual reassessment and evaluation of care based on the following observational guidelines and expected outcomes:

1. Monitor heart rate and quality, respiratory rate and efforts, and colour, and observe behaviours that provide clues to expended effort.
2. Observe nutritional intake, feeding behaviours and weight.
3. Monitor intake, output and weight.
4. Interview and observe behaviours of family.

HYPOXAEMIA

Hypoxaemia refers to an arterial oxygen tension (or pressure) (PaO_2) that is less than normal and can be identified by a decreased arterial saturation or a decreased PaO_2. *Hypoxia* is a reduction in tissue oxygenation that results from low oxygen saturation (SaO_2) and PaO_2, and results in impaired cellular processes. *Cyanosis* is a blue discolouration in the mucous membranes, skin and nail beds of the child with reduced oxygen saturation. It results from the presence of deoxygenated haemoglobin. Cyanosis is usually apparent when arterial oxygen saturations are 80-85% (Nadas, 1992). The presence of cyanosis may not accurately reflect arterial hypoxaemia, because both SaO_2 and amount of circulating haemoglobin are involved.

ALTERED HAEMODYNAMICS

Heart defects that cause hypoxaemia and cyanosis result from desaturated venous blood (blue blood) entering the systemic circulation without passing through the lungs. Three types of defects cause cyanosis in the infant. The first results from severe obstruction to pulmonary blood flow and blood shunting from the right side to the left side of the heart, or *right-to-left shunting*. The second is mixing of arterial and venous blood within the chambers of the heart itself; a single ventricle is an example. The third defect, transposition of the great arteries, presents a unique situation in which the pulmonary and systemic circulations are parallel, rather than in sequence. Fully oxygenated blood returns to the lungs, and desaturated blood returns to the body. Newborns with transposition of the great arteries depend on intracardiac mixing from a patent foramen ovale, septal defect, or ductus arteriosus to allow oxygenation.

CLINICAL MANIFESTATIONS

Over time, two physiological changes occur in the body in response to chronic hypoxaemia: polycythaemia and clubbing. Persistent hypoxaemia stimulates erythropoiesis, resulting in *polycythaemia*, an increased number of red blood cells. Theoretically, a greater number of red blood cells increases the oxygen-carrying capacity of the blood. However, this increased red blood cell formation may result in anaemia if iron is not readily available for the formation of haemoglobin. In addition, polycythaemia increases the viscosity of the blood and tends to crowd out platelets and other coagulation factors. *Clubbing*, a thickening and flattening of the tips of the fingers and toes, is thought to occur because of chronic tissue hypoxia and polycythaemia (Fig. 28-3).

Squatting, most characteristic of children with unrepaired tetralogy of Fallot, is seen in toddlers and older children as an unconscious attempt to relieve chronic hypoxia, especially during exercise. The squatting position is helpful because flexing the legs: (1) reduces the return of venous blood from the lower extremities, which is very desaturated; and (2) increases systemic vascular resistance, which diverts more blood flow into the pulmonary artery. Placing an infant in the knee chest position (recommended during hypercyanotic spells) has the same beneficial haemodynamic effects as squatting. Because of early surgical intervention before walking, squatting is rarely seen.

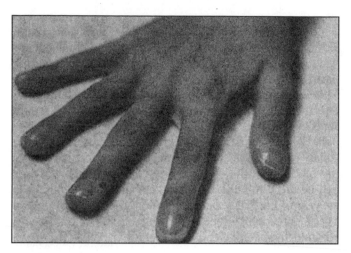

Fig. 28-3 Clubbing of the fingers.

Severe cyanosis (also referred to as blue spells or 'tet' spells because it is often seen in infants with tetralogy of Fallot), may occur in any child whose heart defect includes obstruction to pulmonary blood flow and communication between the ventricles. The infant becomes acutely cyanotic and tachypnoeic because sudden infundibular spasm decreases pulmonary blood flow and increases right-to-left shunting. With other anomalies, an increase in oxygen requirements, which the infant is unable to meet, may cause a spell. Hypoxia causes acidosis, which further increases pulmonary vascular resistance, which further decreases pulmonary blood flow; thus, a vicious cycle ensues. Spells, rarely seen before two months of age, occur most frequently in the first year of life and more often in the morning and may be preceded by feeding, crying or defaecation. Because profound hypoxaemia causes cerebral hypoxia, severe cyanotic spells require prompt assessment and treatment to prevent brain damage or possibly death.

Persistent cyanosis as a result of cyanotic cardiac defects places the child at risk for significant neurological complications. Polycythaemia, and the resultant increased viscosity of the blood, increase the risk of thromboembolic events. Cerebrovascular accidents (CVA) may occur in about 2% of patients; infants with severe cyanosis and iron deficiency anaemia are at greatest risk (Rosenthal, 1989). They may occur spontaneously, but often follow an acute febrile illness, an hypoxic spell, or cardiac catheterization. There is a 2% incidence of brain abscess in this patient population (Newburger, 1992a). Right-to-left shunting of blood in cyanotic heart defects allows bacteria to colonize the brain, which is vulnerable because of hypoxaemia and poor perfusion of the cerebral microcirculation. Rarely seen in children under two years of age, it should be suspected in older children who have pyrexia, headaches, focal neurological signs or seizures. Prompt treatment with antibiotics and surgical drainage is critical, because death or significant neurological impairment may result. Also, children who are cyanotic, especially those with systemic-to-pulmonary shunts, are at increased risk of bacterial endocarditis.

One study highlighted the negative developmental consequences, particularly in the area of motor and cognitive development, that result from chronic hypoxaemia (Neuburger *et al*, 1984).

PROCESS OF DIAGNOSIS

Cyanosis in the newborn can result from cardiac, pulmonary, metabolic or haematological disease, although cardiac and pulmonary causes occur most often. To distinguish between the two, a nitrogen washout test may be helpful. The infant is placed in a 100% oxygen environment, and blood gases are monitored. An accurate history, chest x-ray and, especially, an echocardiogram, contribute to the diagnosis of cyanotic heart disease.

THERAPEUTIC MANAGEMENT

Newborns generally exhibit cyanosis within the first few days of life as the ductus arteriosus, which provided pulmonary blood flow, begins to close. Prostaglandin E_2, which causes vasodilatation and smooth muscle relaxation, thus increasing dilatation and patency of the ductus arteriosus, is administered intravenously to re-establish pulmonary blood flow. The use of prostaglandins has been life-saving for infants with ductus-dependent cardiac defects.

Severe cyanotic spells occur suddenly, and prompt recognition and treatment are essential. Spells are often seen when the child is highly agitated. Treatment of a severe cyanotic spell is outlined in Box 28-1. Morphine, administered intravenously or subcutaneously, is helpful in reducing infundibular spasm. In some instances, propranolol may be given in the interim to prevent infundibular spasm.

The cyanotic infant and child are well hydrated to keep the haematocrit and blood viscosity within acceptable limits to reduce the risk of CVA. Pyrexia is carefully evaluated because bacteraemia can result in bacterial endocarditis. The infant is monitored closely for anaemia because of the risk of CVAs and the reduced arterial oxygen-carrying capacity that occurs. Iron supplementation and possibly blood transfusion are used as needed. Older children and adolescents may require serial phlebotomy to reduce blood viscosity and minimize the risk of

---

◆ **BOX 28-1**

Guidelines for treating severe cyanotic spells

- ◆ Place infant in knee-chest position.
- ◆ Employ calm, comforting approach.
- ◆ Administer 100% oxygen by face mask.
- ◆ Give morphine intraveneously or subcutaneously.
- ◆ Begin intravenous fluid replacement and volume expansion, if needed.
- ◆ Repeat morphine administration.

CVA. The goal is to reduce the haematocrit to approximately 60% by removing small amounts of blood and replacing blood with normal saline or other intravenous solutions to maintain intravascular volume. This procedure is a temporary measure, but may relieve symptoms of dyspnoea, headache, and malaise for short periods and can be repeated every one or two months if polycythaemia is severe.

Respiratory infections or reduced pulmonary function from any cause can worsen hypoxaemia in the cyanotic child. Aggressive chest physiotherapy, administration of antibiotics, and use of oxygen to improve arterial saturations are important interventions.

Palliative surgery

Severely hypoxaemic newborn babies with cardiac defects not amenable to corrective repair may have a palliative surgical procedure called a *shunt.* The shunt serves the same purpose as the ductus arteriosus: to increase blood flow to the lungs through a systemic artery-to-pulmonary artery connection. Currently a *modified Blalock-Taussig shunt* using a Gore-Tex or Impra tube graft to create a communication between the right or left subclavian artery and the pulmonary artery on the same side is the preferred procedure. Because of the higher resistance in the systemic circulation, blood flows from the subclavian artery to the pulmonary artery and to the lungs for oxygenation. This procedure sacrifices the brachial and radial pulse on the affected side, and the hand initially may be slightly cooler and paler until collateral circulation develops. Corrective surgical repair is always preferred to a palliative shunt procedure if it can be performed at low risk. Corrective techniques are described with the cardiac defect.

Following a shunt procedure, the infant must be assessed for signs of increased or decreased pulmonary blood flow. If the shunt is too small or narrow, the newborn may remain severely hypoxaemic, with oxygen saturations below 70%. Surgically revising the shunt or placing an additional shunt may be needed. More often, the shunt is too large and the pulmonary blood flow may be excessive, resulting in signs and symptoms of CHF and oxygen saturations above 85%. The infant may require digoxin and diuretic therapy. Some surgeons place infants on low-dose aspirin therapy for several months to prevent platelet aggregation and subsequent narrowing of the shunt.

IMPLICATIONS FOR NURSING

The general appearance of infants and children with significant cyanosis poses unique concerns. Blue lips and fingernails are obvious signs of their hidden cardiac defect. Clubbing and small, thin stature in older children further indicate severe heart disease. Because body image is a particular concern of adolescents, they will need substantial positive support.

Parents are often fearful of their child's bluish colour, since cyanosis is usually associated with lack of oxygen and severe illness. They also must deal with comments from relatives, friends and strangers about their child's abnormal colour. Parents need a simple explanation of hypoxaemia and cyanosis,

and reassurance that cyanosis does not imply a lack of oxygen to the brain. Parents also should be taught the treatment for severe cyanotic spells.

Dehydration must be prevented in hypoxaemic children, because it potentiates the risk of CVAs. Fluid status is carefully monitored, with accurate intake and output, and daily weight measurements. Nasogastric/nasojejunal feeding or intravenous hydration is given to children unable to take adequate oral fluids. Parents are instructed in the importance of adequate fluid intake and measures to prevent dehydration. An oral electrolyte solution such as Rehydrate or Dioralyte should be available at home if the infant is unable to tolerate the usual formula.

Preventive measures and accurate assessment of respiratory infection are important nursing considerations. Good handwashing and protection from individuals with an obvious respiratory infection are important. Aggressive treatment with antibiotics or antiviral agents as indicated, and supplemental oxygen to decrease hypoxaemia are necessary measures. Infants may need to be nasogastrically fed or given parenteral nutrition if respiratory distress prevents oral feeding.

DEFECTS WITH INCREASED PULMONARY BLOOD FLOW

In this group of cardiac defects, intracardiac communications along the septum or an abnormal connection between the great arteries allows blood to flow from the high-pressure left side of the heart to the lower-pressure right side of the heart (Fig. 28-4). Increased blood volume on the right side of the heart increases pulmonary blood flow at the expense of systemic blood flow. Clinically, patients demonstrate signs and symptoms of CHF. Atrial and ventricular septal defects and patent ductus arteriosus are typical anomalies in this group.

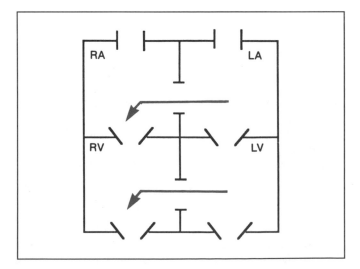

Fig. 28-4 Haemodynamics in defects with increased pulmonary blood flow.

ATRIAL SEPTAL DEFECT

An atrial septal defect (ASD) is an abnormal communication between the two atria resulting from incomplete septation (Fig. 28-5). The defect may be one of three major types:

- **Ostium primum** — opening at the lower end of the septum; may be associated with mitral valve abnormalities.
- **Ostium secundum** — opening near centre of septum.
- **Sinus venosus defect** — opening near junction of superior vena cava and right atrium; may be associated with partial anomalous pulmonary venous connection.

ALTERED HAEMODYNAMICS

Because left atrial pressure slightly exceeds right atrial pressure, blood flows from the left to the right atrium, causing an increased flow of oxygenated blood into the right side of the heart. This volume is well tolerated by the right ventricle because it is delivered under much lower pressure than in a ventricular septal defect. Although there is right atrial and ventricular enlargement, cardiac failure is unusual in an uncomplicated atrial septal defect. Pulmonary vascular changes usually occur only after several decades if the defect is unrepaired.

CLINICAL MANIFESTATIONS

Most children with ASD are asymptomatic. Diagnosis is usually made after discovery of a murmur during routine physical examination.

If an ASD remains unrepaired into adulthood, right and left ventricular hypertrophy will be significant. This may produce atrial arrhythmias, CHF, or emboli formation. These symptoms are usually not apparent until age 20-30 years.

PROCESS OF DIAGNOSIS

The most suggestive signs of ASD are its characteristic murmur. Unless clinical signs suggest pulmonary hypertension, clinical examination combined with echocardiography is sufficient to establish diagnosis.

THERAPEUTIC MANAGEMENT

Because of the risk of CHF and pulmonary vascular obstructive disease later in life, closure of ASD is recommended before school age. Surgical closure is similar to the corrective procedures employed in ventricular septal defect closures. The 1° ASD may require repair or, rarely, replacement of the mitral valve. Surgical closure of all types of ASD is associated with essentially no operative mortality, and postoperative complications are unusual.

VENTRICULAR SEPTAL DEFECT

A ventricular septal defect (VSD) is an abnormal communi-

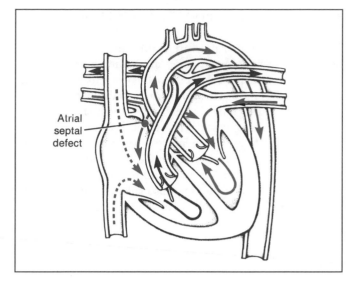

Fig. 28-5 Atrial septal defect. *Red arrows,* saturated blood; *broken red arrows,* desaturated blood; *black arrows,* mixed blood.

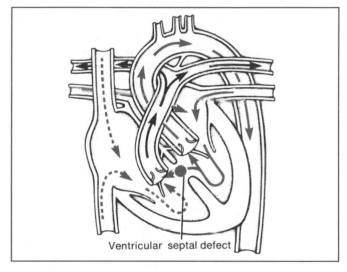

Fig. 28-6 Ventricular septal defect. *Red arrow,* saturated blood; *broken red arrows,* desaturated blood; *black arrows,* mixed blood.

cation between the right and left ventricles resulting from an incomplete septum (Fig. 28-6). VSDs may be classified according to location: membranous (accounting for 80%) or muscular. They are frequently associated with other defects, such as pulmonary stenosis, transposition of the great vessels, patent ductus arteriosus, atrial defects, and coarctation of the aorta. Many VSDs (20-60%) are thought to close spontaneously. Spontaneous closure is most likely to occur during the first year of life in children having small or moderate defects. Closure is a result of growth and proliferation of the muscular septum, apposition of a cusp of the tricuspid valve against the defect, or formation of a membranous diaphragm across the opening (Moller and Neal, 1990).

ALTERED HAEMODYNAMICS

Because of the higher pressure within the left ventricle and because the systemic arterial circulation offers more resistance than the pulmonary circulation, blood flows through the defect into the pulmonary artery. The increased blood volume is pumped into the lungs, which may eventually result in increased pulmonary vascular resistance. Increased pressure in the right ventricle, as a result of left-to-right shunting and pulmonary resistance, causes the muscle to hypertrophy. If the right ventricle is unable to accommodate the increased workload, the right atrium may also enlarge as it attempts to overcome the resistance offered by incomplete right ventricular emptying.

CLINICAL MANIFESTATIONS

The infant with VSD has varying symptoms, depending on age, weight, and size of the defect. Failure to thrive and frequent respiratory infections resulting from increased pulmonary blood flow are the typical course.

One of the characteristic signs of VSD is a loud, harsh murmur. In neonates, the murmur may be absent because of the normally high pulmonary vascular resistance, which tends to equalize the pressure between the two ventricles.

Severe overloading of the right ventricle and occasionally the right atrium causes hypertrophy and an obvious cardiac enlargement. Development of CHF typically occurs.

PROCESS OF DIAGNOSIS

The ECG and echocardiographical findings of right ventricular hypertrophy and cardiomegaly, and prominent pulmonary markings on chest x-ray, usually confirm the diagnosis of VSD. Cardiac catheterization and angiography are necessary to measure pulmonary vascular resistance and precisely define the location and number of VSDs.

THERAPEUTIC MANAGEMENT

Preventing the development of pulmonary vascular obstructive disease demands closure of large VSDs within the first year of life. Early repair prevents progressive respiratory disease.

Surgical closure is accomplished through a sternotomy and using cardiopulmonary bypass. A patch closure is usually performed, but a stitch closure may be used for smaller defects. Surgical closure of membranous VSDs can now be done with a low operative risk in infants, but muscular VSDs continue to have a mortality as high as 30% (Hazinski, 1992). Postoperative complications include residual VSD and conduction disturbances. Advanced pulmonary vascular obstructive disease contraindicates VSD closure. These patients should be considered for an eventual heart-lung transplant.

ATRIOVENTRICULAR SEPTAL DEFECT

Atrioventricular septal defect (AVSD), one anomaly in the group of endocardial cushion defects, results from incomplete fusion of the endocardial cushions during fetal life. The incomplete fusion produces abnormalities in both the atrial and the ventricular septa, as well as in the atrioventricular valve(s). Defects are generally classified as partial (PAVSD), or complete (CAVSD). The most severe form, CAVSD, consists of a single atrioventricular valve common to both right and left atrioventricular chambers. The central communication usually involves a primum ASD above and a large defect in the inlet of the ventricular septum below. It is the most common cardiac defect in children with Down's syndrome (Hoffman, 1990).

PATENT DUCTUS ARTERIOSUS

A patent ductus arteriosus (PDA) is present when the normal fetal structure fails to close completely after birth (Fig. 28-7). In the fetus, most blood entering the pulmonary artery from the right ventricle escapes to the systemic circulation through the normally present ductus arteriosus. This shunt allows more blood to go to the actively growing fetus and less to the virtually nonfunctioning pulmonary system. At birth, closure of the ductus arteriosus normally occurs within hours from exposure of smooth muscle in its vessel wall to increased oxygen tension and little response to the relaxant effect of prostaglandins (Gersony, 1986). Permanent anatomical closure is usually complete towards the end of the first postnatal month. In some infants, this does not occur, and the ductus arteriosus remains patent.

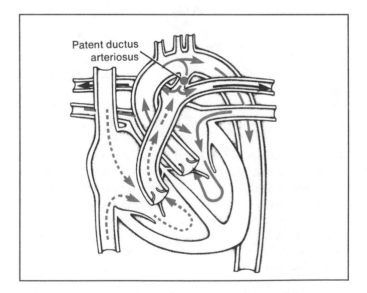

Fig. 28-7 Patent ductus arteriosus. *Red arrows,* saturated blood; *broken red arrows,* desaturated blood; *black arrows,* mixed blood.

ALTERED HAEMODYNAMICS

The haemodynamic consequences of PDA depend on the size of the ductus and the pulmonary vascular resistance. At birth, the resistance in the pulmonary and systemic circulations is almost identical, thus equalizing the resistance in the aorta and pulmonary artery. As the systemic pressure exceeds the pulmonary pressure, blood begins to shunt from the aorta, across the duct, to the pulmonary artery (left-to-right shunt).

The additional blood is recirculated through the lungs and returned to the left atrium and left ventricle. The effect of this altered circulation is increased workload on the left side of the heart, increased pulmonary vascular congestion and possibly resistance, and potentially increased right ventricular pressure and hypertrophy.

CLINICAL MANIFESTATIONS

Some children have no detectable abnormality except for a murmur; others have frequent respiratory infections, signs of CHF, and failure to thrive.

PROCESS OF DIAGNOSIS

Radiological examinations usually demonstrate left atrial and ventricular enlargement, and evidence of increased pulmonary blood flow. The ECG is generally normal, although it may demonstrate left ventricular or biventricular enlargement. An echocardiogram may demonstrate increased pulmonary blood flow and increased venous return. Patients of any age with PDA can undergo surgery without cardiac catheterization, if all the noninvasive findings are typical.

THERAPEUTIC MANAGEMENT

Congestive heart failure is an indication for PDA closure in infancy. In asymptomatic patients, PDA closure can be planned electively and is recommended before age two years. Because of low surgical risk and possible bacterial endocarditis, correction is recommended for all affected children. Surgical intervention involves surgical division or ligation of the patent vessel. Since the defect is outside the heart, cardiopulmonary bypass is not necessary. The risk of surgical PDA closure, excluding premature infants with respiratory distress syndrome, should approach 0% (Adams, Emmanouilides and Riemenschneider, 1989).

In the premature infant with respiratory distress syndrome, indomethacin (a prostaglandin inhibitor) has been used to encourage ductal closure. If this is ineffective, operative closure is suggested and is well tolerated.

In older infants and children, PDA may also be obliterated with an "umbrella" apparatus placed during cardiac catheterization (Roberts, 1989). A double-umbrella device at the tip of the catheter is passed through the PDA to the descending aorta for opening of the distal arms of half the umbrella. The catheter is pulled back through the PDA for opening of the umbrella's proximal arms against the left pulmonary artery side. The entire unit is then released, thus occluding the opening.

OBSTRUCTIVE DEFECTS

Obstructive defects are those in which blood exiting the heart meets an area of anatomical narrowing (stenosis), causing obstruction to blood flow. The pressure in the ventricle and in the great artery before the obstruction is increased, and the pressure in the area beyond the obstruction is decreased. The location of the narrowing is usually near the valve (Fig. 28-8):
- **Valvular** — at the site of the valve itself.
- **Subvalvular** — narrowing in the ventricle below the valve (also referred to as the *ventricular outflow tract*).
- **Supravalvular** — narrowing in the great artery above the valve.

Aortic stenosis, pulmonary stenosis, and coarctation of the aorta (narrowing of the aortic arch) are typical defects in this group. Haemodynamically, there is a pressure load on the ventricle and decreased cardiac output. Clinically, infants and children exhibit signs of CHF. Children with mild obstruction may be asymptomatic. Rarely, as in severe pulmonary stenosis, hypoxaemia may be seen.

COARCTATION OF THE AORTA

Coarctation of the aorta (COA) is a narrowing of the aorta. The position of the narrowing is described as:
- **Preductal** - proximal to the insertion of the ductus arteriosus, usually between that vessel and the left subclavian artery

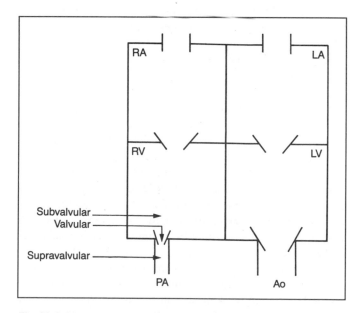

Fig. 28-8 Obstruction to ventricular ejection can occur at the valvular level (shown), below the valve (subvalvular), or above the valve (supravalvular). Pulmonary stenosis is shown here.

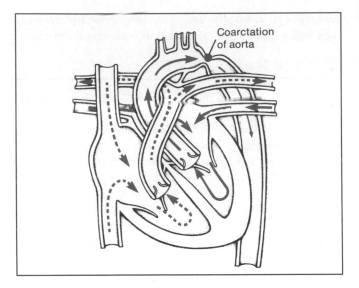

Fig. 28-9 Coarctation of aorta (postductal). *Red arrows*, saturated blood; *broken red arrows*, desaturated blood.

- **Postductal** — distal to the ductus arteriosus (Fig. 28-9).
- **Juxtaductal** — at the level of the ductus arteriosus.

A coexisting bicuspid aortic valve is found in about 50% of patients.

ALTERED HAEMODYNAMICS

The effect of a narrowing within the aorta is increased pressure proximal to the defect and decreased pressure distal to it. In the preductal type of COA, the lower half of the body is supplied with blood by the right ventricle through the ductus arteriosus. In the postductal type, right ventricular outflow cannot maintain blood flow to the descending aorta. Therefore, collateral circulation develops during fetal life to maintain flow from the ascending to the descending aorta.

CLINICAL MANIFESTATIONS

Patients with COA include the symptomatic neonate or infant, and the asymptomatic older child. The neonate or young infant frequently has CHF when admitted to hospital. Often these patients' haemodynamic condition deteriorates rapidly, and they are admitted to the intensive care unit, usually severely acidotic and hypotensive. Mechanical ventilation and inotropic support are often necessary before surgery. In most older children, COA is first recognized at routine physical examination when upper extremity systemic hypertension, weak or absent femoral pulses, and a heart murmur are found. Older children may experience occasional dizziness, headaches, fainting and epistaxis resulting from hypertension. In body areas distal to the defect, blood pressure is decreased. The femoral pulses are weak or absent, the lower extremities may be cooler than the upper ones, and muscle cramps may result during increased exercise from tissue anoxia (a condition called *claudication*).

PROCESS OF DIAGNOSIS

In the neonate and young infant, the chest x-ray usually shows a greatly enlarged heart and congested lung fields. An echocardiogram and Doppler examination confirm the diagnosis. If a question exists about additional intracardiac pathology, a cardiac catheterization is performed.

In older children, the ECG may be normal or may show some degree of left ventricular hypertrophy.

THERAPEUTIC MANAGEMENT

Surgical correction consists of either resection of the coarcted portion with an end-to-end anastomosis of the aorta, or enlargement of the constricted section using a graft of prosthetic material or a portion of the left subclavian artery. Because this defect is outside the heart and pericardium, cardiopulmonary bypass is not required and a thoracotomy incision is used.

Postoperative hypertension is treated with intravenous sodium nitroprusside or amrinone, followed by oral medications, such as captopril, hydralazine, and/or propranolol.

In neonates and infants with isolated COA, hospital mortality is less than 5%, whereas in patients with COA that coexists with complex congenital heart disease, mortality increases significantly. Beyond early infancy, mortality is less than 1% (Moller and Neal, 1990). There is a 5–10% risk of recurrent narrowing in patients who underwent surgical repair as infants (Hellenbrand *et al*, 1990). Percutaneous balloon angioplasty techniques have proved very effective in relieving residual postoperative coarctation gradients.

PULMONARY STENOSIS

Pulmonary stenosis (PS) is a narrowing at the entrance to the pulmonary artery (see Fig. 28-10). The valve may be normal, but the divisions between the cusps are fused so that blood flow through the valve is restricted or the valve may be malformed.

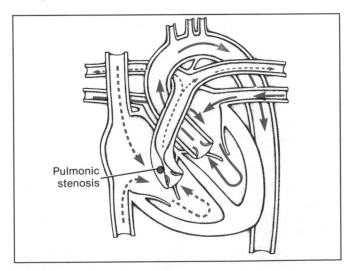

Fig. 28-10 Pulmonary stenosis. *Red arrows*, saturated blood; *broken red arrows*, desaturated blood.

Stenosis may also occur from narrowing in the ventricular outflow tract. Pulmonary atresia is the extreme form of PS in that there is total fusion of the commissures and no blood flows to the lungs. The right ventricle may be hypoplastic.

ALTERED HAEMODYNAMICS

When PS is present, resistance to blood flow causes right ventricular hypertrophy. If right ventricular failure develops, right atrial pressure will increase and this may result in reopening of the foramen ovale, shunting of unoxygenated blood into the left atrium, and systemic cyanosis. If PS is severe, CHF occurs, and systemic venous engorgement will be noted. An associated defect, such as a PDA, partially compensates for the obstruction by shunting blood from the aorta to the pulmonary artery and into the lungs.

CLINICAL MANIFESTATIONS

Symptoms depend on the degree of PS and can range from only a murmur to cyanosis and CHF. Children with moderate defects generally experience dyspnoea and fatigue, especially on exertion, since blood flow to the lungs is insufficient to accommodate demands for increased cardiac output. Occasionally, severe PS is associated with a small right ventricle and an intact ventricular septum. These infants develop a large right-to-left shunt through a foramen ovale; pulmonary blood flow is greatly reduced and acute CHF ensues. Without immediate surgical intervention to increase pulmonary blood flow and relieve right ventricular obstruction, death will occur.

PROCESS OF DIAGNOSIS

An echocardiogram demonstrates the obstruction to the pulmonary artery and any associated defects such as ASD. Cardiac catheterization documents increased pressure in the right side of the heart, and decreased oxygenation in the left side will be noted if a right-to-left shunt is present. X-rays show a normal size heart, usually with normal or decreased pulmonary vascular markings and poststenotic dilatation of the pulmonary artery. An ECG may show several changes, including right atrial and ventricular hypertrophy.

THERAPEUTIC MANAGEMENT

Children with mild degrees of PS may not require invasive intervention, but are followed medically with appropriate antibiotic administration to prevent bacterial endocarditis. Treatment is recommended whenever the child demonstrates a significant pressure gradient across the pulmonary valve, since continued right ventricular hypertension contributes to the development of right ventricular fibrosis.

Critical PS in the infant often requires emergency surgery and carries a higher risk of complications. Although children with severe stenosis may require surgery, many pulmonary defects are being successfully treated with balloon angioplasty.

Through a percutaneous puncture (similar to cardiac catheterization) a catheter is inserted across the stenotic pulmonary valve into the pulmonary artery, and a balloon at the end of the catheter is inflated and rapidly passed through the narrowed opening. The procedure is associated with few complications and has proved highly effective, with a 50-75% reduction in pressure gradient across the pulmonary valve and a low rate of complications (Radtke and Lock, 1990). It is the treatment of choice in most centres and can be done safely in neonates.

In patients requiring surgery, a pulmonary valvotomy is performed. The surgeon works through a small incision in the pulmonary artery. The fused commissures are incised, and the pulmonary artery incision is closed. There is a low risk for both procedures (mortality less than 2%), and the haemodynamic results are excellent. Both balloon dilatation and surgical valvotomy leave the pulmonary valve incompetent because they involve opening the fused valve leaflets; however, these patients are clinically asymptomatic. Long-term problems with restenosis or valve incompetence may occur.

DEFECTS WITH DECREASED PULMONARY BLOOD FLOW

In this group of defects, there is obstruction to pulmonary blood flow and an anatomical defect (ASD or VSD) between the right and left sides of the heart (Fig. 28-11). Because blood has difficulty exiting the right side of the heart via the pulmonary artery, pressure on the right side increases, exceeding left-sided pressures. This allows desaturated blood to shunt right to left, causing desaturation in the left side of the heart and in the systemic circulation. Clinically, these patients are hypoxaemic and usually appear cyanotic. Tetralogy of Fallot and tricuspid atresia are the more common defects in this group.

TETRALOGY OF FALLOT

Tetralogy of Fallot (TOF) is the most common cyanotic heart defect. The anatomical definition includes four defects: (1)

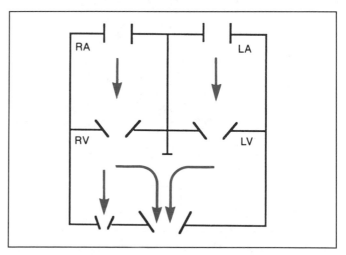

Fig. 28-11 Haemodynamic defects with decreased pulmonary blood flow.

VSD; (2) PS, always subvalvular and often valvular; more accurately called right ventricular outflow tract obstruction; (3) an aorta that overrides the VSD; and (4) right ventricular hypertrophy, which occurs from pulmonary artery obstruction (Fig. 28-12). Wide variation exists in the severity of this defect. Some infants with mild obstruction to pulmonary blood flow have little or no right-to-left shunting and appear pink. The more typical presentation is mild cyanosis at birth, which worsens with age because the PS is progressive, pulmonary blood flow is reduced and the degree of right-to-left shunting increases with time.

Some infants with TOF are extremely cyanotic at birth because of severe obstruction and require immediate intervention to provide pulmonary blood flow.

CLINICAL MANIFESTATIONS

The infant initially may not be cyanotic because the PDA shunts blood to the lungs, bypassing the PS. When the PDA has closed, hypoxaemia and cyanosis become apparent. Cyanosis becomes more severe over time because increasing right ventricular outflow tract obstruction results in decreased pulmonary blood flow and increased right-to-left shunting. Rising haemoglobin and haematocrit concentrations are seen. Severe cyanotic spells may occur with increasing obstruction and infundibular spasm. Squatting is rarely seen because children are usually repaired before age two years. There is a characteristic murmur.

PROCESS OF DIAGNOSIS

A diagnosis is usually made on the history and physical findings alone. However, a cardiac catheterization and/or echocardiogram is performed to evaluate the severity of the anatomical defects and cardiac changes. Laboratory tests determine the degree of polycythaemia and arterial oxygen saturation. Right ventricular hypertrophy is noted on chest x-ray and ECG. The pulmonary arteries vary in size.

THERAPEUTIC MANAGEMENT

The current trend is to repair TOF in infancy. The exact timing depends on the child's overall clinical status and the condition of the pulmonary arteries, but elective repair is usually performed in the first year of life. Indications for repair include increasing cyanosis and the development of severe cyanotic spells. Complete repair involves closure of the VSD and resection of the infundibular stenosis, with a pericardial patch to enlarge the right ventricular outflow tract. The procedure requires a median sternotomy and the use of cardiopulmonary bypass.

In infants who cannot undergo primary repair, a palliative procedure to increase pulmonary blood flow and increase oxygen saturation may be performed. The preferred procedure is the *Blalock-Taussig* or *modified Blalock-Taussig shunt*, which provides blood flow to the pulmonary arteries from the left or right subclavian artery. In general, however, shunts are avoided because they may result in pulmonary artery distortion.

The operative mortality for total correction of TOF is less than 5%. With improved surgical techniques, there is a lower incidence of arrhythmias and sudden death; surgical heart block is rare, even in severely affected infants (Jonas and Lang, 1988).

CARDIAC LESIONS WITH COMMON MIXING

Many complex cardiac anomalies depend on mixing of blood from the pulmonary and systemic circulations within the heart chambers for survival in the postnatal period. Haemodynamically, fully saturated systemic blood flow mixes with the desaturated pulmonary blood flow, causing a relative desaturation of the systemic blood flow. Pulmonary congestion occurs because the differences in pulmonary artery pressure and aortic pressure favour pulmonary blood flow. Cardiac output decreases because of a volume load on the ventricle. Clinically, these patients have a variable picture that combines some degree of desaturation (although cyanosis is not always visible) and signs of CHF.

TRANSPOSITION OF THE GREAT ARTERIES

By definition, transposition of the great arteries (TGA) refers to a condition in which the pulmonary artery leaves the left ventricle and the aorta exits from the right ventricle (Fig. 28-13). This type of circulation is incompatible with extrauterine life, because the body receives only desaturated blood and progressive hypoxaemia will develop. For survival, the parallel circuits must communicate to allow adequate mixing of saturated blood in the pulmonary circulation and desaturated blood

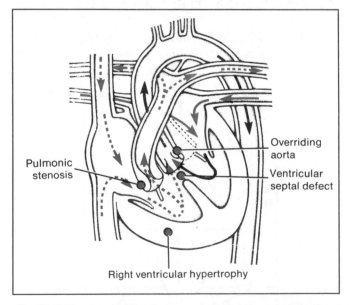

Fig. 28-12 Tetralogy of Fallot. *Red arrows,* saturated blood; *broken red arrows,* desaturated blood; *black arrows,* mixed blood.

Pulmonic stenosis

Overriding aorta

Ventricular septal defect

Right ventricular hypertrophy

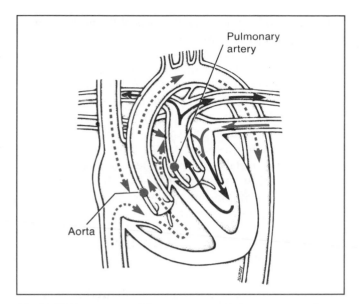

Fig. 28-13 Transposition of the great arteries. *Red arrows*, saturated blood; *broken red arrows*, desaturated blood; *black arrows*, mixed blood.

in the systemic circulation. This is accomplished through associated defects such as septal defects or a PDA.

ASSOCIATED DEFECTS AND HAEMODYNAMICS

The most common defect associated with TGA is a patent foramen ovale. At birth there is also a PDA, although in most instances this closes after the neonatal period. Another associated anomaly may be VSD. Presence of these defects increases the risk of CHF, since they often produce high pulmonary blood flow under high pressure.

CLINICAL MANIFESTATIONS

The severity of the child's condition depends on the amount of blood mixing. Neonates with minimum mixing of systemic and pulmonary venous blood or obstruction to pulmonary blood flow are severely cyanotic at birth. Those with large septal defects or a PDA may be less severely cyanotic, but develop symptoms of CHF during the first weeks of life. In these infants, the only signs at birth may be cyanosis after crying or feeding and progressive tachypnoea. However, severe cyanotic episodes can occur and are thought to result from increased oxygen demand that the cardiovascular system cannot meet.

There is no murmur associated with simple TGA. Cardiomegaly from right and left ventricular hypertrophy may be evident a few weeks after birth. The infant with a large VSD will have symptoms of CHF in the first weeks to month of life.

PROCESS OF DIAGNOSIS

Definitive diagnosis of TGA is made on the findings of two-dimensional echocardiography. Cardiac catheterization may be indicated to define coronary artery anatomy and measure

left-to-right ventricular ratios to determine the left ventricle's ability to assume the work of the systemic circulation.

THERAPEUTIC MANAGEMENT

Both palliative and corrective surgical procedures can be performed for TGA. Whenever possible, primary repair is recommended. The administration of prostaglandin E_2 may be initiated to increase blood mixing if systemic and pulmonary mixing is inadequate to provide an oxygen saturation of 75% or to maintain cardiac output. During cardiac catheterization, a balloon atrial septostomy (Rashkind procedure) may also be performed to increase mixing and maintain cardiac output over a longer period.

Several surgical approaches are available for correction of TGA. The procedure depends on the anatomical defects, the surgeon's preference, and the availability of comprehensive postoperative management. The procedure of choice is the *arterial switch*, which involves transposing the great arteries and mobilizing and reimplanting the coronary arteries. It is a technically challenging procedure, because the coronary arteries must be removed from the aorta before the switch is performed, and then they must be reimplanted into the aorta at its new location. Reimplantation of the coronary arteries is critical to the infant's survival, and they must be reattached without torsion or kinking to provide the heart with its supply of oxygen. The advantage of the arterial switch procedure is the reestablishment of normal circulation, with the left ventricle acting as the systemic pump.

The *Mustard* or *Senning operation* involves the creation of an intra-atrial baffle to tunnel or divert systemic venous blood to the mitral valve (and the left ventricle and pulmonary artery) and divert pulmonary venous blood to the tricuspid valve (and the right ventricle and aorta). Therefore, the procedure does not attempt to transplant the transposed arterial vessels but reverses the function of the atria. An advantage of the Senning operation is the use of the patient's own atrial septum to create the baffle rather than pericardium or prosthetic material, which is used in the Mustard operation. The use of little or no foreign material allows for growth of the biological baffle.

Another surgical option is the *Rastelli procedure*, which is the operative choice in infants with TGA, VSD and severe PS. It involves closure of the VSD with a baffle, directing left ventricular blood through the VSD into the aorta. The pulmonary valve is then closed and a conduit placed from the right ventricle to the pulmonary artery, creating a physiologically normal circulation. Unfortunately, this procedure requires multiple conduit replacements as the child grows.

The optimum time for repair depends on the procedure. The arterial switch can usually be performed safely in the first three weeks to one month of life. The other surgeries are usually performed within the first year of life. Mortality for both the arterial and the atrial switch procedures is less than 5%. However, significant problems occur with late complications following atrial baffle surgery. For example, right ventricular failure, baffle obstructions, and rhythm disturbances occur most often. Only 50% of patients have normal sinus rhythm 10 years after atrial baffle procedures (Castaneda, 1989). Potential complications of the arterial switch include narrowing at the great artery anastomoses or coronary artery insufficiency.

NURSING CARE OF THE FAMILY AND CHILD WITH CONGENITAL HEART DISEASE

When a child is born with a severe cardiac anomaly, the parents are faced with the immense psychological and physical tasks of adjusting to the birth of a child with special needs. Since corrective surgery is being performed at an earlier age, this discussion is primarily directed: (1) towards the family of an infant who has a serious heart defect and requires home care before definitive repair and (2) towards preparation and care of the child and family when heart surgery is performed.

Nursing care of the child with a congenital heart defect begins as soon as the diagnosis is suspected. However, in many instances symptoms that suggest a cardiac anomaly are not present at birth, or are so subtle that they are easily overlooked.

Some heart defects are not evident until the child's growth and/or energy expenditure exceeds the heart's ability to supply oxygenated blood to the tissues. Since the onset of symptoms may be gradual, the child may curtail activity so that the signs of exercise intolerance are less obvious. However, a careful history yields important clues to this change. Most infants suck vigorously and fall asleep after feeding. It is very unusual to hear of a child who prefers to sit rather than crawl or walk, or who falls asleep shortly after beginning a feeding. Likewise, a child who needs frequent rests or naps after limited play periods may also be exhibiting exercise intolerance. Such histories should alert the nurse to assess cardiac function. Other clues are a history of poor weight gain; poor feeding habits, especially the need to pause during feeding; poor suck; difficulty in coordinating sucking, swallowing, and breathing; frequent respiratory infections; cyanosis; and squatting.

Nursing care consists of providing not only direct care to the infant or child, but also indirect care through family members. Cardiac defects are especially frightening to families, because of the serious connotations.

HELP FAMILY ADJUST TO THE DISORDER

Once parents learn of the heart defect, they are initially in a period of shock, followed by high anxiety, especially fear of the child's death. The family needs a period of grief before assimilating the meaning of the defect. Unfortunately, the demands for medical treatment may not allow this, necessitating that the parents be informed of the condition in order to give informed consent for diagnostic/therapeutic procedures. The nurse can be instrumental in supporting parents in their loss, assessing their level of understanding, supplying information

as needed, and helping other members of the health team to understand the parents' reactions.

Severely distressed newborns usually remain in the hospital. This can seriously affect parent-infant bonding unless parents are encouraged to hold, touch, and look at their child. Every effort must be made by health professionals to foster attachment.

A child with CHD may constitute a long-term family crisis. Frequently, the continuing unremitting stresses of care are not fully appreciated by those caring for the family. Even when the child's condition is stabilized or corrected, the family may need to make new adjustments in their life-style. Introducing them to other families with similarly affected children can help them adjust to the daily stresses.

EDUCATE FAMILY ABOUT THE DISORDER

Once parents are ready to hear about the heart condition, it is essential that they be given a clear explanation based on their level of understanding. A simple diagram, pictures, written information or a model of the heart can be most helpful in visualizing the heart and the congenital defect. To prevent confusion, the same type of diagram should be used by all health professionals, and the parents should write down any unclear terms or ask for clarification. Sometimes it is helpful to provide the family with a glossary of frequently used words for reference.

Parents are primarily interested in two types of information: prognosis and surgery. They are frequently upset about indefinite answers to either. The family should be assured that the health care team will be honest in keeping them informed of the child's condition and of decisions regarding future procedures and treatments.

Information given to the child must be tailored to the child's developmental age. Children of all ages need to express their feelings concerning the diagnosis.

HELP FAMILY COPE WITH EFFECTS OF THE DISORDER

Parents also need an explanation regarding the symptoms of the disease. Many children have few symptoms, but may develop CHF. Therefore parents should be aware of early signs of worsening physical status, such as sweating, sudden weight gain, decreased exercise tolerance, poor feeding and increased breathing effort. These symptoms need medical evaluation, but the family should be assured the symptoms usually respond quickly to therapeutic intervention.

Another area of parental concern is the child's level of physical activity. Children do not need to restrict activity, and the best approach is to treat the child normally and to allow self-limited activity.

Children with CHD require good nutrition. The infant may need to be fed small amounts of formula every 2-3 hours to ensure adequate nutrition. If several night-time feedings are required, the nurse should discuss with parents the need to share the responsibility and enlist the help of others whenever possible.

The infant who has more difficulty feeding because of a congenital heart defect should be well supported and in a semi-upright position when fed. This ensures a comfortable position for the infant attempting to coordinate the suck/swallow and breathing process and also decreases the risk of aspiration. Caregivers are encouraged not to interrupt infants who suck vigorously. The infants will pause and pace themselves during the feeding, but they should be stimulated to suck in an attempt to complete the feeding.

The infant with CHD frequently requires caloric supplements, because of the inefficient functioning of the heart and lungs. A diet plan specific to the individual infant's needs is calculated and prescribed by the dietitian in collaboration with the other health personnel.

Children with severe cardiac defects are often anorexic. Encouraging them to eat can be a tremendous challenge.

The family also needs to be knowledgeable regarding the therapeutic management of the disorder, especially the medications the child is receiving. Parents should be taught the correct procedure for giving drugs and cautioned to keep them in a safe place to prevent accidental ingestion.

PREPARE CHILD AND FAMILY FOR SURGERY

Few surgical procedures demand as much planning for preoperative preparation and postoperative care as heart surgery. This discussion focuses on measures specific to the cardiovascular procedure. Technical differences exist between closed- and open-heart surgery. Consequently, there are some additions to physical care postoperatively in open-heart surgery (see chapters 5 and 7).

Several intravenous lines are inserted perioperatively: (1) an ordinary line for infusion of fluids, inserted in a peripheral vein; (2) a venous pressure line, inserted into the right subclavian or jugular vein; and (3) an arterial line for direct measurement of arterial pressure. Younger children need only know the location of each tubing. Older children may appreciate knowing the reason for each infusion, especially when venous and arterial measurements are taken. Since the lines are inserted during surgery, they are not painful, only uncomfortable because of the restricted movement.

The type and size of dressing the child will have after surgery are discussed and can be shown on a doll. Usually one of two types of incisions is made: a *median sternotomy*, which splits the sternum, or a *lateral thoracotomy*, which extends from the midaxillary line to the scapula. Frequently, no sutures are visible because subcuticular, absorbable sutures may be used. If this is done, it should be pointed out to the child and parents, who may fear the incision will open. Sometimes a butterfly incision is used for cosmetic reasons in girls instead of the regular median sternotomy.

The child may be told about chest drains and their purpose in draining fluid from around the heart and lungs. A picture of the equipment used for drainage can be shown to the child, or the setup can be simulated by attaching one end of the tubes

to a doll with a chest dressing and the other end to small bottles. The nurse stresses that the child must move even though the tubes are in place. It can be demonstrated on the doll that the tubing is long enough to permit turning. Since this information may be anxiety producing, it is best left to the end of teaching or eliminated if the child appears too anxious.

An endotracheal (ET) tube is inserted during surgery and may be left in place for ventilatory assistance and tracheobronchial suctioning. The ET tube can be presented as a 'breathing tube' that is placed in the nose or mouth. The nurse explains that while the tube is in, the child will feel it in the throat and will not be able to talk, but nothing is wrong. The child can express desires by pointing or using a picture communication board. The nurse stresses that the tube will be removed as soon as possible, often during the first postoperative day.

The child should be assured that the parents will be there when the child wakes up; they should be allowed to accompany their child to the operating theatre. After all the equipment and procedures have been explained, it is important to talk about 'getting well' and going home. If a doll was used during the preparatory session, the tubes can be removed and the doll can be dressed in regular clothes in anticipation of discharge.

PROVIDE POSTOPERATIVE CARE

Immediate postoperative care is usually in intensive care units. Many of the procedures, such as arterial pressure and central venous pressure (CVP) monitoring and the observations related to vital functions, require additional education and training. However, nurses caring for the child before surgery and during the convalescent period need to be familiar with the major principles of care.

Observe vital signs and arterial/venous pressures

Vital signs and blood pressure are recorded frequently until stable. Heart rate and respirations are counted for one minute, compared with the ECG monitor, and recorded with activity. The heart rate is normally increased after surgery. The nurse observes cardiac rhythm and notifies the medical staff of any changes in regularity. Arrhythmias may occur postoperatively secondary to anaesthetics, acid-base and electrolyte imbalance, hypoxia, surgical intervention or trauma to conduction pathways.

The lungs are regularly auscultated for breath sounds. Diminished or absent sounds most likely indicate an area of atelectasis, which necessitates further medical assessment.

Temperature changes are typical during the early postoperative period. Hypothermia is expected immediately after surgery from hypothermia procedures, effects of anaesthesia, and loss of body heat to the cool environment. During this period, the child is kept warm to prevent additional heat loss. Infants may be placed under radiant heat warmers. During the next 24-48 hours the body temperature may rise as part of the inflammatory response to tissue trauma. After this period, an elevated temperature is most likely a sign of infection and warrants immediate investigation for probable cause.

Intraarterial monitoring of blood pressure is almost always used following open-heart surgery. Residual vasoconstriction after cardiopulmonary bypass makes indirect blood pressure readings less reliable, and intraarterial monitoring permits continuous observation. Continuous blood pressure readings are compared with those taken indirectly with a sphygmomanometer or oscillometry (Dinamap). A discrepancy between the two may indicate a change in peripheral vascular resistance, a malfunction in the electronic device, or human error. The nurse also observes for potential complications of intraarterial monitoring, such as arterial thrombosis, infection, air emboli, or blood loss through the catheter.

The intraarterial line is maintained with a low-rate constant infusion of heparinized saline to prevent clotting.

Intracardiac monitoring lines provide data on cardiac function and output. They are placed intraoperatively and may be present in the left atrium, pulmonary artery, or right atrium. The CVP catheter is inserted into the superior vena cava or inferior vena cava, and the other end is attached to a monitor.

CVP continually changes according to blood volume, heart rate, and myocardial function. If the blood volume decreases, such as in shock, the CVP falls. If the efficiency of the left side of the heart decreases, the resistance to right ventricular ejection will ultimately result in an elevated CVP but decreased intraarterial pressure. CHF and/or hypervolaemia raise the CVP.

The complications of CVP lines are similar to other infusions, with the addition of atrial arrhythmias from irritation of the atrial wall; and haemothorax, pneumothorax, or hydrothorax from accidental puncture as the catheter enters the thorax. The nurse observes for signs and symptoms indicative of each of these risks.

Maintain respiratory status

The child is generally maintained on mechanical ventilation in the immediate postoperative period. When weaning and extubation are completed, humidified oxygen is delivered by mask or head box. The child is encouraged to cough, turn, and deep breathe. Every measure is employed to enhance ventilation and decrease pain, such as splinting of the operative site and use of analgesics. Although crying increases heart rate, it is beneficial in promoting deep respirations.

Chest physiotherapy is given according to need. Since the procedure is uncomfortable, it is important to emphasize to the child the necessity of performing it and to clarify that the percussion, sometimes mistakenly viewed as hitting, is done to loosen secretions in the lungs and is not a punishment. The child is usually comforted by the parents, and if they wish to participate, they can be very helpful in positioning the child.

Suctioning is performed as needed. Deep suctioning is performed carefully to avoid vagal stimulation (cardiac arrhythmias) and laryngospasm, especially in infants. Suctioning is intermittent and maintained for no more than five seconds to prevent depleting the oxygen supply. Heart rate is monitored after suctioning to detect changes in rhythm or rate, especially bradycardia. The child should always be positioned facing the nurse to permit assessment of the child's colour and tolerance to the procedure.

Chest drains are inserted into the pleural and/or mediastinal space during surgery or in the immediate postoperative period to remove secretions and air in order to allow reexpansion of the lung. The chest drain is attached to a water-seal drainage system, which prevents air from travelling up the tube into the pleural space, causing a pneumothorax. The nursing considerations include: (1) do not interrupt water-seal drainage unless the chest tube is clamped, (2) check for tube patency (fluctuation in the water-seal chamber) and (3) maintain sterility.

Drainage is checked hourly for colour and quantity. Immediately postoperatively the drainage may be bright red, but afterward it should be serous. The largest volume of drainage occurs in the first 12-24 hours and is more copious in extensive heart surgery.

Chest x-rays are taken when the drains are inserted to check their location and after they are removed to evaluate the inflation of the lungs. Chest tubes are usually removed on the first to third postoperative day. Lung expansion is demonstrated by decreased fluctuation in the tube and absence of drainage.

Removal of chest drains is a painful, frightening experience. Analgesics such as morphine sulphate (0.1 mg/kg) should be given before the procedure. Children are forewarned that they will feel a sharp, momentary pain. After the suture is cut, the tubes are quickly pulled out at the end of full inspiration to prevent intake of air into the pleural cavity. A purse-string suture (placed when the drains were inserted) is pulled tight to close the opening. A sealing agent may be required if the purse string does not provide good skin closure. The dressing is checked for signs of drainage and any evidence of infection.

Provide maximum rest

After heart surgery, maximum rest should be provided to decrease the workload of the heart and to promote healing. Nursing care is planned according to the child's usual activity and sleep patterns.

Provide comfort

Recent improvements have been made in the management of pain following cardiac surgery. Studies show that adequate analgesia and anaesthesia decreases the body's stress response to surgery and improves postoperative morbidity and mortality (Anand and Hickey, 1992; Wessel, 1993). Continuous intravenous opiate infusions, particularly morphine and fentanyl, are safe and effective methods of pain control (Maguire and Maloney, 1988). Patient-controlled analgesia may be used with children old enough to understand the concept, and epidural morphine is another option (Rosen and Rosen, 1989). Paralysing agents such as atracunium or vecuronium may also be used with the analgesics for children who are very agitated or haemodynamically unstable. Children receiving opiate infusions for a prolonged period are weaned slowly from the medication to prevent withdrawal symptoms.

Duration of pain control and type of pain relief is dictated by the individual child, based on pain assessment.

In addition to pharmacological pain control, every effort is made to minimize the discomfort of procedures, such as using a firm pillow or favourite stuffed animal placed against the chest incision during coughing, and performing treatments *after* pain medication is given, preferably at a time that coincides with the drug's peak effect. Nonpharmacological measures are employed to lessen the perception of pain, and parents are encouraged to comfort their child as much as possible.

Monitor fluids

Intake and output of all fluids must be accurately calculated. Output includes hourly recordings of urine (usually a Foley catheter is inserted and attached to a closed collecting device), drainage from chest and nasogastric tubes, and blood drawn for analysis. Urine is analysed for specific gravity to assess the kidneys' concentrating ability and to assess approximately the body's degree of hydration. Renal failure is a potential risk from a transient period of low cardiac output. The signs of renal failure are decreased urine output (less than 1 ml/kg/hour) and elevated levels of blood urea nitrogen and serum creatinine (Hazinski, 1992).

Fluids are restricted during the immediate postoperative period to prevent hypervolaemia, which places additional demands on the myocardium, predisposing to cardiac failure. Two factors influence increased blood volume. In open-heart surgery, the cardiopulmonary pump is primed with a large volume of fluid (usually electrolyte solution), which may greatly dilute the patient's blood. During circulation through the body, some of this priming fluid diffuses into the interstitial spaces but postoperatively diffuses back into the systemic circulation.

Fluid requirements are based on the child's weight and body surface area. The child is fed as soon as possible. Nasogastric feeding is used if the child is intubated or if the child is unable to complete oral feeds.

Plan for progressive activity

Moderate activity is essential to prevent pulmonary and vascular complications. Initially, turning, coughing and deep breathing are sufficient to promote respiratory expansion. However, passive range of motion exercises, especially to the lower extremities, are instituted to prevent venous stasis.

A progressive schedule of ambulation and activity is planned, based on the child's preoperative activity patterns and postoperative cardiovascular and pulmonary function.

Ambulation is initiated early, depending on the child's condition. The nurse begins ambulation for the child, progressing from sitting on the edge of the bed and dangling the legs to standing up and to sitting in a chair. After ambulation, a rest period is scheduled.

Observe for complications of heart surgery

Several complications can occur after heart surgery, most of which are related to open-heart surgery and use of cardiopulmonary bypass.

Haematological changes

While passing through the heart-lung machine, blood is exposed to substantial trauma by direct contact with oxygen, mechanical action, foreign substances and massive doses of anticoagulants. The result of mechanical trauma is red blood cell haemolysis and potential renal tubular necrosis. Heparinization of the blood during extracorporeal circulation can result in clotting abnormalities from decreased thrombin and prothrombin, decreased platelets, and altered platelet aggregation.

Haemolysis of red blood cells results in blood loss and anaemia, which may require packed red blood cell transfusion. Full blood counts are monitored to identify the severity of the haemolysis. All urine is tested for the presence of blood. If transfusions are required, the child is closely observed for signs of reaction and fluid overload.

Since blood clotting mechanisms are affected, signs of haemorrhage, especially bleeding from the chest drains, and a fall in arterial and venous pressures are important observations. Haemorrhage is more likely to occur in patients who have repair of cyanotic heart defects because of the associated physiological thrombocytopenia.

Cardiac changes

Cardiac failure may result from increased workload on ventricles that have been hypertrophied before surgery. Consequently, signs of heart failure are watched for, including elevation of the CVP.

Low cardiac output syndrome and decreased peripheral perfusion can occur from hypothermia or inability of the left ventricle to maintain systemic circulation. The most important signs of adequate peripheral perfusion are rapid capillary refill, good skin colour, warm extremities, and strong pulses. Evidence of low cardiac output is similar to signs of shock.

Low cardiac output states are aggressively treated with intravenous inotropic medications such as dopamine, dobutamine and amninone. If maximum medical therapy is failing, cardiac assist devices such as the intraaortic balloon pump, ECMO or a ventricular assist device may be used in some centres in certain circumstances. These are new therapies with many complications and mixed results and further study is needed before they are widely used in infants and children (Suddaby and O'Brien, 1993).

Arrhythmias can result from electrolyte imbalance, especially hypokalaemia, and surgical intervention to the septum or myocardium. The heart rate and rhythm are carefully monitored by observing the ECG pattern and the child is assessed for signs of decreased cardiac output. Epicardial pacing wires may be inserted during surgery for managing cardiac arrhythmias postoperatively.

Cardiac tamponade is compression of the heart by blood and other effusion (clots) in the pericardial sac, which severely restricts the normal heart movement. A characteristic sign is *paradoxical pulse pressure*, in which the systolic pressure drops during inspiration because accumulated blood compresses the heart, resulting in a drop in cardiac output. Other signs include a rising venous pressure, falling arterial pressure, narrowing pulse pressure, tachycardia, dyspnoea and cyanosis. Treatment consists of prompt pericardiocentesis to remove the blood or fluid. If active haemorrhage and coagulopathy are present, steps are taken to enhance blood clotting.

Pulmonary changes

Areas of atelectasis are common immediately after surgery as a result of deflation of the lung during cardiopulmonary bypass. Other pulmonary complications include pneumothorax; pulmonary oedema from increased pulmonary blood flow or heart failure; and pleural effusion caused by persistent venous congestion. Signs of pneumothorax are persistent decreased breath sounds, sudden dyspnoea, tachycardia, rapid shallow respirations, cyanosis, and sometimes sharp chest pain. Signs of pulmonary oedema are tachypnoea râles, wheezing, tachycardia, cyanosis, and restlessness. Signs and symptoms of pleural effusions include increased respiratory rate, vomiting, decreased breath sounds, fatigue, irritability and decreased oxygen saturations.

Neurological changes

Cerebral oedema and brain damage may occur during open-heart surgery. Although the exact cause is unknown, it is thought to be a result of tissue ischaemia or emboli. The nurse checks the equal quality of strength and reflexes in both extremities for evidence of paralysis; assesses the pupil size, equality, and reaction to light and accommodation; and assesses the child's orientation to the environment. Any evidence of cerebral damage is immediately reported. The nurse also observes for focal or generalized seizure activity, which may be secondary to electrolyte imbalance.

PROVIDE EMOTIONAL SUPPORT

Children may become depressed after surgery. This is thought to be caused by preoperative anxiety, postoperative psychological and physiological stress, and sensory overstimulation. Typically, the child's disposition improves on leaving the intensive care unit.

Children may also be angry and uncooperative after surgery as a response to the physical pain and to the loss of control imposed by the surgery and treatments. They need an opportunity to express feelings, either orally or through activity. The nurse can be supportive by reassuring children that the procedures that require cooperation, such as coughing and deep breathing, are difficult to perform; by praising them for efforts to cooperate. Children also may express feelings of anger or rejection towards parents. The nurse must reassure parents that this is normal and that with continued support the anger will subside.

The nurse can support the parents by being available for information and explaining all the procedures to them. The first few postoperative days are particularly difficult because parents see their child in pain and realize the potential risks from surgery. They often are overwhelmed by the physical environment of the intensive care unit and feel useless because they can do so little for their child. The nurse can minimize such feelings by including parents in caregiving activities if they wish; by providing information about the child's condition; and by being sensitive to their emotional and physical needs. The importance of their presence in making the child feel more secure is stressed, even if they do not provide physical care.

PLAN FOR DISCHARGE AND HOME CARE

Ideally, discharge planning begins on admission for cardiac surgery and includes an assessment of the parents' adjustment to the child's altered state of health. As mentioned earlier, one of the most common parental reactions is overprotection, and the nurse needs to be aware of times when the family may need help in recognizing the child's improved health status.

The family will need verbal as well as written instructions on medication, nutrition, activity restrictions, subacute bacterial endocarditis, return to school, wound care, and signs and symptoms of infection or complications. Referrals to community agencies may be warranted to assist parents in the transition from hospital to home and to reinforce the teaching.

The parents will also need clear instructions about when to seek medical care, such as for a change in the child's behaviour or an unexplained fever. Follow-up with the cardiologist is also arranged before discharge. Appropriate identification, such as a Medic-Alert bracelet, is indicated for children with a pacemaker or a heart transplant and for those receiving anticoagulation therapy or antiarrhythmic medication.

The nurse also discusses common behaviour disturbances that may occur after discharge, such as nightmares, sleep disturbances, separation anxiety, and overdependence. A supportive, consistent response is essential to allow the child to overcome the surgical experience. The child may work out feelings and fears through therapeutic play, and this should be encouraged.

Although surgical correction of heart defects has improved dramatically, it is still not possible to totally reverse many of the complex anomalies. For many children, repeat procedures are required to replace conduits or grafts or to manage complications, such as restenosis. Consequently, the long-term prognosis is uncertain, and full recovery is not always possible. For these families, medical follow-up and continued emotional support are essential. The nurse can often serve as an important primary health professional and as a resource for referrals when needed.

CARDIAC ARRHYTHMIAS

Cardiac arrhythmias, or abnormal heart rhythms, occur less frequently in children than in adults; however, they are not rare and the incidence is rising. This increase may be attributed to two major factors. First, the survival rate of children under-going complex cardiac surgical procedures is higher, and conduction system damage may be a complication. Second, paediatricians are more aware that certain cardiac arrhythmias in otherwise normal children are important.

CLASSIFICATION

Arrhythmias can be classified according to various criteria, such as effect on heart rate and rhythm:
- **Bradyarrhythmias** — abnormally slow rate
- **Tachyarrhythmias** — abnormally rapid rate
- **Conduction disturbances** — irregular heart rate

Bradyarrhythmias
The most common bradyarrhythmia in children is *complete atrioventricular block (A-V block),* also referred to as complete heart block (Fig. 28-14). This can be either congenital or acquired, as seen in postoperative patients following surgery in the area of the A-V valves and ventricular septum.

Sinus bradycardia in children can be due to the influence of the autonomic nervous system, as with hypervagal tone, or in response to hypoxia and hypotension. Once the infant receives adequate oxygenation and any acidosis is eliminated, the heart rate will often return to baseline. Sinus bradycardias are also known to develop after atrial inversion (baffle) procedures (Mustard or Senning).

Not all bradycardias originate in the sinus node. *Junctional* or *nodal rhythms* are common in the postoperative patient. The impulse for these rhythms originates further down the conduction system, in the A-V node. Identification is marked by absence of P waves on the ECG, and often little change occurs in the heart rate or cardiac output. If there is no significant compromise to the patient's cardiac status, no treatment is necessary.

Tachyarrhythmias
Sinus tachycardia secondary to fever, anxiety, pain, anaemia, dehydration, or any other aetiological factor requiring increased cardiac output should be ruled out first before diagnosing an increased heart rate as pathologic. *Supraventricular tachycardia* (SVT) is one of the most common arrhythmias found in children and refers to a rapid regular heart rate of 200-300 beats/minute (Fig. 28-15). The onset of SVT is often sudden, and the duration is variable. Infants and young children with SVT may be unable to communicate the rapid heart rate, and the clinical course can progress to CHF. Important signs in the infant and young child are poor feeding, extreme irritability, and pallor.

Junctional nodal ectopic tachycardia is a tachyarrhythmia that can result in significant compromise in the paediatric patient. Often the ventricular rate will exceed 250 beats/minute. The onset is characterized by a progressive increase in heart rate, and the duration can range from hours to several days.

Conduction disturbances
Most rhythm disturbances are seen postoperatively in the child undergoing cardiac surgery and are of little significance. A-V blocks are most often related to oedema around the conduction system and resolve without treatment. Temporary epicardial wires are placed in most patients at surgery; if a rhythm disturbance occurs, temporary pacing can be employed. Just before discharge, these are removed by pulling slowly and deliberately down on them from the site of insertion.

PROCESS OF DIAGNOSIS

Several advances in the diagnosis of cardiac arrhythmias have greatly improved the understanding and treatment of these conditions in children. The basic diagnostic procedure is the ECG,

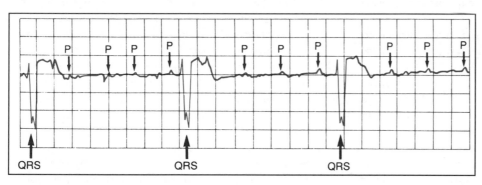

Fig. 28-14 Complete heart block. Note slow rhythm and several P waves not followed by a QRS complex.

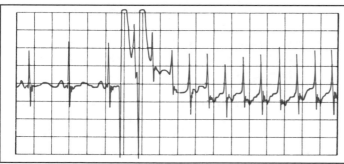

Fig. 28-15 Supraventricular tachycardia (SVT). Note normal sinus rhythm (three PQRST complexes) on the left and the abrupt onset of a very fast rhythm (SVT) on the right.

including 24-hour Holter monitoring. However, more definitive procedures include both noninvasive and invasive techniques.

Electrophysiological cardiac catheterization allows for identification of the conduction disturbance and immediate investigation of drugs that may control the arrhythmia. Patients and families undergoing this procedure are prepared in the same manner as any patient undergoing cardiac catheterization.

THERAPEUTIC MANAGEMENT

Treatment of arrhythmias depends on the cause and severity. Whenever possible, the underlying cause is treated. However, in some cases it is necessary to use antiarrhythmic drugs, with the goal being control, not cure. A permanent pacemaker may be needed in some children. The surgical implantation of a pacemaker is usually a low-risk procedure. Once the wire has been introduced, a small incision is made and a pocket formed under the muscle to house and protect the generator. Continuous ECG monitoring is necessary during the recovery phase to assess pacemaker function.

IMPLICATIONS FOR NURSING

An initial nursing responsibility is recognition of an abnormal heartbeat, either in rate or rhythm. When an arrhythmia is suspected, the apical rate is counted for one full minute and compared with the radial rate. Consistently high or low heart rates should be regarded as suspicious. Accurate nursing assessment, especially in regard to cardiac output, is essential.

The onset and diagnosis of a cardiac arrhythmia are frightening experiences for parents and the older child. Sometimes the arrhythmia rapidly leads to heart failure and an emergency medical crisis. In this situation parents need much support to express their feelings, understand the diagnosis and comply with home therapy, such as daily drug administration. In working with the family, the nurse must not forget the impact of the diagnosis of a heart problem. Often an unspoken fear of potential death exists, even if the arrhythmia is benign, and repeated explanations are needed to allay the anxiety.

A primary focus of nursing care is education of the family about the specific treatment of the arrhythmia. If medication is prescribed, instructions regarding accurate dosage and the importance of administering the correct dose at specified intervals are stressed.

When a pacemaker is implanted, the education of the parents and child includes an explanation of the device, a description of the component parts, the surgical procedure and discharge teaching.

Discharge teaching includes information about the signs and symptoms of infection, general wound care, and any specific limitations to activity. Children with pacemakers should wear a medical alert device, and their parents should have a pacer identification card with specific pacer data in case of an emergency.

In life-threatening arrhythmias, the family needs support and concise information regarding the medical interventions.

KEY POINTS

- Congenital heart disease is the most common form of cardiac disease in children.
- The most common tests used in assessing cardiac function are x-ray, electrocardiography, echocardiography, and cardiac catheterization.
- Cardiac catheterization procedures can be divided into two groups: (1) diagnostic procedures, including angiography, that measure pressures and saturations to establish cardiac diagnosis and (2) interventional procedures, in which catheters or balloon devices are used to correct cardiac defects.
- Several prenatal factors may predispose children to congenital heart disease: maternal rubella during pregnancy, maternal alcoholism, maternal age above 40 years, and maternal insulin-dependent diabetes.
- Congenital heart defects can be divided into four main groups, as determined by haemodynamic patterns: (1) defects that result in increased pulmonary blood flow, (2) obstructive defects, (3) defects that result in decreased pulmonary blood flow, and (4) common mixing.

- Nursing measures in the care of a child with CHF are to assist in improving cardiac function, decrease cardiac demands, reduce respiratory distress, maintain nutritional status, promote fluid loss and provide family support.
- Clinical manifestations of hypoxaemia are cyanosis, polycythaemia, clubbing, and delayed growth and development. The child is at increased risk of hypercyanotic spells, cerebrovascular accidents, brain abscess and bacterial endocarditis.
- Providing postoperative care includes observing vital signs and arterial/venous pressures, maintaining respiratory status, allowing maximum rest, providing comfort, monitoring fluids, planning for progressive activities, giving emotional support, observing for complications of surgery, and planning for discharge and home care.
- Clinical manifestations of CHF are impaired myocardial function (tachyardia, cardiomegaly), pulmonary congestion (dyspnoea, tachypnoea, orthopnoea, cyanosis), and systemic congestion (hepatosplenomegaly, oedema, distended veins).
- Common arrhythmias in children include slow rhythms (bradycardias, heart block) and fast rhythms (sinus tachycardia, supraventricular tachycardia).

REFERENCES

Anand KJS, Hickey PR: Halothane-morphine compared with high-dose sufentanil for anesthesia and postoperative analgesia in neonatal cardiac surgery, *N Eng J Med* 326:1, 1992.

Castaneda AR: Correction of transposition: arterial switch procedure. In Grillo H, editor: *Current therapy in cardiothoracic surgery,* Toronto, 1989, BC Decker.

Gersony WM: Patent ductus arteriosus in the neonate, *Pediatr Clin North Am* 33(3):545, 1986.

Hazinski MF: *Nursing care of the critically ill child,* ed 2, St Louis, 1992, Mosby–Year Book.

Hellenbrand WE *et al:* Balloon angioplasty for aortic recoarchtation: results of valvuloplasty and angioplasty, *Am J Cardiol* 65:793, 1990.

Hoffman JI: Congential heart disease: incidence and inheritance, *Pediatr Clin N Am* 37(1):31, 1990.

Jonas RA, Lang P: Open repair of cardiac defects in neonates and young infants, *Clin Perinatol* 15(3):659, 1988.

Maguire DP, Maloney P: A comparison of fentanyl and morphine use in neonates, *Neonatal Network* 7(1):27, 1988.

Moller JH, Neal WA, editors: *Fetal, neonatal, and infant cardiac disease,* Norwalk, CT, 1990, Appleton & Lange.

Nadas AS: Hypoxemia. In Fyler DC, editor: *Nadas' pediatric cardiology,* Philadelphia, 1992, Hanley & Belfus.

Neuberger JW *et al:* Cognitive function and age at repair of transposition of greater arteries in children, *N Eng J Med* 310:1495, 1984.

Newburger JW: Management of dyslipidemia in childhood and adolescence. In Fyler DC, editor: *Nadas' pediatric cardiology,* Philadelphia, 1992a, Hanley & Belfus.

Radtke W, Lock JE: Balloon dilation, *Pediatr Clin North Am* 37(1):193, 1990.

Roberts PJ: Caring for patients undergoing therapeutic cardiac catheterization, *Crit Care Nurs Clin North Am* 1(2):275, 1989.

Rosen KR, Rosen DA: Caudal epidural morphine for control of pain following open heart surgery in children, *Anesthesiology* 70(3):418, 1989.

Rosenthal A, Dick M: Tricuspid atresia. In Adams FH et al, editors: *Moss' heart disease in infants, children and adolescents,* ed 4, Baltimore, 1989, Williams & Wilkins.

Wessel DL: Hemodynamic responses to perioperative pain and stress in infants, *Crit Care Med* 21(9, suppl):S361, 1993.

FURTHER READING

Diagnostic Procedures

Elixson EM: Hemodynamic monitoring modalities in pediatric cardiac surgical patients, *Crit Care Nurs Clin North Am* 1(2):263, 1989.

Congestive Heart Failure

Dahlmann AR: Captopril, *Neonatal Network* 7(5):41, 1989.

Faxon DP: ACE inhibition for the failing heart: experience, *Am Heart J* 115(5):1085, 1988.

Friedman WF, George BL: Treatment of congestive heart failure by altering loading conditions of the heart, *J Pediatr* 106(5):697, 1985.

Zalzstein E *et al:* Once-daily versus twice-daily dosing of digoxin in the pediatric age group, *J Pediatr* 116(1):137, 1990.

Congenital Heart Disease

Benson DW: Changing profile of congenital heart disease, *Pediatr* 83(5):790, 1989.

Castaneda AR *et al:* Transposition of the great arteries: the arterial switch operation, *Cardiol Clin* 7(2):369, 1989.

Elixson EM, editor: Cardiovascular surgery update: pediatrics, *Crit Care Q* 9(2):entire issue, 1986.

Hellenbrand WE, Mullins CE: Catheter closure of congenital cardiac defects, *Cardiol Clin* 7(2):351, 1989.

Salzer HR *et al:* Growth and nutritional intake of infants with congenital heart disease, *Pediatr Cardiol* 10(1):17, 1989.

Nursing Care

Carroll P: Technical update brief: the child with a chest tube, *Pediatr Nurs* 19(4), 1993.

Foldy SM, Gorman JB: Perioperative nursing care for congenital cardiac defects, *Crit Care Nurs Clin North Am* 1(2):289, 1989.

Hultgren MS: Pulmonary management of children after cardiac surgery, *Crit Care Nurs* 11(1).55, 1991

O'Brien P, Boisvert JT: Discharge planning for children with heart disease, *Crit Care Nurs Clin North Am* 1(2):297, 1989.

Cardiac Dysrhythmias

Alpern D, Uzark K, Dick M: Psychosocial responses of children to cardiac pacemakers, *J Pediatr* 114(3):494, 1989.

Case CL, Trippel DL, Gillette PC: New antiarrhythmic agents in pediatrics, *Pediatr Clin North Am* 36(5):1293, 1989.

Gillette PC *et al:* Dysrhythmias. In Adams FH, Emmanouilides GC, Riemenschneider TA, editors: *Moss' heart disease in infants, children, and adolescents,* ed 4, Baltimore, 1989, Williams & Wilkins.

Higgins SS, Hardy CE, Higashino SM: Should parents of children with congenital heart disease and life-threatening dysrhythmias be taught cardiopulmonary resuscitation? (letter), *Pediatr* 84(6):1102, 1989.

Chapter 29

The Child with Haematological or Immunological Dysfunction

LEARNING OUTCOMES

After studying this chapter you should be able to:

◆ Discuss the components of blood and their varying functions.
◆ Identify common disorders in relation to blood and its functions.
◆ Identify basic nursing considerations which may arise secondary to blood disorders.
◆ Identify further sources of information for yourself and patients regarding various identified blood disorders.
◆ Define the glossary terms.

GLOSSARY

anaemia Reduction of red blood cells or haemoglobin concentration below normal

antigen Substance the body recognizes as foreign that triggers the manufacture of specific antibodies

B-lymphocyte Type of lymphocyte that produces antibodies

basophil Granular leucocyte

coagulation Process of clotting

eosinophil Granular leucocyte

erythrocyte Red blood cell

erythropoiesis Process of red blood cell manufacture

haemoglobin (Hb) Oxygen-carrying, iron-containing pigment in red blood cells

haemolysis The destruction of red blood cells

haemostasis Process whereby bleeding from an injured vessel is stopped

leucocyte General term for the group of cells in the body active in the immune process

lymphocyte One of the major groups of white blood cells

neutrophil Granulocyte that phagocytizes bacteria

phagocytosis Process of ingesting and digesting foreign proteins

plasma Liquid portion of blood

platelet Cellular fragment involved in coagulation

reticulocyte Immature red blood cell

T-lymphocyte Type of lymphocyte active in cellular immunity

thrombocyte Platelet

Disorders related to the blood and/or blood-forming organs in childhood encompass a wide range of diseases and pathological states. Since blood is a multipurpose fluid involved in the functions of so many tissues and organs, either primary or secondary changes in the blood are reflected in the essential functions of these structures.

THE HAEMATOLOGICAL SYSTEM AND ITS FUNCTION

The haematological system, composed of blood and blood-forming tissues, is responsible for a complex system of homeostatic mechanisms. This system produces cells with specific functions, provides for oxygenation and distribution of nutrients and other chemicals to the cells, collects wastes from the cells, and provides immune protection, clotting, and heat regulation.

ORIGIN OF FORMED ELEMENTS

Blood has two major components: a fluid portion called *plasma* and a cellular portion. Plasma is about 90% water and 10% solutes. The principal solutes are albumin, electrolytes and proteins. Among the proteins are clotting factors, globulins, circulating antibodies and fibrinogen. The cellular elements are red blood cells (RBCs, *erythrocytes*), white blood cells (WBCs, *leucocytes*) and platelets *(thrombocytes)*.

The major blood-forming (haemopoietic) organ of the body is the red bone marrow. The lymphatic system plays an important role in regulating blood cells. Lymph nodes regulate the manufacture of WBCs, and the spleen and liver are prime organs for haematopoiesis in the young fetus and cell removal in postnatal life. In the lining of the vascular and lymph channels are cells called macrophages which are capable of phagocytosis (ingestion and digestion of foreign substances), formation of immune bodies, and differentiation into other cells, such as haemocytoblasts, myeloblasts or lymphoblasts.

In infants and young children, all of the bone contains red marrow (so called because of its colour from formation of erythrocytes); however, as bone growth ceases near the end of adolescence, only the ribs, sternum, vertebrae and pelvis continue to produce blood cells. The remainder of the bone marrow becomes yellow from deposition of fat. See Fig. 29-1 for a schematic representation of the development of blood cells.

ERYTHROCYTES

Erythrocytes (red blood cells [RBCs]) are formed from the haemocytoblast in the red bone marrow. As it matures, the RBC loses its nucleus and the cell caves in on both sides, giving the mature *erythrocyte* its characteristic appearance as a biconcave disk. Since the mature RBC does not have a nucleus, it is unable to multiply.

The *reticulocyte* is the last stage of development before the mature erythrocyte. Reticulocytes are slightly larger than erythrocytes, and are used as indicators of active erythropoiesis.

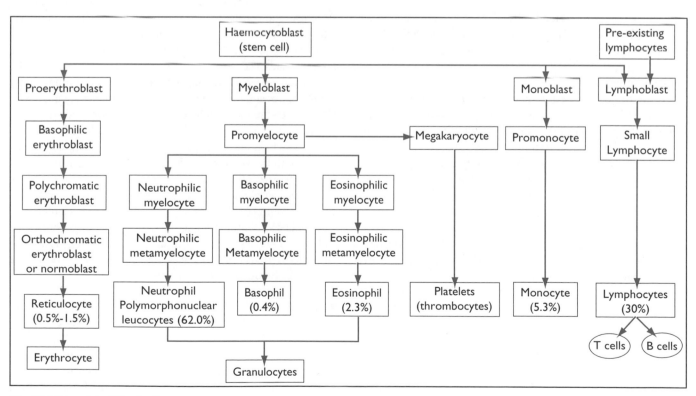

Fig. 29-1 Formation of blood cells.

The usual lifespan of the mature erythrocyte is 120 days. As RBCs grow old, their membranes become fragile and eventually rupture. The contents of the cell are phagocytized by the macrophages in the spleen, liver and bone marrow. The haemoglobin is broken down into the iron-containing pigment haemosiderin and the bile pigments biliverdin and bilirubin. Most of the iron is reused for production of new RBCs or stored in the liver. The bile pigments are excreted by the liver in bile.

Normally, there is a homeostatic balance between the regulation of RBC production and destruction. In states of tissue hypoxia, *erythropoietin* is released by the kidneys into the bloodstream. As a result, the bone marrow is stimulated to produce new RBCs.

Once tissue oxygenation is adequate, the production of erythropoietin ceases. Thus, tissue oxygen requirements control both the stimulation and termination of erythrocyte production. It is important to note that it is the ability of RBCs to transport oxygen to the tissues in response to the needs of the tissues, not the circulating numbers of erythrocytes, that is the basic regulatory mechanism.

The major function of RBCs is to transport haemoglobin (Hb), which in turn carries oxygen to all cells of the body. RBCs' other functions are involved in the transport of waste CO_2 and in the maintenance of blood pH.

The type of Hb in the cells depends on the stage of life. Fetal Hb has a greater affinity for oxygen and is best suited to the fetal environment. During the latter part of pregnancy, the fetus begins developing adult Hb.

LEUCOCYTES

The leucocytes (white blood cells [WBCs]) refer to a number of cells with similar, yet distinct, functions. They are divided into two major classifications — granulocytes and agranulocytes.

Granulocytes

There are three types of granulocytes: *neutrophils, basophils* and *eosinophils*. The name of each of these refers to the characteristic staining property of the granule during laboratory analysis.

The granulocytes, like erythrocytes, are produced in the bone marrow, where they originate from primitive stem cells, which develop into myeloblasts. The differentiation of myeloblasts into various mature WBCs is primarily the result of specialization within the cytoplasm and degeneration of the nucleus. Unlike the erythrocyte, however, all of the WBCs are nucleated.

The agranulocytes comprise two cell types: the *monocytes* and *lymphocytes*. Characteristically, these cells do not develop granules.

The monocytes follow the same sequence of development from the stem cell as the granulocytes (Fig. 29-1). The monocytes, in turn, have the ability to exit the vessels and develop into *macrophages*.

Lymphocytes develop from blast (stem) cells (see Fig. 29-1). The lymphocyte has the potential to develop into T-cells or B-cells.

The exact lifespan of the leucocytes is not as clearly defined as that of the erythrocytes, because their existence in the circulation is primarily for transportation to extravascular areas, where they reside in reservoirs or where they are needed to resist infection.

Granulocytes have a half-life of 6-8 hours in the blood and, after entering the tissues, die over 4-5 days. Agranulocytes live for an extended period, because they remain in inflamed tissue areas longer than the granulocytes.

The regulation of leucocytes is based on the body's need for them. Tissue damage from bacterial or viral agents promotes leucocyte circulation and production.

The leucocytes die as a result of their activity at the site of injury and are phagocytized by other newly formed WBCs. Effective control of the inflammatory process results in a feedback mechanism to the bone marrow and causes lymphogenous organs to cease increased production of WBCs.

Each of the WBCs plays a specific role in the immune process. Neutrophils and monocytes are effective phagocytes and as a result are primarily involved in inflammatory reactions. The functions of lymphocytes in the immune system are discussed on p. 681.

Eosinophils seem to have parasitic properties, and may also function in the immediate type of allergic or anaphylactic hypersensitivity reactions.

Increased numbers of basophils occur during the healing phase of inflammation and during prolonged inflammation.

THROMBOCYTES

Thrombocytes (platelets) are actually small fragments of cells. They are smaller than blood cells, do not possess a cellular structure, and consist of a clear substance containing granules. The origin of platelets is the megakaryocyte.

The lifespan of platelets has been estimated as 8-10 days. The body regulates platelets to maintain a fairly constant level. Platelet production is probably regulated by a hormone, thrombopoietin, but the source and mode of action of this substance are unknown. Old platelets are most likely removed by the liver and spleen.

When there is a break in the continuity of a blood vessel, the platelets, which are normally round or oval disks, come into contact with the wet vessel surface and adhere to the endothelium and to each other. The initial platelets at the site of injury release substances that attract other thrombocytes to the area. This causes a layering of platelets, which eventually forms a plug.

Platelets also influence haemostasis by releasing a substance called *serotonin* at the site of injury. This substance is a vasoconstrictor that produces vascular spasm to decrease the amount of blood flow to the injured area.

ASSESSMENT OF HAEMATOLOGICAL FUNCTION

Several tests can be performed to assess haematological function, including additional procedures to identify the cause of the dysfunction. The full blood count (FBC) is the most common and one of the most valuable tests. Other procedures, such as those related to iron, coagulation and immune status, are discussed throughout the chapter as appropriate.

The FBC is summarized in Table 29-1. The nurse should be familiar with the significance of the findings from the FBC and aware of normal values for age.

RED BLOOD CELL DISORDERS

The most common disorders affecting the blood are those that in some way alter the function or production of RBCs. The

TEST (RANGE)	DESCRIPTION	COMMENTS
Red blood cell (RBC) count (4.0 - 5.2 x 10^{12}/l)	Number of RBCs per mm^3 of blood	Usually reflects level of anaemia
Haemoglobin (Hb) (11.5 - 15.5 g/dl)	Amount of haemoglobin in whole blood	Total Hb dependent on the red cell count and quantity of Hb in each cell
Haematocrit (Hct) (0.35 - 0.45)	Volume of packed RBCs as ratio of whole blood	Indirect measurement of Hb and RBC
Red cell indices a) mean corpuscular volume (MCV 71-95 fl)	Average size of red cells	Good indicator of average red cell size, e.g. microcytic or macrocytic
b) mean corpuscular haemoglobin (MCH 25-33 pg)	Mean weight of Hb in red cells	
c) mean corpuscular haemoglobin concentration (MCHC 31-37 g/dl)	Mean concentration of Hb in red cells	
Reticulocyte count (0.5 - 2%)	Percentage of circulating RBCs which are reticulocytes	Index of bone marrow production of red cells
White blood count (WBC) (4.5 - 13.5 x 10^9/l)	Number of WBCs in the blood	Although total WBC is important; the differential count may be more informative
Differential WBC count in blood	Quantification of WBC subtypes	Values expressed as percentages or absolute values (i.e. percentage x total WBC)
(i) Neutrophils (polymorphs) (30% - 70%; 1.5 - 8.0 x 10^9/l)		Frequently increased in bacterial infections
(ii) Lymphocytes (25% - 70%; 1.5 - 8.0 x 10^9/l)		Involved in immunity and antibody production
(iii) Monocytes (3% - 10%; 0.4 x 10^9/l)		Involved in antigen recognition and inflammatory response
(iv) Eosinophils (2% - 8%; 0.2 x 10^9/l)		Increased in allergic disorders, parasitic infections etc.
(v) Basophils (1% - 3%; 0.1 x 10^9/l)		Histamine release reactions
Platelet count (150 - 400 x 10^9/l)		Cellular fragments in the blood connected with blood clotting
Peripheral blood film	Visualization of the peripheral blood cells for size, shape, morphology	Staining properties of red and white cells in the blood aiding diagnosis of disease

Note: Many haematological parametes are age-dependent. For example, Hb level is highest in the newborn and falls by the age of 2, to rise again until the onset of puberty. Young children tend to have a higher percentage of blood lymphocytes than do adults.

Table 29-1 Tests performed as part of the full blood count (FBC).

following presents an overview of anaemia in general and specific disorders in children that produce an anaemic state.

ANAEMIA

Anaemia is defined as reduction of red cell volume or haemoglobin concentration to levels below normal. It is not a disease itself, but a manifestation of an underlying pathological process. Anaemias are the most common haematological disorders of infancy and childhood.

CLASSIFICATION

Anaemias can be classified using two basic approaches: (1) aetiology or physiology, the causes of erythrocyte and haemoglobin depletion or (2) morphology, the characteristic changes in red cell size, shape and colour. The aetiological approach is more relevant to nurses, because it helps direct the planning of nursing care.

Aetiology

The basic causes of anaemia are: (1) excessive blood loss, (2) increased destruction of RBCs or (3) impaired or decreased rate of production. Each of these causes affects the amount of haemoglobin available to carry oxygen to the cells.

Blood loss

Acute or chronic haemorrhage results in loss of plasma and all formed elements of the blood. After acute haemorrhage, the body replaces plasma within 1-3 days, maintaining blood volume. However, this results in a low concentration of RBCs, which are gradually replaced within 3-4 weeks.

In chronic blood loss, the actual number of RBCs may be normal because of continual replacement. However, insufficient iron is available to form haemoglobin as quickly as it is lost.

Excessive destruction

Excessive destruction or haemolysis of erythrocytes can occur from a variety of causes. One of the most common is a result of a defect within the RBC that shortens the lifespan of the cell so that production cannot keep pace with destruction.

Some conditions cause haemolysis in otherwise normal RBCs. A classic example is blood group incompatibility, such as haemolytic disease of the newborn or consequent to mismatched blood transfusion. Other causes can be toxic drugs, burns, poisonings (such as from lead), and infections such as malaria and splenic sequestration (hypersplenism).

Impaired or decreased production

Decreased production of RBCs can result from either bone marrow failure or deficiency of essential dietary nutrients. Bone marrow failure may be caused by: (1) replacement of bone marrow by fibrosis or by neoplastic cells, such as in leukaemia, (2) depression of marrow activity from irradiation, chemicals or drugs, or (3) interference with bone marrow activity from other systemic diseases, such as severe infection, or chronic renal disease.

Pernicious anaemia develops when the gastric mucosa fails to secrete sufficient amounts of intrinsic factor, which is essential for absorption of vitamin B_{12}. Deprived of vitamin B_{12}, the bone marrow produces fewer but larger (macrocytic) RBCs. These are usually immature and are more rapidly destroyed during circulation. This condition is uncommon in children

The basic physiological defect caused by anaemia is a decrease in the oxygen-carrying capacity of blood and, consequently, a reduction in the amount of oxygen available to the tissues. When anaemia develops slowly, the child may adapt to the declining haemoglobin level.

When the haemoglobin decreases sufficiently to produce clinical manifestations, the signs and symptoms are directly attributable to tissue hypoxia. Muscle weakness, tiredness or pallor are common, but cyanosis is typically not evident.

Central nervous system manifestations include headache, dizziness, irritability, decreased attention span, apathy and depression. Growth retardation, resulting from decreased cellular metabolism and coexisting anorexia, is a common finding in chronic severe anaemia and is frequently accompanied by delayed sexual maturation in older children.

The effects of persistent anaemia on the circulatory system can be profound. Decreased oxygen-carrying capacity of the blood is associated with a compensatory increase in heart rate and cardiac output, and can lead, in severe cases, to cardiac failure precipitated by physical or emotional stress.

PROCESS OF DIAGNOSIS

Diagnosis depends largely on the cause of the anaemia. In general, anaemia may be suspected from findings on the history and physical examination, such as lack of energy, easy fatigability, and pallor, but unless the anaemia is severe, the first clue to the disorder may be alterations in the FBC, such as decreased RBCs, haemoglobin and haematocrit levels.

Various findings on the FBC are also significant, such as increased reticulocytes, which indicate the body's increased demand for RBCs, or changes in the shape of RBCs, such as sickled cells. Rarely, a bone marrow aspiration may be necessary to evaluate the body's ability to produce normal cells, such as in leukaemia and aplastic anaemia.

THERAPEUTIC MANAGEMENT

The objective of medical management is to reverse the anaemia by treating the underlying cause. For example, in nutritional anaemias the specific deficiency is replaced. In instances of severe anaemia, supportive medical care may include oxygen therapy, transfusion of packed red cells, intravenous fluids and rest. In addition to these general measures, more specific interventions may be implemented depending upon the cause.

IMPLICATIONS FOR NURSING

Since anaemia is not a disorder but a symptom of some underlying problem, nursing care is related to determining the cause, fostering appropriate supportive and therapeutic treatments, and decreasing tissue oxygen requirements.

Assessment of the child's physical condition yields valuable evidence regarding the severity of the anaemia, but diagnosis primarily rests on haematological blood studies and a careful history. In interviewing the child and parents, the nurse explores the following areas regarding common causes of childhood anaemia: (1) nutrition, especially dietary intake of iron, (2) past history of chronic, recurrent infection, (3) bowel habits and presence of frank blood in stools (black, tarry stools) and (4) familial history of hereditary diseases, such as sickle cell disease or thalassaemia.

The nursing care of an infant or child with anaemia may involve several approaches. One of the most important is patient education about the process of diagnosis, and nutritional therapy if indicated. Other nursing responsibilities include administration of medications, as well as blood or blood products.

Several blood tests may be needed. If possible, these should be done from one sample to avoid the trauma of repeated venepunctures. The nurse is responsible for preparing the child and family for the tests by: (1) explaining the significance of each test, (2) staying with the child and family during the procedure, and (3) allowing the child to play with the equipment on a doll and/or to participate in the actual procedure; for example, by cleansing the finger with an alcohol swab. The child and family will benefit from the expertise of a play specialist in preparation for any painful procedure. Older children may appreciate the opportunity to observe the blood cells under a microscope or in photographs.

The child's level of tolerance for age-appropriate activities of play is assessed, and adjustments are made to allow as much self-care as possible, without undue exertion. The nurse should observe the child at rest and when active, noting the presence and degree of signs of exertion (e.g., tachycardia, palpitations, tachypnoea, dyspnoea, dizziness, light-headedness and obvious fatigue).

Once a baseline of physical tolerance has been established, the nurse assists the child and family with activities that are physically taxing, such as dressing, feeding or getting out of bed. Scheduling activities throughout the day, with planned rest periods in between, maximizes the child's energy potential without causing undue exertion.

Diversional activities that promote rest, but prevent boredom and withdrawal, are essential. Short attention span, irritability and restlessness are common in anaemia. Therefore, appropriate activities are needed, such as listening to music, watching television, or reading or listening to stories or comics.

Crying and fretfulness increase oxygen needs. Parental/familial presence and involvement in care can help minimize the emotional stress of hospitalization and separation.

Children with anaemia are prone to infection. Infection worsens the anaemia by increasing metabolic needs and, in instances of chronic infection, interferes with erythropoiesis and reduces the survival time of RBCs. Precautions are therefore taken to prevent infection.

Multiple blood samples may present a problem with cumulative blood loss for infants or young children who have severe anaemia. A record should be kept of the volume of blood taken and the nurse should observe for cumulative effects of blood loss, particularly signs of shock and increased hypoxia, which may indicate the need for transfusion.

The main complication of anaemia is cardiac failure, resulting from excessive demands on the heart as a result of increased metabolic needs or of cardiac overload during rapid blood transfusion. Signs and symptoms of heart failure are tachycardia, dyspnoea, moist respirations, cough, shortness of breath and sweating. Packed RBCs are usually administered to prevent circulatory hypervolaemia. When blood transfusions are required in severe anaemia to increase the haemoglobin level, all the precautions for administering blood and observing for signs of transfusion reactions are instituted (Table 29-2).

Oxygen may be administered to provide optimum environmental conditions for haemoglobin saturation. However, oxygen is of limited value because each gram of haemoglobin is able to carry a limited amount of the gas. In addition, prolonged oxygen therapy can decrease erythropoiesis. Therefore, the child is monitored closely for evidence of decreasing benefit from oxygen. One of the first signs of hypoxia is restlessness.

Any blood transfusion carries attendant risks. If the child requires multiple transfusions, the possibility of complications increases. It is critical for the nurse always to be observant for signs indicative of a reaction. Table 29-2 summarizes the major hazards of transfusions, the presenting features commonly associated with each, and nursing responsibilities.

Although haemolytic reactions are rare, ABO incompatibility remains the most common cause of death from blood transfusion. Blood is matched between the donor and recipient for blood groups (A, B, AB or O) and Rh factors (positive or negative).

Besides the nursing precautions and responsibilities outlined in Table 29-2, general guidelines that apply to all transfusions include:

1. Check the identification of the recipient with the donor's blood group and type, regardless of the blood product used.
2. Take vital signs and blood pressure *before* administering blood, to establish baseline data for post-transfusion comparison, then every 15 minutes for one hour while blood is infusing, or according to local policy.
3. Ensure blood products are administered at the prescribed rate.
4. Administer blood through an appropriate filter to eliminate particles in the blood and to prevent the precipitation of formed elements.
5. Start administration of blood within 30 minutes of its arrival from the blood bank; if it is not used, return to blood bank — do not store in the regular unit refrigerator.
6. Infuse a unit of blood (or a specified amount) within 4 hours. If the infusion will exceed this time, the blood should be divded into appropriate-sized quantities by the blood bank, with the unused portion refrigerated under controlled conditions.

COMPLICATION	PRESENTING FEATURES	NURSING INTERVENTION
Immediate reactions		
Haemolytic reactions		
Most severe type, but rare	Chills	Identify donor and recipeint blood types and
Incompatible blood	Shaking	groups before transfusion is begun
Intradonor incompatibility	Fever	
in multiple transfusions	Pain at needle site and along venous tract	Transfuse blood at the prescribed rate; remain with patient
	Nausea/vomiting	Stop transfusion immediately in event of
	Sensation of tightness in chest	signs or symptoms, and notify doctor
	Red or black urine	Save donor blood to re-crossmatch with
	Headache	patient's blood
	Flank pain	Monitor for evidence of shock
	Progressive signs of shock and/or renal failure	Assist in insertion of urinary catheter and monitor hourly outputs. Send sample of patient's blood and urine to laboratory for presence of haemoglobin (indicates intravascular haemolysis)
		Observe for signs of haemorrhage resulting from disseminated intravascular coagulation (DIC)
		Supportive medical therapies to reverse shock
Febrile reactions		
Leukocyte or platelet antibodies	Fever	Leucocyte-poor RBCs are less likely to cause
Plasma protein antibodies	Chills	reaction
		Stop transfusion immediately; report to doctor for evaluation.
Allergic reactions		
Recipient reacts to allergens in	Urticaria	Give antihistamines as prescribed or as prophylaxis
donor's blood	Flushing	to children with tendency towards allergic
	Asthmatic wheezing	reactions
	Laryngeal oedema	Stop transfusions immediately seek urgent medical assistance
		Adrenaline/steroid therapy may be instituted to counteract allergic reactions
Circulatory overload		
Too rapid transfusion (even a	Precordial pain	Transfuse blood at prescribed rate
small quantity)	Dyspnoea	Prevent overload by using packed RBCs or
Excessive quantity of blood	Râles	administering divided amounts of blood
transfused (even slowly)	Cyanosis	Use infusion pump to regulate and maintain
Dry cough	flow rate	
	Distended neck veins	Stop transfusion immediately if signs of overload
		Place child upright with feet in dependent position to increase venous resistance

(cont.)

COMPLICATION	PRESENTING FEATURES	NURSING INTERVENTION

Table 29.2 Nursing care of the child receiving blood transfusions.

COMPLICATION	PRESENTING FEATURES	NURSING INTERVENTION
Air emboli May occur when blood is transfused under pressure	Sudden difficulty in breathing Sharp pain in chest Apprehension	Observe for air infiltration to administration system Clear tubing of air by aspirating air with syringe at the nearest IV port
Hypothermia	Chills Low temperature Irregular heart rate Possible cardiac arrest	Allow blood to warm at room temperature (less than 1 hour) Use an electric warming coil to rapidly warm blood Take temperature if patient complains of chills; if subnormal, stop transfusion
Electrolyte disturbances Hyperkalaemia (in massive transfusions or in patients with renal problems)	Nausea, diarrhoea Muscular weakness Flaccid paralysis Paraesthesia of extremities Bradycardia Apprehension Cardiac arrest	Use washed RBCs or fresh blood if patient at risk Report features to medical staff
Delayed reactions **Transmission of infection** Hepatitis AIDS Malaria Syphilis Bacteria or viruses Other	Signs of infection, e.g., jaundice Toxic reaction: high fever, severe headache or substernal pain, hypotension, intense flushing, vomiting/diarrhoea	Blood is tested for antibodies to HIV, HTLVI, hepatitis C virus, hepatitis B core antigen. In In addition, blood is tested for hepatitis B surface antigen (HBsAg), alanine aminotransferase (ALT), and a serology test is performed for syphilis. Positive units are destroyed. Individuals at risk for carrying certain viruses are deferred from donation. Heat treating of some blood products to destroy HIV also occurs. Report any sign of infection, and, if occurring during transfusion, stop transfusion immediately, and notify doctor
Alloimmunization (Antibody formation) Occurs in patients receiving multiple transfusions	Increased risk of haemolytic, febrile, and allergic reactions	Use limited number of donors Observe carefully for signs of reactions
Delayed haemolytic reaction	Destruction of RBCs and fever 5–10 days after transfusion	Observe for post-transfusion anaemia and decreasing benefit from successive transfusions.

Table 29.2 Nursing care of the child receiving blood transfusions (continued).

7. If a reaction of any type is suspected, stop the transfusion, maintain a patent inravenous line with normal saline and new tubing. Notify the doctor, and do not restart the blood until the child's condition has been medically evaluated.

IRON DEFICIENCY ANAEMIA

Anaemia caused by an inadequate supply of dietary iron is a common nutritional disorder. Factors associated with the development of iron deficiency anaemia include prematurity, low birth weight, late weaning, socioeconomic deprivation, ethnic minority status and food refusal (James and Laing, 1994).

The following discussion is limited to iron deficiency anaemia resulting from inadequate iron in the diet.

At birth, the full-term infant's supply of iron is stored in the circulating haemoglobin of the erythrocytes; the rest is deposited in the liver, spleen and bone marrow. The majority of iron has been transferred from the mother during the last trimester. Maternal iron stores are adequate for the first 5-6 months of life. When dietary intake of iron is not sufficient to meet the infant's growth demands following depletion of fetal iron stores, iron deficiency anaemia results.

The main effect of iron deficiency is decreased haemoglobin and reduced oxygen-carrying capacity of the blood.

CLINICAL MANIFESTATIONS

Clinical manifestations are directly attributed to the reduced amount of oxygen available to tissues, and severity is directly related to the duration of the deficiency.

Although the majority of infants with iron deficiency anaemia are underweight, many are overweight because of excessive milk ingestion. Milk, a poor source of iron, is sometimes given almost to the exclusion of solid foods. Some infants who are fed cow's milk have an increased faecal loss of blood due to milk intolerance. Although chubby, these infants are pale, usually demonstrate poor muscle development, and are prone to infection.

Increasing evidence suggests that long-term iron deficiency, alone or with anaemia, results in impaired cognitive skills, but that this may be reversed with treatment (Jojraninata and Pollitt, 1993).

PROCESS OF DIAGNOSIS

Since iron deficiency primarily affects haemoglobin synthesis, laboratory tests are performed to measure haemoglobin, the morphologic changes in the RBC, and amount of circulating iron (serum ferritin). A stool analysis for occult blood is sometimes performed to rule out chronic faecal blood loss from milk intolerance or structural anomalies such as diverticulitis.

THERAPEUTIC MANAGEMENT

Prevention is the primary goal and is achieved through optimum nutrition and appropriate iron supplementation. The recommendations for feeding include iron supplementation primarily through food sources, except for preterm breastfed infants, whose iron needs may exceed those supplied through human milk. In formula-fed infants, the most convenient and best sources of supplemental iron are iron-fortified milk formula and iron-fortified infant cereal (Walter *et al*, 1993).

After infancy, prevention is accomplished through sound nutritional practices. Unfortunately, this becomes increasingly difficult to ensure during adolescence, when the growth rate is increased and eating patterns are often less than ideal.

Iron deficiency anaemia is usually treated with oral iron supplements. Dietary addition of iron-rich foods is usually inadequate to provide sufficient supplemental quantities of iron. Ideally, the daily dose of iron should be given in two or three divided doses between meals.

Transfusions of placebo red cells are indicated for the severest degree of anaemia, in cases of serious infection, cardiac dysfunction or surgical emergency when anaesthesia is required.

IMPLICATIONS FOR NURSING

The main nursing objective is prevention of nutritional anaemia through parent education. One of the difficulties in terms of infant feeding is encouraging parents to limit the quantity of milk and to introduce solid foods, when they believe milk is best for the infant and equate the resultant weight gain with a 'healthy child'. Although milk is an excellent food, it is deficient in iron, vitamin C, zinc and fluoride. The nurse should emphasize that being overweight is not synonymous with good health.

Educating the child and parents regarding proper administration of oral iron supplements is essential. Several factors affect the absorption of iron, such as stomach acidity. Ideally, iron supplements are administered in two divided doses between meals and are accompanied with a citrus fruit or juice, which helps reduce iron to its most soluble state. Advise parents of expected change in colour of stools (tarry green colour). Place liquid preparations towards the back of the mouth because they will stain teeth temporarily.

Oral iron supplements are available in liquid or tablet form. Because iron ingested in excessive quantities is toxic, even fatal, parents should store it safely away from the reach of children, as with any medication.

Education and support for families whose children are anaemic is often challenging. Meal planning must be based on their budget, family eating pattern, and the child's food preferences. Often, this requires more than a brief discussion about foods high in iron (e.g., meat, fish, egg yolks, green leafy vegetables, legumes, wholegrains, fortified cereals). For teaching to be effective, the nurse may need to offer recipes, assist in planning a shopping list, and investigate food prices for economy. Referral to a paediatric dietitian, where possible, will greatly enhance patient/family education.

SICKLE CELL DISEASE

Sickle cell disease is part of a group of diseases called *haemoglobinopathies*. In these diseases, the normal adult haemoglobin (haemoglobin A or HbA) is partly or completely replaced by a haemoglobin variant, including fetal haemoglobin (HbF). Sickle cell disease includes all the hereditary disorders in which the clinical, haematological, and pathological features are related to the presence of sickle haemoglobin (HbS).

Sickle cell disease is found primarily in the black race, although infrequently it affects people of Mediterranean descent.

MODE OF TRANSMISSION

Sickle cell disease is an autosomal disorder. The expected pattern of transmission from two parents who carry the heterozygous gene HbSA is illustrated in Fig. 12-2.

BASIC DEFECT

The basic defect responsible for the sickling effect of erythrocytes is in the globin fraction of haemoglobin. Haemoglobin S differs from haemoglobin A in the substitution of only one amino acid for another. Under conditions of decreased oxygen tension and lowered pH, the relatively insoluble haemoglobin S changes its molecular structure to form long, slender crystals. The rapid growth of these filamentous crystals causes the formation of crescent- or sickle-shaped red blood cells.

The tendency to sickle is also related to the concentration of haemoglobin within the cell. Since hypertonicity of the blood plasma increases the intracellular concentration of haemoglobin, dehydration promotes sickling. In most instances, the sickling response is reversible under conditions of adequate oxygenation and hydration.

Although the defect is inherited at the time of conception, the sickling phenomenon is usually not apparent until later in infancy because of the presence of fetal haemoglobin (HbF). As long as HbF persists, sickling does not occur. The newborn has from 60-80% fetal haemoglobin, but this rapidly decreases during the first year, so that sickling becomes apparent after four months of age (Sickle Cell Disease Guidance Panel, 1993).

Sickle cell trait

People with sickle cell trait have the same basic defect, but only about 34-45% of the total haemoglobin is haemoglobin S (Pearson, 1984). The remainder is HbA. Normally, these individuals are asymptomatic. However, under conditions of

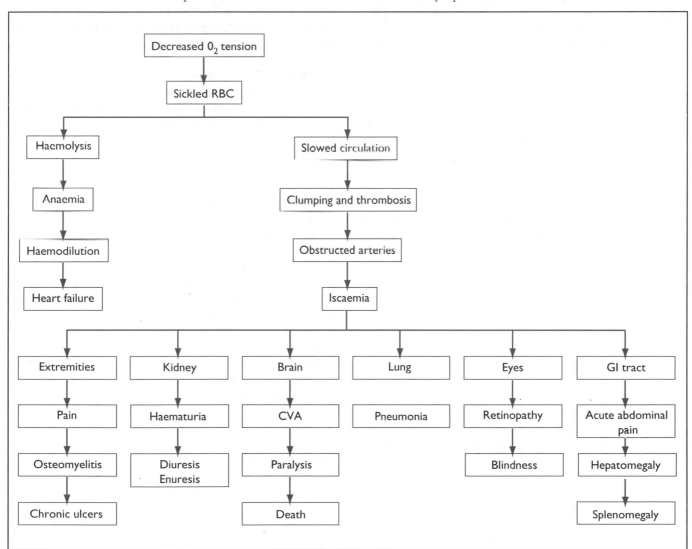

Fig. 29-2 Tissue effects of sickle cell anaemia.

extreme or prolonged deoxygenation, such as strenuous physical exercise, anaesthesia, infection, pulmonary disease, anaemia, high-altitude environments, underwater swimming, or pregnancy, sickling crises may occur. The higher the percentage of haemoglobin S, the more likely the occurrence of symptomatic responses.

CLINICAL MANIFESTATIONS

The changes in sickle cell anaemia are primarily the result of: (1) increased blood viscosity and (2) increased red blood cell destruction (Fig. 29-2). The entanglement and enmeshing of rigid sickle-shaped cells with one another increases blood viscosity. The thickened blood slows the circulation, causing capillary stasis, obstruction and thrombosis. Eventually, tissue ischaemia and necrosis result with pathological changes.

In addition to the effects of sickling on various organ structures, the child with sickle cell anaemia may have a variety of complaints, such as weakness; anorexia; joint, back, and abdominal pain; fever and vomiting. Chronic leg ulcers are common in adolescents and adults. Other generalized effects include growth retardation in both height and weight, delayed sexual maturation, decreased fertility, and priapism (constant penile erection). If the child reaches adulthood, sexual development and adult height are usually achieved.

Sickle cell crises

The clinical manifestations of sickle cell anaemia vary markedly in severity and frequency. The most acute symptoms of the disease occur during periods of exacerbation called *crises*, which are usually precipitated by infection.

Painful crises are the most common. They are the result of sickled cells obstructing the blood vessels, causing occlusion, ischaemia, and potentially necrosis. The major symptoms of this crisis are fever, acute abdominal pain from visceral hypoxia, pain and swelling in the hands and feet, and arthralgia, without an exacerbation of anaemia.

Sequestration crises are caused by the spleen pooling large quantities of blood, causing a precipitous drop in blood volume and ultimately shock. *Aplastic crisis* is diminished red blood cell production, usually triggered by infection.

Another type of bone marrow crisis is *megaloblastic anaemia*, which is attributed to a deficiency of folic acid and/or vitamin B_{12} during periods of pronounced erythropoiesis. Since infection is not always antecedent to aplastic or hypoplastic crises, it is possible that folic acid deficiency is a causative agent.

Haemolytic crisis occurs when there is an even greater rate of red blood cell destruction characterized by anaemia, jaundice and reticulocytosis.

PROCESS OF DIAGNOSIS

Sickle cell anaemia may not be recognized until toddlerhood, during a crisis precipitated by an acute upper respiratory or gastrointestinal infection.

Screening for sickle cell trait has become a controversial subject, since there is no method of preventing the disease other than selective birth procedures.

Specific blood tests are performed to identify the presence of sickle cells in conditions of low blood oxygen. By measuring the percentages of HbA, HbF and HbS, a diagnosis of sickle cell disease or trait can be made.

Screening of newborns can identify children with sickle cell disease or trait. Early diagnosis can facilitate parent education and support, and medical intervention.

THERAPEUTIC MANAGEMENT

There is no cure for sickle cell anaemia, although the role that bone marrow transplant could play is being debated (Davis, 1993). The aims of therapy are: (1) to prevent the sickling phenomenon, which is responsible for the pathological sequelae, and (2) to treat the medical emergency of sickle cell crisis.

Prevention of sickling

Prevention of sickling involves promoting adequate oxygenation and maintaining haemodilution. The successful implementation of these two goals often depends more on nursing intervention than on medical therapies.

Treatment of crisis

More often, medical management is directed at supportive and symptomatic treatment of crises. The main general objectives include: (1) bed rest to minimize energy expenditure and oxygen utilization at the child's discretion, (2) hydration for haemodilution through oral and intravenous therapy, (3) electrolyte replacement, since hypoxia results in metabolic acidosis, which also promotes sickling, (4) analgesics for severe abdominal and joint pain, (5) blood replacement to treat anaemia, and (6) antibiotics to treat any existing infection.

Short-term oxygen therapy may be helpful in severe crises, especially in children with cardiac failure.

Routine transfusions to maintain the haemoglobin above 10 g/dl in children with central nervous system disease can minimize the chances of further neurological problems. The benefits of a regular transfusion programme must be weighed against the associated increased risk of iron overload and alloimunization (Evans, 1989). In the event of surgery, preoperative transfusions are given to prevent anoxia and to suppress the formation of new sickle cells, and postoperatively to replace lost blood.

IMPLICATIONS FOR NURSING

Nursing management of the child with sickle cell anaemia is largely related to teaching and supporting the family, and providing comfort and pain relief to the child during a sickle cell crisis. The disease is usually first recognized when the child is a toddler, and the lifelong care begins with the diagnosis.

Assessment of the child in sickle cell crisis involves all areas and systems that can be affected by circulatory obstruction, including vital signs, neurological signs, vision and hearing, as well as the respiratory, gastrointestinal, renal and musculoskeletal systems. It is also important to assess the location and intensity of pain.

Prevention of crisis

Anything that increases cellular metabolism also results in tissue hypoxia. For the child this includes avoiding: (1) strenuous physical activity, (2) emotional stress, (3) environments of low oxygen concentration, such as high altitudes or nonpressurized aeroplane flights, and (4) known sources of infection. If the child has even a mild infection, the parents must seek medical attention at once.

The importance of haemodilution in preventing sickling has already been discussed. The nurse calculates the child's fluid requirements (approximately 150 ml/kg/day) and assesses the child's usual fluid consumption to evaluate its adequacy, and makes adjustments based on this knowledge. It is not sufficient to advise parents to 'encourage drinking'. They need specific instructions on how many glasses or bottles of fluid are required. Many foods are also a source of fluid, particularly soups, jellies, iced lollies and puddings, and these can be included as liquid sources.

Since the kidneys' ability to concentrate urine is impaired, the child is especially prone to dehydration. Dilute urine is not a valid sign of adequate hydration for children with sickle cell disease. Parents are taught to observe for other indications of fluid loss, such as dry mucous membranes, weight loss, and sunken fontanel in infants.

High fluid intake combined with renal diuresis results in the problem of enuresis. Parents who are unaware of this fact may employ the usual measures to discourage bed-wetting, such as limiting fluids at night, and many resort to punishment to promote bladder control. Reminding the child to urinate frequently during the day, and waking him or her once during the night may prove beneficial if the child's sleep patterns are not disturbed. Parents who are toilet training their toddlers should be aware of the more frequent pattern of urination and increased difficulty in learning control.

Since infection is the major predisposing factor towards development of a crisis, and the body's natural ability to resist infection is compromised, the nurse stresses to parents the importance of adequate nutrition, proper handwashing and isolation from known sources of infection. The last measure must be tempered with an awareness of the child's need to live a normal life. Parents need to be aware of the necessity of seeking prompt medical care at the first sign of any infection.

The family should be taught the signs and symptoms of crises and advised to seek medical attention immediately.

Management of pain is especially difficult and often involves experimenting with various analgesics and schedules. Opiates are usually required to achieve adequate pain relief, and continuous infusion can avoid the peaks and troughs of intermittent administration (Sartori, 1990). Effectiveness can be assessed using age-appropriate pain assessment tools. Patient-controlled analgesia devices have been successfully used by children in painful crisis (Grundy *et al*, 1993).

The use of child-centred behavioural interventions, such as distraction, relaxation and guided imagery, help the child deal with the depression, anxiety and fear that accompany the disease and, consequently, help improve pain relief.

The child should be kept warm. Bed rest is usually well tolerated during a crisis, although actual rest depends on effective analgesia. Although the objective of bed rest is to minimize oxygen consumption, some activity, particularly passive range of motion exercises, is beneficial to promote circulation. The best course of action is to let the child dictate his or her activity tolerance.

Oxygen therapy is administered only if there is hypoxaemia, as inappropriate use can reduce erythropoeisis (Embury *et al*, 1984).

If blood transfusions or exchange transfusions are given, the nurse must observe for signs of transfusion reaction (see Table 29-2).

Intake (especially of intravenous fluids) and output are recorded. The child's weight should be taken on admission, since it serves as a baseline for evaluating hydration. Since diuresis can result in electrolyte loss, the nurse also observes for signs of hypokalaemia. Nurses need to be aware of chest syndrome and stroke, both potentially fatal complications. Once the child's condition has stablized, the family should be helped to identify factors which may have contributed to the onset of the crisis, in an attempt to plan future avoidance strategies (France-Dawson, 1994).

Surgical risks relating to the disease also need to be considered. The main surgical risk is hypoxia from anaesthesia. However, emotional stress, the demands of wound healing, and the possibility of infection potentially increase the sickling phenomenon, both in children with the disease and in those with the trait. The primary nursing objectives are aimed at minimizing each of these threats preoperatively and postoperatively by keeping the child well hydrated, preparing the child psychologically and preventing infection.

Screening and genetic counselling

Screening is recommended during the neonatal period, since early diagnosis allows earlier, more prevention-oriented treatment, such as prophylactic antibiotic therapy and parent education about potential complications.

To be effective, screening must be combined with genetic counselling and long-term follow-up. The nurse plays an important role in conducting family education sessions, following the family in the home, disseminating correct information about the disease and trait to the community, and rendering support to parents of newly diagnosed children. A primary consideration in genetic counselling is informing parents, who both carry the trait, of the chances of having a child with the disease.

Prenatal diagnosis is possible through amniocentesis or chorionic villus sampling. The parents will need ongoing support in their decision to continue with the pregnancy or to terminate it.

Parents are advised to inform all treating practitioners of the child's condition. The use of a MedicAlert bracelet is another way to ensure awareness of the disease.

Parents need to discuss their feelings regarding transmitting a chronic illness to their child. Some parents are able to cope with this fact; some feel great guilt and remorse for giving their child the disease, whereas others regret not knowing they carried the trait. For many parents, the decision regarding subsequent pregnancies is viewed with doubt and ambivalence. The development of multidisciplinary hospital and community sickle cell services offers all members of affected families long-term support.

Agencies that may provide support and advice to families include the Organisation for Sickle Cell Anaemia Research (OSCAR), Sickle Cell Anaemia Relief, and the Sickle Cell Society.

THALASSAEMIA

The term *thalassaemia* is applied to a variety of inherited blood disorders characterized by deficiencies in the rate of production of specific globin chains in haemoglobin. Mediterranean people from Italy, Greece and the Middle East have the highest incidence of the disease. However, the disorder now has a wide geographical distribution, as a result of intermarriages and population migration.

The thalassaemias are classified according to the haemoglobin chain affected and by the amount of the globin chain that is synthesized; for example, if alpha chains are affected, the term α-*thalassaemia* is used. The most common form, β-thalassaemia, will be discussed further.

Silent carriers are individuals who carry the gene, but demonstrate no clinical symptoms. Persons with *thalassaemia trait*, the heterozygous form, usually have mild anaemia, hypochromic and microcytic cells, and elevated HbA_2 and/or HbF. *Thalassaemia intermedia* presents with splenomegaly and severe anaemia. Skeletal deformities, frequent fractures and arthritis complicate the clinical course. The homozygous form, *thalassaemia major*, results in a severe anaemia that is not compatible with life unless transfusion support is given.

MODE OF TRANSMISSION

Thalassaemia is an autosomal-recessive disorder with varying expressivity. Sometimes, the trait is found in only one parent of a child with severe thalassaemia. In this situation, the likelihood is that the other parent carries a gene for some variant of sickle cell anaemia or other haemoglobinopathy.

CLINICAL MANIFESTATIONS

The clinical effects of thalassaemia major are primarily attributable to: (1) defective synthesis of haemoglobin A, (2) structurally impaired red blood cells, and (3) shortened lifespan of the erythrocyte. The onset is usually insidious and not recognized until the latter half of infancy. Signs of anaemia - unexplained fever, poor feeding and a markedly enlarged spleen - particularly in a child of Mediterranean extraction, are descriptive.

Anaemia

Anaemia results from the body's inability to maintain a level of erythropoiesis commensurate with haemolysis. The bone marrow compensates by increasing production of large numbers of immature cells, which have a shortened lifespan.

Anaemia also is exaggerated by aplastic crises after infection, folic acid deficiencies from demands of bone marrow hyperplasia, splenic sequestration, and progressive haemolysis from repeated blood transfusions. The spleen becomes enlarged as a result of extramedullary haemopoiesis and rapid destruction of the defective erythrocytes.

With progressive anaemia, signs of chronic hypoxia, namely, headache, precordial and bone pain, decreased exercise tolerance, listlessness and anorexia, may develop.

Iron overload

Iron accumulates in various tissues of the body. Features of iron overload include endocrine disturbances, especially hypothyroidism, retarded growth and delayed sexual maturation. Diabetes and cardiac failure may also result (Wonke, 1994).

In thalassaemia, excess haemosiderin (the iron-containing pigment from the breakdown of haemoglobin) results from decreased haemoglobin synthesis and increased haemolysis of transfused erythrocytes. Decreased production of haemoglobin results in an excess supply of available iron. In addition, the body probably responds to the anaemia by increasing the rate of gastrointestinal absorption of dietary iron. With the prophylactic use of desferrioxamine to minimize excess iron storage, the characteristic changes in body structures from haemochromatosis have been greatly reduced.

THERAPEUTIC MANAGEMENT

The objective of supportive therapy is to maintain sufficient haemoglobin levels to prevent tissue hypoxia. Transfusions are the foundation of medical management. Recent studies have evaluated the benefits of maintaining the child's haemoglobin level above 10 g/dl, a goal that may require transfusions as often as every 2–4 weeks. The advantages of this therapy include: (1) improved physical and psychological well-being because of the ability to participate in normal activities, (2) decreased cardiomegaly and hepatosplenomegaly, (3) fewer bone changes, (4) normal or near normal growth and development until puberty, and (5) fewer infections (Festa, 1985).

One of the potential complications of frequent blood transfusions is iron overload. To minimize the development of haemosiderosis, desferrioxamine, an iron-chelating agent, is given. To be effective, it must be administered parenterally. The preferred routes are intravenous or subcutaneous, and many children receive home chelation therapy administered by their parents, with the support of community nurses. This intensive therapy allows them to lead a nearly normal life (Piomelli, 1993).

In some children with severe splenomegaly who require repeated transfusions, a splenectomy may be necessary to decrease the disabling effects of abdominal pressure and to increase the lifespan of supplemental red blood cells. A major postsplenectomy complication is severe and overwhelming infection. Therefore, these children are kept on prophylactic antibiotics with close medical supervision for many years, and should receive the pneumococcal and meningococcal vaccines in addition to the regularly scheduled immunizations.

Bone marrow transplantation offers the possibility of cure for some children with thalassaemia, either using marrow from an unaffected sibling, or a matched, unrelated donor (Lucarelli and Wetherall, 1991). However, the potential benefits must be weighed against the risks of the procedure and long-term supportive care may be considered a satisfactory alternative. Children with thalassaemia who undergo allogenic bone marrow transplantation currently have a 59–98% chance of cure (Giardini, 1994; Walters and Thomas, 1994).

IMPLICATIONS FOR NURSING

The objectives of nursing care are to: (1) assist the child in coping with the effects of the illness, (2) support the child's and family's adjustment to a chronic, life-threatening illness and (3) observe for complications of multiple blood transfusions (see Table 29-2).

Basic to each of these goals, is explaining to parents and children the defect responsible for the disorder and its effect on red blood cells. All families with a child who has thalassaemia should be tested for the trait and referred for genetic counselling.

Assist in coping with effects of disorder
Body image alterations, decreased growth and sexual immaturity are frequently difficult adjustment problems for older children. These children feel different from their peers, and the delayed sexual development with ramifications on sexual function is a major issue for the maturing adolescent with an improved life expectancy. Adolescents need an opportunity to express their thoughts and feelings about these complex issues.

With frequent transfusion therapy, there is less restriction imposed on physical activity because of severe anaemia, and these children can pursue activities commensurate with their exercise tolerance. However, the frequency of treatment can interfere with a normal lifestyle. Arranging for blood transfusions and medical supervision at times that interfere least with the child's regular activities, and liaison with the child's school, can promote the child's integration and minimize the disruptive impact of their condition.

Support the family
As with any chronic, life-threatening illness, the needs of the family must be met for optimum adjustment to the stresses imposed by the disorder. These needs are discussed in Chapter 20. A source of information for the family is the Thalassaemia Society UK*. Genetic counselling for the parents and fertile offspring is mandatory, and both prenatal diagnosis and screening for thalassaemia trait are available.

The prognosis for children with thalassaemia major is improving and many children now survive into adulthood. The chief cause of death is heart failure, followed by infection, liver disease and malignancy (Zurlo *et al*, 1989). The nurse must care for families of these children in light of this knowledge, must be willing to discuss the future prospects with the parents and child as appropriate, and must help them plan realistic goals.

APLASTIC ANAEMIA

Aplastic anaemia refers to a condition in which all formed elements of the blood are simultaneously depressed.

Aplastic anaemia can be primary (congenital) or secondary (acquired). Of the congenital variety, one of the best known disorders of which aplastic anaemia is an outstanding feature is *Fanconi anaemia*. The treatment is the same as for other causes of aplastic anaemia. Prognosis is variable, but is better than for acquired types.

The most common causes of acquired aplastic anaemia are:
1. Infection with the human parvovirus (HPV), hepatitis, or overwhelming infection.
2. Irradiation.
3. Drugs, such as the chemotherapeutic agents and several antibiotics, one of the most notable being chloramphenicol.
4. Industrial and household chemicals, including benzene and its derivatives.
5. Idiopathic, in which no identifiable precipitating cause can be found.

The anaemia will not be clinically evident until 6-8 weeks after the bone marrow insult. Therefore, it may be difficult to identify the cause.

CLINICAL MANIFESTATIONS AND PROCESS OF DIAGNOSIS

The clinical manifestations, which include anaemia, leukopenia and decreased platelet count, are usually insidious. The onset is not unlike that seen in leukaemia. Definitive confirmation is based on bone marrow aspiration or biopsy.

Treatment aims to restore function to the marrow and involves two main approaches: (1) immunosuppressive therapy to remove the presumed immunological functions that prolong aplasia and/or (2) replacement of the bone marrow through transplantation. Bone marrow transplantation is the treatment of choice in severe aplastic anaemia when a compatible donor exists. Bone marrow transplantation is associated with a 63% five year survival rate (Pinkel, 1993; Sanders *et al*, 1994).

Currently, antilymphocyte globulin (ALG) is the principal drug treatment for aplastic anaemia. The specific globulin is prepared by immunizing suitable animals, usually horses or rabbits, with human lymphocytes.

Response to immunosuppressive therapy is gradual. Elevations in haemoglobin and red blood cells may take as long as 3-6 months. During this period, the child must be protected from infection and haemorrhage and treated for the pancytopenia with transfusions.

Intravenous immunoglobulin has been used with success in aplastic anaemia of infectious origin (Dwyer, 1992).

Because of the relatively poor prognosis in aplastic anaemia treated with drug therapy, bone marrow transplantation should be considered *early* in the course of the disease if a compatible donor can be found. Transplantation is more successful when performed before multiple transfusions have sensitized the child to leucocyte and HLA antigens.

IMPLICATIONS FOR NURSING

The care of the child with aplastic anaemia is similar to that of the child with leukaemia; that is, preparing the family for the diagnostic and therapeutic procedures, preventing complications from the severe pancytopenia, and emotionally supporting them in terms of a potentially fatal outcome.

During administration of ALG, vigilant attention must be directed to the intravenous infusion to prevent extravasation. To prevent sclerosing from extravasation, a central vein should be used. Because of the child's susceptibility to infection, meticulous care of the venous access catheter is essential. Although anaphylactic reactions to ALG are rare, preparations should be made in advance. The nurse should observe for other reactions. Immediate reactions to ALG are common and include fever and skin rash. Delayed reactions (serum sickness) may also occur within 7-14 days of a course of ALG, and the manifestations are similar to immediate reactions.

DEFECTS IN HAEMOSTASIS

Haemostasis is the process that stops bleeding when a blood vessel is injured. A complex system of clotting, anticlotting, and clot breakdown (fibrinolysis) mechanisms exists in equilibrium to ensure clot formation only in the presence of blood vessel injury and to limit the clotting process to the site of vessel wall injury. Dysfunction in these systems will lead to bleeding or thrombosis. The following discussion focuses on the major conditions that require nursing intervention.

MECHANISMS INVOLVED IN NORMAL HAEMOSTASIS

To understand the role that factor deficiencies play in promoting bleeding tendencies, it is necessary to review the normal coagulation process of blood.

At the time of injury, several events occur at the site of injury to initiate haemostasis. There is local vasoconstriction, compression of the blood vessels by extravasated blood, release of von Willebrand factor (vWF) by endothelial walls, and the presence of collagen that acts as a site for platelet adhesion.

The platelets release a variety of chemicals to stimulate vasoconstriction, vessel repair and to activate and recruit more platelets to the injury site. Receptor sites are located on the platelets for fib-

rinogen and other adhesive proteins, causing the platelets to stick together. As the membrane of the platelet changes, the phospholipids necessary for blood coagulation are exposed, resulting in fibrin production, which secures the platelet plugs to the site.

HAEMOPHILIA

Haemophilia refers to a group of bleeding disorders in which there is a deficiency of one of the factors necessary for coagulation of the blood. Although the symptomatology is similar despite the missing factor, the identification of specific factor deficiencies has allowed definitive treatment with replacement agents. The two most common forms of the disorder are *classic haemophilia* (haemophilia A or factor VIII deficiency) and *Christmas disease* (haemophilia B or factor IX deficiency). The following discussion is primarily concerned with the classic form, which accounts for about 75% of all cases.

Haemophilia is generally classified into three groups according to the severity of factor deficiency as described below; approximately 60-70% of children with haemophilia demonstrate the severe form of the disorder:

Clinical severity	Factor VIII activity	Bleeding tendency
Severe	1%	Spontaneous bleeding without trauma
Moderate	1-5%	Bleeding with trauma
Mild	5-50%	Bleeding with severe trauma or surgery

Haemophilia is transmitted as an X-linked recessive disorder; however, only about 60% of affected children have a positive family history for the disease. The most frequent pattern of inheritance is between an unaffected male and a carrier female.

CLINICAL MANIFESTATIONS

The effect of haemophilia is prolonged bleeding anywhere from or in the body. With severe factor deficiencies, haemorrhage can occur as a result of minor trauma, such as after circumcision, during loss of deciduous teeth, or as a result of a slight fall or bruise.

Subcutaneous and intramuscular haemorrhages are common. *Haemarthrosis*, which refers to bleeding into the joint cavities, especially the knees, elbows and ankles, is the most frequent form of internal bleeding and can result in bone changes and, consequently, disabling deformities. Early signs of haemarthrosis are a feeling of stiffness, tingling or ache in the joint, followed by a decreased ability to move the affected joint. Obvious signs and symptoms are warmth, redness, swelling and severe pain with considerable loss of movement.

Bleeding into the tissue can occur anywhere, but is serious

if it occurs in the neck, mouth or thorax, since the airway can become obstructed. Intracranial haemorrhage can have fatal consequences. Haemorrhage anywhere along the gastrointestinal tract can lead to obstruction, and bleeding into the retroperitoneal cavity is especially hazardous because of the large space for blood to accumulate. Haematomas in the spinal cord can cause paralysis.

PROCESS OF DIAGNOSIS

Diagnosis is usually based on a history of bleeding episodes, evidence of X-linked inheritance, and laboratory findings. Tests that measure platelet function, such as the bleeding time, are all normal in persons with haemophilia, whereas tests that assess clotting factor function may be abnormal.

Carrier detection is possible in classic haemophilia and is an important consideration in families in which female offspring may have inherited the trait. These females may have low Factor VIII levels themselves and be symptomatic. Antenatal diagnosis is possible via amniocentesis or chorionic villus sampling.

THERAPEUTIC MANAGEMENT

The primary therapy for haemophilia is preventing spontaneous bleeding by replacing the missing factor. Vigorous therapy is instituted to prevent chronic crippling effects from joint bleeding.

One of the major concerns with the use of factor replacement is the risk of hepatitis. Improved processing has significantly decreased the risk of disease transmission. Factor VIII manufactured by recombinant DNA is now available; although this eliminates the risk of infection, HIV has been transmitted via contaminated products prior to 1985 in the United Kingdom.

Several other drugs may be included in the therapy plan, depending on the source of the haemorrhage. Corticosteroids are administered to reduce inflammation in the joints; nonsteroidal anti-inflammatory drugs (NSAIDs), such as aspirin and indomethacin should not be used because they inhibit platelet function (and, in the case of aspirin, because of its association with Reye's syndrome in children under 12 years of age). DDAVP is helpful in children who have mild to moderate haemophilia.

Treatment without delay results in more rapid recovery and a decreased likelihood of complications; therefore, most children are treated at home. The family is taught the technique of venepuncture and the administration of the replacement factor. Programmes of prophylactic Factor VIII treatment may be introduced. The child learns the procedure for self-administration between ages 9-12. Home treatment is highly successful, and the rewards, in addition to the immediacy of treatment, are less disruption of family life, fewer school or work days missed, and enhancement of the child's independence and self-esteem.

IMPLICATIONS FOR NURSING

The objectives for nursing care can be divided into immediate needs and long-term goals. Obviously, the most immediate consideration is control of bleeding episodes. However, the ultimate adjustment and prognosis for the child rely heavily on the family's ability to manage the disorder, to learn effective methods of control and prevention, and to balance the need for protection from injury while fostering independence and development.

During infancy and toddlerhood, the normal acquisition of motor skills creates innumerable opportunities for falls, bruises and minor wounds. Restraining the child from mastering motor development can herald more serious long-term problems than allowing the behaviour.

For older children, the family usually needs assistance in preparing for school. A nurse who knows the family can be instrumental in discussing the situation with the school nurse. Activity restrictions must be tempered with sensitivity to the child's emotional and physical needs. As much physical freedom as possible is permitted, although direct contact sports (e.g., rugby, judo, karate), which may risk head or neck injuries, are forbidden.

Oral hygiene and regular dental care is vital. Adolescents also need to be advised to use an electric shaver.

Since any trauma can lead to a bleeding episode, all persons caring for these children must be aware of their disorder. These children should wear MedicAlert identification, and older children should be encouraged to recognize situations in which disclosing their condition is important. Health personnel should take special precautions to prevent the use of procedures such as intramuscular injections or venepunctures. The subcutaneous route is substituted for all normally intramuscular injections, including immunizations.

Early recognition and effective management of bleeding episodes is vital. The earlier a bleeding episode is recognized, the more effectively it can be treated. Children are often aware of internal bleeding before clinical manifestations are evident, and they must be taken seriously when they report their concerns. In addition to the signs of haemarthrosis that have been discussed, the family also needs to be aware of signs and symptoms of internal tissue bleeding which require immediate medical attention: headache, slurred speech, loss of consciousness from bleeding within the brain, and black tarry stools and haematemesis from gastrointestinal bleeding. Factor replacement therapy should be instituted according to established medical protocol.

It is important to prevent the effects of joint degeneration. Repeated haemarthrosis can lead to bone and muscle changes that cause flexion contractures and joint fixation. Obviously, prevention of bleeding is the ideal goal. The physiotherapist plays a vital role in assessing joint function and teaching exercises aimed at achieving normal movement. Factor VIII may be administered prior to physiotherapy treatment, and the child is encouraged to maintain full range of motion in the joint.

The discovery of clotting factor concentrates has greatly changed the outlook for these children. With scheduled infusions of the missing factor, bleeding can be prevented, and the child can live a more normal, unrestricted life. To foster maximum independence, home-care programmes that teach the parent and/or child to administer the drug have been instituted. The nurse skilled in venepuncture techniques is often the person who teaches the families to administer the drug.

Intensive support for the family is essential. Not only is haemophilia a chronic, potentially fatal, hereditary condition, it is also one of unpredictable emergencies that impose additional emotional stress on family members. Children with the moderate or mild form may be undiagnosed until an accident occurs or an elective medical procedure is performed. At other times, parents are aware of the severity of the defect from birth. Whatever the situation, constructive teaching about the disease and measures to control or prevent bleeding must follow a period of parental adjustment to the diagnosis. For the nurse, this involves: (1) carefully listening to the parents' statements regarding their understanding of the condition, (2) being aware of the parents' feelings (particularly the mother's) concerning transmitting the disorder, and (3) assessing factors that affect the family's ability to cope with a crisis, such as marital stability, previous patterns of coping, and the ability to seek out and use help. Genetic counselling is also essential, and should occur as soon as possible after diagnosis. It must include evaluation of parental understanding, counselling about feelings, and transmission of information.

The needs of the family are best met by a multidisciplinary team: paediatrician, haematologist, haemophilia nurse, social worker and physiotherapist. Parent-group discussions are beneficial in addressing those needs and often best met by similarly affected families. Further information for families can be obtained from the Haemophilia Society.

VON WILLEBRAND DISEASE

Von Willebrand disease is a hereditary bleeding disorder characterized by a moderate to severe Factor VIII deficiency, and a reduction in the functional component of the Factor VIII molecule that is required for platelet adhesion to vascular subendothelium (known as von Willebrand factor).

The most characteristic clinical feature of von Willebrand disease is an increased tendency towards bleeding from mucous membranes. The most common symptom is frequent nosebleeds, followed by gingival bleeding, easy bruising, and menorrhagia in females. Unlike haemophilia, it affects both males and females because its inheritance is autosomal dominant. However, the treatment and final outcome are similar in both disorders. Treatment of bleeding is with DDAVP, FVIII, or VW factor.

IMPLICATIONS FOR NURSING

The nursing goals are similar to those for haemophilia, with special considerations related to epistaxis and menorrhagia. Premenstrual administration of DDAVP, tranexamic acid, or use of the contraceptive pill may be used to decrease menstrual flow. Interestingly, these females frequently do not experience excessive bleeding at the time of delivery. This is thought to be because of increased levels of Factor VIII during pregnancy. Decisions regarding childbearing are difficult because of the dominant pattern of inheritance.

IDIOPATHIC THROMBOCYTOPENIC PURPURA

Idiopathic thrombocytopenic purpura (ITP) is an acquired haemorrhagic disorder that results from excessive destruction of platelets. Although the exact cause is unknown, it is believed to be an autoimmune response to disease-related antigens. It is the most commonly occurring thrombocytopenia of childhood.

CLINICAL MANIFESTATIONS

ITP occurs in one of two forms: an acute, self-limiting course or a chronic condition interspersed with remissions. The acute form is most commonly seen after upper respiratory infections or the childhood diseases measles, rubella, mumps and chickenpox. The most common clinical manifestations of either type include easy bruising with petechiae; bleeding from mucous membranes, (e.g., epistaxis, bleeding gums); and internal haemorrhage with evidence of haematuria, haematemesis, melaena, haemarthrosis and menorrhagia; haematomas over the lower extremities that may result in chronic leg ulcers.

PROCESS OF DIAGNOSIS

In ITP the platelet count is below $20 \times 10^9/l$. Although there is no definitive test on which to establish a diagnosis of ITP, several tests are usually performed to rule out other disorders in which thrombocytopenia is a manifestation, such as systemic lupus erythematosus, lymphoma or leukaemia.

THERAPEUTIC MANAGEMENT

Management is primarily supportive, because the course of the disease is self-limiting in most cases. Corticosteroids or intravenous gamma globulin may be given to increase platelet production until spontaneous recovery takes place. Children with chronic ITP have also experienced and sustained a rise in platelet count when treated with ascorbate (a product of ascorbic acid [vitamin C]) (Cohen *et al*, 1993). Children with chronic, symptomatic ITP may require splenectomy.

IMPLICATIONS FOR NURSING

Nursing care is largely supportive. As in any condition with an uncertain outcome, the child and family need emotional support and education. Some of the child's activities may have to be restricted to reduce the risk of serious haemorrhage. Aspirin should not be given.

The family also needs to be aware of signs and symptoms indicating internal bleeding, which, although rare, requires immediate medical attention.

HENOCH-SCHÖNLEIN PURPURA

Henoch-Schönlein purpura (HSP) is a relatively common acquired disorder in children. The aetiology is unknown, but the disease often follows an upper respiratory infection, and allergy or drug sensitivity plays a role in some instances. It is observed more often in white children than in other races, and in boys twice as often as in girls.

The disease is characterized by inflammation of small blood vessels. A generalized vasculitis of dermal capillaries causing extravasation of red blood cells produces the petechial skin lesions.

CLINICAL MANIFESTATIONS

The onset of the disease may be abrupt with simultaneous appearance of several manifestations, or may be gradual with sequential appearance of different manifestations. The primary feature, however, is a symmetrical purpura that involves the buttocks and lower extremities, but may extend to include the extensor surfaces of the upper extremities and, less commonly, the upper trunk and face.

Two-thirds of affected children develop arthritis, ranging from asymptomatic swelling around a single joint to painful tender swelling of several joints, most often the knees and ankles. This resolves in a few days, without permanent damage or deformity.

Two-thirds of the children have gastrointestinal involvement manifested by recurrent colicky midabdominal pain often associated with nausea and vomiting. The stools contain gross or occult blood and mucus.

Renal involvement occurs in up to 50% of affected children and is potentially the most serious long-term complication. Initially, the nephritis is manifested as haematuria, casts and proteinuria. Although the majority of children with renal involvement recover completely, some develop chronic renal disease with eventual renal failure.

PROCESS OF DIAGNOSIS

Diagnosis is usually established on the basis of clinical manifestations. Assessment is made of gastrointestinal and renal involvement.

THERAPEUTIC MANAGEMENT

Management is primarily supportive, with close observation for signs of renal or gastrointestinal manifestations. Oedema, rash, malaise and arthralgia are usually managed with appropriate analgesics.

Most children recover without the need for hospitalization, and in most instances a single acute episode clears spontaneously within one month.

IMPLICATIONS FOR NURSING

Nursing care of the child hospitalized with HSP is primarily supportive, with vigilant observation for signs of complications. Urine and stools are carefully observed for fresh and occult blood.

If the child suffers from joint pain, positioning, careful movement, and administration of analgesics help reduce discomfort. Non-narcotic analgesics also relieve the discomfort of fever and malaise.

Concern about the unsightly appearance of the rash is common. The child and parents can be reassured that it is only a temporary phenomenon, and he or she can be encouraged to wear clothing that helps hide the rash.

DISSEMINATED INTRAVASCULAR COAGULATION

Disseminated intravascular coagulation (DIC) is not a primary disease, but is a secondary disorder of coagulation that complicates several pathological processes (such as hypoxia, acidosis, shock and burns) and many severe systemic disease states (such as congenital heart disease, necrotizing enterocolitis, and gram-negative bacterial sepsis). The disease is characterized by inappropriate systemic activation and acceleration of the normal clotting mechanism.

DIC occurs when the coagulation process is abnormally stimulated, triggering overactivity of: (1) clotting mechanism, leading to widespread thrombus formation and (2) fibrinolysis, causing haemorrhage. Platelets and clotting factors are rapidly destroyed and there is haemolysis of RBCs.

PROCESS OF DIAGNOSIS

DIC is suspected when there is an increased tendency to bleed as from venepuncture or surgical wound, petechiae, bruising, hypotension, or dysfunction of organs due to infarction and ischaemia. Haematological investigations show increased clotting times, a profoundly depressed platelet count, fragmented red blood cells and depleted fibrinogen.

THERAPEUTIC MANAGEMENT

Treatment is directed towards control of the underlying or initiating cause, which in most instances stops the coagulation problem spontaneously. Platelets and fresh frozen plasma may be needed to replace lost plasma components, especially in the child whose underlying disease remains uncontrolled. The administration of heparin to inhibit thrombin formation is most often restricted to severe cases.

IMPLICATIONS FOR NURSING

The goals of nursing care are to be aware of the possibility of DIC in the severely ill child and to recognize signs that might indicate its presence. The child will require close observation and care associated with administration of intravenous fluids, blood products and heparin infusion. Since the child is usually cared for in an intensive care unit, the special needs of the family of a critically ill child must be considered (see Chapter 5).

IMMUNOLOGICAL DEFICIENCY DISORDERS

Several disorders can cause profound, often life-threatening alterations in the body's immune system. Several classifications of immune dysfunction exist. Acquired immune deficiency syndrome (AIDS), severe combined immunodeficiency syndrome (SCIDS), and Wiskott-Aldrich syndrome are the inability of the body to react. An allergy is the overreaction of the immune system to a relatively harmless antigen. The immune response can also be misdirected. In autoimmune disorders, antibodies, macrophages and lymphocytes attack healthy cells.

MECHANISMS INVOLVED IN IMMUNITY

In simple terms, the function of the immune system is to recognize 'self' from 'non-self' and to initiate responses to eliminate the non-self or the foreign substance known as *antigen*.

The protective mechanisms of the body consist of complex, overlapping defence systems. Intact skin serves as the first line of protection for the body. Body secretions such as saliva, sweat and tears contain chemicals that can kill many organisms. The stomach contains acids that can destroy swallowed pathogens which have successfully evaded the mucus of the nose and mouth - organisms trapped in these areas are expelled by sneezing or coughing. If the foreign substance has penetrated these barriers, cellular elements are mobilized.

The functions of the immune system are basically of two types: nonspecific and specific (Fig. 29-3). *Nonspecific immune defences* are activated on exposure to any foreign substance, but react similarly regardless of the type of antigen. The principal activity of this system is *phagocytosis*, the process of ingesting and digesting foreign substances. Phagocytic cells include neutrophils and monocytes (see Fig. 29-3).

Specific defences are those that have the ability to recognize the antigen and respond selectively. The components of adaptive immunity are *humoral immunity* and *cell-mediated immunity*. The cells responsible for these two forms of immunity are the lymphocytes; specifically, B-lymphocytes and T-lymphocytes.

HUMORAL IMMUNITY

Humoral immunity is involved with antibody production and complement, and is concerned with immune processes occurring *outside* the cells, such as on cell surfaces or in body fluids.

The principal cell involved in antibody production is the B-lymphocyte. When challenged with an antigen, B-cells divide and differentiate into *plasma cells*. The plasma cells produce and secrete large quantities of antibodies (immunoglobulins) specific to the antigen.

On initial exposure to an antigen, the B-lymphocyte system begins to produce antibody. This process is referred to as the *primary antibody response*. With subsequent exposure to the antigen, a *secondary antibody response* occurs. An example of the secondary response is consecutive administration of immunizations, often called 'boosters'. Memory B-cells allow the immune system to recognize the same antigen for months or years.

When antibody reacts with antigen, they bind to form an antigen-antibody complex. Antibody aids in the phagocytosis of antigen by sensitizing it in such a manner that it is more readily destroyed by phagocytes, a process known as *opsonization*.

Antibody also activates or fixes complement, the second component of humoral immunity. After being activated by antibody, complement produces a factor that summons T-lymphocytes and macrophages to the antigen site.

CELL-MEDIATED IMMUNITY

Cell-mediated immunity is involved in a variety of specific functions mediated by the T-lymphocyte, and occurs *within* the cell. T-lymphocytes do not carry immunoglobulins. Several T-cell subsets have been identified, including cytotoxic T-cells, helper T-lymphocytes and suppressor T-lymphocytes.

Specific functions of T-lymphocytes include: (1) protection against most viral, fungal and protozoan infections, and slow-growing bacterial infections, such as tuberculosis, (2) rejection of histo-incompatible grafts, (3) mediation of cutaneous delayed hypersensitivity reactions, such as in tuberculin testing, and (4) probably immune surveillance for malignant cells.

The cellular immune response is initiated when a T-lymphocyte is sensitized by antigen. In response to this contact, the T-cell releases numerous humoral factors called *lymphokines*, which eventually bring about death of the antigen.

ACQUIRED IMMUNE DEFICIENCY SYNDROME

Acquired immune deficiency syndrome (AIDS) is a recently recognized disorder. The first published reports of unusual opportunistic infections in previously healthy individuals appeared in 1981; retrospective analysis of data demonstrated the existence of cases since 1978, and possibly before this date. In 1983 and 1984, a retrovirus found in AIDS patients was characterized and named *human immunodeficiency virus* (HIV).

HIV is the causative agent of AIDS. There is currently a move to use the term 'HIV disease', instead of AIDS, to avoid the stigma attached to the term. The virus has been found in almost all body fluids (blood, semen, saliva, vaginal secretions, urine, breast milk and tears), but to date there is evidence that the virus is transmitted through direct contact with blood or blood products, breastfeeding and sexual contact.

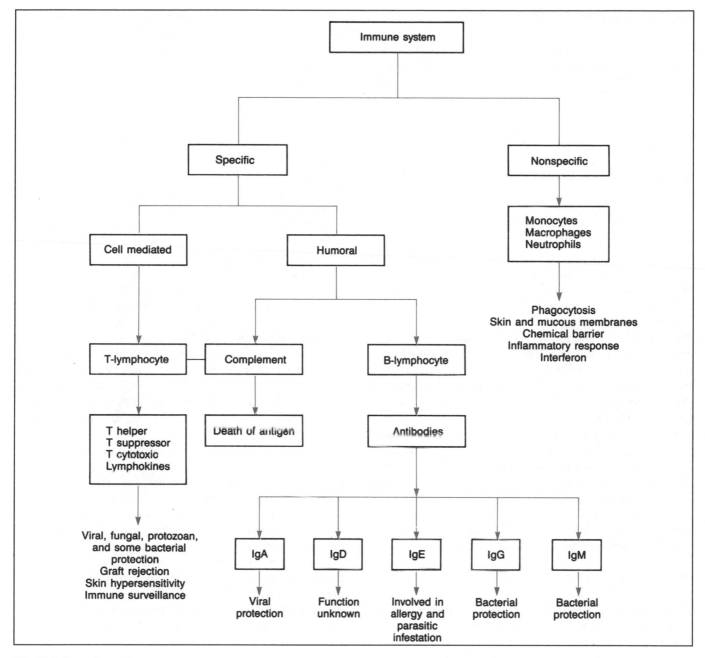

Fig. 29-3 Components of immune system.

There are three groups of children who have contracted HIV: (1) haemophiliacs and others treated with contaminated blood products, (2) those who became infected through intravenous drug use or sexual contact, and (3) children who acquire the virus via vertical transmission (the largest group). In 1993, there were approximately 200 vertically infected children in the UK, found mainly in London (Ades *et al*, 1993).

AIDS is characterized by a generalized dysfunction of the immune system. HIV attacks helper T-cells, where it can either lie dormant or proliferate more virus and eventually inactivate the immune role of the cell in which it resides. In normal individuals, there are more helper than suppressor T-cells, but in people with AIDS there is a reverse helper-to-suppressor ratio.

Abnormal B-cell function is also apparent early in paediatric AIDS, with symptoms of hypergammaglobulinaemia.

CLINICAL MANIFESTATIONS

The definition of paediatric AIDS includes opportunistic infection, recurrent severe bacterial infection, failure to thrive, encephalopathy, malignancy, and lymphoid interstitial pneumonitis (Centers for Disease Control, 1987). Affected children may have some or all of these problems; the pattern of their illness is influenced by the infections to which they have been exposed.

PROCESS OF DIAGNOSIS

The diagnosis is often one of ruling out other probable causes, demonstrating the principal immunological abnormalities in AIDS, establishing a positive antibody to HIV, and testing for the presence of HIV in blood cultures or genetic tests, such as the polymerase chain reaction test which amplifies viral genetic material.

The process of diagnosis in young infants is complicated by the persistence of maternal antibodies to HIV remaining in the baby's system for up to 18 months (European Collaborative Study, 1991).

THERAPEUTIC MANAGEMENT

Currently, there is no cure for HIV disease/AIDS; the disease is progressive and ultimately fatal. Three antiretroviral agents, zidovudine dideoxycytidine (DDC) and didanosine (DDI), are under investigation for the treatment of children with HIV infection. Clinical improvements include weight gain in children with previous growth retardation, a reduction in the size of an enlarged liver and spleen, improvements in IQ scores and other measures of brain function, and improvement in immune system function (Food and Drug Administration, 1990). Treatment is also directed at the prevention and management of the opportunistic infections. The most common infections are chronic candidiasis and pneumocystis carinii pneumonia (PCP). Co-trimoxazole is the drug of choice for PCP prophylaxis, and intermittent intravenous immunoglobulin therapy can provide protection against bacterial and viral infections (Crawley and Gibb, 1993).

Immunization against common childhood illnesses is recommended for all children with HIV infection. Live vaccines should be substituted with inactivated forms.

IMPLICATIONS FOR NURSING

The implications for nursing are caring for the child, preventing the transmission of the virus, and educating the public regarding HIV disease.

The nursing care of the child with HIV disease/AIDS is primarily supportive. Physiological care of the patient is directed at minimal exposure to infections, nutritional support, comfort measures, assessment and recognition of changes in status that may indicate impending sepsis or other complications, and assisting in the treatment of these.

The family of the vertically infected child is faced with multiple problems, affecting every area of their lives. Families require flexible, multidisciplinary care involving hospital and community teams, utilizing the resources of statutory and voluntary sectors (Duggan, 1993). Since the mother is carrying the virus, she may be ill or dying and therefore unable to care for a child. Relatives may assume responsibility for the care of the child. If no extended family is available, early intervention by a social worker can help parents plan for their child's care.

Since the disease is congenitally acquired, the parents may have to deal with feelings of guilt. They will need support throughout the progression of the disease and subsequent bereavement.

Children who have haemophilia represent the second major population of children with HIV disease. They are infected with the virus secondary to treatment of their primary illness. Since haemophilia is inherited, the parents experience guilt, as well as the probable loss of their child. These children are usually older and must deal with peer groups, schools, and the usual developmental tasks of childhood. As these individuals become adolescents and possibly sexually active, they must be taught safer sexual behaviour. Most children who received contaminated Factor VIII in the UK are now, if surviving, of adult age. Blood screening precautions should mean that no new infections in this group should occur in children treated with UK product.

A third group of individuals increasingly infected with HIV is adolescents. Adolescents must be taught about the risks of intravenous drug use and the risks of unprotected sex. The nurse's role as a health educator carries a responsibility to dispel myths about transmission of HIV.

Recommendations for preventing spread of the virus consist of universal precautions, which are the same guidelines for preventing the transmission of other blood-borne diseases, such as hepatitis B virus (see Infection Control, Chapter 8). These precautions should be routinely enforced, regardless of whether a child is known to be infected.

Unfortunately, criticism and ostracism of the child and family persists. In an effort to protect the child and deal with the community's fear, the family may keep the child at home in an atmosphere of overprotection. While certain precautions are justified in limiting exposure to sources of infection, they must be tempered with concern for the child's normal developmental needs.

Confidentiality is a primary consideration — parents have to make choices about sharing information about their child's diagnosis (and often their own). The role of the nurse and the multidisciplinary team is to explore the issues and to support the family's decisions. The Terrance Higgins Trust provides support and advice to families.

SEVERE COMBINED IMMUNODEFICIENCY DISEASE

Severe combined immunodeficiency disease (SCID) is characterized by absence of both humoral and cell-mediated immunity. The consequence of the immunodeficiency is an overwhelming susceptibility to infection and to the *graft-versus-host* reaction, which can occur when any histoincompatible (unmatched) tissue from an immunocompetent donor is infused into the immunodeficient recipient.

CLINICAL MANIFESTATIONS

The most common manifestation is susceptibility to infection early in life, most often by three months of age, when antenatal acquired immunity is exhausted. Specifically, the disorder in children is characterized by chronic infection, failure to completely recover from an infection, frequent reinfection, and infection with unusual agents. In addition, the history reveals no logical source of infection. Failure to thrive is a consequence of the persistent illnesses.

PROCESS OF DIAGNOSIS

Diagnosis is usually based on a history of recurrent, severe infections from early infancy, a familial history of the disorder, and specific laboratory findings, which include lymphocytopenia, lack of lymphocyte response to antigens, and absence of plasma cells in the bone marrow.

THERAPEUTIC MANAGEMENT

The only definitive treatment is a histocompatible bone marrow transplant. The most suitable donor is a sibling with a matched HLA bone marrow. Since the host's immunological system is incompetent, graft rejection is not a problem. However, a graft-versus-host reaction is always a possibility.

Other approaches to SCID are providing passive immunity with intravenous immunoglobulin and maintaining the child in a sterile environment. The latter is effective only if instituted before the existence of any infectious process in the infant, and it represents an extreme effort to prevent life-threatening infections. Other investigational procedures include matched unrelated donor, and mismatch bone marrow transplants.

IMPLICATIONS FOR NURSING

Nursing care depends on the type of therapy used. If bone marrow transplantation is attempted, the care is consistent with that needed for bone marrow transplantation for any condition (see Chapter 30). To prevent infection, all interventions aimed at protecting the immunocompromised child are implemented. However, even with exacting environmental control, these children are prone to opportunistic infection. Chronic fungal infections of the mouth and nails with *Candida albicans* are frequent problems despite vigorous efforts at prevention or treatment. It is important to stress to parents that such conditions are not a result of laxity on their part in preventing them, but are the result of the severe immunological disorder.

Since the prognosis for SCID is very poor if a compatible bone marrow donor is not available, nursing care is directed at supporting the family in caring for a child with a life-threatening illness (see Chapter 21).

WISKOTT-ALDRICH SYNDROME

The Wiskott-Aldrich syndrome is an X-linked recessive disorder characterized by a triad of abnormalities: (1) thrombocytopenia, (2) eczema, and (3) immunodeficiency of selective functions of B- and T-lymphocytes.

The exact defect is unknown. A variety of pathological findings are evident. The platelets are abnormally small in size and have a shortened lifespan. The primary immunological defect consists of the inability of phagocytes to process foreign antigens. As a result, immunologically competent cells fail to produce normal immunoglobulin patterns. Early in life, the immunoglobulin levels may be normal, but later, low levels of IgM are observed.

CLINICAL MANIFESTATIONS

At birth, the major effect of the disorder is bleeding because of the thrombocytopenia. As the child grows older, recurrent infection and eczema become more severe, and the bleeding becomes less frequent. Eczema is typical of the allergic type and readily becomes infected.

PROCESS OF DIAGNOSIS

Diagnosis can usually be made during the neonatal period because of the thrombocytopenia. Specific tests for immunological function confirm the diagnosis. Carrier detection is also possible.

THERAPEUTIC MANAGEMENT

Medical treatment mainly involves: (1) counteracting the bleeding tendencies with platelet transfusions, (2) using intravenous immunoglobulin to provide passive immunity (Dwyer, 1992), and (3) administering prophylactic antibiotics to prevent and control infection. Splenectomy may be performed to reverse the thrombocytopenia, and these children require the same prophylactic measures as any child with asplenia — appropriate immunizations and continuous antibiotics — and, despite their immune deficiency, they are able to mount an adequate immunological response to the inactivated vaccines. When an HLA-matched donor exists, bone marrow transplantation is the treatment of choice.

IMPLICATIONS FOR NURSING

Because of the poor prognosis for these children, the main implication for nursing is supporting the family in the care of a child with a chronic life-threatening illness (see Chapter 21). Physical care is directed at symptom alleviation and preventing or controlling infection. Since eczema is a troublesome problem, nursing measures specific to this condition are especially important. Parents will require genetic counselling to assist in planning future pregnancies. Antenatal testing is also available.

KEY POINTS

◆ Major functions of the haematological system include production of cells, oxygenation, nutrient distribution to the cells, immune protection, collection of wastes from the cells, and heat regulation.

◆ Anaemia is defined as reduction of red cell volume or haemoglobin concentration to levels below normal; disorders are classified either by aetiology/physiology or by morphology.

◆ The nurse's role in treatment of anaemia is to assist in establishing a diagnosis, prepare the child for laboratory tests, decrease tissue oxygen needs, implement safety precautions and observe for complications.

◆ The main nursing goal in preventing nutritional anaemia is parent education regarding correct feeding practices.

◆ Four types of sickle cell crisis are: vaso-occlusive, splenic sequestration, aplastic and hyperhaemolytic.

◆ Nursing care of the child with sickle cell disease is aimed at teaching the family how to recognize and prevent sickling, managing pain during splenic crises, and helping the child and parents adjust to a lifelong, potentially fatal disease.

◆ Nursing care of the child with thalassaemia entails observing for complications of multiple blood transfusions, assisting the child to cope with the effects of illness, and fostering parent-child adjustment to long-term illness.

◆ Common causes of aplastic anaemia include irradiation, drugs, industrial and household chemicals, infections, infiltration and replacement of myeloid elements, and idiopathic conditions.

◆ Nursing care of the child with haemophilia involves preventing bleeding by decreasing the risk of injury, recognizing and managing bleeding, preventing the crippling effects of joint degeneration, and preparing and supporting the child and family for home care.

◆ Paediatric clinical manifestations of HIV disease/AIDS include failure to thrive, interstitial pneumonitis and hepatosplenomegaly. HIV disease remains both a physiological and social disease at present.

REFERENCES

Ades AE *et al:* Vertically transmitted HIV infection in the British Isles, *BMJ* 306:1296, 1993.

Centers for Disease Control: Classification system for HIV infection in children under 13 years of age, *Morbidity Mortality Weekly Report* 15:225, 1987.

Cohen HA *et al:* Treatment of chronic idiopathic thrombocytopenic purpura with ascorbate, *Clin Pediatr* 32(5):300, 1993.

Crawley S, Gibb D: Clinical features and management of HIV infection in children, *Current Paediatr* 3:164, 1993.

Davis S: Bone marrow transplantation for sickle cell disease, *Arch Dis Child* 69:176, 1993.

Duggan C: A family affair: multidisciplinary care for children with HIV and AIDS, *Child Health* 1(1):33, 1993.

Dwyer JM: Manipulating the immune system with immune globulin, *N Engl J Med* 326(2):107, 1992.

Embury SH *et al:* Effects of oxygen inhalation on endogenous erythropoeitin kinetics, erthrpoeisis and properties of blood cells in sickle cell anaemia, *New Eng J Med* 311:291, 1984.

European Collaborative Study: Children born to women with HIV1 infection: natural history and risk of transmission, *Lancet* 337:253, 1991.

Evans J: Practical management of sickle cell disease, *Arch Dis Child* 64:1748, 1989.

Festa RS: Modern management of thalassemia, *Pediatr Ann* 14(9):597, 1985.

Food and Drug Administration: Progress in the use of Zidovudine, *FDA Drug Bull*, p 6, April 1990.

France-Dawson M: Painful crises in sickle cell conditions, *Nurs Stand* 8(45):25, 1994.

Grundy R *et al:* Practical management of pain in sickling disorders, *Arch Dis Child* 69:256, 1993.

James J, Laing G: Iron deficiency anaemia, *Current Paediatr* 4(1):33, 1994.

Jojraninata P, Pollitt E: Reversal of developmental delays in iron deficient infants treated with iron, *Lancet* 341:1, 1993.

Lucarelli G, Wetherall DJ: Bone marrow transplantation for severe thalassaemia, *Br J Haematol* 78:300, 1991.

Pearson HA: Sickle cell syndromes and other hemoglobinopathies. In Miller DR et al, editors: *Blood diseases of infancy and childhood*, ed 5, St Louis, 1984, Mosby–Year Book.

Pinkel D: Bone marrow transplantation in children, *J Pediatr* 122(3):331, 1993.

Piomelli S: Management of Cooley's anaemia, *Baillieres Clin Haematol* 6(1):287, 1993.

Sanders *et al:* Marrow transplant experience for children with severe aplastic anemia, *Am J Pediatr Hematol Oncol* 16(1):43, 1994.

Sartori PC *et al:* Continuous papaveretum infusion for the control of pain in painful sickling crises, *Arch Dis Child* 65:1151, 1990.

Sickle Cell Disease Guidance Panel: *Sickle cell disease: screening, diagnosis, management, and counseling in newborns and infants*, Agency for Health Care Policy and Research, No 93-0562, 1993.

Walter *et al:* Effectiveness of iron-fortified infant cereal in prevention of iron deficiency anemia, *Pediatrics* 91:976, 1993.

Webb D *et al:* Acquired aplastic anaemia—still a serious disease, *Arch Dis Child* 66:858, 1991.

Wonke B: Management of beta thalassaemia major, *Current Paediatr* 4(1):38, 1994.

Zurlo MG *et al:* Survival and causes of death in thalassemia major, *Lancet* 1(8653):27, 1989.

FURTHER READING

Claxton R, Harrison A, editors: *Caring for children with HIV and AIDS,* London, 1991, Edward Arnold.

Franklin I: *Sickle cell disease—a guide for patients, carers and health workers,* London, 1990, Faber & Faber.

Guggan M: Cause and cure for iron deficiency in toddlers, *Health Visitor* 66(7):250, 1993.

May A, Choiseul M: Sickle cell anaemia and thalassaemia: symptoms, treatment and effects on lifestyle, *Health Visitor* 61(7):212, 1988.

McFarlane K: Idiopathic thrombocytopaenic purpura in children, *Paediatr Nurs* 5(5):6, 1993.

Turner T: A helping hand for haemophilia—paediatric haemophilia services, *Nurs Times* 84(49):26, 1988.

Anaemia/Iron Deficiency Anaemia

Barbara JAJ: Infectious complications of blood transfusion: viruses, *BMJ* 300:450, 1990.

Contreras M, Mollison PL: Immunological complications of transfusion, *BMJ* 300:173, 1990.

Miller DR: Anemias: general considerations. In Miller DR *et al.,* editors: *Blood diseases of infancy and childhood,* ed 5, St Louis, 1984, Mosby–Year Book.

Milne RIG: Assessment of care of children with sickle cell disease: implications for neonatal screening programmes, *BMJ* 300:371, 1990.

Oski FA: Iron deficiency—facts and fallacies, *Pediatr Clin North Am* 32(2):493, 1985.

Patterson KL: The childhood anemias, *Pediatr Nurs Update* 1(4):2, 1985.

Sickle Cell Disease

Burghardt-Fitzgerald DC: Pain-behavior contracts: effective management of the adolescent in sickle-cell crisis, *J Pediatr Nurs* 4(5):320, 1989.

Miller ST *et al*: Cerebrovascular accidents in children with sickle-cell disease and alpha-thalassemia, *J Pediatr* 113(5):847, 1988.

Pearson HA *et al*: Developmental pattern of splenic dysfunction in sickle cell disorders, *Pediatr* 76(3):392, 1985.

Phebus CK, Glonger MF, Maciak BJ: Growth patterns by age and sex in children with sickle cell disease, *J Pediatr* 105(1):28, 1984.

Williams S, Maude GH, Serjeant GR: Clinical presentation of sickle cell-hemoglobin C disease, *J Pediatr* 109:586, 1986.

Thalassaemia

Cohen AR, Mizanin J, Schuartz E: Rapid removal of excessive iron with daily high dose intravenous chelation therapy, *J Pediatr* 115(1):151, 1989.

Modell B *et al*: Effect of fetal diagnostic testing on birth rate of thalassemia major in Britain, *Lancet* 2:1383, 1984.

Aplastic Anaemia

Glader BE: Red blood aplasias in children, *Pediatr Ann* (19)3:168, 1990.

Hunter RF, Roth PA, Huang AT: Predictive factors for response to anti-thymocyte globulin in acquired aplastic anemia, *Am J Med* 79(1):73, 1985.

Sanders JE *et al*: Bone marrow transplantation experience for children with aplastic anemia, *Pediatr* 77(2):179, 1986.

Defects in Haemostasis

Buchanan GR *et al*: Hepatitis in household contacts of patients with hemophilia who have received multiple transfusions, *J Pediatr* 108(6):937, 1986.

Bussel JB: Thrombocytopenia in newborns, infants, and children, *Pediatr Ann* 19(3):181, 1990.

Bussel JB *et al*: Treatment of acute idiopathic thrombocytopenia of childhood with intravenous infusions of gammaglobulin, *J Pediatr* 106(6):886, 1985.

Dubansky AS, Oski FA: Controversies in the management of acute idiopathic thrombocytopenic purpura: a survey of specialists, *Pediatr* 77(1):49, 1986.

Rosenblum N, Winter H: Steroid effects on the course of abdominal pain in children with Henoch-Schonlein purpura, *Pediatr* 79(6):1018, 1987.

Shende A: Idiopathic thrombocytopenic purpura in children, *Pediatr Ann* 14(9):609, 1985.

Stuart MJ *et al*: Bleeding time in hemophilia A: potential mechanisms for prolongation, *J Pediatr* 108(2):215, 1986.

Immunological Deficiency Disorders

Committee on Infectious Diseases: Health guidelines for the attendance in daycare and foster care settings of children infected with human immunodeficiency virus, *Pediatr* 79(3):466, 1987.

Fischer GW: Therapeutic uses of intravenous gammaglobulin for pediatric infections, *Pediatr Clin North Am* 35(3):517, 1988.

Flaskerud JH: *AIDS/HIV infection: a reference guide for nursing professionals,* ed 2, Philadelphia, 1991, WB Saunders.

Goodman E, Cohall AT: Acquired immunodeficiency syndrome and adolescents: knowledge, attitudes, beliefs, and behaviors in a New York City adolescent minority population, *Pediatr* 84(1):36, 1989.

Jason JM *et al*: Human immunodeficiency virus infection in hemophilic children, *Pediatr* 82(4):565, 1988.

Selekman J: The multiple faces of immune deficiency in children, *Pediatr Nurs* 16(4):351, 1990.

Todd J: A most intimate foe: how the immune system can betray the body it defends, *Science* 30(2):20, 1990.

USEFUL ADDRESSES

Organisation for Sickle Cell Anaemia Research (OSCAR), Tiverton Road, London N15 6RT.

Sickle Cell Society, 54 Station Road, Halesden, London NW10 4VA.

Sickle Cell Anaemia Relief, PO Box 88, Barking, Essex IGII 8PH.

Thalassaemia Society UK, 107 Nightingale Lane, London N87QY.

Haemophilia Society, 123 Westminster Bridge Road, LondonSE1 7HL.

Terrance Higgins Trust (HIV and AIDS), 52-54 Grays Inn Road, London WCIX 8JO.

Chapter 30

The Child with Cancer

LEARNING OUTCOMES

After studying this chapter you should be able to:

◆ Discuss the aetiology of childhood cancer.
◆ Describe the process of diagnosis and treatment.
◆ Discuss the principles involved in the administration of chemotherapy and radiotherapy.
◆ Discuss new therapies and the process of bone marrow transplantation.
◆ Explain how oncological emergencies may arise and discuss their management.
◆ Demonstrate an awareness of late effects of treatment and how they can be prevented, followed up, and treated.
◆ Identify the key elements in the nursing care of children with cancer.
◆ Describe common types of childhood cancer and summarize the recognized treatment.
◆ Define the glossary terms.

GLOSSARY

biopsy Removal of tissue for examination

biotherapy Treatment that uses BRM to combat malignancy

BMD Bone marrow depression

BMT Bone marrow transplantation

carcinogen Substance that causes cancer

chemotherapy Treatment with chemical substances having a specific effect on a disease

classification Identification of specific characteristics of a disease

GVHD Graft-versus-host disease

immunosuppression Inhibition of antibodies to antigens that may be present

limb salvage Preservation of the limb with removal of a tumour

malignancy A cancerous condition

metastasis A second lesion developing away from the primary lesion

myelosuppression Reduction in the blood-forming cells made in the bone marrow

neoplasm A mass of newly formed tissue

oncology The study of cancer

radiotherapy Treatment by means of irradiation

staging Defining the phase of a disease

tumour lysis Rapid breakdown of malignant cells

aring for children with cancer presents unique challenges to nurses. Despite the dramatic improvements in survival, the needs of families are tremendous as they cope with a serious physical illness and the fear that their child may not survive. Nurses must maintain an up-to-date knowledge bank on which to base their practice in a rapidly developing field, and develop the interpersonal and educational skills to provide support throughout the acute and chronic phases of illness.

This chapter is primarily concerned with the physical problems associated with several types of childhood cancer. The general psychological needs of these children and their families are discussed in Chapter 20, in terms of chronic illness, and Chapter 21 with regard to life-threatening conditions.

CANCER IN CHILDREN

Cancer is the leading cause of death from disease in children aged 0-16 years and the second cause of death from all causes, exceeded only by road accidents. Cancer affects one child in 650, with about 1,200 new cases being diagnosed every year in the UK. For children in all age groups, leukaemia is the most common cancer, followed by brain tumours.

The most significant aspect of childhood cancer is the improved prognosis during the last three decades. Currently, more than 65% of all children with malignant neoplasms treated at major cancer centres will become long-term survivors (Robinson, 1993).

AETIOLOGICAL FACTORS

Low doses of radiotherapy have been associated with childhood cancer and some children appear to have a genetic predisposition to the disease. Children with Down's syndrome in particular have an increased risk of developing leukaemia (Poplack, 1993). The link between environmental radiation from nuclear power plants and increased incidence of leukaemia is, as yet, unsubstantiated (Bithall *et al*, 1994).

Children with immune deficiencies, or children whose immune system has been suppressed, such as following organ transplantation, are at a greater risk of developing various cancers. There is an increased risk of secondary cancers in some children successfully treated for their primary malignancy. This is becoming of major concern, as more intensive treatment regimens are now being used.

ASSESSMENT

When a child is suspected of having cancer, extensive diagnostic procedures are carried out to locate the primary site and any evidence of metastases. In addition to the initial workup, diagnostic tests are repeated regularly to assess the effectiveness of treatment. Consequently, the child is subjected to numerous noninvasive and invasive procedures, many of which cause considerable discomfort and anxiety; therefore, these children require much preparation and emotional support. The following is an overview of the more typical diagnostic procedures.

HISTORY AND PHYSICAL EXAMINATION

The history and physical examination are often the first indication of the presence of cancer. Vague complaints, such as fatigue, pain in a limb, night sweats, anorexia, headache and general malaise, may be the earliest signs and need to be taken seriously.

LABORATORY TESTS

Any number of laboratory tests may be performed, but most often a full blood count and chemistry, and urinalysis will be done. Malignancies of the blood-forming organs manifest signs early, and these frequently cause changed elements in the blood and increased production of immature cells. Since many of the chemotherapeutic agents depress bone marrow function, repeated blood counts are a constant feature of follow-up care.

Blood chemistry yields important information concerning renal function, liver function and electrolyte balance. Evaluation of renal and liver function is important not only for the detection of cancer or metastases to these organs, but also for monitoring during treatment because of the extra burden placed on these systems to metabolize and excrete the chemotherapeutic drugs.

A lumbar puncture (LP) is a routinely performed in leukaemia, brain tumours, and other cancers that may metastasize to the spinal cord and brain. (An LP is also performed to administer intrathecal drugs, such as methotrexate and cytosine arabinoside, when this mode of administration is part of the treatment protocol.)

IMAGING TECHNIQUES

Advances in imaging procedures have greatly aided in the diagnosis of solid tumours and have minimized the need for invasive techniques. In addition to x-rays, sophisticated imaging techniques such as computerized tomography (CT), ultrasound, nuclear scan, and magnetic resonance imaging (MRI) are carried out.

BIOPSY

As part of the diagnostic evaluation, biopsies are essential to determine the classification and stage of the disease. While the classification of the tumour may not change, the stage frequently does and is usually directly related to prognosis (the higher the stage, the poorer the prognosis).

Biopsies may be performed during surgical removal of the tumour. In the case of lymphomas, surgery may be performed specifically to obtain tissue samples of the spleen and involved lymph nodes. Easily accessed nodes, such as those in the cervical or axillary region, may be removed for biopsy.

Bone marrow studies are performed to assess the extent of disease in haematological disorders or when metastases are suspected.

TREATMENT

Because of the relatively small number of children with cancer, the UKCCSG (United Kingdom Children's Cancer Study Group) and the MRC (Medical Research Council) established collaborative groups of paediatric oncologists from different regions of the United Kingdom to systematically pool their information regarding treatment and other aspects of cancer care. Based on the evaluation of using different types of treatment, these experts plan and initiate comparative clinical trials or studies. During the past 30 years, the use of clinical trials and new protocols have been responsible for major advances in the approaches to cancer treatment.

SURGERY

The main goal of surgery, besides obtaining biopsies, is to remove all traces of tumour and restore normal body functioning. Surgery is most successful when the tumour is encapsulated and localized. It may only be palliative if the cancer has spread to other sites.

The recent trend is towards more conservative surgical excision. For example, in some types of bone cancer, such as osteosarcoma, patients are successfully treated with resection of the diseased portion of the bone, rather than amputation. There is an increasing emphasis on the use of combination drug therapy and radiotherapy after limited surgical intervention. Chemotherapy is frequently given before surgical removal to reduce tumour size and to monitor the response to drug treatment.

CHEMOTHERAPY

Chemotherapy, the use of drugs with antineoplastic capabilities, may be the primary form of treatment, or it may be used as an adjunct to surgery and/or radiotherapy. Although several agents have been found to be effective in treating different forms of cancer, the remarkable survival rates have been the result of improved combination drug regimens. Combining drugs allows for optimum cell-cycle destruction with minimal toxic effects and decreased resistance by the cancer cells to the agent.

The use of venous access devices, especially indwelling atrial catheters and implantable infusion ports, has greatly facilitated safe and effective drug administration with minimal discomfort for the child. Continuous infusions over an extended period using syringe pumps have made possible the administration of certain drugs, with less toxicity than when the drug is administered intermittently (Mioduszewski and Zarbo, 1987).

Chemotherapeutic agents are classified according to their cytotoxic action. The principal drugs used in the treatment of childhood cancer are summarized in Table 30-1. Unfortunately, the drugs are not selectively cytotoxic for malignant cells; therefore, other cells with a high rate of proliferation, such as the bone marrow, hair, skin, and epithelial cells of the gastrointestinal tract, are also affected. Frequently, the problems related to the destruction of these normal cells require more nursing intervention than the disease itself.

NURSING ALERT

Precautions in administering and handling chemotherapeutic agents

Many chemotherapeutic agents are vesicants (sclerosing agents) that can cause severe cellular damage if even minute amounts of the drug infiltrate surrounding tissue. Chemotherapeutic drugs must be given through a free-flowing intravenous line. The infusion is stopped *immediately* if any sign of infiltration (pain, stinging, swelling or redness at needle site) occurs. Only nurses experienced with chemotherapeutic agents should administer vesicants. Guidelines are available in individual units and must be followed meticulously, in order to prevent tissue damage to patients. Interventions for extravasation vary, but each nurse should be aware of local policies and implement them at once.

When chemotherapeutic and immunological agents are given, the child must be observed for 20 minutes after the infusion for signs of anaphylaxis (cyanosis, hypotension, wheezing, severe urticaria). Emergency equipment must be available.

If a reaction is suspected, the drug is discontinued, the intravenous line is flushed with saline, and the child's vital signs and subsequent responses are monitored.

Handling chemotherapeutic agents may present risks to handlers, especially if they are pregnant, although the exact degree of risk is not known.

RADIOTHERAPY

Radiotherapy is frequently used in the treatment of childhood cancer, usually in conjunction with chemotherapy and/or surgery. It can be used for curative purposes and is often employed for palliation to relieve symptoms by shrinking the size of the tumour. Recent advances in radiation therapy have optimized its beneficial effects and minimized many of the undesirable side effects (Tait, 1992), although high-dose radiation is associated with many serious late effects.

The acute untoward reactions from radiotherapy depend primarily on the area to be irradiated. Total-body irradiation (TBI) is associated with the most severe reactions and is employed in preparation for bone marrow transplantation.

Table 30-2 summarizes the acute effects of chemotherapy and radiation therapy, and nursing interventions that may be helpful in lessening or preventing them.

BIOLOGICAL THERAPIES

In recent years, much research has focused on biological therapy — the use of biological response modifiers (BRMs) to treat cancer. BRMs are agents or interventions that modify the relationship between tumour and host by therapeutically

AGENT ADMINISTRATION[b, f]	SIDE EFFECTS AND TOXICITY[c, d]	COMMENTS AND SPECIFIC NURSING[f] CONSIDERATIONS
Alkylating agents		
Cyclophosaphamide PO, IV, IM	N/V (3-4 hours later) (severe at high doses) BMD (10-14 days later) Alopecia Haemorrhagic cystitis Severe immunosuppression Stomatitis (rare) Hyperpigmenatation Transverse ridging of nails Infertility	Give dose early in day to allow adequate fluids afterward Maintaing fluid intake before administering drug and for 2 days after to prevent chemical cystitis; encourage frequent voiding even during night Warn parents to report signs of burning on urination or haematuria Test all urine passed for presence of blood
Ifosfamide IV	Haemorrhagic cystitis BMD (10-14 days later) Alopecia Neurotoxicity – lethargy, disorientation, somnolence, seizures (rare)	Mesna is given to reduce haemorrhagic cystitis Hydrate as with cyclophosphamide Myelosuppression less severe than with cyclophosphamide
Melphalan PO, IV	N/V (severe) BMD (2-3 weeks later) Diarrhoea Alopecia	Vesicant Give over 1 hour
Procarbazine PO	N/V (moderate) BMD (3–4 weeks later) Lethargy Dermatitis Myalgia Arthralgia Less commonly: Stomatitis Neuropathy Alopecia Diarrhoea	Central nervous system depressants (phenothiazines, barbiturates) enhance central nervous system symptoms Monoamine oxidase (MAO) inhibition sometimes occurs; therefore all other drugs are avoided unless medically approved; red wine, broad beans, broad bean pods, and yeast extracts (e.g., Marmite) are avoided

(cont.)

Table 30.1 Summary of chemotherapeutic agents used in the treatment of childhood cancers.
[a] Table includes principal drugs used in the treatment of childhood cancers. Several other conventional and investigational chemotherapeutic agents may be employed in the treatment regimen.
[b] IV, intravenous; IT, intrathecal; PO, by mouth; IM, intramuscular; SC, subcutaneous.
[c] N/V, nausea and vomiting. Mild = < 20% incidence; moderate = 20–70% incidence; severe = >75% incidence.
[d] BMD, bone marrow depression
[e] Vesicants (sclerosing agents) can cause severe cellular damage if even minute amounts of the drug infiltrate surrounding tissue. Only nurses experienced with chemotherapeutic agents should administer vesicants. The drugs must be given through a free-flowing intravenous line. The infusion is stopped *immediately* if any sign of infiltration (pain, stinging, swelling, or redness at needle site) occurs.
Interventions for extravasation vary, but each nurse should be aware of the local policies and impplement them at once.
[f] Abbreviation for a chemical compound.

Dacarbazine IV	N/V (especially after first dose) (severe) BMD (7-14 days later) Alopecia Flu-like syndrome Burning sensation in vein during infusion (not extravasation)	Vesicant[e] (less sclerosive) Must be given cautiously in patients with renal dysfunction
Cisplatin IV	Renal toxicity (severe) N/V (1-4 hours later) (severe) BMD (mild, 2-3 weeks later) Ototoxicity Electrolyte disturbances, especially hypomagnesium, hypocalcaemia, hypokalaemia, and hypophosphataemia Anaphylactic reactions may occur	Renal function must be assessed before giving drug Must maintain hydration before and during therapy (specific gravity of urine is used to assess hydration) Mannitol may be given IV to promote osmotic diuresis and drug clearance Monitor intake and output Monitor for signs of ototoxicity (e.g., ringing in ears), ensure that routine audiogram is done before treatment for baseline and routinely during treatment Monitor for signs of electrolyte loss, i.e. hypomagnesium - tremors, spasm, muscle weakness, lower extremity cramps, irregular heartbeat, convulsions, delirium Have emergency drugs at bedside[g]
Carboplatin IV	Similar to cisplatin but less oto/nephrotoxic BMD mainly united to thrombocytopenia.	
Alkalating agents Chlorambucil PO	N/V (mild) BMD (7-14 days later) Diarrhoea Dermatitis Less commonly may be hepatotoxicity	Usually slow onset of side effects; side effects related to high doses

(cont.)

Table 30.1 Summary of chemotherapeutic agents used in the treatment of childhood cancers *(continued)*.
[g] Emergency drugs include oxygen and parenteral preparations of adrenaline 1:1000, diphenhydramine or similar antihistamine, aminophylline, corticosteroids, and vasopressors.

Antimetabolites

Cytosine arabinoside IV, IM, SC, IT	N/V (mild) BMD (7-14 days later) Mucosal ulceration Immunosuppression Hepatitis (usually subclinical)	Crosses blood-brain barrier Use with caution in patients with hepatic dysfunction
5-Azacytidine IV	N/V (moderate) BMD 7-14 days later) Diarrhoea	Infuse slowly via IV drip to decrease severity of N/V
Mercaptopurine (6-MP) PO	N/V (mild) Diarrhoea Anorexia Stomatitis BMD (4-6 weeks later) Immunosuppression Dermatitis Less commonly may be hepatic dysfunction	6-MP is an analogue of xanthine; therefore allopurinol delays its metabolism and increases its potency, necessitating a lower dose (0.3 to 0.25) of 6-MP

Methotrexate (MTX) PO,
IV, IM, IT
May be given in conventional
doses (mg/m^2) or high doses (g/m^2)
	N/V
	Diarrhoea
	Mucosal ulceration (2-5 days later)
	BMD (10 days later)
	Immunosuppression
	Dermatitis
	Photosensitivity
	Alopecia (uncommon)
	Toxic effects include:
	Hepatitis (fibrosis)
	Osteoporosis
	Nephropathy
	  Pneumonitis (fibrosis)
	   Neurologic toxicity with IT use -
	   pain at injection site
		Side effects and
		toxicity are dose related
		Potency and toxicity
		increased by reduced
		renal function,
		salicylates,
		sulfonamides, and
		aminobenzoic acid;
		avoid use of these
		substances
		High-dose therapy:
		  Folinic acid or
		  leucovorin decreases
		  cytotoxic action of
		  MTX; used as an
		  antidote for overdose
		  and to enhance normal
		  cell recovery following
		  high-dose therapy; avoid
		  use of vitamins containing
		  folic acid during
		  MTX therapy unless
		  prescribed by doctor
		  Report signs of neurotoxicity

6-Thioguanine (6-TG) PO	N/V (mild)
	BMD (7-14 days later)
	Stomatitis
	Rarely:
	  Dermatitis
	  Photosensitivit
	  Liver dysfunction
		Side effects are
		unusual

(cont.)

Table 30.1 Summary of chemotherapeutic agents used in the treatment of childhood cancers *(continued)*.

Plant alkaloids

Vincristine IV	Neurotoxicity - paraesthesia (numbness); ataxia; weakness; footdrop; constipation (paralytic ileus); hoarseness (vocal cord paralysis); abdominal, chest, and jaw pain; mental depression Fever N/V (mild) BMD (minimal; 7-14 days later) Alopecia	Vesicant[e] Report signs of neurotoxicity (individuals with underlying neurological problems may be more prone to neurotoxicity) Monitor stool patterns closely; administer stool softener Excreted pimarily by liver into bilary system; administer cautiously to anyone with biliary disease
Vinblastine IV	Neurotoxicity (same as for vincristine but less severe) N/V (mild) BMD (especially neutropenia; 7-14 days later) Alopecia	Same as for vincristine
VP-16-213 IV, O	N/V (mild to moderate) BMD (7-14 days later) Alopecia Hypotension with rapid infusion Bradycardia Diarrhoea (infrequent) Stomatitis (rare) May reactivate erythema of irradiated skin (rare) Allergic reaction with anaphylaxis possible.	Give as slow IV infusion Have emergency drugs available at bedside[g]

Antibiotics

Actinomycin-D (ACT-D) IV	N/V (2-5 hours later) (moderate) BMD (especially platelets; 7-14 days later) Immunosuppression Mucosal ulceration Abdominal cramps Diarrhoea Anorexia (may last a few weeks) Alopecia Acne Erythema or hyperpigmentation of previously irradiated skin Fever Malaise	Vesicant[e] Enhances cytotoxic effects of radiation therapy but increases toxic effect May cause serious desquamation of irradiated tissue
Doxorubicin IV	N/V (moderate)	Vesicant[e]

(cont)

Table 30.1 Summary of chemotherapeutic agents used in the treatment of childhood cancers *(continued)*.

	Stomatitis	(extravasation may
	BMD (7-14 days later)	*not* cause pain)
	Fever, chills	Warn parents that
	Local phlebitis	drug causes urine to
	Alopecia	turn red (for up to 12
	Cumulative-dose toxicity:	days after administration);
	Cardiac abnormalities	this is normal, not haematuria
	Heart failure	
Daunorubicin IV	Similar to doxorubicin	Similar to doxorubicin
Bleomycin IV, IM, SC	Allergic reaction – fever, chills, hypotension, anaphylaxis	Should give test dose (SC) before
	Fever (nonallergic)	therapeutic dose
	N/V (mild)	administered
	Stomatitis	Have emergency
	Cumulative dose effects include:	drugs[g] at bedside
	Skin – rash, hyperpigmentation, thickening,	Hypersensitivity
	ulceration, peeling, nail changes, alopecia	occurs with first one
	Lungs – pneumonitis with infiltrate that	to two doses
	can progress to fatal fibrosis	Concentration of drug in skin and lungs accounts for toxic effects

Hormones

Corticosteroids (prednisolone most frequently used) PO; also IM or IV but rarely used	For short-term use, no acute toxicity	Explain expected effects, especially
	Usual side effects are mild; moon face,	especially in terms
	fluid retention, weight gain, mood changes,	of body Image,
	increased appetite, gastric irritation, insomnia,	increased appetite, and
	susceptibility to infection	personality changes
		Monitor weight gain
		Recommend moderate salt restriction
		Administer after food or milky drink
		May need to disguise bitter taste
		(crush tablet and mix with
		syrup, jam, ice cream, or
		other highly flavoured substance
		Observe for potential
		infection sites; usual
		inflammatory response and
		fever are absent
	Long term effects of chronic steroid	Same as for short-
	administration are mood changes,	term use; in addition,
	hirsutism, trunk obesity, thin extremities,	encourage foods high
	muscle wasting and weakness, osteoporosis,	in potassium
	poor wound healing, bruising, potassium loss	(bananas, raisins,
	gastric bleeding, hypertension, diabetes mellitus,	prunes, coffee, chocolate)
	growth retardation	Test stools for occult blood
		Monitor blood pressure
		Test urine for sugar

(cont.)

Table 30.1 Summary of chemotherapeutic agents used in the treatment of childhood cancers *(continued)*.

		Observe for signs of abrupt steroid withdrawal; flu-like symptoms, hypotension, hypoglycaemia, shock
Enzymes		
L-Asparaginase IV, IM	Allergic reactions (including anaphylactic shock)	Have emergency
	Fever	drugs at bedside[g]
	N/V (mild)	Record signs of
	Anorexia	allergic reaction, such
	Weight loss	as urticaria, facial
	Toxicity:	oedema, hypotension,
	Liver dysfunction	or abdominal cramps
	Hyperglycaemia	Check weight daily
	Renal failure	
	Pancreatitis	
Nitrosoureas		
Carmustine IV	N/V (2-6 hours later) (severe)	Prevent extravasation; contact with
Lomustine PO	BMD (3-4 weeks later)	skin causes brown spots
	Burning pain along IV infusion (usually due to alcohol diluent)	Oral form – give 4 hours after meals when stomach is empty
	BCNU – flushing and facial burning on infusion	Reduce IV burning by diluting drug and infusing slowing via IV drip
	Alopecia	Crosses blood-brain barrier
Other Agents		
Hydroxyurea PO	N/V (mild)	Must be given cautiously in patients
	Anorexia	with renal dysfunction
	Less commonly:	
	Diarrhaea	
	BMD	
	Mucosal ulceration	
	Alopecia	
	Dermatitis	

Table 30.1 Summary of chemotherapeutic agents used in the treatment of childhood cancers (*continued*).

changing the host's biological response to tumour cells. BRMs may affect the host's immunological mechanisms (immunotherapy), have direct antitumour activity, or have other biological effects (Yasko and Dudjak, 1990).

Much of the current work in biotherapy is directed towards the use of *monoclonal antibodies* in diagnosis and treatment of cancers. Through a complex process, special cells are fused to form a hybrid clone that produces antibodies that recognize a single specific antigen, hence the term *monoclonal antibody* ('mono' meaning one and 'clone' meaning exact duplicate). These clones are then frozen, maintained in culture, or grown as tumours in mice to produce large quantities of the antibody in ascites fluid (Weinberg and Parkman, 1989).

Peripheral blood stem cell transplants (PBSCT) have only recently been developed and have been made possible by the use of haematopoietic growth factors such as granulocyte macrophage colony stimulating factor (GMCSF). These growth factors, which can be produced in the laboratory, occur naturally in the body and control the production of new blood cells in the bone marrow. Growth factors can be injected to stimulate the bone marrow to produce large numbers of new immature normal cells, which spill out into the bloodstream and can then be extracted from it. They can be returned to the patient after high dose treatment, either as PBSCT or to augment an autologous bone marrow transplant (Mitchell *et al*, 1994).

Growth factors may also be administered following high dose chemotherapy to reduce the duration of neutropenia, and thus the risk of infection.

BONE MARROW TRANSPLANTATION

Another approach to the treatment of childhood cancer is bone marrow transplantation (BMT). Candidates for transplantation are children who have malignancies that are unlikely to be cured by other means. BMT allows for lethal doses of chemotherapy, often combined with radiation therapy, to be given in order to rid the body of all cancer cells. Once the body is free of malignant cells, and the immune system is suppressed to prevent rejection of the transplanted marrow, the donor marrow cells or the cells previously stored from the patient's own marrow are given to the patient by intravenous transfusion. The newly transfused marrow will then begin to produce functioning, nonmalignant blood cells.

Presently, three types of transplants may be done:
- **Allogeneic,** which involves matching a histocompatible donor, usually a sibling, with the recipient; may also involve a matched unrelated donor (MUD).
- **Autologous,** which uses the patient's own marrow or stem cells from peripheral blood (PBSCT).
- **Syngeneic,** which uses marrow from an identical twin.

The most common type of bone marrow transplantation is allogeneic. The selection process of a suitable donor and the potential complications in transplantation are related to the human leukocyte antigen (HLA).

SITE/EFFECTS	NURSING INTERVENTIONS	SITE/EFFECTS	NURSING INTERVENTIONS
Gastrointestinal tract		**Head**	
Nausea/vomiting	Give regular antiemetic Measure amount of emesis to prevent dehydration	Nausea/vomiting (from stimulation of vomiting centre in brain)	Same as for gastrointestinal tract
Anorexia	Encourage fluids and foods best tolerated, usually light, soft diet and small, frequent meals	Alopecia	Same as for skin Encourage regular dental care, fluoride treatments
	Minor weight loss	Potential effects	
Mucosal ulceration	Use frequent mouthwashes and oral hygiene to prevent mucositis	Parotitis	May need analgesics to relieve discomfort
		Loss of taste	
Diarrhoea	Can be controlled with antispasmodics and kaolin preparations Observe for signs of dehydration	Xerostomia (dry mouth)	Combat severe dryness of mouth with oral hygiene and liquid diet
		Urinary bladder	
		Rarely cystitis	More likely to occur with concomitant use of cyclophosphamide Encourage liberal fluid intake and frequent voiding Evaluate for haematuria
Skin			
Alopecia (within 2 weeks; begins to regrow by 3-6 months)	Introduce idea of wig Stress necessity of scalp hygiene and need for head covering in cold weather		
Dry or moist desquamation	Do not refer to skin change as a 'burn' (implies use of too much radiation) Keep skin clean Wash daily, using water Do not remove skin marking for radiation fields Avoid exposure to sun For dryness, apply lubricant For desquamation, consult dermatologist	**Bone marrow**	
		Myelosuppression	Observe for pyrexia Avoid use of suppositories rectal temperatures Observe signs of anaemia Observe signs of low platelets

Table 30.2 Early side effects of radiotherapy

The importance of HLA matching is to prevent the serious complication known as *graft–versus–host disease (GVHD)*. Since the child's immune system is essentially rendered 'nonfunctional' prior to the transplant, there is little difficulty with bone marrow rejection by the recipient. However, the donor's marrow has a normal, competent immune system, and may contain antigens not matched to the recipient's antigens, which begin attacking body cells. The more closely the HLA systems match, the less likely GVHD is to develop.

Although the actual transplant procedure is simple, prevention of complications is less so. During the aplastic phase, and for the 10- to 20-day period after transplantation, before the new marrow engrafts, the child is extremely susceptible to infection. The potential benefits and risks to each individual child must be considered before embarking on any transplant procedure (Treleaven and Barrett, 1992).

COMPLICATIONS OF THERAPY

Although tremendous advances have been achieved through current modes of cancer therapy, the successes are not without consequences. Numerous side effects are expected with chemotherapy and radiotherapy, and these are discussed under Nursing Care of the Child with Cancer. Other complications that are less frequently seen, but generally more serious and possibly permanent, are described here.

PAEDIATRIC ONCOLOGICAL EMERGENCIES

Life-threatening conditions may develop in children with cancer as a result of aggressive treatment modalities or from the malignancy itself. Rapid tumour lysis can be potentially dangerous, leading to hyperuricaemia, hypocalcaemia, hyperphosphataemia and hyperkalaemia (Mahon and Casperson, 1993). This occurs when massive cellular damage from cytotoxic therapy releases large amounts of uric acid, which can accumulate and precipitate in the renal tubules, eventually causing tubular obstruction (tumour lysis syndrome). Allopurinol prevents the metabolic breakdown of xanthine to uric acid and should be administered to prevent such an emergency in the newly diagnosed or relapsed patient receiving high dose chemotherapy.

Obstruction may create an emergency for a child with cancer. Space-occupying lesions (especially from Hodgkin's disease and non-Hodgkin's lymphoma [NHL]), located in the chest may cause superior vena cava obstruction, leading to airway compromise and potentially to respiratory failure. Children may have a mass obstructing the spinal cord, as manifested by symptoms ranging from tingling to paraesthesias, and loss of bowel and bladder control. Children with brain tumours may develop symptoms ranging from increased intracranial pressure to respiratory compromise and herniation, depending on the location and size of the tumour (Heideman *et al*, 1993).

Infections in the immunocompromised child can constitute an emergency situation. Gram-negative sepsis can result in numerous complications, including disseminated intravascular coagulation (DIC), created by a bacteria or fungus causing damage to the endothelial system. As a result, life-threatening haemorrhage or leukocytosis may occur.

LONG-TERM SEQUELAE OF TREATMENT

Vigorous treatment of childhood cancers has resulted in dramatically improved survival rates. It is estimated that by the year 2000 one young person in 1,000 will have survived childhood cancer (Meadows and Hobbie, 1986). However, treatment programmes combining surgery, irradiation and chemotherapy are not without their complications. Some may occur immediately, such as loss of a limb from surgical amputation. Others may occur much later. Concern regarding the late effects of treatment is increasing, because of the greater number of children who are cured and surviving into adulthood (Morris-Jones, 1991). Table 30-3 shows that few organs are exempt from the toxicity of cancer treatment. Although many factors influence the development of late effects from radiation or chemotherapy, some of the more important ones include the total cumulative dose given, the age of the child (the younger the child, the more radiosensitive the body organs), and the location of the tumour. As a general principle, cytotoxic therapy is more harmful to rapidly growing tissue than to slowly growing tissue.

NURSING CARE OF THE CHILD WITH CANCER

The child with cancer presents a challenge to the nurse providing care for hospitalized children, as well as children returning to the outpatient setting.

Nursing care of children with cancer is directly related to the regimen of therapy. Education is a constant feature of the nursing role, especially in terms of new treatments, clinical trials and home care. It is important that the family are given as much support as possible and that emphasis is placed on returning to 'normality'.

PREVENTION OF COMPLICATIONS OF MYELOSUPPRESSION

A delicate balance must be maintained between killing malignant cells and preserving healthy cells. Supportive therapy is critical when normal tissues are damaged. Some types of malignancies (leukaemia, lymphoma) and most of the chemotherapeutic agents cause myelosuppression. The reduced numbers of blood cells result in secondary problems of infection, bleeding tendencies and anaemia. Supportive care involves both medical and nursing management.

Infection

A life-threatening complication of treatment for childhood cancer is overwhelming infection secondary to neutropenia. The nurse caring for the child with a fever must be aware of the signs and symptoms of septic shock (see Chapter 24).

The child is most susceptible to overwhelming infection during three phases of the disease: (1) at the time of diagnosis and relapse when the cancer process has replaced normal leukocytes, (2) during immunosuppressive therapy, and (3) after prolonged antibiotic therapy, which predisposes the child to the growth of resistant organisms.

The child with fever is evaluated for potential sites of infection, such as from a needle puncture, central line site, mucosal ulceration, anal fissures, minor abrasion, or skin tears (e.g., a hangnail). Although the body may not be able to produce an adequate inflammatory response to the infection, and the usual clinical signs of infection may be partially expressed or absent, fever will occur. Therefore, temperature is monitored closely. To identify the source of infection, blood, stool, urine and nasopharyngeal cultures, and chest x-ray films may be taken. If a **neutropenic** child develops a fever, treatment is initiated immediately, with intravenous broad-spectrum antibiotics.

The first defence against infection is prevention. When the child is hospitalized, all measures to control transfer of infection are instituted, such as the use of a private room, restriction of all visitors and health personnel with active infection, and strict handwashing technique with an antiseptic solution. The use of protective (reverse) isolation is controversial;

SYSTEMIC EFFECTS/ CLINICAL MANIFESTATION	ASSOCIATED MODE OF TREATMENT
Central nervous system (CNS)	
Leukoencephalopathy (syndrome ranging from lethargy, dementia, and seizures to quadriplegia and death)	Methotrexate and/or CNS irradiation
Mineralizing microangiopathy (headaches, focal seizures, incoordination, gate abnormalities)	Methotrexate and/or CNS irradiation
Peripheral neuropathy (footdrop, incoordination)	Vincristine
Cognitive deficits (intelligence, nonlanguage skills)	Intrathecal chemotherapy and/or cranial irradiation (especially before age 3 years)
Cardiovascular	
Cardiomyopathy (tachycardia, tachypnoea, dyspnoea, shortness of breath, oedema, palpitations)	Anthracyclines (doxorubicin and daunorubicin) and/or irradiation to heart High dose cyclophosphamide
Pericardial damage (pleural effusion, cardiomegaly)	Mediastinal irradiation
Respiratory	
Pneumonitis (dyspnoea, nonproductive cough, fever)	Lung irradiation, alkylating agents, possibly bleomycin, vinblastine, cisplatin
Pulmonary fibrosis (dyspnoea, restrictive ventilation, decreased exercise tolerance)	
Gastrointestinal	
Chronic enteritis (colic, abdominal pain, vomiting, diarrhoea, constipation, bleeding)	Abdominal irradiation, methotrexate, cytosine arabinoside
Hepatic fibrosis (jaundice, hepatomegaly)	Methotrexate, 6-mercaptopurine
Urinary	
Haemorrhagic cystitis (chronic microscopic haematuria to gross haemorrhage)	Cyclophosphamide; cisplatin; irradiation, especially in combination with anthracyclines
Bladder fibrosis (decreased bladder capacity, ureteral reflux)	
Tubular necrosis (decreased creatinine clearance)	Cisplatin

(cont.)

Table 30-3 Late effects of cancer treatment.

Endocrine	
Growth retardation (abnormal growth velocity)	Irradiation to the thyroid, pituitary gland,
Thyroid dysfunction	testes, ovaries
Gonadal dysfunction (see Reproductive)	
Reproductive	
Possible gonadal damage - both sexes (amenorrhoea, de-creased sperm counts, increased follicle-stimulating and luteinizing hormones (FSH, LH), decreased testosterone/oestrogen)	Alkylating agents Irradiation to the pituitary gland, testes, ovaries
Skeletal	
Linear growth retardation (short stature)	Irradiation, long-term steroids
Spinal deformities, scoliosis, kyphosis, asymmetric growth, pathological fractures	Irradiation
Immune	
Asplenia (overwhelming infection, fever)	Splenectomy (Hodgkin's disease)
Sensory organs	
Cataracts (opacity over pupil)	Cranial irradiation, high-dose steroids
Hearing (decreased hearing associated with high-frequency loss)	Cisplatin
Additional effects	
Dental problems	
Increased caries, periodontal disease, hypoplastic teeth, hypodontia (delayed or absent tooth development)	Irradiation to maxilla and mandible
Second malignancies	
Bone and soft tissue tumours	Irradiation, alkylating agents
Leukaemia	
Nonlymphocytic leukaemia	

Table 30-3 Late effects of cancer treatment (*continued*).

however, research provides evidence that protective isolation does *not* decrease the risk of infection nor improve survival (Frenck, Kohl and Pickering, 1991) (recommendations will vary according to local treatment centre policy).

Prevention of infection continues after discharge from hospital. However, social restriction must be tempered with the child's need for resuming normal activity. The child should be encouraged to return to school as soon as possible.

Nutrition is another important component of infection prevention. An adequate protein-calorie intake provides the child with better defences against infection, and increased tolerance to chemotherapy and irradiation. However, providing optimum nutrition during periods of anorexia and vomiting from chemotherapy is a tremendous challenge. Every effort is made to encourage the child to eat (see Feeding the Sick Child, Chapter 8). Nasogastric feeds or total parenteral nutri-

tion are instituted if necessary, and meticulous care is implemented to prevent infection.

Immunizations

Measles and chickenpox can be potentially fatal for immunocompromised children. Viral replication following the administration of live vaccine for polio, measles, rubella and mumps can also cause serious disease in immunocompromised children who receive them. The *inactivated* poliovirus vaccine should be given to immunosuppressed children and their household contacts in place of the routine immunization with the oral poliovirus. Children who have not received chemotherapy for at least one year can be given live vaccines. Children who are immunosuppressed can receive varicella (chickenpox) immunoglobulin (ZIG), but should receive it within 48 hours of exposure.

Haemorrhage

Before the use of transfused platelets, haemorrhage was a leading cause of death in children with some types of cancer. Now, most bleeding episodes can be prevented or controlled with judicious administration of platelets.

Since infection increases the tendency to haemorrhage, and bleeding sites become more easily infected, special care is taken to avoid performing skin punctures whenever possible. When fingerpricks, venepunctures, intramuscular injections and bone marrow aspirations are performed, an aseptic technique must be employed with continued observation for bleeding.

Meticulous mouth care is essential, since gingival bleeding with resultant mucositis is a frequent problem. Since the rectal area is prone to ulceration from various drugs, strict hygiene is essential. To prevent additional trauma, rectal temperatures and suppositories are avoided. Frequent turning, the use of a flotation or alternating-pressure mattress, and sheepskin under bony prominences prevent development of pressure sores.

The child with a platelet count of less than 20 x 10⁹/l should be assessed closely for signs of active bleeding. Petechiae are often one of the first signs of a low platelet count.

Children at home who have low platelet counts are advised to avoid those activities that might cause injury or bleeding, such as riding bicycles or skateboards, roller skating and contact sports. These restrictions can be terminated once the platelet count rises.

Anaemia

Initially anaemia may be profound, due to the complete replacement of the bone marrow by cancer cells. During induction therapy, blood transfusions with packed red cells may be necessary to raise haemoglobin to levels approaching 10 g. The usual precautions in caring for the child are instituted (see Chapter 29).

Anaemia is also a consequence of drug induced myelosuppression. Although not as severely affected as the white blood cells, erythrocyte production may be delayed. Since children have an amazing capacity to withstand low haemoglobin levels, the best approach is to allow the child to regulate activity with reasonable adult supervision. It may be necessary for the parents to alert the schoolteacher to the child's physical limitations regarding strenuous activity.

MANAGEMENT OF PROBLEMS RELATED TO IRRADIATION AND DRUG TOXICITY

Irradiation and chemotherapy present several challenges to providing effective care. The complexity of the treatment protocols alone is often overwhelming to families. In addition, each therapy is associated with several predictable side effects. The following is a discussion of common problems and appropriate interventions.

Nausea and vomiting

The nausea and vomiting that occur shortly after administration of several of the drugs, and as a result of cranial or abdomina radiation, can be profound. Although several antiemetic agents are available, no product is uniformly successful in controlling the vomiting. For mild to moderate vomiting, antiemetics such as prochlorperazine or metoclopramide may be effective. Unfortunately, both drugs can cause several side effects in children, particularly extrapyramidal reactions.

A drug that has yielded promising results is THC (delta-9-tetrahydrocannabinol), the active component of marijuana. Synthetic cannabinoids are now being used in children undergoing chemotherapy.

Ondansetron, a 5-HT3 receptor antagonist, is probably the most effective antiemetic presently available (Pinkerton *et a*, 1990); unfortunately, the cost of this drug still limits its use.

The most beneficial regimen for antiemetic control has been the administration of the antiemetic *before* the chemotherapy begins (30 minutes to one hour before) and regular (not PRN) administration every two, four, or six hours for at least 24 hours after chemotherapy. There is some evidence that beginning antiemetic therapy up to 24 hours before the chemotherapy adds additional effectiveness (Williams *et al*, 1989). The goal is to prevent the child from ever experiencing nausea or vomiting, and to prevent the development of anticipatory symptoms.

Anorexia

Loss of appetite is a direct consequence of the chemotherapy and/or radiation. It is a major problem for parents, because it is the one area they feel responsible for, particularly when so many other facets of care are outside their control.

The following theories have been postulated to explain persistent anorexia: (1) a physical cause related to the cancer that is nonspecific; (2) a conditioned aversion to food from nausea and vomiting during treatment; (3) stress in the environment, related to eating and/or to the child's condition; and (4) depression. When loss of appetite and weight persists, the nurse should investigate the family situation to determine if any of these variables are contributing to the problem. To prevent conditioned aversion to food, it is best to offer few foods and no favourite foods before chemotherapy.

Mucosal ulceration

One of the most distressing side effects of several drugs is gastrointestinal mucosal cell damage, which results in ulcers anywhere along the alimentary tract. Oral ulcers (stomatitis) are red, eroded, painful areas in the mouth and/or pharynx (see also Stomatitis, Chapter 16). They greatly compound anorexia, because eating is extremely uncomfortable. When oral ulcers develop, the following interventions are helpful: (1) a bland, moist, soft diet; (2) use of soft sponge toothbrush; and (3) frequent mouthwashes, according to local policy. Although local anaesthetics are effective in temporarily relieving pain, many children dislike the taste and numb feeling they produce.

An unclean mouth is a potential source of infection and a sore mouth can be extremely distressing. Mouth care must be carried out carefully and regularly, and children should have a dental assessment prior to commencing treatment.

Protocols for oral care during myelosuppression vary according to the institution. Chlorhexidine gluconate is used at many institutions because of its dual effectiveness against candidal as well as bacterial infections. *Candida* prophylaxis using antifungal agent is routinely used in patients with prolonged myelosuppression.

Administering mouth care is particularly difficult in infants and toddlers. A satisfactory method of cleaning the mouth is to wrap a piece of gauze around a gloved finger, soaked with the appropriate solution. Forceps should never be used. Mouth care should be done routinely after meals and at bedtime, and as often as every 2-4 hours to rid mucosal surfaces of debris, which becomes an excellent medium for bacterial and fungal growth.

Difficulty in eating is a major problem with stomatitis and may warrant hospitalization if the child refuses fluids. The child will usually choose the foods that are best tolerated. Surprisingly, some children prefer salty foods to more bland ones. Drinking can usually be encouraged if a straw is used to bypass the ulcerated oral mucosa.

Rectal Ulceration

If rectal ulcers develop, meticulous toilet hygiene after each bowel movement is vital to reduce the risk of infection. The use of stool softeners is necessary to prevent further discomfort. The child may voluntarily avoid defaecation to prevent discomfort. Rectal thermometers and suppositories are avoided because they may further traumatize the area.

Neurological problems

Vincristine, and to a lesser extent vinblastine, can cause various neurotoxic effects, one of the more common of which is severe constipation and possible paralytic ileus from decreased bowel innervation. Constipation is further aggravated by opioids. Bowel movements must be carefully documented and parents should be advised to report any problems or changes in stool habits. Physical activity and stool softeners are helpful in preventing constipation, but laxatives or enemas may be necessary to stimulate evacuation. Dietary changes such as increased fibre are not advised, because the increased bulk tends to increase faecal distention and discomfort without producing the necessary mechanical stimulation.

Footdrop, weakness and numbing of the extremities may cause difficulty in walking or fine hand movement. The nurse should look for these problems and warn parents of these side effects, which are reversible once the drug is stopped.

A neurological syndrome (postirradiation somnolence) may develop 5-8 weeks after central nervous system irradiation and may last from 4-15 days. It is characterized by somnolence with or without fever, anorexia, and nausea and vomiting. Parents should be warned of the possibility of such symptoms and encouraged to seek medical evaluation, since somnolence may be an early indicator of long-term neurological sequelae after cranial irradiation.

Alopecia

Hair loss is a side effect of several chemotherapeutic drugs and cranial irradiation. Not all children lose their hair during drug therapy; however, retaining hair is the exception rather than the rule. It is better to warn children and parents of this side effect, than to allow them to think that it is only a remote possibility.

The family should know that the hair falls out in clumps, causing patchy baldness. To lessen the trauma of seeing large amounts of hair on bed linen or clothing, the child and family may decide to cut the hair short. Families should also be aware that wigs are available and that hair regrows in 3-6 months. The hair frequently is darker, thicker and curlier than before.

If the child chooses not to wear a wig, attention to some type of head covering is important, especially in cold or sunny climates. Scalp hygiene is also important. The scalp should be washed regularly, as with any other body part, but soap and friction must be avoided during cranial irradiation.

BONE MARROW TRANSPLANTATION

The needs of the family are great when bone marrow transplantation is expected. These children may be hospitalized for many weeks and are usually in a medical centre that specializes in this procedure. Because of the risk of infection, the unit may employ strict protective isolation, including laminar airflow to filter the air. Consequently, the child is faced with the additional trauma of isolation (see also Chapter 5) and must adhere to strict guidelines on personal hygiene.

The side effects and complications of the intense conditioning regimens are a challenge to nursing care. Such problems can be divided into three groups: (1) immediate (e.g., severe mucositis, parotitis, nausea, vomiting and diarrhoea), (2) intermediate (e.g., hair loss, interstitial pneumonia, drowsiness at 4-6 weeks) and (3) late effects (e.g., cataracts, sterility, growth impairment).

The four weeks post transplant are the most hazardous to children as they have no neutrophils or platelets, and the risk of haemorrhage and infection are great. Cytomegalovirus (CMV) can cause a potentially life-threatening pneumonia. Graft-versus-host disease (GVHD) where the T-lymphocytes in the donor's marrow recognize the host as a foreign protein and attack it, is another serious complication with a high mortality rate. It can affect the skin, gastrointestinal tract, liver, heart and lungs, lymphoid tissue and bone marrow. It is characterized by a hardening of the tissues and drying of the mucous membranes. Treatment involves the use of steroids, azathioprine or cyclosporine. During BMT, families will clearly be concerned about successful engraftment and fear of fatal complications. Consequently, nurses involved with the child and family need to provide sensitive care and to maintain a supportive attitude during the many crises that may arise.

FAMILY EDUCATION

Nurses working with children who have cancer play a significant supportive role in helping the family understand the various therapies, preventing or managing expected side effects or toxicities, and observing for late effects of treatment.

Instruction regarding home care frequently involves teaching about medication schedules, observation for side effects or toxicities that require further evaluation, measures to prevent or manage these problems, and care of special devices such as central venous catheters. Compliance is a very important issue; poor adherence to drug regimens may result in relapse (Davies, Lennard, and Lilleyman, 1993). Every effort must be made to ensure that the family understands the importance of adhering to the prescribed treatment schedule (see Chapter 8). The role of the paediatric oncology outreach nurse specialist has greatly enhanced support and education for families in the home setting.

THE CHILDHOOD CANCER SURVIVOR

With ever-increasing numbers of childhood cancer survivors, the legacy of their diagnosis and treatment becomes apparent. As they grow toward adulthood, these children and their families require complex care to meet their specific physical and psychosocial needs. A multidisciplinary teamwork approach is being developed in many specialist centres to meet these needs.

IMPLICATIONS FOR NURSING

Clinics designed to follow children who survive childhood cancer have become an essential part of the paediatric oncology service, and the nurse has a major responsibility within that setting.

Four systems, in particular, may develop complications unique to these children, and require careful assessment following therapy for cancer: (1) the central nervous system, (2) endocrine system, (3) reproductive system, and (4) skeletal system.

Nurses caring for young children with cancer must be aware of the impairment caused by treatment with cranial irradiation and intrathecal chemotherapy. Intellectual and motor function may be impaired because of interference with neural development before maturation of the brain is complete. Assessment of children who have received cranial radiation and intrathecal chemotherapy must incorporate an extensive neurological evaluation which includes cognitive function.

Radiation therapy to growing bones or reproductive glands responsible for growth-related hormones can delay or stunt growth. Nurses must document growth by assessing height and weight at each visit. Any decrease in growth velocity should be further evaluated. Further assessment includes documenting parental heights, obtaining a wrist x-ray film to predict further growth potential, and assessing gonadal development and pituitary function.

Radiation therapy and the alkylating agents can cause hormonal dysfunction, decreased fertility and sterility. The potential for gonadal dysfunction depends on the child's age, sex, type of treatment, and the duration and total doses of treatment. Nursing assessment must begin with careful documentation of the child's sexual development. Assessment of delayed or absent sexual development is discussed in Chapter 18.

Sterility or infertility can cause much distress and sensitive counselling will be required. Sperm banking for adolescent boys should be used prior to commencing treatment, if possible.

Radiation therapy to developing bone and cartilage may cause numerous abnormalities. Assessment includes close observation of the irradiated bone for defects, such as spinal kyphoscoliosis, leg length discrepancy, and skull and facial disfigurement.

Irradiated bones are more fragile and may fracture easily, have functional limitations, and may heal slowly in the presence of infection. Osteoporosis may develop. Children who have received radiation therapy to the mandibular area are at risk of dental caries, arrested tooth development and incomplete dental calcification. A careful assessment of the oral cavity in children who have received radiation therapy to the mandible is performed at each clinic visit.

In addition to physical effects, there is also concern for the psychological sequelae of surviving cancer (Eiser and Havermans, 1994). Long-term survivors have reported that their illness disrupted school attendance, resulted in academic difficulties, and altered future plans and peer relationships. While most youngsters adapted well, some developed emotional problems, specifically, symptoms related to depression and/or alcoholism (Lansky *et al*, 1985).

Regardless of the level of functioning at the time of cure, having cancer is a stressful experience, and nurses can play an important part in supporting and educating children and young people regarding the long-term effects of treatment.

CANCERS OF THE BLOOD AND LYMPH SYSTEMS

Leukaemias, Hodgkin's disease, and lymphomas arise in the blood and lymph systems. Children with all of these cancers have benefitted from improved methods of treatment in recent years, and a significant proportion of affected children will be long-term survivors.

LEUKAEMIAS

Leukaemia is a broad term given to a group of malignant diseases of the bone marrow and lymphatic system. It accounts for about one-third of childhood cancer and 80% of these are of the acute lymphoblastic type (ALL). Current 5-year survival rates for children with ALL approach 70%.

Morphology

Leukaemia is classified according to its predominant cell type and level of maturity, as described by the following:

- **Lympho** — for leukaemias involving the lymphoid or lymphatic system.
- **Myelo** — for those of myeloid (bone marrow origin).
- **Blastic and acute** — for those involving immature cells.
- **Cytic and chronic** — for those involving mature cells.

PATHOLOGICAL AND RELATED CLINICAL MANIFESTATIONS

Leukaemia is an unrestricted proliferation of immature white blood cells in the blood-forming tissues of the body (Fig. 30-1). The resultant pathology and clinical manifestations of the disease are caused by infiltration and replacement of any tissue of the body with nonfunctional leukaemic cells (blasts). Highly vascular organs, such as the spleen and liver, are the most severely affected.

Bone marrow dysfunction

In all types of leukaemia, the proliferating cells depress bone marrow production of the formed elements of the blood by competing for and depriving the normal cells of the essential nutrients for metabolism. The three main consequences are: (1) *anaemia* from decreased erythrocytes, (2) *infection* from neutropenia, and (3) *bleeding* from decreased platelet production.

The most frequent presenting signs and symptoms of leukaemia are a result of infiltration of the bone marrow. These include fever, pallor, fatigue, anorexia, haemorrhage (usually petechiae), and bone and joint pain. In the presence of neutropenia, the body's normal bacterial flora can become aggressive pathogens. Any break in the skin is a potential site of infection. Frequently, vague abdominal pain is caused by areas of inflammation from normal flora within the intestinal tract.

Disturbance of involved organs

The testes, spleen, liver and lymph glands may demonstrate marked infiltration, enlargement and eventually fibrosis with leukaemic cells.

Another important site of involvement is the central nervous system. Initially, leukaemic cells do not tend to invade this area, probably as a result of the protective blood-brain barrier. However, this normal protective mechanism also prevents the antileukaemic drugs, with the exception of a few agents, from entering the brain in sufficient therapeutic doses to be effective. Before prophylactic use of cranial irradiation and intrathecal methotrexate, central nervous system involvement was frequent in children who survived six months or more.

PROCESS OF DIAGNOSIS

Leukaemia is usually suspected from the history, physical manifestations, and a peripheral blood count that contains immature blast cells, frequently combined with low blood counts. Definitive diagnosis is based on bone marrow aspiration or biopsy. Typically, the bone marrow is hypercellular with primarily blast cells. Once the diagnosis is confirmed, a lumbar puncture is performed to determine if there is any central nervous system involvement.

THERAPEUTIC MANAGEMENT

Treatment of ALL involves the use of chemotherapeutic agents with or without cranial irradiation in three phases: (1) *induction*, which achieves a complete remission or disappearance of observable leukaemic cells; (2) CNS prophylactic therapy; and (3) continuing therapy, *maintenance with intensification* (**consolidation**). Throughout treatment, children are prescribed prophylactic co-trimoxazole to minimize the risk of developing *Pneumocystis carinii* pneumonia which can be potentially fatal for these children, due to prolonged immunosuppression.

CNS prophylaxis

Treatment for the central nervous system involves prophylactic treatment with cranial irradiation, and intravenous and/or intrathecal administration of chemotherapy. Because of concern regarding late endocrine and neuropsychological effects, cranial irradiation is generally reserved for high-risk patients and/or those with central nervous system disease (Chessels, 1994).

Bone marrow transplantation

Bone marrow transplants have been used successfully in treating some children with acute lymphocytic leukaemia (ALL) and acute myeloid leukaemia (AML). In general, bone marrow transplantation is not recommended for children with ALL during the first remission because of the excellent results possible with chemotherapy. Because of the poorer prognosis in children with AML, transplantation may be considered during first remission (Vega *et al*, 1987). Transplantation may be indicated in second remission for children in the 'better risk' categories who relapse after initial treatment.

Acute myeloid leukaemia

With AML the drug therapies differ from those used for lymphoid leukaemia. Treatment for AML is far more intensive than for ALL; high doses of chemotherapy are administered over a period of approximately six months, resulting in prolonged periods of profound neutropenia.

IMPLICATIONS FOR NURSING

Nursing care of the child with leukaemia is directly related to the regimen of therapy. Secondary complications that necessitate supportive physical care are caused by myelosuppression, drug toxicity and leukaemic infiltration. General aspects of care appropriate for the child with leukaemia have been discussed under Nursing Care of the Child with Cancer. Psychological interventions appropriate for children with leukaemia during significant phases of therapy are discussed in Chapter 21.

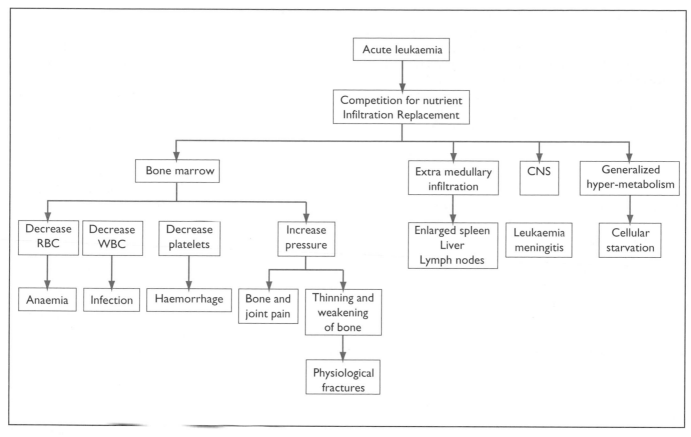

Fig. 30-1 Principal sites of tissue involvement in leukaemia.

LYMPHOMAS

The lymphomas are a group of neoplastic diseases that arise from the lymphoid and haematopoietic systems. They are usually divided into Hodgkin's disease and non-Hodgkin's lymphoma (NHL), and are subdivided according to tissue type and extent of disease (staging). Although Hodgkin's disease is extremely rare before five years of age, there is a striking increase between the ages of 15-19 years, when it occurs with almost the same frequency as leukaemia.

HODGKIN'S DISEASE

Hodgkin's disease originates in the lymphoid system and primarily involves the lymph nodes. It predictably metastasizes to non-nodal or extralymphatic sites, especially the spleen, liver, bone marrow, lungs and mediastinum.

CLINICAL STAGING AND PROGNOSIS

Accurate staging of the extent of disease is the basis for treatment protocols and expected prognosis.

Prognosis for patients with Hodgkin's disease has improved dramatically in the past few years, largely as a result of the sys-

tematic staging procedure and improved treatment protocols. The prognosis is excellent in children with localized disease. Even in children with disseminated disease, long-term remissions are possible in more than one-half of the patients. Overall, the cure rate is as high as 90% (Thompson, 1991). Unfortunately, a number of children may have late recurrences of the original disease or may develop a second malignancy, especially osteosarcoma, soft tissue sarcoma, thyroid carcinoma or leukaemia.

CLINICAL MANIFESTATIONS

Hodgkin's disease is characterized by painless enlargement of lymph nodes. The most common finding is enlarged, firm, non-tender, movable nodes in the supraclavicular area.

Other signs and symptoms depend on the extent and location of involvement. Systemic symptoms include low-grade and/or intermittent fever, anorexia, nausea, weight loss, night sweats or pruritus. Generally, such symptoms indicate advanced lymph node and extralymphatic involvement.

DIAGNOSTIC EVALUATION

The history and physical examination often yield important clues to the disease, such as fevers, night sweats or weight loss, and enlarged lymph nodes, spleen, or liver. Because of the multiple organs that can become involved, diagnosis consists of several tests to confirm the presence of Hodgkin's disease and to assess the extent of involvement for accurate staging. Tests include full blood count, liver function tests, urinalysis and erythrocyte sedimentation rate. Computed tomography (CT) of the chest, liver, spleen and bone is done to detect metastases. Biopsy is essential to diagnosis and staging. The enlarged lymph node is excised and analyzed for histological type.

THERAPEUTIC MANAGEMENT

The primary modes of therapy are radiation and chemotherapy. Each may be used alone or in combination. The decision is based on the clinical staging. The goal of treatment is obviously a cure; however, aggressive therapy increases the chances of complications in the disease-free state and can seriously compromise the quality of life. One of the major concerns with combined radiation and antineoplastic drug therapy is the serious late effects in children with an excellent prognosis, and follow-up care of children taken off therapy is essential to identify relapse, as well as second malignancies (Tucker *et al*, 1988).

IMPLICATIONS FOR NURSING

Nursing care involves the same objectives as for patients with other types of cancer. Since this is most often a disease of adolescents and young adults, the nurse must have an appreciation of their psychological needs and reactions during the diagnostic and treatment phases.

Explain treatments and side effects

The most common side effect of radiation is malaise, which may result from damage to the thyroid gland, causing hypothyroidism. Lack of energy is particularly difficult for adolescents, because it prevents them from keeping up with their peers. Sometimes adolescents will push themselves to the point of physical exhaustion rather than admit fatigue and succumb to the decreased activity tolerance. Follow-up care is essential to diagnose hypothyroidism early and to institute thyroid replacement therapy.

An area of concern for adolescents is the high risk of sterility from irradiation and chemotherapy. Both irradiation to the gonads and drugs, particularly procarbazine and alkylating agents, may lead to infertility, although sexual function is not altered. Younger females are more likely to retain ovarian function.

NON-HODGKIN'S LYMPHOMA

Histological classification of childhood NHL is strikingly different from that of Hodgkin's disease and from adult NHL in several respects (Sandlund, Hutchinson, and Crist, 1991):
- The disease is usually diffuse rather than nodular.
- The cell type is either undifferentiated or poorly differentiated.
- Dissemination occurs earlier, more often, and more rapidly.

STAGING AND PROGNOSIS

Non-Hodgkin's lymphoma is heterogeneous, exhibiting a variety of morphological, cytochemical and immunological features, not unlike the diversity seen in leukaemia. Classification is based on the pattern of histological presentation; namely, nodular (circumscribed) or diffuse (spread out). Immunologically, these cells are also classified as T-cells, B-cells (an example of which is Burkitt's lymphoma), or null cells, which lack specific immunological properties.

The clinical staging system used in Hodgkin's disease is of little value in NHL. Favourable prognosis is defined by: (1) lymph node involvement only and limited to one or two adjacent lymphatic regions (excluding the mediastinum); (2) an extranodal site in the nasopharynx, oropharynx or other isolated extranodal site, with or without regional lymphadenopathy; or (3) gastrointestinal involvement, with or without regional lymphadenopathy, limited to the mesentery (Magrath, 1993). The use of aggressive combination chemotherapy has had a major impact on the survival rates of children with NHL. The most effective treatment regimens result in cure in almost all children with limited disease involvement.

CLINICAL MANIFESTATIONS

Clinical manifestations depend on the anatomical site and extent of involvement. Many of those seen in Hodgkin's disease may be present in NHL, although rarely does a single symptom give rise to the diagnosis. Rather, metastases to the bone marrow or central nervous system may produce signs and symptoms typical of leukaemia. Lymphoid tumours compressing various organs may cause intestinal or airway obstruction, cranial nerve palsies, or spinal paralysis.

The exception to the usual presentation of NHL is Burkitt's lymphoma, a type of cancer that is rare in the United Kingdom, but endemic in parts of Africa. It is a rapidly growing neoplasm that is most commonly seen as a mass in the jaw, abdomen or orbit.

PROCESS OF DIAGNOSIS

Current recommendations for staging include a surgical biopsy for histopathological confirmation of disease with immuno-phenotyping and cytogenetics evaluation; bone marrow aspiration; radiological studies, especially CT scans of the lungs and gastrointestinal organs; and lumbar puncture.

THERAPEUTIC MANAGEMENT

The present treatment protocols for NHL include an aggressive approach using chemotherapy. At present, the differentiation between lymphoblastic lymphoma and all other lymphomas is widely used as a way to categorize patients for specific treatment regimens (Magrath, 1993).

IMPLICATIONS FOR NURSING

Nursing care of the child with NHL is very similar to the care discussed in the section, Nursing Care of the Child with Cancer. Because of the intensive chemotherapy protocol, nursing care is primarily directed towards managing the side effects of these agents.

NERVOUS SYSTEM TUMOURS

Two major forms of childhood cancer are derived from neural tissue. Brain tumours are the most common solid tumours that occur in children and are second only to leukaemia as a form of cancer. Neuroblastomas are the most common malignant tumours of infancy and are second only to brain tumours as the type of solid malignancy seen during the first ten years (Fernbach and Vietti, 1991). Both of these tumours have presented difficulties in identifying successful modes of treatment and have not demonstrated the dramatic improvements in survival seen in many other forms of cancer.

BRAIN TUMOURS

Most brain tumours (about 60%) are *infratentorial* (below the tentorium cerebelli), which means that they occur in the posterior third of the brain, primarily in the cerebellum or brain stem. This anatomical distribution accounts for the frequency of symptoms resulting from increased intracranial pressure. A smaller number are *supratentorial*, or within the anterior two thirds of the brain, mainly the cerebrum.

Because the neoplasms can arise from any cell within the cranium, it is possible to have tumours originating from the nerve cells, neuroepithelium, glia, cranial nerves, blood vessels, pineal gland and hypophysis. Within each of these structures, specific cells may be involved to provide a histological classification of the major tumours found in children.

CLINICAL MANIFESTATIONS

The signs and symptoms of brain tumours are directly related to their anatomical location and size, and to some extent, the age of the child. In infants, whose sutures are still open, virtually no early detectable symptoms develop. It is not until spinal fluid obstruction causes markedly increased head size that a lesion may be suspected. Head circumference allows for detection of increased intracranial pressure. Because the tumour typically grows to a large size before being diagnosed, prognosis in infants is generally poorer than in older children.

Even in older children, clinical manifestations may be nonspecific. However, the most common symptoms are headache, especially on awakening, and vomiting that is not related to feeding and is attributable to increased intracranial pressure.

PROCESS OF DIAGNOSIS

Diagnosis of a brain tumour is based subjectively on presenting clinical signs and objectively on neurological tests. Because the signs and symptoms are vague and easily overlooked, early diagnosis necessitates a high index of suspicion during history taking. Several tests may be employed in the neurological evaluation, but the most common diagnostic procedure is computed tomography (CT).

Magnetic resonance imaging (MRI) permits early diagnosis of brain tumours, as well as assessment of tumour growth during or following treatment. Definitive diagnosis is based on tissue specimens obtained during surgery.

THERAPEUTIC MANAGEMENT

Treatment may involve the use of surgery, radiotherapy and chemotherapy. All three may or may not be used, depending on the type of tumour. The treatment of choice is total removal of the tumour without residual neurological damage. Patients with the most complete tumour removal have the greatest chance of survival. Several surgical advances have allowed the biopsy and removal of tumours in areas previously considered too dangerous for traditional operative techniques. *Stereotactic surgery* involves the use of CT and MRI in conjunction with other special computer techniques to represent the size and shape of the tumour in three dimensions.

Radiotherapy is used to treat most tumours and to shrink the size of the tumour. The use of chemotherapy is controversial. However, if effective chemotherapy regimens are found, radiotherapy could be delayed, or even omitted, reducing the related morbidity (Pinkerton, Cushing, and Sepion, 1994). In addition, other drugs, such as corticosteroids, may be needed to manage complications, such as brain oedema.

The problems of treatment and relatively poor prognosis, especially in infants and young children, are compounded by the serious late effects of all three modes of therapy.

IMPLICATIONS FOR NURSING

Nursing care of the child with a brain tumour involves: (1) assessing for signs and symptoms related to the tumour, (2) preparing the child and parents for the diagnostic tests and operative procedure, (3) preventing postoperative complications, (4) planning for discharge, and (5) promoting a return to optimum functioning. The principles of care are similar, regardless of the type of intracranial lesion. Since a brain tumour is a potentially fatal diagnosis, the nurse is urged to incorporate the psychological interventions discussed in Chapter 21.

The realm of possible consequences following the diagnosis of a brain tumour is vast. They are not discussed here. Rather, the reader is urged to refer to other sections of the text that deal with possible outcomes, such as the paralysed, visually impaired, or unconscious child, or the care of a child with a ventricular shunt, epileptic disorder or meningitis. Numerous physical problems can occur with progression of the tumour that may necessitate the nurse to teach the family appropriate home care to allow the child the highest quality of life for the longest period of time. (See discussion of discharge planning and home care in Chapter 5.)

NEUROBLASTOMA

Neuroblastoma originates from embryonic neural crest cells that normally give rise to the adrenal medulla and the sympathetic ganglia. Consequently, the majority of the tumours arise from the adrenal gland or from the retroperitoneal sympathetic chain. The primary site is within the abdomen. Other sites may be within the head, neck, chest or pelvis.

CLINICAL MANIFESTATIONS

The signs and symptoms of neuroblastoma depend on the location and stage of the disease. Most presenting signs are caused by compression of adjacent structures. With abdominal tumours the most common presenting sign is a firm, nontender, irregular mass in the abdomen that crosses the midline (in contrast to Wilms' tumour, which is usually confined to one side).

Distant metastasis frequently causes supraorbital ecchymosis, periorbital oedema, and proptosis (exophthalmos) from invasion of retrobulbar soft tissue. Lymphadenopathy, especially in the cervical and supraclavicular areas, may also be an early presenting sign. Bone pain may or may not be present with skeletal involvement. Vague symptoms of widespread metastases include pallor, weakness, irritability, anorexia and weight loss.

Other primary tumours may cause significant clinical effects, such as neurological impairment from an intracranial lesion, respiratory obstruction from a thoracic mass, or varying degrees of paralysis from compression of the spinal cord.

PROCESS OF DIAGNOSIS

Diagnostic evaluation is aimed at locating the primary site and areas of metastases. A skeletal survey; skull, neck, chest, abdominal, and bone CT scans; ultrasound; and a bone marrow test are used to locate a tumour mass and/or metastases. Neuroblastomas, particularly those arising on the adrenal glands or from a sympathetic chain, excrete the catecholamines adrenaline and noradrenaline. Analyzing the breakdown products that are normally excreted in the urine, namely, vanillylmandelic acid (VMA) and homovanillic acid (HVA), permits detection of a suspected tumour both before and after medical/surgical intervention.

STAGING AND PROGNOSIS

In recent years, there has been an attempt to classify tumours according to stages in order to establish improved criteria for treatment and prognosis at the time of diagnosis and surgery.

An international system of staging for neuroblastoma has been developed (Brodeur *et al*, 1988).

Unfortunately, most children with neuroblastoma have metastatic disease at the time of diagnosis; the first signs being caused by involvement in the nonprimary site, usually the lymph nodes, bone marrow, skeletal system, the skin or liver. For this reason, prognosis for neuroblastoma is poor, but the age of the child and the stage of the disease at diagnosis are important prognostic factors. Neuroblastoma is one of the few tumours that may demonstrate spontaneous regression (especially Stage IV-S), possibly as a result of maturity of the embryonic cell or development of an active immune system.

In recent years, considerable controversy has developed regarding the use of mass screening for neuroblastoma in infants (Parker *et al*, 1992). Whether the cost/benefit ratio of screening for this rare tumour in infants is worthwhile remains to be seen (Murphy *et al*, 1991).

THERAPEUTIC MANAGEMENT

Accurate clinical staging is important for establishing initial treatment. Therefore, surgery is employed both to remove as much of the tumour as possible and to obtain biopsies. In Stages I and II, complete surgical removal of the tumour is the treatment of choice.

Chemotherapy is the mainstay of therapy for extensive local or disseminated disease. If the tumours respond to chemotherapy, surgical removal of the primary is attempted at a later date.

The precise role of radiotherapy is unclear. It does not appear to be of any benefit in children with Stage I and II disease; it is commonly used with Stage III disease although it may not improve survival expectancy; and it may make a large tumour operable. The potential for targeted radiotherapy using ^{131}I MIBG (metaiodobenzylguanadine), which is selectively taken up by neuroblastoma cells, is currently under evaluation (Lashford *et al*, 1992). It offers palliation for metastatic lesions in bones, lungs, liver or brain.

IMPLICATIONS FOR NURSING

Nursing considerations are similar to those discussed previously in the section, Nursing Care of the Child with Cancer, including psychological and physical preparation for diagnostic and operative procedures, prevention of postoperative complications for abdominal, thoracic or cranial surgery, and explanation of chemotherapy and radiotherapy and their side effects.

Since this tumour carries a poor prognosis for many children, every consideration must be given the family in terms of coping with a life-threatening illness (see Chapter 21). Because of the high degree of metastasis at the time of diagnosis, many parents suffer much guilt for not having recognized signs earlier. Often, the guilt is expressed as anger towards professionals for not diagnosing it sooner. Parents need much support in dealing with these feelings and expressing them to the appropriate people.

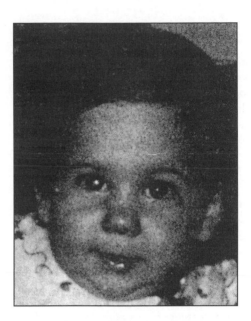

Fig. 30-2 Cat's eye reflex. Whitish appearance of lens is produced as light falls on tumour mass in right eye.

BONE TUMOURS

Malignant bone tumours represent less than 5% of all malignant neoplasms but are more common in children than in adults. The peak ages during childhood are 15-19 years. The sexes are affected equally until puberty, at which time the ratio approaches 2:1 in favour of males. This propensity for males with a peak incidence during adolescence is thought to result from the accelerated growth rate of osseous tissue.

GENERAL CONSIDERATIONS

Neoplastic disease can arise from any tissues involved in bone growth, such as the osteoid matrix, bone marrow elements, fat, blood and lymph vessels, nerve sheath, and cartilage. In children, the two types that account for 85% of all primary malignant bone tumours are osteogenic sarcoma and Ewing's sarcoma. They have several characteristics in common, which are discussed in the following sections.

CLINICAL MANIFESTATIONS

Most malignant bone tumours produce localized pain in the affected site, which may be severe or dull and may be attributed to trauma or the vague complaint of 'growing pains'. The pain is often relieved by a flexed position, which relaxes the muscles overlying the stretched periosteum. Frequently, it draws attention when the child limps, curtails physical activity, or is unable to hold heavy objects.

PROCESS OF DIAGNOSIS

Diagnosis begins with a thorough history and physical examination. A primary objective is to rule out causes such as trauma or infection. Careful questioning regarding pain is essential in attempting to determine the duration and rate of tumour growth. Physical assessment focuses on functional status of the affected area, signs of inflammation, size of the mass, involvement of regional lymph nodes, and any systemic indication of generalized malignancy, such as anaemia, weight loss and frequent infection.

Definitive diagnosis is based on radiological studies, particularly CT, to determine the extent of the lesion; radioisotope bone scans to evaluate metastases; and either needle or surgical bone biopsy to determine the histological pattern. Radiological findings are characteristic for each type of tumour. In osteogenic sarcoma, needle-like new bone formation growing at right angles to the diaphysis (shaft) produces a 'sunburst' appearance. In Ewing's sarcoma, the deposits of new bone in layers under the periosteum produce an 'onion skin' appearance. In both types of bone tumours, soft tissue infiltration may be apparent.

Lung tomography is usually a standard procedure, since pulmonary metastases are the most common complication of primary bone tumours.

PROGNOSIS

A better understanding of the biology of neoplastic growth has resulted in more aggressive treatment and improved prognosis. The natural history of osteogenic sarcoma and Ewing's sarcoma suggests that multiple submicroscopic foci of metastatic disease are present at the time of diagnosis, despite no clinical evidence of localized involvement. Before the use of aggressive multimodal therapy, pulmonary metastases invariably appeared in 6-24 months in patients with osteogenic sarcoma who were treated with surgical excision of the tumour. Now, with surgery for osteosarcoma or intensive radiotherapy for Ewing's sarcoma combined with chemotherapy, survival statistics are improving for both types of bone cancer. Survival rates differ according to the specific treatment protocols and are influenced by several factors, such as the site of the primary tumour, especially in Ewing's sarcoma, and the presence or absence of metastatic disease at diagnosis. However, approximately 60% of children with either type of bone cancer can be expected to be long-term survivors (Jaffe, 1991b).

OSTEOGENIC SARCOMA

Osteogenic sarcoma (osteosarcoma) is the most common bone cancer in children. Its peak incidence is between 10-25 years of age. It presumably arises from bone-forming mesenchyma, which gives rise to malignant osteoid tissue. Most primary tumour sites are in the metaphysis (wider part of the shaft, adjacent to the epiphyseal growth plate) of long bones, especially in the lower extremities. More than one-half occur in the femur, particularly the distal portion, with the rest involving the humerus, tibia, pelvis, jaw and phalanges.

THERAPEUTIC MANAGEMENT

Optimum treatment of osteosarcoma is controversial. The traditional approach has consisted of radical surgical resection or amputation of the affected area, followed by intensive chemotherapy. Another surgical approach for selected patients are limb salvage procedures, which involve en bloc resection of the primary tumour with internal prosthetic replacement of the involved bone. For example, with osteosarcoma of the distal femur, a total femur and joint replacement is performed. The disfigurement of amputation is avoided, but internal prostheses in growing children require repeated surgical intervention to maintain function (Craft, 1991). Frequently, children undergoing a limb salvage procedure will receive preoperative chemotherapy in an attempt to decrease tumour size and make surgery more manageable (Simon, 1988; Simon *et al*, 1989).

Chemotherapy now plays a vital role in treatment and may be employed both before and after surgery. When pulmonary metastases are found, thoracotomy and chemotherapy have resulted in prolonged survival and potential cure. These combined-modality approaches have significantly improved the prognosis in osteosarcoma.

IMPLICATIONS FOR NURSING

Nursing care depends on the type of surgical approach. Obviously, the family may have more difficulty adjusting to an amputation than a limb salvage procedure. In either instance, preparation of the child and family is critical. Straightforward honesty is essential in gaining the cooperation and trust of the child.

Sometimes children have many questions about the prosthesis, limitations on physical ability, and prognosis in terms of cure. For those who wish for information, it may be helpful to introduce them to someone who has had a similar operation before surgery or to show them pictures of the prosthesis. Teenagers are quite likely to be angry and withdrawn, and may require a great deal of emotional support.

If an amputation is performed, the child is usually fitted with a temporary prosthesis immediately after surgery, which permits early functioning and fosters psychological adjustment. During hospitalization, the child begins physiotherapy to become proficient in the use and care of the device.

Phantom limb pain may develop following amputation. This symptom is characterized by sensations such as tingling, itching, and more frequently pain felt in the amputated leg.

Discharge planning must begin early during the postoperative period. Once the child has begun physiotherapy, the nurse should consult with the physiotherapist and practitioner to evaluate the child's physical and emotional readiness to re-enter school.

The family and child need much support in adjusting not only to a life-threatening diagnosis but also to alteration in body form and function. Since loss of a limb constitutes a grieving process, those caring for the child need to recognize that the reactions of anger and depression are normal and necessary. Often, parents view the anger as a direct affront to them for allowing the amputation to occur, or they see the depression as rejection.

EWING'S SARCOMA

Ewing's sarcoma arises in the marrow spaces of the bone rather than from osseous tissue. The tumour originates in the shaft of long and trunk bones, most often affecting the femur, tibia, fibula, humerus, ulna, vertebra, scapula, ribs, pelvic bones and skull. It occurs almost exclusively in individuals under age 30, with the majority between 4-25 years of age.

THERAPEUTIC MANAGEMENT

Surgical amputation is not routinely recommended. The treatment of choice is intensive irradiation of the involved bone, combined with chemotherapy.

IMPLICATIONS FOR NURSING

The psychological adjustment to Ewing's sarcoma is typically less traumatic than to osteogenic sarcoma because of the preservation of the affected limb. Many families accept the diagnosis with a sense of relief in knowing that this type of bone cancer does not necessitate amputation, and initially they may not be aware of the damaging effects on the irradiated site. High-dose radiotherapy often causes a skin reaction of dry or moist desquamation followed by hyperpigmentation. The child should wear loose-fitting clothes over the irradiated area to minimize additional skin irritation. Because of increased sensitivity, the area is protected from sunlight and sudden changes in temperature, such as from heating pads or ice packs. The child is encouraged to use the extremity as tolerated. An active exercise programme may be planned by the physiotherapist to preserve maximum function.

OTHER SOLID TUMOURS

In addition to the cancers already discussed, several other types of solid tumours may occur in children. Wilms' tumour, rhabdomyosarcoma and retinoblastoma are unique in that they tend to be diagnosed early, typically before five years of age. Wilms' tumour and retinoblastoma are also unusual in that they are among the few types of cancer that may occur in both hereditary and nonhereditary forms.

WILMS' TUMOUR

Wilms' tumour, or nephroblastoma, is the most frequent intraabdominal tumour of childhood and the most common type of renal cancer. The peak incidence is at three years of age.

CLINICAL MANIFESTATIONS

The most common presenting sign is a swelling or mass within the abdomen. The mass is characteristically firm, non-tender, confined to one side, and deep within the flank. Parents usually discover the mass during routine bathing or dressing of the child.

Other clinical manifestations are the result of compression from the tumour mass, metabolic alterations secondary to the tumour, or metastases. Haematuria occurs in less than one-quarter of children with Wilms' tumour. Anaemia, usually secondary to haemorrhage within the tumour, results in pallor, anorexia and lethargy. Hypertension, probably caused by secretion of excess amounts of renin by the tumour, occurs occasionally. Other effects of malignancy include weight loss and fever. If metastases have occurred, symptoms of lung involvement, such as dyspnoea, cough, shortness of breath, and pain in the chest, may be evident.

PROCESS OF DIAGNOSIS

In a child suspected of having Wilms' tumour, special emphasis is placed on the history and physical examination for the presence of congenital anomalies. Specific tests include chest x-ray, abdominal ultrasound, CT, haematological and biochemical studies, and urinalysis.

STAGING AND PROGNOSIS

Wilms' tumour occurs more frequently in the left kidney, which is advantageous because surgically this kidney is easier to manipulate and remove. Although the tumour may become quite large, it remains encapsulated for an extended period.

The histology of the tumour cells is identified and classified according to two groups: favourable histology (FH) and unfavourable histology (UH). Only about 12% of Wilms' tumours demonstrate UH, which is associated with a poorer prognosis and demands a more aggressive treatment protocol, regardless of the clinical stage.

Survival rates for Wilms' tumour are the highest among all childhood cancers. Children with localized tumour (Stages I and II) have a 90% chance of cure with multimodal therapy.

THERAPEUTIC MANAGEMENT

The tumour, affected kidney, and adjacent adrenal gland are removed. Great care is taken to keep the encapsulated tumour intact, since rupture can seed cancer cells throughout the abdomen, lymph channel, and bloodstream. The other kidney is carefully inspected for evidence of disease or dysfunction. Regional lymph nodes are inspected and a biopsy is performed when indicated.

If both kidneys are involved, the child may be treated with radiotherapy and/or chemotherapy preoperatively to shrink the tumour, allowing more conservative therapy. In some cases a partial nephrectomy is performed on the less affected kidney, with a total nephrectomy on the opposite side. Bilateral nephrectomy is considered as a last resort.

Postoperative chemotherapy is indicated for all children with Wilms' tumour. Radiotherapy is indicated for residual abdominal disease or lung metastases.

IMPLICATIONS FOR NURSING

The nursing care of the child with Wilms' tumour is similar to that of other cancers treated with surgery, irradiation and chemotherapy. However, there are some significant differences.

Preoperative care

As with many of the other cancers, the diagnosis of Wilms' tumour is a shock. Frequently, the child has no physical indication of the seriousness of the disorder other than a palpable abdominal mass. As it is the parents who usually discover the mass, the nurse needs to take into account their feelings regarding the diagnosis. Whereas some parents are grateful for the detection of the tumour, others feel guilty for not finding it sooner, or feel angry towards the practitioner for missing it on earlier examinations.

The preoperative period is usually one of swift diagnosis, and surgery is carried out as soon as possible. In addition to the usual preoperative observations, blood pressure is monitored, since hypertension from excess renin production is a possibility.

Since radiotherapy and chemotherapy are usually begun immediately after surgery, parents need an explanation of what to expect.

Postoperative care

Despite the extensive surgical intervention necessary in many children with Wilms' tumour, the recovery period is usually rapid. The major nursing responsibilities are those following any abdominal surgery. These children are at risk from intestinal obstruction from vincristine-induced paralytic ileus, radiation-induced oedema, and postsurgical adhesion formation. It is therefore important that gastrointestinal activity, such as bowel movements, bowel sounds, distention and vomiting, are monitored. Other considerations are frequent evaluation of blood pressure and observation for signs of infection and chest physiotherapy.

Because the child is left with only one kidney, certain precautions are recommended to prevent injury to the organ, including avoiding contact sports or any activity that has a high risk potential. Urinary tract infections should be prevented with good hygiene, especially in girls, and adequate fluid intake. Prompt detection and treatment of any genitourinary signs or symptoms is mandatory.

RHABDOMYOSARCOMA

Soft tissue sarcomas are the fourth most common type of solid tumours in children. These malignant neoplasms originate from undifferentiated mesenchymal cells in muscles, tendons, bursae and fascia, or in fibrous, connective, lymphatic or vascular tissue. They derive their name from the specific tissue(s) of origin, such as myosarcoma (*myo* = muscle). Rhabdomyosarcoma (*rhabdo* = striated) is the most common soft tissue sarcoma in children. Because striated (skeletal) muscle is found almost anywhere in the body, these tumours occur in many sites, the most common of which are the head and neck. The disease occurs in children in all age groups, but most commonly in children younger than five years of age.

CLINICAL MANIFESTATIONS

The initial signs and symptoms are related to the site of the tumour and compression of adjacent organs. Some tumour locations, particularly the orbit, produce symptoms early in the course of the illness and contribute to rapid diagnosis and improved prognosis. Other tumours, such as those of the retroperitoneal area, produce no symptoms until they are large, invasive and widely metastasized. In some instances a primary tumour site is never identified.

PROCESS OF DIAGNOSIS

Unfortunately, many of the signs and symptoms attributable to rhabdomyosarcoma are vague and frequently suggest a common childhood illness, such as 'earache' or 'runny nose'.

Radiographic studies to isolate a tumour site are performed, accompanied by chest x-ray examinations, CT, bone surveys and bone marrow aspiration to rule out metastases. A diagnostic lumbar puncture is indicated for head and neck tumours. An excisional biopsy is done to confirm histological type.

STAGING AND PROGNOSIS

Careful staging is extremely important for planning treatment and determining prognosis. With the change in treatment from radical surgery or radiotherapy to a multimodal approach, survival rates for all stages have increased considerably.

Data suggest that children who remain disease free for two years are probably cured; however, if relapse occurs, the prognosis for long-term survival is extremely poor (Raney *et al*, 1993).

THERAPEUTIC MANAGEMENT

Since this tumour is highly malignant, with metastases frequently occurring at the time of diagnosis, aggressive combination therapy is recommended. In the past, radical surgical removal of the tumour was the treatment of choice, but with improved survival from combined chemotherapy and radiation, surgery plays a lesser role. Complete removal of the primary tumour is advocated whenever possible. However, only biopsy is required in certain tumour locations, such as those of the orbit when followed by radiation and chemotherapy.

IMPLICATIONS FOR NURSING

The nursing responsibilities are similar to those for other types of cancer, especially that for solid tumours when surgery is employed.

RETINOBLASTOMA

Retinoblastoma is a congenital malignant tumour arising from the retina. It is a relatively rare tumour, and can be inherited. It may be present at birth or may arise in the retina during the first two years of life. The average age of the child at the time of diagnosis is 17 months.

CLINICAL MANIFESTATIONS

Retinoblastoma has few grossly obvious signs. Typically, it is the parent who first observes a whitish 'glow' in the pupil, known as the *cat's eye reflex* or *leukokoria*. The reflex represents visualization of the tumour as the light momentarily falls on the mass (Fig. 30-2). When a tumour arises in the macular region (area directly at the back of the retina when the eye is focused straight ahead), a white reflex may be seen when the tumour is quite small. It is best observed when a bright light is shining towards the child as the child looks forward. It is sometimes accidentally discovered by parents when taking a photograph of their child using a flash attachment.

The next most common sign is strabismus resulting from poor fixation of the visually impaired eye, particularly if the tumour develops in the macula, the area of sharpest visual acuity. Blindness is usually a late sign, but it is not always obvious unless the parents consciously observe for behaviours indicating loss of sight, such as bumping into objects, slowed motor development or turning of the head to see objects lateral to the affected eye.

PROCESS OF DIAGNOSIS

The first step in diagnosis is carefully listening to and recognizing the significance of reports from family members regarding suspected abnormalities within the eye. Parental remarks that in any way suggest the presence of such findings must be taken seriously and investigated. Distant metastases are rare, but if suspected, a bone marrow aspiration, bone survey, and lumbar puncture may be performed.

STAGING AND PROGNOSIS

Staging of retinoblastomas is done under indirect ophthalmoscopy before surgery to determine accurately tumour size and location (Grabowski and Abramson, 1991). Cure rates for survival are much better than for retention of useful vision. The overall five-year survival rate is 85-90% for unilateral and bilateral tumours (Donaldson and Smith, 1989).

Of major concern in long-term survivors is the development of secondary tumours, especially osteogenic sarcoma. Children with bilateral disease (hereditary form) are more likely to develop secondary cancers than children with unilateral disease. It is thought that these individuals are predisposed to developing cancer, and radiation increases their risk.

THERAPEUTIC MANAGEMENT

Treatment of retinoblastoma depends chiefly on the stage of the tumour at diagnosis. In general, unilateral localized retinoblastomas are treated with irradiation. The aim of radiotherapy is to preserve useful vision in the affected eye and eradicate the tumour.

Other approaches towards treating small, localized tumours involve: (1) *radiotherapy utilizing surface applicators* (surgical implantation of a cobalt 60 applicator on the sclera until the maximum radiation dose has been delivered to the tumour), and (2) *photocoagulation* (use of a laser beam to destroy retinal blood vessels that supply nutrition to the tumour).

With advanced tumour growth, especially optic nerve involvement, enucleation of the affected eye is the only treatment option. The use of chemotherapy in advanced disease is controversial and has not shown improved survival. In the case of central nervous system disease, intrathecal chemotherapy may be administered (Donaldson and Egbert, 1993).

With bilateral disease, every attempt is made to preserve useful vision in the less affected eye with enucleation of the severely diseased eye. When bilateral tumours are found very early, enucleation may be prevented with only the use of radiotherapy to both eyes.

IMPLICATIONS FOR NURSING

The care of the child with retinoblastoma involves much attention to aspects of diagnosis, treatment protocols, and possible hereditary factors. Nursing objectives include: (1) identifying signs of retinoblastoma, (2) preparing the family for diagnostic/therapeutic procedures and home care, and (3) providing emotional support. The importance of recognizing possible early signs and appreciating their significance has already been discussed.

Prepare the family for diagnostic/therapeutic procedures and home care

Since the tumour is usually diagnosed in infants or very young children, most of the preparation for diagnostic tests and treatment involves parents. After indirect ophthalmoscopy, the child may not see very clearly, or the eyes may be sensitive to light because of pupillary dilation. Parents are made aware of these normal reactions before the procedure.

When enucleation is necessary, the child and family need to be prepared for the child's facial appearance. An eye patch is in place, and the child's face may be oedematous. Parents often fear seeing the surgical site because they imagine a cavity in the skull. Once the child is fitted for a prosthesis, usually within three weeks, the facial appearance returns to normal. Parents will need instruction regarding care of the surgical site and preparation for any additional therapy. They will also require help with the care and safety of the prosthesis.

Support the family

The diagnosis of retinoblastoma presents some special concerns in addition to those created by any type of cancer. Families with a history of the disorder may feel great guilt for transmitting the defect to their offspring. In families with no history of retinoblastoma, the discovery of the diagnosis is a shock, frequently complicated by guilt for not having found it sooner. Since parents frequently are the first to observe the cat's eye reflex, they may feel angry at themselves or others, especially professionals, for delaying a more thorough examination.

Other concerns are also related to the hereditary aspects of the disease. Of great importance to parents is the recurrence risk of retinoblastoma in their subsequent offspring and in the offspring of the surviving affected child. With improving prognosis for these children, the necessity of genetic counselling is assuming greater importance.

These families are also encouraged to seek regular follow-up for the affected child, to detect possible subsequent, or secondary, tumours. All subsequent offspring of unaffected parents and survivors should undergo regular indirect ophthalmoscopy under anaesthesia to detect retinoblastoma at its earliest stage.

KEY POINTS

◆ Criteria used to determine cure of cancer include cessation of therapy for a minimum of five years, continuous freedom from clinical and laboratory evidence of cancer, and minimal or no risk of relapse.

◆ Although the cure rate for most types of childhood cancer has improved, the late effects of treatment are of increasing concern.

◆ Determination of malignancy and metastases is made by history and physical examination, laboratory tests, imaging techniques and biopsy.

◆ The major modes of cancer therapy are surgery, chemotherapy, radiotherapy, immunotherapy and bone marrow transplantation.

◆ Types of bone marrow transplants are allogeneic, autologous and syngeneic.

◆ Nursing goals in the care of the child with cancer are to prepare the family for diagnostic and therapeutic procedures, prevent complications of myelosuppression (infection, haemorrhage, anaemia), manage problems of irradiation and drug toxicity, and provide continued emotional support.

◆ Leukaemia is the most common form of childhood cancer. Current five-year survival rates exceed 60% in major research centres, and the majority of these children will be cured.

◆ The traditional approach to treatment of osteosarcoma has been radical surgical resection or amputation followed by chemotherapy. Limb preservation to prevent amputation is now playing an increasing role.

◆ Wilms' tumour shows an increased incidence among siblings and identical twins, demonstrating a hereditary predisposition.

REFERENCES

Abernathy E: Biotherapy: an introductory overview, *Oncol Nurs Forum* 14(6):13, 1987.

Bithall JF *et al:* Distribution of childhood leukaemias and non-Hodgkin's lymphoma near nuclear installations in England and Wales, *BMJ* 309:501, 1994.

Brodeur GM *et al:* International criteria for diagnosis, staging, and response to treatment in patients with neuroblastoma, *J Clin Oncol* 6(12):1874, 1988.

Chessels JM: Central nervous system directed therapy in acute lymphoblastic leukaemia, *Balliere Clin Haematol* 7(2):349, 1994.

Craft AN: Prosthetic replacement for surgery for bone tumoursæ cure at less cost? *Br J Cancer* 63:173, 1991.

Davies HA, Lennard L, Lilleyman JS: Variable mercaptopurine metabolism in children with leukaemia: a problem of compliance? *BMJ* 306:1239, 1993.

Donaldson SS, Egbert PR: Retinoblastoma. In Pizzo PA, Poplack DG: *Principles and practice of pediatric oncology*, ed 2, Philadelphia, 1993, JB Lippincott.

Eiser C, Havermans T: Long term social adjustment after treatment for childhood cancer, *Arch Dis Child* 70:66, 1994.

Fernbach DJ, Vietti TJ, editors: General aspects of childhood cancer. In Fernbach DJ, Vietti TJ, editors: *Clinical pediatric oncology*, ed 4, St Louis, 1991, Mosby.

Frenck R, Kohl S, Pickering LK: Principles of total care: infections in children with cancer. In Fernbach DJ, Vietti TJ, editors: *Clinical pediatric oncology*, ed 4, St Louis, 1991, Mosby.

Grabowski EF, Abramson DH: Retinoblastoma. In Fernbach DJ, Vietti TJ, editors: *Clinical pediatric oncology*, ed 4, St Louis, 1991, Mosby.

Heideman RL *et al:* Tumors of the central nervous system. 1993. In Pizzo PA, Poplack DJ, editors: *Principles and practice of pediatric oncology*, ed 2, Philadelphia, 1993, JB Lippincott.

Jaffe N: Osteosarcoma, *Pediatr Rev* 12(11):333, 1991b.

Lansky SB *et al*: Late effects: psychosocial, *Clin Oncol* 4(2):239, 1985.

Lashford *et al:* A phase I/II study of ^{131}I metaiodobenzylguanadine in chemo-resistant neuroblastoma: a UKCCSG investigation, *J Clin Oncol* 11:1478, 1992.

Magrath IT: Malignant non-Hodgkin's lymphomas. In Pizzo PA, Poplack DJ, editors: *Principles and practice of pediatric oncology*, ed 2, Philadelphia, 1993, JB Lippincott.

Mahon SM, Casperson DS: Pathophysiology of hypokalemia in patients with cancer: implications for nurses, *Oncol Nurs Forum* 20(6):937, 1993.

Meadows AT, Hobbie WW: The medical consequences of cure, *Cancer* 58:524, 1986.

Mioduszewski J, Zarbo AG: Ambulatory infusion pumps: a practical view at an alternative approach, *Semin Oncol Nurs* 3(2):106, 1987.

Mitchell PLR *et al:* Peripheral blood stem cells to augment autologous bone marrow transplantation, *Arch Dis Child* 70:237, 1994.

Morris-Jones PH: The late effects of cancer therapy in childhood, *Br J Cancer* 64:1, 1991.

Murphy SB *et al:* Do children benefit from mass screening for neuroblastoma? *Lancet* 337:344, 1991.

Parker L *et al*: Screening for neuroblastoma in the North of England, *BMJ* 305:1260, 1992.

Pinkerton CR, Cushing P, Sepion B: *Childhood cancer management: a practical handbook*, London, 1994, Chapman & Hall.

Pinkerton CR *et al*, 5 - HT$_3$ antagonist ondansetron - an effective outpatient treatment, *Arch Dis Child* 65:822-825, 1990.

Raney RB *et al:* Rhabdomyosarcoma and the undifferentiated sarcomas. In Pizzo PA, Poplack DJ, editors: *Principles and practice of pediatric oncology*, ed 2, Philadelphia, 1993, JB Lippincott.

Robinson LL: General principles of the epidemiology of childhood cancers. In Pizza PA, Poplack DG, editors: *Principles and practice of pediatric oncology*, ed 2, Philadelphia 1993, JB Lippincott.

Sandlund JT, Hutchinson RE, Crist WM: Non-Hodgkin's lymphoma. In Fernbach DJ, Vietti TJ, editors: *Clinical pediatric oncology*, ed 4, St Louis, 1991, Mosby.

Simon MA: Limb salvage for osteosarcoma, *J Bone Joint Surg* 70A:307, 1989.

Tait D: Minimization and management of morbidity from radiotherapy. In Plowman PN, Pinkerton CR: *Paediatric oncology: clinical practice and controversies*, London, 1992, Chapman & Hall.

Thompson EI: Hodgkin's disease. In Fernbach DJ, Vietti TJ, editors: *Clinical pediatric oncology,* ed 4, St Louis, 1991, Mosby.

Treleaven J, Barrett J: *Bone marrow transplantation in practice,* Edinburgh, 1992, Churchill Livingstone.

Tucker MA *et al*: Risk of second cancers after treatment for Hodgkin's disease, *N Engl J Med* 318(2):76, 1988.

Weinberg KI, Parkman R: Interface between immunodeficiency and pediatric cancer. In Pizzo PA, Poplack DG: *Principles and practice of pediatric oncology,* Philadelphia, 1989, JB Lippincott.

Williams CJ *et al*: Comparison of starting antiemetic treatment 24 hours before or concurrently with cytotoxic chemotherapy, *BMJ* 298:430, 1989.

Yasko JM, Dudjak LA: *Biological response modifier therapy: symptom management,* Pittsburgh, 1990, Cancer Educational and Support Services.

FURTHER READING

Cancer in Children

Association of Pediatric Oncology Nurses: Scope of practice, *J Assoc Pediatr Oncol Nurs* 7(1):22, 1990.

Draper G, Stiller C: Cautious optimism, *Paediatr Nurs* 1(3):22, 1989.

Hockenberry MJ, Coody DK: *Pediatric oncology and hematology: perspectives on care,* St Louis, 1986, Mosby–Year Book.

Lewis I: Building on success, *Paediatr Nurs* 1(2):12, 1989.

Muir KR *et al*: Shared care in paediatric oncology, *J Cancer Care* 1(1):15, 1992.

Oakhill A: *The supportive care of the child with cancer,* London, 1988, Butterworth.

Outcome standards of pediatric oncology nursing practice, *J Assoc Pediatr Oncol Nurs* 7(1):24, 1990.

Thompson J: *The child with cancer: nursing care,* London, 1990, Scutari.

Willoughby M, Siegal SE: *Haematology and oncology—paediatrics 1,* London, 1982, Butterworth.

Chemotherapy

Garvey FC: Current and future nursing issues in the home administration of chemotherapy, *Semin Oncol Nurs* 3(2):142, 1987.

Lind J, Bush NJ: Nursing's role in chemotherapy administration, *Semin Oncol Nurs* 3(2):83, 1987.

Priestman TJ: *Cancer chemotherapy: an introduction,* London, 1989, Springer-Verlag.

Rogers B, Emmett EA: Handling antineoplastic agents: urine mutageneity in nurses, *Image J Nurs Scho* 19(3):108, 1987.

Bone Marrow Transplantation

Atkins DM, Patenaude AF: Psychosocial preparation and follow-up for pediatric BMT patients, *Am J Orthopsychiatry* 57(2):246, 1987.

Durbin M: Bone marrow transplantation: economic, ethical, and social issues, *Pediatr* 82(5):774, 1988.

Gottlieb SE, Portnoy S: The role of play in a pediatric bone marrow transplantation unit, *Child Health Care* 16(3):177, 1988.

Hann IM: Bone marrow transplantation, *Curr Opin Pediatr* 2:143, 1990.

Nims JW, Strom S: Late complications of bone marrow transplant recipients: nursing care issues, *Semin Oncol Nurs* 4(1):47, 1988.

Long-Term Sequelae of Treatment

D'Angio G: Cure is not enough: late consequences associated with radiation treatment, *J Assoc Pediatr Oncol Nurs* 5(4):20, 1988.

Green DM: *Long term complications of therapy for cancer in childhood and adolescence,* Baltimore, 1989, Johns Hopkins University Press.

Hoffman B: Cancer survivors at work: job problems and illegal discrimination, *Oncol Nurs Forum* 16(1):39, 1989.

Meadows AT: Second malignant neoplasms in childhood cancer survivors, *J Assoc Pediatr Oncol Nurs* 6(1):7, 1989.

Moore IM, Kramer J, Ablin A: Late effects of central nervous system prophylactic leukemia therapy on cognitive functioning, *Oncol Nurs Forum* 13(4):45, 1986.

Ochs J, Mulhern RK: Late effects of antileukemic treatment, *Pediatr Clin North Am* 35(4):815, 1988.

Peckham VC: Learning disorders associated with the treatment of cancer in childhood, *J Assoc Pediatr Oncol Nurs* 5(4):10, 1988.

Takaue Y, *et al*: Second malignant neoplasms in treated Hodgkin's disease, *Am J Dis Child* 140(1):49, 1986.

Vanderwal R, Nims J, Davies B: Bone marrow transplantation in children: nursing management of late effects, *Cancer Nurs* 11(3):132, 1988.

Symptom Management

Eland JM: Pharmacologic management of acute and chronic pediatric pain, *Issues Compr Pediatr Nurs* 11:93, 1988.

Frick SB *et al*: Chemotherapy-associated nausea and vomiting in pediatric oncology patients, *Cancer Nurs* 11(2):118, 1988.

Hamner SB, Miles MS: Coping strategies in children with cancer undergoing bone marrow aspirations, *J Assoc Pediatr Oncol Nurs* 5(3):11, 1988.

Ohanian NA: Informational needs of children and adolescents with cancer, *J Assoc Pediatr Oncol Nurs* 6(3):94, 1989.

Robertson WW: Orthopedic interventions for problems associated with the treatment of cancer in childhood, *J Assoc Pediatr Oncol Nurs* 6(1):12, 1989.

Wickham R: Managing chemotherapy-related nausea and vomiting: the state of the art, *Oncol Nurs Forum* 16(4):563, 1989.

Yasko JM: Control of anticipatory nausea and vomiting, *Issues Oncol Nurs* 4(3):4, 1987.

Yasko JM, Greene P: Coping with problems related to cancer and cancer treatment, *CA* 37(2):106, 1987.

Young JA, Eslinger P, Galloway M: Radiation treatment for the child with cancer, *Issues Compr Pediatr Nurs* 12(2/3):159, 1989.

Leukaemias/Lymphomas

Davies B: Sibling bereavement, *Seminars Oncol Nurs* 9(2):107, 1993.

Dickens M: *Miracles of courage—how families meet the challenge of a child's critical illness,* Devon, 1987, David & Charles.

Dixon DM, Dominic K: Left out in the cold, *Paediatr Nurs* 5(3):28, 1993.

Evans M: Teenagers and cancer, *Paediatr Nurs* 5(1):14, 1989.

Pearce G, O'Keefe A: Childhood cancer: psychological needs—are they being met? *J Cancer Care* 1(1):3, 1992.

Chapter 31

The Child with Cerebral Dysfunction

LEARNING OUTCOMES

After studying this chapter you should be able to:

◆ Describe the various methods of assessment of cerebral function.
◆ List 10 specific neurological investigations.
◆ Devise a care plan for the unconscious child that includes physical, psychological, social and spiritual needs.
◆ Discuss the possible effects of a major head injury on the physical and cognitive development of the child.
◆ List the signs and symptoms of bacterial meningitis.
◆ List the different types of brain tumours and current treatments.
◆ Define the different types of seizure disorders.
◆ Devise a care plan for a child with hydrocephalus requiring insertion of a ventriculo-peritoneal shunt.
◆ Define the glossary terms.

GLOSSARY

ACTH Adrenocorticotropic hormone

aura A sensation, as of warmth or light, that may precede an attack of migraine or an epileptic seizure

conciousness The ability to respond to sensory stimuli and to have subjective experiences

concussion A transient and reversible neuronal dysfunction

convulsion Involuntary muscular contraction and relaxation

GCS Glasgow Coma Scale

Head injury Any pathological process involving the scalp, skull, meninges or brain as a result of mechanical force

PaCO$_2$ Arterial carbon dioxide pressure

PaO$_2$ Arterial oxygen pressure

postictal Period following a convulsion

seizure A sudden attack

SIADH Syndrome of inappropriate antidiuretic hormone

eural control between children and their environment is made possible by the nervous system. Any
disturbance in this system can produce alterations in the way
in which the system receives, integrates and responds to stimuli
entering the system.

Children are constantly changing as their systems develop
and mature, and neurodevelopmental milestones represent the
transition of immature primitive reflexes to mature activity.
This chapter is concerned primarily with alterations in consciousness caused by trauma, hypoxia, infectious processes and
seizure activity.

CEREBRAL STRUCTURE AND FUNCTION

The nervous system is composed of three intimately connected and functioning parts: (1) the central nervous system (CNS),
composed of two cerebral hemispheres, the brainstem, the cerebellum and the spinal cord; (2) the peripheral nervous system,
which consists of the cranial nerves that arise from or travel to
the brainstem and the spinal nerves that travel to or from the
spinal cord, which may be motor (efferent) or sensory (afferent);
and (3) the autonomic nervous system (ANS), composed of the
sympathetic and parasympathetic systems, which provide automatic control of vital functions (Table 31-1).

CENTRAL NERVOUS SYSTEM

The bony skull forms the strongest covering and provides the
primary protection to the brain. It is an expandable structure
in the infant and young child, but becomes rigid in the older
child and adolescent. Blood is supplied to the dura mater by
the middle meningeal artery, a branch of the external carotid
artery. It enters the skull at a point inferior to the temporal
bone, then branches over the surface of the dura, usually
encased in a groove in the temporal and parietal bones.
Damage to this artery or its branches is a frequent cause of
an epidural haematoma.

STRUCTURE	DESCRIPTION	FUNCTION	DYSFUNCTION
Cerebrum	Two hemispheres divided arti-ficially into lobes Upper parts divided anteriorly and posteriorly by longitudi-nal fissure Lower parts joined centrally by block of fibres, the cor-pus callosum	Centre for consciousness, thought, memory, sensory input, motor activity	Pressure or damage produces signs and symptoms spe-cific to involved areas
Frontal lobes	Most anteriorly located of all lobes that end posteriorly at fissure of Rolando	Posterior portion contains cells that control motor ac-tivity throughout body Basis for social interaction Recognition of cause-and-effect relationships, abstract thinking, expressive lan-guage	Injury or damage to anterior portion may cause person-ality changes, altered intel-lectual functioning Impaired movement of body part directly related to mo-tor centre for that part Memory deficits Language deficits
Parietal lobes	Situated posterior to fissure of Rolando	Important for appreciation of sensation, somatic interpre-tation and integration	Language dysfunction Aphasia, apraxia, motor and sensory loss to lower ex-tremities, atopognosia
Occipital lobe	At posterior base of skull Most posteriorly placed lobe	Receives stimuli for vision Spatial orientation Visual recognition	Injury produces impaired vi-sion, functional blindness

Table 31-1 Structure and function of the brain.

STRUCTURE	DESCRIPTION	FUNCTION	DYSFUNCTION
Cerebrum *(cont.)*			
Temporal lobes	Situated anterior to occipital lobe and inferior to parietal lobes	Receives and interprets stimuli for taste, vision, sound, smell Converts crude visual impressions into recognizable images	Injury or destruction causes inability to interpret meanings of sensory experiences
	Point where temporal, parietal, and occipital lobes converge	Primary interpretive area	Impairment causes inability to interpret sensory stimuli; difficulty in understanding higher levels of meaning of body sensory experiences
	Point where temporal, parietal, and frontal lobes converge	Centre for speech, hearing, receptive language	Impairment produces aphasia Hearing dysfunction
Cerebellum	Located just below posterior part of cerebrum and separated from it by tentorium Contains two lateral lobes joined by midline portion, the vermis	Necessary for refinement and coordination of all muscle movements, including walking, talking, control of muscle tone and balance	Dysmetria, ataxia, dysarthria, hypotonia, nystagmus, dystonia Rest tremor
Basal ganglia	Situated deeply within cerebral hemispheres on either side of midline	Unconscious or automatic control of lower motor centres Excitation causes inhibition of muscle tone throughout body	Chorea, athetosis Dystonia Rest tremors
Diencephalon	Situated between cerebrum and mesencephalon	Contains diffuse fibres that compose reticular activating system	Stupor
Thalamus	Rounded mass forms most of lateral wall of third ventricle and part of floor of lateral ventricles	Major relay station for sensory impulses to cerebral cortex Activates cerebral cortex	Impaired consciousness
Hypothalamus	Lies beneath thalamus Forms floor of third ventricle	Vital control centre for involuntary functions (e.g., blood pressure, satiety, hunger, rage, feeding, water conservation, temperature, sleep regulation, libido) Controls secretion of tropic hormones	Impairment causes alterations in vegetative functions Somnolence, coma Anorexia, loss of weight, fever, diabetes insipidus, loss of libido Endocrine disorders

(cont.)

Table 31-1 Structure and function of the brain (continued).

STRUCTURE	DESCRIPTION	FUNCTION	DYSFUNCTION
Brainstem	Extends from cerebral hemi sphere to spinal cord	All cranial nerves (except I) arise from brainstem	Stupor, coma
Mesencephalon- (mid-brain)	Lies below inferior surface of cerebellum and above pons	Main connection between forebrain and hindbrain Contains nuclei for cranial nerves III, IV, part of V	Impaired consciousness No independent movement or verbal response Decerebrate posturing Neurological hyperventilation
	Ventral portion composed of cerebral peduncles	Control of eye movement	Impaired function of muscles supplied by these nerves
Pons	Located just above medulla oblongata	Contains pneumotaxic centre - control of respiration	Deep, rapid, or periodic breathing
		Cranial nerves V through VIII	Impaired function of muscles supplied by these nerves
Medulla	Forms attachment of brain to spinal cord Separated from pons by horizontal groove	Contains vital centres, including respiratory and vasomotor cranial nerves IX, X, XI, XII	Impaired vital functions No response to any stimuli Ataxic (Biot) breathing Flaccid muscle tone Deep tendon, gag, corneal reflexes absent

Table 31-1 Structure and function of the brain (continued).

BRAIN COVERINGS

Within the skull, the brain is covered and protected further by three membranes, the *meninges* — the dura mater, arachnoid membrane and pia mater. The tough outer membrane, the *dura mater,* is a double layer that serves as the outer meningeal layer and the inner periosteum of the cranial bones, separated by the *epidural space.* The dura is closely attached to the skull in infancy, causing slower spread of blood in epidural haemorrhage. This adherence explains why epidural haemorrhages are uncommon in the first two years of life.

The middle meningeal layer, the *arachnoid membrane,* is a delicate, avascular, weblike structure that loosely surrounds the brain. Between the arachnoid and the dura mater lies the *subdural area,* a potential space that normally contains only enough fluid to prevent adhesion between the two membranes. During cerebral trauma, however, the fine blood vessels that bridge the subdural space are stretched and ruptured, causing venous blood to escape and spread freely. The subdural space is small in children; therefore, small amounts of blood can increase intracranial haemorrhage significantly.

The innermost covering layer, the *pia mater,* is a delicate transparent membrane that, unlike the other coverings, adheres closely to the outer surface of the brain, conforming to the folds (gyri) and furrows (sulci). Within the pial layer lie the arteries and veins of the brain. Between the pia mater and the arachnoid membrane is the *subarachnoid space.* Cerebrospinal fluid (CSF) fills the entire subarachnoid space surrounding the brain and spinal cord, which acts as a protective cushion for the brain tissue. Further protection is provided by fibrous filaments known as *arachnoid trabeculae,* which help anchor the brain. When the head receives a blow, these attachments allow the arachnoid to slide on the dura, preventing excessive movement.

INCREASED INTRACRANIAL PRESSURE (ICP)

The brain, tightly enclosed in the solid bony cranium, is well protected, but highly vulnerable to pressure that may accumulate within the enclosure.

Early signs and symptoms of increased ICP are often subtle and assume many patterns, such as personality changes, irritability, and fatigue (Box 31-1). In older children, subjective symptoms are headache, especially when lying flat (e.g., on awakening in the morning) or when coughing, sneezing or bending over, and nausea and vomiting. The child may complain of double vision or blurred vision with movement of the head. Seizures are not uncommon. In children whose cranial sutures have not closed, there is an increase in the head circumference and bulging fontanelles. Cranial sutures may become diastatic, or split, and head circumference can enlarge until the child is five years of age if the pathology progresses slowly. As pressure increases, pupils become progressively sluggish in reaction, eventually to become fixed and dilated,

---

◆ BOX 31-1

Signs of increased intracranial pressured (ICP) in infants and children

Infants

Tense, bulging fontanel; lack of normal pulsations

Separated cranial sutures

Macewen (cracked-pot) sign

Irritability

High-pitched cry

Increased occipitofrontal circumference (OFC)

Distended scalp veins

Changes in feeding

Cries when held or rocked

'Setting sun' sign

Children

Headache

Nausea

Vomiting — often without nausea

Diplopia, blurred vision

Seizures

Personality and Behaviour Signs

Irritability (toddlers), restlessness

Indifference, drowsiness, or lack of interest

Decline in school performance

Diminished physical activity and motor performance

Increased complaints of fatigue, tiredness; increased time devoted to sleep

Significant weight loss possible from anorexia and vomiting

Memory loss if pressure is greatly increased

Inability to follow simple commands

Progression to lethargy and drowsiness

Late Signs

Lowered level of consciousness

Decreased motor response to command

Decreased sensory response to painful stimuli

Alterations in pupil size and reactivity

Sometimes decerebrate or decorticate posturing

Cheyne-Stokes respirations

Papilloedema

---

sometimes referred to as 'blown'. The level of consciousness progressively deteriorates from drowsiness to eventual coma.

ALTERED STATES OF CONSCIOUSNESS

Consciousness implies awareness — the ability to respond to sensory stimuli and to have subjective experiences. There are two aspects of consciousness: *alertness,* an arousal-waking state including the ability to respond to stimuli, and *cognitive power,* including the ability to process stimuli and produce verbal and motor responses.

An altered state of consciousness usually refers to varying states of unconsciousness that may be momentary or may last for hours, days or indefinitely. *Unconsciousness* is depressed cerebral function — the inability to respond to sensory stimuli and to have subjective experiences. *Coma* is defined as a state of unconsciousness from which the patient cannot be aroused, even with painful stimuli.

LEVEL OF CONSCIOUSNESS

Assessment of level of consciousness (LOC) remains the earliest indicator of improvement or deterioration in neurological status. LOC is determined by observations of the child's responses to the environment. Other diagnostic tests, such as motor activity, reflexes and vital signs, are more variable and do not necessarily directly parallel the depth of the comatose state.

COMA ASSESSMENT

Several scales have been devised in an attempt to standardize the description and interpretation of the degree of depressed consciousness. The most popular of these is the Glasgow Coma Scale (GCS), which consists of a three-part assessment: eye opening, verbal response and motor response. The GCS requires observational skills and is readily reproducible between observers. A paediatric version recognizes that expected verbal and motor responses must be related to the child's age. When assessing LOC in young children, it is often useful to have a parent present to help elicit a useful response. An infant or child may not respond in an unfamiliar environment or to unfamiliar voices. Children older than three years of age should be able to give their name, although they may not be aware of place or time.

Numerical values, 1-5, are assigned to the levels of response in each category. The sum of these numerical values provides an objective measure of the patient's LOC. The lower the score, the deeper is the coma. A normal person would score the highest, 15; a score of eight or below is generally accepted as a definition of coma; the lowest score, three, indicates deep coma or death.

The GCS in itself is not sufficient to determine the responses of all children. For example, a quadriplegic child can score very low, but be cerebrally intact because the child cannot respond to commands physically. However, the GCS provides a more objective method for evaluating the state of consciousness in most cases. Any child less than three years of age who cries is assigned a full verbal score. Severely injured children (GCS of eight or less) may have a consistent grading of motor response, verbal response and eye opening.

GCS is a useful predictor of outcome, particularly in the group of children who are admitted with a GCS score of five or more and who subsequently do not deteriorate. In one study the presence of abnormal plantar and pupillary light reflexes predicted an outcome of death or severe disability (Grewal and Sutcliffe, 1991).

NEUROLOGICAL EXAMINATION

The purpose of the neurological examination is to establish an accurate, objective baseline of neurological function. Therefore, it is essential that the neurological examination be documented in a fashion that is *reproducible*. In this way, a comparison of baseline, previous and current findings allows the observer to detect subtle changes in the neurological status that might not be evident otherwise. Descriptions of behaviours should be simple, objective, and easily interpreted: "Drowsy but awake and conversationally rational/oriented", "Sleepy but arousable with vigorous physical stimuli. Pressure to nail bed of right hand results in upper extremity flexion/lower extremity extension".

Vital signs, observation of posture and movement (both spontaneous and elicited), eye examination, CN testing, and reflex testing provide valuable clues regarding the LOC, the site of involvement, and the probable cause, although they do not necessarily parallel the depth of a comatose state.

VITAL SIGNS

Pulse, *respiration*, and *blood pressure* provide information regarding the adequacy of circulation and the possible underlying cause of altered consciousness. *Autonomic activity* is most intensively disturbed in deep coma and in brainstem lesions. *Body temperature* is often elevated, and sometimes the elevation may be extreme. Coma of a toxic origin may produce hypothermia. High temperature is most frequently a sign of an acute infectious process or heat stroke, but may be caused by ingestion of some drugs, especially salicylates, alcohol, and barbiturates, or intracranial bleeding. A fever sometimes follows a cerebral seizure.

The pulse is variable and may be rapid, slow and bounding, or feeble. Blood pressure may be normal, elevated or decreased. The Cushing reflex or pressor response that causes a slowing of the pulse and an increase in blood pressure is uncommon in children; when it occurs, it is a very late sign. Vital signs are also affected by medications. For assessment purposes, *changes* in pulse and blood pressure are more important than the direction.

Respirations are more often slow, deep and irregular. Slow and deep breathing is often seen in the heavy sleep caused by sedatives, after seizures or in cerebral infections. Slow, shallow breathing may result from sedatives or narcotics. Hyperventilation (deep and rapid respirations) is usually the result of

metabolic acidosis or abnormal stimulation of the respiratory centre in the medulla caused by salicylate poisoning, hepatic coma or Reye's syndrome.

SKIN

The skin may offer clues to the cause of unconsciousness. The body surface should be examined for the presence of injury, needle marks, petechiae, bites and ticks. Evidence of toxic substances may be found on the hands, face, mouth and clothing — especially in small children.

EYES

Pupil size and reactivity are assessed. Pupils either react or do not react to light. Pinpoint pupils are commonly observed in poisoning, such as opiate or barbiturate poisoning, or in brainstem dysfunction. Widely dilated and reactive pupils are often seen after seizures and may involve only one side. Dilated pupils may also be caused by eye trauma. Widely dilated and fixed pupils suggest paralysis of third CN secondary to pressure from herniation of the brain through the tentorium. A unilateral fixed pupil usually suggests a lesion on the same side. Bilateral fixed pupils usually imply brainstem damage, if present for more than five minutes. Dilated and nonreactive pupils are also seen in hypothermia, anoxia, ischaema, poisoning with atropine-like substances, or prior instillation of mydriatic drugs. The sudden appearance of a fixed and dilated pupil is a neurosurgical emergency.

Some of the therapies used (e.g., barbiturates) can alter pupil size and reaction. The description of eye movements should indicate whether one or both eyes are involved and how the reaction was elicited. The parents should be asked if the child has a strabismus. A pre-existing strabismus will cause the eyes to appear normal under compromise.

Funduscopic examination reveals additional clues. *Papilloedema*, if it develops at all, will not be evident early in the course of unconsciousness, because papilloedema takes 24-48 hours to develop. The presence of preretinal (subhyaloid) haemorrhages in children is almost invariably the result of acute trauma with intracranial bleeding, usually subarachnoid or subdural haemorrhage.

MOTOR FUNCTION

Observation of spontaneous activity, posture and response to painful stimuli provides clues to the location and extent of cerebral dysfunction. Even subtle movements (e.g., the outturning of a hip) should be noted and the child should be observed for other signs. Asymmetric movements of the limbs or absence of movement suggests paralysis. In hemiplegia, the affected limb lies in external rotation and will fall uncontrollably when lifted and allowed to drop. These observations should be described rather than labelled. In the deeper comatose states there is little or no spontaneous movement and the musculature tends to be flaccid. There is considerable variability in the motor behaviour in lesser degrees of coma. For example, the child may be relatively immobile or restless and hyperkinetic; muscle tone may be increased or decreased. Tremors, twitching and spasms of muscles are common observations. The patient may display purposeless plucking or tossing movements. Combative or negativistic behaviour is not uncommon. Hyperactivity is more common in acute febrile and toxic states than in cases of increased ICP. Convulsions are common in children and may be present in coma as a result of any cause.

THE CHILD WITH CEREBRAL COMPROMISE

Cerebral compromise as a result of physical injury, infection, near-drowning or toxic injury may result in varying states of consciousness. Nursing actions are directed primarily towards detection of possible alterations in condition and prevention of further damage to the various systems and tissues.

NURSING CARE OF THE UNCONSCIOUS CHILD

The unconscious child requires continuous nursing attendance with observation, recording and evaluation of changes in objective signs. These observations provide valuable information regarding the patient's progress. Often, they serve as a guide to diagnosis and treatment. Therefore, careful and detailed observations are essential for the patient's welfare. In addition, vital functions must be maintained and complications prevented through conscientious and meticulous nursing care. The outcome of unconsciousness may be early and complete recovery, death within a few hours or days, persistent and permanent unconsciousness, or recovery with varying degrees of residual mental and/or physical disability.

Emergency measures are directed towards ensuring a patent airway, stabilization of the spine when indicated, treatment of shock, and reduction of ICP (if present). Delayed treatment often leads to increased damage. As soon as emergency measures have been implemented - in many cases concurrently - therapies for specific causes are begun. Because nursing care is closely related to the medical management, both are considered here.

ASSESSMENT

Continual observation of LOC, pupillary reaction, and vital signs is essential to management of CNS disorders. Regular assessment of neurological signs is a vital part of nursing comatose children. Vital signs are taken and recorded regularly. The frequency depends on the cause of coma, the status, and the progression of cerebral involvement. Intervals may be as frequent as every 15 minutes or as long as every two hours. Significant alterations are reported immediately. Temperature is taken every 2-4 hours, depending on the patient's condition. An elevated temperature may occur in children with CNS dys-

function; therefore, a light covering is sufficient.

The LOC is assessed periodically, including size, equality, and reaction of pupils to light and signs of meningeal irritation, such as nuchal rigidity. This also includes response to vocal commands, spontaneous behaviour, resistance to care, and response to painful stimuli. Motions of any type, changes in muscle tone or strength, and body position are noted.

Pain management for the comatose child requires astute nursing observation and management. Signs of pain include changes in behaviour (e.g., increased agitation and rigidity, and alterations in physiological parameters); usually increased heart rate, respiratory rate and blood pressure; and decreased oxygen saturation. Since these findings are not specific for pain, the nurse should observe for their appearance during times of induced or suspected pain and their disappearance following the inciting procedure or the administration of analgesia. A pain assessment record should be used to document indications of pain and the effectiveness of interventions (see Pain Assessment, Chapter 5).

Sedatives are usually avoided, but may be indicated when extreme agitation or restlessness may result in further damage. If so, chloral hydrate or triclofos are preferred. These drugs are less likely to produce respiratory depression, but produce no analgesia. However, favourable results are achieved with the administration of codeine and acetaminophen, which are analgesics.

Anticonvulsants, primarily phenytoin or phenobarbitone, are ordered for control of seizure activity.

RESPIRATORY MANAGEMENT

Respiratory effectiveness is the primary concern in care of the unconscious child, and establishment of an adequate airway is *always* the first priority.

Children in lighter stages of coma may be able to cough and swallow, but those in deeper states of coma are unable to handle secretions, which tend to pool in the throat and pharynx. Dysfunction of CN IX and X places the child at risk of aspiration and cardiac arrest; therefore the child is positioned to prevent aspiration of secretions, and the stomach is emptied to reduce the likelihood of vomiting. In infants, blockage of air passages from secretions can happen in seconds. In addition, upper airway obstruction from laryngospasm is a frequent complication in comatose children.

A temporary airway can be used for the child who is suffering a temporary loss of consciousness, such as after a seizure or anaesthesia. For children who remain unconscious for a time, a nasotracheal or orotracheal tube is inserted to maintain the open airway and to facilitate removal of secretions. A tracheostomy is performed in cases in which laryngoscopy for introduction of an endotracheal tube would be difficult or dangerous. Suctioning is used only as needed to clear the airway, exerting care to prevent increasing ICP. Respiratory status is observed and evaluated regularly. Signs of respiratory embarrassment may be an indication for ventilatory assistance.

When the respiratory centre is involved, mechanical ventilation is usually indicated. Chest physiotherapy is carried out on a regular basis, and the child's position is changed at least every two hours to prevent pulmonary complications.

NUTRITION AND HYDRATION

Fluids and calories are supplied initially by the intravenous route. An intravenous infusion is started early, and the type of fluid administered is determined by the general condition of the patient. Fluid therapy requires careful monitoring and adjustment based on neurological signs and electrolyte determinations. Often, comatose children are unable to cope with the same amounts of fluid they could tolerate at other times, and overhydration must be avoided to prevent fatal cerebral oedema.

Later, nutrition is provided in a balanced formula given by nasogastric or gastrostomy tube. The nasogastric tube is usually taped in place with care to prevent pressure on the nares. Most children have continuous feedings, but if bolus feedings are used, the tube is rinsed with water after each feeding. Tubes are replaced according to unit policy. Nostrils are alternated with each replacement to prevent nasal irritation and pressure. Overfeeding should be avoided to prevent vomiting with its attendant danger of aspiration. Stomach contents are aspirated and measured before feeding to ascertain the amount remaining in the stomach. If the residual volume is excessive (depending on the size of the child), the dietitian and doctor should be consulted regarding alteration of the formula composition to provide the needed calories and nutrients in a smaller volume. The aspirated contents should always be replaced.

Hydration is maintained in the same manner. When cerebral oedema is a threat, fluids may be restricted to reduce the chance of fluid overload. Skin and mucous membranes are examined for signs of dehydration. Observation for signs of altered fluid balance related to abnormal pituitary secretions is a part of nursing care.

MEDICATIONS

The cause of unconsciousness determines specific drug therapies. Children with infectious processes are given antibiotics appropriate to the disease and the infecting organism, and corticosteroids are prescribed for inflammatory conditions and oedema. Cerebral oedema is an indication for osmotherapy with osmotic diuretics (e.g., mannitol), diuretics (e.g., frusemide), and/or hypertonic glucose solution. Sedatives are often indicated for extreme restlessness, agitation and hyperresponsiveness to stimuli. Sedatives or anticonvulsants are prescribed for seizure activity. Analgesics are prescribed to control pain.

NURSING ALERT

When used for seizures, phenytoin should be administered slowly, but infused completely in one hour (the drug tends to precipitate). Too rapid administration may cause cardiac arrhythmias.

ELIMINATION

A retention catheter is usually inserted in the older child, and a plastic collection bag is placed on the infant or small child. Long-term use of collection bags creates excoriation problems, however. The child who formerly had bowel and bladder control is generally incontinent.

HYGIENE

Routine measures for cleansing and maintaining skin integrity are an integral part of nursing care of the unconscious child. Skinfolds require special attention to prevent excoriation. The child who is unable to move is prone to develop tissue breakdown and pressure necrosis; therefore, the child is placed on a resilient appliance (e.g. alternating-pressure and water-filled mattresses) to prevent pressure on prominent areas of the body. The goal is prevention by regular change of position and inspection of vulnerable areas, such as the ankle, trochanter, and shoulder. Since unconscious children undergo numerous invasive procedures, these skin sites require special assessment and intervention to promote healing and to prevent infection. Bed linen and any clothing are kept dry and free of wrinkles. If the child requires surgery or radiography, the nurse checks all dressings, bony sites, catheters and intravenous access lines.

Mouth care is performed at least twice daily, since the mouth tends to become dry or coated with mucus. The teeth are carefully brushed with a soft toothbrush or cleaned with gauze saturated with saline twice daily. Lips are coated with ointment, or other preparations to protect them from drying, cracking or blistering.

The deeply comatose child is also prone to eye irritation. The corneal reflexes are absent; therefore, the eyes are easily irritated or damaged by linen, dust or other substances that may come in contact with them. There is excessive dryness as a result of decreased secretions, especially if the child is undergoing osmotherapy to reduce or prevent brain oedema, and incomplete closure of the eyes. The eyes should be examined regularly and carefully for early signs of irritation or inflammation. Artificial tears (methylcellulose) are placed in the eyes every 1-2 hours. Sometimes, eye dressings may be needed to protect the eyes from possible damage.

POSITIONING AND EXERCISE

The unconscious child is positioned to prevent aspiration of saliva, nasogastric secretions, and vomitus and to minimize ICP. The head of the bed is elevated, and the child is placed in a side-lying or semiprone position. A small, firm pillow is placed under the head, and the uppermost limbs are flexed and supported with pillows. The weight of the body should not rest on the dependent arm. In the semiprone position the child lies with the dependent arm at the side behind the body, the opposite side supported on pillows, and the uppermost arm and leg flexed and resting on the pillows. This position prevents undue pressure on the dependent extremities. The dependent position of the face encourages drainage of secretions and prevents the flaccid tongue from obstructing the airway.

Normal range of motion exercises help to maintain function and prevent contractures of joints. Exercises should be done gently and with full range of motion. Footboards can be used to help prevent footdrop; splinting may be needed to prevent severe contractures of wrist, knee or ankle in decerebrate children.

STIMULATION

Sensory stimulation is important in the care of the unconscious child, just as it is in the care of the alert child. For the temporarily unconscious or semiconscious child, sensory stimulation helps to arouse the child to the conscious state and orient the child in terms of time and place. Auditory and tactile stimulation are especially valuable. Tactile stimulation is not appropriate for the child in whom it may elicit an undesirable response. However, for other children tactile contact often has a relaxing and calming effect. When the child's condition permits, holding or rocking the child has a soothing effect and provides the body contact needed by young children.

The auditory sense is often present in a state of coma. Hearing is the last sense to be lost and the first one to be regained; therefore, the child should be spoken to as any other child. Conversation around the child should not include thoughtless or derogatory remarks. A radio playing soft music, a music box, or a record player is frequently used to provide auditory stimulation. Singing the child's favourite songs or reading a favourite story is a tactic used to maintain the child's contact with a familiar world. Having parents tape songs or stories provides a continuous source of familiar stimulation. Above all, it is important to remember that this is a child who has all the needs of any ill child.

FAMILY SUPPORT

Dealing with the parents of an unconscious child is especially difficult. They may demonstrate all the guilt, fear, hostility and anxiety of any parent of a seriously ill child (see Chapter 21). In addition, these parents are faced with the uncertain outcome of the cerebral dysfunction. The fear of death, mental retardation or other permanent disability is present. Nursing intervention with parents depends on the nature of the pathological condition, the personality of the parents, and the parent-child relationship before injury or illness (Mercer, 1994).

HEAD INJURIES

The Children's Head Injury Trust (1988) states:

More than 40,000 children each year in the UK alone are admitted to hospital with head injuries. Many are of a serious nature with consequences which will trouble the children for the rest of their lives. More regularly, and in increasing numbers, children with severe head injury and brain damage are surviving, and swelling the numbers of children and adults who must address their future limited by the residual handi-caps: handicaps which are largely unseen and which are little understood or appreciated by the community at large.

PATHOPHYSIOLOGY

Head injury can be defined as any pathological process involving the scalp, skull, meninges or brain, as a result of mechanical force. Head injuries can be regarded as localized or generalized. In localized injuries the force is spent on a local area of both skull and underlying tissues; in generalized injuries the force is transmitted to the entire skull, causing independent movement, distension and damage.

Patients with mild head injuries have a GCS score of 13-15; those with moderate head injuries have a GCS score of 9-12. A GCS score of 8 or less indicates severe injury.

Concussion

The most common head injury is concussion, a transient and reversible neuronal dysfunction with instantaneous loss of awareness and responsiveness from trauma to the head that persists for a relatively short time - usually minutes or hours. It is generally followed by amnesia for the moment of the injury, and by amnesia of a variable period before the injury. This post-traumatic amnesia is characteristic, and reflects the extent and severity of injury to the brain after blunt trauma. Post-traumatic amnesia consists of two parts: (1) retrograde amnesia, the period of time before impact for which the patient has no memory, and (2) anterograde amnesia, the period of memory loss after injury. Amnesia in both these periods tends to lessen with time, although there is some permanent amnesia.

Contusion and laceration

The terms *contusion* and *laceration* are used to describe visible bruising and tearing of cerebral tissue. Contusions represent petechial haemorrhages along the superficial aspects of the brain at the site of impact (coup injury) and/or a lesion remote from the site of direct trauma (contrecoup injury). In serious accidents, there may be multiple sites of injury.

The major areas of the brain susceptible to contusion or laceration are the occipital, frontal and temporal lobes. Also, the irregular surfaces of the anterior and middle fossae at the base of the skull are capable of producing bruises or lacerations on forceful impact. Contusions may cause focal disturbances in strength, sensation or visual awareness. The degree of brain damage in the contused areas varies according to the extent of vascular injury. Signs will vary from mild, transient weakness of a limb, to prolonged unconsciousness and paralysis. However, the signs and symptoms may be clinically indistinguishable from concussion.

As a rule, contusions are less common in infants and young children than in adults with comparable trauma, and contrecoup injuries are relatively rare in infants. However, infants who are roughly shaken (whiplash-shake syndrome) can sustain profound neurological impairment, seizures, retinal haemorrhages, and intracranial subarachnoid or subdural haemorrhages. In addition to these classic injuries, high cervical spinal cord haemorrhages and contusions can occur (Zapp *et al*, 1992).

Cerebral lacerations are generally associated with penetrating or depressed skull fractures. However, they may occur without fracture in small children. When brain tissue is actually torn, with bleeding into and around the tear, usually more severe and prolonged unconsciousness and paralysis occur, leaving permanent scarring and some degree of disability.

Fractures

Skull fractures are found in more than 25% of children who are seen with head injuries (Mealey, 1988). However, the immature skull, because of its flexibility, is able to sustain a greater degree of deformation than the adult skull before it incurs a fracture. It requires substantial force to produce a fracture in the skull of an infant. A fracture may occur with little or no brain damage. Conversely, severe and fatal brain injury can take place without fracture. The undersurface of the skull contains grooves in which the meningeal arteries lie. A fracture that runs through one of these grooves may tear the artery and produce severe and damaging haemorrhage. The types of fractures that occur are linear, depressed, compound, basilar and diastatic. As a rule, the faster the blow, the greater the likelihood of a depressed fracture; a low-velocity impact tends to produce a linear fracture.

COMPLICATIONS

The major complications of trauma to the head are haemorrhage, infection, oedema, and herniation through the tentorium. Infection is always a hazard in open injuries, and oedema is related to tissue trauma. Vascular rupture may occur even in minor head injuries, causing haemorrhage between the skull and cerebral surfaces. Compression of the underlying brain produces effects that can be rapidly fatal or insidiously progressive.

Subdural haemorrhage

Presenting signs of acute haematoma include evidence of increased ICP, such as increased head size and bulging fontanels (in the infant), retinal haemorrhages, extraocular palsies (especially CN VI), hemiparesis, quadriplegia and sometimes elevated temperature. Older children may display an unsteady gait, and papilloedema is usually present. Since papilloedema is a late sign of increased ICP, it constitutes an emergency. In infants, the bleeding may be extensive enough to lower the haematocrit significantly and may be observed before any change in LOC in fast-expanding lesions.

Repeated subdural taps often provide relief in the infant. Surgical evacuation of the haematoma is the treatment of choice in the older child and is frequently required in infants.

Structural complications may occur as the result of head injuries. Hydrocephalus is seen when there has been subarachnoid haemorrhage or infection. Focal deficits, including optic atrophy, CN palsies, motor deficits, diabetes insipidus or aphasia may be seen. The type of residual effect depends on the location and nature of the trauma. True mental retardation occurs only after severe injuries.

PROCESS OF DIAGNOSIS

A severe head injury, such as one sustained in a fall from a significant height or in a motor vehicle accident, requires prompt evaluation and treatment. Since head injuries are frequently accompanied by injuries in other areas (spine, viscera, extremities), the examination is performed with care to avoid further damage. Box 31-2 lists manifestations of head injury.

Over 75% of children who die as a consequence of head injury have evidence of ischemic brain damage (Noah *et al*, 1992). Because little can be done about the original primary insult, care of the secondary brain injuries remains the goal in the management of the injured child.

Initial assessment

Priorities in the initial phase in the care of a child with a head injury include assessment of the ABCs (airway, breathing, circulation); assessment for spinal cord injury; evaluation for shock; a neurological examination, especially LOC; pupillary symmetry and response to light; and seizures. The assessment is carried out quickly in relation to vital signs. Excited and irri-

---

◆ **BOX 31-2**

Clinical manifestations of acute head injury

Minor Injury
May or may not lose consciousness
Transient period of confusion
Somnolence
Listlessness
Irritability
Pallor
Vomiting (one or more episodes)

Signs of Progression
Altered mental status (e.g., difficulty rousing child)
Mounting agitation
Development of focal lateral neurological signs
Marked changes in vital signs

Severe Injury
Signs of increased ICP **(see Box 31-1)**
  Increased head size (infant)
  Bulging fontanel (infant)
Retinal haemorrhage
Extraocular palsies (especially CN VI)
Hemiparesis
Quadriplegia
Elevated temperature (sometimes)
Unsteady gait (older child)
Papilloedema (older child)

Associated Signs
Skin injury (to area of head sustaining injury)
Other injuries (e.g., to extremities)

table children may have a rapid pulse, may hyperventilate, appear pale and feel clammy shortly after an injury. Deep, rapid, periodic or intermittent and gasping respirations, wide fluctuations or noticeable slowing of the pulse, and widening pulse pressure or extreme fluctuations in blood pressure are signs of brainstem involvement. It is important to note that marked hypotension may represent internal injuries.

Ocular signs such as fixed and dilated pupils, fixed and constricted pupils, and pupils that are poorly reactive or unreactive to light and accommodation indicate increased ICP or brainstem involvement. It is important to remain with the patient who demonstrates fixed and dilated pupils, since these are ominous signs with the probability of respiratory arrest. Dilated, nonpulsating blood vessels indicate increased ICP before the appearance of papilloedema. Retinal haemorrhages are seen in acute head injuries. Observation of asymmetric pupils or one dilated, unreactive pupil in a comatose child is a neurosurgical emergency that may require evacuation of an epidural haematoma. Bleeding from the nose or ears (although uncommon in children) needs further evaluation, and a watery discharge from the nose (rhinorrhoea) that is positive for glucose suggests leaking of CSF from a skull fracture.

Temperature may be moderately elevated for 1-2 days following an initial mild hypothermia after injury. A persistent fever may indicate subarachnoid haemorrhage or infection.

Special tests

After a thorough clinical examination, a variety of diagnostic tests are helpful in providing a more definitive diagnosis of the type and extent of the trauma. Where available, CT is especially valuable in diagnosis of neurological trauma and usually makes other diagnostic procedures unnecessary (Blevins, 1992). CT is indicated for a deteriorating state while the patient is under observation, for persistent somnolence, or for vomiting that does not abate within 12 hours.

THERAPEUTIC MANAGEMENT

Most children with mild to moderate concussion who have not lost consciousness can be cared for and observed at home after careful examination reveals no serious intracranial injury. Parents are instructed to check the child every two hours to determine any changes in responsiveness. The sleeping child should be wakened to see if the child can be roused normally. Parents are advised to maintain contact with the attending doctor, who usually wishes to examine the child again in 1-2 days. The manifestations of epidural haematoma in children do not generally appear until 24 hours or more after injury.

Maintaining contact with the parents for continued observation and re-evaluation of the child, when indicated, facilitates early diagnosis and treatment of possible complications such as haematoma, hydrocephalus, cysts and post-traumatic seizures. Children with minor injuries who live far from medical facilities or whose parents or caregivers are not deemed reliable in observing their condition are generally hospitalized for 24-48 hours for observation.

Children with severe injuries, those who have lost consciousness for more than a few minutes, and those with prolonged and continued seizures or other focal or diffuse neurological signs must be hospitalized until their condition is stable and their neurological signs have diminished. The child is kept on nil by mouth or restricted to clear liquids, if able to take fluids by mouth, until it is determined that vomiting will not occur. Intravenous fluids are indicated for the child who is comatose and for the child with persistent vomiting.

The volume of intravenous fluid is carefully monitored to avoid aggravating any cerebral oedema and to minimize the possibility of overhydration in case of SIADH (syndrome of inappropriate antidiuretic hormone). However, damage to the hypothalamus or pituitary gland may produce diabetes insipidus with its accompanying hypertonicity and dehydration. Fluid balance is closely monitored by daily weight, accurate intake and output measurement, and serum osmolality to detect early signs of water retention, excessive dehydration, and states of hypertonicity or hypotonicity.

Restlessness can be satisfactorily managed, if necessary, with codeine phosphate or chloral hydrate, and headache is usually controlled with codeine or DF118. Anticonvulsants are used for seizure control and frequently in cases of suspected contusion or laceration. Antibiotics are administered if there are lacerations, CSF leakage, or excessive cerebral tissue damage. Prophylactic tetanus toxoid is given as appropriate. Cerebral oedema is managed as described for the unconscious child.

Surgical intervention

Scalp lacerations are sutured after careful examination of underlying bone. Torn dura is sutured, as well. Depressed fractures require surgical elevation and removal of bone fragments. A skull fracture depressed more than the thickness of the skull or an intracranial haematoma causing more than a 5 mm midline shift are indications for surgery. 'Ping-pong ball' skull fractures in very young infants can correct themselves within a few weeks or may require surgical elevation.

Prognosis

The outcome of craniocerebral trauma depends on the extent of injury and complications. However, the outlook is generally more favourable for children than for adults. More than 90% of children with concussions or simple linear fractures recover without symptoms after the initial period. The incidence of fatalities and neurological sequelae is lower in children, even in those with severe head injuries. The prognosis for recovery is primarily related to the duration of coma and the degree of injury (Eiben *et al*, 1984).

The concern regarding outcome is increasingly focused on cognitive, emotional and/or mental problems. Recent studies indicate that children experience a higher frequency of psychological disturbances following head injury, whereas adults are more prone to complaints of a physical nature. Children who suffer even minor head injuries may exhibit unacceptable behaviour, poor attention span, impaired self-control, difficulty managing stress or frustration, oversensitivity, irritability, mental inconsistency, personality changes, headaches and memory impairment (Boll, 1985; Eisenberg and Briner, 1989; Jacobson *et al*, 1986).

Children may be more vulnerable than adults to long-term cognitive and behavioural dysfunction after diffuse brain injury. Even with recovery, the effects of brain injury on a child's potential can never be known.

True coma (not obeying commands, eyes closed, and not speaking) usually does not exceed more than 2 weeks. A child's eventual outcome can range from brain death to a persistent vegetative state to complete recovery. However, even the best recovery may be associated with personality changes, including mood liability, loss of confidence, and impaired short-term memory, headaches, and subtle cognitive impairments. Many children are left with significant disabilities after head-injury that appear months later as learning difficulties, behavioural changes, or emotional disturbances (Reynolds, 1992).Generally within six months to one year after the injury, 90% of the long-term neurological outcome has been achieved.

IMPLICATIONS FOR NURSING

The hospitalized child requires careful neurological assessment and evaluation. Frequent nursing assessments can provide information needed to establish a correct diagnosis, identify signs and symptoms of increased ICP, determine clinical management and prevent many complications.

The child is placed on bed rest, usually with the head of the bed elevated slightly. Appropriate safety measures, such as cot sides kept up for older children and seizure precautions for children of all ages, are implemented. The extremely restless child may require that hard surfaces be padded and restraint used to prevent the possibility of further injury. Specially made beds are now available for this contingency. Care is individualized according to the specific needs of the child. Children may be restless and irritable, but more often their reaction is to fall asleep when left undisturbed. A quiet environment helps reduce the restlessness and irritability. Bright lights shining directly into the child's face are irritating. This often makes checking the pupil responses more difficult to perform and more aggravating to the child.

Frequent examinations of vital signs, neurological signs, and LOC are extremely important nursing observations. When possible, they should be performed by a single observer in order to better detect subtle changes that may indicate worsening of neurological status. Pupils are checked for size, equality, reaction to light, and accommodation. After the initial elevations usually seen after injury, the vital signs generally return to normal unless there is brainstem involvement. An axillary temperature is the safest method of measuring temperature, since seizures are not uncommon and vomiting is a frequent response in children, especially when the child is disturbed.

The most important nursing observation is assessment of the child's LOC. Alterations in consciousness appear earlier in the progression of an injury than alterations of vital signs or focal neurological signs. Some expected responses may be mis-

interpreted as deviations from the normal. Frequent examinations of alertness are fatiguing to the child; therefore, the child often desires to fall asleep, which may be confused with depressed consciousness. When left alone, the child promptly dozes. It is not uncommon to observe ocular divergence through the partially closed eyelids.

Observations of position and movement provide additional information. Any abnormal posturing is noted, as well as whether or not it occurs continuously or intermittently. Questions nurses might ask themselves include:
- Are the child's hand grips strong and equal in strength?
- Are there any signs of decerebrate or decorticate posturing?
- What is the child's response to stimulation?
- Is movement purposeful, random or absent?
- Are movement and sensation equal on both sides or restricted to one side only?

The child may complain of headache or other discomfort. The child who is too young to describe a headache will be irritable and resist being handled. The child who suffers from vertigo will often assume a position and vigorously resist being moved. Forcible movement causes the child to vomit and display spontaneous nystagmus. Seizures, relatively common in children at the time of injury, may be of any type but are more often generalized regardless of the type of injury. Any seizure activity should be carefully observed and described in detail. Children in postictal states are more lethargic with sluggish pupils.

Drainage from any orifice is noted. Bleeding from the ear suggests the possibility of a basal skull fracture. The amount and characteristics of the drainage are observed, and since the auditory canal may be a source of infection, dry, sterile cotton gauze can be placed loosely at the orifice and changed when soiled. Suctioning through the nose is contraindicated, since there is a high risk of secondary infection and the probability of the catheter entering the brain substance through a fracture.

Head trauma is frequently accompanied by other undetected injuries; therefore, any bruises, lacerations, or evidence of internal injuries or fractures of the extremities are noted and reported. Associated injuries are evaluated and treated appropriately.

The child with normal LOC is usually allowed clear liquids unless fluid is restricted. If the child has an intravenous infusion, it is maintained as prescribed. The diet is advanced to that appropriate for the child's age, as soon as the condition permits. Intake and output are measured and recorded, and incontinence of bowel or bladder is noted in the child who has been toilet trained.

The child should be observed for unusual behaviour, but interpretation of behaviour should be made in relation to the child's normal behaviour. For example, urinary incontinence during sleep would be of no consequence in a child who routinely wets the bed, but would be highly significant for a child who is always dry. In addition, a child who is subject to nightmares might cry out and demonstrate agitated behaviour at night. Parents are valuable resources in evaluating objectively behaviours of their children. Information obtained from parents at or shortly after admission is helpful in evaluating the child's behaviour; for example, the ease with which the child is normally roused, the usual sleeping position, how much the child sleeps during the day, motor activity the child is capable of (rolling over, sitting up, climbing), hearing and visual acuity, appetite, and manner of eating (spoon, bottle, cup). There would be less concern about a child who falls asleep several times during the day if this particular type of behaviour is consistent with the child's usual behaviour.

When the child is discharged, the parents are advised of probable post-traumatic symptoms that may be expected, such as behavioural changes, sleep disturbances, phobias and seizures. They should understand observations that should be made and how to contact the doctor, nurse or health clinic in case the child develops unusual signs or symptoms. The importance of follow-up evaluation should be emphasized.

Rehabilitation of brain-injured children is begun as soon as feasible, and usually involves the family and a rehabilitation team (Scott-Jupp, 1992). Careful assessment of the child's capabilities, limitations, and probable potential is made as early as possible and appropriate interventions are implemented to maximize the residual capacities. Useful contacts include the Children's Head Injury Trust and Headway.

INTRACRANIAL INFECTIONS

The nervous system and its coverings are subject to infection by the same organisms that affect other organs of the body. However, the nervous system is limited in the ways in which it responds to injury. Infectious processes share virtually the same clinical and pathological features. They differ primarily in the growth and virulence of the specific organism. Laboratory studies are needed to identify the causative agent. The inflammatory process can affect the meninges *(meningitis)*, brain *(encephalitis)* or spinal cord *(myelitis)*.

Most children with acute febrile encephalopathy have either bacterial meningitis or viral meningitis as their underlying cause (Rubenstein, 1992). Meningitis can be caused by a variety of organisms, but the three main types are:

1. **Bacterial,** or pyogenic, caused by pus-forming bacteria, especially the meningococcus, pneumococcus, and influenza bacilli.
2. **Tuberculous,** caused by the tubercle bacillus.
3. **Viral,** or aseptic, caused by a wide variety of viral agents.

BACTERIAL MENINGITIS

Bacterial meningitis is a potentially fatal disease and, although the advent of antimicrobial therapy has had a marked effect on the course and prognosis, it remains a significant cause of illness in the paediatric age groups. Its importance lies primarily in the frequency with which it occurs in infancy and childhood, and the unnecessarily high death rates and residual damage caused by undiagnosed and untreated or inadequately treated cases. Ninety percent of cases occur in children between the ages of one month and five years; infants 6-12 months of age are at greatest risk (Krugman *et al*, 1985).

AETIOLOGY

Bacterial meningitis can be caused by any of a variety of bacterial agents. *Haemophilus influenzae* (type B) (Hib), *Streptococcus pneumoniae*, and *Neisseria meningitidis* (meningococcus) organisms are responsible for bacterial meningitis in 95% of children older than two months. *H. influenzae* is the predominant organism in children three months to three years of age, but is rare in infants younger than three months, who are apparently protected by passively acquired bactericidal substances, and in children older than five years, who are beginning to acquire this protection. With the routine use of *H. influenzae* type B vaccines, the aetiology of bacterial meningitis is changing.

CLINICAL MANIFESTATIONS

The clinical manifestations of acute bacterial meningitis depend to a large extent on the age of the child. The picture is also influenced to some degree by the type of organism, the effectiveness of therapy for antecedent illness, and whether it occurs as an isolated entity or as a complication of another illness or injury.

Children and adolescents

The illness is likely to be abrupt, with fever, chills, headache and vomiting that are associated with or quickly followed by alterations in sensorium. Often the initial sign is a seizure, which may recur as the disease progresses. The child is extremely irritable and agitated, and may develop photophobia, delirium, hallucinations, aggressive or maniacal behaviour, or drowsiness, stupor and coma. Sometimes, the onset is slower, frequently preceded by several days of respiratory or gastrointestinal symptoms. Occasionally, a prior infection treated with antibiotics masks or delays the signs of meningitis.

The child resists flexion of the neck, and as the disease progresses, the neck stiffness becomes marked until the head is drawn into extreme overextension (opisthotonos). Kernig and Brudzinski signs are positive. Reflex responses are variable, although they show hyperactivity. The skin may be cold and cyanotic with poor peripheral perfusion.

Other signs and symptoms may appear that are peculiar to individual organisms. Petechial or purpuric rashes usually indicate a meningococcal infection, especially when the eruption is associated with a shock-like state. Joint involvement is seen in meningococcic and *H. influenzae* infection. A chronically draining ear commonly accompanies pneumococcal meningitis. *E. coli* infection may be associated with a congenital dermal sinus that communicates with the subarachnoid space.

Infants and young children

The classic picture of meningitis is rarely seen in children between three months and two years of age. The illness is characterized by fever, poor feeding, vomiting, marked irritability and frequent seizures, which are often accompanied by a high-pitched cry. A bulging fontanel is the most significant finding; nuchal rigidity, and Brudzinski and Kernig signs are helpful in diagnosis (Clinical Diagnosis of Meningitis in Children, 1993).

Neonates

Meningitis in newborn and premature infants is extremely difficult to diagnose. The vague and nonspecific manifestations, characteristic of all neonatal sepsis, bear little resemblance to the findings in older children. These infants are usually well at birth, but within a few days begin to look and behave poorly. They refuse feeds, have poor sucking ability, and may vomit or have diarrhoea. They display poor tone, lack of movement and a poor cry. Other nonspecific signs that may be present include hypothermia or fever (depending on the maturity of the infant), jaundice, irritability, drowsiness, seizures, respiratory irregularities or apnoea, cyanosis, and weight loss. The full, tense, and bulging fontanel may or may not be present until late in the course of the illness, and the neck is usually supple. Untreated, the child's condition will decline to cardiovascular collapse, seizures and apnoea.

Complications

The incidence of complications from acute bacterial meningitis has been significantly reduced with early diagnosis and vigorous antimicrobial therapy. If infection extends to the ventricles, thick pus, fibrin, or adhesions may occlude the narrow passages, thereby obstructing the flow of CSF to cause obstructive hydrocephalus. Subdural effusions occur frequently, and thrombosis may occur in meningeal veins or venous sinuses. Destructive changes may take place in the cerebral cortex, and brain abscesses may form by direct extension of the infection or by vascular dissemination. Extension of the infection to the areas of the cranial nerves or compression necrosis from increased pressure may cause deafness, blindness, or weakness or paralysis of facial or other muscles of the head and neck.

One of the most dramatic and serious complications usually associated with meningococcal infections is meningococcal septicaemia or meningococcaemia. When the onset is severe, sudden and rapid (fulminate), it is known as the Waterhouse-Friderichsen syndrome. The syndrome is characterized by overwhelming septic shock, disseminated intravascular coagulation (DIC), and massive bilateral adrenal haemorrhage. Meningococcaemia requires immediate emergency treatment, hospitalization, and intensive care. The mortality is as high as 85% (Jenkins, 1992).

THERAPEUTIC MANAGEMENT

Acute bacterial meningitis is a medical emergency that requires early recognition and immediate institution of therapy to prevent death and to avoid residual disabilities. The initial therapeutic management includes:

• Isolation precautions

• Initiation of antimicrobial therapy
• Maintenance of optimum hydration
• Maintenance of ventilation
• Reduction of increased ICP
• Management of bacterial shock
• Control of seizures
• Control of extremes of temperature
• Correction of anaemia
• Treatment of complications

The child is isolated from other children, usually in an intensive care unit, for close observation. An intravenous infusion is started as soon as the lumbar puncture has been completed in order to facilitate the administration of antimicrobial agents, fluids, anticonvulsive drugs, and blood if needed. The child is placed on a cardiac monitor.

Drugs

Until the causative organism is identified, the choice of antibiotic is based on the known sensitivity of the organism most likely to be the infective agent in any given situation, and the probable interactions with the specific patient. Except under special circumstances, the drugs are administered intravenously throughout the course of treatment. The drugs are given in large doses, and the period of therapy is determined by CSF findings and the child's clinical condition. Appropriate antibiotics are administered following identification of the causative organism.

Nonspecific measures

Maintaining hydration is a prime concern. Intravenous fluids and the type and amount of fluid are determined by the patient's condition. The optimum hydration involves correction of any fluid deficits, followed by low maintenance levels to prevent cerebral oedema. If indicated, measures are employed to reduce ICP. Increased ICP seen with CNS infections commands attention because of the severe reduction of cerebral perfusion pressure (CPP) in children suffering from bacterial meningitis in the early period, herpes encephalitis, and postinfectious encephalitis with severe status epilepticus.

Complications are treated appropriately, such as aspiration of subdural effusion in infants and heparin therapy for children who develop disseminated intravascular coagulation syndrome. Shock, if it occurs in the child, is managed by restoration of blood volume and maintenance of electrolyte balance. Seizures occur in affected children during the first few days of treatment. These are controlled with appropriate anticonvulsants.

Lumbar puncture is carried out as needed to determine the effectiveness of therapy. The patient is evaluated neurologically during the convalescent period and at regular intervals during the succeeding year.

Prognosis

The age of the child, the rapidity of diagnosis after onset, and the adequacy of therapy are important in the prognosis of bacterial meningitis. The mortality of neonatal meningitis is approximately 50%, although late-onset β-haemolytic streptococcal meningitis carries a 15-20% case fatality. With *H. influenzae* disease and meningococcal meningitis, the mortality rate is 5-10%, and with pneumococcal meningitis in infancy and childhood, about 20%.

Sequelae of bacterial meningitis are seen most frequently when the disease occurs in the first two months of life and least often in children with meningococcal meningitis. The residual deficits in infants are primarily a result of communicating hydrocephalus and the greater effects of cerebritis on the immature brain. In older children, the residual effects are related to the inflammatory process itself or result from vasculitis associated with the disease. Evaluation of CN VIII is needed for at least a six-month follow-up period to assess for possible hearing loss.

Prevention

According to the Health Education Authority 1992 findings:

Each year about 1300 children in the United Kingdom are infected by Hib. Over half of these children develop Hib meningitis. Hib is the commonest cause of bacterial meningitis in children under 4 years old. Most children with the infection become very ill and have to go to hospital. Each year around 65 die and about 150 are left with permanent brain damage.

Hib immunization is given as a separate injection at the same time as diphtheria, pertussis and tetanus. There are no serious side effects. One child in 10 has some redness and swelling, usually no larger than approximately 2 cm across, after the injection. Since it was first used, more than 25 million doses have been given nationwide without serious side effects. Children should receive injections for Hib at the ages of two, three, and four months (Health Education Authority, 1992).

IMPLICATIONS FOR NURSING

Nurses should take necessary precautions to protect themselves and others from possible infection. Parents are taught the proper procedures and supervised in their application.

The room should be kept as quiet as possible and environmental stimuli kept at a minimum, since most affected children are sensitive to noise, bright lights, and other external stimuli. Most children are more comfortable without a pillow and with the head of the bed slightly elevated. A side-lying position is more often assumed because of nuchal rigidity. The nurse should avoid actions, such as lifting the child's head, that cause pain or increase discomfort. Measures are employed to ensure safety, since the child is often restless and subject to seizures.

The nursing care of the child with meningitis is determined by the child's symptoms and treatment. Observation of vital signs, neurological signs, level of consciousness, urine output, and other pertinent data is carried out at frequent intervals, and all children are observed carefully for signs of increased ICP, shock or respiratory distress.

Fluids and nourishment are determined by the child's status. The child with insufficient gag reflex is usually given nothing by mouth. Other children are allowed clear liquids initially and progressed to a diet suitable for their age. Careful monitoring and recording of intake and output are needed to determine deviations that might indicate impending shock or increasing fluid accumulation, such as cerebral oedema or subdural effusion.

One of the most difficult problems in nursing care of children with meningitis is maintaining the intravenous infusion for the length of time needed to provide adequate antimicrobial therapy (usually ten days). Since continuous intravenous fluids are usually not necessary, a heparin lock device is used.

BRAIN ABSCESS

Brain abscesses are the most common form of intracranial suppurative process in children. Intracranial abscesses form when pyogenic organisms gain access to nervous tissue by way of the bloodstream from foci of infection or from direct inoculation of organisms from meningitis, penetrating trauma or surgical procedures. The majority of cases spread from secondary ear, nose or throat sources; meningitis, sepsis or cyanotic congenital heart disease.

Antibiotic therapy is effective during abscess formation. Successful management consists of surgical drainage of a localized infection and antibiotic therapy. Where possible, the source of the infection is eradicated.

A decline in mortality has been documented with the advent of CT scanning (Tekkok and Erbergl, 1992). The progression of the disease and the child's mental status before admission continue to be prognostic factors.

Nursing care is similar to that for the child with increased ICP. Support of the child and family is essential since the prognosis for mortality and death remain high.

ENCEPHALITIS

Encephalitis is an inflammatory process of the CNS producing altered function of various portions of the brain and spinal cord. Encephalitis can be caused by a variety of organisms, including bacteria, spirochaetes, fungi, protozoa, helminths and viruses.

The clinical features of encephalitis are similar regardless of the agent involved. Manifestations can range from a mild benign form that resembles aseptic (non-bacterial) meningitis, lasting a few days and being followed by rapid and complete recovery, to a fulminating encephalitis with severe CNS involvement. Treatment is primarily supportive, including conscientious nursing care, control of cerebral manifestations, and adequate nutrition and hydration, with observation and management as for other disorders involving cerebral injury. Neurological monitoring, administration of medicines, and support of the child and parents are the major aspects of care.

EPILEPSY: CLASSIFICATION

There are many different types of epileptic seizures, and each has unique characteristics. They are classified on the basis of careful clinical description of the attacks in conjunction with results of physical examination and EEG analysis. The onset of a seizure is abrupt, paroxysmal, and transitory, and signs are highly variable. The International Classification of Epileptic Seizures divides seizures into two major categories: partial seizures and generalized seizures (Box 31-3).

PARTIAL SEIZURES

Partial seizures are caused by abnormal electrical discharges from epileptogenic foci limited to a more or less circumscribed region of the cerebral cortex. There is usually evidence that the irritating focus of the seizure is secondary to an underlying condition that causes damage to brain tissue. Focal lesions include scars from previous craniocerebral trauma, atrophy, malformations or tumours. Focal seizures may arise from any area of the cerebral cortex, but the frontal, temporal, and parietal lobes are most often affected. The area of cerebral involvement is reflected by clinical manifestations.

Partial seizures are categorized as: (1) those with elementary or simple symptoms, (2) those with associated impairment of consciousness, and (3) those with impaired consciousness and that spread to become generalized. The hallmark of partial seizures is the onset in a portion of one cerebral hemisphere, as evidenced by focal spikes or sharp waves on the EEG.

Simple partial seizures

Focal seizures are characterized by localized motor symptoms; somatosensory, psychic, autonomic symptoms; or a combination of these. The abnormal discharges remain unilateral. The most common motor seizure in children is the aversive seizure, in which the eye or eyes and head turn away from the side of the focus. In some children, the upper extremity towards which the head turns is abducted and extended, and the fingers are clenched, giving the impression that the child is looking at the closed fist. The child may be aware of the movement or may lose consciousness simultaneously with assuming the position.

A common form is the sylvian seizure, in which there are tonic-clonic movements involving the face, salivation and arrested speech. These are most common during sleep. On rare occasions, children display the *Jacksonian* march, an orderly, sequential progression of clonic movements that begin in a foot, hand or face and, as electrical impulses spread from the irritable focus to contiguous regions of the cortex, move or 'march' body parts activated by these cerebral regions. Motor seizures are particularly common in hemiplegic children. The movements, which are usually clonic, begin in the hemiplegic hand, spread to the entire affected side and, in many cases, become generalized seizures. Postictal weakness is common after this type of seizure.

Special sensory seizures are characterized by various sensations, including numbness, tingling, prickling, paraesthesia, or pain that originates in one area (e.g., face or extremities) and spreads to other parts of the body. Visual sensations or formed images may be manifestations. Motor phenomena such as posturing or hypertonia may accompany sensory seizures. Special sensory seizures are uncommon in children under eight years of age.

Complex partial seizures

Partial seizures with complex symptoms are the most difficult to recognize and are among those most difficult to control. Because they involve more organized and higher-level cerebral function as well as sensory and motor function, they have been termed *psychomotor seizures*. The attack is characterized by a period of altered behaviour for which the individual is amnesic and during which he or she is unable to respond to the environment. Although children do not lose consciousness during an attack, they have no recollection of their behaviour during the seizure. Drowsiness or sleep usually follows the seizure. Confusion and amnesia may be prolonged.

◆ **BOX 31-3**

International classification of epileptic seizures

I. Partial seizures (seizures beginning locally)
  A. Simple partial seizures (with elementary symptomatology; consciousness unimpaired)
    1. With motor symptoms
    2. With somatosensory or special sensory symptoms
    3. With autonomic symptoms
    4. Compound forms (with psychic symptoms)
  B. Complex partial symptomatology (temporal lobe or psychomotor seizures; generally with impaired consciousness)
    1. With impairment of consciousness only
    2. With cognitive symptomatology
    3. With affective symptomatology
    4. With psychosensory symptomatology
    5. With psychomotor symptomatology
    6. Compound forms
  C. Partial seizures, secondarily generalized
II. Generalized seizures (bilaterally symmetric; without local onset; with impairment of consciousness)
  A. Tonic-clonic (grand mal) seizures
  B. Tonic seizures
  C. Clonic seizures
  D. Absence (petit mal) seizures
  E. Atonic seizures
  F. Myoclonic seizures
  G. Infantile spasms
  H. Akinetic seizures
III. Unilateral seizures (those involving one hemisphere)
IV. Unclassified epileptic seizures (due to incomplete data)

Modified from Commission on Classification and Terminology of the International League Against Epilepsy, 1981.

Psychomotor seizures are observed more often in children from three years of age through adolescence. These seizures may begin with an *aura*, complex sensory phenomena associated with the beginning of a seizure reflect the complicated connections and integrative functions of that area of the brain. The most frequent sensation is a strange feeling in the pit of the stomach that rises towards the throat. This feeling is often accompanied by odd or unpleasant odours or tastes, complex auditory or visual hallucinations, or ill-defined feelings of elation or strangeness (e.g., *déjà vu*, a feeling of familiarity in a strange environment). Small children may emit a cry or attempt to run for help as a manifestation of an aura. Strong feelings of fear and anxiety and a distorted sense of time and self may be mental symptoms associated with an episode.

A variety of patterns of motor behaviour may be observed during a psychomotor attack. The attacks are usually stereotypical and recur in a similar manner with each subsequent seizure. It is sometimes difficult to determine whether the manifestations are related to a seizure disorder or to a nonconvulsive behavioural disturbance. The child may suddenly cease activity, appear dazed, stare into space, become confused and apathetic, and become limp, stiff, or display some form of posturing. The primary feature may be confusion, and the child may perform purposeless, complicated activities in a repetitive manner (automatisms), such as walking, running, kicking, laughing, or speaking incoherently, most often followed by postictal confusion or sleep. The predominant observations may be oropharyngeal activities (e.g., lip smacking, chewing, drooling, swallowing) and nausea or abdominal pain followed by stiffness, a fall, and postictal sleep. Rarely, children manifest auras such as rage or temper tantrums, and aggressive acts are uncommon during a seizure. See Box 31-3 for a comparison of simple partial, complex partial, and absence seizures.

GENERALIZED SEIZURES

Generalized seizures without a focal onset appear to arise in the reticular formation, and the clinical observations indicate that the initial involvement is from both hemispheres. Loss of consciousness occurs and is the initial clinical manifestation. Unlike partial seizures that become generalized, there is no aura. Attacks occur at any time, day or night, and the interval between attacks may be minutes, hours, weeks or even years. Most affected persons first experience seizures in childhood, and children whose seizures begin before the age of four years have mental retardation, and behavioural and learning problems more frequently than those whose seizures begin later.

Tonic-clonic seizures
The generalized tonic-clonic seizure, traditionally known as *grand mal*, is the most common and most dramatic of all seizure manifestations of childhood. The seizure usually occurs without warning. There is a rolling of the eyes upward and immediate loss of consciousness. If the child is standing, he or she falls to the floor or ground. The child stiffens in a generalized and symmetric tonic contraction of the entire body musculature. The arms usually flex, whereas the legs, head and neck extend. The child may utter a peculiar piercing cry produced as the jaws clamp shut and the thoracic and abdominal muscles contract, forcing air through tightly closed vocal cords. This tonic phase lasts approximately 10-20 seconds, during which the child is apnoeic and may become cyanotic. Autonomic stimulation causes increased salivation.

The tonic rigidity is replaced by violent jerking movements as the trunk and extremities undergo rhythmic contraction and relaxation of the clonic phase. During this time, the child may foam at the mouth and be incontinent of urine and faeces. As the attack ends, the movements become less intense and occur at longer intervals until they cease entirely. The clonic phase generally lasts about 30 seconds, but can vary from only a few seconds to half an hour or longer. A series of seizures at intervals too brief to allow the child to regain consciousness between the time one attack ends and the next begins is known as *status epilepticus*. This requires emergency intervention. A succession of interrupted seizures can lead to exhaustion, respiratory failure and death.

In the postictal state, children appear to relax but may remain semiconscious and difficult to rouse. They may awaken in a few minutes, but remain confused for several hours. They are poorly coordinated, with mild impairment of fine motor movements. Children may have visual and speech difficulties and may vomit or complain of severe headache. When left alone, they usually sleep for several hours. On awakening they are fully conscious, but usually feel tired and complain of sore muscles and headache, but have no recollection of the entire event.

Absence seizures
Absence seizures, traditionally called *petit mal* or *lapses*, are characterized by a brief loss of consciousness with minimal or no alteration in muscle tone and may go unrecognized because the child's behaviour is changed very little. Attacks almost always first appear during childhood. In most instances, the onset occurs between 4-12 years of age. Attacks are rarely detected before age five, usually cease at puberty, but may be seen in adults. They are more common in girls than in boys.

During these brief seizure episodes, there are lapses of unconsciousness and the child may appear inattentive or daydreaming. The child's schoolwork may deteriorate, and the child may become very frustrated and develop behaviour problems. It is important that the absence seizure be distinguished from daydreaming and attention deficit hyperactivity disorder (ADHD), which also exhibits inattentiveness or short attention span. An early diagnosis of the absence seizure supported with an EEG is essential. A seizure can be induced by asking the child to hyperventilate during the EEG, thus differentiating it from daydreaming or ADHD (Middleton, 1993).

During adolescence, a child with absence seizures may cease having seizures, which is sometimes referred to as 'growing out of the seizure'. In other cases, the youngster may develop tonic-clonic seizures or simple partial seizures.

The EEG is obtained for all children with convulsive manifestations and is the most useful tool for evaluating seizure disorders. The EEG is carried out under varying conditions - with the child asleep, awake, awake with provocative stimulation (flashing lights, noise), and hyperventilating. Stimulation elicits abnormal electrical activity, which is recorded on the EEG.

THERAPEUTIC MANAGEMENT

The objective of treatment of convulsive disorders is to: (1) control the seizures or to reduce their frequency, (2) discover and correct the cause when possible, and (3) help the child who has recurrent seizures to live as normal a life as possible. Seizures of a recurrent nature are treated as soon as the diagnosis is established. If the seizure activity is a manifestation of an infectious, traumatic or metabolic process, the seizure therapy is instituted as a part of the general therapeutic regimen. Seizure control is considered to prevent secondary brain cell injury from the neuronal discharge and hypoxia.

Drug therapy

It is known that persons predisposed to epilepsy have seizures when their basal level of neuronal excitability exceeds a critical point or threshold; no attack occurs if the excitability is maintained below this threshold. The administration of anticonvulsant drugs serves to raise this threshold and prevent seizures. Consequently, the primary therapy for convulsive disorders is the administration of the appropriate anticonvulsant drug or combination of drugs in a dosage that provides the desired effect without causing undesirable side effects or toxic reactions. Anticonvulsant (anti-epileptic) drugs are believed to exert their effect primarily by reducing the responsiveness of normal neurons to the sudden, high-frequency nerve impulses that arise in the epileptogenic focus. Thus, the convulsive seizure is effectively suppressed; the abnormal brain waves may or may not be altered. However, complete control can be achieved only in 70-80% of children with epilepsy, and 20-30% of children prove more difficult to control. Some success has been achieved in treating infantile spasms with ACTH. Hyperkalaemia can be a late side effect of this therapy.

Therapy is begun with a single drug known to be effective for the child's particular type of seizure, and the dosage is gradually increased until the seizures are controlled or until the child develops signs of toxicity. If the drug is effective, but does not sufficiently control the seizures, a second drug is added in gradually increasing doses. Once seizures are controlled, the drug or drugs are usually continued for at least 2 years.

Periodic re-evaluation of the drug is important to assess the continued effectiveness and to alter the dosage if indicated. The dosage will need to be increased as the child grows. Blood levels often prove valuable in determination of optimum dosage levels (see Box 31-4). Blood cell counts, urinalysis and liver function tests are obtained at frequent intervals in children receiving particular anticonvulsant medications. Repeat EEGs are generally obtained every 1.5-2 years .

Blood levels are particularly unreliable in patients receiving sodium valproate. Optimal serum concentration is uncertain, as blood levels vary throughout the day and a single specimen is unreliable. Several studies have reported poor interpatient correlation between dosage and plasma level, particularly in young children and patients/clients receiving multiple antiepileptic drug therapy (Bruni *et al*, 1978).

The most accurate evaluation of plasma levels of sodium valproate requires an average estimation based on several determinations during the course of 24 hours (Loiseau, 1984). If only a single estimate is made it is vital that this is taken at a fixed time in relation to dosing and meals if it is to be of any comparative value with subsequent measurements.

Withdrawal of anti-epileptic therapy follows a predesigned protocol, usually begun when the child has been seizure-free for at least two years with a normal EEG. Relapse in children may be related to factors such as neurological deficit or a positive family history for epilepsy. Recurrence is most likely within the first year after discontinuance of the medication.

When a medication is discontinued, the dosage should be reduced gradually over 1-2 weeks. Sudden withdrawal of a drug can cause an increase in the number and severity of seizures, often precipitating status epilepticus. If the time for reducing the medication coincides with puberty or, in younger children, occurs during periods when the child is subject to frequent infections, the drug is continued for a longer period.

Complications of drug therapy

Side effects of continued use of anticonvulsant medications are sometimes distressing to the child and the family. Most side effects are transient and dose related, but warrant immediate attention of health care personnel. Drug reactions require clinical evaluation and serum drug levels. Combination therapy, such as with barbiturates and carbamazepine, can potentiate drug levels. Careful monitoring is necessary to avoid toxicity. It is also important to be aware that phenytoin causes gingival hyperplasia, which can be cosmetically undesirable. Frequent gum massage and careful attention to good oral hygiene are recommended. Ataxia and rashes often disappear when drug dosages are reduced. Depression, which has been reported in children with epilepsy who are taking barbiturate anticonvulsants, can be relieved by changing drugs.

More troublesome, however, is the accumulating evidence indicating that anticonvulsant therapy may have detrimental effects on behaviour and mental function (Engel, 1989).

In children with epilepsy surgery is reserved for those who suffer from repetitive incapacitating (refractory) seizures present for an extended period without evidence of remission. The epileptogenic area should be in a surgically removable and functionally silent region of the brain. Since a very extensive medical (such as invasive EEG monitoring), psychosocial, and psychometric evaluation is required, prospective candidates should be able to understand, cooperate, and tolerate the testing (Hodges and Root, 1991).

Status epilepticus

Status epilepticus is defined as a continuous seizure that lasts more than 30 minutes or as serial seizures from which the child does not regain a premorbid level of consciousness. The initial treatment is directed towards support and maintenance of vital functions, including maintaining an adequate airway, administration of oxygen, and hydration, and followed by intravenous administration of either diazepam or phenobarbitone. Concurrent intravenous loading with phenytoin is usually necessary for sustained control of seizures.

The child must be closely monitored during administration to detect early alterations in vital signs that may indicate impending cardiac arrest or respiratory depression. When diazepam is ineffective, phenobarbitone, often in extremely high levels that may require respiratory support, is given intravenously as the initial medication. Patients who do not respond to drug therapy may require the use of intravenous and/or general anaesthesia, or thiopentone.

Status epilepticus is a medical emergency requiring immediate intervention to prevent permanent injury to the brain. Equally imperative to halting the tonic-clonic movement is correct diagnosis of the underlying problem. The outcome is related to the aetiology and duration of the status epilepticus (Davidson, 1993).

The prognosis following treatment for status epilepticus is more favourable than previously reported. Most children will probably have no intellectual impairment. Children who do have cognitive deficits or who die are likely to have preceding developmental delay, neurological abnormality, or concurrent serious illness (Verity, Ross, and Golding, 1993).

NURSING CARE OF THE CHILD WITH EPILEPSY

Nursing care of the child with a convulsive disorder involves both acute care during a seizure and long-term management. A child with epilepsy and the family require continuous and consistent support in dealing with the stigma associated with a seizure disorder. Education can decrease the psychological conflicts that persist with the burden of epilepsy. Educating

---

◆ BOX 31-4

Value of blood tests for different anticonvulsant drugs

Drug	Need for Blood Tests
Phenytoin	Essential
Carbamazepine	Useful
Ethonisimide	Useful
Phenobarbitone	Sometimes useful
Primidone	Not often useful
Sodium valproate	Not often useful
Clonazepam	Not often useful
Vigabatrin	Not often useful

From Oxley and Smith, 1991.

---

the child, family and community are key nursing functions (Appleton, 1993).

Assessment

An important nursing function during a seizure is observing the seizure and describing its pertinent features. Any alterations in behaviour and characteristics of the attack, such as sensory-hallucinatory phenomena (e.g., an aura), motor effects (e.g., eye movements, muscular contractions, laterality, complex activities), alterations in consciousness, and postictal state are noted and recorded (Shantz, 1993).

Generalized seizures and others with dramatic manifestations are easily detected, but absence seizures present more difficulties. They are easily misinterpreted as inattention. Any unusual behaviour, even seemingly inconsequential behaviour such as a momentary interruption of activity, staring, or mental blankness, should be described. The more detailed these descriptions, the more valuable they are for assessment. The nurse notes the time that the seizure began and times the length of the seizure. This is especially important if the child becomes cyanotic.

History taking is a vital tool for identifying factors that aid in establishing a cause of the seizures. Interviewing the child and the family helps to elicit problems related to the psychological impact of the disorder on their lives.

Implications for Nursing

The child must be protected from injury during the seizure, and nursing observations made during the attack provide valuable information for diagnosis and management of the disorder.

It is impossible to halt a seizure once it has begun, and no attempt should be made to do so. The nurse must remain calm, stay with the child, and prevent the child from sustaining any harm during the attack. If possible, the child should be isolated from the view of others by closing a door or pulling screens. A seizure can be very upsetting to the child, other visitors, and their families. If other people are present, they should be assured that the affected child is in no danger, and after the attack they can be provided with a simple explanation to meet their needs.

The convulsing child should not be moved or forcefully restrained, and force should not be exerted in an attempt to place a solid object between the teeth. A standing child whom the nurse is able to reach in time, or a child who is seated in a chair (including a wheelchair), should be eased to the floor immediately. After the attack, the child should be placed on its side in bed or a similar place to allow the child to sleep. A side-lying position can prevent a hypotonic tongue from occluding the airway. If the child is at school or away from home, the parents should be contacted so that the child can be taken home to rest.

Children who are known to have convulsive attacks or who are under observation for seizures will require special precautions. The extent of these measures will depend on the type and frequency of the seizure. Children who are subject to daily seizures should not be permitted to engage in activities in which they might be injured, such as climbing. If necessary, additional protection can be provided by lightweight bicycle helmets. These children should have siderails on beds with the hard surfaces padded if there is danger that they could hurt themselves.

Children who have infrequent seizures or who are relatively free of seizures will have few restrictions on their activities. However, some precautions are implemented; for example, the bed should be protected with a waterproof mattress or sheeting.

Changes in personality, indifference to school activities and family, hyperactivity, or even psychotic behaviour may sometimes be observed. The potential effects of anticonvulsants on learning and behaviour should be considered. Progressive intellectual deterioration in a child with epilepsy requires investigation of present medication plus the role of the underlying cerebral pathology.

The degree to which activities are restricted is individualized for each child and depends on the type, frequency, and severity of the seizures; the child's response to therapy; and the length of time the seizures have been controlled. Normal healthy activities are encouraged for children, and participation in competitive sports is determined on an individual basis. With encouragement, most older children can accept the restrictions placed on activities. Climbing trees or structures from which the child might fall and be seriously injured is not usually permitted. The well-controlled child can ride a bicycle or swim if accompanied by a companion (Kemp, 1993). Few other restrictions should be placed on children regarding sports and peer activity, to reduce the likelihood of needlessly accentuating differences.

Because the child is encouraged to attend school and other normal activities, the school nurse and the teacher should be made aware of the child's condition and the therapy. They can help to ensure regularity of medication and any special care the child might need. The child's teacher should be instructed regarding care of the child during a seizure so that he or she can act in a calm manner to ensure the child's welfare and to influence the attitudes of the child's classmates.

FEBRILE CONVULSIONS

Febrile convulsions are transient disorders of children that occur in association with a fever. They are one of the most common neurological disorders of childhood, affecting about 3% of children. Most febrile convulsions occur after six months of age and usually before age three years, with increased frequency in children younger than 18 months. They are unusual after five years of age. Boys are affected about twice as often as girls, and there appears to be an increased susceptibility in families, indicating a possible genetic predisposition.

The cause of febrile convulsions is still uncertain. They are associated with disease outside the CNS and are usually generalized, brief, and self-limited. A history and physical assessment usually rule out CNS disease. In most children, the height and rapidity of the temperature elevation seem to be factors. The fever usually exceeds 38.8 °C and occurs during the temperature rise rather than after a prolonged elevation. Sometimes it constitutes the dramatic beginning of an illness. Febrile convulsions usually accompany an upper respiratory or gastrointestinal infection, and 25% of children with simple febrile convulsions have a recurrence of the seizure with subsequent infections. Since fevers are almost impossible to prevent in children, efforts are directed towards preventing an increase in the temperature.

Treatment consists of controlling the convulsions with phenobarbital or diazepam in appropriate dosage, and reducing the temperature by administration of paracetamol or paracetamol syrup. Whether or not to implement continuous prophylactic anticonvulsant therapy in children who have experienced their initial febrile convulsion is still controversial. At present, anticonvulsant therapy is recommended for children with febrile convulsions who are at increased risk for developing sequelae. Little risk of neurological deficit, mental retardation or altered behaviour has been observed as sequelae of febrile convulsions.

Febrile convulsions are divided into two categories: simple and complex. Simple febrile convulsions are brief, last from 10-15 minutes and are generalized. Complex febrile convulsions are prolonged and may have focal features. The chance of developing chronic seizure disorder is increased in children who have a prolonged convulsion, those with focal convulsions, those who have a near relative who experiences convulsions, and those with an abnormal EEG. Recurrences are more likely when the first seizure occurs in the first year of life. Seventy-five percent of recurrences take place within one year of the first febrile convulsion and almost 90% within two years of onset.

KEY POINTS

- The central nervous system (CNS) is composed of the brain and spinal cord. Brain, blood and cerebrospinal fluid (CSF) maintain an equilibrium inside the skull; and disturbance of these components creates disequilibrium.
- Level of consciousness (LOC) is the most important indicator of neurological health; altered levels include sleep, confusion, delirium, pseudowakeful states and comatose states.
- Complete neurological examination includes LOC; posture; motor, sensory, cranial nerve (CN), and reflex testing; and vital signs.
- Nursing care of the unconscious child focuses on respiratory management, neurological assessment, increased intracranial pressure (ICP) monitoring, supplying adequate nutrition and hydration, drug therapy, promoting elimination, hygienic care, positioning and exercise, stimulation, and family support.
- Primary head injury involves features that occur at the time of trauma, including fractured skull, contusions, intracranial haematoma and diffuse injury. Secondary complications include hypoxic brain damage, increased ICP, infection, cerebral oedema and post-traumatic syndromes.
- The young child's response to head injury is different because of the following features: larger head size, expandable skull, larger amount of blood volume to the brain, small subdural spaces, and thinner, softer brain tissue.
- Fractures resulting from head injuries may be classified as linear, depressed, compound, basilar and diastatic.
- Nursing care of the child with meningitis includes administration of antibiotics, prevention of self-infection, removal of environmental stimuli, correct positioning, vital signs monitoring, intravenous therapy, and promoting fluid, nutritional status, and supportive care of the family.
- Encephalitis may result from direct invasion of the CNS by a virus or from postinfectious involvement of the CNS after viral disease.
- A seizure is a symptom of underlying pathology and is manifest by sensory-hallucinatory phenomena, motor effects, sensorimotor effects and loss of consciousness.

REFERENCES

Appleton RE: Special link—epilepsy clinical nurse specialist, *Nurs Times* 89(19):40, 1993.

Blevins SH, Benson S: A better way to get kids through scans, *RN* 55(10):40-44, 1992.

Boll T: Minor head injury in children, out of sight but not out of mind, *J Clin Child Psychol* 12:74, 1985.

Bruni J: Steady state kinetics of valproic acid in epileptic patients, *Clin Pharmacol Ther* 24(3):324, 1978.

Clinical diagnosis of meningitis in children, *Emerg Med* 25(4)175, 1993.

Commission on Classification and Terminology of the International League Against Epilepsy: proposal for revised clinical and electroencephalographic classification of epileptic seizures, *Epilepsia* 22:489, 1981.

Davidson DLW: The need for guidelines on the use of rectal diazepam, *Seizure* 2:1, 1993.

Eiben CF *et al*: Functional outcome of closed head injury in children and young adults, *Arch Phys Med Rehabil* 65:168, 1984.

Eisenberg H, Briner A: Late complication of head injury. In McLaurin R, editor: *Pediatric neurosurgery*, Philadelphia, 1989, WB Saunders Co.

Engel J: *Seizures and epilepsy*, Philadelphia, 1989, FA Davis.

Grewal M, Sutcliffe AJ: Early prediction of outcome following head injury: an assessment of the value of GCS score trend and abnormal plantar and pupillary light reflexes, *J Pediatr Surg* 26:1161, 1991.

Health Education Authority: Protect yor child with new Hib immunisation, London 1992, HEA.

Hodges K, Root L: Surgical management of intractable seizure disorders, *J Neurosci Nurs* 24(6):340, 1991.

Jacobson MS *et al*: Follow-up of adolescent trauma victims: a new model of care, *Pediatr* 77:236, 1986.

Jenkins TL: Fulminant meningococcemia in pediatric patients: nursing considerations, *Pediatr Nurs* 18(6):629, 1992.

Kemp AM: Epilepsy in children and the risk of drowning, *Arch Dis Child* 68:684, 1993.

Loiseau: National use of valproate: indications and drug regimen in epilepsy, *Epilepsia* 25(suppl):565, 1984.

Mealey J: Skull fractures. In Eichelberger M, Paatsch G, editors: *Pediatric trauma care*, Rockville, MD, 1988, Aspen.

Mercer A: Psychological approaches to children with life threatening conditions and their families, *ACPP Review and Newsletter* 16(2):56, 1994.

Middleton DB: After a child's first seizure, *Emerg Med* 25(4):181-191, 1993.

Muira H: Plasma levels and pharmokinetics of antiepileptic drugs in children, *Folia Psychiatr Neurol* 35:305, 1981.

Noah ZL *et al*: Management of the child with severe brain injury, *Crit Care Clin* 8(1):59-77, 1992.

Oxley J, Smith J, editors: *The epilepsy reference book*, ed 1, London, 1991, Faber & Faber.

Rubenstein JS: Acute pediatric CNS infections. In Fuhrman BP, Zimmerman JJ, editors: *Pediatric Critical Care*, St Louis, 1992, Mosby.

Reynolds E: Controversies in caring for the child with a head injury, *MCN* 17:246-251, 1992.

Scott-Jupp R: Rehabilitation and outcome after severe head injury, *Arch Dis Child* 67:222, 1992.

Tekkok IH, Erbergi A: Management of brain abscess in children: review of 130 cases over a period of 21 years, *Child Nerve Syst* 8(7):411-416, 1992.

Verity CM, Ross EM, Golding J: Outcome of childhood status epilepticus and lengthy febrile convulsions: findings of national cohort study, *BMJ* 307:225-228, 1993.

Zepp F *et al*: Battered child syndrome, Neuropediatrics 23(4): 188,1992.

FURTHER READING

General

James HE: Neurologic evaluation and support in the child with an acute brain insult, *Pediatr Ann* 15:16, 1986.

McKellar A: Head injuries in children and implication for their prevention, *J Pediatr Surg* 24:577, 1989.

Molmar GE *et al*: Pediatric rehabilitation: brain damage causing disability, *Arch Phys Med Rehabil* 70:166, 1989.

Neurological Assessment

Hellier A, Ptak H, Cerrito M: CATS inside my brain: children's understanding of the cerebral computed tomography scan procedure, *Child Health Care* 14:211, 1986.

Hershey BL, Zimmerman RA: Pediatric brain computed tomography, *Pediatr Clin North Am* 32:1477, 1985.

Kryba FN, Ogburn-Russell L, Rutledge JN: Magnetic resonance imaging: the latest in diagnostic technology, *Nurs '87* 17(1):45, 1987.

Moore PC: When you have to think small for a neurological exam, *RN* 51(6):38, 1988.

Reilly PL *et al*: Assessing the conscious level in infants and young children, *Childs Nerv Syst* 4:31, 1988.

Increased Intracranial Pressure

Boortz-Marx R: Factors affecting intracranial pressure: a descriptive study, *J Neurosurg Nurs* 17:89, 1985.

Jess LW: Assessing your patient for increased ICP, *Nurs '87* 17(6):34, 1987.

Brain Death

Elliott J, Smith DR: Meeting family needs following severe head injury: a multidisciplinary approach, *J Neurosurg Nurs* 17:111, 1985.

Myer EC: Determination of brain death in infants and children, *Curr Opin Pediatr* 1:315, 1989.

Head Injury

Bagnato SJ, Feldman H: Closed head injury in infants and preschool children: research and practice issues, *Inf Young Child* 2(1):1, 1989.

Billmire ME, Myers PA: Serious head injury in infants: accident or abuse? *Pediatr* 75:340, 1985.

Gordon VL: Recovery from a head injury: a family process, *Pediatr Nurs* 15:131, 1989.

Hobdell EF *et al*: The effect of nursing activities on the intracranial pressure of children, *Crit Care Nurse* 9(6):75, 1989.

Johnson SLJ: Post-traumatic tremor in head-injured children, *Arch Dis Child* 67:227, 1992.

Martin KM: Predicting short-term outcome in comatose head-injured children, *J Neurosci Nurs* 19:9, 1987.

Sherman DW: Managing acute head injury, *Nurs '90* 20(4):47, 1990.

Worthington J: The impact of adolescent development on recovery from traumatic brain injury, *Rehabil Nurs* 14:118, 1989.

Near-Drowning

Butler S: Out of the water, but not out of the woods, *RN* 51(6):26, 1988.

Shovein J *et al*: Near drowning, *Am J Nurs* 89:680, 1989.

Wintemute GJ, Wright MA: Swimming pool owners' opinions of strategies for prevention of drowning, *Pediatr* 85:63, 1990.

Wintemute GJ *et al*: Drowning in childhood and adolescence: a population based study, *Am J Public Health* 77:830, 1987.

Intracranial Infections

Bonadio WA, Mannenbach M, Krippendorf R: Bacterial meningitis in older children, *Am J Dis Child* 144:463, 1990.

Coderre C: Meningitis: danger when the diagnosis is viral, *RN* 52(8):50, 1989.

Dagbjartsson A, Ludvigsso P: Bacterial meningitis: diagnosis and initial antibiotic therapy, *Pediatr Clin North Am* 34:219, 1987.

Johnson DL *et al*: Treatment of intracranial abscesses associated with sinusitis in children and adolescents, *J Pediatr* 113:15, 1988.

Spaniolo AM, Van Antwerp C: Case study of a child with meningococcemia, *J Pediatr Nurs* 1:396, 1986.

Epilepsy

Appleton RE: Infantile spasms, *Arch Dis Child* 69:614, 1993.

Ashkenasi A, Snead OC: Epileptic syndromes in children and their therapy, *Curr Opin Pediatr* 1:269, 1989.

Austin JK: Predicting parental anticonvulsant medication compliance, *J Pediatr Nurs* 4:88, 1989.

Austin JK, McDermott N: Parental attitude and coping behavior in families of children with epilepsy, *J Neurosci Nurs* 20:174, 1988.

Dreyfuss FE: Classification of epileptic seizures, *Pediatr Clin North Am* 36:265, 1989.

Duchowny MS: Surgery for intractable epilepsy: issues and outcome, *Pediatr* 84:886, 1989.

Lacey DJ: Status epilepticus, *J Clin Psychiatry* 49:33, 1988.

Schwartz R *et al*: Ketogenic diets in the treatment of epilepsy: short-term clinical effects, *Dev Med Child Neurol* 31:145, 1989.

Tse AM: Seizures and societal attitudes: a teaching tool for children, siblings, classmates, parents, and classroom teachers, *Issues Compr Pediatr Nurs* 9:299, 1986.

Vining EP: Educational, social, and life-long effects of epilepsy, *Pediatr Clin North Am* 36:449, 1989.

Other Seizures

Bonadia WA: Febrile convulsion is a common pediatric disorder, *Pediatr Emerg Care* 4:229, 1988.

Hirtz DG: Generalized tonic-clonic and febrile seizures, *Pediatr Clin North Am* 36:365, 1989.

Meningitis

Mellor DH: The place of computed tomography and lumbar puncture in suspected bacterial meningitis, *Arch Dis Child* 67:1417, 1992.

Chapter 32

The Child with Endocrine Dysfunction

LEARNING OUTCOMES

After studying this chapter you should be able to:

◆ Define normal growth.
◆ List the possible determinants of the normal growth pattern.
◆ List and describe the possible causes of short stature.
◆ Define what a hormone is and how it works.
◆ Explain the meaning of target organ.
◆ State causes of over- or undersecretion of the endocrine hormones in relation to altered physiology.
◆ Describe the psychological and social effects of over- or undersecretion of hormones on the child and family.
◆ Be aware of the types of treatment, facilities and advice available to families.
◆ Recognize and describe a child's experience of an endocrine disorder.
◆ Describe how nurses can help the child and family to manage the disorder more effectively.
◆ Define the glossary terms.

GLOSSARY

allele The different forms of a gene; alleles that occur at the same position on a chromosome pair may produce different effects during development

Chvostek sign Facial muscle spasm elicited by tapping the facial nerve in the region of the parotid gland

gluconeogenesis Formation of glucose from molecules that are not themselves carbohydrates (e.g., amino acids, lactate, and glycerol portion of fats)

glycogenolysis Breakdown of glycogen to glucose

Trousseau sign Carpal spasm elicited by pressure applied to nerves of the upper arm

The major chemical regulators of the body are internal secretions and their secreting cells, known as the endocrine system. The function of the endocrine system is to secrete intracellularly synthesized hormones into the circulation, where they are transported to nearby or distant sites to stimulate, catalyse or serve as pacemaker substances for metabolic processes.

This chapter is primarily concerned with problems associated with oversecretion or undersecretion of the major hormones or defective responses.

THE ENDOCRINE SYSTEM

The endocrine system consists of three components: (1) the *cell*, which sends a chemical message by means of a hormone; (2) the *target cells*, or *end organs*, which receive the chemical message; and (3) the *environment* through which the chemical is transported (blood, lymph, extracellular fluids) from the site of synthesis to the sites of cellular action.

The endocrine glands, which are distributed throughout the body, are listed in Box 32-1.

HORMONES

A hormone is a complex chemical substance, produced and secreted into body fluids by a cell or group of cells, that exerts a physiological controlling effect on other cells. Some are *local hormones*, creating their effect near the point of secretion.

◆ **BOX 32-1**

Endocrine glands

Pituitary gland (hypophysis cerebri) — a pea-sized gland that lies within a deep bony depression at the base of the cranium, the sella turcica, and is attached to the hypothalamus on the undersurface of the brain by a slender infundibulum or pituitary stalk

Thyroid gland — two large lateral lobes and a connecting portion, the isthmus, situated on the anterior aspect of the neck just below the larynx

Parathyroid glands — four or five (there may be more or less) small, round bodies attached to the posterior surfaces of the lateral lobes of the thyroid gland

Adrenal glands — pyramid-shaped glands situated atop the kidneys, fitting like caps over these organs

Ovaries — glands located in the female pelvis on each side of the uterus at the fimbriated end of the uterine (fallopian) tubes

Testes — oval-shaped glands situated within the male scrotum

Islets of Langerhans — small clusters of endocrine cells within the pancreas situated between the acinar or exocrine-secreting portions of the gland

---

General hormones are produced in one organ or part of the body and are carried through the bloodstream to a distant part, or parts, of the body where they initiate or regulate physiological activity of an organ or group of cells.

CONTROL OF HORMONE SECRETION

Regulation of hormonal secretion is based on negative feedback. As a general rule, endocrine glands have a tendency to oversecrete their particular hormones. However, once the physiological effect of the hormone has been achieved, this information is transmitted to the producing gland, either directly or indirectly, to inhibit further secretion. If the gland undersecretes, the inhibition is relieved, and the gland increases production of the hormone. As a result, the hormone is secreted according to the amount needed. This is the primary function of the tropic hormones.

The endocrine gland primarily responsible for stimulation and inhibition of target glandular secretions is the *anterior pituitary*, or 'master gland'. *Tropic* (which literally means 'turning') hormones secreted by the anterior pituitary regulate the secretion of hormones from various target organs (Fig. 32-1). As blood concentrations of the target hormones reach normal levels, a negative message is sent to the anterior pituitary to inhibit release of the tropic hormone. For example, thyroid-stimulating hormone (TSH) responds to low levels of circulating thyroid hormone (TH). As blood levels of thyroid hormone reach normal concentrations, a negative feedback message is sent to the anterior pituitary, resulting in diminished release of thyroid-stimulating hormone.

The pituitary gland is, in turn, controlled by either hormonal or neuronal signals from the hypothalamus. Two types of substances are secreted from the hypothalamus: (1) *releasing hormones* and (2) *inhibitory hormones*, which are secreted within the hypothalamus and transported by way of the pituitary portal system to the anterior pituitary, where they stimulate the secretion of tropic hormones. Pituitary hormones that lack feedback control from the product of a target tissue (growth hormone, prolactin and melanocyte-stimulating hormone) require hypothalamic inhibitors and stimulators for their control.

Not all hormones depend on other hormones for their release. For example, insulin is secreted in response to blood glucose concentrations. Other glandular hormones that are not under the control of the pituitary gland are glucagon, parathyroid hormone (PTH), antidiuretic hormone (ADH) and aldosterone.

DISORDERS OF PITUITARY FUNCTION

Deficiencies of the anterior pituitary hormones may be the result of organic defects or of idiopathic aetiology. They may occur as a single hormonal problem or in combination with other hormonal deficiencies. The clinical manifestations

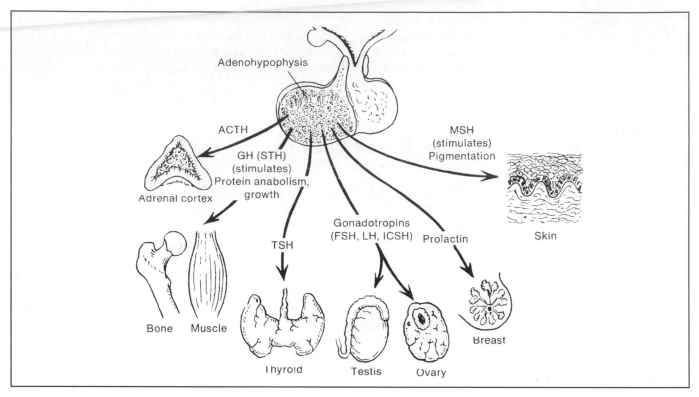

Fig. 32-1 Anterior pituitary hormones and their target organs and tissues. See text for discussion. (From Anthony CP, Thibodeau GA: Textbook of anatomy and physiology, ed 10, St Louis, 1979, Mosby–Year Book)

depend on the hormones involved and the age of onset. If the tropic hormones are involved, the resulting disorder reflects the altered stimulus to the target gland. For example, if thyroid-stimulating hormone is deficient, thyroid hormone is also deficient, and the child displays the manifestations of hypothyroidism.

HYPOPITUITARISM

Hypopituitarism is diminished or deficient secretion of pituitary hormones. The consequences of the condition depend on the degree of dysfunction and lead to gonadotropin deficiency with absence or regression of secondary sex characteristics; somatotropin deficiency, in which children display retarded somatic growth; thyrotropin deficiency that produces hypothyroidism; and corticotropin deficiency, which results in manifestations of adrenal hypofunction. Hypopituitarism can result from any of the conditions listed in Box 32-2.

The most common organic cause of pituitary hyposecretion is tumours in the pituitary or hypothalamic region, especially the craniopharyngiomas. These tumours usually invade the anterior and posterior pituitary lobes and the hypothalamus, causing panhypopituitarism. The child may have shown growth retardation for quite some time before developing any symptoms or signs of increased intracranial pressure, local compression or the destructive effects of the tumour.

Idiopathic hypopituitarism is usually related to growth hormone (GH) deficiency, which inhibits somatic growth in all cells of the body. Although children with hypopituitarism

---

◆ **BOX 32-2**

Aetiology of hypopituitarism

Aplasia or hypoplasia
  Developmental defects
  Idiopathic — sporadic; genetic
Destructive lesions
  Trauma — perinatal; child abuse; basal skull fracture
  Infiltrative lesions — tumours; tuberculosis; toxoplasmosis;
  haemochromatosis; sarcoidosis
Irradiation — CNS; eye; middle ear
Autoimmune hypophysitis
Surgery - removal of pharyngeal pituitary; ablation of craniopharyngioma or other tumour
  Vascular — aneurysm; infarct
Functional deficiency
  Psychosocial dwarfism
  Anorexia nervosa

---

are normal at birth, they show growth patterns that progressively deviate from the normal growth rate, often beginning in infancy (Wit and van Uneu, 1992). The chief complaint in most instances is short stature. Of those who seek help, boys outnumber girls three to one. The extent of idiopathic GH deficiency may be complete or partial, but the cause is unknown. It is frequently associated with other pituitary hormone deficiencies, such as deficiencies of TSH and ACTH; thus, it is theorized that the disorder is probably secondary to hypothalamic deficiency. It has also been observed that there is a higher than average frequency in some families, which indicates a possible genetic aetiology or possible psychosocial factors in several instances (Skuse, 1989; Stanhope, Wilks and Hamil, 1994).

CLINICAL MANIFESTATIONS

The usual presenting complaint is short stature. These children generally grow normally during the first year and then follow a slowed growth curve that is below the third percentile. The children tend to be overweight for height and frequently have increased subcutaneous fat distribution.

Skeletal proportions are normal for the age, but these children appear younger than their chronological age (Fig. 32-2) and have a doll-like or 'cherubic' facial appearance. They are no less active than other children if directed to size-appropriate sports such as swimming, wrestling, gymnastics, soccer or ballet. Bone age is nearly always retarded, but is closely related to height age — the degree of retardation depends on the duration and extent of the hormonal deficiency.

Most of these children have normal intelligence. In fact, during early childhood they often appear precocious in their learning, because their ability seems to exceed their small size. These children are usually not pushed to perform at their chronological age, but at their height age. However, emotional problems are not uncommon, especially as they near puberty, when their smallness becomes increasingly apparent compared with their peers.

PROCESS OF DIAGNOSIS

Only a small number of children with delayed growth or short stature have hypopituitary dwarfism. In the majority of instances, the cause is constitutional delay. The process of diagnosis is aimed at isolating organic causes.

A complete diagnostic assessment should include a family history, a history of the child's growth patterns and previous health status, physical examination, radiological surveys and endocrine studies.

Family history
A family history is of utmost importance in relating short stature to genetic background. Children with constitutional delays frequently are the products of parents who experienced similar slow growth patterns and delayed sexual maturation. A small percentage of those with hypopituitarism demonstrate an autosomal-recessive inheritance pattern. Height and weight of siblings should be compared with the child's growth patterns at comparable age periods.

Child's history
The child's history should include a thorough prenatal history to rule out maternal disorders that may have influenced growth,

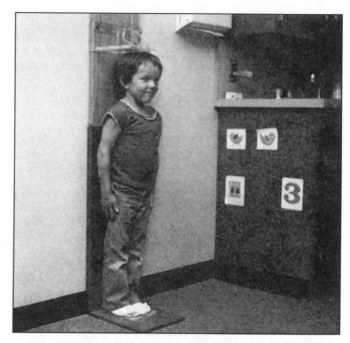

Fig. 32-2 Ten-year-old child with growth hormone deficiency. Height is 108 cm.

such as malnutrition, alcohol or smoking. Birth height and weight should be compared with gestational age. Children with hypopituitarism are usually of normal size and gestational age at birth. Whenever possible, the child's growth patterns since birth should be evaluated, especially growth velocity, as compared with standard measurements. The age of onset of short stature provides a significant diagnostic clue.

The child's past health history is investigated for evidence of chronic illness that may have influenced growth patterns. Signs and symptoms suggesting a tumour, such as visual disturbances, headache, and signs of increasing intracranial pressure, are important. Such symptoms often precede retarded growth but may not have been regarded as significant. With lesions involving the hypothalamus, the history may also reveal characteristic manifestations of dysfunction such as somnolence, thermodysregulation, epilepsy, and hyperphagia, resulting in obesity. Since a craniopharyngioma can affect the secretion of any of the pituitary hormones, assessment for hypothyroidism, hypoadrenalism and hypoaldosteronism should also be included.

Physical examination
Accurate measurement of height and weight, and comparison with standard growth charts are essential (Fry, 1994). Other measurements may include sitting height, leg length and head circumference. Sexual development should be assessed and compared with age-appropriate development. Observation of general appearance yields valuable clues. A funduscopic examination and testing for visual acuity should be performed to detect evidence of ocular damage from a tumour.

Radiological surveys

A skeletal survey in children younger than three years of age, and radiological examination of the wrist for centres of ossification in older children, may be important in evaluating growth. Computed tomography, radionuclear scans or carotid angiograms may be needed to establish diagnosis and localisation of lesions in the head.

Endocrine studies

Definitive diagnosis is based on absent or subnormal reserves of pituitary GH. Since GH levels are normally so low in children that differentiation from abnormal concentrations is unreliable, GH secretion should be stimulated, followed by measurement of blood levels (Brook and Hindmarsh, 1991; Shah *et al*, 1992; Ghigo *et al*, 1994; Ilondo *et al*, 1990).

THERAPEUTIC MANAGEMENT

Treatment of GH deficiency caused by organic lesions is directed towards correction of the underlying disease process (e.g., surgical removal or irradiation of a tumour). The definitive treatment of GH deficiency is replacement of GH. This is successful in 80% of affected children. Human-derived GH (hGH), obtained from human cadavers, is no longer available because of some reported adverse effects (Brown, 1988; Fradkin, 1993). Creutzfeldt-Jakob disease, a rare neurodegenerative condition, was reported in some patients after administration of the natural form of GH (Brown, Gajdusek, and Gibbs, 1985). Biosynthetic GH prepared by recombinant DNA technology is now available and is the therapy of choice.

Children who respond to the therapy typically increase their growth rate from 3.5-4.0 cm/year before treatment to 8-10 cm/year during the first year of therapy. This is the initial period of 'catch-up' growth, when height velocity may increase two- or four-fold. Young children usually respond better than adolescents, obese children better than thin children, and severely GH-deficient children better than those with partial deficiencies (Underwood *et al*, 1986). Treatment does not appear to make up a deficit in *prognosis* of eventual height that is already present at diagnosis; however, it does prevent further loss of stature (Bundak *et al*, 1988). Therefore, early diagnosis is important to successful therapy.

The decision to stop GH therapy is made jointly by the child, family and health care team. Radiological evidence of epiphyseal closure is a criterion for ending therapy. Dosage is increased as the time of epiphyseal closure nears, in order to gain the best advantage of the GH. Children with other hormone deficiencies require replacement therapy to correct the specific disorders. The sex hormones are usually begun during adolescence to promote normal sexual maturation.

IMPLICATIONS FOR NURSING

The principal implication for nursing is identifying children with growth problems. Despite the fact that the majority of growth problems are not a result of organic causes, any delay in normal growth and sexual development poses special emotional adjustments for these children.

The nurse may be a key person in helping to establish a diagnosis. For example, if serial height and weight records are not available, the nurse can question parents about the child's growth in comparison with that of siblings, peers or relatives. Investigating clothing sizes is often helpful in determining growth at different ages. Parents of these children frequently comment that the child wore out clothes before growing out of them or that, if the clothing fit the body, it often was too long in the sleeves or legs.

Because the behavioural or physical changes that suggest a tumour are insidious, they are frequently overlooked. It is important to correlate the onset of any positive findings with the initial evidence of growth retardation.

Part of a nurse's role in helping establish a diagnosis is assisting with diagnostic tests. Preparation of the child and family is especially important if several tests are being performed.

Child and family support

Once a diagnosis is made confirming an organic cause of the problem, the parents and child need an opportunity to express their thoughts and feelings. Family members may feel anger and resentment towards members of the health staff for not detecting the problem sooner. Parents may experience guilt for not seeking medical attention earlier, especially if the child had been miserable from experiencing ridicule and criticism from peers. Each family member needs a sympathetic listener who is aware of his or her needs. Appropriate emotional support from the nurse can include an affirmation of each person's justified feelings, such as anger or guilt, and emphasis on the treatment plan and prospects for improvement in the future.

Children undergoing hormone replacement require additional support. Therapy for GH deficiency requires daily subcutaneous injections. Nursing functions include family education concerning medication preparation and storage, injection sites, injection technique and syringe disposal. Administration of GH is facilitated by family routines that include a specific time of day for the injection. This is usually the evening, to mimic the pattern of normal production of growth hormone. Starcharts and stickers are a helpful means of promoting compliance in younger children. Pen injector devices help children take control of their treatment.

Even when hormone replacement is successful, these children attain their eventual adult height at a slower rate than their peers; therefore, they need assistance in setting realistic expectations regarding the future and the careers on offer to them.

Since these children appear younger than their chronological age, others frequently relate to them in infantile or childish ways. They should wear styles that accentuate their actual age, not their size. If abilities and strengths are emphasized rather than physical size, such children are more likely to develop a positive self-image. Professionals and families may find the Child Growth Foundation a useful resource.

PITUITARY HYPERFUNCTION

Excess growth hormone before closure of the epiphyseal shafts results in proportional overgrowth of long bones, until the individual reaches a height of 2.4 m or more. Vertical growth is accompanied by rapid and increased development of muscles and viscera. Weight is increased, but is usually in proportion to height. Proportional enlargement of head circumference also occurs and may result in delayed closure of the fontanels in young children. Children with a pituitary secreting tumour may also demonstrate signs of increasing intracranial pressure, especially headache.

If hypersecretion of GH occurs after epiphyseal closure, growth is in the transverse direction, producing a condition known as *acromegaly*. Typical facial features include overgrowth of head, lips, nose, tongue, jaw, and paranasal and mastoid sinuses; separation and malocclusion of the teeth in the enlarged jaw; disproportion of the face to the cerebral division of the skull; increased facial hair; thickened, deeply creased skin; and increased tendency towards hyperglycaemia and diabetes mellitus.

PROCESS OF DIAGNOSIS

Diagnosis is based on a history of excessive growth during childhood. Radiological studies may reveal a tumour in an enlarged sella turcica, normal bone age, enlargement of bones (such as the paranasal sinuses), and evidence of joint changes. Endocrine studies to confirm excess of other hormones, specifically thyroid, cortisol and sex hormones, should also be included in the differential diagnosis.

THERAPEUTIC MANAGEMENT

If a lesion is present, surgical treatment by cryosurgery or hypophysectomy is performed to remove the tumour whenever feasible. Other therapies aimed at destroying pituitary tissue include external irradiation and radioactive implants.

IMPLICATIONS FOR NURSING

The primary implication for nursing is early identification of children with excessive growth rates. Although medical management is unable to reduce growth already attained, further growth can be retarded, and the earlier the treatment, the more control there is in predetermining a normal adult height. Nurses in ambulatory settings who are frequently involved in growth screening should refer children who demonstrate excessive linear growth for a medical assessment. They should also observe for signs of a tumour, especially headache, and evidence of concurrent hormonal excesses, particularly the gonadotropins, which cause signs of precocious puberty.

Children with excessive growth rates require as much emotional support as those with short stature. However, girls may suffer from the effects of excessive height much more than boys. Children and their parents need an opportunity to express their feelings. The nurse can help these children overcome problems such as social isolation, low self-esteem and conflicts over body image, especially during adolescence, when they are larger than their peers.

PRECOCIOUS PUBERTY

Manifestations of sexual development before age nine in boys or age eight in girls are considered precocious and should be investigated. Early sexual development can have several causes and may result from a disorder of the gonad, the adrenal gland, or the hypothalamic-pituitary gonadal axis. The disorder is nine times more common in girls than in boys (Silver, Gotlin, and Klingensmith, 1984).

TRUE PRECOCIOUS PUBERTY

True, or complete, precocious puberty is always isosexual. It results from premature activation of the hypothalamic-pituitary-gonadal axis, which produces early maturation and development of the gonads with secretion of sex hormones, development of secondary sex characteristics, and sometimes production of mature sperm or ova. True precocious puberty may be caused by a variety of organic brain lesions, such as tumours, congenital lesions or postinflammatory disorders, but in most instances no cause can be identified. These cases are termed *functional idiopathic* or *constitutional precocious puberty*.

PRECOCIOUS PSEUDOPUBERTY

Precocious pseudopuberty, or incomplete puberty (also called pseudosexual precocious puberty), differs from true sexual precocity in that there is no early secretion of gonadotropin. Most cases result from early overproduction of sex hormone, usually caused by a tumour of the ovary or testis, a tumour or hyperplasia of the adrenal gland, or exogenous sources of androgens or oestrogens. There is no maturation of the gonads, but there is appearance of secondary sex characteristics. Unlike true sexual precocity, precocious pseudopuberty may be heterosexual. A tumour of the adrenal gland in a girl can cause early and inappropriate female development (e.g., clitoral enlargement and masculinization).

Isolated manifestations that are usually associated with puberty may be seen as variations in normal sexual development. They appear without other signs of pubescence and are probably caused by unusual end organ sensitivity to prepubertal levels of oestrogen or androgen. Included are:
- **Premature thelarche** — development of breasts in prepubertal females.
- **Premature pubarche** (premature adrenarche) — early development of sexual hair.

THERAPEUTIC MANAGEMENT

Treatment of precocious pseudopuberty is directed towards the specific cause, when known. Precocious puberty of central (hypothalamic-pituitary) origin is managed with daily subcutaneous or monthly injections of a synthetic analogue of luteinizing hormone-releasing hormone (LHRH), which regulates pituitary secretions. This therapy slows the prepubertal growth to normal rates in affected children. Treatment is discontinued at a chronologically appropriate time, allowing pubertal changes to resume.

IMPLICATIONS FOR NURSING

Psychological support and guidance of the child and family are the most important aspects of management. Although the majority of children do not display behaviour problems, girls with true precocious puberty have a high incidence of problem behaviour, primarily social difficulties related to age/appearance dyssynchrony and moodiness (Sonis, 1985).

Parents need a detailed explanation and reassurance of the benign nature of the condition. Dress and activities for the physically precocious child should be appropriate to the chronological age. Heterosexual interest is not usually advanced beyond the child's chronological age, and parents need to understand that the child's mental age is congruent with the chronological age, and that the child's normal, overt manifestations of affection are age appropriate and do not represent sexual advances.

Despite the early sexual development, maturation of the gonads and the appearance of secondary sexual characteristics proceed normally. The most difficult time for the child is usually the school years before adolescence. After puberty, physical differences from peers are no longer present.

Although the child's heterosexual behaviour is appropriate for the chronological age, the nurse should emphasize to parents that the child is fertile. Usually, no form of contraception is necessary, unless the child is sexually active. In this situation, proper counselling is important because forms of birth control such as oestrogen pills will prematurely initiate epiphyseal closure, resulting in stunted linear growth.

DIABETES INSIPIDUS

The principal disorder of posterior pituitary hypofunction is diabetes insipidus (DI) (sometimes called neurogenic DI) resulting from hyposecretion of antidiuretic hormone (ADH), or vasopressin, and producing a state of uncontrolled diuresis. This disorder is not to be confused with nephrogenic DI, a rare hereditary disorder affecting primarily males, caused by unresponsiveness of the renal tubules to the hormone.

Neurogenic DI may result from several different causes. Primary causes are familial or idiopathic; of the total groups, approximately 45-50% are idiopathic. Secondary causes include trauma (accidental or surgical), tumours, granulomatous disease, infections (meningitis or encephalitis), or vascular anomalies (aneurysm).

CLINICAL MANIFESTATIONS

The cardinal signs of DI are polyuria and polydipsia. In the older child, excessive urination accompanied by a compensatory insatiable thirst may be so intense that the child does little more than go to the toilet and drink fluids. Not infrequently, the first sign is enuresis. In infants, the initial symptom is irritability that is relieved with feedings of water, but not milk. Infants also are prone to dehydration, electrolyte imbalance, hyperthermia, azotaemia and potential circulatory collapse.

Dehydration is usually not a serious problem in older children, who are able to drink larger quantities of water. However, any period of unconsciousness, such as after trauma, may be life threatening because the voluntary demand for fluid is absent. During such instances, careful monitoring of urine volumes, specific gravities, blood osmolarity concentration and intravenous fluid replacement is essential to prevent dehydration.

PROCESS OF DIAGNOSIS

The simplest test used to diagnose this condition, the Water Deprivation Test, is restriction of oral fluids and observation of consequent changes in urine volume and concentration. Normally, reducing fluids results in concentrated urine and diminished volume. In DI, fluid restriction has little or no effect on urine formation, but causes weight loss from dehydration. Accurate results from this procedure require strict monitoring of urine output, measurement of urine concentration (specific gravity or osmolality), and frequent checks of weight, thirst drive and vital signs. A weight loss between 3-5% indicates significant dehydration and requires termination of the fluid restriction.

If this test is positive, the child should be given a test dose of injected aqueous vasopressin (DDAVP), which should alleviate the polyuria and polydipsia. Unresponsiveness to exogenous vasopressin usually indicates nephrogenic DI.

An important diagnostic consideration is to differentiate DI from other causes of polyuria and polydipsia. Other tests used in the diagnostic assessment include a skull radiograph film to detect a tumour, kidney function tests and blood electrolyte levels, and specific endocrine studies to isolate associated problems. In rare instances, a psychological consultation may be warranted to confirm the possibility of compulsive water drinking related to psychogenic causes such as Munchausen's syndrome by proxy (Meadow, 1982, 1985; Rosenberg, 1987).

THERAPEUTIC MANAGEMENT

The usual treatment is hormone replacement with an intranasal spray of desmopressin acetate (DDAVP). It is also available in tablet form.

Some 'breakthrough' urination is allowed during the evening hours, as a precaution against overmedication.

IMPLICATIONS FOR NURSING

The initial objective is identification of the disorder. Since an early sign may be sudden enuresis in a child who is toilet trained, excessive thirst with bed-wetting is an indication for further investigation. Another clue is persistent irritability and crying in an infant that is relieved only by bottle-feedings of *water*.

After confirmation of the diagnosis, parents need a thorough explanation regarding the condition with specific clarification that DI is a different condition from diabetes mellitus. They must realize that treatment is lifelong. The child should be actively involved in taking his or her own medication, if able to do so.

For emergency purposes, these children should wear MedicAlert tags. Older children should carry the nasal spray with them for temporary relief of symptoms. School personnel need to be aware of the problem in order to give the child unrestricted use of the lavatory. Failure to permit this may result in embarrassing accidents that often result in the child's unwillingness to attend school.

Children receiving DDAVP need to be observed for possible overdose of the drug. The signs of overdosage are those of water intoxication.

DISORDERS OF THYROID FUNCTION

The thyroid gland secretes two types of hormones: (1) *thyroid hormone*, which consists of the hormones *thyroxine (T4)* and *triiodothyronine (T3)*, and (2) *thyrocalcitonin*. The secretion of thyroid hormones is controlled by thyroid-stimulating hormone (TSH) from the anterior pituitary, which in turn is regulated by thyrotropin-releasing factor (TRF) from the hypothalamus as a negative feedback response. Consequently, hypothyroidism or hyperthyroidism may result from a defect in the target gland, or from a disturbance in the secretion of TSH or TRF. Since the functions of T_3 and T_4 are qualitatively the same, the term *thyroid hormone (TH)* will be used throughout the discussion.

The synthesis of TH depends on available sources of dietary iodine and tyrosine. The thyroid is the only endocrine gland capable of storing excess amounts of hormones for release as needed. During circulation in the bloodstream, T_4 and T_3 are bound to carrier proteins (thyroxine-binding globulin [TBG]). They must be unbound before they are able to exert their metabolic effect.

The main physiological action of thyroid hormone is to regulate the basal metabolic rate and thereby control the processes of growth and tissue differentiation.

Thyrocalcitonin helps maintain blood calcium levels by decreasing the calcium concentration. Its effect is the opposite of parathyroid hormone (also known as parathormone) in that it inhibits skeletal demineralization and promotes calcium deposition in the bone.

JUVENILE HYPOTHYROIDISM

Hypothyroidism, a deficiency in secretion of thyroid hormones, is one of the most common endocrine problems of childhood. It may be either congenital or acquired.

Beyond infancy, primary hypothyroidism may be caused by several defects. For example, a congenital hypoplastic thyroid gland may provide sufficient amounts of TH during the first year or two, but may be inadequate when rapid body growth increases demands on the gland.

Clinical manifestations depend on the extent of dysfunction and the age of the child at the onset. The presenting symptoms are: (1) decelerated growth from chronic deprivation of thyroid hormone or (2) thyromegaly. Impaired growth and development are less when hypothyroidism is acquired at a later age and, since brain growth is nearly complete by 2-3 years of age, mental retardation or neurological sequelae are not associated with juvenile hypothyroidism. Other manifestations are myxoedematous skin changes (dry skin, puffiness around the eyes, sparse hair), constipation, sleepiness, and poor memory and concentration.

Therapy is thyroid hormone replacement. The same treatment is used in infants, although the prompt treatment needed for infants is not required for children. In children with severe symptoms, the restoration of euthyroidism is achieved more gradually with administration of increasing amounts of L-thyroxine over 4-8 weeks

IMPLICATIONS FOR NURSING

Cessation or retardation of growth in a child whose growth has previously been normal should alert the observer to the possibility of hypothyroidism. Following diagnosis and implementation of thyroxine therapy, the importance of compliance and periodic monitoring of response to therapy should be stressed to parents. Children should learn to take responsibility for their own health, as soon as they are able, after discussion with the family and medical professionals.

GOITRE

A goitre is an enlargement or hypertrophy of the thyroid gland. It may occur in deficient (hypothyroid), excessive (hyperthyroid), or normal (euthyroid) thyroid hormone secretion. It can be congenital or acquired and can be palpated in about 5% of school-aged children (Mahoney, 1987). Congenital disease usually occurs as a result of maternal administration of antithyroid drugs and/or iodides during pregnancy. Acquired disease can result from increased secretion of pituitary TSH in response to decreased circulating levels of TH or from infiltrative neoplastic or inflammatory processes. In areas where dietary iodine (essential for TH production) is deficient, goitre can be endemic.

Enlargement of the thyroid gland can be mild and therefore noticeable only when there is an increased demand for TH (e.g., during periods of rapid growth). Enlargement of the thyroid at birth can be sufficient to cause severe respiratory distress. Sporadic goitre is usually caused by lymphocytic thyroiditis, and intrinsic biochemical defects in the synthesis of the hormones are associated with goitres. Thyroid hormone replacement is necessary to treat the hypothyroidism and to reverse the thyroid-stimulating hormone effect on the gland.

IMPLICATIONS FOR NURSING

Identification of large goitres is facilitated by their obvious appearance. Smaller nodules may be evident only on palpation. Nurses in ambulatory settings need to be aware of the possibility of goitres and must report such findings to a doctor. Benign enlargement of the thyroid gland may occur during adolescence and should not be confused with pathological states. Nodules rarely are caused by a cancerous tumour, but always require evaluation.

LYMPHOCYTIC THYROIDITIS

Lymphocytic thyroiditis (Hashimoto disease, juvenile autoimmune thyroiditis) is the most common cause of thyroid disease in children and adolescents, and accounts for the largest percentage of juvenile hypothyroidism. The disease is four to seven times more common in girls than in boys and four times more common in white than in black people (Fink and Beall, 1982). Although it can occur during the first three years of life, it more frequently appears after age six. It reaches a peak incidence at adolescence (DiGeorge, 1987), and there is evidence that the disease is self-limited.

CLINICAL MANIFESTATIONS

The presence of the enlarged thyroid gland is usually detected by the doctor or children's nurse practitioner during a routine examination, although it may be noted by parents when the child swallows. In most children, the entire gland is enlarged symmetrically (but may be asymmetric), and is firm, freely movable and non-tender. There may be manifestations of moderate tracheal compression (sense of fullness, hoarseness, and dysphagia), but it is extremely rare for nontoxic diffuse goitre to enlarge to the extent that its size causes mechanical obstruction. Most children are euthyroid, but some display symptoms of hypothyroidism. Others have signs suggestive of hyperthyroidism, such as nervousness, irritability, increased sweating or hyperactivity.

PROCESS OF DIAGNOSIS

Thyroid function tests are usually normal, although TSH levels may be slightly or moderately elevated. With progressive disease, the T_4 decreases followed by a decrease in T_3 levels and an increase in TSH. The majority of children have serum antibody titres to thyroid antigens.

THERAPEUTIC MANAGEMENT

In many cases the goitre is transient and asymptomatic, and regresses spontaneously within one or two years. Therapy of nontoxic diffuse goitre is usually simple, uncomplicated and effective. Oral administration of TH will decrease the size of the gland significantly. It provides the feedback needed to suppress TSH stimulation, and the hyperplastic thyroid gland gradually regresses in size. Surgery is contraindicated in this disorder. Untreated patients should be evaluated periodically.

IMPLICATIONS FOR NURSING

Nursing care consists of identifying children with thyroid enlargement, reassuring them that the condition is probably only temporary, and reinforcing instructions for thyroid therapy.

HYPERTHYROIDISM

The largest percentage of hyperthyroidism in childhood is caused by Graves disease, usually associated with an enlarged thyroid gland and exophthalmos (protruding eyeballs). Most cases of Graves disease occur in children aged 6-15, with a peak at 12 and 14 years of age, but may be present at birth in children of thyrotoxic mothers. The incidence is five times higher in girls than in boys.

The hyperthyroidism of Graves disease is apparently caused by an autoimmune response to TSH receptors, but no specific aetiology has been identified. There is definitive evidence for familial association with a high concordance incidence in twins.

CLINICAL MANIFESTATIONS

The development of manifestations is highly variable. Signs and symptoms develop gradually, with an interval between onset and diagnosis of approximately 6-12 months. The principal clinical features are excessive motion—irritability, hyperactivity, short attention span, tremors—insomnia and emotional lability. Gradual weight loss, despite a voracious appetite, is observed in half of the cases. Linear growth and bone age are usually accelerated. Muscle weakness often occurs. Hyperactivity of the gastrointestinal tract may cause vomiting and frequent stooling. Cardiac manifestations include a rapid, pounding pulse, even during sleep; widened pulse pressure; systolic murmurs and cardiomegaly. Dyspnoea occurs during slight exertion, such as climbing stairs. The skin is warm, flushed and moist. Heat intolerance may be severe and is accompanied by diaphoresis. The hair is unusually fine and unable to hold a wave.

Exophthalmos is observed in many children. As protrusion of the eyeball increases, the child may not be able to completely cover the cornea with the lid. Visual disturbances may include blurred vision and loss of visual acuity.

PROCESS OF DIAGNOSIS

Presence of a thyroid mass in a child requires a thorough history, including inquiry into prior irradiation to the head and neck. Diagnosis is established on the basis of increased levels of T_4 and T_3. TSH is suppressed to unmeasurable levels.

THERAPEUTIC MANAGEMENT

Therapy for hyperthyroidism is controversial, but all methods are directed towards retarding the rate of hormone secretion. The three acceptable modes available are: (1) the antithyroid drugs, which interfere with the biosynthesis of thyroid hormone, including propylthiouracil (PTU), (2) subtotal thyroidectomy, and (3) ablation with radioiodine (^{131}I-iodide). Each is effective, but each has advantages and disadvantages.

While affected children exhibit signs and symptoms of hyperthyroidism, their activity should be limited to classwork only. Vigorous exercise is restricted until thyroid levels are decreased to normal or near normal values.

Thyrotoxicosis

Thyrotoxicosis (thyroid 'crisis' or thyroid 'storm') may occur from sudden release of the hormone. Although unusual in children, a crisis can be life-threatening. These 'storms' are evidenced by acute onset of severe irritability and restlessness, vomiting, diarrhoea, hyperthermia, hypertension, severe tachycardia, and prostration. There may be rapid progression to delirium, coma and even death. A crisis may be precipitated by acute infection, surgical emergencies or discontinuation of antithyroid therapy. Treatment, in addition to antithyroid drugs, is administration of ß-adrenergic blocking agents (propranolol), which provide relief from the adrenergic hyperresponsiveness that produces the disturbing side effects of the reaction. Therapy is usually required for 2-3 weeks.

IMPLICATIONS FOR NURSING

The initial nursing objective is identification of children with hyperthyroidism. Since the clinical manifestations often appear gradually, the goitre and ophthalmic changes may not be noticed, and the excessive activity may be attributed to behavioural problems.

Much of children's care is related to treating physical symptoms before a response to drug therapy is achieved. A regular routine is beneficial in providing frequent rest periods, minimizing the stress of coping with unexpected demands, and meeting the children's needs promptly.

The child may benefit from a shortened school day. Despite the excessive activity of these children, they tire easily, experience muscle weakness, and are unable to relax to recoup their strength.

Heat intolerance may produce considerable family conflict. Preferring a cooler environment than others, the child is likely to open windows, complain about the heat, wear minimal clothing, and kick off blankets while sleeping. Although the child should dress in accordance with climatic conditions, the use of light cotton clothing in the home, good ventilation, frequent baths, and adequate hydration is helpful in providing comfort.

Dietary requirements should be adjusted to meet the child's increased metabolic rate. Although the need for calories is increased, these should be provided in wholesome foods rather than 'junk' foods. The child may require vitamin supplements to meet the daily requirement. Rather than three large meals, the child's appetite may be better satisfied by five or six moderate meals throughout the day.

Once therapy is instituted, the drug regimen is explained, emphasizing the importance of observing for side effects of antithyroid drugs. Untoward effects of propylthiouracil and related compounds include urticarial rash, fever, arthritis or arthralgia.

Surgical care

If surgery is anticipated, iodine is usually administered for a few weeks before the procedure.

DISORDERS OF PARATHYROID FUNCTION

The parathyroid glands secrete parathormone, the main function of which, along with vitamin D and calcitonin, is homeostasis of serum calcium concentration and the mineralization of bone. Secretion of PTH is controlled by a negative feedback system involving the serum calcium ion concentration. Low ionized calcium levels stimulate PTH secretion, causing absorption of calcium by the target tissues. High ionized calcium concentrations suppress PTH.

HYPOPARATHYROIDISM

Two classic forms of hypoparathyroidism are observed during childhood: *autoimmune hypoparathyroidism*, in which there is deficient production of PTH, and *pseudohypoparathyroidism*, in which production of PTH is increased, but end-organ responsiveness to the hormone is deficient. The presenting signs or symptoms are similar.

Autoimmune hypoparathyroidism may occur as a component of multiglandular failure, usually related to autoimmune phenomena. Familial hypoparathyroidism is inherited as an autosomal recessive trait, with early onset, usually in the first month of life.

Hypoparathyroidism can also occur secondary to other causes. Postoperative hypoparathyroidism may follow thyroidectomy with acute or gradual onset and may be transient or permanent. Two forms of transient hypoparathyroidism may be present in the newborn, both of which are the result of a relative PTH deficiency. One type is caused by maternal hyperparathyroidism or maternal diabetes mellitus. A more common, later, form appears almost exclusively in infants fed a milk formula with a high phosphate to calcium ratio.

CLINICAL MANIFESTATIONS

Children with pseudohypoparathyroidism are short with round faces, short thick necks, and short and stubby fingers and toes with dimpling of the skin over the knuckles. None of these are observed in hypoparathyroidism. In both types, the skin can be dry, scaly and coarse with skin eruptions, the hair is often brittle, and the nails are thin and brittle with characteristic transverse grooves. Subcutaneous soft tissue calcifications appear in pseudohypoparathyroidism, but not in idiopathic hypoparathyroidism. Dental and enamel hypoplasia occur in both types.

Tetany, convulsions, carpopedal spasm, muscle cramps and twitching, paraesthesias, and laryngeal stridor are often the initial symptoms in both types. Mental retardation is a prominent feature of pseudohypoparathyroidism and may also occur in idiopathic hypoparathyroidism, but is less frequent in later onset disease and with early diagnosis and treatment. Swings of emotion, loss of memory, depression and confusion can occur. Papilloedema may be seen in the idiopathic disease, but is rare in pseudohypoparathyroidism. Since hypoparathyroidism results in decreased bone resorption and inactive osteoclastic activity, skeletal growth is retarded.

PROCESS OF DIAGNOSIS

The diagnosis of hypoparathyroidism is made on the basis of clinical manifestations associated with decreased serum calcium and increased serum phosphate. Levels of plasma PTH are low in idiopathic hypoparathyroidism, but high in pseudohypoparathyroidism. End-organ responsiveness is tested by the administration of PTH with measurement of urinary cyclic AMP. Kidney function tests are included in the differential diagnosis to rule out renal insufficiency. Although bone radiographs are usually normal, they may demonstrate increased bone density and suppressed growth.

THERAPEUTIC MANAGEMENT

The objective of treatment is to maintain normal serum calcium and phosphate levels with minimum complications. Long-term management consists of administration of massive doses of vitamin D, and oral calcium supplementation. Blood calcium and phosphate are monitored frequently until the levels have stabilized; they are then monitored monthly and less often until the child is seen at six-month intervals. Renal function, blood pressure, and serum vitamin D levels are measured every six months. Serum magnesium levels are measured every 3-6 months to permit detection of hypomagnesaemia, which may raise the requirement for vitamin D.

IMPLICATIONS FOR NURSING

The initial objective is recognition of hypocalcaemia. Unexplained convulsions, irritability, gastrointestinal symptoms (diarrhoea, vomiting, cramping), and positive signs of tetany should lead the nurse to suspect this disorder. Much of the initial nursing care is related to the physical manifestations and coping with seizures and safety precautions. Injectable calcium gluconate should be at hand for emergency use.

HYPERPARATHYROIDISM

Hyperparathyroidism is rare in childhood, but can be primary or secondary. The most common cause of primary hyperparathyroidism is adenoma of the gland. The most common causes of secondary hyperparathyroidism are chronic renal disease. The common factor is hypercalcaemia.

CLINICAL MANIFESTATIONS

The manifestations of primary hyperparathyroidism are grouped according to the system involved (Box 32-3).

PROCESS OF DIAGNOSIS

Blood studies to identify any alterations in calcium/phosphate ratio are routinely performed. Measurement of PTH, as well as several tests to isolate the cause of the hypercalcaemia, such as renal function studies, should be included. Other procedures used to substantiate the physiological consequences of the disorder include electrocardiography and radiological bone surveys.

THERAPEUTIC MANAGEMENT

Treatment depends on the cause of hyperparathyroidism. The treatment of primary hyperparathyroidism is surgical removal of the tumour or hyperplastic tissue. Treatment of secondary hyperparathyroidism is directed at the underlying contributing cause, which subsequently restores the serum calcium balance. However, in some instances the underlying disorder

---

◆ BOX 32-3

Manifestations of primary hyperparathyroidism

Gastrointestinal — nausea, vomiting, abdominal discomfort, and constipation

Central nervous system — delusions, confusion, hallucinations, impaired memory, lack of interest and initiative, depression, and varying levels of consciousness

Neuromuscular — weakness, easily fatigued, muscle atrophy (especially proximal muscles of the lower limbs), twitching of the tongue, paraesthesias in extremities

Skeletal — vague bone pain, subperiosteal resorption of phalanges, spontaneous fractures, and absence of lamina dura around the teeth

Renal — polyuria and polydipsia, renal colic, and hypertension

is irreversible, such as in chronic renal failure. In this instance, treatment is aimed at raising serum calcium levels in order to inhibit the stimulatory effect of low levels on the parathyroids. This includes oral administration of calcium salts, high doses of vitamin D to enhance calcium absorption, a low-phosphate diet, and administration of a phosphorus-mobilizing aluminium hydroxide to reduce phosphate absorption.

IMPLICATIONS FOR NURSING

The initial nursing objective is recognition of the disorder. Since secondary hyperparathyroidism is a consequence of chronic renal failure, the nurse is always alert to signs that suggest this complication.

Much of the initial nursing care is related to the physical symptoms and prevention of complications. To minimize renal calculi formation, hydration is essential.

Children with renal rickets (osteodystrophy) may wear splints to minimize skeletal deformities. If the child is confined to bed, the nurse should discuss the proper use of orthopaedic appliances with the physiotherapist.

The diet needs supervision to ensure compliance with low-phosphate foods, particularly dairy products. The nurse should instruct parents regarding foods that need to be avoided and the necessity of administering calcium and vitamin D.

DISORDERS OF ADRENAL FUNCTION

The adrenal glands consist of two distinct portions: the cortex (outer section) and the medulla (inner core). Each portion produces different hormones.

ADRENAL HORMONES

The adrenal cortex secretes the hormones, collectively known as steroids, that are essential to life. The medulla produces the catecholamines, adrenaline and noradrenaline. Since these chemicals are also produced by the sympathetic nervous system, absence of the adrenal supply is not incompatible with life.

ADRENAL CORTEX

The cortex secretes three groups of hormones that are classified according to their biological activity: (1) glucocorticoids (cortisol, corticosterone), (2) mineralocorticoids (aldosterone), and (3) sex steroids (androgens, oestrogens and progestins). The glucocorticoids and mineralocorticoids influence metabolic regulation and stress adaptation. The sex steroids influence sexual development, but are not essential because the gonads secrete the major supply of these hormones.

ADRENAL MEDULLA

The adrenal medulla secretes the catecholamines adrenaline and noradrenaline. Both hormones have essentially the same effects on different organs as those caused by direct sympathetic stimulation, except that the hormonal effects last several times longer. Their major actions are outlined in Box 32-4.

Although the catecholamines evoke similar responses from target sites, there are some important differences. Adrenaline has a greater effect on cardiac activity than noradrenaline, but it causes only weak constriction of the blood vessels in muscles in comparison to the effect of noradrenaline. As a result, noradrenaline elevates blood pressure, whereas adrenaline increases cardiac output. Another important difference is their effect on metabolism. Adrenaline increases the metabolic rate to a much greater extent than noradrenaline.

Control of secretion of catecholamines, primarily in response to physiological or emotional stress, is through the hypothalamus.

Catecholamine-secreting tumours are the primary cause of adrenal medullary hyperfunction. In children, the most common neoplasms of this type are phaeochromocytoma, neuroblastoma and ganglioneuroma.

ACUTE ADRENOCORTICAL INSUFFICIENCY

The acute form of adrenocortical insufficiency (adrenal crisis) may result from several causes during childhood. Although it is a rare disorder, some of the common aetiological factors include haemorrhage into the gland from trauma, which may be caused by a prolonged, difficult labour; fulminating infections, such as meningococcaemia, which result in haemorrhage and necrosis (Waterhouse-Friderichsen syndrome); abrupt withdrawal of exogenous sources of cortisone or failure to increase exogenous supplies during stress; or as a result of congenital adrenogenital hyperplasia of the salt-losing type.

CLINICAL MANIFESTATIONS

Early symptoms of adrenocortical insufficiency include increased irritability, headache, diffuse abdominal pain, weakness, nausea and vomiting, diarrhoea and fever. The child

---

◆ BOX 32-4

Physiological effects of catecholamine secretion

Increased cardiac activity
Vasoconstriction of blood vessels (elevation of blood pressure)
Increased rate and depth of respirations
Bronchial dilation
Inhibition of gastrointestinal activity
Increased muscular contraction
Pupillary dilation
Increased metabolic rate
Heightened sensory awareness
Diaphoresis

is in a shock-like state with a weak, rapid pulse, decreased blood pressure, shallow respirations, cold clammy skin and cyanosis. Circulatory collapse is the end result.

In the newborn, adrenal crisis is accompanied by extreme hyperpyrexia, tachypnoea, cyanosis and convulsions. Usually there is no evidence of infection or purpura.

PROCESS OF DIAGNOSIS

There is no rapid, definitive test for confirmation of acute adrenocortical insufficiency. Routine procedures such as measurement of plasma cortisol levels are too time-consuming to be practical. Therefore, diagnosis is usually made based on clinical presentation, especially when a fulminating sepsis is accompanied by haemorrhagic manifestations and signs of circulatory collapse despite adequate antibiotic therapy. Since there is no real danger in administering a cortisol preparation for a short period, treatment should be instituted immediately. Improvement with this therapy confirms the diagnosis.

THERAPEUTIC MANAGEMENT

Treatment involves initial intravenous replacement of cortisol, replacement of body fluids to combat dehydration and hypovolaemia, administration of glucose solutions to correct hypoglycaemia, and specific antibiotic therapy in the presence of infection. If haemorrhage has been severe, whole blood may be replaced. In the event that these measures do not reverse the circulatory collapse, vasopressors are used for elevation of blood pressure.

Once the child's condition is stabilized, oral doses of cortisone, fluids and salt are given. To maintain sodium retention, aldosterone is replaced by synthetic salt-retaining steroids.

IMPLICATIONS FOR NURSING

Because of the abrupt onset and potentially fatal outcome of this condition, prompt recognition is essential.

Once the acute phase is over and the hypovolaemia is corrected, the child is started on oral fluids, and regraded slowly to prevent vomiting.

The nurse should observe for signs of hypokalaemia, such as cardiac irregularities and muscle weakness. The condition is rapidly corrected with intravenous and oral potassium replacement.

The sudden, severe nature of this disorder necessitates a great deal of emotional support for the child and family. The child may be in an intensive care unit where the surroundings are strange and frightening. Despite the need for emergency intervention, the nurse must be sensitive to the family's psychological needs and prepare them for each procedure. Since recovery within 24 hours is often dramatic, the nurse should keep the parents informed of the child's condition.

CHRONIC ADRENOCORTICAL INSUFFICIENCY

Chronic adrenocortical insufficiency (Addison's disease) is rare in children. When it does occur, it is usually caused by a destructive lesion of the adrenal glands, neoplasms, or an idiopathic cause. At one time, tuberculosis was the leading cause of adrenal gland destruction.

Evidence of this disorder is usually gradual in onset, since 90% of adrenal tissue must be nonfunctional before signs of insufficiency are manifest. However, during periods of stress, when demands for additional cortisol are increased, symptoms of acute insufficiency may appear in a previously well child. The cardinal signs and symptoms are listed in Box 32-5.

Definitive diagnosis is based on measurements of functional cortisol reserve. The cortisol and urinary 17-hydroxycorticosteroid levels are low and fail to rise while plasma ACTH levels are elevated with corticotropin (ACTH) stimulation, the definitive test for the disease.

THERAPEUTIC MANAGEMENT

Treatment involves replacement of glucocorticoids (cortisol) and mineralocorticoids (aldosterone). Some children are able to be maintained solely on oral supplements of cortisol (cortisone or hydrocortisone preparations) with a liberal intake of salt. During stressful situations, such as infection, emotional upset or surgery, the dosage must be tripled to accommodate the body's increased need for glucocorticoids. Failure to meet this requirement will precipitate an acute crisis. Overdosage produces appearance of cushingoid signs.

◆ BOX 32-5

Cardinal signs of chronic adrenocortical insufficiency

Muscular weakness and mental fatigue, which are aggravated by slight additional exertion or minor illness

Pigmentary changes of previous scars, palmar creases, mucous membranes, and hair; hyperpigmentation over pressure points (elbows, knees, or waist); or, less frequently, loss of pigmentation (vitiligo)

Weight loss resulting from dehydration and anorexia from impaired gastrointestinal functioning (decreased hydrochloric acid)

Hypotension and small heart size, which predispose to dizziness and syncopal (fainting) attacks

Irritability, apathy and negativism

Signs of hypoglycaemia, such as headache, hunger, weakness, trembling, and sweating; other signs seen in some children are recurrent unexplained convulsions, an intense craving for salt, and acute abdominal pain

Children with more severe states of chronic adrenal insufficiency require mineralocorticoid replacement to maintain fluid and electrolyte balance.

IMPLICATIONS FOR NURSING

Once the disorder is diagnosed, parents need guidance concerning drug therapy. They must be aware of the continuous need for cortisol replacement. Sudden termination of the drug, because of inadequate supplies or inability to ingest the oral form because of vomiting, places the child in danger of an acute adrenal crisis. Therefore parents should always have a spare supply of the medication in the home. Ideally, they should have the intravenous hydrocortisone preparation in the home and written instructions for emergencies, and have been instructed in proper technique for intramuscular injection of the drug in case of a crisis. As was mentioned earlier, unnecessary administration of cortisone will not harm the child but, if needed, may be life-saving. The child should wear a MedicAlert tag to permit medical personnel to adjust requirements during emergency care. If there is evidence of acute insufficiency, contact the general practitioner immediately.

Parents also need to be aware of side effects of the drugs. Undesirable side effects of cortisone include gastric irritation, which is minimized by ingestion with food or the use of an antacid; increased excitability and sleeplessness; weight gain that may require dietary management to prevent obesity; and, rarely, behavioural changes, including depression or euphoria.

The side effects of mineralocorticoids are primarily caused by overdosage and include generalized oedema, which is first noticed around the eyes; hypertension, which may cause headaches; cardiac arrhythmias; and signs of hypokalaemia.

CUSHING SYNDROME

Cushing syndrome is a characteristic group of manifestations caused by excessive circulating free cortisol. It can result from a variety of aetiologies, which generally fall into one of four categories (Box 32-6).

◆ **BOX 32-6**

Aetiology of Cushing syndrome

Pituitary — Cushing syndrome with adrenal hyperplasia, usually attributed to an excess of ACTH

Adrenal — Cushing syndrome with hypersecretion of glucocorticoids, generally the result of adrenocortical neoplasms

Ectopic — Cushing syndrome with autonomous secretion of ACTH, most often caused by extrapituitary neoplasms

Iatrogenic — Cushing syndrome, frequently the result of administration of large amounts of exogenous corticosteroids

---

Cushing syndrome is uncommon in children. When seen, it is often caused by excessive or prolonged steroid therapy that produces a cushingoid appearance. This condition is reversible once the steroids are gradually discontinued. Abrupt withdrawal will precipitate acute adrenal insufficiency. Gradual withdrawal of exogenous supplies is necessary to allow the anterior pituitary an opportunity to secrete increasing amounts of adrenocorticotropic hormone to stimulate the adrenals to produce cortisol.

CLINICAL MANIFESTATIONS

The clinical manifestations are numerous, due to the widespread actions of cortisolone (Fig. 32-3). Changes in physical appearance occur early in the disorder and are of considerable concern to older children. The physiological disturbances, such as hyperglycaemia, susceptibility to infection, hypertension and hypokalaemia, may have life-threatening consequences unless recognized early and treated successfully.

PROCESS OF DIAGNOSIS

Several tests are helpful in confirming excess cortisol levels. They include fasting blood glucose levels for hyperglycaemia, scrum electrolyte levels for hypokalaemia and alkalosis, 24-hour urinary levels of elevated 17-hydroxycorticoids and 17-

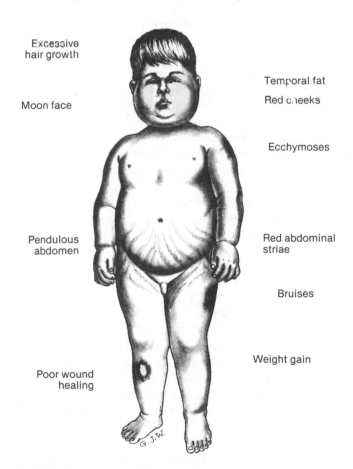

Excessive hair growth

Moon face

Temporal fat

Red cheeks

Ecchymoses

Pendulous abdomen

Red abdominal striae

Bruises

Weight gain

Poor wound healing

Fig. 32-3 Characteristics of Cushing syndrome.

ketosteroids, and radiological studies of bone for evidence of osteoporosis and imaging of the skull for enlargement of the sella turcica. Another procedure used to establish a more definitive diagnosis is the dexamethasone (cortisone) suppression test. Administration of an exogenous supply of cortisone normally suppresses adrenocorticotropic hormone production. However, in individuals with Cushing syndrome, cortisol levels remain elevated. This test is helpful in differentiating between children who are obese and those who appear to have cushingoid features.

THERAPEUTIC MANAGEMENT

Treatment depends on the cause. In most cases, surgical intervention involves bilateral adrenalectomy and postoperative replacement of the cortical hormones (the therapy for this is the same as that outlined for chronic adrenal insufficiency). If a pituitary tumour is found, surgical extirpation or irradiation may be chosen. In either of these instances, treatment of panhypopituitarism is with hormone replacement.

IMPLICATIONS FOR NURSING

Nursing care also depends on the cause. When cushingoid features are caused by steroid therapy, the effects may be lessened with administration of the drug early in the morning and on an alternate-day basis. Giving the drug early in the day maintains the normal diurnal pattern of cortisol secretion. If given during the evening, it is more likely to produce symptoms, because endogenous cortisol levels are already low and the additional supply exerts more pronounced effects. An alternate-day schedule allows the anterior pituitary an opportunity to maintain more normal hypothalamic-pituitary-adrenal control mechanisms (i.e., growth).

If an organic cause is found, nursing care is related to the treatment regimen. Although a bilateral adrenalectomy permanently solves one condition, it reciprocally produces another syndrome.

Postoperative complications of adrenalectomy are related to the sudden withdrawal of cortisol. The nurse should observe for signs of a shock-like state, especially hypotension and hyperpyrexia.

CONGENITAL ADRENOGENITAL HYPERPLASIA

Disorders caused by excessive secretion of androgens by the adrenal cortex are known variously as *congenital adrenogenital hyperplasia (CAH), adrenocortical hyperplasia (ACH), adrenogenital syndrome (AGS),* and *congenital adrenocortical hyperplasia (CAH).* Hyperfunction of the adrenal gland can occur from several causes, such as a virilizing adrenal tumour. However, in children the most common cause is congenital adrenogenital hyperplasia, an inborn deficiency of various enzymes nec-

essary for the biosynthesis of cortisol. Congenital adrenogenital hyperplasia is inherited as an autosomal-recessive disorder or may result from a tumour or maternal ingestion of steroids.

CLINICAL MANIFESTATIONS

Excessive androgens cause masculinization of the urogenital system during the twelfth and twentieth weeks of fetal development. The most pronounced abnormalities occur in females, who are born with varying degrees of ambiguous genitalia (pseudohermaphroditism). Masculinization of external genitalia causes the clitoris to enlarge so that it appears as a small phallus. Fusion of the labia produces a sac-like structure resembling the scrotum without testes. However, no abnormal changes occur in the internal sexual organs, although the vaginal orifice is usually closed by the fused labia.

In males, enlargement of the genitals (macrogenitosomia precox) and frequent erections are the principal signs.

Untreated congenital adrenogenital hyperplasia results in early sexual maturation, with enlargement of the external sexual organs; development of axillary, pubic and facial hair; deepening of the voice; acne; and marked increase in musculature with changes toward an adult male physique. However, in contrast to precocious puberty, breasts do not develop in the female, and she remains amenorrhoeic and infertile. In the male, the testes remain small and spermatogenesis does not occur. In both sexes, linear growth is accelerated and epiphyseal closure is premature, resulting in short stature by the end of puberty.

PROCESS OF DIAGNOSIS

Clinical diagnosis is initially based on congenital abnormalities that lead to difficulty in assigning sex to the newborn, and on signs and symptoms of adrenal insufficiency or hypertension. Definitive diagnosis is confirmed by evidence of increased 17-ketosteroid levels in most types of congenital adrenogenital hyperplasia. Usually, the level of 17-hydroxycorticoids is low or near normal. In complete 21-hydroxylase deficiency, blood electrolytes demonstrate loss of sodium and chloride, and elevation of potassium. In older children, bone age is advanced and linear growth is increased. Chromosome typing for positive sex determination and to rule out any other genetic abnormality (e.g., Turner syndrome) is always done in any case of ambiguous genitalia.

Another test that can be used to visualize the presence of pelvic structures is ultrasonography, and a sinogram. It is especially useful in congenital adrenogenital hyperplasia, because it readily identifies the absence or presence of female reproductive organs in a newborn or in a child with ambiguous genitalia. Because it yields immediate results, it has the advantage of determining the child's gender long before the more complex laboratory results for chromosomal analysis or steroid levels are available.

THERAPEUTIC MANAGEMENT

The initial medical objective is to confirm the diagnosis and to assign a sex to the child. In both sexes, cortisone is administered to suppress the abnormally high secretions of adrenocorticotropic hormone. If this is begun early enough, it is very effective. Cortisone depresses the secretion of adrenocorticotropic hormone by the adenohypophysis, which in turn inhibits the secretion of adrenocorticosteroids, which stems the progressive virilization. The signs and symptoms of masculinization in the female gradually disappear, and excessive early linear growth is slowed. Puberty occurs normally at the appropriate age.

The recommended oral dosage is divided, to simulate the normal diurnal pattern of adrenocorticotropic hormone secretion. Since these children are unable to produce cortisol in response to stress, it is necessary to increase the dosage during episodes of infection, fever or other stresses. Acute emergencies require immediate intravenous or intramuscular administration of hydrocortisone. Children with the salt-losing type of congenital adrenogenital hyperplasia require aldosterone replacement, and supplementary dietary salt. Frequent laboratory tests are conducted to assess the effects on electrolytes, hormonal profiles and renin levels. These are tapered, from weekly to monthly.

Depending on the degree of masculinization in the female, reconstructive surgery may be required to reduce the size of the clitoris, separate the labia, and create a vaginal orifice. This should be done after the infant is physically able to withstand the procedure and before she is old enough to be aware of the abnormal genitalia (usually preschool). Plastic surgery is generally done in stages and yields excellent cosmetic results. Reports concerning sexual satisfaction after partial clitoridectomy indicate that the capacity for orgasm and sexual gratification is not necessarily impaired.

IMPLICATIONS FOR NURSING

Of major importance is recognition of ambiguous genitalia in newborns. If there is any question regarding assignment of sex, the parents need to be told immediately, in order to prevent the embarrassing situation of informing family members of the child's sex and then having to change the announcement.

Parents need an explanation regarding this disorder that will help them explain it to others. Before confirmation of the diagnosis and sex of the child, the nurse should refer to the infant as 'child' or 'baby' rather than 'he' or 'she' and definitely not 'it'. When referring to the external genitalia, it is preferable to refer to them as sex organs and to emphasize the similarity between the penis/clitoris and scrotum/labia during fetal development. In this way, it can be explained that the sex organs were overdeveloped because of too much male hormone secretion. Using a correct vocabulary allows parents to explain the abnormalities to others in a straightforward manner, just as if the defect involved the heart or an extremity.

It is also important to stress that sex assignment and rearing depend on psychosocial influences, not on genetic sex hormonal influences during fetal life. Parents often fear that the infant will retain 'male behavioural characteristics' because of prenatal masculinization and will not be able to develop female characteristics. It is also beneficial to mention that ambiguous genitalia have no relationship with homosexual or bisexual activity later in life.

In general, rearing the genetically female child as a female is preferred, because of the success of surgical intervention and the satisfactory results with hormones in reversing virilism and providing a prospect of normal puberty and the ability to conceive. This is in contrast to the choice of rearing the child as a male, in which case the child is sterile and may never be able to function satisfactorily in heterosexual relationships.

As soon as the sex is determined, parents should be informed of the findings and encouraged to choose an appropriate name, and the child should be identified as a male or female, with no reference to ambiguous sex. Suggesting ways to avoid questioning remarks from visitors, such as changing the child's nappy in a separate room, is also helpful. If surgery is anticipated, showing parents before and after photographs of reconstruction helps to reinforce the expected cosmetic benefits.

Nursing considerations regarding cortisol and aldosterone replacement are the same as those that are discussed for chronic adrenocortical insufficiency. However, since parents may be overwhelmed with the diagnosis and obvious abnormalities at the time of birth, they may not hear all the discharge instructions regarding the medication schedule. Written instructions in the parent-held records are important and reassuring to the family. A follow-up visit by a children's liaison nurse, health visitor, or someone from the Parent Help Support Group for Congenital Adrenal Hyperplasia may be helpful (details are available from the Child Growth Foundation).

A dilemma often arises, however, regarding what these children should know about their condition, especially gender identification. Because the knowledge that one has been reared opposite to the genetic gender can initiate profound psychological problems, it is recommended that children not be told this fact but rather be given an explanation regarding their physical disabilities, such as infertility, and the need for hormone replacement and plastic surgery. Parents, in turn, must believe that these children have been raised according to their 'true sex', which is absolutely honest, since sex is not solely a biological entity but an expression of multiple environmental influences.

Since the hereditary form of adrenogenital hyperplasia is an autosomal-recessive disorder, parents should be referred for genetic counselling before conceiving another child. The nurse's role is to ensure that parents understand the probability of transmitting the trait or disorder with each pregnancy. Affected offspring also require genetic counselling, since both sexes are generally able to reproduce.

HYPERALDOSTERONISM

Excessive secretion of aldosterone may be caused by an adrenal tumour or, in some types of adrenogenital syndromes, may be the result of enzymatic deficiency. The signs and symptoms are caused by increased sodium levels, water retention, and potassium loss. Hypervolaemia causes hypertension and resultant headaches.

The clinical diagnosis is suspected when there are findings of hypertension, hypokalaemia, and polyuria that fail to respond to antidiuretic hormone administration. Renin and angiotensin titres are abnormally low. Urinary levels of 17-hydroxycorticosteroids and 17-ketosteroids are normal in primary hyperaldosteronism caused by an aldosterone-secreting tumour, but are usually abnormal in adrenogenital syndrome.

THERAPEUTIC MANAGEMENT

Temporary treatment of the disorder involves replacement of potassium and administration of spironolactone, a diuretic that blocks the effects of aldosterone, thereby promoting excretion of sodium and water while preserving potassium. Definitive treatment is similar to that for chronic adrenocortical insufficiency.

IMPLICATIONS FOR NURSING

An important nursing consideration is recognition of the syndrome, particularly in children who demonstrate high blood pressure. After the diagnosis, nursing care should be related to the treatment regimen.

PHAEOCHROMOCYTOMA

Phaeochromocytoma is an adrenal tumour characterized by secretion of catecholamines. The tumour most commonly arises from the chromaffin cells of the adrenal medulla. Approximately 10% of these tumours are located in extra-adrenal sites. In children, they are frequently bilateral or multiple and are generally benign. Often, there is a familial transmission of the condition as an autosomal-dominant trait that tends to favour males.

CLINICAL MANIFESTATIONS

The clinical manifestations of phaeochromocytoma are caused by an increased production of catecholamines, producing hypertension, tachycardia, headache, decreased gastrointestinal activity with resultant constipation, increased metabolism with anorexia, weight loss, hyperglycaemia, polyuria, polydipsia, hyperventilation, nervousness and diaphoresis. In severe cases, signs of congestive heart failure are evident.

PROCESS OF DIAGNOSIS

The clinical manifestations mimic those of other disorders, such as hyperthyroidism. Therefore, several tests specific to these conditions may be performed as part of the differential diagnosis. In only a small number of instances is a palpable tumour suggestive of the diagnosis. Definitive tests include measurement of urinary levels of the catecholamine metabolites.

THERAPEUTIC MANAGEMENT

Definitive treatment consists of surgical removal of the tumour(s). The major complications that can occur during surgery are severe hypertension, tachyarrhythmias and hypotension. Stabilization of the blood pressure before, during and after the operation is highly critical, but a successful anaesthetic technique for this is available and used, thus reducing complication risks.

IMPLICATIONS FOR NURSING

An initial nursing objective is identification of children with this disorder. Outstanding clues are hypertension and hypertensive attacks. Therefore, a careful history of the onset of symptoms and association with stressful events is helpful in distinguishing between an organic and a psychological cause for the symptoms.

Preoperative nursing care involves frequent monitoring of vital signs and observing for evidence of hypertensive attacks and congestive heart failure.

The environment is made conducive to rest and reducing emotional stress. This requires adequate preparation during hospital admission and before surgery. Parents are encouraged to stay with their child and to participate in daily care. Play activities need to be tailored to the child's energy level, but must not be overly strenuous or challenging, since these can increase metabolic rate and promote frustration and anxiety.

DISORDERS OF PANCREATIC HORMONE SECRETION

The islets of Langerhans of the pancreas have three major functioning cells: the alpha cells, which produce glucagon, the beta cells, which produce insulin, and the delta cells, which produce somatostatin. Glucagon causes an increase in blood glucose by stimulating the liver and other cells to release stored glucose (glycogenolysis). Glucagon acts as an emergency supplier of glucose whenever the blood glucose falls too low, and is believed to function more independently when insulin is lacking. Somatostatin, although secreted by the islet cells, is found in greater supply in the hypothalamus, where it prevents the release of growth hormone. In the islets of Langerhans, somatostatin is believed to regulate the release of insulin and glucagon. This discussion of disorders of pancreatic hormone secretion is limited to diabetes mellitus.

DIABETES MELLITUS

Diabetes mellitus (DM) is the commonest endocrine disorder in childhood and is almost always insulin-dependant (Type I). It is a disorder of carbohydrate metabolism in which sugars in the body are not oxidized to produce energy. This is due to the lack of the hormone insulin. Diabetes mellitus affects about 2% of the population in the UK.

The disease is rare in infancy, and children younger than school age have a low incidence rate. However, a recent study showed the incidence of diabetes in school-aged children is increasing and that onset is occurring at an even younger age. The peak incidence is reached during early adolescence.

CLASSIFICATION

DM can be classified as *idiopathic* or *secondary*. Secondary DM can be precipitated by exogenous factors and is usually (but not always) reversible when the primary disorder is treated.

Idiopathic DM can be classified into two major groups, and characteristics of insulin-dependent DM (IDDM, or Type I) and non-insulin-dependent DM (NIDDM, or Type II) are outlined in Table 32-1.

CHARACTERISTICS	TYPE I (IDDM)	TYPE II (NIDDM)
Age of onset	Less than 20 years	Over 40 years
Type of onset	Abrupt	Gradual
Sex ratio	No sex difference	Females outnumber males
Percentage of population	5-8%	85-90%
Hereditary:		
Family history	Sometimes	Frequency
HLA	Associations	No associations
Twin concordance	25-50%	90-100%
Ethnic distribution	Primary whites	Common to all
Presenting symptoms	Three Ps* common	May be none
Nutritional status	Underweight	Overweight
Insulin (natural):		
Pancreatic content	Usually 0	Over 50% normal
Serum insulin	Low to absent	High or low
Primary resistance	Minimum	Marked
Islet cell antibodies	80-85%	Less than 5%
Metabolic control	Difficult	Usually easy
Stability	Unstable	Stable
Therapy:		
Insulin	Always	20-30% of patients
Oral agents	Ineffective	Often effective
Diet only	Ineffective	Often effective
Chronic complications	Greater than 80%	Variable
Ketoacidosis	Common	Infrequent

*Polyuria, polydipsia, and polyphagia.

Table 32.1 Comparison of characteristics of types I and II diabetes mellitus.

AETIOLOGY

IDDM is an autoimmune disease that arises when a person with a genetic predisposition is exposed to a precipitating event, usually a viral infection. Islet cells appear to be particularly susceptible to either direct viral damage or chemical insult. The virus serves as a 'trigger'.

Genetic factors

IDDM is not inherited, but heredity is unquestioned as a prominent factor in the aetiology. There are more than 40 rare genetic syndromes of which diabetes is a major feature (Nora and Fraser, 1989). No simple Mendelian pattern is found for DM.

CLINICAL MANIFESTATIONS

The symptomatology of diabetes is more readily recognizable in children than in adults, so it is surprising that the diagnosis may sometimes be missed or delayed. Diabetes is a great imitator; influenza, gastroenteritis and appendicitis are the conditions most often diagnosed, only to find that the disease was really diabetes. Diabetes should be suspected in families with a strong family history of diabetes.

The sequence of chemical events that take place results in hyperglycaemia and acidosis, which in turn produce weight loss, polyphagia, polydipsia and polyuria - the cardinal symptoms of the disease.

Frequently identified symptoms of overt diabetes include enuresis, change in temperament and unusual fatigue. Abdominal discomfort is also common. Other symptoms include dry skin, blurred vision, boils, abscesses and urinary tract infections.

At diagnosis, the child may be *hyperglycaemic*, with elevated blood glucose levels and glucose in the urine; *ketotic*, with ketones measurable in the blood and urine, with or without dehydration; or suffering from *diabetic ketoacidosis*, with dehydration, electrolyte imbalance and acidosis.

PROCESS OF DIAGNOSIS

Three groups of children who should be considered as possibly diabetic are (1) children who have glycosuria, polyuria, and a history of weight loss or failure to gain despite a voracious appetite; (2) those with transient or persistent glycosuria; and (3) those who display manifestations of metabolic acidosis, with or without stupor or coma. In every case, diabetes must be considered if there is glycosuria, with or without ketonuria, in association with otherwise unexplained hyperglycaemia.

A random (nonfasting) venous whole blood or plasma glucose of >10 or >11.1 mmol/l, respectively, is diagnostic of diabetes in the presence of other symptoms of the condition.

Serum insulin levels may be normal or moderately elevated at the onset of diabetes; delayed insulin response to glucose indicates the presence of prediabetes.

THERAPEUTIC MANAGEMENT

Current recommendations stress the need for consistent support for the family and child with IDDM. This is achieved through a multidisciplinary team approach from a full supporting diabetic team consisting of a paediatrician, children's specialist diabetes nurse, paediatric dietitian and, if possible, a psychologist. In order to minimize mismanagement of diabetic problems, close liaison and educational support should be given to other carers and people, such as school teachers, by the diabetic team.

Careful juggling of the diabetes and the child's and family's lifestyles can be problematic. A comprehensive, ongoing educational programme tailored to suit individual needs is important to help achieve good metabolic control and to reduce the risk of diabetic complications, especially during adolescence.

Insulin therapy

The majority of children are treated with human insulin injection: insulin dosage is tailored to each child based on home blood glucose monitoring. The goal of insulin therapy is to maintain near normal blood glucose values.

Insulin preparations

Soluble insulin (rapid-acting) is best administered subcutaneously at least 20–30 minutes before meals. This allows sufficient time for absorption and results in a significantly more reduced postprandial rise in blood glucose than if the meal were eaten immediately following the insulin injection. Some authorities advocate multiple injections throughout the day, rather than the twice-daily regimen; that is, a once-daily dose of long-acting insulin to simulate the basal insulin secretion and injections of rapid-acting insulin before each meal. A multiple daily injection (MDI) programme is particularly suitable for the child whose DM is difficult to manage, has a varied lifestyle, or who is undergoing an adolescent growth spurt.

Monitoring control

Monitoring the effectiveness of insulin therapy is a vital part of management. It is the only way to determine the amount of insulin needed by a child at any given time. Several measurements are used to evaluate the glucose levels as a basis for insulin administration and regulation.

Urine testing

Urine tests for glucose have many limitations. There is poor correlation between simultaneous glycosuria and blood glucose concentration, as it depends upon the renal threshold. However, urine testing for ketones remains a cornerstone of home management. It is recommended that urine be tested for ketones during an illness, periods of poor control and whenever blood glucose is 17 mmol/l or higher, as these factors may indicate the need for more insulin.

Blood glucose monitoring

Home blood glucose monitoring (HBGM) has improved diabetes management and is used successfully by children from the onset of their diabetes. By testing their own blood, children are able to change their insulin regimen to maintain their glucose level at near normal levels (the normal range of blood glucose is 4–8 mmol/l). The optimal method of assessing control is testing four times a day: once before each meal and again before going to bed.

Glycosylated haemoglobin

The measurement of glycosylated haemoglobin (haemoglobin A_{1c}) levels is an index of mean blood glucose over the preceding 6–10 weeks. The test is a satisfactory method for assessing control, detecting incorrect testing, monitoring effectiveness of changes in treatment, defining patients' goals, and detecting nonadherence.

Diet

Essentially, the nutritional needs of children with diabetes are no different from those of healthy children, except for deletion of concentrated sugar. Children with diabetes need no special foods or supplements. They need sufficient calories to balance daily expenditure for energy and to satisfy the requirement for growth, development and activity. Unlike the healthy child whose insulin is secreted in response to food intake, insulin injected subcutaneously has a relatively predictable time of onset, peak effect, duration of action, and absorption rate depending on the type of insulin used. Consequently, the timing of food consumption must be regulated to correspond to the time and action of the insulin prescribed, if possible.

Meals and snacks should ideally be eaten at the same times each day, to space out the carbohydrate, enabling better control of blood glucose levels and minimizing the risk of hypoglycaemia.

Food intake may be planned in a variety of ways, but is based on a balanced diet. The family may follow the exchange system. The exchange system indicates the amount (portion size) of each food by volume or weight and is prescribed in terms of the number of 'exchanges' from each food group that constitutes each meal and snack.

Concentrated sweets are eliminated. Dietary fibre is important in dietary planning because of its influence on digestion, absorption and metabolism of many nutrients. It has been found to diminish the rise in blood sugar after meals. Correctly used, the diet allows for flexibility.

Exercise

Exercise is encouraged. Exercise lowers blood sugar levels, depending on the intensity and duration of the activity. However, in most instances children's activities are unplanned, and the resulting decrease in blood sugar can be compensated for by providing extra snacks before (and, if prolonged, during) the activity.

Physical training tends to increase tissue sensitivity to insulin, even in the resting state. Vigorous muscular contrac-tion increases regional blood flow and accelerates the absorption and circulation of insulin that is injected into the area, which can contribute to development of hypoglycaemia. If exercise involving leg muscles is planned, it is recommended that nonexercised sites (arm or abdomen) should be used for insulin injection.

Children who regularly participate in organized sports are advised to adjust their insulin dosage in anticipation of sustained physical activity. Optimum adjustments for each child are determined primarily by trial and error.

Hypoglycaemia

The most common causes of hypoglycaemia are bursts of physical activity without additional food, or delayed, omitted or incompletely consumed meals. Sometimes the reaction from sustained exercise may occur several hours after the exercise. Occasionally, hypoglycaemic reactions occur unexpectedly and without apparent cause. They may be the result of an inadvertent or deliberate error in insulin administration.

The signs and symptoms of hypoglycaemia are caused by both increased adrenergic activity and impaired brain function. The increased adrenergic nervous system activity plus increased secretion of catecholamines produce nervousness, pallor, tremulousness, palpitations, sweating and hunger. Weakness, dizziness, headache, drowsiness, mood changes, loss of coordination, convulsions and coma are more severe responses and reflect central nervous system glucose deprivation and the body's attempts to elevate the serum glucose levels.

It is often difficult to distinguish between hyperglycaemia and a hypoglycaemic reaction. Since the symptoms are similar and usually begin with changes in behaviour, the simplest way to differentiate between the two is to test the blood glucose level. Blood glucose is low in hypoglycaemia, but significantly elevated in hyperglycaemia. Urinary ketones may be present following hypoglycaemia, due to starvation ketone production. In doubtful situations, it is safer to give the child some simple carbohydrate. This will help alleviate the symptoms in the case of hypoglycaemia, but will do little harm if the child is hyperglycaemic.

Children are usually able to detect the onset of hypoglycaemia, but some are too young to implement treatment. Parents should become adept at recognizing the onset of symptoms — for example, a change in a child's behaviour such as tearfulness or euphoria. In the majority of cases, 10-15 g of simple carbohydrate, such as honey or liquid glucose, will elevate the blood glucose level and alleviate the symptoms. The simpler the carbohydrate, the more rapidly it will be absorbed. The rapid-releasing sugar is followed by a complex carbohydrate such as a slice of bread or a digestive biscuit.

For a mild reaction, milk or fruit juice is a good food to use in children, as is cola (100 ml) and Lucozade™ (60 ml). All children with diabetes should carry with them glucose tabs (Dextrosol™ or glucose tablets, 10 g = 3 tablets), or some sugar cubes.

It is better to overtreat than to undertreat. The treatment may be repeated in 10-15 minutes if the initial response is not satisfactory.

An insulin reaction is often the most feared aspect of diabetes, since severe brain symptoms may develop. The treatment of choice for severe hypoglycaemia is 10% (2 ml/kg maximum) glucose administered intravenously.

Glucagon is sometimes prescribed for home treatment of hypoglycaemia. It is packaged as an emergency kit containing a syringe with a vial of diluent and a vial of powder, which are mixed up and reconstituted for use. It is administered subcutaneously. It functions by releasing stored glycogen from the liver and requires about 15-20 minutes to elevate the blood glucose level.

Illness management

Illness alters diabetes management, and maintaining control is usually related to the seriousness of the illness. In the well-controlled child, an illness will run its course as it does in the unaffected child. The goal during an illness is to maintain normal glucose level while recognizing and treating urinary ketones. Frequent monitoring of blood glucose and urine for ketones is important. Some hyperglycaemia and ketonuria are expected in most illnesses, even with diminished food intake, and are an indication for increased insulin. Insulin should never be omitted during an illness, although dosage requirements may increase, decrease, or remain unchanged, depending on the severity of the illness and the child's appetite. In the presence of nausea or decreased appetite, simple carbohydrates may be substituted for carbohydrate-containing exchanges in the meal plan. Fluids are encouraged to prevent dehydration and to flush out ketones.

New data support the concept that life expectancy in the child with diabetes is lengthened if the body is maintained in as normal a physiological state as possible. Complications are associated with both control and duration of diabetes. A healthy lifestyle, a balance of adequate rest and exercise, and good nutrition along with close management of the disease will help promote the child's future health as an adult.

Surgery

The physiological and emotional stresses related to surgery require careful adjustment of insulin. Since the child receives intravenous glucose during surgery and the stress of the surgery itself will also raise the blood glucose level, the risk of an insulin reaction is very slight. Regular insulin should be continued until the child is able to tolerate oral feedings and a return to the routine pattern of insulin administration.

THERAPEUTIC MANAGEMENT: DIABETIC KETOACIDOSIS

Diabetic ketoacidosis (DKA), the most complete state of insulin deficiency, is a life-threatening situation. Management consists of rapid assessment, adequate insulin to reduce the elevated blood glucose level, fluids to overcome dehydration, and electrolyte replacement.

Fluid and electrolyte therapy

All patients with diabetic ketoacidosis suffer from dehydration (10% of total body weight in severe ketoacidosis) due to the osmotic diuresis, accompanied by depletion of electrolytes. Serum pH and bicarbonate reflect the degree of acidosis. Prompt and adequate fluid therapy restores tissue perfusion and suppresses the elevated levels of stress hormones.

Insulin

The preferred method for administering insulin to the child with ketoacidosis is a continuous infusion of low-dose insulin consisting of a 0.1 U/kg priming dose followed by 0.1 U/kg/hour. This appears to be an efficient, simple and physiologically sound form of therapy (Sperling, 1984). The insulin is added to 0.9% normal saline, and some of the mixture is run through the intravenous tubing to saturate the insulin-binding sites that exist on the plastic tubing. It has been found that plastic tubing and in-line filters can chemically bind to significant amounts of insulin, thereby reducing the amount of the medication reaching the bloodstream. The infusion is titrated using a 'sliding scale' to lower the blood glucose about 4 mmol/l/hour to obtain a blood glucose level of approximately 10–12 mmol/l. The insulin infusion is then continued until the pH and serum bicarbonate are normal. Subcutaneous insulin is then instituted using a sliding scale of insulin.

IMPLICATIONS FOR NURSING: ACUTE CARE

Children with DM may be admitted to the hospital at the time of their initial diagnosis, during illness or surgery, or for episodes of ketoacidosis which may be precipitated by any of a variety of factors. Most children are able to keep the disease under control with periodic assessment and adjustment of insulin, diet and activity as needed under the supervision of a paediatric team. Under most circumstances these children can be managed very well at home and require hospitalization only for a serious illness or upset.

However, a small number of children with diabetes exhibit a degree of metabolic lability and have repeated episodes of diabetic ketoacidosis that require hospitalization, which interferes with education and social development. These children appear to display a characteristic personality structure. They tend to be unusually passive and nonassertive and to come from families that are inclined to smooth over conflicts without resolution. Children in this type of setting experience fluctuating emotions with little, if any, opportunity or ability to resolve them. This can lead to erratic blood glucose results and poor metabolic control.

Helping any child develop into a secure, stable young adult is important. For the child with diabetes, pressures imposed by the medical profession and peers can make this harder.

Hospital management

The child with diabetic ketoacidosis requires specialist, high dependency nursing care. Careful and accurate records should be maintained, including vital signs (pulse, respiration, temperature, blood pressure), intravenous fluids, electrolytes, insulin (needed and given), blood glucose levels (a strict record), and intake and output. A urine collection device or retention catheter is used to obtain the urine measurements, which include volume, specific gravity, and glucose and ketone values. The level of consciousness is assessed and recorded at frequent intervals. The comatose child generally regains consciousness fairly soon after initiation of therapy, but is managed as any unconscious child during that time.

When the critical period is over, the task of regulating insulin dosage to diet and activity is begun. The same meticulous records of intake and output, urine glucose and ketone levels, and insulin administration are maintained. Where possible, all children should be actively involved in their own care and are given responsibility for keeping the intake and output record, testing the blood and urine, and, when appropriate, administering their own insulin. The British Diabetic Association's Youth Department is a good source of information and is able to put families in touch with each other.

Concepts of child and family education

The setting for the educational process can facilitate the learning process. There are times in the educational process when individual instruction is needed, but contact with other children and/or parents can assist in adjustment to the reality of the disease and the implications of having a chronic condition. Supplementary material such as audiovisual aids enhances the learning process and promotes retention of information (Brown, 1991).

Child and family support

The parents and other family members of the child with newly diagnosed DM experience various emotional responses to the crises, just as the physiological responses affect the child. There is often a large element of guilt on the parents' side about the child developing diabetes. The continuous pressure and task of handling the disease is taxing to the most stable family, and can be very emotionally draining.

Adolescents appear to have most difficulty adjusting. Adolescence is a time when there is much stress towards being 'perfect' and being like their peers and, no matter what others say, having diabetes is being different. Diabetes can be a powerful tool that they can use to manipulate others within the family, friends and professionals.

Denial is sometimes expressed by omitting insulin, not performing tests, and eating incorrectly, as well as faking results and hypoglycaemic episodes. It is often difficult for the adolescent to know what to tell friends who doubt that they have the disease, and how to tell them. The diabetic team psychologist could help them do this.

Activity holidays and other special groups are very useful for the child and family (Moran, 1985).

The diabetic team should be able to work in partnership with the child and family to meet their needs. They need to receive consistent support, praise and encouragement for efforts made to control and cope with the condition in order to minimize the risk of future complications. It is important for the parents to recognize that as children grow and develop, they are children first and children with diabetes second.

KEY POINTS

- ◆ Pituitary dysfunction is manifest primarily by growth disturbance.
- ◆ Disorders of thyroid function include hypothyroidism, autoimmune thyroiditis, goitre and hyperthyroidism.
- ◆ Therapy for hyperthyroidism is directed at retarding the rate of hormone secretion and may include drug therapy, thyroidectomy or radioiodine therapy.
- ◆ Disorders of adrenal function include acute adrenocortical insufficiency, chronic adrenocortical insufficiency, Cushing syndrome, congenital adrenogenital hyperplasia and hyperaldosteronism.
- ◆ Four categories of Cushing syndrome are pituitary, adrenal, ectopic and iatrogenic.
- ◆ Management of congenital adrenogenital hyperplasia includes assignation of a sex according to genotype, administration of cortisone, and, possibly, reconstructive surgery.
- ◆ Childhood diabetes mellitus is categorized as insulin-dependent, non-insulin-dependent, and maturity-onset diabetes of youth.
- ◆ The focus of diabetes management is insulin replacement, diet and exercise.
- ◆ Education of families includes explanation of diabetes, meal planning, administering insulin injections, monitoring, general hygienic practices, promoting exercise, record keeping and observing for complications.

REFERENCES

Brook CGD, Hindmarsh PC: Tests for growth hormone secretion, *Arch Dis Child* 66:85, 1991.

Brown F: An alternative education, *Nurs Stand* 5(30):54, 1991.

Brown P: Human growth hormone therapy and Creutzfeldt-Jakob disease: a drama in three acts, *Pediatr* 81:85, 1988.

Brown P, Gajdusek DC, Gibbs CJ: Potential epidemic of Creutzfeldt-Jakob disease from human growth hormone therapy, *N Engl J Med* 313:728, 1985.

DiGeorge AM: The endocrine system. In Behrman RE, Vaughan VC, *Textbook of Paediatrics*, ed 13, Philadelphia, 1987, WB Saunders Co.

Fink JN, Beall GN: Immunological aspects of endocrine diseases, *JAMA* 248:2696-2700, 1982.

Fradkin E *et al:* Risk of leukemia after treatment with pituitary growth hormone, *JAMA* 270(23):2829, 1993.

Fry T: Monitoring children's growthæ introducing the new child growth standards, *Prof Care Mother Child* 4(8):231, 1994.

Ghigo E *et al:* Glucagon stimulates GH secretions after intramuscular but not intravenous administration: evidence against the assumption that glucagon per se has a GH-releasing activity, *J Endocrinol Invest* 17:849, 1994.

Ilondo MM *et al:* Serum growth hormone levels measured by radioimmunoassay and radioreceptor assay: a useful diagnostic tool in children with growth disorders? *J Clin Endocrinol Metab* 70:1445, 1990.

Lamont G: Growth disorders and the role of the specialist nurse, *Paediatr Nurs* 4(8):23, 1992.

Mahoney CP: Differential diagnosis of goiter, *Pediatr Clin North Am* 34:891-905, 1987.

Meadow R: Munchausen syndrome by proxy, *Arch Dis Child* 57:92, 1982.

Meadow R: Management of Munchausen syndrome by proxy, *Arch Dis Child* 60:385, 1985.

Moran MM: Diabetes camps: management guidelines, *Pediatr Nurs* 11:183, 1985.

Nora JJ, Fraser FC: *Medical Genetics*, Philadelphia PA, 1989, Lea & Febiger.

Reiter EO et al: Childhood thyromegaly: recent developments, *J Pediatr* 99:507, 1981.

Rosenberg DA: Web of deceit: a literature review of Munchausen syndrome by proxy, *Child Abuse Negl* 11:547, 1987.

Rosenfield R: Androgen disorders in children: too much, too early, too little, or too late, *Pediatrics in Review* 5(5):147, 1983.

Shah A, Stanhope R, Matthew D: Hazards of pharmacological tests of growth hormone secretion in childhood, *BMJ* 304:173, 1992.

Sherwood MC et al: Diabetes insipidus and occult intracranial tumours, *Arch Dis Child* 61:1222, 1986.

Silver HK, Gotlin RW, Klingensmith GJ, editors: Endocrine disorders. In Kempe CH, Silver HK, O'Brien D: *Current paediatric diagnosis and treatment*, ed 8, Los Altos, CA, 1984, Lange Medical Publications.

Skuse D: Emotional abuse and delay in growth, *BMJ* 299:26, 1989.

Sonis WA et al: Behavior problems and social competence in girls with true precocious puberty, *J Pediatr* 106:156, 1985.

Sperling MA: Diabetic ketoacidosis, *Pediatr Clin North Am* 31:591, 1984.

Stanhope R, Wilks Z, Hamil G: Psychosocial aspects of growth. Failure to growæ lack of food or lack of love? *Prof Care Mother Child* 4(8):234, 1994.

Underwood LE et al: Growth hormone levels during sleep in normal and growth hormone deficient children, *Pediatr* 48:946, 1971.

Wheeler MD, Styne DM: Diagnosis and management of precocious puberty, *Pediatr Clin N AM* 37(6):1255, 1990.

Wit JM, van Uneu H: Growth of infants with neonatal growth hormone deficiency, *Arch Dis Child* 67(7):920, 1992.

FURTHER READING

Pituitary Dysfunction

Bercu BB: Growth hormone treatment and the short child: to treat or not to treat? *J Pediatr* 110:991, 1987.

Brook CGD: *Clinical paediatric endocrinology*, ed 2, London, 1989, Blackwell Scientific.

Brook CGD: Who's for growth hormone? *BMJ* 304:131, 1992.

Costin G, Kaufman FR: Growth hormone secretory patterns in children with short stature, *J Pediatr* 110:362, 1987.

Lamont G: Growth disorders and the role of the specialist nurse, *Paediatr Nurs* 4(8):23, 1992.

Saggese G, Cesaretti G: Criteria for recognition of the growth-inefficient child who may respond to treatment with growth hormone, *Am J Dis Child* 143:1287, 1989.

Stern M, Zaiken H: Assessing the child with short stature, *Pediatr Nurs* 11:106, 1985.

Disorders of Thyroid Function/Disorders of the Parathyroid Gland

Gorton C, Sadeghi-Nejd A, Senior B: Remission in children with hyperthyroidism treated with propylthiouracil, *Am J Dis Child* 141:1084, 1987.

Adrenal Dysfunction

Lee PDK, Winter RJ, Green OC: Virilizing adrenocortical tumors in childhood: eight cases and a review of the literature, *Pediatr* 76:437, 1985.

Pescovitz OH: Precocious puberty, *Pediatrics in Review* 11(8):229, 1990.

Sanford SJ: Dysfunction of the adrenal gland: physiologic considerations and nursing problems, *Nurs Clin North Am* 15:481, 1980.

Diabetes Mellitus: General

Brown F: An alternative education, *Nurs Stand* 3(30):54, 1991.

Diabetes Control and Complications Trial Research Group: The effect of intensive treatment of diabetes on the development and progression of long term complications in insulin dependent diabetes mellitus, *New Eng J Med* 329:683, 1993.

Ingersoll GM *et al:* Cognitive maturity and self-management among adolescents with insulin-dependent diabetes mellitus, *J Pediatr* 108:620, 1986.

Kans HMJ *et al*, editors: Diabetes care and research in Europe. *The St Vincent declaration programme*, Geneva, 1992, World Health Organization.

Royal College of Nursing (Diabetes Nursing Forum): *Guidelines on the use of blood glucose monitoring equipment by nurses in clinical areas,* London, 1991, RCN.

Shaw V, Lawson M, editors: *Clinical paediatric dietetics,* London, 1994, Blackwell Scientific.

Sonksen P *et al*: *Diabetes at your fingertips,* London, 1991, Class.

Stillitoe R: *Psychology and diabetes,* London, 1988, Chapman & Hall.

Tanner JM: *Foetus into man—physical growth from conception to maturity,* ed 2, Ware, 1989, Castlemead.

Tattershall R, Gale E: *Diabetes: clinical management,* Edinburgh, 1990, Churchill Livingstone.

Diabetes Mellitus: Testing and Monitoring

Cradock S: Blood glucose monitoring—why test? *Diabetic Nurs* 1(2):5, 1989.

Davis SG *et al*: In-hospital bedside blood glucose monitoring: the importance of a quality control program, *J Pediatr Nurs* 4:353, 1989.

Polish IB *et al*: Nonsocomial transmission of hepatitis B virus associated with use of a spring-loaded finger-stick device, *New Eng J Med* 326:721, 1992.

Strumph PS, Odoroff CL, Amatruda JM: The accuracy of blood glucose testing by children, *Clin Pediatr* 27:188, 1988.

Diabetes Mellitus: Therapeutic Management

Chase HP *et al*: Cyclosporine A for the treatment of new-onset insulin-dependent diabetes mellitus, *Pediatr* 85:241, 1990.

Gavin JR: Diabetes and exercise, *AJN* 88:178, 1988.

Hahn K: Teaching patients to administer insulin, *Nurs '90* 20(4):70, 1990.

USEFUL ADDRESSES

British Diabetic Association (BDA), 10 Queen Anne Street, London WM 0BD.

Child Growth Foundation, 2 Mayfield Avenue, Chiswick, London W4 1PW.

Chapter 33

The Child with Musculoskeletal or Articular Dysfunction

LEARNING OUTCOMES

After studying this chapter you should be able to:

- Assess the child with trauma.
- Discuss the effects and management of the immobilized child.
- Discuss the aetiology of childhood fractures and describe the types of fractures found in children.
- Discuss bone healing and the implications for nursing.
- Describe the types of immobilization devices used for childhood fractures.
- Discuss musculoskeletal dysfunction and appropriate medical and nursing management.
- Describe and discuss childhood orthopaedic infections.
- Describe and discuss the management of juvenile arthritis.
- Define the glossary terms.

GLOSSARY

Compartment syndrome Increased pressure within an enclosed space which compromises muscles and nerves within the space

Greenstick fracture An incomplete fracture similar to the break observed when a green stick is broken

Non-accidental injury A traumatic non-accidental incident which produces physical injury in a child

SUFE Slipped upper femoral epiphysis

Traction A forward force applied to a part of the body

The musculoskeletal system is composed of a variety of structures. The skeleton, or bony framework, provides the support; the muscles, tendons, ligaments and joints allow for active movement. The bulk of musculoskeletal problems are related to traumatic injuries, which are common in childhood. The first part of this chapter is devoted to the problem of immobility and trauma, particularly musculoskeletal trauma. The remainder of the chapter deals with less common skeletal and articular disorders.

THE CHILD AND TRAUMA

Trauma is the leading cause of death in children over the age of one year and is an important cause of disability during childhood and adolescence. Most injuries are relatively minor, cause little disruption in the daily life of the child and produce only minor discomfort. However, accidental injury is the leading cause of death in the paediatric age group.

TRAUMA MANAGEMENT

In order to provide optimum care for trauma victims, community resources for children must be available and appropriately organized for rapid transit, skilled care and specialized facilities.

EPIDEMIOLOGY OF TRAUMA

Many aspects of injury are affected by the developmental stage of the child in both the type of injury that is incurred and the physiological response to injury.

Accidental injury

Children's everyday activities include vigorous play, such as climbing, falling, running into immovable objects, and receiving blows to any part of their bodies. All of these activities make them prone to injury.

Young children and teenagers usually do not calculate risks as they learn to manipulate their environment and achieve developmental goals. Therefore, accidents are a part of most childhood experiences. Fortunately, when children fall or are hit, their body resilience protects them from incurring serious damage to soft tissue, the musculoskeletal system, or other body organs. Children's bones are more flexible than adults', and therefore do not offer the rigid resistance to external forces that are likely to cause fractures.

Non-accidental injury (NAI)

Unfortunately, careless handling of an infant or child (in some instances intentional physical abuse) is not uncommon in our society. A multitude of different types of bone and soft tissue injuries are inflicted on children by adults. Small children, who are unable to protect themselves, are most vulnerable. It is estimated that perhaps 25% of fractures in children under three years of age are the result of child abuse. A traumatic incident that produces physical injury to an infant or child may be the outcome of an accident that was no one's fault or may be associated with child abuse. A well-documented history is essential to determine the cause of the injury.

Birth injuries

During the birth process, fractures, dislocations and/or nerve damage may be sustained. These injuries most often occur when the baby is large, the presentation is breech, or forceful extraction is used because of fetal distress. The two most common types of musculoskeletal injuries incurred during birth are fractured clavicle and brachial plexus injury.

Childhood characteristics

Certain developmental characteristics of children at various ages render them more susceptible to injury. For example, the large head of infants and toddlers predisposes them to head injury, especially in falls. Also, the relatively large spleen and liver, and the broad costal arch make these organs prone to direct trauma. Because of their light weight and small size, infants and small children are easily thrown around in a moving vehicle.

Later, in school-aged children and adolescents, whose bone growth outstrips muscle growth, difficulty controlling movement can contribute to physical injury.

PREVENTION OF INJURY

Hazardous environmental factors play a major role in the number of serious accidents incurred by children. Stairways without handrails or a gate at the top, cluttered walkways, waxed floors or throw rugs can contribute to a severe fall. Playground equipment should be checked periodically for hazards, and play areas should be supervised.

Musculoskeletal trauma is most likely to occur in contact sports, with sprains being common. Certain contact sports, such as football or rugby, tend to produce joint damage, especially knee injuries. Severe hyperflexion of the neck from diving, trampoline activities, or football produces spinal cord injury and quadriplegia. Protective head and shoulder gear is helpful, but youngsters usually do not consistently wear appropriate protection unless they are well supervised.

For children riding in a car, an effective infant or child car seat is a must to avoid their being thrown during a sudden stop or collision.

ASSESSMENT OF TRAUMA

The site of the injury usually influences the order of priority of interventions when instituting emergency care. The safety of both the victim and the 'Good Samaritan' rescuers must be considered in order to prevent further injury. The major reason for thinking through steps to be taken in an emergency before the actual incident occurs, is to have a mental repertory of pre-planned actions available at a stimulus-response level.

◆ Emergency Treatment

Trauma

Make certain that the child and rescuer are not in immediate danger of additional trauma.

Do not move child unless absolutely necessary.

Keep child flat unless injury or symptoms specifically indicate otherwise:

  Head injury – elevate head slightly.

  Vomiting – carefully turn head to side.

Apply ABCs of emergency management;

  Airway – ensure open airway.

  Breathing – promote breathing; if not breathing, begin pulmonary resuscitation.

  Circulation – check pulse; if no pulse, begin chest compression.

Assess for extent of injury.

Stop bleeding with direct pressure to the wound or at appropriate bleeding point(s):

  Elevate injured part.

  Apply sterile or clean dressing.

Use tourniquets only when bleeding cannot be stopped by any other means:

  Release tourniquet pressure every 15-20 minutes.

  Notify person(s) taking over care of the child of the presence of tourniquet(s).

  Do not remove tourniquet until a doctor is present.

Assess for further injury.

Determine state of consciousness:

  Talk to child.

  Observe child's behaviour.

If present, do not remove objects protruding from child's body.

Check for evidence of decreased motor or sensory function in extremities:

  Infant and young child – observe spontaneous movement in extremities.

  Older child – ask if able to wiggle extremities.

Evaluate pain – present, absent; severe, mild.

  Attempt to alleviate with nonpharmacological techniques.

Assess pulses in extremity distal to the injury.

  Check colour and temperature of extremities.

Manage any injuries appropriately (e.g., splint fractures) (see Emergency Treatment: Fracture, p. 777).

Identify child.

Obtain information regarding the injury from witnesses, if any.

Call ambulance or transport to nearest facility.

NOTE: If spinal cord injury is suspected, do not move child unless absolutely necessary for the child's safety.

EMERGENCY MANAGEMENT

Guidelines for care of the child at the scene of the injury are outlined under Emergency Treatment. The first concerns are always for *airway, breathing,* and *circulation* (ABC), after which other injuries are managed as indicated by the assessment. Severe bleeding is treated by removing gross debris from the wound, such as glass, but not if a large object is impaled in the victim. In this situation, the wound is covered with a sterile or clean dressing, and direct pressure is applied over the wound or at appropriate pressure points.

Assessment of the child involves observation from head to toes, because infants and young children are unable to communicate except by crying and other behaviours.

A spinal cord injury is suspected if there is loss of sensation or motor function. In this case, a child is moved only if remaining in the present position is a threat to safety; if so, the child is carried in log fashion with the head and neck held firmly in a neutral position. No attempt should be made to transport the child until adequate help can be obtained to keep the body in straight alignment throughout and after the repositioning.

NURSING ALERT

Pain at the level of the injury, local muscle spasms and sensorimotor loss are the outstanding features of spinal cord injury.

The child should be identified as soon as feasible by anyone who knows the child. It is important to determine if the child has any existing health problems that might have implications for the circumstances of the injury and for therapeutic management. Any witnesses are asked for details about the incident to aid in assessment of the child's emotional responses.

In situations of severe injury, the emergency medical team will be needed to treat shock and to transport the child adequately to the nearest accident and emergency department.

SYSTEMATIC ASSESSMENT

The first priority on admission to an accident and emergency department is rapid assessment of the ABC status (airway, breathing, and circulation). Since the overwhelming majority of childhood injuries are the result of blunt-impact trauma, multiple organ involvement is a common finding; therefore, it is essential to perform a systematic assessment of the trauma victim. The most efficient method consists of a head-to-toe assessment (Box 33-1).

THE IMMOBILIZED CHILD

Immobilization is a major therapy for injuries to soft tissues, long bones, ligaments, vertebrae and joints. Restriction of motion for a period of time at the site at which muscle or bone integrity has been disrupted allows tissue and bone to heal. However, prolonged immobilization, whether for therapy or because of disability, can produce severe complications, many of which are preventable (see Fig. 33-1).

◆ **BOX 33-1**

Guidelines for assessing trauma

Head

Observe for level of consciousness.

Feel the head — palpate for depression or swelling over the cranium; feel the facial bones for depression or pain.

Observe for bruises, petechiae of skin and conjunctiva, singed hair, extraocular movement, pupil size and reactivity.

Observe the palate and mobility of the maxilla if child is cooperative.

Observe for drainage from ears and nose.

Neck

Observe status of neck veins (distended with chest injury), swelling, bruising, deformity of thyroid cartilage, penetrating wounds.

Palpate cervical spine (maintaining traction and neutral position), thyroid for tenderness, position of trachea, evidence of subcutaneous emphysema, carotid pulses.

Auscultate for bruits.

Chest

Observe symmetry of respiratory movement, flail segment, bruising, penetrating wounds.

Palpate clavicles, sternum, thoracic spine, subcutaneous emphysema; compress rib cage for local tenderness.

Auscultate for diminished breath sounds (haemothorax or pneumothorax), shifted or muffled heart sounds, pericardial rub.

Abdomen

Observe for distention, bruising, penetrating wounds, blood at the meatus or perineum.

While patient is quiet, palpate the bladder gently; compress the pelvic brim.

Auscultate for diminished bowel sounds, bruits.

Extremities

Observe for perfusion, gross deformity, spontaneous movement.

Palpate pulses at ankles, wrists, groin; palpate for local bone tenderness and sensation.

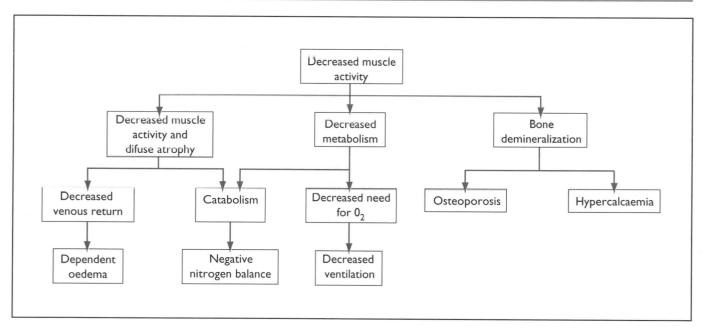

Fig. 33-1 Effects of immobilization.

IMMOBILIZATION

One of the most difficult aspects of illness is the immobility it often imposes on a child. Children's natural tendency to be mobile influences all elements of growth and development — physical, social, psychological and emotional. Children are immobilized only when necessary and for the shortest time possible.

AETIOLOGY OF IMMOBILIZATION

Children who are forced to remain inactive, because of physical limitations or therapy, display the multiple effects of restricted movement. Reasons for immobility include: congenital defects (e.g., spina bifida); degenerative disorders (e.g., muscular dystrophy); and infections or accidents that impair the integumentary system (severe burns), the musculoskele-

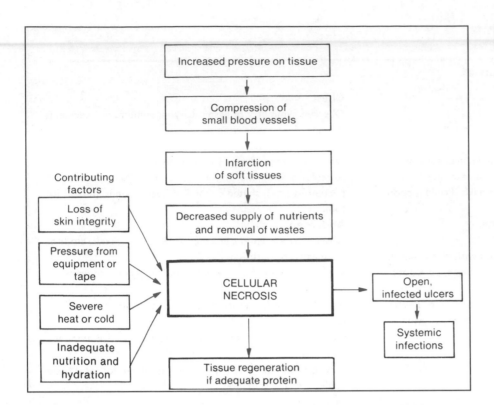

Fig. 33-2 Sequence of events in tissue breakdown.

tal system (fractures, osteomyelitis) or the neurological system (spinal cord injury, polyneuritis, head injury). Sometimes therapies, such as traction and spinal fusion, are also responsible for prolonged immobilization.

Integumentary system

Circulation to the skin is reduced during inactivity and may be further impeded by dependent oedema. Circulation is especially compromised in places where the bone surface is near the skin, such as areas over the sacrum, occiput, trochanter and ankle, and continued impairment causes rapid necrosis with ulcer formation. Mechanical irritation from appliances, such as straps, rods and ropes, and the friction of bedclothes during turning or other movement can produce skin breakdown. Healing capacity is also impaired by poor circulation, negative nitrogen balance and anaemia. Immobilization often makes it difficult to carry out adequate cleansing and hygienic measures, which may also contribute to tissue breakdown in areas that are difficult to reach (see Fig. 33-2). Children with sensory deficit should be guarded against extremes of heat and cold in direct contact with the skin.

Cellular breakdown caused by prolonged pressure can be identified by several characteristics. Prolonged redness (more than 30 minutes) indicates that a pressure area is developing and treatment should be instituted. Other signs of tissue ischaemia include local increase in temperature over the area, blistering, swelling, or dark purple or black discolouration. The pressure area may be limited to the skin and subcutaneous layer, or may be deeper with widespread underlying tissue destruction.

Neurosensory system

Preventing pressure on vulnerable areas and avoiding unnatural positions of flexion and extension that apply inappropriate pressure on nerves and blood vessels reduce the likelihood of compression injury. Periodic active and/or passive plantar flexion and dorsiflexion of the feet and hands will stimulate circulation and keep nerves from becoming pinched.

PSYCHOLOGICAL EFFECTS OF IMMOBILIZATION

Children perceive restraint by people or inanimate objects as either comforting or stressful. Adult controls on behaviour often provide children with a sense of security in frightening situations or when they fear loss of control. On the other hand, forced inactivity deprives them of one of their most valuable means for dealing with stress. Children who are confined to bed may become victims of their fears and fantasies, without the physical means for stress reduction.

Active children have many opportunities for input from a wide variety of settings. When they are immobilized by disease or as a part of a treatment regimen, they experience diminished environmental stimuli with a loss of tactile input and an altered perception of themselves and their environment. This sensory deprivation frequently leads to a feeling of isolation, boredom and being forgotten, especially by peers.

Physical interference with the activity of infants and young children gives them a feeling of helplessness. There appears to be a significant relationship between physical restraint and the incidence of language problems. Children who are restrained by casts, splints, or straps during the first three years of life have more difficulty with language than children whose activities are unrestricted. Language delay is even more marked in children with neurological impairment.

The struggle for independence is thwarted by imposed immobility. For example, for toddlers, exploration and imitative behaviours are essential to developing a sense of autonomy. To children, the inability to move is threatening to self-preservation and reactivates the struggle between activity and passivity, and between dependence and independence.

Behavioural changes are noted when children experience prolonged sensory deprivation. Some of these behaviours are demonstrated by a higher than normal level of anxiety (Box 33-2). Children seek attention by reverting to earlier developmental behaviours, such as wanting to be fed, bed-wetting and baby talk. In many ways, immobilized children are realistically dependent on others; therefore, intelligent and sensitive care is required to prevent major developmental regressions during the period of immobility.

Limbs in casts or traction transmit less than normal sensory data. The presence of sensory impairment may be a concomitant problem of the involved part. Numbness or loss of feeling markedly alters proprioception. Children who have limited ability to feel others touching them not only experience less tactile stimuli in a physical sense, but are also deprived of warm, loving feelings that arise from being touched. The loss of feeling derived from touch can further add to their sense of being isolated and unwanted.

Children may react to immobility by active protest, anger and aggressive behaviour, or they may become quiet, passive and submissive. Often, children believe that the immobilization is a justified punishment for misbehaviour. Children should be allowed to discharge their anger, but it should be within the limits of safety to their self-esteem and not damaging to the integrity of others. For example, providing an object to attack, rather than a person or a valued possession, is safe and therapeutic.

The most difficult situations are those involving major injuries and diseases that produce a disfigurement or a severe loss of function that directly affects children's self-image, such as burns, amputation or the sudden catastrophic effects of an accident that leaves healthy, athletic children paralysed for life. Feelings of anger and hostility are difficult for children to express when they are at the mercy of the environment. They dare not speak out against or defy the authorities on whom they depend so completely. Consequently, their aggression may be masked by cheerfulness or rigidity. When they are unable to express their anger, the aggression is often displayed inappropriately through regressive behaviour and outbursts of crying or temper tantrums over insignificant irritations.

EFFECT ON FAMILIES

Catastrophic illness or disability severely taxes the resources of the family. The following are commonly occurring problems:
1. Financial strains may decrease or totally eliminate the family's resources.
2. The focus of attention is placed, at least temporarily, on the affected member; therefore, other members of the family may feel neglected or their needs may not be met.
3. The family may have difficulty accepting the child's altered body image.
4. Individual family members may be unable to express their feelings and may become immobilized in the face of the crisis.
5. Parents often experience a sense of guilt over their child's immobilization. Failure to protect their child, from their perception, forms the basis of their inability to cope.

The family's needs may require the services of other professionals, such as a social worker, psychiatrist or marriage counsellor. In preparation for discharge, home visits are advisable and home management is frequently planned weeks in advance of the actual discharge. This includes special considerations for cultural, economic, physical and psychological needs. A child with a severe disability is very dependent, and caregivers need rest periods to revitalize themselves. Individual and group counselling is beneficial for pre-problem-solving situations and provides an emotional support system. Parent groups are also helpful and often allow nonthreatening social contact. The families of children with permanent disabilities need long-term resources, since some of the most difficult problems arise as they try to sustain high-quality care for many years.

IMPLICATIONS FOR NURSING

Assessment of the child who is immobilized as a result of an injury or a degenerative disease not only includes the injured part (e.g., fracture or damaged joint), but also the other systems that may be affected secondarily — the circulatory, renal, respiratory, muscular and gastrointestinal systems. In long-term

---

◆ **BOX 33-2**

Behavioural Changes in Immobilized Children

Higher than normal level of anxiety leads to:
  Restlessness
  Difficulty with problem solving
  Inability to concentrate on activities
  Depression
  Regression
  Egocentrism
Monotony leads to:
  Sluggish intellectual responses
  Sluggish psychomotor responses
  Decreased communication skills
  Increased fantasizing
  Hallucinations

---

immobilization, there also may be neurological impairment and metabolic changes in electrolytes (especially calcium), nitrogen balance and general metabolic rate.

Frequent position changes help prevent dependent oedema and fluid movement to third spaces, and stimulates circulation, respiratory function, gastrointestinal motility and neurological sensations.

Each metabolic disturbance is treated specifically. Metabolism is increased by activity within the limitations of the disability and capabilities of the child. High-protein, high-calorie foods are encouraged for correction of negative nitrogen balance. It is desirable to determine the child's favourite foods and to allow the family to bring special foods from home. Sometimes, supplementary nasogastric feedings or parenteral nutritional support may be needed.

Diet modification for the child with increased serum calcium presents problems, because the dairy foods that children often desire are high in this mineral. The primary nursing measure for hypercalcaemia is conscientious hydration and active remobilization as soon as possible.

Adequate hydration promotes bowel and kidney function, and helps prevent complications in these systems. It is important to determine the words the child uses for elimination. Embarrassment can be avoided by a mutually satisfactory communication system. Whenever possible, the child should be helped into a sitting position to use a suitable urinal or a bedpan. Providing privacy for toileting and encouraging the child to participate in solving toileting problems will increase the chances of a successful programme.

Children should be encouraged to be as active as their condition and restrictive devices allow. Those who are unable to move will need passive exercise and movement.

Play is the most useful tool of nursing, and activities which are selected on the basis of interest, ability and limitations, should include some form of physical activity that encourages the use of uninvolved muscles and joints. Any activity that is tolerated (e.g., turning in bed or changing position of a bed in the room) helps alter the monotony of immobilization, and dissipates tension and frustration.

Using dolls to illustrate and explain the restraining method is a valuable tool for small children. Placing a cast, tubing or other restraining equipment on the doll offers the child a non-threatening opportunity to express, through the doll, feelings concerning the restrictions and feelings towards the nurse and other health providers. It also provides a means for anticipatory teaching and explanation of needed restraining devices (see Chapter 5).

Self-care to the maximum extent is usually well received by children. They can help plan their daily routine, select their diet (when possible), and choose the clothes they are to wear, including innovative adornment, such as a favourite T-shirt, or other items of apparel that express each child's autonomy and individuality.

It is important for children to understand behavioural limitations or rules, and their questions should be answered. For example, they need to know the reasons for medical, nursing, occupational and physical therapies, and to know that schedules are necessary. Most of children's activity of daily living centres around play; therefore, therapies that incorporate this concept are more likely to gain their cooperation.

Visits from significant persons, such as family members and friends, offer occasions for emotional support and also provide opportunities for learning how to care for the child. The needs of a child with severe disability can be very complex, and family members require time to assimilate the teachings and demonstrations needed to understand their child's situation and care.

Some privacy is needed, particularly by the teenager, and most long-term health care facilities recognize that rooms shared by two to four youngsters are better environments for habilitation or rehabilitation. When room-mates are selected according to age and companionship, a chance is available to test out thoughts and feelings safely with others. If a traumatic incident caused the child's disability, guilt feelings may be displayed overtly or masked behind regressive or aggressive behaviour. The feeling that "I must have been bad to receive this fate" is common, and honest feedback stating, "It just happened — it was an accident", needs repeating many times. Additional aspects of grieving are involved if there was a loss of another person in the accident.

For a child with greatly restricted movement (e.g., a child with quadriplegia or a child with a large bilateral hip spica cast), nursing care is a challenge. These situations require long-term care either in the hospital or at home. Wherever the care occurs, consistent planning and coordination of activities with professionals and significant others are vital. Nursing assessment includes psychosocial data as well as physical manifestations, since long-term immobilization has a profound effect on the child and the family.

The effectiveness of nursing interventions is determined by continual reassessment and evaluation of care based on the following observational guidelines and expected outcomes:

1. Observe vital signs, neurological signs and respiratory, gastrointestinal and renal functioning; inspect skin; observe effects of correct functioning of equipment and appliances (restraints, traction, cast, braces).
2. Observe child's behaviour; engage in dialogue to elicit feelings, concerns and interests.
3. Observe the child's activities and interests.
4. Interview child and family regarding their feelings and concerns; observe family interaction at home, if possible.

MOBILIZATION DEVICES

Children usually respond well to mobilization and require little encouragement; however, they need instruction in the correct use of appliances, their operation, and precautions for their safe usage.

BRACES

Paralysed or markedly weakened extremities can sometimes be stabilized by braces that facilitate walking. Some are designed to stabilize the extremities and offer support during ambulation. Special joint hinges permit the hip, knee and ankle to flex during sitting, whereas the leg is held rigid during ambulation. Meticulous skin care and wearing protective clothing under the brace are necessary. Braces for the growing child will need frequent adjusting and replacement by the orthotist, if long-term use is necessary.

A brace is frequently used to support the spine and trunk during ambulation in conditions such as scoliosis and spinal cord injury. The brace must fit each body curvature to avoid undue pressure on tissues and imbalance between muscle groups. Bony prominences where the brace has contact, such as along the spine, chin and iliac crests, are observed closely for pressure or irritation and are padded as necessary. A corset with metal stays may provide the needed torso support, especially for a paraplegic child. Generally, the corset is more comfortable than the brace, and presents fewer problems with dressing. Specialized devices can be used to provide upright mobility in small children with lower limb paralysis who shift body weight to achieve locomotion.

Parallel bars

Parallel bars provide secure handrails on both sides of children as they learn to walk again, with or without braces. As they become more proficient, a walker with or without wheels is substituted for the bars and children are no longer confined to a limited territory. Children then progress to crutches if their age and condition permit.

CRUTCHES AND STICKS

Crutches are used when children are not allowed to bear weight or can only place part of their body weight on an extremity, such as most lower leg injuries. *Axillary* crutches are used infrequently as temporary assistance. *Forearm* crutches are the usual selection for children who anticipate permanent use, such as paraplegic children who are able to use braces. For children with limited hand and arm strength or function, *trough* crutches allow the weight to be assumed by the elbow. For habilitating small children, special crutches stabilized with three or four legs provide the needed stability for a child to maintain an upright position and learn to walk.

Children must be properly fitted for the crutch or stick to prevent poor posture and crutch pressure on the axilla during ambulation. Measuring for crutches and teaching crutch and stick use are usually assumed by the physiotherapist.

Bed exercises for strengthening arms and shoulders are important if immobilization has been prolonged.

SPECIAL BEDS

Older quadriplegic children often require a special bed to immobilize the head and spine during the early phases of spinal cord injury care. Some rehabilitation units use a regular bed for the patient in cervical traction, whereas others use a Stryker frame or one of the Roto-Rest beds. Whatever special bed is used, the success of its use is greatly influenced by the prepa-

ration of the child. Explanations of how the bed works (and, when possible, showing the child someone being turned in the bed) are needed.

A Stryker frame employs two frames, one anterior and one posterior, to turn the child horizontally. The Stryker wedge frame was designed to allow prone-supine turning by one person, but for safety, two appropriately qualified people are used for turning a child in a Stryker frame. Cervical traction can easily be attached to the stationary frame and presents no discomfort when turning, as long as the weights are prevented from swinging. Before turning, the child's arms and legs are aligned within the frame and straps are wrapped around the entire 'sandwich' of frames. All of the skin areas should be checked with each turning.

The Roto-Rest bed operates electrically; with the entire body securely immobilized by firm bolsters, the person is slowly and constantly rotated from side to side. Traction can be attached to this bed, and various parts can be removed to permit care and physiotherapy. The continuous changes of position decrease the problems of pressure areas and promote venous circulation. The bed has a major advantage over a Stryker frame for teenagers with tracheostomies or other conditions that do not allow placing them in the prone position. The bed is made in an adult size and is suited only for large children.

WHEELCHAIRS

Wheelchairs are used temporarily or permanently as a means of transportation. A wheelchair should fit the child and should contain any adaptations needed, such as an elevating leg rest or reclining back. The child is taught how to transfer in and out of the chair and how to propel it safely. Detachable or rotating armrests, which permit easy transfer in and out, are needed for children with spinal cord injuries.

Other desirable features are detachable and swing-away footrests and detachable desk arms. Elevating leg rests are required for children who are prone to contractures, and a reclining back rest is needed for those who may have poor trunk balance. A proper cushion with adequate padding should be provided for the child who has decreased sensation. Hand rim and brake lever projections are helpful for the child with upper extremity weakness. Children with paraplegia will require upper arm strengthening exercises and instruction on transfer techniques before wheelchair mobilization.

Various motorized chairs are available for marked upper extremity weakness, and mouth- or cheek-operated models are available for children who do not have the use of upper extremities, so that children can operate them independently.

THE CHILD WITH A FRACTURE

The musculoskeletal system, like all the body systems of the newborn, is immature, and the specific functions of the system develop slowly so that the muscles, bones, tendons and ligaments can function in an integrated fashion to perform complex tasks.

The epiphysis, located at the ends of long bones, consists of layers of cartilage, subchondral bone and sponge-like cancellous bone. Situated between the diaphysis and epiphysis is the epiphyseal plate, which plays a major role in the longitudinal growth of the developing child. The periosteum, the thin, tough membrane covering all bones, contains blood vessels that nourish the living bone. Damage to this thin membrane can be a major problem in bone growth and healing.

FRACTURES

Bones fracture when the resistance of the bone against the stress being exerted yields to the stress force. Fractures are a common injury at any age, but are more likely to occur in children and the elderly.

AETIOLOGY

The causes of fracture injuries in children are those described for general traumatic injuries in childhood. Fractures in infancy are more often the result of birth trauma or child abuse. Aside from motor vehicle accidents, true accidents rarely occur in infancy; therefore, injury in children in that age group warrants further investigation. In any small child, radiological evidence of old fractures at various stages of healing is, with few exceptions, an indication of physical abuse. Rarely, the cause may be defects in bone development, as seen in *osteogenesis imperfecta*. Most often, however, early bone trauma in infants consists of periosteal bleeding in the long bones of arms and legs, usually caused by rough handling, twisting and pulling, which is not evident on radiological examination until 3-6 weeks after the injury.

Fractures of the forearm are common bone injuries in childhood and are usually caused when the child extends the palm of the hand to break a fall. The force resulting from a fall on the outstretched hand progresses up the length of the extremity with the possibility of injury to finger, wrist, elbow, shoulder and/or clavicle. The clavicle is a bone frequently broken in children; approximately one-half of clavicle fractures occur in children under ten years of age. Many occur at birth. Hip fractures are rare in children and require a great deal of violence to produce. A femoral neck or shaft fracture may be sustained in children 6-7 years of age as a result of pedestrian-motor car accidents, because their hip height is on the same level as a motor car bumper. In older children, knee and lower limb injuries are common.

At all ages, motor vehicle accidents are a frequent cause of bone injury. Most children who are hit by a motor car are 4-7 years of age. A triad of injuries must be kept in mind when making an assessment of injuries: (1) the child's femur, which is at the level of the bumper, is fractured; (2) the bonnet of the motor car produces injuries to the child's chest and trunk; and (3) a contralateral head injury is usually sustained when the child is thrown to the ground by the impact. Therefore, a child with any of these injuries, who was struck by a motor car, should be examined for evidence of the other two.

Types of fractures

A fractured bone consists of fragments - the fragment closer to the midline (the proximal fragment), and the fragment farthest from the midline (the distal fragment). When fracture fragments are separated, the fracture is *complete;* when fragments remain attached, it is said to be *incomplete*

All fractures affect the entire cross-section of the bone. The twisting of an extremity, while the bone is breaking, results in the spiral break. If the fracture does not produce a break in the skin, it is a *simple,* or *closed,* fracture. *Open,* or *compound,* fractures are those with an open wound through which the bone is or has protruded. If the bone fragments cause damage to other organs or tissues (e.g., the lung or bladder), the injury is said to be *complicated.* When small fragments of bone are broken from the fractured shaft and lie in the surrounding tissue, the fracture is called *comminuted.* This type of fracture is rare in children. The types of fractures that occur most often in children are shown in Fig. 33-3 and described in Box 33-3.

Epiphyseal injuries

The weakest point of long bones is the cartilage growth plate or epiphyseal plate. Consequently, this is a frequent site of damage during trauma. When fracture lines deviate from a transverse direction through the degenerating cells, more serious damage to the epiphysis and the plate may occur. Figure 33-4 illustrates the types of epiphyseal injuries in order of increasing risk of permanent epiphyeseal damage and possible growth disturbances.

Detection of epiphyseal injuries is sometimes difficult, and they may be mistaken for dislocations or ligamentous injuries. Fractures involving the epiphysis or epiphyseal plate present special problems in determining whether or not bone growth will be affected. Early and correct assessment is essential to minimize the incidence of longitudinal growth problems and angular deformities.

CLINICAL MANIFESTATIONS

Children demonstrate the usual signs of injury — generalized swelling, pain or tenderness, and diminished functional use of the affected part. There may be bruising, severe muscular rigidity and sometimes crepitus (a grating sensation at the fracture site).

Vascular injury is most likely to occur with supracondylar fractures of the humerus and femur. Femoral and popliteal vessels and the sciatic nerve are prone to trauma in femoral fractures; humeral fractures may cause damage to the medial, ulnar or radial nerves and to the brachial artery.

NURSING ALERT

The five 'Ps' of ischaemia from a vascular injury — pain, pallor, pulselessness, paraesthesia and paralysis — should be kept in mind when making an assessment.

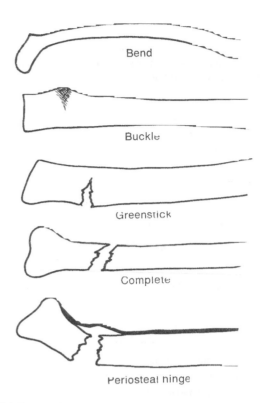

Fig. 33-3 Types of fractures in children.

PROCESS OF DIAGNOSIS

A medical history is often lacking for childhood injuries. Infants are unable to communicate, and older children are unreliable informants. In cases of child abuse, parents may give false information deliberately in order to protect themselves.

Radiography

Radiological examination is the most useful diagnostic tool for assessing skeletal trauma. The calcium deposits in bone make the entire structure radiopaque. Ossification centres alter the appearance of the bone, and much of the skeleton of infants and young children is composed of radiolucent growth cartilage that does not appear on radiographs. In addition, the epiphyseal cartilage and undisplaced separations of the epiphysis, which often occur, are not easily detected on radiographs.

Many practitioners obtain a film of the uninjured limb for a direct comparison to help identify minor alterations in alignment and configuration of the epiphysis, and associated injuries that might be missed. Radiographs are taken after fracture reduction and in some situations may be taken during the healing process to determine satisfactory progress.

Blood studies

Severe soft tissue, muscle and bone injury results in a destruction of red blood cells with an increase in bilirubin and a decrease in the haemoglobin or haematocrit reading. Serum levels of creatine, alkaline phosphatase, serum glutamic-oxaloacetic transaminase (SGOT) and lactic dehydrogenase (LDH) may increase in proportion to the amount of muscle damage.

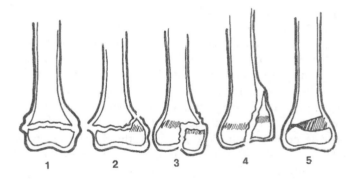

Fig. 33-4 Types of epiphyseal injuries in order of increasing risk.

A normal physiological response to tissue injury is the inflammatory process with a slight elevation of white blood cells, especially neutrophils. When infection occurs, the increase in leukocytes is anticipated and the accompanying symptoms of fever and lethargy develop.

THERAPEUTIC MANAGEMENT

The goals of fracture management are:
1. To regain alignment and length of the bony fragments (reduction) and to correct deformity.
2. To retain alignment and length (immobilization).
3. To restore function to the injured parts.

In children, the bone fragments are usually realigned and immobilized by traction or by closed manipulation and casting until adequate callus is formed. Weight bearing and active movement for the purpose of regaining function can begin after the fracture site is stable. The child's natural tendency to be active is usually sufficient to restore normal mobility. Open reduction is seldom required and is limited to fractures that cannot be maintained by conservative methods, and when there is interposed tissue or injury to arteries or nerves. Surgical reductions are more likely to delay normal healing and may predispose to nonunion.

Children are most frequently hospitalized for fractures of the femur and the supracondylar area of the distal humerus. If simple reductions cannot be achieved, or a neurovascular problem is detected after injury, observation in hospital is indicated. The method of fracture reduction is determined by several criteria (Box 33-4).

Problems associated with fracture injury involve both the doctor and the nurse in their management (Box 33-5). Specific interventions and nursing responsibilities in the general management are directed towards restoring bone integrity and functional use, and are discussed in relation to the major modalities of fracture immobilization — casting and traction (see also Emergency Treatment).

Surgical intervention

When surgical intervention is necessary to realign a fracture, the child needs physical and psychological preparation. Preoperative teaching is the same as for any other surgical procedure. Orthopaedic surgery uses a variety of rods, screws, staples and plates. The child needs to know about these unfamiliar objects and how they will appear when he or she returns from the procedure. Fixating devices are made of substances that do not act as foreign proteins to the body and therefore are not rejected. Usually, the rods are driven down the shaft of the long bones, whereas screws and plates are attached to the side of the bone shaft. Postoperatively, the bone healing takes place with callus formation just as it does in a new fracture. Generally, the child with an internal fixation device sits in a chair and walks with a walker or crutches within a few days. The most common postoperative complication is infection. The nurse's responsibility includes close monitoring of neurovascular changes in the involved extremity and the prevention of postanaesthesia problems.

THE CHILD IN A CAST

The completeness of the fracture, the type of bone involved, and the amount of weight that can be placed on the limb influence how much of the extremity must be included in the cast to immobilize the fracture site completely. In most situations, the joints above and below the fracture are immobilized to eliminate the possibility of movement that might cause displacement at the fracture site. Four major categories of casts are used for immobilization of fractures: *upper extremity* to immobilize wrist and/or elbow, *lower extremity* to immobilize ankle and/or knee, *spinal* and *cervical* for immobilization of the spine, and *spica casts* to immobilize the hip and knee.

◆ **BOX 33-4**

Criteria for determining use of reduction method for fractures

Age of child
Degree of displacement
Amount of overriding
Degree of oedema
Condition of skin and soft tissue
Sensation and circulation distal to fracture

◆ **BOX 33-5**

Problems associated with fracture injury

Control of pain, haemorrhage, and oedema
Relief of muscle spasms
Realignment of fracture fragments
Promotion of bone healing
Immobilization of fracture until adequate healing has begun
Prevention of secondary complications
Limitation of disuse syndrome
Restoration of function

◆ *Emergency Treatment*

Fracture
Assess extent of injury — 5 'Ps':
  Pain and point of tenderness
  Pulse — distal to the fracture site
  Pallor
  Paraesthesia — sensation distal to the fracture site
  Paralysis — movement distal to the fracture site
Determine the mechanism of injury.
Move injured part as little as possible.
Cover open wounds with sterile or clean dressing.
Immobilize the limb, including joints above and below fracture site; do not attempt to reduce fracture or push protruding bone under the skin.
Soft splint (pillow or folded towel).
Rigid splint (rolled newspaper or magazine).
Uninjured leg can serve as splint for leg fracture if no splint available.
Reassess neurovascular status.
Apply traction if circulatory compromise is present.
Elevate the injured limb if possible.
Apply cold to the injured area.
Call ambulance or transport to medical facility.
Always be alert to the possibility of other more serious injuries.

Casting materials

Casts are constructed from gauze strips and bandages impregnated with plaster of Paris or synthetic lighter-weight and water-resistant materials (e.g., fibreglass and polyurethane resin). Table 33-1 compares the relative merits of plaster and synthetic casts.

Cast application

There are several methods of holding a child during cast application. Special cast tables that hold the child's body are used for applying large hip spica casts. If possible, children should be allowed to play with a small doll that has a cast so that they understand what will be done. Before the cast is applied, the extremities are checked for any abrasions, cuts or other alterations in the skin surface and for the presence of rings or other items that might cause constriction from swelling; such objects are removed. Identification bands are placed on a noninjured extremity if hospitalization is anticipated.

A tube of stockinet is stretched over the area to be casted, and bony prominences are padded with soft cotton sheeting. Dry rolls of gauze impregnated with plaster of Paris are immersed in a bucket of tepid water with the open end of the roll downward to allow soaking of the bandage. The wet plaster rolls are put on in a bandage fashion and moulded to the extremity. A heat-producing chemical reaction occurs between the plaster and water as the plaster becomes a crystalline gypsum. During application of the cast, the underlying stockinet is pulled over the raw edges of the cast and secured with a layer of wet plaster 1.2-2.5 cm below the rim to form a smooth, padded edge to protect the skin.

IMPLICATIONS FOR NURSING

The complete evaporation of the water from the hip spica cast can take 24-72 hours when traditional types of plaster materials are used. Drying occurs within 30 minutes with new quick-drying substances. Turning the child at least every two hours will help to dry the cast evenly. The cast must remain uncovered to allow it to dry from the inside out.

A wet cast should be supported by a pillow covered with plastic and should be handled by the palms of the hands to prevent indenting the cast and creating pressure areas/plaster sores. A dry plaster of Paris cast produces a hollow sound when tapped with the finger. Suspected plaster sores should be reported so a window can be made in the cast to observe the site.

During the first few hours after a cast is applied, the chief concern is that the extremity may continue to swell to the extent that the cast becomes a tourniquet, shutting off circulation and producing neurovascular complications. A measure for reducing the likelihood of this potential problem is to elevate the body part, thereby increasing venous return. If oedema is excessive, casts are bivalved; that is, cut to make anterior and posterior halves that are held together with an elastic bandage. The cast and the involved extremity are observed frequently for neurovascular integrity and any signs of compromise. Permanent muscle and tissue damage can occur within six hours (McCullough and Evans, 1985), for

which nurses can be held liable (Northrup and Kelly, 1987).

When plastering an extremity that has sustained an open fracture, a window is often left over the wound area to allow for observation and for dressing of the wound. A surgical reduction is usually plastered as for a closed fracture. For the first few hours after surgery, there may be substantial bleeding that will soak through the cast. Periodically, the circumscribed blood-stained area should be outlined with a black felt-tip pen and the time indicated to provide a guide for assessing the amount of bleeding.

When the child is discharged home, parents need instructions on drying and caring for the cast and checking for signs and symptoms that indicate the cast is too tight (see Parent Guidelines). They should also be told to take the child to the health professional for attention if the cast becomes too loose, since a loose cast no longer serves its purpose.

Parent Guidelines

Cast Care

Keep the casted extremity elevated on pillows or similar support for the first day, or as directed by the health professional.

Avoid indenting the cast until it is thoroughly dry.

Observe the extremities (fingers or toes) for any evidence of swelling or discolouration (darker or lighter than a comparable extremity) and contact the health professional if noted.

Check movement and sensation of the visible extremities frequently.

Follow health professional's orders regarding any restriction of activities.

Restrict strenuous activities for the first few days.

   Engage in quiet activities, but encourage use of muscles.

   Move the joints above and below the cast on the affected extremity.

Encourage frequent rest for a few days, keeping the injured extremity elevated while resting.

Avoid allowing the affected limb to hang down for any length of time.

   Keep an injured upper extremity elevated (e.g., in a sling) while upright.

   Elevate a lower limb when sitting and avoid standing for too long.

Do not allow the child to put anything inside the cast.

   Keep small items that might be placed inside the cast away from small children.

Keep a clear path for ambulation.

   Remove toys, hazardous floor rugs, pets or other items over which the child might stumble.

Use crutches appropriately if lower limb fracture.

   The crutches should fit properly, have a soft rubber tip to prevent slipping, and be well padded at the axilla.

	PLASTER OF PARIS	SYNTHETIC
Composition and preparation	Cotton tape permeated with calcium sulphate crystals that interlock as tape dries (tepid water-activated)	1. Polyester/cotton tape permeated with polyurethane resin (cool water-activated) 2. Knitted fibreglass tape with polyurethane resin (tepid water-activated or photoactivated) 3. Knitted thermoplastic polyester fabric (hot water-activated)
Setting time	3 to 8 minutes	3 to 15 minutes
Drying time	10 to 72 hours (varies with cast size)	5 to 30 minutes (varies with type of cast)
Indentations	Slow drying time increases possibility	Rapid drying time reduces likelihood of indentations; allows rapid use
Weight	Relatively heavy; bulky; difficulty wearing regular clothing	Lightweight; less bulky; can wear with regular clothing; allows for greater range of activity
Conformity	Moulds readily to body part	Does not mould easily to body parts; unsuitable for small children or severely displaced fractures
Surface	Smooth exterior; does not scratch clothing or furniture;	Rough exterior; very sharp edges can snag clothing or abrade skin
Cost	Relatively inexpensive; an advantage if cast changes anticipated	Expensive; cost three to seven times that of plaster casts
Stability	Relatively stable; must keep cast dry	Very stable but should be kept dry; clean with small amount of mild soap and water; dry with towel followed by blow dryer on cool or warm setting
Miscellaneous	Child may feel uncomfortable warming or burning sensation under cast while drying (chemical reaction) Skin under cast may become irritated Cast must be protected when around water (bathing)	Special aids may be required for application or removal of some types Increased activity may displace fracture Skin under cast may become macerated from inadequate drying after water immersion

Table 33-1 Comparison of plaster of Paris and synthetic cast.

Cast removal

Cutting the cast to remove it or to relieve tightness is a frightening experience for children. They fear the sound of the cast cutter and are terrified that their flesh, as well as the cast, will be cut. Since it works by vibration, a cast cutter cuts only the hard surface of the cast. The vibration also generates heat that may be felt by the child. Preparation for the procedure will help reduce anxiety, especially if a trusting relationship has been established between the child and the nurse. Children need continual reassurance that all is going well and that their behaviour is accepted.

Home care for children in casts creates problems of various magnitude, especially with large casts (e.g., a hip spica). Commonplace situations become problematic; for example, returning the child home safely and comfortably. Standard seat belts and car seats are not readily adapted for use by children in casts. Sitting can be impossible in a spica cast, and leg casts require extra space in a small room, under a table or in a bathroom. Children in spica casts usually find the prone position easier for self-feeding from a small table placed next to the dining table or on the floor. Beanbags are used to aid comfort. The conventional toilet is almost impossible for a child in a spica cast. Small bedpans or other containers offer alternatives for elimination.

After the cast is removed, the skin surface will be caked with desquamated skin and sebaceous secretions. Simple soaking in a bathtub is usually sufficient for their removal. Application of olive oil or lotion provides lubrication and comfort. Parents and child should be instructed not to pull or forcibly remove this material with vigorous scrubbing, because this may cause excoriation and bleeding.

THE CHILD IN TRACTION

Bone fragments that cannot be aligned initially by simple traction and stabilization with a cast require the extended pulling force offered by continuous traction. Traction also may be used for other purposes (Box 33-6).

PURPOSES OF TRACTION

When forces having both direction and magnitude act on an object at the same point simultaneously from opposite directions, the object either changes its state of rest or motion, or remains in equilibrium. The use of traction in the management of fractures is the direct application of these forces to produce equilibrium at the fracture site. A forward force (traction) is produced by attaching weight to the distal bone fragment, which is balanced by the backward force of the muscle pull (countertraction) and the frictional force between the patient and the bed. The two essential components of traction are forward traction and countertraction.

To reduce or realign a fracture site, traction is provided by weights applied to the distal bone fragment; body weight provides countertraction. By adjusting the line of pull upward or downward or by adducting or abducting the extremity, the operator uses these forces to align the distal and proximal bone fragments. To attain equilibrium, the amount of forward force is adjusted by adding weight to or subtracting weight from the traction, and/or countertraction can be increased by elevating the foot of the bed to create a greater gravitational pull to the backward force.

The three primary purposes of traction for reduction of fractures are:

1. To fatigue the involved muscle and reduce muscle spasm so that bones can be realigned
2. To position the distal and proximal bone ends in desired realignment to promote satisfactory bone healing
3. To immobilize the fracture site until realignment has been achieved and sufficient healing has taken place to permit casting or splinting

The realignment of the fragments is a gradual process that is achieved more rapidly in infants, who have limited muscle tone, than in muscular teenagers. The desired line of pull and callus formation are checked periodically by radiological examination. The traction pull, to some degree, immobilizes the fracture site; however, adjunctive immobilizing devices such as splints or casts are sometimes used with skeletal traction.

TYPES OF TRACTION (GENERAL)

The pull needed for traction can be applied to the distal bone fragment in several ways (Box 33-7).

The type of traction applied is determined primarily by the age of the child, the condition of the soft tissues, and the type and degree of displacement of the fracture. Fractures most commonly treated by application of traction are those involving the humerus, femur and vertebrae.

UPPER EXTREMITY TRACTION

Treatment of fractures of the humerus by traction is accomplished by either: (1) overhead suspension, in which the arm, bent at the elbow, is suspended vertically by skin or skeletal attachment and traction is applied to the distal end of the humerus, or (2) Dunlop traction, in which the arm is suspended horizontally, using either skin or skeletal attachment.

Fractures of the humerus, which are usually the result of a fall with the arm in extension, frequently involve the supracondylar portion. There are three major complications associated with this injury: Volkmann ischaemic contractures; traumatic injury to the median, ulnar or radial nerves; and angulation deformities. The fracture must be carefully reduced, usually with the child under anaesthesia, and because of the danger of complications, children with closed reduction of supracondylar fractures are usually hospitalized for overnight observation. In severely malaligned fractures, closed reduction with the child under anaesthesia is followed by application of skin or skeletal traction for 2-3 weeks, after which a long arm cast is applied for an additional 2-3 weeks.

LOWER EXTREMITY TRACTION

The frequent site for a femoral fracture is in the middle third of the shaft. In a fracture in the lower third of the shaft, the

---

◆ BOX 33-6

Purposes of traction

To realign bone fragments

To provide rest for an extremity

To help prevent or improve contracture deformity (e.g., in children with spasticity)

To correct a deformity

To treat a dislocation

To allow preoperative or postoperative positioning and alignment

To provide immobilization of specific areas of the body

To reduce muscle spasms (rare in children)

To maintain reduction of a problematic inguinal hernia in infants

pull of the gastrocnemius muscle causes the distal fragment to become downwardly displaced. The severity of the fracturing force and the ability of the muscles to hold the fracture out of alignment will determine the fracture type and the amount of overriding of the fragments. The periosteum may remain intact, which helps maintain alignment.

Fractures of the femur can often be reduced with early application of a hip spica cast in young children. When traction is required, several types may be employed, based on the initial assessment.

Bryant traction ('gallows' traction)

Adhesive traction strips are applied to the child's legs and secured with elastic bandages wrapped from the foot to the groin (Fig. 33-5). Both of the child's hips are flexed at a 90-degree angle with the knees in extension and the legs suspended by pulleys and weights. The child's weight supplies the countertraction; therefore, the buttocks are slightly elevated off the bed. The ankle bones are protected with stockinet or cotton wadding and foam. This type of traction is used for children younger than two years of age.

Bryant traction is unsuitable for older children or children with spasticity, and is usually limited to children who weigh less than 12-14 kg and are under two years of age, because of the risk of postural hypertension. The child's position needs to be monitored, and the alignment of the fracture is checked by periodic radiographs with needed traction adjustments made by the operator. Remodelling and callus formation occur rapidly within 2-3 weeks.

A specific complication of overhead traction is impairment of circulation. This is especially a problem in Bryant traction because of the gravitational vascular draining of the elevated extremities, the possible tourniquet effect of the bandages, and the effect of the traction, which can trigger vasospasms.

A child younger than two years of age normally has the hips in flexion most of the time; therefore, the mild contracture that might develop from this position is easily corrected. The youngster is permitted sufficient room between the foot and the traction foot plate to move the foot and prevent ankle problems. The legs must be maintained perpendicular to the trunk, and the buttocks should not be allowed to rest on the mattress.

Straight leg or 'buck' extension

Buck extension (Fig. 33-6) is a type of skin traction with the legs in an extended position, but it differs from Bryant traction in that the hips are not flexed. The postural hypertension that could develop as a result of Bryant traction is avoided, and this traction allows for greater mobility.

Hamilton-Russell traction

Hamilton-Russell traction (Fig. 33-7) uses skin traction on the lower leg and a padded sling under the knee. Two lines of pull, one along the longitudinal line of the lower leg and one perpendicular to the leg, are produced. This combination of pulls allows realignment of the lower extremity and immobilizes the hip and knee in a flexed position. Because the traction is set up to have two ropes pulling in the same direction at the foot plate, the traction pull will be twice the amount of weight at the end of the bed. For example, 2.3 kg of weight produces 4.5 kg of pull.

'90°-90°' traction

One type of skeletal traction is 90°–90° traction (90-90 traction) (Fig. 33-8). The lower leg is put in a boot cast or supported in a sling, and a skeletal Steinmann pin or Kirschner wire is placed in the distal fragment of the femur. This traction:

- Achieves the desired line of pull for reducing the fracture by means of the skeletal traction.
- Allows a 90-degree flexion of both the hip and the knee.
- Supports the lower extremity in a desired position with good venous return.
- Provides adequate immobilization of the fracture site.

◆ BOX 33-7

Types of traction

Manual traction — traction applied to the body part by the hand placed distally to the fracture site. Nurses frequently provide manual traction during cast application.

Skin traction — pull applied directly to the skin surface and indirectly to the skeletal structures. The pulling mechanism is attached to the skin with adhesive material or an elastic bandage. Both types are applied over soft, foam-backed traction straps to distribute the traction pull.

Skeletal traction — pull applied directly to the skeletal structure by a pin, wire or tongs inserted into or through the diameter of the bone distal to the fracture.

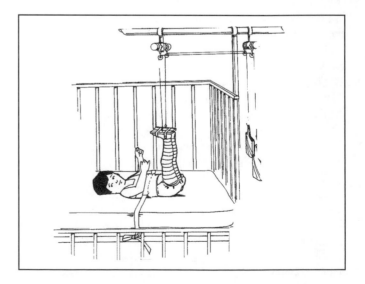

Fig. 33-5 Bryant traction ('gallows' traction excludes the weights).

Balance suspension traction

Balance suspension traction (Fig. 33-9) may be used with or without skin or skeletal traction. Unless used with another traction, the balanced suspension merely suspends the leg in a desired flexed position to relax the hip and hamstring muscles and does not exert any traction directly on a body part. A Thomas splint extends from the groin to midair above the foot, and a Pearson attachment supports the lower leg.

The Pearson attachment will stay wherever positioned. This traction requires very careful checking of splints and ropes to make certain that no slippage or fraying has occurred. However, the most common traction for primary school-aged children with femoral shaft fractures is straight leg skin traction using a Thomas splint.

CERVICAL TRACTION

The cervical area is a vulnerable site for flexion or extension injuries to muscle, vertebrae and/or the spinal cord. Cervical muscle trauma without other complications is treated with a cervical soft or hard collar to relieve the weight of the head from the fracture site. Intermittent cervical skin traction might be employed with a head halter and weight to decrease muscle spasms.

When a child displaces or fractures a cervical vertebra, it is necessary to reduce and immobilize the site with cervical skeletal traction. The spinal cord runs through the intravertebral canal, and dislocation or fracture of the vertebrae can also cause spinal cord trauma.

Physical examination, especially a neurological assessment, and radiological studies are essential diagnostic aids to determine:
• Presence of vertebral fracture.
• Degree of vertebral dislocation.
• Displacement of intravertebral disc.
• Compression of spinal cord and other neurological structures.
• Sensory, motor and autonomic nerve deficits.

Cervical traction is usually accomplished by insertion of Crutchfield or Barton tongs through burr holes in the skull. If the injury has been limited to a vertebral fracture without neurological deficit, a halo cast can be applied to permit earlier ambulation.

IMPLICATIONS FOR NURSING

To assess the child in traction, it is essential to know the purpose for which the traction is applied. Regular assessment of both the child and the traction apparatus is required.

Evaluating the therapeutic effects and possible negative consequences is essential to good patient care. Many of the nursing problems associated with a child in traction are related to immobility. However, there are several physical needs that require attention and vigilance.

In addition to routine skin observation and care, children in skeletal traction will need special skin care at the pin site.

When children are first placed in traction, they may have increased discomfort as a result of the traction pull fatiguing the muscle. Analgesics and muscle relaxants should be given during this phase of care. An explanation should be given according to each child's level of development about what is happening and why the child must remain in the device.

Some devices assist children in performing activities independently. An overhead trapeze (often referred to as a 'monkey pole'), which they can use to help lift themselves, facilitates hygiene and repositioning, and provides exercise for uninvolved muscles.

The effectiveness of nursing interventions is determined by continual reassessment and evaluation of care based on the following observational guidelines and expected outcomes:
1. Perform routine assessment of the child and traction.
2. Perform assessment for circulation, skin integrity, neurological function, and evidence of infection.

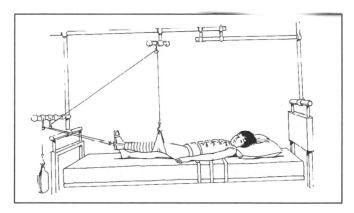

Fig. 33-7 Hamilton-Russell traction.

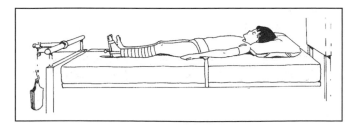

Fig. 33-6 Straight leg or 'buck' extension traction.

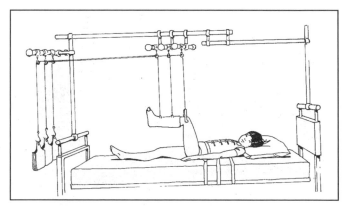

Fig. 33-8 '90-90' traction.

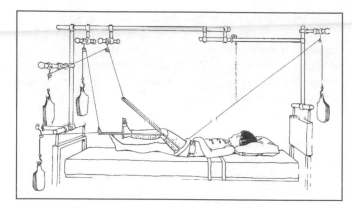

Fig. 33-9 Balance suspension with Thomas ring splint and Pearson attachment.

3. Observe types of activity in which child engages; observe for visitors and interaction with other patients and staff.
4. Interview child and family regarding feelings and concerns.

FRACTURE COMPLICATIONS

In addition to problems related to immobilization, the major complications of fractures include the following areas: circulatory impairment, nerve compression, compartment syndrome, Volkmann's ischaemic contracture, epiphyseal damage, nonunion, malunion, infection, renal calculi, and pulmonary embolus. These are described below.

Major complications associated with fractures may be immediately detected. For example, the fracture may be associated with damage to internal organs, as can occur with skull, chest or pelvic fractures. Alternatively, the fracture itself may initiate a life-threatening situation, such as haemorrhage, oligaemic shock, infection in compound injuries, electrolyte shifts, protein breakdown, and other metabolic responses of trauma (McCrae, 1990). In addition, gross psychological disturbance may be provoked by recall of the incident which caused the fracture.

The specific complications of fractures include areas discussed below.

CIRCULATORY IMPAIRMENT

If the trauma or immobilizing device restricts veins or arteries in the affected extremity, bone healing will be seriously impaired. Careful assessment of the pulses, skin colour and temperature is an important nursing responsibility. After injury, swelling of tissues occurs more rapidly in the child than in the adult. In the upper extremity, brachial, radial, ulnar and digital pulses are felt. In the leg, femoral, popliteal, posterior tibial and dorsalis pedis pulses are checked.

Closely associated with an inadequate blood supply is a low haematocrit value, which can result from the initial blood loss or surgically induced anaemia. Although the blood flow may be adequate, a lowered amount of haemoglobin will not provide a sufficient supply of oxygen for tissue repair.

NERVE COMPRESSION SYNDROMES

Nerve damage can take place at the time of injury, develop in the process of realignment, or be a complication of an immobilizing apparatus. The syndromes are classified according to the anatomical area affected and can involve the median (carpal tunnel syndrome), ulnar (at wrist or elbow), radial, posterior tibial (tarsal tunnel syndrome), common peroneal, or sciatic nerves. Peroneal nerve damage can result in footdrop, and radial nerve impairment produces wristdrop.

Treatment is alleviation of pressure on the nerve. The practitioner determines whether correcting the alignment will alleviate pressure on the nerve or if surgical intervention is necessary. At times, sensory or motor changes indicate ischaemia, and the treatment is correction of the vascular disturbance.

COMPARTMENT SYNDROMES

A *compartment* is a group of muscles surrounded by tough, inelastic fascial tissue. The compartment syndrome occurs when increased pressure within this closed space increases and compromises circulation to the muscles and nerves within the space. Muscles and nerves of both upper and lower extremities are enclosed within such compartments. The most frequent causes of compartment syndrome are tight dressings or casts, haemorrhage, trauma, burns, surgery, and extravasation of IV fluids into soft tissues.

Signs and symptoms of compartment syndrome reflect a deficit or deterioration of neuromuscular status in the anatomical area surrounding the involved structures. These include motor weakness and pain or discomfort out of proportion to the injury and unrelieved by pain medication. Tenseness may be noted on palpation of the area. Treatment of compartment syndrome warrants immediate relief of pressure, which sometimes requires fasciotomy.

Volkmann contracture

Volkmann contracture (ischaemic muscular atrophy) is a serious, persistent flexion contraction of the forearm and hand caused by massive infarction of muscle. Pressure from a cast, a tight bandage, or from swelling from the injury in the area of the elbow begins with arterial occlusion and then progresses to muscle anoxia and reflex vasospasms. Finally, the lack of blood supply leads to muscle necrosis and replacement with fibrous tissue.

The neuromuscular symptoms are severe pain, pallor or cyanosis, oedema, absence of pulses in the extremity, and loss of sensitivity. Unrelieved, the occlusive hypoxic process can cause contracture if ischaemia lasts as little as six hours. If not treated, the contracture leads to severe deformity and paralysis.

The immediate treatment is to remove any mechanically obstructive materials, such as tight bandages, and extend the joint to free blood vessels. If the symptoms do not improve an emergency fasciotomy, sometimes preceded by arteriography, may be the only way to restore blood supply.

EPIPHYSEAL DAMAGE

Growth of bone originates from the epiphyseal plate, and damage to this structure could result in an unequal extremity length. Surgical intervention to the epiphysis on the affected extremity, or to the epiphyseal line on the opposite extremity, is the usual treatment.

NONUNION

When inadequate reduction, poor immobilization, or a damaged or softened cast cannot maintain the bone fragments in correct alignment for repair, bone healing is impaired. The factors most likely to interfere with bone healing and cause delayed union or nonunion are: (1) separation of bone fragments at fracture site, (2) loss of haematoma, (3) interposition of tissue between bone fragments, (4) loss of bone tissue, especially from necrosis, (5) infection, (6) poor nutrition and (7) interruption of blood supply.

The haematoma, which becomes the matrix for bone deposition in the break, must be free of infection or bits of adipose or connective tissue. The constant supply of nutrients and bone-forming cells brought to the area by way of the bloodstream provides the vital ingredients for repair.

Sometimes, artificial means are employed to facilitate bone healing. Bone grafting becomes necessary when bone nonunion occurs. The donor sites are usually the tibia or the iliac crest. Bleeding of bone ends may need to be artificially stimulated, and at times holes are drilled near the bone ends in an attempt to increase circulation. Postsurgical immobilization of the recipient area is crucial to a successful graft.

MALUNION

Malunion is fracture union with increased angulation or deformity at the fracture site. It can be detected at any stage in the healing process or after complete healing. Unsatisfactory reduction is the usual reason for malunion. A cast or splint that allows fracture movement will also likely result in malunion. Periodic radiological examinations will help detect this complication and avoid its becoming a major problem over a long period.

Correction of the malunion, when healing is near completion, requires surgical intervention.

INFECTION

Osteomyelitis, infection of the bone, is often secondary to a bloodstream infection, but is a potential problem in open fractures or when bone surgery has been performed. Any bacterial organism can cause this infectious process; however, *Staphylococcus aureus* is the most frequent pathogen.

KIDNEY STONES

Although uncommon in children, renal calculi are a poten-

tial risk whenever the child has a limb that is non-weight bearing for a long time, especially if the circumstances also produce urinary stasis. Preventive measures for renal calculi are to maintain good hydration, to mobilize the child as much as possible, and to check closely the amount and characteristics of urinary output. Any urinary tract infection should be treated promptly with appropriate antimicrobials and urine acidification, because the nucleus of the calculi is often composed of bacterial debris or calcium and the buildup of stone is precipitated by alkaline urine.

PULMONARY EMBOLI

Blood, air, or fat emboli can be a hazard to the child with a fracture. As postinjury bleeding and clotting occur, a small piece of the clot can travel to vital organs, such as the lung, heart or brain, and produce a life-threatening vascular obstruction and ischaemia. Generally, the pulmonary system is the most frequent site for emboli deposition, but it may not occur until 6-8 weeks after the injury.

Fat emboli are the greatest threat to an individual with multiple fractures, particularly in fractures of the long bones such as the femur. Fat droplets from the marrow are transferred to the general circulation by means of the venous-arterial route, where they can be transported to the lung or brain. This type of emboli phenomenon occurs within the first 24 hours, generally in the second 12 hours after the injury occurs. Adolescents are the usual victims in the paediatric age groups.

Emboli in the vital organs produce the classic symptoms of shock. Petechial haemorrhages of the chest and shoulders are the outstanding signs that differentiate this condition from other kinds of shock. Deep breathing, coughing and mechanical respiratory assistance are important to maintain adequate alveolar gas exchange. An intravenous infusion is established to treat the shock and administer medications such as heparin and corticosteroids.

AMPUTATION

A child may be born with the congenital absence of a body part, have a traumatic loss of an extremity, or need a surgical amputation for a pathological condition such as osteogenic sarcoma. With today's surgical technology and the quick thinking of bystanders who save a traumatically amputated body part, some children have had fingers and arms sewn back on with variable degrees of functional use regained.

Surgical amputation or the surgical repair of a permanently severed limb focuses on constructing an adequately nourished stump. A smooth, healthy, padded stump, free of nerve endings, is important in prosthesis fitting and for subsequent ambulation.

IMPLICATIONS FOR NURSING

Stump shaping is done postoperatively with special elastic bandaging using a figure-8 bandage or a stump sock, which applies pressure in a cone-shaped fashion. This technique decreases stump oedema, controls haemorrhage, and aids in developing desired contours so that the child will bear weight on the posterior aspect of the skin flap rather than on the end of the stump. Stump elevation may be used during the first 24 hours, but after this time the extremity should not be left in this position because contractures in the proximal joint will develop and seriously hamper ambulation.

For older children and adolescents, arm exercises and bed pushups, as well as parallel bars, which are used in prosthesis-training programmes, help to build up the arm muscles necessary for walking with crutches.

Depending on the age, children or their parents will need to learn stump hygiene, including careful soap and water washing every day and checking for skin irritation, breakdown or infection. A tube of stockinette or talcum powder is used to slide the prosthesis on more easily. A careful skin check must be done every time the prosthesis is removed, and prosthesis tolerance time must be adjusted to prevent skin breakdown.

For children who have had an amputation, phantom limb sensation is an expected experience because the nerve-brain connections are still present. Gradually, these sensations fade. Preoperative discussion of this phenomenon will aid a child to understand these 'unusual feelings' and not to hide the experiences from others.

INJURIES AND HEALTH PROBLEMS RELATED TO SPORTS PARTICIPATION

Every sport has some potential for injury to the participant — whether the youngster engages in serious competition or participates for pure enjoyment. Serious injury is not limited to the athlete who competes in rough contact sports; a large number of severe or fatal injuries occur to those who are not physically prepared for the activity.

The awkward and inexperienced youngster suffers more injury than the more skilled and experienced one. More injuries occur during recreational sports participation than in organized athletic competition.

Not only does the activity itself pose a hazard of greater or lesser degree, but the environment and the sports or recreational equipment present additional risks.

PREPARATION FOR SPORTS

Physical strength, coordination, endurance and size vary considerably among youngsters who wish to compete against each other. Sports competition between young people who differ markedly in strength and agility is unfair and hazardous. Matching of candidates for sports should be made relative to physical maturity, height, weight, and physical fitness and skills, particularly in a sport involving rigorous body contact. Age is a less important consideration.

The role of health professionals in relation to sports injuries is directed towards prevention, treatment and rehabilitation.

Of these, the area of prevention is perhaps the most important. To this end, children who are actively involved in athletic programmes need: medical evaluation as a prerequisite to participation; education in sports skills with correct training and conditioning methods; omission of tactics that are dangerous beyond the ordinary risk associated with the specific sport; use of appropriate protective equipment, properly maintained and suited to the individual; and an environment with maximum provision for safety and availability of first-aid and medical services.

TYPES OF INJURY

The injuries sustained in sports or recreational activities can involve any part of the body and extend from relatively minor cuts, bruises and abrasions to totally incapacitating central nervous system injuries or death.

A variety of injuries can result when an external force is exerted with severe stress on tissue, muscle and skeletal structures. The body structures attempt to accommodate the force, but when they are unable to do so, injuries occur. Two general types of injury are recognized: (1) *acute overload*, which includes injuries such as dislocations, sprains and muscle pulls, and (2) *chronic overload (overuse syndrome)*, which includes stress fractures, tendinitis, bursitis and fasciculitis. More than 95% of sports injuries involve the soft tissues, not the bony skeleton.

Acute overload injuries occur suddenly during an activity and produce immediate symptoms. They can be caused by a blow or by overstretching, twisting or otherwise causing a sudden stress to tissues.

CONTUSIONS

Contusions are probably the most common sports injuries. A contusion is damage to the soft tissue, subcutaneous structures and muscle. The tearing of these tissues and small blood vessels, and the inflammatory response, lead to haemorrhage, oedema and associated pain when the youngster attempts to move the injured part. The escape of blood into the tissues will be observed as bruising.

Immediate treatment consists of cold application, as in the treatment of sprains described previously. Return to participation is allowed when the strength and range of motion of the affected extremity are equal to those of the opposite extremity.

Although not always directly related to sports, crush injuries occur in children when they trap or hit their fingers. A severe crush injury involves the bone, with swelling and bleeding beneath the nail (subungual) and sometimes laceration of the pulp of the distal phalanx. The subungual haematoma can be released by drilling holes at the proximal end of the nail. The time-honoured method of applying a heated paper clip or needle to melt the nail is highly effective and causes few problems. However, any procedure should be performed with aseptic technique. If the bone is fractured, any communication with the skin essentially renders it an open, or 'compound', fracture.

DISLOCATIONS

Dislocations are less common in children than in older persons, but some types are peculiar to the younger age groups. Before final closure of the epiphyses, injuries to the joints are more likely to cause epiphyseal separation than dislocation. For example, shoulder dislocation occurs most often in older adolescents, and dislocation unaccompanied by fracture is rare. Dislocation of the phalanges is the most common type seen in children, followed by elbow dislocations. Injury to the hip causes dislocation more frequently than femoral neck fracture (often experienced by persons in the older age groups).

In children younger than five years of age, the hip is usually dislocated by a fall, but trauma is minimal because of the largely cartilaginous acetabulum and general joint laxity. Children with naturally lax joints, such as children with Down's syndrome, are more prone to recurrent dislocation of the hip.

A dislocation occurs when the force of stress on the ligament is so great as to displace the normal position of the opposing bone ends or the bone end to its socket.

Simple dislocations should be reduced as soon as possible with the child under sedation and often local anaesthesia. An unreduced dislocation will be complicated by increased swelling, making reduction difficult and increasing the risk of neurovascular problems. Reduction is accomplished by simple traction and slight flexion followed by immobilization in a splint for 10-16 days or up to three weeks or more for healing of torn ligaments.

PATELLA

The patella is always dislocated laterally. This may result from injury or may be recurrent in nature. Most dislocations are reduced spontaneously by a companion, but recurrent dislocations may require surgery to secure the patella.

RADIAL HEAD

This common injury — caused by a sudden longitudinal pull — results in subluxation or partial dislocation of the load of the radius in the elbow. Firm finger pressure on the forearm returns the bone structures to normal alignment. A click is heard and normal function is restored, usually within the hour.

SPRAINS AND STRAINS

These common injuries occur particularly among athletic youngsters and cause varying degrees of tissue damage. The terms are used interchangeably by the lay population, and initial first aid treatment is identical. The terms do, however, represent different injuries, as is discussed below.

SPRAINS

A sprain occurs when trauma to a joint is so severe that a ligament is partially or completely torn or stretched by the force created as a joint is twisted or wrenched. Sprains are classified according to degree of injury (Box 33-8).

The presence of joint laxity is the most valid indicator of the severity of a sprain. There is a rapid onset with swelling, often diffuse, accompanied by immediate disability and appreciable reluctance to use the injured joint.

STRAINS

A strain is a microscopic tear to the musculotendinous unit and has features in common with sprains. The area is painful to touch and is swollen. Most strains are incurred over time, rather than suddenly, and the rapidity of the appearance provides clues regarding severity. In general, the more rapidly the strain occurs, the more severe the injury. When the strain involves the muscular portion, there is more bleeding, often palpable soon after injury and before oedema obscures the haematoma.

THERAPEUTIC MANAGEMENT

The first 6-12 hours is the most critical period for virtually all soft tissue injuries. Basic principles of managing sprains and other soft tissue injuries are summarized in the acronyms RICE or ICES:

R — rest	I — ice
I — ice	C — compression
C — compression	E — elevation
E — elevation	S — support

Soft tissue injuries should be iced immediately. This is best accomplished with crushed ice wrapped in a towel or encased in a screw-top ice bag or plastic bag (e.g., a resealable storage bag). A wet elastic wrap is applied to provide compression and to keep the ice pack in place. A single layer of the wrap is placed over the injured area to protect the skin under the ice pack, and the remainder of the bandage secures the pack in place.

◆ BOX 33-8

Classification of sprains

Grade I: Mild injury; involves overstretching or microscopic tearing but without haemorrhage or increased instability of the involved joint. Swelling may develop later.

Grade II: Moderate injury; involves partial, overt tearing of the ligament with at least some ligamentous continuity remaining; usually immediate pain and swelling with decreased function.

Grade III: Severe injury; total loss of ligamentous continuity, that is, disruption of one or more ligaments or the musculotendinous unit. Pain is immediate, but subsides because none of the pain fibres is being stretched. Swelling may be minimal because haemorrhage extravasates outside of the area into soft tissues.

Nine to 15 minutes of ice exposure produces a deep-tissue vasodilation without increased metabolism. Ice therapy should never be applied for more than 30 minutes (Dyment, 1988). However, the effects last up to seven hours.

Elevating the extremity uses gravity to facilitate venous return and reduce oedema formation in the damaged area. The point of injury should be kept several centimetres above the level of the heart for therapy to be effective.

OVERUSE SYNDROME

Bursae, tendons, muscles, ligaments, joints and bones are all subject to overuse caused by repetitive microtrauma. Often associated with young athletes, common overuse disorders include plantar fasciitis and Osgood-Schlatter disease.

STRESS FRACTURES

With intensity and duration of training many young athletes suffer stress fractures, especially after a recent increase in training regimens. They occur as a result of repeated muscle contraction and are seen most often in repetitive weight-bearing sports such as running, gymnastics and basketball. They occur less often in swimmers (upper extremity). The sites in order of frequency are the tibia (50%), metatarsals (18%), fibula (12%), femur (6%) and other (less than 1%) (Orava, 1980).

The most important clinical sign is pain over the involved bony surface. Diagnosis is established on the basis of clinical observation. Occasionally, a bone scan may be needed.

THERAPEUTIC MANAGEMENT

Development of inflammation is common to all overuse syndromes; therefore, the management is directed towards rest or alteration of activities, physiotherapy and medication. Rest is the primary therapy, usually interpreted as reduced activity and use of alternative exercise — *not* bed rest or immobilization with casting. The primary purpose is to alleviate the repetitive stress that initiated the symptoms.

HEALTH CONCERNS ASSOCIATED WITH SPORTS

Several health concerns that are related to sports activities may affect athletic performance and/or the physical well-being of the participant. These are:
- Nutrition—a well balanced diet must be accompanied by adequate hydration. Competitive sports participation should be combined with sound professional dietary advice and supervision.
- Exercise-related menstrual dysfunction—this includes delayed menarche, hypooestrogenic bone loss, and stress-related fractures.
- Drug misuse—young sports competitors may be tempted to abuse substances, such as psychomotor stimulants (e.g.,

amphetamines) or anabolic steroids, to enhance individual performance.
- Sudden death—either through injury; underlying medical conditions, such as cardiac abnormalities (e.g., hypertropic cardiomyopathy); or environmental causes, such as heat stroke or hypothermia. Adequate medical support and supervision of young sports competitors is essential.

MUSCULOSKELETAL DYSFUNCTION

The disorders affecting the skeletal structures and associated musculature are primarily congenital, traumatic, secondary to metabolic dysfunction, or idiopathic in origin. Some appear at any age, such as fractures, whereas others have a predilection for a different stage of the childhood span of growth and development.

TORTICOLLIS

Torticollis (wry neck) is a congenital or acquired condition in which the neck is flexed and turned to the affected side as a result of shortening of the sternocleidomastoid muscle. In early infancy a firm, non-tender mass may be felt in the midportion of the muscle. The mass regresses and is replaced by fibrous tissue. If the condition remains untreated, there is permanent limitation of neck movement, and the head and face become asymmetric, probably related to impaired blood supply to the depressed side of the head.

If stretching exercises are unsuccessful, surgical release of the sternocleidomastoid muscle may be needed.

PERTHES DISEASE

Perthes disease is a self-limited disorder in which there is aseptic necrosis of the femoral head. The disease affects children 3-12 years old, but most cases occur in males between 4-8 years old as an isolated event. In approximately 10-15% of cases the involvement is bilateral.

PATHOPHYSIOLOGY

The pathological events seem to take place in four stages (Box 33-10). The entire process may encompass as little as 18 months or may continue for several years. The reformed femoral head may be severely altered or may appear entirely normal.

CLINICAL MANIFESTATIONS

The onset is insidious and the history may reveal only intermittent appearance of a limp on the affected side or a symptom complex including hip soreness, ache, or stiffness that can be constant or intermittent. There may be a vague history of trauma. The diagnosis is established by radiological examination and bone scan.

THERAPEUTIC MANAGEMENT

Since deformity occurs early in the disease process, the aim of treatment is to keep the head of the femur 'contained' in the acetabulum, which serves as a mould to preserve the spherical shape of the head and to maintain a full range of motion. Activity causes microfractures of the soft, ischaemic epiphysis, which tend to induce synovitis, stiffness and adductor contracture (Staheli, 1986). The initial therapy is rest, and non-weight bearing, which helps reduce inflammation and restore motion.

Containment can be accomplished by non-weight-bearing devices, such as an abduction brace, leg casts, or a leather harness sling, that prevent weight bearing on the affected limb; by various weight-bearing appliances such as abduction-ambulation braces or casts after a period of bed rest and traction; and by surgical reconstruction and containment procedures. Surgical correction returns the child to normal activities in 3-4 months.

The disease is self-limited, but the ultimate outcome of therapy depends on early and efficient treatment and the age of onset of the disorder. The later the diagnosis is made, the more femoral damage has occurred before treatment is implemented. In most cases, the prognosis is good.

IMPLICATIONS FOR NURSING

School nurses are often the first health professionals to identify affected children and to refer them for medical evaluation. They are also persons on whom the child and family can rely to help them understand and adjust to the therapeutic measures. Since most care of these children is conducted on an outpatient basis, the major emphasis of nursing care is teaching the family about the care and management of the corrective appliance selected for therapy. The family needs to learn the purpose, function, application and care of the corrective device and the importance of compliance in order to achieve the desired outcome.

◆ BOX 33-9

Stages of Perthes disease

Stage I: Aseptic necrosis or infarction of the femoral capital epiphysis with degenerative changes producing flattening of the upper surface of the femoral head — the *avascular stage.*
Stage II: Capital bone absorption and revascularization with fragmentation (vascular resorption of the epiphysis) that gives a mottled appearance on radiographs — the *fragmentation, or revascularization, stage.*
Stage III: New bone formation, which is represented on radiographs as calcification and ossification or increased density in the areas of radiolucency; this filling-in process appears to take place from the periphery of the head centrally — the *reparative stage.*
Stage IV: Gradual reformation of the head of the femur without radiolucency and, it is hoped, to a spherical form — the *regenerative stage.*

Suitable activities including swimming must be devised to meet the needs of the child in the process of developing a sense of initiative or industry. Activities that meet the creative urges are well received. This is also an opportune time to encourage the child to begin a hobby such as collections, model building or crafts.

SLIPPED UPPER FEMORAL EPIPHYSIS

Slipped upper femoral epiphysis, or *coxa vara,* refers to the spontaneous displacement of the proximal femoral epiphysis in a posterior and inferior direction. It develops most frequently shortly before or during accelerated growth and the onset of puberty, and is most frequently observed in obese children. Bilateral involvement has been reported variously as 16-40%.

CLINICAL MANIFESTATIONS

The following different varieties of clinical behaviour have been observed: (1) an episode of trauma in which the epiphysis is acutely displaced in a previously functional joint; (2) gradual displacement without definite injury with progressively increased hip disability; (3) intermittent bouts of displacement alternating with periods of well-being with gradual appearance of symptoms associated with ambulation (e.g., external rotation); and (4) a combined gradual and traumatic displacement, in which there is gradual slippage with further displacement caused by injury.

Slipped femoral epiphysis is suspected when an adolescent or preadolescent youngster, especially one who is obese or tall and lanky, begins to limp and complains of pain in the hip continuously or intermittently. The pain is frequently referred to the groin, anteromedial aspect of the thigh, or the knee. Physical examination reveals early restriction of internal rotation on adduction and external rotation deformity, with loss of abduction and internal rotation as the severity increases. The diagnosis is confirmed by radiological examination.

THERAPEUTIC MANAGEMENT

The treatment varies with the degree of displacement, but involves surgical stabilization and correction of deformity. In mild cases, simple pin fixation is sufficient. More extensive displacement requires skeletal traction followed by pin fixation or osteotomy. The prognosis depends on the degree of deformity and the occurrence of complications, such as avascular necrosis and cartilaginous necrosis. As in other disorders, early diagnosis and implementation of therapy increase the likelihood of a satisfactory cure.

IMPLICATIONS FOR NURSING

Nursing care is the same as that for a child in a cast or a child in traction, discussed previously in this chapter.

KYPHOSIS AND LORDOSIS

The spine, consisting of numerous segments, can acquire deformation curves of three types: kyphosis, lordosis and scoliosis (Fig. 33-10).

KYPHOSIS

Kyphosis is an abnormally increased convex angulation in the curvature of the thoracic spine (Fig. 33-10, *B*). It can occur secondary to disease processes such as tuberculosis, chronic arthritis, osteodystrophy, or to compression fractures of the thoracic spine. The most common form of kyphosis is 'postural'. Children, especially during the time when skeletal growth outpaces growth of muscle, are prone to exaggeration of a tendency toward kyphosis. They assume bizarre sitting and standing positions. This is particularly common in self-conscious adolescent girls who assume a round-shouldered slouching posture in the attempt to hide their developing breasts and increasing height.

Postural kyphosis is almost always accompanied by a compensatory postural lordosis, an abnormally exaggerated concave lumbar curvature. Treatment consists of postural exercises to strengthen shoulder and abdominal muscles, and bracing for more marked deformity. Unfortunately, treatment is difficult because of the nature of the adolescent personality. The best approach is to emphasize the cosmetic value of corrective therapy and to place the responsibility on the adolescent for carrying out an exercise programme at home with regular visits to and assessments by a therapist.

Most adolescents respond well to selected sports as a supplement to regular exercise. Boys prefer weight lifting (preferably performed from a prone or supine position on a bench) and track sports. Girls respond well to dancing classes (ballet or modern dancing). Swimming is excellent and has the added advantages of exercising all muscles, eliminating gravity, and teaching breath control.

LORDOSIS

Lordosis is an accentuation of the lumbar curvature beyond physiological limits (Fig. 33-11, *C*). It may be a secondary complication of a disease process, the result of trauma, or idiopathic. Lordosis is a normal observation in toddlers and, in

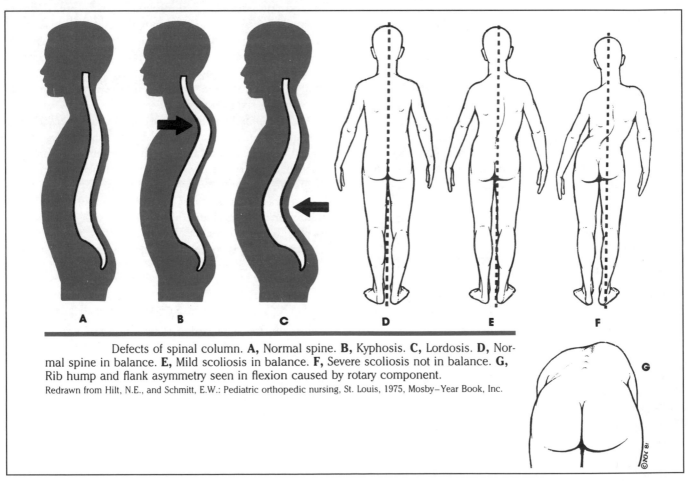

Defects of spinal column. **A,** Normal spine. **B,** Kyphosis. **C,** Lordosis. **D,** Normal spine in balance. **E,** Mild scoliosis in balance. **F,** Severe scoliosis not in balance. **G,** Rib hump and flank asymmetry seen in flexion caused by rotary component.
Redrawn from Hilt, N.E., and Schmitt, E.W.: Pediatric orthopedic nursing, St. Louis, 1975, Mosby–Year Book, Inc.

Fig. 33-10 Defects of spinal column. **A,** Normal spine. **B,** Kyphosis. **C,** Lordosis. **D,** Normal spine in balance. **E,** Mild scoliosis in balance. **F,** Severe scoliosis not in balance. **G,** Rib hump and flank asymmetry seen in flexion caused by rotary component. (Redrawn from Hilt NE, Schmitt EW: *Pediatric orthopedic nursing*, St Louis, 1975, Mosby–Year Book)

older children, is often seen in association with flexion contractures of the hip, obesity, congenital dislocated hip, slipped femoral capital epiphysis, and acondroplastic dwarfism. During the pubertal growth spurt, lordosis of varying degrees is observed in teenagers, especially girls. In obese children the weight of the abdominal fat alters the centre of gravity, causing a compensatory lordosis. Unlike kyphosis, severe lordosis is usually accompanied by pain.

Treatment involves management of the predisposing cause when possible, such as weight loss and correction of deformities. Postural exercises and/or support garments are helpful in relieving symptoms in some cases; however, these do not usually effect a permanent cure.

SCOLIOSIS

Scoliosis, the most common spinal deformity, is a lateral curvature of the spine usually associated with a rotary deformity (produced by rotation of affected vertebrae) that eventually causes cosmetic and physiological alterations in the spine, chest and pelvis. It can appear at any age, but is more frequent in adolescent girls during their growth spurt.

AETIOLOGY

Structural scoliosis is characterized by changes in the spine and its supporting structures that cause loss of flexibility and non-correctable deformity. The spine fails to straighten on side bending, and a truly structural deformity displays a rotational deformity not observed in functional curvatures. Structural scoliosis may be congenital or may be a secondary defect associated with other disorders, especially neuromuscular disease or paralysis. In 70% of cases, it is 'idiopathic' without apparent cause.

CLINICAL MANIFESTATIONS

Idiopathic scoliosis is seldom apparent before ten years of age and is most noticeable at the beginning of the preadolescent growth spurt. Parents will often bring a child for evaluation because of 'ill-fitting' clothes such as uneven pant lengths or uneven skirt hems. There is rarely discomfort and there are few outward signs until the deformity is well established. Early detection and treatment are essential to successful management.

PROCESS OF DIAGNOSIS

Diagnosis is made by observation and radiological examination. The undressed child viewed from the posterior side will often reveal primary curvature and a compensatory curvature that places the head in alignment with the gluteal fold (Fig. 33-11, *E*). In uncompensated scoliosis the head and hips are not in alignment (Fig. 33-11, *F*). In advanced cases with rotary deformity, rib hump and flank asymmetry are observed when the child bends from the waist unsupported with the arms (Fig.

33-11, *G*). A clinical deformity can be documented by placing a scoliometer, a modified inclinometer, across the back at the point of maximum deformity while the child is in the forward-bent position (Bunnell, 1984). Radiographs taken in the standing position establish the degree of spinal curvature.

THERAPEUTIC MANAGEMENT: NONOPERATIVE

A thorough examination, history and assessment of the child are carried out in order to evaluate the status of the deformity, factors contributing to the defect, and factors that may influence the outcome of therapy. Treatment is best undertaken in a centre in which a team is available that specializes in management of scoliosis. Current management involves straightening and realignment of the vertebrae by either external (bracing) or internal (surgical) fixation techniques. Although there is some question regarding whether or not bracing is effective in preventing progression of curvatures (Miller, Nachemson, and Schultz, 1984), it still remains the primary mode of therapy for minor curvatures. Bracing is not curative, but may slow the progression of the deformity until the spine has reached the more adult size.

THERAPEUTIC MANAGEMENT: OPERATIVE

Surgical intervention may be required for correction. The indications for surgery are:

- **Physiological** — pulmonary function is diminished considerably, approximately 50%.
- **Functional** — children with neurological disabilities have difficulty sitting or walking because of imbalance.
- **Cosmetic** — some children whose curvature is amenable to bracing are unable to use that therapy because of a self-image problem.
- **Pain** — although rare in children, some older youngsters may have chronic discomfort from sitting on one buttock continually; pressure sores become a problem.

With few exceptions, the techniques consist of spinal realignment and straightening by way of external or internal fixation and instrumentation combined with bony fusion (arthrodesis) of the realigned spine. The degree of curvature and the cause determine the decision for surgery. Bracing and exercise have been universally disappointing in curves greater than 40 degrees, and paralytic and congenital curves, which will eventually progress, are best treated with early surgical stabilization. Age of the child and location of the curvature influence the decision for surgery, and any curve that does not respond to more conservative measures requires surgical correction.

Harrington instrumentation

The most frequently performed operative techniques for correction of the deformity involve the implantation of a rigid metal appliance. The *Harrington distraction* system consists of a metal rod applied to the *concave* side of the scoliotic curve, with cannulated hooks attached to the vertebra at each end of the curve. The spine is straightened by progressive distraction between the hooks in a manner similar to the mechanism of a motor car jack. The *Harrington compression* system employs compression to the *convex* curve of the spine posteriorly by means of hooks attached to either end of the curve and a semi-rigid, threaded rod. Progressive compression is applied to the convexity by advancing small nuts along the threaded rod from opposite directions, shortening the distance between the hooks. The two techniques are frequently used in combination. Chips and strips of bone (from ileum or tibia) are placed across prepared vertebrae to provide fusion to the involved portion of the vertebral column.

Following Harrington instrumentation, the child is immobilized on a Stryker frame or is 'log-rolled' on an ordinary hospital bed. The child must remain absolutely flat until the brace is applied. When the child has sufficiently recovered from the surgery, usually after 8-12 days, an immobilizing plaster jacket is applied from occiput to pelvis, which is changed at three months and maintained for a total of six months. Further immobilization with a removable cast may be required for sites with delayed healing. Regular follow-up management is continued at three- to six-month intervals for 3-5 years.

Luque segmental instrumentation

The Luque segmental spinal instrumentation provides segmental stability by the use of wires and flexible L-shaped rods. By way of a posterior approach, wires are threaded beneath the laminae of each vertebra and tightened around the rods resting along the transverse processes so that the spinal column is stabilized by transverse traction on each vertebra. The spine is fused with a bone graft taken from the iliac crest. The advantages to this procedure are that the patient can walk within a few days and that no postoperative immobilization is required. The disadvantage is a possibility of spinal nerve damage.

Dwyer instrumentation

The Dwyer instrumentation and fusion technique involves transfixing cannulated screws to each vertebra in the curvature, then threading a titanium cable through the cannulae of the screw heads. When satisfactory correction is achieved, the screw heads are crimped to the cable, and bone chips (obtained from the iliac bone) are placed between adjacent vertebral bodies to facilitate fusion. Tension is then applied to the cable to maintain alignment. This procedure requires an anterior approach, but because the cable does not provide rigid fixation, a supplemental fusion via a posterior approach is usually needed. The Dwyer procedure is performed less frequently in children with idiopathic scoliosis, but is well suited to treatment of spina bifida. Children post Dwyer instrumentation normally require initial management in the ICU.

Other

Other surgical procedures have been tried and proved successful in selected cases. Many of the current procedures combine features of the methods previously described. Various modifications of the Harrington procedure are used. One that is used infrequently combines the Harrington and Dwyer (Zielke) procedures. A newer approach uses the distraction force of the Harrington rods plus the strength of Luque segmentation (Cotrel-Dubousset procedure).

IMPLICATIONS FOR NURSING

Treatment for scoliosis extends over a significant portion of the affected child's period of growth. In adolescents, this period is the one in which their identity, physical and psychological, is formed. For some youngsters, much of this time is spent in the hospital setting immobilized in complex, unattractive appliances. For those treated on an outpatient basis, it means a modified lifestyle and being 'different' from their peers, even though they are usually able to engage in many activities enjoyed by other youngsters.

Assessment

One of the major functions of nurses is to learn to detect the presence of scoliosis. For example, in structural scoliosis one shoulder will remain higher than the other when the child bends forward and is observed from behind.

When the child first faces the prospect of a prolonged period in a brace, cast or other device, the therapy programme and the nature of the device must be explained thoroughly to the child and parents so that they will have an understanding of the anticipated results, how the appliance corrects the defect, the freedoms and constraints imposed by the device, and what they can do to help achieve the desired goal. The management involves the skills and services of a team of specialists, including the orthopaedist, physiotherapist, anaesthetist, orthotist (a specialist in fitting orthopaedic braces), nurse, social worker and sometimes a pulmonary specialist.

It is difficult for a child to be restricted at any phase of development, but the teenager needs continual positive reinforcement, encouragement, and as much independence as can be safely assumed during this time. Although adolescents cope well for the first year or two after casting, problems may arise as the time extends. Nurses need to be aware of this and must be prepared to provide support and encouragement if problems arise (Davis and Lewis, 1984). Guidance and assistance regarding anticipated problems, such as selection of clothing and participation in social activities, are appreciated by adolescents. Socialization with peers should be encouraged and every effort expended to help the adolescent feel attractive and worthwhile.

Preoperative care

The child hospitalized for surgical management requires preparation for the procedures involved, which are puzzling and often frightening to very young patients. They need to know what is going to happen, and should be given a full explanation of why the procedure is necessary and the potential outcome of the surgery.

Postoperative care

Postoperatively, patients may be monitored in an intensive care unit. They may be placed on an egg-crate mattress to prevent pressure areas, and the child with Harrington instrumentation is often placed on a Stryker frame, which facilitates care and lessens the possibility of damage to the fusion and indwelling instruments from twisting the spine, and the possibility of 'popping out' the rods. Nurses who work with these appliances should become familiar with their mechanism before assuming responsibility for patient care. The child who is not on a Stryker frame must be carefully log rolled when turned. It is essential that the child remains flat at all times.

In addition to the usual postoperative assessments — of wound, circulation, and vital signs — the neurological status of the patient requires special attention, especially that of the extremities. Prompt recognition of any neurological impairment is imperative, because delayed paralysis may develop that requires removal of the instrumentation. The patient is encouraged to exercise by contracting and relaxing the thigh and calf muscles periodically.

There is usually some degree of paralytic ileus following the procedure; therefore, nursing includes care of the nasogastric intubation and assessment for returning bowel function. Because of the extensive blood loss during the surgical procedure and renal hypoperfusion, observation of urinary output is especially important, and the child normally has an indwelling urinary catheter.

The child is at risk of feeling considerable pain for the first few days following surgery, and requires frequent administration of pain medication (see Pain Management, Chapter 5). Because of the anterior approach, patients with Dwyer instrumentation also require thoracotomy care in addition to the care related to the fusion and realignment procedures.

Children with a Luque procedure are kept flat for 12 hours before logrolling is begun. The head of the bed can be elevated on the second day and range of motion exercises begun. Activity is begun by instructing the patient to roll from a side-lying position to a sitting position on the surgeon's instructions. Next, walking slowly with the aid of a safety belt and walker is allowed, and finally unassisted ambulation, which is usually achieved by the sixth day.

All patients are started on physiotherapy as soon as they are able, beginning with a range of motion exercises. Self-care in activities of daily living, such as washing and eating, is always encouraged. Throughout the hospitalization, diversionary activities and contact with family and friends are an important part of nursing care and planning.

The family is encouraged to become involved with the patient's care to facilitate the transition from hospital to home management. Family members learn to apply and care for the brace or learn cast care, with special attention to jagged edges on the cast, padding of the appliance, and daily skin checks for reddened areas, especially in areas such as under the arms or over the hips. They may need assistance in modifying the environment for limited ambulation and acquiring needed home care items such as an egg-crate mattress, straight-backed chair and a raised toilet seat. The child and family need to learn efficient ways to move and to carry out various activities of daily living. The diet may require modification. Overeating and constipation can be problems related to limited activity.

An organization which provides education and services to both families and professionals is the Scoliosis Association (UK).

The effectiveness of nursing interventions is determined by continual reassessment and evaluation of care based on the following observational guidelines and expected outcomes:

1. Observe and interview the child relative to problems and solutions experienced.
2. Observe the child for evidence of proper usage of the method of management and signs of complications (e.g., skin irritation).
3. Observe and interview the child and family regarding their feelings and concerns.

ORTHOPAEDIC INFECTIONS

Infections of bones and joints are not uncommon and often pose a problem with diagnosis because of their similarity of symptoms. The most frequently observed infection is osteomyelitis, and in populations where tuberculosis is endemic, this disease is encountered increasingly in nursing practice.

OSTEOMYELITIS

Osteomyelitis, an infectious process of bone, can occur at any age but occurs most frequently between ages 5-14 years. It is twice as common in boys as in girls.

AETIOLOGY

Any organism can cause osteomyelitis, and there is some relationship between the age of the child and the type of organism responsible. In older children, staphylococci are the most common organisms, approximately 80% of which are *Staphylococcus aureus;* in younger children other organisms predominate, especially *Haemophilus influenzae.* One report describes *Pseudomonas aeruginosa* osteomyelitis acquired from puncture wounds. The organism was present in the soles of the sneakers the children were wearing (Fisher, Goldsmith, and Gilligan, 1985). In children with sickle cell anaemia, *Salmonella* organisms are frequently responsible for osteomyelitis.

Osteomyelitis can be acquired from *exogenous* or *haematogenous* sources. Exogenous osteomyelitis is acquired by invasion of the bone by direct extension from the outside as a result of a penetrating wound, open fracture, contamination during surgery, or secondary extension from an overlying abscess or burn.

Haematogenous spread of organisms from a pre-existing focus is the most common source of infection. Common sources of foci include furuncles, skin abrasions, impetigo, upper respiratory tract infection, acute otitis media, tonsillitis, abscessed teeth, pyelonephritis or infected burns. Other factors that predispose to development of osteomyelitis are poor physical condition, poor nutrition, and surroundings that are not hygienic.

PATHOPHYSIOLOGY

Infective emboli from the focus of infection travel to the small end arteries in the bone metaphysis, where they set up an infectious process. The infection does not spread to the epiphysis, since it has a blood supply separate from the metaphysis. The infectious process leads to local bone destruction and abscess formation. The abscess, with its collected necrotic debris, exerts pressure within the rigid, unyielding bone and ruptures into the subperiosteal space, where the pressure lifts and strips the periosteum. The infection spreads beneath the periosteum, causing thrombosis of vessels and adding further to the bony necrosis.

In infants and very young children, the elevated periosteum attempts to wall off the infection by forming new bone — *involucrum*. Underneath, the cortex, deprived of blood supply, dies, and the necrotic bone that cannot be absorbed continues to produce more intraosseous tension and necrosis.

CLINICAL MANIFESTATIONS

Signs and symptoms of *acute* haematogenous osteomyelitis begin abruptly and build up to a maximum intensity during the first few days of the disease, usually less than one week. There is frequently a history of trauma to the affected bone.

Children with acute osteomyelitis can appear very ill. They may be irritable and restless with elevated temperature, rapid pulse and dehydration. There is usually localized tenderness, increased warmth and diffuse swelling over the involved bone. The extremity is painful, especially on movement. The child holds it in semiflexion, and the surrounding muscles are tense and resist passive movement. Most cases involve the femur or tibia and, to a lesser extent, the humerus and hip. In infants, the diagnosis is more difficult because of the lack of systemic symptoms. The disorder may involve multiple bones or joints because of the difficulty in confining an infectious process in children in this age group.

In *subacute* haematogenous osteomyelitis, symptoms have been present for a longer period and the child sometimes has been treated with antibiotics, often for another infection, which modify the clinical symptoms. In some instances, the infection may produce a walled-off abscess rather than a spreading infection.

PROCESS OF DIAGNOSIS

In acute osteomyelitis, there is marked leukocytosis and an elevated erythrocyte sedimentation rate. Blood culture is usually positive during the early stage, but radiological findings are often negative or show only soft tissue swelling for 10-14 days. After this time, the radiological findings reveal new bone formation. Computed tomography may reveal bone changes at an early stage, and scintigraphy (radioisotope scanning) reveals a greater uptake of radionucleotides in osteomyelitic bone than in normal bone.

Similar symptoms are observed in rheumatic fever, rheumatoid arthritis, leukaemia and other malignant lesions, cellulitis, erysipelas and scurvy. Sometimes, the osteomyelitis may be unrecognized if it occurs as a complication of a severe toxic and debilitating illness.

THERAPEUTIC MANAGEMENT

As soon as blood cultures have been drawn, prompt and vigorous intravenous antibiotic therapy is initiated. The choice is influenced by age, and the dosage determined is sufficient to ensure high blood and tissue levels. Since most cases of osteomyelitis are caused by staphylococci, large doses of benzyl penicillin are administered and supplemented by methicillin or flucloxacillin. In children younger than three years of age, the infectious agents are more likely to be penicillin-resistant staphylococci or gram-negative organisms; therefore, the agents of choice are usually methicillin, fusidic acid, or clindamycin in conjunction with ampicillin. Neonates in whom coliform organisms are likely to be involved are given kanamycin or gentamicin in addition to ampicillin. In selected cases, some antibiotics may be administered orally following a short, intensive intravenous course.

When the infective agent is identified, the appropriate antibiotic is usually continued for at least 3-4 weeks, but the length of therapy is determined by the duration of symptoms, the initial response to treatment, and the sensitivity of the organism in the specific case. Because of prolonged high-dose therapy, it is important to monitor haematological, renal, hepatic and other organ systems that might be adversely affected by the drugs (e.g., ototoxic).

Antibiotic therapy is accompanied by local treatment. The child is placed on complete bed rest, and immobilization of the affected extremity, which may require a splint or bivalved cast, is continued throughout therapy to limit the spread of infection and, when it is a complication of a fracture, to maintain alignment of bone fragments. Weight bearing on the nonfractured leg is prohibited to avoid the possibility of pathological fracture.

Opinions differ regarding surgical intervention, but many advocate sequestrectomy and surgical drainage to decompress the metaphyseal space before pus erupts and spreads to the subperiosteal space to form abscesses that strip the periosteum from bone or form draining sinuses. When these complications occur, a chronic infection usually persists. When surgical drainage is carried out, polyethylene tubes are placed in the wound. One tube instils an antibiotic solution directly into the infected area by gravity; the other, connected to a suction apparatus, provides drainage.

IMPLICATIONS FOR NURSING

During the acute phase of illness, any movement of the affected limb will cause discomfort to the child; therefore, the child is positioned comfortably with the affected limb supported. Moving and turning are carried out carefully and gently to minimize discomfort. The child may require pain medication or sedation. Vital signs are taken and recorded frequently, and measures are implemented to reduce a significant temperature elevation.

Antibiotic therapy requires careful observation and monitoring of the intravenous equipment and site. Since more than one antibiotic is usually administered, the compatibility of the drugs must be determined and care taken to avoid mixing noncompatible drugs.

Children with an open wound need scrupulous wound and skin precautions to minimize infection both to themselves and to other patients. Antibiotic solution administered directly into the wound is most efficiently accomplished with a regular intravenous infusion set-up that is prepared and regulated as any intravenous infusion. The drainage tubes are connected to wall suction for continuous removal. Intake and output are measured and recorded, and the character of the wound drainage is noted. The amount and character of drainage on the wound dressing are also noted.

Casts are sometimes employed for immobilization and, if so, routine cast care is carried out. The extremity is examined for sensation, circulation and pain, and the area over the inflammation is usually left open for observation. The affected area, casted or uncasted, is assessed for colour, swelling, heat, movement and tenderness.

The child usually has a poor appetite and may be subject to vomiting. Nourishment in the form of high-calorie liquids such as fruit juices and jellies should be encouraged until the child begins to feel better. Adequate nutrition enhances and expediates healing.

When the acute stage subsides, children begin to feel better, the appetite improves, and they become interested in their surroundings and relationships. They wish to move about in bed and are allowed to do so. However, weight bearing on the affected limb is not permitted until healing is well under way in order to avoid pathological fractures. Diversional and constructive activities become important nursing interventions.

As the infection subsides, physiotherapy is instituted to ensure restoration of optimum function. The child is usually discharged with oral antibiotics, and progress is followed closely for some time.

SEPTIC (SUPPURATIVE, PYOGENIC, PURULENT) ARTHRITIS

Infection of the joints, like infection of bone, usually develops through haematogenous dissemination from another focus; occasionally, it may result from direct extension of a soft tissue infection. Joint infections occur predominantly in males, especially adolescents. In infancy, however, the incidence in boys and girls is more nearly equal. Any joint may be involved, but the hip, knee, shoulder and other large joints are more commonly affected. Usually, only one joint is involved.

The signs and symptoms of suppurative arthritis, unlike osteomyelitis, are usually characteristic. The presence of a warm and tender joint, painful on even gentle pressure, is sufficient to differentiate it from osteomyelitis, in which gentle passive motion is tolerated. When superficial joints are involved, they are exquisitely painful and swollen; deep-seated joints show little superficial evidence. In most instances, there is history of a traumatic injury to the affected joint.

THERAPEUTIC MANAGEMENT

Treatment consists of open surgical drainage of hip and shoulder joint disease, and repeated needle aspirations of the joint space in other joints. The goals are: (1) to cleanse the joint to avoid destruction of articular cartilage, (2) to decompress the joint to avoid interference with the blood supply to the epiphysis, (3) to eradicate the infection with adequate antibiotic therapy, and (4) to prevent secondary bone infection and haematogenous spread. Therapy is similar to that for osteomyelitis: intravenous antibiotic therapy, relief of pain, immobilization of the joint, and prohibition of weight bearing until healing is complete. Nursing care is the same as that for osteomyelitis.

TUBERCULOSIS

Tubercular infection of the bones is acquired by haematogenous dissemination from a primary tubercular focus. The most common sites in infants and small children are the carpals and phalanges and corresponding bones of the feet. One or several bones may be involved, with spindle-shaped swelling and tenderness as soft tissues are affected. The process, relatively painless, persists with intermittent symptoms for several months and may leave a permanent deformity. Affected areas are immobilized with a splint or cast, and appropriate drug therapy instigated.

SKELETAL AND ARTICULAR DYSFUNCTION

There are a variety of disorders involving bones. Fractures of bones are relatively common in childhood. Rickets is less common, but is still a preventable disease in most instances. Uncommon disorders of bone and connective tissue, such as arachnodactyly (Marfan syndrome) and achondroplasia, do not cause immobilization. Bone tumours (see Chapter 30) are dreaded diseases, and bone infections are responsible for significant morbidity. There are other rare disorders, but only one — osteogenesis imperfecta — is elaborated further.

OSTEOGENESIS IMPERFECTA (BRITTLE BONE DISEASE)

Osteogenesis imperfecta (OI) is a group of heterogenous inherited disorders of connective tissue characterized by connective tissue and bone defects, including one or more of the following: varying degrees of bone fragility leading to fractures, blue sclerae, progressive bone deformities, presenile hearing loss, and dentinogenesis imperfecta, hypoplastic teeth with an opalescent blue or brown discolouration. The inheritance pattern is autosomal dominant in the majority of cases, although the most severe form demonstrates autosomal-recessive inheritance.

THERAPEUTIC MANAGEMENT

The treatment of OI is primarily supportive. The goals of a rehabilitation approach to management are directed to preventing: (1) positional contractures and deformities, (2) muscle weakness and osteoporosis, and (3) malalignment of lower extremity joints prohibiting weight bearing.

Surgery is sometimes used to help treat the manifestations of the disease. Surgical techniques are used to correct deformities that interfere with bracing, standing or walking. For the child with recurrent fractures, inserting an intermedullary rod provides stability to bones. Unfortunately, the rods must be replaced as the child grows; otherwise, fractures may occur through the unprotected portion of the bone.

IMPLICATIONS FOR NURSING

Infants and children with this disorder require careful handling to prevent fractures. They must be supported when they are turned, positioned, moved and fondled. Even changing a nappy may cause a fracture in severely affected infants. These children should never be held by the ankles during a nappy change, but should be gently lifted by the buttocks.

One of the most distressing features of OI is its frequent confusion with child abuse. Numerous fractures and easy bruising characteristic of OI are signs usually observed in child abuse; parents must often deal with accusations of abuse until a correct diagnosis is made. This is very traumatic for parents; therefore, they need considerable nonjudgemental support during this time.

Both parents and the affected child need education regarding the child's limitations, as well as guidelines in planning suitable activities that promote optimum development and protect the child from harm. Realistic occupational planning and genetic counselling are part of the long-term goals of care. Educational materials and information can be obtained from the Brittle Bone Society. This organization also has a network that can put a family in contact with other families with a similar problem.

JUVENILE CHRONIC ARTHRITIS

Clinically and pathologically, juvenile chronic arthritis (JCA) is an inflammatory disease with unknown inciting agents and a slight tendency to occur in families. Both infectious and autoimmune theories have been presented, but there is no convincing evidence to establish either one as an aetiological agent. There are two peak ages of onset: between 2-5 and between 9-12 years of age. Females are affected by JCA somewhat more frequently than males. In many instances, the disease remains undiagnosed for years.

JCA is, in many ways, similar to the adult disease, but there are many features that are distinct. A distinguishing feature is its tendency to occur in the prepubertal child. Characteristics of JCA include negative results in the latex fixation test in 90% of cases; classic symptoms of spiking fever, skin rash, or pericarditis in 5-10% of cases; tendency to be very mild in 70% of cases, with few joints involved; development of iridocyclitis as a complication in 8-20% of milder forms; and 'burning itself out' over 2-3 years in milder forms and over 8-10 years in most other forms.

CLINICAL MANIFESTATIONS

Whether a single joint or multiple joints are involved, stiffness, swelling and loss of motion develop in the affected joints. They are swollen and warm to the touch but seldom red. The swelling results from oedema, joint effusion and synovial thickening. The affected joints may be tender and painful to the touch, or may be relatively painless. The limited motion early in the disease is the result of muscle spasm and joint inflammation; later it is caused by ankylosis or soft tissue contracture. Morning stiffness or 'gelling' of the joint(s) is characteristic and present on arising in the morning or after inactivity. Infections, injuries, or surgical procedures often precipitate a flare-up of the arthritis; therefore, prompt recognition and treatment of infections are necessary.

Growth may be retarded during periods of active disease, usually with growth spurts during remissions. In severe, long-standing cases, growth is significantly retarded. Corticosteroid therapy is also a contributing factor. There may be growth disturbances, either overgrowth or undergrowth, adjacent to the inflamed joints — for example, altered leg length after knee involvement, and micrognathia (receding chin) from temporomandibular arthritis.

JCA is a variable disease and is now recognized to pursue three major disease courses: *systemic onset*, *monoarticular* or *pauciarticular* (involving few joints, usually less than five), and *polyarticular* (simultaneous involvement of four or more joints).

PROCESS OF DIAGNOSIS

The diagnosis of JCA is one of exclusion, that is, differentiation from a variety of disorders with similar manifestations at the onset of the disease. Radiological findings are variable, but the earliest manifestations are widening joint spaces followed by gradual evidence of fusion and articular destruction. There may be evidence of soft tissue swelling, osteoporosis and periostitis around affected joints.

There are no specific diagnostic tests for JCA. The erythrocyte sedimentation rate may or may not be elevated, depending on the degree of inflammation present. Leukocytosis is generally present in the early stages of classic systemic disease. The latex fixation test, the most common test used to detect the presence of rheumatoid factor in adults, is negative in 90% of juvenile cases. Rheumatoid factors are found in some children, usually those with disease of later onset.

Antinuclear antibodies are found in three-quarters of rheumatoid factor-positive and in one-quarter of rheumatoid factor-negative children and in pauciarticular type I diseases, but not in children with systemic onset or pauciarticular type II disease. There is a strong relationship between the presence of antinuclear antibodies and chronic iridocyclitis, but no relationship to the severity of the disease.

THERAPEUTIC MANAGEMENT

There is no specific cure for JCA. The major goals of therapy are to: (1) preserve joint function, (2) prevent physical deformities, and (3) relieve symptoms without iatrogenic harm. This involves both initial and long-term planning, parent and patient education and counselling, physiotherapy and occupational therapy, good health and nutritional education and management, specific drug therapy, orthopaedic consultation, and periodic eye examination (Brewer and Arroyo, 1986).

Whenever possible, children are treated at home under the supervision of the health team, and intermittent treatment by qualified professionals is administered. Hospitalization may be needed during severe exacerbations or when intercurrent illness warrants. Iridocyclitis, which is unique to JCA, can occur and requires the attention of an ophthalmologist.

Drugs
A variety of antirheumatic drugs is available, and most are effective in suppressing the inflammatory process and relieving pain. The drugs may be given alone or in combination.

NSAIDs
The primary group of drugs prescribed for JCA are the nonsteroidal anti-inflammatory drugs (NSAIDs). These include aspirin, tolmetin sodium, ibuprofen, naproxen, declofenac sodium, and mefenamic acid. All these drugs act in a similar manner, and none is superior to the others in producing the desired effects — analgesic, antipyretic, and anti-inflammatory. Reduction in fever takes place in hours, relief of pain occurs in a matter of hours or days (more often in weeks, however), but the anti-inflammatory effect (reductions in swelling, pain on motion, tenderness, and limitation of motion of involved joints) does not occur for 30-37 days (Brewer and Arroyo, 1986). Consequently, these drugs should not be discontinued without an adequate trial period. Sometimes, several drugs are tried before one or two are found that are effective and safe for any given child.

Since there is a narrow margin between effective and toxic doses, the levels are monitored regularly until the dosage is sufficient to maintain the optimum level and a satisfactory clinical response. The total daily dose is divided into four doses to be administered with each meal and at bedtime. Some find better compliance when the drug is given only twice daily.

SAARDs
The second group of drugs used to treat JCA are the slower-acting antirheumatic drugs (SAARDs). These include gold,

D-penicillamine, and hydroxychloroquine. SAARDs may be added to the regimen when one or two NSAIDs have been ineffective. Injectable gold is the initial SAARD used. The weekly injections can be a problem with young children, but cooperation is important. Auranofin is one oral gold preparation available in the UK. Hydroxychloroquine and chloroquine have a similar action to gold or penicillamine, and are better tolerated (British National Formulary, 1994).

Other drugs
Cytotoxic drugs such as cyclophosphamide, azathioprine, chlorambucil, and methotrexate are reserved for patients with severe debilitating disease and who have responded poorly to NSAIDs and SAARDs.

Corticosteroids are the most potent anti-inflammatory agents available. However, they do not cure the disease or prevent joint damage, and their chronic side effects are undesirable. They are administered in the lowest effective dose, given on alternate days rather than daily, and used for the shortest period possible. Indications for daily corticosteroid (prednisone) therapy are life-threatening disease (e.g., pericarditis), incapacitating systemic disease unresponsive to other anti-inflammatory therapy, and iridocyclitis.

Physical management
Programmes of physical management are individualized for each child and designed to reach the ultimate goal—preserving function and/or preventing deformity. Physiotherapy is directed towards specific joints, focusing on strengthening muscles, mobilizing restricted joint motion, and preventing or correcting deformities; occupational therapy assumes responsibility for generalized mobility and performance of activities of daily living.

Surgery
The benefits of synovectomy, an established preventive and therapeutic procedure in adults, are questionable in the child with rheumatoid arthritis. It is used primarily in pauciarticular disease. Joint replacement is proving successful in older children, but is reserved until the child is fully grown. The cooperation of the child is imperative. Joint fusion is sometimes used.

IMPLICATIONS FOR NURSING

Assessment
Nursing children with JCA involves assessment of their general health, the status of involved joints, and children's emotional response to all ramifications of the disease: pain, physical restrictions, therapies and self-concept.

The effects of the disease are manifest in every aspect of a the child's life, including participation in physical activities, social experiences and personality development. Much of the children's adjustment to the stresses and demands of the disease, and the level of functioning they achieve, are directly related to the reaction and support they receive from their family and the health professionals concerned.

Relieve pain

The pain of JCA is related to several aspects of the disease — severity, functional status, individual pain threshold, family variables and psychological adjustment. Although complete pain relief would be highly desirable, it is probably unrealistic. The aim is to provide as much relief as possible with anti-inflammatory medication and other therapies to help children tolerate the pain and cope as effectively as possible (Lovell and Walco, 1989).

Promote general health

A well-balanced diet and assessment of nutritional status are integral parts of health supervision. The discomfort and increased need for rest may create problems of weight control. Excess weight causes additional strain on inflamed joints, especially those of the lower extremities. Excessive fatigue and overexertion should be avoided by regular periods of rest, especially during acute flare-ups of arthritis. Symptoms may exacerbate during a viral illness.

Posture and body mechanics are important for children with JCA, both when they are at rest and when they are active. They must have a firm mattress to maintain good alignment of spine, hips and knees, and no pillow or a very thin one. Children who are confined to bed either at home or in the hospital may require supports or splints to maintain positioning.

School-aged children are encouraged to attend school, even on days when there may be some pain or discomfort. The aid of the school nurse is enlisted so that a child is permitted to take the prescribed medication at school and to arrange for rest in the nurse's office during the day. It is important that the child attend school to learn skills and engage in social interaction, especially if the JCA continues to limit physical skills.

Facilitate compliance

The child and family are involved in the therapeutic plan. They need to know the purpose and correct use of splints and appliances, and the medication regimen. The family is instructed regarding administration of medications, as well as the value of a regular schedule of administration to maintain a satisfactory drug level in the body. If evidence of drug toxicity is noted, the family is instructed to stop the medication and notify the health professional. The UK Committee on the Safety of Medicines (CSM) has considered available evidence on possible links between Reye's syndrome and aspirin use by feverish children, and recommends that aspirin should no longer be given to children under 12 years unless specifically indicated.

Encourage heat and exercise

Heat has been shown to be beneficial to children with arthritis. Moist heat is best for relieving pain and stiffness, and the most efficient and practical method is in the bathtub. The temperature and duration of the bath are specified by the therapist, but usually do not exceed ten minutes at 37.8°C. Sometimes hydrotherapy, paraffin bath, or hot packs may be used as needed for temporary relief of acute swelling and pain. Hot packs are easily applied at home using a Turkish towel wrung out after being immersed in hot water or heated in a microwave oven, applied to the area, and covered with plastic for 20 minutes. Painful hands or feet can be immersed in a pan of water for ten minutes two or three times daily in addition to tub baths.

Activities of daily living provide satisfactory exercise for older children to maintain maximum mobility with minimum pain. These children should be encouraged in their efforts and patiently allowed to dress and groom themselves, to assume daily tasks, and to care for their belongings. It is often difficult for stiff fingers to manipulate buttons, comb or brush hair, and turn taps, but parents and other caregivers should try not to offer assistance to them. In addition, children should learn and understand why others do not help them. Many helpful devices, such as self-adhering fasteners, tongs for manipulating difficult items, and grab bars installed in bathrooms for safety, can be employed to facilitate tasks. A raised toilet seat often makes the difference between dependent and independent toilet use.

Arthritis Care provides services for both parents and professionals, and nurses should refer families to these agencies as an added resource.

The child

JCA affects every aspect of the child's daily life. The physical pain and limitations interfere with performance of normal tasks and provision of self-care. Even simple tasks, such as dressing, hair combing, use of the bathroom, cutting food, climbing stairs, manipulating doors and taps, and using public transportation, are difficult or impossible. There may be school difficulties related to transportation to and from school, stairs, and loss of time as a result of exacerbations and hospitalization. Physical limitations interfere with participation in many activities, both curricular and extracurricular, which limits peer contacts and interaction, and increases social isolation. These problems are especially critical for adolescents, for whom peer acceptance and relationships are so vital to personality development. These children increasingly turn to solitary activities and to the family at a time when they are expected to move into greater independence and relationships with peers.

The effectiveness of nursing interventions is determined by continual reassessment and evaluation of care based on the following observational guidelines and expected outcomes:

1. Observe child's behaviour and employ pain assessment and management techniques.
2. Conduct routine assessment of child's general health.
3. Observe the child during planned and unplanned activities, assess mobility of joints, and observe the use of prescribed appliances.
4. Observe child's ability to perform activities of daily living.
5. Observe and interview child and family regarding feelings and concerns.

THERAPEUTIC MANAGEMENT

The objectives of medical treatment are: (1) to reverse the autoimmune and inflammatory processes and (2) to prevent exacerbations and complications. Therapy involves the use of specific and supportive medications and regulation of activity and diet.

Drugs

The principal drugs used to control inflammation are the corticosteroids, administered in doses sufficient to suppress symptoms, then tapered to the lowest suppressive dose.

Another group of drugs effective in relieving the dermatological, arthritic, and renal symptoms of the disease are antimalarial preparations, such as hydroxychloroquine and chloroquine.

NSAIDs, such as aspirin, relieve muscle and joint pains and reduce tissue inflammation. Drugs used to control various complications include anticonvulsants, antihypertensives, and antibiotics. The selection of appropriate medication in each of these categories is essential, since many of them greatly aggravate the disease process and affect renal function.

KEY POINTS

- Trauma is the leading cause of death in children and is caused by accidental injury, child abuse injury and birth injuries.
- The major consequences of immobilization are loss of muscle strength, endurance, and muscle mass; bone demineralization leading to osteoporosis; loss of joint mobility; and contractures.
- Features of children's fractures not observed in the adult include presence of growth plate, thicker and stronger periosteum, porosity of bone, more rapid healing and less stiffness.
- Types of fractures seen in children are bends, buckle, greenstick and complete.
- Goals of fracture management in children are to regain alignment and length of the bony fragments, retain alignment and length, and restore function to injured parts.
- The method of fracture reduction is determined by the age of the child, degree of displacement, amount of overriding, amount of oedema, condition of skin and soft tissues, sensation, and circulation distal to fracture.
- Participation in sports predisposes adolescents to acute injuries, such as contusions, dislocations, sprains, and strains, and overuse syndromes, such as stress fractures.
- Health concerns associated with sports are related menstrual dysfunction, drug misuse and sudden death.
- Osteomyelitis is acquired by direct or secondary invasion or haematogenous spread of infectious organisms.
- Goals of therapy for juvenile chronic arthritis are to preserve joint function, prevent physical deformities, and relieve symptoms without iatrogenic harm.

REFERENCES

Brewer EJ, Arroyo M: Use of nonsteroidal anti-inflammatory drugs in children, *Pediatr Ann* 15:575, 1986.

Bunnell WP: An objective criterion for scoliosis screening, *J Bone Joint Surg* 66-A:1381, 1984.

Cohen FL: *Clinical genetics in nursing practice*, Philadelphia, 1984, JB Lippincott.

Davis SE, Lewis SA: Managing scoliosis: fashions for the body and mind, *MCN* 9:186, 1984.

Dyment PG: Initial management of minor acute soft-tissue injuries, *Pediatr Ann* 17:99, 1988.

Fisher MC, Goldsmith JF, Gilligan PH: Sneakers as a source of Pseudomonas aeruginosa in children with osteomyelitis following puncture wounds, *J Pediatr* 106:607, 1985.

Lovell DJ, Walco GA: Pain associated with juvenile rheumatoid arthritis, *Pediatr Clin North Am* 36:1015, 1989.

McCullough FL, Evans LM.: Assessment of neurovascular status in children, *Orthop Nurs* 4(4):19, 1985.

McCrae R: *Practical fracture treatment*, London, 1990, Churchill Livingstone.

Miller JAA, Nachemson AL, Schultz AB: Effectiveness of braces in mild idiopathic scoliosis, *Spine* 9:632, 1984.

Northrup CE, Kelly ME: *Legal issues in nursing*, St Louis, 1987, Mosby–Year Book.

Orava S: Stress fractures, *Br J Sports Med* 14:40, 1980.

Staheli LT: The hip. In Gellis SS, Kagan BM: *Current pediatric therapy 12*, Philadelphia, 1986, WB Saunders.

FURTHER READING

General

Brady M, Grey M: Growing pains: a myth or a reality, *J Pediatr Health Care* 3:219, 1989.

Dandy D: *Essential orthopaedics and trauma*, ed 2, London, 1993, Churchill Livingstone.

Dudek G: Nursing update: hypophosphatemic rickets, *Pediatr Nurs* 15:45, 1989.

Huckstep RL: *A simple guide to orthopaedics*, London, 1993, Churchill Livingstone.

Mason KJ: Pediatric orthopaedics: developmental norms, *Orthop Nurs* 8(4):45, 1989.

Meadow SR, Smithelis RW: *Lecture notes on paediatrics*, ed 6, London, 1991, Blackwell Scientific.

Trauma

Alexander R *et al*: Serial abuse in children who are shaken, *Am J Dis Child* 144:58, 1990.

Betz C: Injury: our children's greatest health problem, *J Paed Nurs* 8(6):353, 1993.

Butler K: Nurse-aid. Management of children 1: accidents, *BJN* 3(11):579, 1994.

Harris BH *et al*: The crucial hour, *Pediatr Ann* 16:301, 1987.

Jamison DW: When emergency care is up to you, *RN* 50(4):26, 1987.

Leyendecker M *et al*: Rescuing a multiple trauma victim, *Nurs '89* 19(10):54, 1989.

Partridge C: Spinal cord injuries: aspects of psychological care, *BJN* 3(1):12, 1994.

Immobilization

Olson EV: The hazards of immobility, *Am J Nurs* 90:43, 1990.

Rubin M: The physiology of bed rest, *Am J Nurs* 88:50, 1988.

Willey T: High-tech beds and mattress overlays, *Am J Nurs* 89:1142, 1989.

Fractures

Adams JC, Hamblen DL: *Outline of fractures,* ed 10, London, 1992, Churchill Livingstone.

Cochran S: Open fracture, *Nurs '87* 17(5):33, 1987.

Cuddy CM: Caring for a child in a spica cast: a parent's perspective, *Orthop Nurs* 5(3):17, 1986.

Evans B: Nurse-aid. Management of fractures 2, *BJN* 2(8):432, 1993b.

Evans B: Nurse-aid. Management of fractures 3, *BJN* 2(10):539, 1993c.

Feller NG, Stroup K, Christian L: Helping staff nurses become mini-specialists, *Am J Nurs* 89:991, 1989.

Gamron R: Taking the pressure out of compartment syndrome, *Am J Nurs* 88:1076, 1988.

Lavin RJ: The high-pressure demands of compartment syndrome, *RN* 52(2):22, 1989.

McCullough FL: Skeletal trauma in children, *Orthop Nurs* 8(2):41, 1989.

Mead M, Morgan M: Fractures, sprains and soft tissue injuries. In Mead D, Sibert J: *The injured child: an action plan for nurses,* London, 1991, Scutari.

Morean S: *Plaster casting: patient problems and nursing care,* Oxford, 1989, Heinemann.

Morris L *et al*: Special care for skeletal traction, *RN* 51(2):24, 1988.

Morris L *et al*: Nursing the patient in traction, *RN* 51(1):26, 1988.

Rang M, Wright J: Pitfalls in fractures, *Pediatr Ann* 18:53, 1989.

Redheffer GM, Bailely M: Assessing and splinting fractures, *Nurs '89* 19(6):51, 1989.

Amputation

Miller RA, Evans WE: Immediate postop prosthesis, *Am J Nurs* 87:310, 1987.

Varni JW *et al*: Family functioning, temperament, and psychologic adaptation in children with congenital or acquired limb deficiencies, *Pediatr* 84:323, 1989.

Disorders Related to Sports

American Academy of Pediatrics, Committee on Sports Medicine: Amenorrhea in adolescent athletes, *Pediatr* 84:394, 1989.

American Academy of Pediatrics, Committee on Sports Medicine: Knee brace use by athletes, *Pediatr* 85:228, 1990.

Backous DD *et al*: Soccer injuries and their relation to physical maturity, *Am J Dis Child* 142:839, 1988.

Council on Scientific Affairs: Drug abuse in athletes, *JAMA* 259:1703, 1988.

Goldberg B *et al*: Injuries in youth football, *Pediatr* 81:255, 1988.

Krowchuk DP *et al*: High school athletes and the use of ergogenic aids, *Am J Dis Child* 143:486, 1989.

McLain LG, Reynolds S: Sports injuries in a high school, *Pediatr* 84:446, 1989.

Nickerson HJ *et al*: Causes of iron deficiency in adolescent athletes, *J Pediatr* 114:657, 1989.

Pratt M: Strength, flexibility, and maturity in adolescent athletes, *Am J Dis Child* 143:560, 1989.

Rowland TW, Kelleher JF: Iron deficiency in athletes, *Am J Dis Child* 143:197, 1989.

Yelverton GA: Anabolic steroids, *Pediatr Nurs* 15:63, 1989.

Scoliosis

Bridwell KH: Cotrel-Dubousset instrumentation, *Orthop Nurs* 7(1):11, 1988.

DiRaimondo CV, Green NE: Brace-wear compliance in patients with adolescent idiopathic scoliosis, *J Pediatr Orthop* 8:143, 1988.

Jacobs-Zacny JM, Horn MJ: Nursing care of adolescents having posterior spinal fusion with Cotrel-Dubousset instrumentation, *Orthop Nurs* 7(1):17, 1988.

Johnson JB, Killman-Young J: Adolescence, anxiety, and adaptation: preparing for posterior spine fusion with instrumentation, *J Pediatr Nurs* 3:348, 1988.

Rauen KK, Ho M: Children's use of patient-controlled analgesia after spine surgery, *Pediatr Nurs* 15:589, 1989.

Voznak L: My life with scoliosis, *Orthop Nurs* 7(1):22, 1988.

Orthopaedic Infections

Barton LL, Dunkle LM, Habib FH: Septic arthritis in childhood, *Am J Dis Child* 141:898, 1987.

Juvenile Chronic Arthritis

Mortensen ME, Rennebohm RM: Clinical pharmacology and use of non-steroid anti-inflammatory drugs, *Pediatr Clin North Am* 36:1113, 1989.

Ignatavicius DD: Meeting the psychosocial needs of patients with rheumatoid arthritis, *Orthop Nurs* 6(3):16, 1987.

Rosenberg AM: Advanced drug therapy for juvenile rheumatoid arthritis, *J Pediatr* 114:171, 1989.

Scott JT: *Copeman's textbook of the rheumatic diseases,* vols I & II, ed 6, London, 1990, Churchill Livingstone.

Southwood TR *et al*: Unconventional remedies used for patients with juvenile arthritis, *Pediatr* 85:150, 1990.

Winkel MF: Juvenile rheumatoid arthritis—parent support group: do parents perceive a need? *Pediatr Nurs* 14:131, 1988.

Chapter 34

The Child with Neuromuscular Dysfunction

LEARNING OUTCOMES

After studying this chapter you should be able to:

- Describe the classification and diagnosis of a range of muscular dysfunctions
- Differentiate upper motor and lower motor neurone disorders
- Discuss the therapeutic management of children with cerebral palsy
- Outline the role of the professions allied to medicine in the overall management of children with neuromuscular dysfunctions
- Plan nursing care for children with all types of neuromuscular lesions
- Define the glossary terms

GLOSSARY

ataxia Unsteadiness, incoordination

athetosis Slow, twisting movement of limbs

atrophy Wasting

choreiform Involuntary, jerky (movements)

dysarthria Imperfect articulation

dyskinesia Abnormal involuntary movement

dystonia Abnormal muscle tone producing involuntary movements and posture

hypertrophy Thickening

hypertonia Increased muscle tension

hypotonia Decreased muscle tension

moro Reflex; outstretching and curling-in of limbs if head falls back

paraplegia Paralysis of lower limbs

plantar flexion Downward turning of toes

quadriplegia Paralysis of all four limbs; often greater involvement of legs than arms

spasticity Increased muscle tone producing rigidity if severe

Disorders of muscle or muscle innervation interfere with physical movement and are, in most instances, more difficult to manage than those involving traumatic injury as discussed in the early segments of Chapter 33. This chapter is primarily concerned with impairment of innervation to muscles and, to a lesser extent, with muscle pathology.

NEUROMUSCULAR DYSFUNCTION

Weakness or abnormal performance of skeletal muscle may represent a defect in the muscle itself or may reflect a pathological disorder at some point along the neural pathway from the cortex of the brain to the neuromuscular junction.

Some clinical features are shared by muscle disease, *myopathy*, which differs in many ways from muscle dysfunction resulting from disorders of neuronal structures — the brain, cranial nerve nuclei, long nerve tracts, anterior horn cells of the spinal cord, and peripheral nerves. The motor unit consists of the lower motor neuron, the neuromuscular junction, and the muscle fibres it supplies (Fig. 34-1). The upper motor neuronal pathways from the cerebrum to the lower motor neuron are described as: (1) pyramidal — those with fibres extending from the cortex, coming together in the medulla, crossing from one side to the other, then extending down the cord to synapse with anterior horn motor neurons; and (2) extrapyramidal — a complex network of motor neurons that comprise relays between motor areas of the cortex, basal ganglia, thalamus, cerebellum and brainstem.

CLASSIFICATION AND DIAGNOSIS

The site of pathological disturbance determines the type of muscular dysfunction. In general, *upper motor neuron* lesions produce weakness associated with spasticity, increased deep tendon reflexes and abnormal superficial reflexes. The primary disorder of upper motor neuron dysfunction is cerebral palsy. Lesions of *lower motor neurons* interrupt the reflex arc, causing weakness and atrophy of the skeletal muscles involved, with associated hypotonia or flaccidity, which eventually progress to atrophy with varying degrees of contracture deformity. A disorder of the *extrapyramidal pathway* and the cerebellum rarely produces muscle weakness.

Lower motor neuron involvement is usually symmetrical (except that of poliomyelitis and single peripheral nerve disease). Disorders of the pyramidal tract are more often asymmetrical. Muscle wasting is characteristic of lower motor neuron lesions and more marked than in diseases of muscles. Hereditary factors and metabolic disease are more often responsible for muscular weakness and atrophy of gradual onset. Deep tendon reflexes are briskly active in upper motor neuron disease, are diminished or absent in lower motor neuron disease, and depend on the progress of muscle degeneration in the myopathies.

CLASSIFICATION

The most useful classification of neuromuscular disorders is one that defines the site of origin of the pathological lesion: the anterior horn cells of the spinal cord, the peripheral nerves, the neuromuscular junction, and the muscles.

Diseases of anterior horn cells

Diseases and disorders that affect the anterior horn cells are the result of destruction or atrophy of the anterior horn of the spinal column with the inability to transfer impulses from sensory neurons to motor neurons. Enteroviruses are prominent aetiological agents that selectively affect anterior horn cells. Degeneration of the anterior horn cells is caused by inherited disorders, primarily the spinal muscular atrophies.

Neuropathies

Disorders affecting peripheral nerves may be *mononeuropathies*, involving a single nerve and the muscles it innervates, or *polyneuropathies*, which involve multiple nerves and the muscles

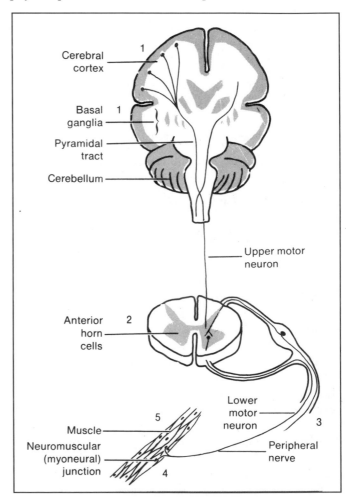

Fig. 34-1 Site of origin for neuromuscular disorders. *1*, Cerebral palsy; *2*, poliomyelitis, spinal muscular atrophy; *3*, mononeuropathies, polyneuropathies; *4*, myasthenia gravis, neurotoxic disorders; *5*, muscular dystrophies.

they supply. Neuropathies are caused by several hereditary diseases, traumatic injury, infections, poisons and (secondarily) some metabolic diseases. Examples of acute and chronic polyneuropathies are infectious polyneuritis and peroneal muscular atrophy, respectively.

Neuromuscular junction disease

Disorders involving a neurochemical deficiency interfere with transmission of nerve impulses to muscles at the neuromuscular junction. Normally, nerve impulses are transmitted to skeletal muscles across the neuromuscular junction by acetylcholine. This is accomplished in three steps: (1) acetylcholine is released from vesicles in the terminal nerve endings; (2) it then diffuses across the junction and contacts receptor sites in the muscle membrane, stimulating the muscle to contract; and (3) it is removed by the action of cholinesterase. Interference at any of these three steps will block transmission of nerve impulses and prevent muscular contraction.

Diseases of muscles

Disorders that affect the muscles directly may be a result of inflammatory, degenerative or metabolic causes. Chief among these are the muscular dystrophies.

DIAGNOSTIC TOOLS

To aid in differentiating between diseases with similar manifestations, several diagnostic tools are used.

The *electromyogram* (EMG) measures the electrical potentials generated in individual muscles. A fine, sterile needle electrode is inserted into the muscle. The electrical activity generated in the skeletal muscles is measured during rest and during contraction.

Nerve conduction velocity: the velocity of electrical impulse conduction along motor or sensory nerves is frequently measured in conjunction with electromyography. Certain diseases affect the peripheral nerves, prolonging the conduction time from the point of stimulation of the nerve to the muscle.

Muscle biopsy is the most useful laboratory examination to confirm and classify muscle disorders. *Serum enzyme measurement* of creatine kinase is also helpful in diagnosis.

HYPOTONIA

Decreased muscle tone in an infant is not an unusual observation in the neonatal period and is one of the most common presenting symptoms in neuromuscular disorders.

CLINICAL MANIFESTATIONS

Hypotonia, sometimes called the *floppy infant syndrome*, is marked by diminished muscle tone and weakness in both spontaneous and passive motion, and in reflex testing. The infant, when placed in a supine position, assumes a characteristic 'frog posture' or lies in some other unusual position at rest (see Fig.

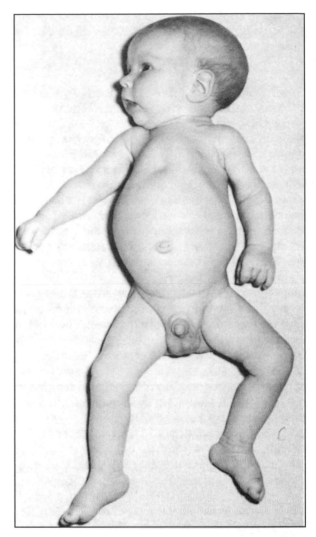

Fig. 34-2 Patient with Werdnig-Hoffmann disease lying in typical posture of abduction of legs at hips and flexion of knees. Arms are flexed slightly with little movement at shoulders. Movements of fingers and toes are present. Pectus excavatum deformity of chest is common and is the result of unopposed diaphragmatic breathing. (From Swaiman KF, Wright FS: *The practice of pediatric neurology*, ed 2, St Louis, 1982, Mosby–Year Book)

34-2). When held in the horizontal position the hypotonic infant droops over the supporting hand with head and extremities hanging loosely, resembling an inverted 'U' (see Fig. 34-3). The muscles feel flabby when palpated, and there is marked head lag when the infant is pulled to a sitting position. Poor sucking may be noted.

THERAPEUTIC MANAGEMENT AND IMPLICATIONS FOR NURSING

The management of these infants is determined by the cause of the hypotonia. It is a nursing responsibility to record and report findings that suggest hypotonia in an infant so that further evaluation can be carried out.

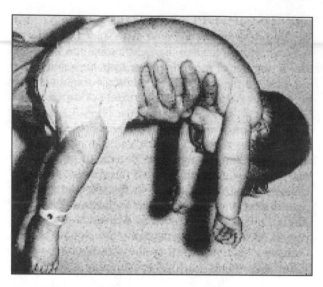

Fig. 34-3 Hypotonicity demonstrated by horizontal suspension in an infant with Werdnig-Hoffmann disease. (From Swaiman KF and Wright FS: *The practice of pediatric neurology*, ed 2, St Louis, 1982, Mosby-Year Book Inc.)

CEREBRAL PALSY

Cerebral palsy (CP) is a nonspecific term applied to disorders characterized by impaired movement and posture, of early onset. It is nonprogressive and may be accompanied by intellectual and language deficits. It is the most common permanent physical disability of childhood, and studies suggest that the incidence is approximately two in every 1,000 live births (Healy and Smith, 1988; Nelson, 1989).

AETIOLOGY

Damage is usually caused by ischaemia and/or asphyxia in the antenatal, perinatal or postnatal period. Premature infants are particularly vulnerable and the increased prevalence of CP (approximately 20% since the 1960s) probably reflects the improved survival of very low birth weight babies (Bhushan, Paneth, and Keily, 1993).

CLINICAL MANIFESTATIONS

The alert observer may suspect CP when a child demonstrates some of the following groups of manifestations.

Delayed gross motor development
This is a universal manifestation of CP. The child shows a delay in all motor accomplishments, and the discrepancy between motor ability and expected achievement tends to increase with successive developmental milestones as growth advances. It is especially significant if other developmental behaviour, such as language and social awareness, are normal.

Abnormal motor performance
Neuromotor dysfunction is particularly evident in motor per-

formance. An early sign is preferential unilateral hand use that may be apparent at about six months of age. Hand dominance does not normally develop until at least the second year. Children with hemiplegia have an asymmetrical crawl, using the unaffected arm and leg to propel themselves on either the buttocks or the abdomen. Spasticity may cause the child to stand or walk on the toes. Uncoordinated or involuntary movements are characteristic of dyskinetic CP, and facial grimacing and writhing movements of the tongue, fingers, and toes are signs of athetosis. Other significant signs of motor dysfunction are poor sucking and feeding difficulties.

Alterations of muscle tone
Increased or decreased resistance to passive movements is a sign of abnormal muscle tone; the child may feel stiff on handling or dressing; when pulled to a sitting position, the child may extend the entire body, rigid and unbending at the hip and knee joints. This is an early sign of spasticity.

Abnormal postures
Children with spastic CP assume abnormal postures at rest or when their position is changed. In the supine position, spasticity is evident by scissoring (legs in crossed position, knees, hips and ankles stiff) and extension of legs and with the feet plantar flexed. This posture is exaggerated when others try to make the child bear weight. Spasticity may be mild or severe, depending on the degree of impairment. The hemiparetic child may rest with the affected arm adducted and held against the torso, with the elbow pronated and slightly flexed, and the hand closed.

Reflex abnormalities
Persistence of primitive infantile reflexes is one of the earliest clues to CP; for example, asymmetric tonic neck reflex or the persistence of the Moro, plantar and palmar grasp reflexes.

Associated disabilities
Some of the disabilities associated with CP are visual impairment, hearing impairment, communication and speech difficulties, seizures and intellectual impairment.

Learning disability
One-third of children with CP have normal intelligence (fewer have high normal or superior intelligence compared with the normal population); one-third have mild learning problems; and one-third have moderate or severe learning disability. As a group, children with athetosis and ataxia are intellectually superior to those with other types of CP.

Attention deficit — hyperactivity disorder
The primary presenting symptoms are poor attention span, marked distractibility and hyperactivity.

Seizures
Seizures are more likely to accompany postnatally acquired hemiplegia. They are an unusual finding with athetosis and

diplegia. The most common type is generalized tonic-clonic seizure, and the peak incidence of commencement is between two and six years of age.

Sensory impairment

Abnormalities of vision occur more often in CP, and hearing loss is frequently an associated disability.

CLINICAL CLASSIFICATION

CP has been classified in several ways. The most useful classification is based on the nature and distribution of neuromuscular dysfunction (Hughes and Newton, 1992).

Spastic cerebral palsy

The most common clinical type, spastic CP, presents with increased reflexes, increased muscle tone and (often) weakness.

Dyskinetic cerebral palsy

Dyskinesia implies abnormal involuntary movements, which disappear in sleep and are aggravated by stress. The major manifestation is athetosis involving all extremities, the trunk, neck, facial muscles and tongue. Imperfect articulation (dysarthria) makes it difficult to understand what the child is saying.

Involuntary movements may take on choreiform (involuntary, irregular, jerking movements) and dystonic (disordered muscle tone) manifestations that increase in intensity under emotional stress and during adolescence.

Ataxic cerebral palsy

The least common type of CP, ataxia, is caused by a defect in the cerebellum or its pathways. It is characterized by nonprogressive failure of muscle coordination and by irregular muscle action. Affected children have a wide-based gait and perform rapid, repetitive movements poorly.

Mixed-type cerebral palsy

A combination of spasticity and athetosis is described as mixed-type CP. Many affected children are severely disabled. This combination is sometimes observed after traumatic postnatal head injury or asphyxia.

PROCESS OF DIAGNOSIS

The neurological examination and history are the primary modalities for diagnosis. A thorough knowledge of normal variations of motor development is required for detecting abnormal progress, and a careful history is elicited to detect possible aetiological factors. The child's spontaneous movements and behaviour are observed, including posture and attitude. Muscle size, function and tone are also observed.

Supplementary diagnostic tests may be used, such as electroencephalography, tomography and screening for metabolic defects. The possibility of slowly progressive degenerative disease and early onset, slow-growing brain tumours must be ruled out.

THERAPEUTIC MANAGEMENT: GENERAL CONCEPTS

The goals of therapy for children with CP are early recognition and promotion of an optimum developmental course to enable affected children to attain their potential within the limits of their brain dysfunction. The disorder is permanent, and therapy is chiefly symptomatic and preventive. To be effective, it requires the services of an organized team of health professionals that considers: (1) the nature of the physical disability, (2) defects associated with the disorder, and (3) the interpersonal and social influences encountered by the affected child.

The broad aims of therapy are: (1) to establish locomotion, communication and self-help; (2) to gain optimum appearance and integration of motor functions; (3) to correct associated defects as effectively as possible; and (4) to provide educational opportunities adapted to the needs and capabilities of the child. Each child is evaluated and managed on an individual basis. The plan of therapy may involve a variety of settings, facilities and specially trained people, including the parents. The scope of the child's needs may require, in addition to the paediatrician and nurse, professionals such as a psychologist and/or psychiatrist, orthopaedic surgeon, physiotherapist, teacher, social worker, speech therapist, neurologist, orthotist, audiologist, occupational therapist and dietitian.

Mobilizing devices

Children can be enabled to mobilize with the aid of tripods, frames and 'Kay-Posture Walkers' (which encourage an upright posture while providing stability from behind). Wheelchairs can be customized to meet the needs and preferences of older children (see Mobilization Devices, Chapter 33).

Surgery

Orthopaedic surgery may be required to decrease or abolish spastic muscle imbalance. This includes tendon lengthening procedures (especially heel-cord lengthening), release of spastic wrist flexor muscles, and correction of hip and adductor muscle spasticity or contracture to improve locomotion (Dormans, 1993). Selective dorsal rhizotomy has provided marked improvement in some children with CP (Park and Owen, 1992). However, achieving the benefits from the surgery requires intensive physiotherapy and family commitment; botulinum toxin has been used with some success in postponing or abolishing the need for surgery (Calderon-Gonzalez *et al*, 1994; Cosgrove *et al*, 1994).

Medication

Drugs such as baclofen and dantrolene (skeletal muscle relaxants) may be of some benefit, although doses that reduce spasticity may bring side effects of drowsiness, or hypotonia which prevents weight-bearing.

Antiepileptic medications, such as sodium valproate, carbamazepine and others, are administered to children who have troublesome seizures.

Technical aids

A variety of technical aids are available to improve the functioning of children with CP. For example, there are specially designed electromechanical toys that use biofeedback, operated from a head unit. In the same way, devices can facilitate communication with voice synthesizers or message-printers.

Many other electronic devices allow independent functioning and enable persons with CP eventually to function in their own homes and places of work.

Other considerations

Care of visual and auditory deficits requires the attention of appropriate specialists, and speech therapy involves the services of a speech therapist. Dental care is especially important for children with CP and is too frequently overlooked.

THERAPEUTIC MANAGEMENT: PHYSIOTHERAPY

Physiotherapy is one of the most frequently used conservative treatment modalities. It requires the specialized skills of a qualified therapist with an extensive repertoire of exercise methods who can design a programme to stimulate each child to achieve functional goals.

There are several methods of physiotherapy or physical education currently in use and many combine aspects of different schools of thought. All forms, however, require a high degree of commitment from the family.

Passive exercises and stretching are important; for example, stretching of the gastrocnemius muscle and its tendon to help prevent tightness and spasticity, which lead to toe walking and equinus position of the ankle. Prevention of contracture deformity is a prime function of physiotherapy.

Occupational therapy

Training in manual skills and activities of daily living should proceed along developmental lines and according to the child's functional level. Sitting, balance, crawling and walking are encouraged at appropriate ages. When standing is attempted, therapy may be needed to strengthen and improve balance, which is sometimes facilitated by the use of splints, callipers and other ambulation aids.

Play is a valuable tool in a therapeutic programme and is selected to combine therapy with the child's ability and interest. This often requires a great deal of ingenuity and inventiveness from those involved in the child's care. Young preschool children with all forms of delayed development benefit from the Portage scheme. This is taught to parents in the home, and sets realistic goals, suggests ideas on how to achieve them, and the order in which they should be learned (Bluma, 1976). The importance of parents feeling they are actively working to help their child, and the regular progress reports by the Portage worker, emphasize the positive aspects of a situation in which negatives seem to be more obvious.

The child may need considerable help (and patience) in learning to feed, dress and care for personal hygiene. These are the earliest and most important tasks on which to concentrate.

Speech training under the supervision of a speech therapist is begun early, before the child learns poor habits of communication. Parents and others can help by following the directions of the speech therapist and by talking to the child slowly and using pictures or handling objects about which the adult is speaking. Feeding techniques, such as encouraging the child to use the lips and tongue in eating, help to facilitate speech; for example, placing food at the side of the tongue, first on one side then on the other; making the child use the lips to take food from a spoon, rather than placing it directly on the tongue; and avoiding using the teeth to remove the food from the utensil. If severe dysarthria prevents articulate speech and the child has reasonable intelligence, nonverbal communication is taught, using Makaton signing, Bliss symbolic boards and other methods (Walker and Armfield, 1981).

As the child progresses from simple feeding and self-care activities, training is extended to include other tasks that are within the child's developmental and functional capabilities, such as cooking or typing. It should be remembered that children should not be expected to learn a task until they are at the developmental stage at which it would normally be accomplished. Any accomplishment promotes self-reliance and self-esteem for healthier personality development.

Education

As in all aspects of care, educational requirements are determined by the child's needs and potential. Children with mild physical disability, normal intelligence, and no associated learning disability should attend mainstream school with the help of a full- or part-time welfare assistant. When attendance at mainstream classes is not appropriate, children may be taught in special units within the mainstream school or in schools for children with special needs, depending on the child's requirement and the schools available in his or her community.

Recreation

Recreational activities are also a necessary part of growing up. Some children and adolescents with CP can compete in athletic and artistic endeavours, and there are many games and pastimes that are suited to their capabilities. There are increasing, though still inadequate, numbers of holiday schemes and sports facilities for disabled children and adults. Details can be obtained from SCOPE (formerly the Spastics Society).

IMPLICATIONS FOR NURSING

Nurses and health visitors in a community setting, especially those in schools, GP practices and clinics, are more likely to become involved with a family in which there is a child with CP. Both the child and the family need the help, support and encouragement that nurses are prepared to offer, and nurses can be involved in all aspects of the child's management. Nurses who know the family and their special needs and problems are in the best position to provide guidance and support.

Assessment

Early recognition of CP is often a result of alert observation by the nurse. Unusual manifestations in a newborn can be signs of a variety of conditions, but an infant who displays poor feeding, rigidity, tenseness or hypotonia merits closer scrutiny. Delayed attainment of developmental milestones is one of the most valuable clues to recognizing CP.

Planning

Nursing objectives for the child with CP include:
1. Establish locomotion and communication.
2. Encourage self-help.
3. Facilitate acquisition of educational opportunities adapted to the needs and capabilities of the child.
4. Promote a positive self-image in the child.
5. Support the family in its efforts to meet the needs of the child.
6. Care for the child during hospitalization.

Implementation

Nurses working with children need to be well acquainted with normal child growth and development, and with the tools of assessment. The earlier any deviation from normal is detected, the better the outlook for optimum developmental attainment. Nurses who are acquainted with services and facilities can refer the family to qualified practitioners.

Physiotherapists will teach parents how to position children for various activities and how to carry out appropriate exercises.

Although practical advice is important, the nurse or physiotherapist should offer suggestions at a pace that can be absorbed by the parents, to avoid making them feel inadequate in their parenting abilities. The parents are given positive feedback for their observations of the infant, the progress *they* note, and how *they* differentiate the child's needs.

Sometimes, parents need support simply because the demands made on them are very fatiguing. It is better for parents of young children with CP to reduce the *quantity* of involvement with their children, rather than reduce the *quality* of the interactions.

Probably the nursing interventions most valuable to the family are support and help in coping with the emotional aspects of the disorder (see Chapter 20). Initially, the parents need supportive counselling directed towards understanding the implications of the diagnosis and the feelings that it engenders. Later, they need clarification regarding what they can expect from the child and from health professionals. Having a child with CP implies numerous problems of daily management and changes in family life.

There are constant demands, sometimes with few rewards, and the day-by-day changelessness of these demands is frustrating for parents. The nurse needs to support the parents in their frustration, their problem solving, their concerns, their approaches to helping the child, and their lack of gratification, as well as the positive approaches they use. Siblings of a child with a disability are affected and may respond to the presence of the child with overt or less evident behavioural problems. The family needs a relationship with nurses who can provide continued contact, support and encouragement.

Parents can also find help and solace from parent groups with whom they can share problems and concerns, and from whom they can derive comfort and practical information. The national organizations, SCOPE and Contact-a-Family, have branches in most communities. The addresses of the nearest branches can be obtained from a local telephone directory or Social Services department. The associations provide a variety of services for children and families. There are also several excellent books available to guide parents and nurses who work with the child with CP. Children with disabilities, and their families, are also entitled to Disability Living Allowance which helps with the increased financial demands for things such as transport and extra help with childcare.

Hospitalized child

CP is not a disorder that requires hospitalization; consequently, many nurses are not accustomed to handling these children. The basic concept to keep in mind when caring for such children is that they are, first of all, children who happen to be afflicted with a disorder that limits their capacities in performing some activities of daily living and, for some, communicating with others. They should be approached and treated the same as any child in the hospital. Frequently people tend to 'talk down' to them and do things for them that they are perfectly capable, although not as adeptly as children without a disability, of doing for themselves. This is especially humiliating to a teenager who values independence and self-esteem.

Evaluation

The effectiveness of nursing interventions is determined by continual reassessment and evaluation of care based on the following observational guidelines and expected outcomes:
1. Observe the child's movements and speech.
2. Observe the child's activities, especially those related to self-care.
3. Interview the family regarding the child's activities and school attendance.
4. Observe the child's interactions with others and the choice of activities; interview the child regarding feelings and concerns.
5. Interview the family regarding their feelings and concerns and observe the members' interaction with the child.
6. Observe the child's behaviour and responses during hospitalization.

SPINAL MUSCULAR ATROPHY

The spinal muscular atrophies are a group of disorders characterized by progressive weakness and wasting of skeletal muscle caused by degeneration of anterior horn cells in the spinal cord and the cells of the motor nuclei in the brainstem. They are inherited as autosomal recessive traits (Gordon, 1991).

Type 1 (Werdnig-Hoffman Disease)

This group comprises the infants who acquire the disease *in utero* or during the first three months of life. The infant is inactive and lies in the frog position (Fig. 34-2); active movement is limited to fingers and toes. Breathing is diaphragmatic with sternal recession caused by intercostal muscle paralysis. The cry and cough are weak and secretions tend to pool in the pharynx. The face, however, is alert, and sensation and intellect are normal. These infants achieve no motor milestones, and die from respiratory failure or infection; usually by the age of 18 months.

Type 2 (Intermediate SMA)

This group comprises infants who attain early milestones up to sitting; normal standing posture does not develop. The progressive degeneration appears to stabilize between the ages of 1-2 years, but the effects of increasing growth causes deformities, as do contracture formations. Death can occur in childhood, but most children affected survive to early middle age.

Type 3 (Chronic Spinal Muscular Atrophy/Kugelberg-Welander Disease)

This group has an insidious course. The onset can occur at any time from 2-17 years of age. Some children lose the ability to walk 8-9 years after the onset of symptoms, but many can still walk after 20 years or more. Many affected people have a normal life expectancy.

THERAPEUTIC MANAGEMENT

The diagnosis is established from electromyography demonstrating a denervation pattern and is sometimes confirmed by muscle biopsy. Treatment is symptomatic and, in Types 2 and 3, preventive; primarily prevention of infection and treating orthopaedic problems, the most serious of which is scoliosis (Granata *et al*, 1993). Many children benefit from powered chairs, lifts and accessible environmental controls. Vigorous antibiotic therapy and chest physiotherapy are implemented during upper respiratory tract infections. Nasogastric feeding in babies with Werdnig-Hoffman Disease is usually necessary, as choking and tiring on sucking easily occur.

IMPLICATIONS FOR NURSING

The infant or small child with extensive paralysis requires frequent change of position to prevent physical injury and complications, especially pneumonia. The pharynx requires frequent suctioning to remove secretions, and feeding must be carried out slowly and carefully to prevent aspiration. Since these children are intellectually normal, verbal, tactile and auditory stimulation are important aspects of care.

Children who are able to sit require proper support and attention to alignment, to prevent deformities and other complications. Children who survive beyond infancy will need attention to educational needs and opportunities for social interaction with other children. Parents of a child with a chronic or potentially fatal illness require a great deal of support and encouragement (see Chapters 20 and 21). The parents of children with a genetically transmitted disorder also should be encouraged to seek genetic counselling.

INFECTIOUS POLYNEURITIS (GUILLAIN-BARRÉ SYNDROME)

Infectious polyneuritis, also known as infectious neuronitis and Guillain-Barré syndrome (GBS), is probably the most common form of polyneuritis. It is an acute polyneuropathy in which motor dysfunction predominates over sensory disturbance. It may occur at any age.

The precise aetiological agent is unknown; it has been suggested that it may be a toxic sequela of an original infection, an activated latent virus, or a manifestation of an acute infection. It may also be associated with *Mycoplasma* and *Pneumocystis* infections, or gram-negative organisms.

CLINICAL MANIFESTATIONS

The paralytic manifestations of GBS are usually preceded by a mild influenza-like illness or sore throat. The onset can be rapid, reaching peak activity within 24 hours, or a gradual progression of symptoms over days or weeks. Neurological symptoms initially involve muscle tenderness, sometimes accompanied by paraesthesia and cramps. Proximal muscle weakness progressing to paralysis usually occurs before distal weakness, and there is a tendency towards symmetrical involvement. In most patients, paralysis ascends from the lower extremities, frequently involving the muscles of the trunk, including the respiratory muscles, upper extremities, and those supplied by cranial nerves.

Tendon reflexes are depressed or absent, and paralysis is flaccid. Paralysis may involve facial, pharyngeal and laryngeal muscles. Evidence of intercostal and phrenic nerve involvement includes breathlessness in vocalizations and shallow, irregular respirations. There may be variable degrees of sensory impairment. Most patients complain of muscle tenderness or sensitivity to slight pressure. Urinary incontinence or retention and constipation are frequently present.

Course and prognosis

The general health of the child and the extent of paralysis influence the outcome of the illness. Almost all deaths are caused by respiratory failure; therefore, early diagnosis and access to respiratory support are especially important. Muscle function begins to return two days to two weeks after the onset of symptoms, and recovery is complete in most cases. The rate of recovery is usually related to the degree of involvement, and may extend from a few weeks to months. The greater the degree of paralysis, the longer the recovery phase.

THERAPEUTIC MANAGEMENT

Treatment of Guillain-Barré syndrome is symptomatic. Corticosteroid therapy has been of benefit in the early stages (Vallee *et al*, 1993). Respiratory and pharyngeal involvement requires assisted ventilation. Recent studies indicate that plasma exchange (plasmapheresis) may be beneficial both in shortening the length of illness and lessening the long-term disability (Jansen *et al*, 1993), and intravenous infusions of immunoglobulins appear to have had impressive results in some cases (Abdelkarim, 1994; Rantala *et al*, 1991).

IMPLICATIONS FOR NURSING

Nursing care is essentially supportive and is the same as that required for quadriplegia from any cause. The emphasis of care is on close observation, to assess the extent of paralysis, and prevention of complications.

During the acute phase of the disease, the child's condition should be carefully observed for possible difficulty in swallowing and for respiratory involvement. Vital signs and level of consciousness are monitored frequently. For the child who develops respiratory distress, the care is the same as for any child requiring mechanical ventilation (see Chapter 26).

Throughout the recovery phase, special emphasis is placed on prevention of complications, including good postural alignment, frequent change of position to avoid pressure sores, and passive physiotherapy. Children with oral and pharyngeal involvement are fed via a nasogastric tube to ensure adequate nutrition. Bowel and bladder care is needed to avoid constipation and urine retention.

Later, as the disease stabilizes and recovery begins, an active physiotherapy programme is implemented to prevent contracture deformities and to facilitate muscle recovery.

Throughout the course of the illness, child and parent support is paramount. The usual rapidity of the paralysis and the long period of recovery tax the emotional reserves of all family members. The parents and child benefit from repeated reassurance that recovery is occurring and from realistic information regarding the possibility of permanent disability. In the event of a residual disability, the family needs assistance in accepting and adjusting to the loss of function (see Chapter 20). The Guillain-Barré Syndrome Support Group, is an organization devoted to support, education and research.

MYASTHENIA GRAVIS

Myasthenia gravis (MG) is relatively uncommon in childhood. Juvenile MG appears to be identical to that seen in adults and usually has its onset after age ten years, but it may appear as early as age two years. Girls are affected six times as often as boys. Juvenile and adult forms of the disease are autoimmune disorders associated with attack of circulating antibodies on the acetylcholine receptors on the muscle end plate, blocking their function.

CLINICAL MANIFESTATIONS

The most common symptoms are general paralysis of the optic muscles with ptosis and diplopia. Difficulty in swallowing, chewing and speaking are also prominent, accompanied by weakness and paralysis of all skeletal muscles. The signs and symptoms are more pronounced in the late afternoon and evening. They are relieved by rest and made worse by exercise and stress.

PROCESS OF DIAGNOSIS

The diagnosis is made on the basis of the characteristic distribution of muscle weakness and the progressive weakness on repeated or sustained muscular contraction. The diagnosis is established by observation of the response to the anticholinesterase drugs. Intravenous administration of a small test dose of edrophonium produces a beneficial effect in one minute, but lasts for less than five minutes. Electrophysiological studies are helpful in diagnosis and help document transmission failure at the neuromuscular junction. Antibodies to human muscle acetylcholine are detected in serum of almost all affected persons, although not invariably at the outset of the disease.

THERAPEUTIC MANAGEMENT

Treatment consists of the oral administration of anticholinesterase drugs, the least toxic of which is pyridostigmine. The dosage is gradually increased until a satisfactory result is obtained. The child must be observed for signs of parasympathetic stimulation from over medication. These include lacrimation, salivation, abdominal cramps, sweating, diarrhoea, vomiting, bradycardia and weakness of respiratory muscles.

Other therapies, directed at the immunological mechanism, are necessary for children who do not respond to anticholinesterase drugs alone; thymectomy is performed, particularly if there is thymus enlargement (Adams, 1990); plasmapheresis is used for short-term intensive intervention or, in more intractable cases, as a regular therapeutic manoeuvre while awaiting the impact of the immunosuppression by prednisolone and azathioprine, which usually takes at least six months (Badurska, Ryniewicz, and Strugalska, 1992).

The prognosis of juvenile MG is relatively good. However, the course of the disease can be marked by fluctuating remissions and exacerbations.

IMPLICATIONS FOR NURSING

These children need continuous medical and nursing supervision. The parents are taught the importance of accurate administration of medications, with special emphasis on recognizing side effects with the dangers of choking, aspiration, and respiratory distress.

NEONATAL MYASTHENIA GRAVIS

A *transient* form of MG occurs in approximately 15% of infants born to mothers with myasthenia gravis who may not be aware that they have the disease. These infants display generalized weakness and hypotonia at birth: there is no evidence of neurological damage, and the symptoms usually disappear within 2-4 weeks.

Persistent neonatal MG is a familial abnormality of neuromuscular transmission. It appears indistinguishable from the transient form, but the mother usually does not have the disease. The disease persists throughout life, and more than one sibling may be affected, which suggests a genetic aetiology. Sex distribution is equal. The disorder is relatively resistant to drug therapy, and the eyelid and extraocular muscles seem to be the muscles most severely affected.

The prognosis in persistent neonatal MG is usually good. Although there is gradual worsening of symptoms with age, the life span is not affected significantly.

SPINAL CORD INJURIES

Spinal cord injuries with major neurological involvement are not a common cause of physical disability in childhood. The principles of management and nursing care apply to all spinal cord lesions, regardless of aetiology, particularly myelomeningocele, the most common cause of paraplegia in the paediatric age group.

In addition to care related to the immobilized child (see Chapter 33), children with damage to the spinal cord present other problems. A high level of paraplegia may create major problems in the ability to sit upright without support, whereas children with paraplegia with lower level injuries can walk with minimum assistance (see Table 34-1). The extent of paralysis is determined by both neurological and clinical assessment. Although the majority of children with spinal cord injuries are paraplegic, many are quadriplegic. Some children with quadriplegia are able to move only their face and neck muscles, whereas others are able to lift and bend their arms, but are unable to perform fine hand movements. Almost every physiological system is disrupted in a child with high-level quadriplegia. Not only are the central and peripheral nerves impaired, but there is also autonomic nervous system dysfunction. Vital structures such as blood vessels, lungs, bladder and bowel are affected.

AETIOLOGY

The most common cause of serious spinal cord damage in children is congenital defects of the spinal cord (e.g., myelomeningocele). Postnatal causes are primarily accidental injury and birth trauma.

Mechanisms of injury

Falling from heights occurs less often in children than in adults, but vertebral compression of the spine from blows to the head or buttocks occurs in water sports, falls from horses or other athletic injuries. Birth injuries may occur in breech delivery from traction force on the cord during delivery of the head and shoulders. Infants sustain cervical cord damage (as well as brain and eye damage, mental retardation, and death) when they are shaken; a common feature of non-accidental injury. Infants have very weak neck muscles, and during vigorous shaking their heavy heads wobble rapidly back and forth.

CLINICAL MANIFESTATIONS

As a result of pathological responses to the initial trauma, spinal cord injury causes three stages of response; therefore, the extent and severity of damage cannot be determined at first. Immediate loss of function is caused by both anatomical and impaired physiological function, and improvement may not be evident for weeks or even months.

First stage
Manifestation of the initial response to acute injury is flaccid paralysis below the level of the damage. Local effects of cord oedema and ischaemia produce a physiological transection with or without an anatomical severance. Manifestations include absence of reflexes at or below the cord lesion with flaccidity or limpness of the involved muscles, loss of sensation and motor function, and autonomic dysfunction (symptoms of hypotension, low or high body temperatures, and loss of bladder and bowel control).

These symptoms occur soon after the injury and last 1-6 weeks with much autonomic reflex cord function returning in about three weeks. The length of this stage indicates to some degree the extent of later recovery. In general, the shorter the duration of spinal shock, the more neurological recovery can be anticipated. Problems related to this first stage are the serious consequences of prolonged immobility: atrophy of both paralysed and noninvolved muscles, calcium loss from bone, atonic bladder and urinary retention, risk of skin breakdown, reduced cardiac output and plasma volume, and respiratory compromise (especially with high involvement).

Second stage
Except in the situations previously mentioned, flaccid paralysis is replaced by spinal reflex activity and increasing spasticity or, in partial lesions, greater or lesser degree of neurological recovery. Diagnosis may be confused in infants, since spinal reflexes in paralysed limbs may be misinterpreted as the normal movements in the infant. Even minor stimuli, such as rubbing the mattress, are sufficient to elicit spinal reflexes. Concurrent crying may also lead to the erroneous impression that sensation is intact. Reflex withdrawal or extension of the limb after tactile or pinprick stimulus confirms a diagnosis.

Problems related to spasticity include contractures (especially of the hip adductor, hip and knee flexor muscles, and heel cords). The atonic bladder becomes hypertonic, and, instead of continuous dribbling, urine is expelled involuntarily at intervals by reflex action.

Third stage
In the final stage, neurological signs are stabilized in terms of loss and recovery of function. The major emphasis is on rehabilitation. A problem unique to injury in childhood is pro-

HIGHEST INTACT CORD SEGMENT	FUNCTIONAL CAPACITY	FUNCTIONAL GOALS
C1-3 Muscle innervation: None below chin, including phrenic nerve to diaphragm	No voluntary control below chin Respiratory paralysis complete May cause bradycardia or tachycardia, vomiting	Artificial ventilation; can be taught glossopharyngeal breathing to be used for short periods Electric wheelchair Adaptive equipment for special tasks in bed or wheelchair using mouth stick
C4 (high quadriplegia) Muscle innervation: Intact sternocleidomastoid, trapezius, upper cervical paraspinous muscles	No voluntary function of upper extremities, trunk or lower extremities All neck movements Ventilator dependent	Electric wheelchair Externally powered devices and adaptive equipment for special tasks in bed or wheelchair with mouth stick, such as turning pages, using electric typewriter Totally dependent for activities of daily living
C5 Muscle innervation: Partial deltoid, biceps, major muscles of rotator cuffs at shoulders Diaphragm	Abduction, flexion, and extension of arm Flexion and extension of forearm Unable to roll over or attain sitting position Abdominal respiration Poor respiratory reserve	Electric wheelchair Requires attendant to assist in moving and transfer to wheel chair Adaptive devices for self-feeding, grooming, using electric typewriter Vocational potential with adaptive devices
C6 Muscle innervation: Pectoralis major, serratus anterior, latissimus dorsi muscles Complete deltoid and brachioradialis muscles Partial triceps muscle	Significant increase in function over that with lesion at C5 level Adduction and medial rotation of arm Wrist extension Good elbow flexion	Cuff strapped to hand permits use of implements for self-care and other activities Able to assist in dressing and transfer Hand rim extension permits independence in wheelchair
C7 Muscle innervation: Triceps and finger flexor and extensor-muscle	With elbow stabilized in extension and intact shoulder depressor muscles able to lift body weight	Almost complete independence within limitations of wheelchair

(Cont.)

Table 34-1 Functional significance of spinal cord lesions (Continued).

HIGHEST INTACT CORD SEGMENT	FUNCTIONAL CAPACITY	FUNCTIONAL GOALS
C7 (continued) Shoulder depressor muscles Still nerve disruption to intercostal muscles	Grasp and release still weak; dexterity lacking	Requires some assistance in transfer and lower extremity dressing Hand splints helpful Can roll over in bed, sit up in bed, and eat independently Homebound employment possible Outside work usually not feasible
T1-10 (high paraplegia) Muscle innervation: Full innervation of upper extremity muscles Considerable energy expenditure to put	Full use of upper extremities, including, intrinsic muscles of hand Trunk balance poor May have difficulty in lifting sufficiently to put on lower extremity clothing on long leg braces with extensive attachments	Completely wheelchair dependent Trunk balance benefits from training Able to drive car with hand controls May be braced for standing May hold job away from home Cannot manage public transportation
T10-12 Muscle innervation: Full abdominal and upper back muscle control	Good trunk balance Good respiratory reserve Can accomplish moderate hiphiking using external oblique and latissimus dorsi muscles	Ambulation with bilateral long braces using four-point or swing-through crutch gait Usually able to negotiate kerbs Some able to use public transportation Few vocational limitations as long as does not require much walking or standing
L3 or below Muscle innervation: Quadriceps muscle Partial gluteus and hamstring muscles	May be lumbar lordosis Floppy ankles	Ambulates well, often with short leg braces with or without stick Difficulty in getting out of wheelchair May never require wheelchair

Table 34-1 Functional significance of spinal cord lesions (continued).

gressive spinal deformity, usually not seen in adults or in adolescents, near the end of the growth period. Scoliosis develops in the major percentage of children with high thoracic and cervical lesions, and is almost certain to occur in children with quadriplegia whose injury occurred in infancy or early childhood. Consequently, affected infants and children are placed in carefully constructed trunk supports. Proper immobilization during vertebral healing helps prevent progressive deformity.

PROCESS OF DIAGNOSIS

A history of the nature of the injury provides valuable clues regarding the possible type of damage incurred and direction for further assessment without the risk of additional damage (see Table 34-1). A complete neurological examination is performed to determine if damage was incurred and, if so, the level and extent of any nerve impairment. Hot and cold water, a tuning fork, and cotton wool may also be used to determine specific sensory loss. Proprioception (knowing where one's extremities are) is a vital sense for ambulating safely.

Radiological examination is important for localizing the lesion, but the nature of the spine in childhood frequently creates difficulty in interpretation. Radiographs must be taken carefully and with sufficient help to prevent further damage to the spine. Several people may be needed to log roll the patient and to support the head during turning or transfer.

THERAPEUTIC MANAGEMENT

The management of the child with spinal cord injury is complex. Initial care begins at the scene of the accident; therefore, education and training of rescue personnel in stabilization and transfer techniques to prevent or reduce the severity of injury is important; no one should be allowed to move the child unless he or she is able to do so carefully. Because of the complexity and relative infrequency of these injuries, it is usually recommended that these children be transferred to a spinal injury centre for care by specially trained personnel.

Management during the first stage is primarily supportive, with efforts directed towards preventing further neuronal damage, avoiding complications, and maintaining vital functions. Children with cervical lesions often have compromised respiratory function and may require ventilatory assistance. Cervical lesions may require skeletal traction or other devices to maintain position, and corticosteroids are administered in an attempt to prevent destructive oedema. Operative intervention may be necessary to remove bone fragments and debris, but routine surgical exploration usually is not recommended.

The focus of the second phase is primarily rehabilitative and is aimed at returning the patient to the home and community. The focus is on maximizing the potential for self-help, education, and, for the older child, vocational counselling.

Prognosis

The ultimate outlook for spinal cord function after injury depends on the completeness of the cord transection, the site of injury, and the complicating damage to the neuronal tissue.

In general, recovery from thoracic lesions is usually hopeless for motor function, and victims are relegated to life in a wheelchair. Cervical injuries are variable in extent of damage. Incomplete lesions produce hemiplegia, and complete transection implies some involvement of all limbs from partial use of upper extremities to complete paralysis, including the need for artificial maintenance of respiration. Lumbar injury may involve partial or complete loss of function in lower limbs and bladder.

IMPLICATIONS FOR NURSING

The nursing care of the paralysed child is complex and challenging. As a member of acute care and rehabilitation teams, the nurse is involved in all aspects of care. Ideally, initial care takes place in a special intensive care unit with personnel trained to handle spinal cord injuries, and nursing management is concerned primarily with prevention of complications and maintenance of functions.

Once the acute period is over, the lesion is usually static and nonprogressive, regardless of whether the paralysis is secondary to trauma, congenital defects, infection, treated tumour or surgery. The nurse is a member of a team of specialists, including doctors from several specialty areas, physiotherapists and occupational therapists, psychologists, social workers and teachers. Each team member has a unique contribution to make, and mutual agreement for specific areas of responsibility and evaluation of progress are determined during regularly scheduled team conferences.

Respiratory care

The child with a high-level injury (quadriplegia) will require continuous ventilatory assistance. In most instances, a tracheostomy is the method of choice for greater ease in clearing secretions and for less trauma to tissues for long-term ventilator dependence.

Children with lesions below the C4 level are seldom ventilator dependent, but their vital capacity is significantly reduced. They should be positioned for optimum chest expansion, and a variety of breathing exercises and assistive devices are used to stimulate deep breathing. Chest physiotherapy is performed several times daily, and nebulized oxygen may be needed occasionally.

The cough reflex is markedly diminished and, together with weak intercostal muscles, the youngster may have difficulty with secretions. Increasing the elastic qualities of the lung by exercise will help to achieve a productive cough.

Temperature regulation

Temperature regulation usually creates few problems, although environmental conditions can influence body temperature. Clothing and blankets are added or removed according to the body temperature. An elevated temperature that cannot be corrected by environmental measures should be investigated, urinary tract or upper respiratory tract infection being possible causes.

Skin care

Initially, the child is turned every two hours around-the-clock by specially trained personnel. A pressure-relieving mattress is kept underneath the child, and the skin is thoroughly inspected every four hours for signs of pressure, especially over bony prominences such as the sacrum, scapulae, heels and occiput when the child is in a supine position; the trochanters and the lateral aspect of the ankles, heels and knees when in a side-lying position; and the ischial tuberosities when in a sitting position. The common type of pressure lesion begins in deeper tissues and is visible on the surface only at a later stage; therefore, areas that feel firm, irregular, warm or appear to be only slightly reddened require careful evaluation. Keeping the skin clean and dry is particularly important in these children, especially those who are incontinent.

Physiotherapy

Maintaining good body alignment, preventing pressure from bed linen, providing proper support, and applying splints as ordered and padded booties to hold the feet in the correct position are important in daily care. Passive exercises are carried out under the guidance of a physiotherapist. In children with upper motor neuron involvement, the spasticity that develops may require administration of an antispasmodic drug, usually baclofen.

During the period of immobilization, unless there are contraindications, exercises are aimed at maintaining and increasing the strength of the child's intact musculature. Upper extremity strengthening is especially important to the paraplegic child who must rely on these muscle groups for turning, transferring, dressing, crutch walking and other activities. Children are usually eager to use their muscles and respond to interesting and innovative activities.

Neuropathic bladder

When the nerve supply to the bladder is compromised it often results in disturbance of normal function. This can lead to a flaccid or atonic bladder which does not contract and empty in the normal way, resulting in over-distention and overflow incontinence. It is important to recognize and treat this problem by regularly emptying the bladder using the clean intermittent catherization technique. This reduces the risk of infection, protects the kidneys and promotes continence (Hunt de la, 1989).

In some patients, including those with upper motor neurone lesions, a hyperreflexic bladder may be present. Here, the bladder contracts periodically by reflex, but the emptying may be incomplete and may result in residual urine causing infection, vesicoureteric reflux and kidney dilation and scarring. Clean intermittent catherization and medications such as oxybutynin (an anticholinergenic agent), may form part of the management, but in some children lower urinary tract surgery is required to protect renal function.

All children who present with a neuropathic bladder should be under the care of a paediatric urologist who will make regular assessments including urodynamic studies, thus ensuring correct management and minimizing the risk of loss of renal function.

Bowel training

Successful bowel training is easier to institute than bladder management. The aim is to control defaecation until an appropriate time and place are found. A diet with sufficient roughage for adequate stool bulk and insertion of a glycerin or bisacodyl suppository at a convenient time, either morning or evening, are often all that are necessary to induce a bowel movement within a short time. The probability of an accident between times is diminished once the bowel is completely evacuated.

Stool softeners, such as lactulose, are usually prescribed, and manual anal stimulation may help initiate evacuation, especially in spastic paraplegia. Sometimes, an oral laxative such as senokot may be necessary. Once an appropriate regimen is established, little modification is required.

Remobilization

As soon as the condition warrants, the child is moved from a reclining to an erect position. An upright position must be accomplished gradually, by increasing the angle until the vertical angle is reached.

Many devices help children increase their mobility and function. The child with some limb function progresses to parallel bars and then to a walker; the child with quadriplegia learns to use a wheelchair - among the most valuable aids available to the child with a spinal cord injury. Selection of a wheelchair should be made carefully in relation to where it will be used, architectural barriers, and the functional capacity of the child. For children with upper limb involvement, a variety of motorized wheelchairs are used, but the more complex they are, the greater their cost, weight and tendency to break down. Wheelchair tolerance is gained over a period of time, accompanied by measures to prevent pressure sores.

A variety of braces and other appliances can be adapted for use by many children. The primary purpose of lower limb bracing in the child with a spinal cord injury is for ambulation, although correction of deformities may be attempted.

Children, with their natural and overwhelming propensity for mobility, usually attain or may even surpass the maximum expectation in ambulation. However, as they approach adulthood, the increasing weight and energy cost usually cause them to resort to predominant use of the wheelchair for mobility and the pursuit of more intellectual and vocational interests. Wheelchair mobility has the advantages of requiring no more energy than normal walking and allowing the person with paraplegia to maintain the speed of other pedestrians on level ground.

Physical rehabilitation

The major aims of physical rehabilitation are to prepare the child and family to resume life at home and in the community. Members of the complex rehabilitation team work collaboratively to identify the child's problems and to plan realistic interventions. Integration of activities is coordinated by one team member, most often a specialist in physical medicine and rehabilitation. Training in the rehabilitation centre involves maximum achievement commensurate with each child's physical capacities. Instruction for home routine is stressed and includes all the precautions and management implemented in the hospital, such as skin care, nutrition, bladder and bowel training, and an exercise programme.

Physical rehabilitation of children with quadriplegia takes approximately six months; children with paraplegia can achieve these goals in 1-3 months, but require constant vigilance to avoid complications. Emotional adjustments take longer, especially in older children and adolescents. In most children the outlook is favourable unless life-threatening consequences of urinary pathology are severe or if emotional adjustment is poor.

Psychosocial rehabilitation

Early acquired or congenital disability is usually more readily accepted by children than paralysis that appears later in childhood. Rehabilitation includes not only the child's emotional responses, but also those of the people who maintain the closest contacts with the child. As with any disability, children should be treated as normally as possible and encouraged in developmental tasks at the age at which they would normally be expected to acquire abilities and perform activities. However, goals must be realistic, and children should not be forced beyond their capabilities.

Severe depression can be emotionally and intellectually immobilizing, but it indicates that the child is no longer hiding behind denial. In rehabilitation, it is desirable for the child to begin to express negative feelings towards the situation, since these feelings, redirected by efforts of the rehabilitation team, are the ones that will motivate the child towards learning a new way of life.

The needs of youngsters who are permanently disabled must be re-evaluated periodically by the rehabilitation team, including the youngsters and their families. As young adults, these teenagers may not be financially independent, which alters the choice of occupation or profession.

The outlook for children with spinal cord injury is favourable for integration into society. Increasing awareness of the needs of persons with disabilities has removed many structural and occupational barriers. The success of a rehabilitation programme is not judged by how well children manage within the rehabilitation setting, but by how well they function in the outside world. In addition to agencies that offer assistance to children with disabilities in general, some agencies provide specific assistance to the paralysed, including children. The Royal Association for Disability and Rehabilitation (RADAR) and The Disabled Living Foundation supply information, hope, peer support and practical advice.

Sexuality

The problems of self-esteem are particularly marked when children with a spinal cord injury reach puberty, and are likely to be even more intense if the disability occurs during adolescence. Sexual development and awareness, and changing perceptions of body image, are prominent aspects of adolescence. A loss in these areas is a severe blow to these youngsters. Development of secondary sex characteristics does not seem to be altered by spinal cord injury, and it is now believed that with comprehensive rehabilitation, well-motivated young people can look forward to successful participation in marital and family activities.

In females, if the injury occurs after the onset of menstruation, there is usually a temporary cessation and irregularity in menstrual flow, but in the majority menstruation usually resumes. Ovulation and conception are possible, but females will not experience vulval or clitoral orgasms, although they can learn to use other erogenous zones for a sexual experience. This is important to emphasize in sex education, because many females have the misconception that because they lack sensation, they are unable to conceive.

As soon as adolescent males become aware of their functional loss, they will be concerned about sexual capacities, regardless of the type of sexual activities experienced before the spinal cord injury. The practitioner will provide them with information about what can be expected regarding erection, ejaculation and other sexual experiences. The health professional should take the initiative in discussing sexuality with youngsters and their families. Parents of younger children will want to know about their children's sexual and reproductive potential. As their interest and understanding increase, children need to know the specifics of physiology, prognosis, and sexual techniques related to their particular problems.

Most rehabilitation teams have an active programme in sexual counselling to help youngsters learn intimacy and how to function sexually within their limitations. Through individual and group counselling they gain new attitudes concerning sexuality experiences, exclusive or inclusive of intercourse.

MUSCULAR DYSFUNCTION

Skeletal muscles are subject to many disorders that cause degeneration of muscle fibres with subsequent loss of function. In most instances, there is fibrous connective tissue replacement of muscle fibres, proximal muscles are affected more severely than distal ones, and the lower limbs are affected to a greater extent than the upper. Children with muscle disease characteristically develop a waddling gait and have difficulty running, climbing and rising from a sitting position. Innervation is not affected.

Diseases of skeletal muscles can be inflammatory (such as polymyositis), the result of endocrine dysfunction (such as hypothyroidism and hyperthyroidism), or caused by congenital defects (such as absence of muscle, periodic paralysis, and the various muscular dystrophies and myotonias).

In addition to the electromyogram, measurement of serum enzyme activity is often helpful in differential diagnosis of muscle disease. The intracellular enzyme creatine kinase is present in muscle tissues and very few other organs and is released in large amounts in some diseases of muscles, such as muscular dystrophy. Creatine kinase is not elevated in neuropathic disease. Although the treatment in many muscle disorders is palliative and symptomatic, rather than curative, an accurate diagnosis is essential for rehabilitation, planning treatment in those amenable to specific therapy, and genetic counselling.

JUVENILE DERMATOMYOSITIS

Dermatomyositis is a multisystem inflammatory disorder of unknown aetiology and is often difficult to distinguish from muscular dystrophy. There is proximal limb and trunk muscle weakness, and loss of reflexes. Neck muscles are frequently affected, and the child may have difficulty lifting his or her head or supporting it in an upright position. Muscles tend to be stiff and sore, and chewing may be difficult. Soft palate dysfunction may make speech difficult and may interfere with breathing. Distal muscle strength and reflex response remain unaffected. Dermatomyositis, frequently classified as a collagen disease, is characterized by red, indurated skin lesions over the cheeks and nose, and a violet discolouration of the eyelids. The skin over extensor muscle surfaces may be erythematous, scaly and atopic.

Dermatomyositis usually responds to corticosteroid therapy with or without high dose intravenous gammaglobulin therapy; with early and vigorous treatment most affected children eventually recover (Collet *et al*, 1994). Physiotherapy is essential to prevent contracture deformity and to rebuild muscle strength. Bracing or splinting may be needed. Although the prognosis for survival has improved, it remains a serious illness that can be fatal.

MUSCULAR DYSTROPHIES

The muscular dystrophies (MDs) constitute the largest and most important single group of muscle diseases of childhood. They all have a genetic origin in which there is gradual degeneration of muscle fibres. They are characterized by progressive weakness and wasting of symmetrical groups of skeletal muscles, with increasing disability and deformity. In all forms of muscular dystrophy, there is insidious loss of strength, but each differs in regard to muscle groups affected, age of onset, rate of progression, and inheritance patterns.

The basic defect in muscular dystrophy is unknown. Serum creatine kinase is consistently increased in affected individuals, which assists in diagnosis and affords a means for early detection of the disorder in asymptomatic children in families at risk. Electromyography (EMG) and muscle biopsy are important diagnostic procedures and, if available, muscle ultrasound, which shows echogenicity in diseased muscles.

Treatment of the muscular dystrophies consists mainly of providing supportive measures, including physiotherapy, orthopaedic procedures to minimize deformity, and assisting the affected child in meeting the demands of daily living.

The major forms of muscular dystrophy are summarized in Table 34-2.

DUCHENNE MUSCULAR DYSTROPHY

The most severe and the most common muscular dystrophy of childhood is Duchenne. An X-linked inheritance pattern is identified in 50% of cases; the remainder appear as sporadic cases and probably represent fresh mutations. As in all X-linked disorders, males are affected almost exclusively, though less severely-affected female carriers are now being recognized. The incidence is approximately 1:3,500 male births (Thomas and Dubowitz, 1989; Multicentre Study Group, 1992). Box 34-1 describes the characteristics of DMD.

Recent studies indicate that dystrophin, a protein product in skeletal muscle, is absent from the muscle of children with DMD, although it is present in reduced amounts or abnormal in character in children with Becker MD, a milder variant (Hoffman, Brown and Kunkel, 1987).

CLINICAL MANIFESTATIONS

Evidence of muscle weakness usually appears during the third year, although there may have been a history of delay in motor development, particularly walking. Difficulties in running, riding a bicycle, and climbing stairs are usually the first symptoms noted. Later, abnormal gait on a level surface becomes apparent. In the early years, rapid developmental gains may mask the progression of the disease. Questioning of parents may reveal that the child has difficulty rising from a sitting or supine position. Occasionally, enlarged calves may be noticed by parents.

Typically affected males have a waddling gait and lordosis, fall frequently, and develop a characteristic manner of rising from a squatting or sitting position on the floor (Gower sign) (Fig. 34-4). Muscles, especially of calves, thighs and upper arms, become enlarged from fatty infiltration and feel unusually firm or woody on palpation. The name *pseudohypertrophy* is derived from this muscular enlargement. Profound muscular atrophy occurs in later stages, and as the disease progresses, contractures and deformities involving large and small joints are common complications. Ambulation becomes impossible between 8-12 years of age. Upper limb involvement follows; facial, oropharyngeal and respiratory muscles are spared until the terminal stages of the disease. Ultimately, the disease process involves the diaphragm and auxiliary muscles of respiration, and cardiomegaly is common. The cause of death is usually respiratory tract infection or cardiac failure.

Mild mental retardation is commonly associated with muscular dystrophy. The mean intelligence quotient is about 20 points below the normal, and significant learning problems are present in 25% of these children.

◆ **BOX 34-1**

Characteristics of Duchenne muscular dystrophy

Early onset, usually between 3-5 years of age
Progressive muscular weakness, wasting, and contractures
Calf muscle hypertrophy in most cases
Loss of independent ambulation between 8-12 years of age
Slowly progressive generalized weakness during teenage years
Relentless progression until death from respiratory or cardiac failure

PRIMARY MYOPATHY INHERITANCE PATTERN	AGE OF ONSET	INITIAL MANIFESTATIONS	PROGRESSION	THERAPY
Duchenne X-linked recessive; sporadic	Early childhood; aged 1-3 years	Lordosis Waddling gait Difficulty in rising from floor and climbing stairs Fat deposits replace wasted gastrocnemius muscles	Rapid Ultimately involves all voluntary muscles Death usually occurs between ages 15 and 25 years	Supportive Physio-therapy to prevent disuse atrophy of unaffected muscles
Becker X-linked recessive; sporadic	Between 4-25 yrs	Mild proximal pelvic girdle weakness Calf muscle pain	Slow; loss of independent ambulation after approx. 25 years from onset; lifespan slightly reduced	Supportive
Limb-girdle Autosomal recessive (usually)	Usually over age 8 years	Weakness and wasting initially of pelvic, knee and calf muscles	Variable but usually slow Most become incapacitated within 20 years of onset, in some, disability may remain slight	Supportive Physio-therapy to prevent disuse atrophy of unaffected muscles
Facioscapulohumeral (Landouzy-Dejerine) Autosomal dominant;	Early adolescence; over age 8 years	Lack of facial mobility Difficulty in raising arms over head Forward slope of shoulders	Very slow May be intervals with no progression Considerable disability in time but lifespan unaffected	Supportive

Table 34-2 Characteristics of the major muscular dystrophies.

Complications

The major complications of muscular dystrophy include contractures, disuse atrophy, infections, obesity and cardiopulmonary problems.

Contracture deformities of hips, knees and ankles occur from early selective muscle involvement and often exaggerate the weakness. Passive and active stretching under the supervision of a physiotherapist are helpful. Scoliosis caused by muscle imbalance is common and tends to progress. Bracing with a rigid corset may be needed for support and spinal fusion is performed in some boys.

Atrophy of disuse from prolonged inactivity occurs readily when children are immobilized or confined to bed with illness, injury or surgery, and efforts should be made to avoid any need for prolonged bed rest. A daily goal for well children should be at least three hours of ambulation when disability is moderate, to maintain muscle strength. When ambulation is lost, the use of standing frames and corrective seating, regularly adjusted to suit the young person's shape and size, are used to lessen the inevitable risk of progressive scoliosis.

Infections become increasingly frequent. Consequently, even minor upper respiratory tract infections may become serious problems in these children. Prompt and vigorous antibiotic therapy, supplemented by postural drainage and chest physiotherapy, is effective. Because these children are unable to cough, secretions collect easily.

Obesity is a frequent complication that contributes to premature loss of ambulation. Proper dietary intake and a diver-

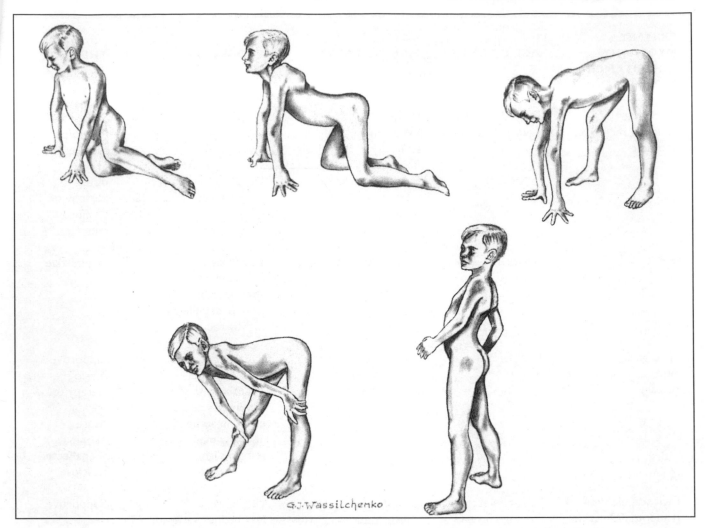

G.J.Wassilchenko

Fig. 34-4 Child with Duchenne muscular dystrophy attains standing posture by assuming a kneeling position, then gradually pushing his torso upright (with knees straight) by 'walking' his hands up his legs (Gower sign). Note marked lordosis in upright position.

sified recreational programme help reduce the likelihood of obesity and enable children to maintain ambulation and functional independence for a longer time.

Cardiac manifestations are usually late events, but may occur in ambulatory children. The most significant of these, cardiac failure, is difficult to correct in advanced cases, but treatment with digoxin and diuretics is often beneficial in the early stages of the disease.

PROCESS OF DIAGNOSIS

The disease is confirmed by serum enzyme measurement, muscle ultrasound (if available), EMG, and muscle biopsy. The serum creatine kinase is extremely high, even in the first two years of life before the onset of clinical weakness. EMG readings show a decrease in amplitude and duration of motor unit potentials. Biopsy reveals degeneration of muscle fibres with fibrosis and fatty tissue replacement, and absence of dystrophin. About two-thirds of affected boys are found to have a deletion of the Duchenne gene when DNA tests are done on blood samples; at present this is useful for genetic counselling and may, in future, enable diagnosis to be made on blood sampling alone.

Some success has been reported in antenatal diagnosis of DMD but is subject to uncertainties (Beiber and Hoffman, 1990).

THERAPEUTIC MANAGEMENT

There is no effective treatment for muscular dystrophy. Increased muscle bulk and muscle power have been reported following a course of corticosteroid (Mendell *et al,* 1989; Brooke *et al,* 1987). At present, the beneficial effects from administration of corticosteroids seem to be outweighed by the side effects. However, future refined regimens may give some hope of interim beneficial effect while possibilities of cellular or gene replacement therapy are being developed.

Maintaining function in unaffected muscles for as long as possible is the primary goal. It has been found that children who remain as active as possible are able to avoid wheelchair confinement for a longer period. Early recourse to a wheelchair accelerates deconditioning and promotes the development of lower limb contractures. Maintenance of function includes physiotherapy, surgery to release contracture deformities, and bracing and spinal surgery for scoliosis (Scott *et al*, 1993). Genetic counselling is recommended for parents, female siblings, and maternal aunts and their female offspring.

IMPLICATIONS FOR NURSING

The care and management of a child with muscular dystrophy involves the combined efforts of a comprehensive health team. Nurses can help clarify the roles of these health professionals to the family and others. The major emphasis of nursing care is to assist the child and family to cope with the progressive, incapacitating, and fatal nature of the disease; to help design a programme that will afford a greater degree of independence and reduce the predictable and preventable disabilities associated with the disorder; and to assist them to deal constructively with the limitations the disease imposes on their daily lives.

Working closely with other team members, nurses help the family to develop the child's self-help skills to give him or her the satisfaction of being as independent as possible for as long as possible. Parents must be helped to develop a balance between limiting the child's activity because of muscular weakness and allowing him or her to accomplish things alone. This requires continual evaluation of the child's capabilities, which are often difficult to assess. Fortunately, most children with muscular dystrophy instinctively recognize the need to be as independent as possible and strive to become so.

Practical difficulties faced by families are physical limitations of housing and mobility. Families often live in houses or flats that are unsuited to wheelchairs (e.g., no street-level entrance, upstairs bedrooms and bathrooms). Many of these families have no independent means of transportation. Assisting with these problems involves a team approach.

Parents' social lives are also restricted, and the family's activities must be continually modified to the needs of the affected child or children (see Chapter 20). Consequently, parents, too, tend to lead more isolated lives. When the child becomes increasingly helpless, the family may need some respite care and nurses can assist with decision making and support the family in this area.

Each child's therapy programme is tailored to individual needs and capabilities, and families should be active participants and assist with the physiotherapy. Many parents erroneously believe that by exerting sufficient effort, the child can overcome the weakness and prevent progression of the disease process; they may need advice on what level of exercise is helpful and when it becomes counter-productive in terms of the child's other needs.

No matter how successful the programme and how well the family adapts to the disorder, superimposed on the physical and emotional problems associated with a child with a long-term disability is the constant presence of the ultimate outcome of the disease. All the manifestations seen in the child with a fatal illness are encountered in these families (see Chapter 21). The guilt feelings of the mother may be particularly pronounced in this disorder, because of the mother-to-son transmission of the defective gene.

Nurses and specialist family care workers are especially valuable health professionals as they come to know the family and the family's problems (Walker, 1991). They can be alert to problems and needs of the families and make necessary referrals when supplementary services are indicated. The Muscular Dystrophy Group of Great Britain and Northern Ireland has branches in most communities to provide assistance to families in which there is a member or members with muscular dystrophy.

KEY POINTS

◆ Upper motor neuron lesions produce weakness associated with spasticity, increased deep tendon reflexes, and abnormal superficial reflexes; lower motor neuron lesions interrupt the reflex arc, causing weakness and atrophy of the skeletal muscles.

◆ Clinical manifestations of cerebral palsy include delayed gross motor development, abnormal motor performance, alterations of muscle tone, abnormal postures, reflex abnormalities, and associated problems such as learning disability, seizures, attention deficit disorder and sensory impairment.

◆ Werdnig-Hoffmann disease is characterized by progressive weakness and wasting of skeletal muscles caused by degeneration of anterior horn cells.

◆ Nursing care of the child with Guillain-Barré syndrome consists of monitoring vital signs, ensuring alignment and positioning, physiotherapy, and support of the family.

◆ Primary management of myasthenia gravis is oral administration of anticholinesterase drugs.

◆ Spinal cord injuries usually involve the following four interre-

lated pathological changes: cellular damage to cord tissue, haemorrhage and vascular damage, structural changes of white and grey matter related to vascular disruption, inflammation and oedema, and local biochemical response to trauma.

◆ Therapeutic management of spinal cord injury is directed towards preventing further neuronal damage, avoiding complications and maintaining vital functions.

◆ Goals of rehabilitation in spinal cord injury are to maximize function, assist the child and family in realistic goal setting, and help the child cope with stigma and build self-esteem and confidence.

◆ Muscular dystrophies are the largest and most important group of muscular dysfunctions in childhood.

◆ Major complications of Duchenne muscular dystrophy include contractures, disuse atrophy, infections, obesity and cardiopulmonary problems.

REFERENCES

Abdelkarim A Al-Qudah: Immunoglobulins in the treatment of Guillain-Barrç syndrome in early childhood, *J Child Neurol* 9(2):178, 1994.

Adams C et al: Thymectomy in juvenile myasthenia gravis, *J Child Neurol* 5(3):316, 1990.

Badurska B, Ryniewicz B, Strugalska H: Immunosuppressive treatment for juvenile myasthenia gravis, *European J Pediatr* 151(3):215, 1992.

Bhushan V, Paneth N, Keily JL: Impact of improved survival of very low birth weight infants on recent secular trends in the prevalence of cerebral palsy, *Pediatr* 91(6):1094, 1993.

Beiber FR, Hoffman EP: Duchenne and Becker muscular dystrophies: genetics, prenatal diagnosis, and future prospects, *Clin Perinatol* 17(4):845, 1990.

Bluma S et al: *Portage guide to early education*, Windsor, 1976, NFER-Nelson.

Brooke MH et al: Clincial investigation of Duchenne muscular dystrophy: interesting results in a trial of prednisone, *Arch Neurol* 44:82, 1987.

Calderon-Gonzalez R et al: Botulinum toxin A in management of cerebral palsy, *Pediatr Neurol* 10(4):284, 1994.

Collet E et al: Juvenile dermatomyositis: treatment with intravenous gammaglobulin, *Br J Dermatol* 130(2):231, 1994.

Cosgrove et al: Botulinum toxin in the management of lower limb cerebral palsy, *Devel Med Child Neurol* 36(5)386, 1994.

Dormans JP: Orthopedic management of children with cerebral palsy, *Pediatr Clin North Am* 40(3):645, 1993.

Gordon N: The spinal muscular atrophies, *Devel Med Child Neurol* 33(10):934, 1991.

Granata C et al: Spine surgery in spinal muscular atrophy: long-term results, *Neuromuscular Disorders* 3(3):207, 1993.

Healy A, Smith B: Cerebral palsy: setting the stage for the future, *Contemp Pediatr* 5(2):44, 1988.

Hoffman EP, Brown RH, Kunkel LM: Dystrophin: the protein product of the Duchenne muscular dystrophy locus, *Cell* 51:919, 1987.

Hughes I, Newton R: Genetic aspects of cerebral palsy, *Devel Med Child Neurol* 34(1):80, 1992.

Hunt de la MN et al: Intermittent catherisation for neuropathic urinary incontinence, *Arch Dis Child* 64(6):821, 1989.

Iannaccone ST et al: Current status of Duchenne muscular dystrophy, *Pediatr Clin North Am* 39(4):879, 1993.

Jansen PW et al: Guillain-Barrç syndrome in childhood: natural course and efficacy of plasmapheresis, *Pediatr Neurol* 9(1):16, 1993.

Mendell JR et al: Randomized, double-blind six-month trial of prednisone in Duchenne's muscular dystrophy, *N Engl J Med* 320:1592, 1989.

Multicentre Study Group: Diagnosis of Duchenne and Becker muscular dystrophies by polymerase chain reaction, *JAMA* 267(19):2609, 1992.

Nelson KB: Cerebral palsy. In Swaiman KF: *Pediatric neurology*, St. Louis, 1989, Mosby–Year Book Inc.

Park TS, Owen JH: Surgical management of spastic diplegia in cerebral palsy, *N Engl J Med* 326(11):745, 1992.

Rantala H et al: Occurrence, clinical manifestations, and prognosis of Guillain-Barrç, *Arch Dis Child* 66(6):706, 1991.

Scott J et al: Spinal fusion in Duchenne muscular dystrophyæfixation and fusion to the sacropelvis? *J Pediatr Orthoped* 13(6):752, 1993.

Thomas NH, Dubowitz V: Muscular dystrophy and other muscle disorders, *Curr Opin Pediatr* 1:296, 1989.

Vallee I et al: Intravenous immune globulin is also an effective therapy of acute Guillain-Barrç syndrome in affected children, *Neuropediatr* 24(4):235, 1993.

Walker C: *Lifethreatening illness (Spring update)*, London, 1991, NAWCH.

Walker M, Armfield A: What is the makaton vocabulary, *Special Education: Forward Trends* 8(3):16, 1981.

FURTHER READING

General

Aicardi J: *Diseases of the nervous system in childhood*, London, 1992, MacKeith Press.

Brett EM: *Paediatric neurology*, ed 2, Edinburgh, 1991, Churchill Livingstone.

Evans OB: *Manual of child neurology*, Edinburgh, 1987, Churchill Livingstone.

Gordon N, McKinlal I: *Neurologically handicapped children: treatment and management (books 1 and 2)*, Oxford, 1986, Blackwell Scientific.

Hosking G: *An introduction to paediatric neurology*, London, 1985, Faber & Faber.

McCarthy GT: *Physical disability in childhood*, Edinburgh, 1992, Churchill Livingstone.

Menkes JH: *Textbook of child neurology*, ed 4, Philadelphia, 1990, Lea & Febinger.

Cerebral Palsy

Cottam PJ, Sutton A: *A system for overcoming motor disorder*, London, 1986, Croom Helm.

Edmond A et al: Cerebral palsy in two national cohort studies, *Arch Dis Child* 64(6):848, 1989.

Kuban KC, Leviton A: Medical progress: cerebral palsy, *New Eng J Med* 330(3):188, 1994.

MacGregor D: The cerebral palsies of childhood, *Med International* 100:4184, 1992.

Robinson ROH et al: Conductive education at the Peto Institute, Budapest, *BMJ* 299(6708):1145, 1989.

Stanton M: *Cerebral palsy: a practical guide*, London, 1992, Optima.

Neuromuscular Dysfunction

Barden C et al: An unusual neurologic problem: Werdnig-Hoffman disease, *Crit Care Nurs* 10(10):60, 1990.

Heckmatt J: Nocturnal hypoventilation in children with non-progressive neuromuscular disease, *Peds* 83(2):250, 1989.

Kleyweg RP et al: The natural history of Guillain-Barré syndrome in 18 children and 50 adults, *J Neurol Neurosurg Psychiatr* 52(7):853, 1989.

Newsom-Davies J: Myasthenia gravis, *Med International* 100:4168, 1992.

Spinal Cord Injury

Chadwick AT, Oestring HH: Caring for patients with spinal cord injuries, *Nurs* 19(11):53, 1989.

Deegan S: Close to normality, *Nurs Times* 87(44):65, 1991.

Dewis ME: Spinal cord injured adolescents and young adults: the meaning of body changes, *J Adv Nurs* 14(5):389, 1989.

Laskowski-Jones L: Acute SCI—how to manage the damage, *Am J Nurs* 12:23, 1993.

Mostyn CM: Educating Jamie, *Nurs Times* 83(41):36, 1987.

Partridge C: Spinal cord injuries: aspects of psychological care, *Br J Nurs* 3(1):12, 1994.

Sinclair GM: *Nursing the neurosurgical patient*, Oxford, 1991, Butterworth & Heinemann.

Muscular Dysfunction

Bowman JE: Screening newborn infants for Duchenne muscular dystrophy, *BMJ* 306(6874):349, 1993.

Bushby KMD: Recent advances in understanding muscular dystrophy, *Arch Dis Child* 67(10):1310, 1992.

Dubowitz V: *A colour atlas of muscle disorders in childhood*, London, 1989, Wolfe.

Emery A: *Muscular dystrophy: the facts*, Oxford, 1994, Oxford University Press.

Hilton T *et al*: End of life care in Duchenne muscular dystrophy, *Pediatr Neurol* 9(3):165, 1993.

Rodillo E *et al*: Respiratory muscle training in Duchenne muscular dystrophy, *Arch Dis Child* 64(5):736, 1989.

Smith RA *et al*: Early diagnosis and secondary prevention of Duchenne muscular dystrophy, *Arch Dis Child* 64(6):787, 1989.

USEFUL ADDRESSES

Contact a family, 170 Tottenham Court Road, London W1P OHA.

Disabled Living Foundation, Unit 12, City Forum, 250 City Road, London EC1V 8AF.

Guillain-Barré Syndrome Support Group, Lincolnshire County Council Offices, Eastgate, Sleaford, Lincs NG 34 7EB.

Royal Association for Disability and Rehabilitation (RADAR), 250 City Road, London EC1V 8AF.

Scope (formerly the Spastics Society), 12 Park Crescent, London W1N 4EQ.

Index

A

ABC 708
Abdomen, acute 571
Abdominal distention 564, 573
Abdominal pain 564
  infant 264—265
ABO incompatibility 193–195
Abortion 346
Absence seizures 676–677
Abused child 79–80
  see also Child abuse
Accident and Emergency
  anaphylaxis 84, 85
  burnout 83
  categories of attenders 78
  child abuse 79–80
  death of child 81
  department 78–87
  emergency nurse
  practitioners 86
  environment 78
  nursing requirements 78, 79
  primary care 86
  resuscitation 84–85
  statistics 78
  sudden infant death 81–82
  therapeutic play 78–79
  triage 83–84, 85
Accidents
  in hospital 110
  incidences of 79
  non-accidental injury 79–80
  poisoning 80–81
  prevention 169–171
  social class 79
  statistics 78, 80
  see also Safety
  see also Injuries; Trauma
Acidosis
  burns 468
  shock 459
Acid balance
  imbalance 442–443
Acne 335–336
Acromegaly 687
Action for Sick Children's Charter 28
Addison's disease 694–695
Adolescence 353–368
  behavioural problems 80–81, 354–367
  chronic illness 378
  communication 135–136
  disability 378

physical health 335–348
Adolescent unit 72
Adrenal crisis 693–694
Adrenocortical insufficiency
  acute 693–694
  chronic 694–695
Adrenogenital hyperplasia 696–697
Aetiology unknown
  disorders of 271–273
AIDS 346–347, 626–628
Airway 518, 520
  obstruction 519,522
  trauma patient 708
Allergy
  anaphylactic shock 460–461
  food 84
Allis sign 237
Allitt case 283, 284
Alopecia, cancer therapy 646
Amblyopia 423
Amelia 240
Amenorrhoea 343–344
Amputation 723–724
Anaclitic depression 50
Anaemia 612–615
  aplastic 621–622
  cancer therapy 645
  classification 612
  Fanconi 621
  iron deficiency 615–616
  leukaemia 648
  pernicious 612
  preterm 218
  sickle cell 616–620
  thalassaemia 620–621
  thermal injuries 467
Anaesthetic
  before procedure 102
Analgesia 93–95
  balanced 93
  brachial plexus block 93
  caudal extradural block 93
  epidural infusions 93
  nonpharmacological methods 95
  nurse controlled 95
  patient controlled 94–95
  peripheral nerve block 93
    before procedure 102
  World Health Organization
    analgesic ladder 93
  see also Pain management
Anaphylaxis 84, 460–461

management of 85
Anencephaly 233
Animal bites 317
Anisometropia 423
Anorectal malformations 245–246
  classification of 245
Anorexia, cancer treatment 645
Anorexia nervosa 356–359
Anterior horn cell disease 740
  spinal muscular atrophy 745–746
Anticonvulsant drug therapy 677
  blood values for 678
Antipyretic 109
Apgar score 199
Aplastic anaemia 621–622
Apnoea 84, 516
  infant 273–274
  preterm infant 208–209
Apnoea monitors 274
Appendicitis, acute 570–571
Appetite, loss of 108
Area Child Protection Committee 280
Arnold-Chiari malformation 230, 233
Arteriopuncture 510
Arthritis
  septic 733
  juvenile chronic 734–737
Asphyxiation 541
Aspiration
  foreign bodies 169, 541–542
    prevention 169
  of medication 116, 117
  pneumonia 542
Assessment
  cardiac function 584–587
  gastrointestinal 563–564
  high-risk newborn 199–200
  nursing 127–126
  recording 128
Association for spina bifida and hydro-cephalus 233
Asthma 84
  bronchial 546–552
  exercise induced 549
Atrial septal defect 593
Atrioventricular block 605
Atrioventricular septal
  defect 594
Attention deficit-hyperactivity
  disorder 323–327
Autism, infantile 274–275
Autonomy 6, 387